Every Decker book is accompanied by a CD-ROM.

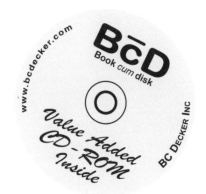

The disk appears in the front of each copy, in its own sealed jacket. Affixed to the front of the book will be a distinctive Bc̄D sticker **"Book *cum* disk."**

The disk contains the complete text and illustrations of the book, in fully searchable PDF files. The book and disk are sold *only* as a package; neither is available independently, and no prices are available for the items individually.

BC Decker Inc is committed to providing high-quality electronic publications that complement traditional information and learning methods.

We trust you will find the book/CD package invaluable and invite your comments and suggestions.

Brian C. Decker
CEO and Publisher

Burket's
Oral Medicine
Diagnosis & Treatment

Tenth Edition

Burket's
Oral Medicine
Diagnosis & Treatment
Tenth Edition

MARTIN S. GREENBERG, DDS
Professor and Chairman of Oral Medicine
Associate Dean of Hospital Affairs
School of Dental Medicine
University of Pennsylvania
Chief of Oral Medicine
University of Pennsylvania Medical Center
Philadelphia, Pennsylvania

MICHAEL GLICK, DMD
Professor
Department of Diagnostic Sciences
New Jersey Dental School
Newark, New Jersey

2003
BC Decker Inc

BC Decker Inc
P.O. Box 620, L.C.D. 1
Hamilton, Ontario L8N 3K7
Tel: 905-522-7017; 800-568-7281
Fax: 905-522-7839; 1-888-311-4987
E-mail: info@bcdecker.com
www.bcdecker.com

© 2003 BC Decker Inc

Previous edition copyright 1994

02 03 04 05 / GSA / 9 8 7 6 5 4 3 2 1

ISBN 1-55009-186-7

Printed in Spain

Sales and Distribution

United States
BC Decker Inc
P.O. Box 785
Lewiston, NY 14092-0785
Tel: 905-522-7017; 800-568-7281
Fax: 905-522-7839; 888-311-4987
E-mail: info@bcdecker.com
www.bcdecker.com

Canada
BC Decker Inc
20 Hughson Street South
P.O. Box 620, LCD 1
Hamilton, Ontario L8N 3K7
Tel: 905-522-7017; 800-568-7281
Fax: 905-522-7839; 888-311-4987
E-mail: info@bcdecker.com
www.bcdecker.com

Foreign Rights
John Scott & Company
International Publishers' Agency
P.O. Box 878
Kimberton, PA 19442
Tel: 610-827-1640
Fax: 610-827-1671
E-mail: jsco@voicenet.com

Japan
Igaku-Shoin Ltd.
Foreign Publications Department
3-24-17 Hongo
Bunkyo-ku, Tokyo, Japan 113-8719
Tel: 3 3817 5680
Fax: 3 3815 6776
E-mail: fd@igaku-shoin.co.jp

U.K., Europe, Scandinavia, Middle East
Elsevier Science
Customer Service Department
Foots Cray High Street
Sidcup, Kent
DA14 5HP, UK
Tel: 44 (0) 208 308 5760
Fax: 44 (0) 181 308 5702
E-mail: cservice@harcourt.com

Singapore, Malaysia, Thailand, Philippines, Indonesia, Vietnam, Pacific Rim, Korea
Elsevier Science Asia
583 Orchard Road
#09/01, Forum
Singapore 238884
Tel: 65-737-3593
Fax: 65-753-2145

Australia, New Zealand
Elsevier Science Australia
Customer Service Department
STM Division
Locked Bag 16
St. Peters, New South Wales, 2044
Australia
Tel: 61 02 9517-8999
Fax: 61 02 9517-2249
E-mail: stmp@harcourt.com.au
www.harcourt.com.au

Mexico and Central America
ETM SA de CV
Calle de Tula 59
Colonia Condesa
06140 Mexico DF, Mexico
Tel: 52-5-5553-6657
Fax: 52-5-5211-8468
E-mail: editoresdetextosmex@prodigy.net.mx

Argentina
CLM (Cuspide Libros Medicos)
Av. Córdoba 2067 - (1120)
Buenos Aires, Argentina
Tel: (5411) 4961-0042/(5411) 4964-0848
Fax: (5411) 4963-7988
E-mail: clm@cuspide.com

Brazil
Tecmedd
Av. Maurílio Biagi, 2850
City Ribeirão Preto – SP – CEP: 14021-000
Tel: 0800 992236
Fax: (16) 3993-9000
E-mail: tecmedd@tecmedd.com.br

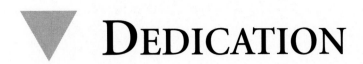

DEDICATION

This book is dedicated to the memory of Drs. Vernon J. Brightman, Irwin Ship, and S. Gary Cohen whose friendship, advice, and expertise continue to be greatly missed.

And
To my wife, Patti, and children, Deborah and Daniel.

Martin S. Greenberg

And
To my wife, Patricia, and children, Noa, Jonathan, and Gideon.

Michael Glick

Contents

▼ PART IV   PRINCIPLES OF MEDICINE

PREFACE

This year celebrates the 50th anniversary of the publication of the first edition of Lester Burket's classic text, *Oral Medicine: Diagnosis and Treatment*. The tenth edition is accompanied by a change in publisher, a new coeditor, and the addition of several authors. New chapters on topics of growing importance in oral medicine such as transplantation and geriatrics have been added, many chapters were entirely rewritten, and the remainder of the text has been significantly revised, reorganized, and updated. These major changes were necessary to reflect the increasing complexity and sophistication of this expanding field.

One man essentially wrote the first edition of the text. The present text includes the work of 30 authors who have been carefully selected for their expertise and clinical experience in specific areas of oral medicine or medicine. This book remains at its core a book for students, residents, and clinicians who require up-to-date information and a rational approach to the diagnosis and comprehensive management of the oral medicine patient. The text applies the latest available basic and clinical science information to the chairside and bedside.

Part I describes modern methods of evaluation, including a totally new chapter "Maxillofacial Imaging" by Sharon Brooks, who emphasizes the practical use of CT and MRI in clinical practice to supplement the use of standard dental imaging. "Diagnosis and Medical Risk Assessment" has been expanded, with the help of Michael Siegel; it provides a foundation for understanding subsequent chapters that focus on pathologic conditions and specific medical conditions.

Part II consists of six chapters describing oral mucosal and salivary gland disease. The chapters on salivary gland disease and on red and white lesions are entirely new, written by experienced clinicians that have made significant contributions to the field, such as Philip Fox, Sol Silverman, and Donald Cohen. Margaret Grisius and Indraneel Bhattacharyya also have made major contributions.

The chapters on oral cancer by Joel Epstein and those on ulcerative and vesiculobullous lesions contain major revisions to reflect the important new information such as diagnostic molecular techniques and immunodiagnostic techniques that has revolutionized these fields. Use of new therapy for oral mucosal diseases is highlighted.

Part III contains completely new chapters on temporomandibular disorders and orofacial pain, topics of major importance to clinicians and students of oral medicine. The efforts of Bruce Blasberg have helped to make these chapters a major contribution to the understanding of these controversial and rapidly changing fields.

The impact of medical conditions and diseases on the provision of dental care has changed dramatically since the previous edition. Consequently, a major emphasis of the tenth edition is the update of chapters addressing medical issues. Several of the medical chapters have been written by practicing physicians in collaboration with oral health care providers. The different perspective of medical providers such as Mark Lepore, Robert Anolik, Frank Silvestry, Elizabeth Tarka, Irving Herling, and Susan Silverton has given this edition a more practical approach based on the experience of these expert clinicians.

"Diseases of the Respiratory Tract" has been completely rewritten, as has "Diseases of the Cardiovascular System." Both of these chapters describe numerous conditions of importance to oral health care providers and offer practical recommendations on dental care for patients with asthma, hypertension, or bacterial endocarditis prophylaxis.

Major revisions highlighting the impact of oral health care for patients with gastrointestinal diseases, renal disease, hematologic diseases, bleeding and clotting disorders, and immunologic diseases is provided by Michael Siegel, Jed Jacobson, Robert Braun, Scott DeRossi, Katharine Ciarrocca, Lauren Patton, and Adi Garfunkel, all prominent clinicians in the field of oral medicine.

In the completely new chapter on transplant medicine by Thomas Sollecito, a complex subject is explained in a simple and practical manner, which assures both safe and appropriate care for patients before and after having endured solid organ and hematopoietic stem-cell transplants.

John Molinari, a world-renowned authority on infectious diseases, has made a significant contribution to a completely new chapter on hepatitis C virus, tuberculosis, HIV disease, and water-borne diseases of particular interest to oral health care providers. These specific infectious diseases were chosen for their great continuous impact on both the practice of infection control and provision of oral health care for infected patients.

Brian Mealey, one of the foremost oral health experts in this field, has contributed a separate chapter on diabetes mellitus, while Susan Silverton has updated her contribution on endocrine disease. Jonathan Ship, a major contributor to our present knowledge of oral health among older individuals, has provided a completely new chapter on geriatrics and oral medicine.

Lastly, the authors wish to thank the many individuals without whose help this text would not be possible, particularly Mrs. Hazel Dean and Kimmy Rolfe whose expertise, experience, and attention to detail help make our ideas a reality.

Martin S. Greenberg
Michael Glick

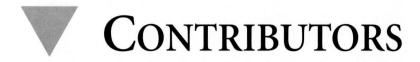

CONTRIBUTORS

Robert Anolik, MD
Allergy and Asthma Specialists, PC
Blue Bell, Pennsylvania

Indraneel Bhattacharyya, DDS, MSD
Department of Oral Biology
University of Nebraska
Lincoln, Nebraska

Bruce Blasberg, DMD, FRCD(C)
Department of Oral Biological and Medical
    Sciences
University of British Columbia
Vancouver, British Columbia

Robert J. Braun, DDS, MS
Department of Oral Medicine
Temple University
Philadelphia, Pennsylvania

Vernon J. Brightman, DMD, MDSc, PhD
Department of Oral Medicine
University of Pennsylvania
Philadelphia, Pennsylvania

Sharon L. Brooks, DDS, MS
Department of Oral Medicine/
    Pathology/Oncology
University of Michigan School of Dentistry
Ann Arbor, Michigan

Katharine N. Ciarrocca, DMD, MSEd
Department of Oral Medicine
University of Pennsylvania
Philadelphia, Pennsylvania

Donald M. Cohen, DMD, MS, MBA
Department of Oral and Maxillofacial Surgery
    and Diagnostic Sciences
University of Florida College of Dentistry
Gainesville, Florida

S. Gary Cohen, DMD
Department of Oral Medicine
University of Pennsylvania
Philadelphia, Pennsylvania

Scott S. DeRossi, DMD
Department of Oral Medicine
University of Pennsylvania
Philadelphia, Pennsylvania

Joel B. Epstein, DMD, MSD, FRCD(C)
Department of Oral Medicine
University of Washington
Seattle, Washington

Lewis R. Eversole, DDS, MSD
Department of Pathology and Medicine
University of the Pacific
San Francisco, California

Philip C. Fox, DDS
Department of Oral Medicine
Carolinas Medical Center
Charlotte, North Carolina

Adi Garfunkel, DDS
Department of Oral Medicine
Hebrew University
Jerusalem, Israel

Michael Glick, DMD
Department of Diagnostic Sciences
New Jersey Dental School
Newark, New Jersey

Martin S. Greenberg, DDS
Department of Oral Medicine
University of Pennsylvania
Philadelphia, Pennsylvania

Margaret M. Grisius, DDS
Department of Oral Medicine
University of Pennsylvania
Philadelphia, Pennsylvania

Irving M. Herling, MD
Cardiovascular Division
University of Pennsylvania
Philadelphia, Pennsylvania

Jed J. Jacobson, DDS, MS, MPH
Delta Dental Plans of Michigan,
    Indiana, and Ohio
Lansing, Michigan

Mark Lepore, MD
Allergy and Asthma Specialists, PC
Blue Bell, Pennsylvania

Brian Mealey, DDS, MS
Department of Periodontics
Wilford Hall Medical Center
Lackland AFB, Texas

John A. Molinari, PhD
Department of Biomedical Sciences
University of Detroit Mercy School of Dentistry
Detroit, Michigan

Lauren L. Patton, DDS
Department of Dental Ecology
University of North Carolina School of
    Dentistry
Chapel Hill, North Carolina

Jonathan A. Ship, DMD
Department of Oral Medicine
New York University College of Dentistry
New York, New York

Michael A. Siegel, DDS, MS
Department of Oral Medicine and Dermatology
University of Maryland, Baltimore
Baltimore, Maryland

Sol Silverman Jr, DDS, MS
Department of Stomatology
University of California School of Dentistry
San Francisco, California

Susan F. Silverton, MD, PhD
University of Nevada School of Dentistry
Las Vegas, Nevada

Frank E. Silvestry, MD
Cardiovascular Division
University of Pennsylvania
Philadelphia, Pennsylvania

Thomas P. Sollecito, DMD
Department of Oral Medicine
University of Pennsylvania
Philadelphia, Pennsylvania

Elizabeth A. Tarka, MD
Cardiovascular Division
University of Pennsylvania
Philadelphia, Pennsylvania

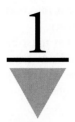

1

THE PRACTICE OF ORAL MEDICINE

MARTIN S. GREENBERG, DDS

▼ ORAL MEDICINE IN THE HOSPITAL
Requesting Information
Answering Consultations

▼ MANAGEMENT OF DENTAL PATIENTS WITH
SEVERE MEDICAL PROBLEMS

The field of oral medicine consists chiefly of the diagnosis and medical management of the patient with complex medical disorders involving the oral mucosa and salivary glands as well as orofacial pain and temporomandibular disorders. Specialists trained in oral medicine also provide dental and oral health care for patients with medical diseases that affect dental treatment, including patients receiving treatment for cancer, diabetes, cardiovascular diseases, and infectious diseases. All dentists receive predoctoral training in these fields, but the complex patient requires a clinician with specialized training in these fields. The American Academy of Oral Medicine defines the field as follows:

Oral medicine is the specialty of dentistry that is concerned with the oral health care of medically compromised patients and with the diagnosis and nonsurgical management of medically related disorders or conditions affecting the oral and maxillofacial region. Oral medicine specialists are concerned with the nonsurgical medical aspects of dentistry. These specialists are involved in the primary diagnosis and treatment of oral diseases that do not respond to conventional dental or maxillofacial surgical procedures. The practice of oral medicine will provide optimal health to all people through the diagnosis and management of oral diseases. Fundamental to this vision are the following:

1. Recognition of the interaction of oral and systematic health
2. Integration of medical and oral health care
3. Management of pharmacotherapeutics necessary for treatment of oral and systemic diseases
4. Investigation of the etiology and treatment of oral diseases through basic science and clinical research
5. Research, teaching, and patient care

6. Provision of care for medically complex patients and for those undergoing cancer therapy
7. Prevention, definition and management of the following disorders:
   —Salivary gland disease
   —Orofacial pain and other neurosensory disorders
   —Disorders of the oral mucosa membranes

The Third World Workshop on Oral Medicine (Chicago, 1998) was charged with updating and summarizing the state of the field in four major areas: (1) diseases of the oral mucosa, (2) infectious diseases of the orofacial region, (3) orofacial pain, and (4) salivary gland and chemosensory disorders. The American Board of Oral Medicine, the group charged with approving programs in the field, has fully or preliminarily approved approximately 10 postdoctoral residency programs in the United States. The graduates of these programs are found in universities, medical centers, and private practices throughout the country and provide needed oral health consultation services to local dentists and physicians.

▼ ORAL MEDICINE IN THE HOSPITAL

The hospital is frequently the setting for the most complex cases in oral medicine. Hospitalized patients are most likely to have oral or dental complications of bone marrow transplantation, hematologic malignancies, poorly controlled diabetes, major bleeding disorders, and advanced heart disease. The hospital that wishes to provide the highest level of care for its patients must have a dental department.

The hospital dental department should serve as a community referral center by providing the highest level of dental treatment for patients with severe systemic disease and management of the most medically complex patients is best performed in the hospital because of the availability of sophisticated diagnostic and life-sustaining equipment and the proximity of expert consultants in all areas of health care.

Hospital patients with oral medical problems may be seen by the dentist in three ways:

1. The patient may be admitted as an inpatient to the dental service. This is done most frequently for patients who require dental care and who also have severe medical problems.
2. The patient may be seen as a hospital outpatient. This is the common procedure for the majority of patients with diagnostic problems of the oral mucosa, jaws, and salivary glands.
3. The patient may be seen by consultation at the request of another department of the hospital. Some of the most difficult and unusual problems evaluated by the hospital dentist are seen as consultations.

Examples of problems or needs that are rarely seen in outpatient practice but are commonly seen in hospitalized patients are oral ulcers, oral bleeding, and oral infection secondary to blood dyscrasias or chemotherapy; acute parotitis in debilitated patients; dental care to prevent osteoradionecrosis

prior to radiotherapy; and dental care to prevent infection prior to organ transplantation or open heart surgery.

To handle consultations properly, the dentist must be familiar with the proper method of requesting and answering consultations. Hospitals may differ in the form used, but there is a universally accepted method that should be followed.

Requesting Information

The standard format used to request medical information from other departments is simple. The difficulty arises in deciding what medical information is necessary for a particular patient. This requires experience as well as knowledge of how a medical problem may change dental treatment.

When requesting information from other departments, it is necessary to write only two or three sentences containing the following data: age and sex of the patient, dental treatment to be performed, and medical information required. A typical consultation request is as follows:

> The patient is a 35-year-old male who requires multiple dental extractions under local anesthesia. A history of a possible heart murmur was elicited. Is a murmur present, and if so, is it functional or organic?

Two points can be made concerning the above theoretic consultation request to a cardiologist. First, *the request is brief*. Detailed descriptions of the nuances of dental therapy are unnecessary, but information regarding surgery or extensive treatment should be included. Second, *the request is specific*. The cardiologist is asked for medical information concerning the presence of an organic heart murmur. He or she is not asked to give "clearance" for treatment. When a request sent to a physician asks vague questions such as "Is it all right to treat the patient?" the physician may not understand the information required and may send a vague or noncommittal reply. These vague replies are often stored in a patient's chart as alleged legal protection, but they rarely assist the dentist in treating the patient effectively. The chief rule in requesting a consultation is be aware of what medical information is required, and request the specific information, not "clearance."

Answering Consultations

There is a standard format that should be followed when answering consultations from other hospital departments. Consultations that are answered only by short phrases such as "denture adjusted" or "tooth extracted" are unsatisfactory since the physician who hospitalized the patient for a medical problem is not given sufficient information. This information may be important in the management of the patient. Below is an uncomplicated consultation concerning a patient who developed dental pain while being hospitalized for a medical problem.

> The patient is a 55-year-old male who was hospitalized 5 days ago because of an acute onset of severe chest pains. A diagnosis of acute myocardial infarction was made, and the

patient is now being treated with complete bed rest and heparin. The patient began complaining of pain in the maxillary left molar region yesterday. He states that the pain is made worse when cold fluids are placed into his mouth. Examination at bedside shows no asymmetries, masses, or lesions of the neck, skin of the face, or salivary glands. There are two marble-sized left submandibular lymph nodes that are not tender and that are freely movable. The patient states that they have been present, unchanged in size, for many years. The temporomandibular joint is normal. The left buccal mucosa has a small 5 mm × 3 mm shallow ulcer opposite the maxillary first molar. There is no induration present around the ulcer. This same tooth has a large carious lesion and a sharp edge of enamel. No other dental or oral mucosal lesions are noted.

Impressions:

1. Dental pain secondary to pulpitis of a maxillary molar. There is no indication that this is referred chest pain, especially since cold locally applied exacerbates the pain.
2. Traumatic ulcer of buccal mucosa secondary to sharp tooth.

Recommendations:

1. Place sedative temporary filling in tooth and smooth rough edge at bedside to minimize stress to patient at this time.
2. Follow oral ulcer for healing; should see significant healing within 1 week or will re-evaluate to exclude carcinoma.
3. After acute phase of myocardial infarction, permanently treat tooth. Observe patient to ascertain whether pain disappears with above management or whether further treatment is necessary. Recommend minimal treatment at this time because of medical condition and anticoagulant therapy.

Note that the following outline was used in answering the above sample consultation.

1. Brief summary of pertinent information from the patient's medical chart
2. History of oral complaint
3. Examination findings
4. Impressions and/or differential diagnosis
5. Recommendations for treatment

A brief summary has several functions. First, the consultation becomes a complete entity; when another clinician reads the consultation, he or she will immediately understand the case. Second, a consulting dentist must read the medical chart before making a diagnosis or recommending treatment. A patient with oral lesions may also have skin, genital, anal, or eye lesions that will make the diagnosis easier. The chart will often have information such as physical or laboratory findings that will affect the type of dental treatment that should be recommended.

Having to write an intelligent opening statement encourages a rushed clinician to read the entire chart before writing the consultation. A good medical summary makes it clear to the requesting physician that the dentist has read the chart and has taken its contents into consideration when making recommendations.

The second portion of the consultation is a summary of examination findings. It should contain comments regarding the neck, face, salivary glands, temporomandibular joint, oral mucosa, gingiva, and teeth. A description of abnormalities—not a diagnosis—should be made in this section. The diagnosis may be wrong, but at least an accurate description of the condition is available for reference when the patient is examined at a later date. It is also important to remember not to use dental jargon or symbols when writing consultations; it is easier, but the physician may not understand their meaning.

The last portion of the consultation is labeled "Recommendations" and is an important procedure in hospital etiquette. All treatment for a hospitalized patient must be approved by the admitting clinician, who is ultimately responsible for the patient. Therefore, recommendations for treatment are made by the dentist, but the admitting physician has the authority to accept or reject them.

▼ MANAGEMENT OF DENTAL PATIENTS WITH SEVERE MEDICAL PROBLEMS

For several reasons, a dentist may choose to hospitalize a patient with severe medical problems. Important considerations are the availability of emergency resuscitation supplies; nursing care before and after the dental procedure; consultations with other medical disciplines; clinical laboratory facilities before and after the dental procedure; and operating rooms and anesthesiologists. Several medical insurance plans now cover hospitalization for patients with severe medical problems who are admitted for dental treatment.

Once the dentist decides that a patient should be treated in a hospital, the dentist should consider whether the dental procedure should be done on an inpatient or outpatient basis. The reason for using the hospital determines this choice. For example, if the hospital is being used for a patient with severe heart disease because of the resuscitation equipment available, hospitalization before and after the procedure may be unnecessary, and outpatient hospital management will accomplish the objectives. Conversely, a patient with hemophilia may require factor concentrates to elevate factor VIII levels prior to oral surgery. In this case, the hospital setting becomes more important for preoperative management and postoperative observation than for the procedure.

The dentist may choose to hospitalize patients for dental treatment of the following disorders:

1. Bleeding disorders due to hereditary disease, bone marrow suppression or extensive liver disease
2. Susceptibility to shock due to adrenocortical insufficiency or uncontrolled diabetes
3. Severe cardiovascular disease
4. Susceptibility to infection due to primary or secondary immunodeficiency

5. Need of heavy sedation or general anesthesia
6. Neuromuscular or other physical disability requiring special dental equipment for proper management

Most hospitals allow single-day admissions and have day surgery or short procedure units. Such a schedule is convenient for patients who require heavy sedation or general anesthesia but who do not require extensive pre- or postoperative care.

Dental patients who are admitted to the hospital should have a complete medical history and a head and neck examination noted on the chart by a member of the dental staff. Most hospitals require a physical examination by a physician or an oral surgeon, but this does not excuse the hospital dentist from writing a history and regional examination findings on the chart. There are many 2-year general-practice residencies and some oral medicine specialty programs that train dentists to perform competent screening and complete physical examinations.

Dentists who admit patients to a hospital may not be able to perform a complete physical examination, but they must be capable of understanding the implications of the physician's examination and its relationship to the dental procedure to be performed. If the physician writes "PMI 6th ICS AAL gr iv/vi systolic ⓜ in mitral region radiating to axilla" under "heart examination," the dentist should understand that the heart is enlarged and that a probable organic murmur is present. In

this case, further evaluation such as a cardiology consultation may be necessary before dental surgery is performed.

The hospital dentist should write the necessary orders for patients he or she admits, including orders regarding diet, frequency of vital signs, bed rest, medications, and laboratory tests. The dentist should be able to interpret the results of the tests he or she orders.

In summary, the hospital dentist is responsible for the total welfare of the hospitalized patients he or she admits. The dentist may be unable to treat all problems that arise, but he or she must know whom to consult to treat these problems. The dentist must also be trained to answer complex consultations regarding oral disease that are requested from other departments.

Hospital general-practice residency programs in dentistry train residents in physical diagnosis, laboratory diagnosis, and advanced oral medicine, to help them manage dental patients with severe medical problems. Residencies in oral medicine train dentists to provide oral health and dental care for patients with complex medical disorders as well as difficult diagnostic problems of the mouth and jaws. The future of dentistry and oral medicine in the hospital rests with the men and women being trained in these programs. Their training not only will benefit the dental profession but (more important) will also raise the level of oral health care available to patients with compromised health.

2

Evaluation of the Dental Patient: Diagnosis and Medical Risk Assessment

Michael Glick, DMD

Michael A. Siegel, DDS, MS

Vernon J. Brightman, DMD, MDSc, PhD

Objectives for the health status of the US population for the early twenty-first century have already been published by the US Department of Health and Human Services.[1] Three sweeping goals have been introduced: (1) an increase in the span of healthy life; (2) the reduction of health disparities; and (3) universal access to preventive services. These are commendable goals that need to be achieved for a rapidly aging population that is suffering from an increased incidence of medical and physical disabilities requiring improved access to medical services.

The mean age for individuals in the United States in 1998 was 36.2 years, with 12.7% of the population over 65 years of age. However, by 2015, the number of Americans over the age of 65 years will have increased by almost 16%, compared to the number of such Americans in 1998.[2] The increase will be even more dramatic among African Americans, who will show an increase of 20%. Many different factors contribute to this extended survival trend, including better nutrition, healthier lifestyles, life modifications that directly reduce risks of developing specific diseases, and more advanced medical technologies and therapies (such as advanced imaging modalities, gene therapy, and organ transplantation that will enable survival for medically complex patients). This trend is also a reflection of longer survival among younger individuals with chronic debilitating conditions. The gathering of relevant patient-specific medical information for the purpose of the provision of oral health care needs to reflect continuous social changes as well as changes in medical management. Social changes (such as changing sexual practices), access to dental and medical care, and the insurance industry affect every aspect of health care delivery. Dental therapy must be modified to accommodate these social changes to ensure that patients can receive affordable care that is specifically designed to their needs.

The oral health status of Americans is undergoing changes. Because more people are going to retain their dentition, the use of dental services will increase.[3] The need for preventive dental care is predicted to increase while the need for direct restorative intervention will decrease among the younger patient population. However, this will not be the case with the aging adult population. These patients will have a continuous need to improve masticatory function while still demanding superior esthetic results. Furthermore, recent information suggests that there is a more intimate relationship between oral and systemic health.[4] Thus, the challenge facing dentists in the twenty-first century is a rapidly growing population of patients who have chronic medical conditions, take multiple medications, yet still require routine, safe, and appropriate oral health care. This chapter addresses the rationale and method for gathering relevant medical and dental information (including the examination of the patient) and the use of this information for dental treatment. This process can be divided into the following four parts:

1. Taking and recording the medical history
2. Examining the patient and performing laboratory studies
3. Establishing a diagnosis
4. Formulating a plan of action (including dental treatment modifications and necessary medical referrals)

It is of interest to note that by the end of the initial history and physical examination in medical practices, the diagnosis has been correctly established in almost 90% of cases.[5]

▼ MEDICAL HISTORY

Methods and Problems

Obtaining a medical history is an information gathering process for assessing a patient's health status. The medical history comprises a systematic review of the patient's chief or primary complaint, a detailed history related to this complaint, information about past and present medical conditions, pertinent social and family histories, and a review of symptoms by organ system. The medical history also includes biographic and demographic data used to identify the patient. An appropriate interpretation of the information collected through a medical history achieves three important objectives: (1) it enables the monitoring of medical conditions and the evaluation of underlying systemic conditions of which the patient may or may not be aware; (2) it provides a basis for determining whether dental treatment might affect the systemic health of the patient; and (3) it provides an initial starting point for assessing the possible influence of the patient's systemic health on the patient's oral health and/or dental treatment.

Over the years, a number of techniques have been used by the health care community to gather the pertinent information that constitutes the medical history. There is no one universally accepted method; rather, individual approaches are tailored to specific needs. The nature of the patient's dental visit (ie, initial, emergency, elective continuous care, or recall) often dictates how the history is taken. The different formats include self-administered pre-printed forms filled out by the patient, direct interview of the patient by the clinician, or a combination of both. All of these methods have benefits and drawbacks.

The use of self-administered screening questionnaires is the most commonly used method in dental settings (Figure 2-1). Such questionnaires have been used in medical practices for more than 50 years. The classic Cornell Medical Index contained 176 questions.[6] The challenge in modern dentistry, as well as in medicine, is to use a questionnaire that has enough questions to cover the essential information but is not too long to deter a patient's willingness and ability to fill it out.

Pre-printed self-administered health questionnaires are readily available and standardized, are easy to administer, and do not require significant "chairside" time. They also give the clinician a starting point from which to conduct more in-depth medical queries. Unfortunately, they are restricted to the questions chosen on the form and are therefore limited in scope. The questions on the form can be misunderstood by the patient, resulting in inaccurate information, and they require a specific level of reading comprehension. As pre-printed forms cover broad areas without necessarily focusing on particular problems pertinent to an individual patient's specific medical condition, the use of these forms requires that the provider have enough background knowledge to understand why the questions on the forms are being asked. Furthermore, the provider needs to realize that a given standard history form necessitates timely and appropriate follow-up questions, especially when positive responses have been elicited.

A definite routine for performing and recording the history and examination should be established and conscientiously followed.[7] This not only minimizes the chance of overlooking important data but frequently results in the attainment of pertinent information that the patient does not consider to be related to the present illness (eg, symptoms or functional changes in more distant parts of the body) or that may be evidence of other problems of even more significance to the patient's well-being than is the particular problem he or she brings to the dentist.

Due to the drawbacks of pre-printed forms, clinicians are also required to gather more data by directly interviewing patients with medical problems. Based on the clinician's knowledge of the natural history and presentations of oral and systemic disease, he or she may need to encourage the patient to provide greater detail about selected symptoms (eg, onset, progression, response to treatment, and other associated symptoms and events). Proper follow-up questions (from the information given by the patients on pre-printed forms) and the direct-query method of gathering information provide clinicians with more patient-specific information and provide the

Date _____ Chart No. _____

University Of Pennsylvania School Of Dental Medicine
Health Questionnaire

Name _____ Male __ Female __

Address _____

City _____ State _____

Zip Code_____ Home Phone (_____)_____

Occupation _____ Work Phone (_____)_____

Employer _____ Date of Birth _____

Social Security Number_____

Person to contact in case of emergency _____

Relation to the patient _____ Daytime telephone no. _____

Medical doctor's name _____ **Phone no.** _____

Address_____ **Date of last visit** _____

My major dental problem or reason for seeking treatment is _____

This questionnaire will be used by your dentist to help treat you safely. Please answer all questions as accurately as possible.

Do you have a history of any of the following? (Please check yes or no)

	Yes	No		Yes	No
High blood pressure / Hypertension			Anemia		
Heart murmur			Bleeding disorder		
Rheumatic fever			Kidney disease		
Mitral valve prolapse			Renal dialysis		
Angina pectoris / Chest pain			Organ transplant		
Heart attack			Cancer		
Prosthetic (artificial) heart valve			Radiation therapy		
Irregular/rapid heart beat			Chemotherapy		
Pacemaker/Implanted defibrillator			Epilepsy / Seizure		
Heart disease			Stomach ulcer		
Heart or bypass surgery			Colitis / Intestinal problems		
Stroke			Arthritis		
Emphysema			Artificial joints		
Asthma			Sexually transmitted disease		
Diabetes			AIDS/HIV		
Thyroid disease			Tuberculosis (TB)		
Liver disease			Psychiatric treatment		
Hepatitis / Jaundice			Allergy to latex		

Have you ever taken an appetite suppressant? (Such as Fen-Phen)   ___ Yes ___ No

Do you use tobacco?   ___ Yes ___ No

Do you use alcohol?   ___ Yes ___ No

Do you use recreational drugs?   ___ Yes ___ No

For women only: Are you pregnant?   ___ Yes ___ No

Do you have any other medical problems not listed above? _____

_____

Over Please

FIGURE 2-1 Self-administered health questionnaire.

Please List:			
Medications	Allergies	Surgeries/Operations (Type and Year)	Hospitalizations

To the best of my knowledge, all of the preceding answers are true and correct. If I ever have any changes, I will inform the dental student or instructor at my next appointment.

Patient's Signature _____

FIGURE 2-1   Self-administered health questionnaire.

added advantages of fostering a good patient-provider relationship. This direct contact between provider and patient also provides an opportunity for patient education, allows patients to relate their expectations and fears of dental procedures, and offers providers an opportunity to discuss the importance of accurate medical information and its relevance to dental care. It also allows the clinician to assess subtle patient posturing that might suggest hesitation or a reluctance to reveal information. The clinician's manners and demeanor (including his or her friendliness, empathy, openness, and nonjudgmental attitude) during this process often determine patient satisfaction and compliance.[8] The clinician's ability to put patients at ease will come into play during the initial medical interview. To facilitate this process, the clinician should exhibit an attentive posture, maintain eye contact, make the patient understand that the clinician understands the patient's specific oral health problem, and recognize the patient's emotional disposition toward dental care. The most effective history-taking technique relies on establishing a dialogue between patient and clinician, which should provide both with an opportunity to satisfy the separate agendas each brings to the interview. Although the clinician will have a scripted agenda, it is important that time be given for the patient to tell his or her "story."

It must be understood that patients can only provide data related to their medical status relative to their own knowledge base and willingness to provide the information. In one study, 65% of a group of diabetic patients who reported having a heart murmur actually had no evidence of cardiovascular disease, leading the authors to conclude that a self-reported history of heart disease should not be the sole criterion for antibiotic premedication.[9] In most cases, patients' desire for privacy is the most compelling reason not to divulge medical information to their dentist.[10] A further barrier is patients' reluctance

to provide medical information to their dentist when they do not perceive that the information is relevant to their dental care. Thus, patient education, as well as the fostering of an environment where patients feel comfortable to inform providers of their medical status, needs to be encouraged. Ultimately, however, patients cannot be considered as having provided an accurate and comprehensive assessment of their medical status.

All medical information obtained in a dental care setting is considered confidential and constitutes a legal document. While it is appropriate for the patient to fill out a history form in the waiting room, any discussion of the patient's responses must take place in a safeguarded setting. Furthermore, access to the written record must be limited to office personnel who are directly responsible for the patient's care. Any other release of private information should be approved, in writing, by the patient and retained by the dentist as part of the patient's medical record.

Many medical conditions are associated with slow and gradual changes that may progress to severe debilitating diseases. Early detection and intervention may abate the progression of the disease or even result in complete resolution; equally important is the monitoring of patients' compliance with medical treatment guidelines and medications. Thus, oral health care providers should update a patient's medical history on a timely basis. Changes in a patient's health status or medication regimen should be reviewed at each office visit prior to initiating dental care.

The barriers to obtaining a complete medical history by preprinted forms followed by appropriate in-depth questions or by direct query of patients include (but are not limited to) time constraints imposed by busy practices, the unwillingness of patients to reveal aspects of their medical status, and the impatience of the dentist with listening to patients, as well as a variety of religious and moral issues that may arise. For example, patients of certain religious beliefs may refuse transfusions during surgical procedures, and individuals who are intravenous drug users may be at risk for infectious diseases, which must be considered during the provision of even routine dental care. However, the main limitation of gathering any medical information is the depth of the medical knowledge of the individual asking the questions. Thus, the information provided by the patient needs to be reviewed by a knowledgeable individual.

Consultations (usually with a patient's physician) are initiated when additional medical information is necessary to assess a patient's medical status. These can be done verbally or in a written format. Any verbal and written communication should be documented in the patient's record. It is important to communicate with other medical health care workers in a set and predetermined fashion. A consultation letter should identify the patient and contain a brief overview of the patient's pertinent medical history and a request for specific medical information (see "Problem-Oriented Record," later in this chapter). Although a physician's advice and recommendation may be helpful in managing a dental patient, the provision of safe and appropriate dental care is the responsibility of the practicing dentist. Thus, the essence of a medical consultation is to obtain necessary medical information with which the oral health care provider can decide how to treat his or her patient.

Components

The components of a medical history may vary slightly, but most medical histories contain specific information under specific headings. Information on the health of the patient can be arbitrarily divided into objective and subjective information. The objective information consists of an account of the patient's past medical history, as well as information gained by physical and supplementary examination procedures (ie, signs). The subjective information (ie, symptoms) is a report of the patient's own sensory experience but can also be secondhand, as in the case of children or others unable to communicate for themselves. This secondhand information is often used to confirm and supplement a patient's description of his or her complaint.

BIOGRAPHIC AND DEMOGRAPHIC INFORMATION

The recording of the patient's name, address, and telephone number; identification number (eg, social security number); age (date of birth); sex; race or ethnicity; name, address, and telephone number of a friend or next of kin; name, address, and telephone number of the referring dentist or physician, as well as that of the physician(s) and dentist(s) whom the patient consults for routine problems; and insurance and billing data is usually handled by clerical personnel and is readily computerized. The clinician should confirm the accuracy of these data in an informal fashion as the interview proceeds.

CHIEF COMPLAINT AND HISTORY OF THE PRESENT ILLNESS

The chief complaint is established by asking the patient to describe the problem for which he or she is seeking help or treatment. The chief complaint is recorded in the patient's own words as much as possible and should not be documented in technical (ie, formal diagnostic) language unless reported in that fashion by the patient; this may give the dentist some insight into the patient's "dental intelligence quotient." Patients may or may not volunteer a detailed history of the problem for which they are seeking treatment, and additional information usually needs to be elicited by the examiner. The patient's responses to these questions constitute the history of the present illness (HPI). A typical description of the chief complaint of a patient presenting for emergency dental care might be the following: This 32-year-old white male presents for emergency dental care, complaining that "I have been having pain in my lower left back tooth for the last 2 weeks, and it needs to be taken out." Questioning during the HPI will center around the offending tooth in the mandibular left posterior sextant. The astute clinician will note that this patient may not realize that this particular tooth can be retained and can then inform the patient of appropriate treatment options once more historical and diagnostic data have been collected.

The HPI is the course of the patient's chief complaint: when and how it began; what exacerbates and what ameliorates the complaint (when applicable); if and how the complaint has been treated, and what was the result of any such treatment; and what diagnostic tests have been performed. Direct and specific questions are used to elicit this information and should be recorded in the patient record in narrative form, as follows:

1. When did this problem start?
2. What did you notice first?
3. Did you have any problems or symptoms related to this?
4. What makes the problem worse or better?
5. Have the symptoms gotten better or worse at any time?
6. Have any tests been performed to diagnose this complaint?
7. Have you consulted other dentists, physicians, or anyone else related to this problem?
8. What have you done to treat these symptoms?

In the example of the 32-year-old patient with pain in the mandibular left sextant described above, the HPI may be documented as follows:

The discomfort began acutely 2 weeks ago while the patient was chewing ice. This discomfort was first noted as a sharp pain and a cracking sound. The patient claims that a piece of his tooth came out. The patient complains of subsequent extreme sensitivity to hot and cold stimuli that does not linger once the stimulus is removed. The patient avoids this area of his mouth and does not have any pain unless the tooth is exposed to thermal stimuli. He is a patient of record in this practice and has been out of town, so he has not sought care elsewhere. When asked, he claims that he desires to have his tooth extracted because of the discomfort. When he was advised that it may be possible to completely relieve his discomfort and retain his tooth, he commented, "let me know what this will involve."

PAST DENTAL HISTORY

Despite its frequent omission from the dental record, the past dental history (PDH) is one of the most important components of the patient history. This is especially evident when the patient presents with complicating dental and medical factors such as restorative and periodontal needs coupled with a systemic disorder such as diabetes. Significant items that should be recorded routinely are the frequency of past dental visits; previous restorative, periodontic, endodontic, or oral surgical treatment; reasons for loss of teeth; untoward complications of dental treatment; fluoride history, including supplements and the use of well water; attitudes towards previous dental treatment; experience with orthodontic appliances and dental prostheses; and radiation or other therapy for oral or facial lesions. Information on the general features of past treatment (rather than specific and detailed tooth-by-tooth descriptions) are needed at this time. In regard to radiation or other therapy for oral or facial lesions, exact information is needed about the date and nature of diagnosis; the type and anatomic location of treatment; and the names, addresses, and telephone numbers of the physicians and dentists involved and the facility (hospital or clinic) where the treatment was given. Likewise, clear details of any previous untoward complications of dental treatment must be recorded or must be obtained subsequently if not immediately available from the patient.

PAST MEDICAL HISTORY

The past medical history (PMH) includes information about any significant or serious illnesses a patient may have had as a child or as an adult. The patient's present medical problems are also enumerated under this category. The PMH is usually organized into the following subdivisions: (1) serious or significant illnesses, (2) hospitalizations, (3) transfusions, (4) allergies, (5) medications, and (6) pregnancy.

Serious or Significant Illnesses. The patient is asked to enumerate illnesses that required (or require) the attention of a physician, that necessitated staying in bed for longer than 3 days, or for which the patient was (or is being) routinely medicated. In the dental context, specific questions are asked about any history of heart, liver, kidney, or lung diseases; congenital conditions; infectious diseases; immunologic disorders; diabetes or hormonal problems; radiation or cancer chemotherapy; blood dyscrasias or bleeding disorders; and psychiatric treatment. These questions also serve to remind the patient about medical problems that can be of concern to the dentist and are therefore worthy of reporting.

Hospitalizations. A record of hospital admissions complements the information collected on serious illnesses and may reveal significant events such as surgeries that were not previously reported. Hospital records are often the dentist's best source of accurate documentation of the nature and severity of a patient's medical problems, and a detailed record of hospitalizations (ie, name and address of the hospital, dates of admission, and reason for the hospitalization) will assist in securing such information.

Transfusions. A history of blood transfusions, including the date of each transfusion and the number of transfused blood units, may indicate a previous serious medical or surgical problem that can be important in the evaluation of the patient's medical status; in some circumstances, transfusions can be a source of a persistent transmissible infectious disease.

Allergies. The patient's record should document any history of classic allergic reactions, such as urticaria, hay fever, asthma, or eczema, as well as any untoward or adverse drug reaction (ADR) to medications, local anesthetic agents, foods, or diagnostic procedures. Events reported by the patient as fainting, stomachache, weakness, flushing, itching, rash, or stuffy nose, and events such as urticaria, skin rash, acute respiratory difficulties, erythema multiforme, and the symptoms of serum sickness should be differentiated from psychological reactions or aversions (side effects) to particular medications or foods. For example, a patient who claims to be allergic to penicillin should be questioned as to the type of reaction to determine if it is toxic in nature (nausea and vomiting) or truly allergic (urticaria, pruritus, respiratory distress, or anaphylaxis). It is good practice to record that a patient has no known drug allergies (NKDA).

It is particularly important to document any allergy to latex.[11,12] Allergic reactions to latex are becoming more prevalent, and because of the routine use of latex gloves by oral health care workers, it is imperative to elicit such information prior to instituting a clinical examination.[13] Atopic individuals, patients who have urogenital anomalies, and those with certain disorders such as spina bifida are predisposed to latex allergy.[14]

Medications. An essential component of a medication history is a record of all the medications a patient is taking. Identification of medications helps in the recognition of drug-induced (iatrogenic) disease and oral disorders associated with different medications,[15] and in the avoidance of untoward drug interactions when selecting local anesthetics or other medications used in dental treatment. The types of medications, as well as changes in dosages over time, often give an indication of the status of underlying conditions and diseases. For this purpose, the clinician carefully questions the patient about any prescription or over-the-counter (OTC) medications, "alternative" medications, and other health care products the patient is currently taking or has taken within the previous 4 to 6 weeks. The name, nature, dose, and dosage schedule of each is recorded. *Physicians Desk Reference (PDR)*[16] (for prescription drugs), *PDR for Nonprescription Drugs and Dietary Supplements*,[17] *Drug Information Handbook for Dentistry*,[18] *Physicians' GenRx*,[19] *Martindale: the Extra Pharmacopoeia*,[20] and *Facts and Comparison*[21] describe and illustrate the medications commonly used in the United States and overseas and should be consulted when the identity or mode of action of a particular medication is unknown. Similarly, assistance can be obtained from the prescribing physician or from a pharmacist, who usually has rapid access to computerized drug information such as the Micromedex computerized clinical information system (CCIS) (Micromedex, Inc., Denver, Colo.).[22]

Pregnancy. Knowing whether or not a woman of childbearing age is pregnant is particularly important when deciding to administer or prescribe any medication (Table 2-1).

The benefit versus the potential risk of any procedure involving exposure of the pregnant patient to ionizing radiation must be considered. In this context, a patient who believes she could be pregnant but who lacks confirmation by pregnancy test or a missed menstrual period should be treated as though she were pregnant. The number of times a woman has been pregnant (gravida [G]), given birth (para [P]), and had an abortion (A) is usually recorded in the form of GxPxAx. For example, "G3P2A0" refers to a woman during her third pregnancy, with two previous live births and no history of abortion (either elective or spontaneous).

SOCIAL HISTORY

Different social parameters should be recorded. These include marital status (married, separated, divorced, single, or with a "significant other"); place of residence (with family, alone, or in an institution); educational level; occupation; religion; travels abroad; tobacco use (past and present use and amount); alcohol (ETOH) use (past and present use and amount); and recreational drug use (past and present use, type, and amount). When obtaining the social history, the clinician should take into account the patient's chief complaint and PMH in order to gather specific information pertinent to the patient's dental management. For example, the social history can be quite limited for a healthy patient who needs only a single restorative procedure; however, an extensive social history may be necessary for a patient with a positive history of hepatitis C who continues to use intravenous drugs.

FAMILY HISTORY

Serious medical problems in immediate family members (including parents, siblings, spouse, and children) should be listed. Disorders known to have a genetic or environmental basis (such as certain forms of cancer, cardiovascular disease including hypertension, allergies, asthma, renal disease, stomach ulcers, diabetes mellitus, bleeding disorders, and sickle cell anemia) should be addressed. Also noted are whether parents, siblings, or offspring are alive or dead; if dead, the age at death and cause of death are recorded. This type of information will alert the clinician to the patient's predisposition to develop serious medical conditions.[23]

There are also several inherited anomalies and abnormalities that can affect the oral cavity.[24] Many, such as congenitally missing lateral incisors, amelogenesis imperfecta, ectodermal dysplasia and cleft lip and/or palate, may have a direct impact on the type of dentistry indicated.

REVIEW OF SYSTEMS

The review of systems (ROS) is a comprehensive and systematic review of subjective symptoms affecting different bodily systems (Table 2–2). The value of performing a ROS together with the physical examination has been well established.[25,26] The clinician records both negative and positive responses. Direct questioning of the patient should be aimed at collecting additional data to confirm or rule out those disease processes that have been identified by the clinician as likely explanations for the patient's symptoms. This type of questioning may also alert the clinician to underlying systemic conditions that were not fully described in the PMH. Furthermore, the ROS will help to monitor changes in medical conditions. The design of the ROS is aimed at categorizing each major system of the body so as to provide the clinician with a framework that incorporates many different anatomic and physiologic expressions reflective of the patient's medical status. The ROS includes general categories, to allow for completeness of the review. A complete ROS includes the following categories:

1. General
2. Head, eyes, ears, nose, and throat (HEENT)
3. Cardiovascular
4. Respiratory
5. Dermatologic
6. Gastrointestinal
7. Genitourinary
8. Gynecologic
9. Endocrine
10. Musculoskeletal
11. Hematologic-lymphatic
12. Neuropsychiatric

Numerous examples can be provided to underscore the importance of the ROS. Seemingly unrelated systemic disorders that significantly affect a patient's dental care may be disclosed. A woman may disclose a history of hoarseness (throat category), which, when coupled with a history of smoking and

---

TABLE 2-1 Drug Categories for Pregnant Patients

Category	Risks or Adverse Effects
A	No risk demonstrated in any trimester
B	No adverse effects in animals; no human studies available
C	Given only after risks to fetus are considered; animal studies have shown adverse reactions; no human studies available
D	Definite fetal risks; may be given despite risks if needed for life-threatening conditions
X	Absolute fetal abnormalities; not to be used anytime during preganancy

TABLE 2-2   Review of Systems

Organ or System	Symptoms
General	Weight changes, malaise, fatigue, night sweats
Head	Headaches, tenderness, sinus problems
Eyes	Changes in vision, photophobia, blurring, diplopia, spots, discharges
Ears	Hearing changes, tinnitus, pain, discharge, vertigo
Nose	Epistaxis, obstructions
Throat	Hoarseness, soreness
Respiratory	Chest pain, wheezing, dyspnea, cough, hemoptysis
Cardiovascular	Chest pain, dyspnea, orthopnea (number of pillows needed to sleep comfortably), edema, claudication
Dermatologic	Rashes, pruritus, lesions, skin cancer (epidermoid carcinoma, melanoma)
Gastrointestinal	Changes in appetite, dysphagia, nausea, vomiting, hematemesis, indigestion, pain, diarrhea, constipation, melena, hematochezia, bloating, hemorrhoids, jaundice
Genitourinary	Changes in frequency, urgency, dysuria, hematuria, nocturia, incontinence, discharge, impotence
Gynecologic	Menstrual changes (frequency, duration, flow, last menstrual period), dysmenorrhea, menopause
Endocrine	Polyuria, polydipsia, polyphagia, temperature intolerance, pigmentations
Musculoskeletal	Muscle and joint pain, deformities, joint swellings, spasms, changes in range of motion
Hematologic/lymphatic	Easy bruising, epistaxis, spontaneous gingival bleeding, increased bleeding after trauma, swollen or enlarged lymph nodes
Neuropsychiatric	Syncope, seizures, weakness (unilateral and bilateral), changes in coordination, sensations, memory, mood, or sleep pattern, emotional disturbances, history of psychiatric therapy

neck lymph node examination, may uncover a cancer of the throan. A woman complaining of burning in her mouth might advise her dentist that she is taking a broad-spectrum antibiotic for a urinary tract infection (genitourinary category); this information might allow the dentist to determine that the antibiotic is the underlying cause of an oral fungal infection and to provide the patient with appropriate care. By carefully questioning the patient about each system listed above (and listed more specifically in Table 2-2), the dental practitioner can assess what the impact of systemic disorders will be on the patient's dental management.

▼ EXAMINATION OF THE PATIENT

General Procedure

The examination of the patient represents the second stage of the diagnostic procedure. An established routine is mandatory. A thorough and systematic inspection of the oral cavity and adnexal tissues minimizes the possibility of overlooking previously undiscovered pathologies. The examination is most conveniently carried out with the patient seated in a dental chair, with the head supported. When dental charting is involved, having an assistant record the findings saves time and limits cross-contamination of the chart and pen. Before seating the patient, the clinician should observe the patient's general appearance and gait and should note any physical deformities or handicaps.

The routine oral examination (ie, thorough inspection, palpation, auscultation, and percussion of the exposed surface structures of the head, neck, and face; detailed examination of the oral cavity, dentition, oropharynx, and adnexal structures, as customarily carried out by the dentist) should be carried out at least once annually or at each recall visit. Laboratory studies and additional special examination of other organ systems may be required for the evaluation of patients with orofacial pain or signs and symptoms suggestive of otorhinologic or salivary gland disorders or pathologies suggestive of a systemic etiology. A less comprehensive but equally thorough inspection of the face and oral and oropharyngeal mucosae should also be carried out at each dental visit. The tendency for the dentist to focus on only the tooth or jaw quadrant in question should be strongly resisted. Each visit should be initiated by a deliberate inspection of the entire face and oral cavity prior to the scheduled or emergency procedure. The importance of this approach in the early detection of head and neck cancer and in promoting the image of the dentist as the responsible clinician of the oral cavity cannot be overemphasized (see Chapter 8, Oral Cancer).

Examination carried out in the dental office is traditionally restricted to that of the superficial tissues of the oral cavity, head, and neck and the exposed parts of the extremities. On occasion, evaluation of an oral lesion logically leads to an inquiry about similar lesions on other skin or mucosal surfaces or about the enlargement of other regional groups of lymph nodes. Although these inquiries can usually be satisfied directly by questioning the patient, the dentist may also quite appropriately request permission from the patient to examine axillary nodes or other skin surfaces, provided the examination is carried out competently and with adequate privacy for the patient. A male dentist should have a female assistant present in the case of a female patient. Female dentists should have a male assistant present in the case of a male patient. Similar precautions should be followed when it is necessary for a patient to remove tight clothing for accurate measurement of blood pressure. Facilities for a complete physical examination, however, are not traditionally available in dental offices and clinics, and a complete physical examination should not be attempted when facilities are lacking or when custom excludes it.

In the case of hospitalized inpatients, dental staff are delegated to carry out preoperative complete physical examinations of the patients they have admitted for operating room procedures and general anesthesia. Instruction in the procedures for carrying out and recording the complete physical examination (ie, examination of heart, lungs, abdomen, extremities, central and peripheral nervous systems, special sensory functions, and musculoskeletal system) is therefore part of the postdoctoral training of oral surgery, oral medicine, and hospital dentistry residents. For details of this examination, readers are referred to the many available texts on physical diagnosis.[27–31]

The degree of responsibility accorded to the dentist in carrying out a complete physical examination varies from hospital to hospital and from state to state. The dentist's involvement may range from permission to examine extraoral structures for educational purposes only, to permission to carry out certain parts of the complete physical examination under the supervision of a physician who reviews and certifies the findings, to full privileges and responsibility for conducting necessary physical examinations before and after general anesthesia or surgical procedures.

The examination procedure in dental office settings includes the following:

1. Registration of vital signs (respiratory rate, temperature, pulse, and blood pressure).

2. Examination of the head, neck, and oral cavity, including salivary glands, temporomandibular joints, and lymph nodes
3. Examination of cranial nerve function
4. Special examination of other organ systems
5. Requisition of laboratory studies

Vital Signs

Vital signs (respiratory rate, temperature, pulse, and blood pressure) are routinely recorded as part of the examination (Table 2-3). In addition to being useful as an indicator of systemic disease, this information is essential as a standard of reference should syncope or other untoward medical complications arise during patient treatment.

RESPIRATORY RATE

Normal respiratory rate during rest is 14 to 20 breaths per minute. Any more rapid breathing is called tachypnea and may be associated with underlying disease and or elevated temperature.

TEMPERATURE

The dental patient's temperature should be taken when systemic illness or systemic response secondary to dental infection (eg, bacteremia) is suspected. The normal oral (sublingual) temperature is 37°C (98.6°F), but oral temperatures < 37.8°C (100°F) are not usually considered to be significant. Studies of sublingual, axillary, auditory canal, and rectal temperatures in elderly patients indicate that these traditionally accepted values differ somewhat from statistically determined values.[32–34] Recent drinking of hot or cold liquids or mouth breathing in very warm or cold air may alter the oral temperature. Also, severe oral infection may alter the local temperature in the mouth without causing fever. When it is important to determine the patient's general temperature, it is necessary to determine the temperature with other means. Digital thermometers used in the auditory canal are popular and accurate.

TABLE 2-3 Vital Signs

	Normal	Tachypnea		
Respiratory rate	14–16 breaths/min	> 20 breaths/minute		
	Oral	**Axillary**	**Rectal**	**Aural**
Normal temperature	98.6F/37.0C	97.6F/36.3C	99.6F/37.7C	99.6F/37.7C
	Brady cardia	**Normal**	**Tachycardia**	
Pulse rate	< 60 beats per minute	60-100 beats/minute	> 100 beats/minute	
	Regular	**Regular irregular**	**Irregular irregular**	
Pulse rhythm	Evenly spaced beats. May vary slightly with respiration.	Regular pattern with skipped beats.	No pattern. Chaotic.	

bpm = beats per minute.

PULSE RATE AND RHYTHM

Always determine the patient's pulse rate and rhythm (see Table 2-3). The normal resting pulse rate is between 60 and 100 beats per minute (bpm). A patient with a pulse rate >100 bpm (tachycardia), even considering the stress of a dental office visit,[35–37] should be allowed to rest quietly away from the dental operatory to allow the pulse to return to normal before the start of dental treatment. If the patient's pulse rate remains persistently high, medical evaluation of the tachycardia is appropriate because severe coronary artery disease or myocardial disease may be present. Note that the pulse rate normally rises about 5 to 10 bpm with each degree of fever. Rates that are consistently < 60 bpm (bradycardia) warrant medical evaluation although sinus bradycardia, a common condition, can be normal.

Although a healthy person may have occasional irregularities or premature beats (especially when under stress) a grossly irregular pulse can indicate severe myocardial disease (arrhythmia or dysrhythmia), justifying further cardiac evaluation before dental treatment is instituted. Cardiac consultation is necessary for the accurate interpretation of most pulse rate abnormalities.

Pulse rate abnormalities may be regular or irregular. Irregular rate abnormalities may be divided further into regularly irregular and irregularly irregular abnormalities.

It is usually unnecessary to measure the patient's respiratory rate in the dental office unless cardiopulmonary disease is suspected or general anesthesia or another type of sedation is planned. However, the examiner should note whether the patient is breathing very rapidly, is short of breath, or is dyspneic. These symptoms alone may indicate the presence of pulmonary or cardiac disease, anemia, or acute anxiety.

BLOOD PRESSURE

Many dental procedures are stressful to the patient and may cause an elevation of the blood pressure (Table 2-4).[38] Also, accidental intravascular injection or rapid absorption (eg, injection into a venous plexus) of local anesthetics containing epinephrine may cause a transient rise in the blood pressure. Dental treatment for patients with hypertension is discussed in Chapter 13, Disease of the Cardiovascular System. Syncope due to anxiety or medications is usually associated with systemic hypotension.

If a patient is receiving treatment for hypertension or if the patient does not regularly visit a physician, blood pressure should be measured before instituting dental treatment. The routine recording of blood pressure in the dental office has been demonstrated to be a valuable method of medical case finding.[39,40]

Blood pressure should be measured with appropriate equipment and in a standardized fashion[41,42] (Table 2-5). Although sphygmomanometers are the most accurate devices, validated electronic devices or aneroid sphygmomanometers with appropriately sized cuffs are sufficient for blood pressure screening in dental settings. Finger monitors should not be used.[43]

Electronic devices are usually accurate to within 3% of a manual sphygmomanometer. Their ease of use in comparison with manual sphygmomanometers is a great advantage and encourages increased use. Both blood pressure and pulse are recorded, but irregular rhythms cannot be detected. To detect potential deviations, electronic devices should occasionally be calibrated against a manual sphygmomanometer.

Faulty technique will produce errors.[44] If the cuff is applied too loosely, if it is not completely deflated before applying, or if it is too small for the patient's arm, the pressure readings obtained will be erroneously high and will not represent the pressure in the artery at the time of measurement. The one factor mentioned above that is not within the province of the practitioner to change is the arm size. The width of the cuff should be about 40% of the diameter of the patient's arm, and the bladder length should encircle about 80% of the arm. For patients with unusually large arms, it may be appropriate to use a "thigh" cuff. If a thigh cuff is not available, keep in mind that the readings will be too high. If the cuff is deflated too rapidly (>2–3 mm Hg per heartbeat), the recorded systolic pressure will be erroneously low, and the diastolic pressure will register as too high.

Head, Neck, and Oral Cavity (Including Salivary Glands Temporomandibular Joint, Lymph Nodes, and Cranial Nerve Function)

The ability to perform a thorough physical examination of the superficial structures of the head, neck, and oral cavity is essential for all dentists and any clinician involved in diagnosing and treating oral disease. This examination should be carried out on all new dental patients and repeated at least yearly on patients of record. To perform this examination procedure successfully, the examiner needs the following:

1. Adequate knowledge of the anatomy of the region to be able to recognize normal structures and their common variations
2. A well-practiced technique for displaying all of the skin and mucosal surfaces of the head, neck, and oral cavity with minimal discomfort to the patient and a routine

---

TABLE 2-4 Blood Pressure Values

Category	Systolic Blood Pressure (mm Hg)	Diastolic Blood Pressure (mm Hg)
Nonhypertensive		
Optimal	< 120 and	< 80
Normal	< 130 and	< 85
High normal	130–139 or	85–89
Hypertensive		
Stage 1	140–149 or	90–99
Stage 2	160–179 or	100–109
Stage 3	≥ 180 or	≥ 110

Adapted from The Sixth Report of the Joint National Committee on Prevention, Detection, Evaluation, and Treatment of High Blood Pressure.[41]

TABLE 2-5 Proper Technique of Blood Pressure Measurement

1. Patient should refrain from smoking or ingesting products containing caffeine within 30 minutes of the blood pressure measure.

2. Seat patient with his or her back supported, arms bare over the biceps and supported at heart level.

3. Patient should rest for 5 minutes in the chair prior to the measure.

4. The bladder of the cuff should encircle at least 80% of the arm.

5. Place the bladder centered over the brachial artery, with the cuff's lower border 1 to 2 inches above the elbow crease in the anticubital fossa.

6. Palpate the radial pulse.

7. Place a stethoscope on the brachial artery, and listen.

8. Inflate the bladder up to about 20 to 30 mm Hg above the point at which the pulse is no longer palpable (palpable systolic pressure).

9. Both systolic (first appearance of sound or the initial return of palpation of the radial artery) and diastolic (disappearance of sound) blood pressure should be recorded.

10. Two or more readings separated by 2 minutes should be averaged. If the two readings differ by more than 5 mm Hg, two additional readings should be done and averaged.

Adapted from The Sixth Report of the Joint National Committee on Prevention, Detection, Evaluation, and Treatment of High Blood Pressure.

that ensures the systematic examination of all the tissues that can be approached in this way

3. Knowledge of the variety of disease processes that can affect the superficial structures of the head, neck, and oral cavity

4. The ability to succinctly record (in writing) both normal and abnormal findings noted during the examination

The order of examination is a matter of individual choice, but an established and reproducible routine is desirable. Ideally, necessary intraoral and bite-wing radiography should be available when the systematic examination of the oral cavity is carried out. Examination gloves, tongue blades or dental hand mirrors, a dental explorer and periodontal probe, gauze pads, a dental chair, a lamp or flashlight (for illuminating the oral cavity), and a stethoscope are the basic equipment needed.

The examination routine encompasses the following eight steps:

1. Note the general appearance of the individual and evaluate emotional reactions and the general nutritional state. Record the character of the skin and the presence of petechiae or eruptions, as well as the texture, distribution, and quality of the hair. Examine the conjunctivae and skin for petechiae, and examine the sclerae and skin for evidence of jaundice or pallor. Determine the reaction of the pupils to light and accommodation, especially when neurologic disorders are being investigated.

2. Palpate for adenopathy. The superficial and the deep lymph nodes of the neck are best examined from behind the patient, with the patients's head inclined forward sufficiently to relax the tissues overlying the lymph nodes. Look for distention of the superficial veins as well as for evidence of thyroid enlargement (see also the section on neck and lymphnodes). Palpate any swellings, nodules, or suspected anatomic abnormalities.

3. Examine in sequence the inner surfaces of the lips, the mucosa of the checks, the maxillary and mandibular mucobuccal folds, the palate, the tongue, the sublingual space, the gingivae, and then the teeth and their supporting structures. Last, examine the tonsillar and the pharyngeal areas and any lesion, particularly if the lesion is painful. Any noted asymmetry should be investigated further.

4. Completely visualize the smooth mucosal surfaces of the lips, cheeks, tongue, and sublingual space by using two tongue depressors or mirrors. Perform a more detailed examination of the teeth and supporting tissues with the mouth mirror, the explorer, and the periodontal probe.

5. Have the patient extend the tongue for examination of the dorsum; then have the patient raise the tongue to the palate to permit good visualization of the sublingual space. The patient should extend the tongue forcibly out to the right and left sides of the mouth to permit good visualization of the sublingual space and to permit careful examination of the left and right margins. A piece of gauze wrapped lightly around the tip of the tongue helps when manually moving the patient's tongue. Examine the tonsillar fossae and the oropharynx.

6. Use bimanual or bi-digital palpation for examination of the tongue, cheeks, floor of the mouth, and salivary glands. Palpation is also useful for determining the degree of tooth movement. Two resistant instruments, such as mirror handles or tongue depressors, placed on the buccal and lingual surfaces of the tooth furnish more accurate information than when fingers alone are directly employed.

7. Examine the teeth for dental caries, occlusal relations, possible prematurities, inadequate contact areas or restorations, evidence of food impaction, gingivitis, periodontal disease, and fistulae.

8. After the general examination of the oral cavity has been completed, make a detailed study of the lesion or the area involved in the chief complaint.

A list of normal anatomic structures that may be identified by superficial examination of the head, neck, and oral cavity is provided in Table 2-6. No attempt is made to identify each

TABLE 2-6   Normal Anatomic Structures That May Be Identified by Superficial Physical Examination of the Head, Neck, and Oral Cavity

Head: extraoral structures

  Face

    Skin

    Nose (alae, external nares, nasal mucosa)

    Eyes (pupils, palpebral and bulbar conjunctivae, irises, lacrimal caruncle, lacrimal glands and duct orifices, orifice of the nasolacrimal duct, eyebrows, eyelashes, commissures)

    Jaws (mandibular border, angle, symphysis, condyle and coronoid processes; malar process, maxilla, infraorbital foramen, mental foramen, lingual notch, maxillary sinuses)

    Masticatory muscles (temporalis, masseter, buccinator)

    Parotid gland

    Muscles of expression (obicularis oris, depressor and levator anguli oris, obicularis oculi)

    Distribution of branches of the facial nerve

    External carotid, lingual, and temporal pulses

  Scalp and cranium (frontal, occipital, and temporal bones; mastoid process; nuchal point; frontal sinuses; cranial aponeurosis; insertion of temporal muscle)

  Ears (pinna, external auditory meatus and canal, tragus, helix)

Neck (anterior, posterior, and submaxillary triangle; sternocleidomastoid; platysma; digastric and mylohyoid muscles; thyroid and cricoid cartilages; trachea; wings of hyoid bone; thyroid gland; anterior and posterior cervical lymph nodes; submandibular lymph nodes; sternal notch and clavicles; first cervical vertebra (atlas), carotid pulse)

Relationships: mesial, distal, anteroposterior, buccal, facial, labial, vestibular, lingual, palatal, coronal, sagittal, lateral, interproximal, gingival, incisal, occlusal

Head: intraoral structures

  Lips (skin and mucosal surfaces, vermilion border, commissures, oral vestibule, minor salivary glands, labial frenum)

  Checks (buccinator muscle, buccal fat pad, buccal frenum, occlusal line [linea alba], orifice and papilla of parotid gland duct [Stensen's duct], minor salivary glands, Fordyce's granules, buccal vestibule)

  Tongue (dorsum [anterior two-thirds and posterior one-third]; filiform, fungiform, vallate, and voliate papillae; foramen cecum; lymphoid follicles of posterior one-third; ventral surface, including mucosa, fimbriated folds, superficial veins and varicosities, anterior lingual glands [Blandin and Nuhn's glands] and ducts)

  Floor of mouth (plicae submandibularis [sublingual folds], submandibular duct [Wharton's duct], and orifice of submandibular and sublingual gland ducts [sublingual caruncle]; lingual vestibule; genial tubercles; mylohyoid ridge; lingual nerve)

  Palate (hard and soft palates, reflecting line, foveae palatini, maxillary tuberosity, pterygoid hamulus, tensor palati muscle, anterior and posterior palatine canals, uvula)

  Gingivae (marginal gingivae, attached keratinized [alveolar] and nonkeratinized [areolar] gingivae, gingival sulcus, interdental papillae)

  Retromolar region (retromolar pad, external oblique ridge, palatoglossal arch [anterior pillar of fauces], pterygomandibular ligament, retromolar triangle, stylohyoid ligament

  Pharynx (palatine tonsils, palatopharyngeal arch [posterior pillar of fauces], tonsillar crypts, posterior pharyngeal wall, lateral pharyngeal wall, orifice of eustachian tube and posterior nares, larynx, pyriform fossa, epiglottis, internal pterygoid muscle, Waldeyer's ring, lingual tonsils, adenoids)

  Teeth: chart the designation and name of each tooth

---

structure during a routine head and neck examination. However, the ability to recognize all of these structures is basic to performing a physical examination of this region in which asymmetries, swellings, discolorations, changes in texture, and tender areas may have to be differentiated from normal structures. Abnormalities that should be specifically sought and noted are discussed below, under the specific regions covered by the oral examination.

FACIAL STRUCTURES

Observe the patient's skin for color, blemishes, moles, and other pigmentation abnormalities; vascular abnormalities such as angiomas, telangiectasias, nevi, and tortuous superficial vessels; and asymmetry, ulcers, pustules, nodules, and swellings. Note the color of the conjunctivae. Palpate the jaws and super-

ficial masticatory muscles for tenderness or deformity. Note any scars or keloid formation.

LIPS

Note lip color, texture, and any surface abnormalities as well as angular or vertical fissures, lip pits, cold sores, ulcers, scabs, nodules, keratotic plaques, and scars. Palpate upper lip and lower lip for any thickening (induration) or swelling. Note orifices of minor salivary glands and the presence of Fordyce's granules.

CHEEKS

Note any changes in pigmentation and movability of the mucosa, a pronounced linea alba, leukoedema, hyperkeratotic patches, intraoral swellings, ulcers, nodules, scars, other red or white patches, and Fordyce's granules. Observe openings of Stensen's ducts and establish their patency by first drying the mucosa with gauze and then observing the character and extent of salivary flow from duct openings, with and without milking of the gland. Palpate muscles of mastication.

MAXILLARY AND MANDIBULAR MUCOBUCCAL FOLDS

Observe color, texture, any swellings, and any fistulae. Palpate for swellings and tenderness over the roots of the teeth and for tenderness of the buccinator insertion by pressing laterally with a finger inserted over the roots of the upper molar teeth.

HARD PALATE AND SOFT PALATE

Illuminate the palate and inspect for discoloration, swellings, fistulae, papillary hyperplasia, tori, ulcers, recent burns, leukoplakia, and asymmetry of structure or function. Examine the orifices of minor salivary glands. Palpate the palate for swellings and tenderness.

THE TONGUE

Inspect the dorsum of the tongue (while it is at rest) for any swelling, ulcers, coating, or variation in size, color, and texture. Observe the margins of the tongue and note the distribution of filiform and fungiform papillae, crenations and fasciculations, depapillated areas, fissures, ulcers, and keratotic areas. Note the frenal attachment and any deviations as the patient pushes out the tongue and attempts to move it to the right and left.

Wrap a piece of gauze (4 cm × 4 cm) around the tip of the protruding tongue to steady it, and lightly press a warm mirror against the uvula to observe the base of the tongue and vallate papillae; note any ulcers or significant swellings. Holding the tongue with the gauze, gently guide the tongue to the right and retract the left cheek to observe the foliate papillae and the entire lateral border of the tongue for ulcers, keratotic areas, and red patches. Repeat for the opposite side, and then have the patient touch the tip of the tongue to the palate to display the ventral surface of the tongue and floor of the mouth; note any varicosities, tight frenal attachments, stones in Wharton's ducts, ulcers, swellings, and red or white patches. Gently palpate the muscles of the tongue for nodules and tumors, extending the finger onto the base of the tongue and pressing forward if this has been poorly visualized or if any ulcers or masses are suspected. Note tongue thrust on swallowing.

FLOOR OF THE MOUTH

With the tongue still elevated, observe the openings of Wharton's ducts, the salivary pool, the character and extent of right and left secretions, and any swellings, ulcers, or red or white patches. Gently explore and display the extent of the lateral sublingual space, again noting ulcers and red or white patches.

GINGIVAE

Observe color, texture, contour, and frenal attachments. Note any ulcers, marginal inflammation, resorption, festooning, Stillman's clefts, hyperplasia, nodules, swellings, and fistulae.

TEETH AND PERIODONTIUM

Note missing or supernumerary teeth, mobile or painful teeth, caries, defective restorations, dental arch irregularities, orthodontic anomalies, abnormal jaw relationships, occlusal interferences, the extent of plaque and calculus deposits, dental hypoplasia, and discolored teeth.

TONSILS AND OROPHARYNX

Note the color, size, and any surface abnormalities of tonsils and ulcers, tonsilloliths, and inspissated secretion in tonsillar crypts. Palpate the tonsils for discharge or tenderness, and note restriction of the oropharyngeal airway. Examine the faucial pillars for bilateral symmetry, nodules, red and white patches, lymphoid aggregates, and deformities. Examine the postpharyngeal wall for swellings, nodular lymphoid hyperplasia, hyperplastic adenoids, postnasal discharge, and heavy mucous secretions.

SALIVARY GLANDS

Note any external swelling that may represent enlargement of a major salivary gland. A significantly enlarged parotid gland will alter the facial contour and may lift the ear lobe; an enlarged submandibular salivary gland (or lymph node) may distend the skin over the submandibular triangle. With minimal manipulation of the patient's lips, tongue, and cheeks, note the presence of any salivary pool, and note whether the mucosa is moist, covered with scanty frothy saliva, or dry.

To evaluate parotid gland function, dry the cheek mucosa around the orifice of each parotid duct, and massage or "milk" the gland and duct externally, observing the amount and character of any excreted material. With a normal gland, clear and freely flowing saliva will be readily apparent; a limited flow (usually only one or two drops) of viscous saliva, cloudy or frankly purulent discharges, or the absence of flow are abnormal and indicate the need for additional evaluation of the salivary glands. When salivary flow is reduced, there may be a brief flow of viscous or cloudy saliva, followed by a small amount of apparently normal saliva; this emphasizes the need for careful observation of the initial flow. Psychic stimuli (such as asking the patient to think of a cold refreshing lemon drink on a hot day) may also be used to increase the flow of parotid saliva during the examination. Palpate any suspected parotid swelling externally at this time, recording texture and any tenderness or nodularity; distinguish parotid enlargement from hypertrophy and spasm of the masseter muscle.

For the submandibular and sublingual glands, use bimanual palpation (insert the gloved index finger beside the tongue in the floor of the mouth and locate the two salivary glands and any enlarged submandibular lymph nodes, using a second finger placed externally over the gland); note the location, texture, and size of each gland and any tenderness or nodules. Dry the orifices of both Wharton's ducts and note the amount and character of the excreted saliva as one and then the other submandibular glands and ducts are "milked." Palpate Wharton's duct on each side for any salivary calculi. When either the parotid or the submandibular/sublingual salivary flow appears minimal, flow may often be stimulated by either gustatory stimuli (such as lemon juice swabbed on the tongue dorsum) or painful stimuli (eg, pricking the gingiva with an explorer). With stimulation of the salivary flow, minor salivary gland function can be demonstrated by the appearance of multiple small beads of saliva on the dried upper- and lower-lip mucosa. (See Chapters 9, Salivary Gland Disease and 3, Maxillofacial Imaging for descriptions of more detailed evaluation of salivary function and imaging of the salivary glands.)

TEMPOROMANDIBULAR JOINT

Observe deviations in the path of the mandible during opening and closing, as well as the range of vertical and lateral movement.[45] Palpate the joints, and listen for clicking and crepitus during opening and closing of the jaw; use a stethoscope to characterize and locate these sounds accurately. Note any tenderness over the joint or masticatory muscles (temporalis, masseter) while palpating externally and over the lateral pterygoid and buccinator muscles (distal and lateral to upper molar teeth) and the medial pterygoid muscle (pterygomandibular ligament and medial aspect of anterior faucial pillar) with the patient's mouth open. Explore the anterior wall of the external auditory meatus for tenderness and pain that are usually associated with capsulitis. (See Chapter 10, Temporomandibular Disorders for descriptions of more detailed evaluation and imaging of the temporomandibular joint.)

NECK AND LYMPH NODES

Examination of the neck is a natural extension of a routine dental examination and includes examination of the sub-mandibular and cervical lymph nodes (draining the oropharynx and other tissues of the head and neck and anastomosing with lymphatics from the abdomen, thorax, breast, and arm), the midline structures (hyoid bone, cricoid and thyroid cartilages, trachea, and thyroid gland), and carotid arteries and neck veins.[46] (Examination of the submandibular and sublingual salivary glands was described in the preceding section.) With the patient's neck extended, note the clavicle and the sternomastoid and trapezius muscles, which define the anterior and posterior triangles of the neck. Palpate the hyoid bone, the thyroid and cricoid cartilages, and the trachea, noting any displacement or tenderness. Palpate around the lower half of the sternomastoid muscle, and identify and palpate the isthmus and wings of the thyroid gland below and lateral to the thyroid cartilage, checking for any nodularity, masses, or tenderness. If local or generalized thyroid enlargement is suspected, check to ascertain whether the mass moves up and down with the trachea when the patient swallows. Observe the external jugular vein as it crosses the sternomastoid muscle, and with the patient at an angle of approximately 45° to the horizontal, note any distension and or pulsation in the vein. Distension of >2 cm above the sternal notch is abnormal; in severe right-sided heart failure, distension as far as the angle of the mandible may be seen. Place the diaphragm of the stethoscope over the point of the carotid pulse, and listen for bruits or other disturbances of rhythm that may indicate partial occlusion of the carotid artery.

Palpate for lymph nodes in the neck (Figure 2-2), commencing with the most superior nodes and working down to the clavicle. Palpate anterior to the tragus of the ear for preauricular nodes; at the mastoid and base of the skull for

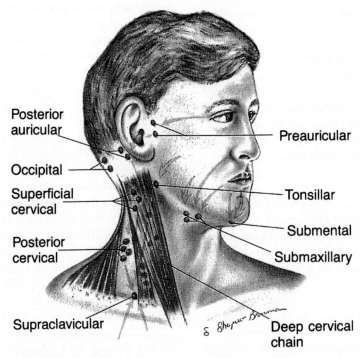

FIGURE 2-2 Lymph nodes of the head and neck.

posterior auricular and occipital nodes; under the chin for the submental nodes; and further posterior for submandibular and lingual-notch nodes (usually palpated when the submandibular salivary gland is examined). The superficial cervical nodes lie above the sternomastoid muscle; the deep cervical nodes lie between the sternomastoid muscle and cervical fascia. To examine the latter, ask the patient to sit erect and to turn his or her head to one side to relax the sternomastoid; use thumb and fingers to palpate under the anterior and posterior borders of the relaxed muscle, and repeat the procedure on the opposite side. Next, palpate the posterior cervical nodes in the posterior triangle close to the anterior border of the trapezius muscle. Finally, check for supraclavicular nodes just above the clavicle, lateral to the attachment of the sternomastoid muscle.

Normal lymph nodes may be difficult to palpate; enlarged lymph nodes (whether due to current infection, scarring from past inflammatory processes, or neoplastic involvement) are usually readily located. Many patients have isolated enlarged and freely movable submandibular and cervical nodes from past oral or pharyngeal infection. Nodes draining areas of active infection are usually tender; the overlying skin may be warm and red, and there may be a history of recent enlargement. Nodes enlarged as the result of metastatic spread of a malignant tumor have no characteristic clinical appearance and may be small and asymptomatic or grossly enlarged. Classically, nodes enlarged due to cancer are described as "fixed to underlying tissue" (implying that the tumor cells have broken through the capsule of the lymph node or that necrosis and inflammation have produced perinodular scarring and adhesions), but this feature will usually be absent except with the most aggressive or advanced tumors. Gradually enlarging groups of nodes in the absence of local infection and inflammation are a significant finding that suggests either systemic disease (eg, infectious mononucleosis or generalized lymphadenopathy associated with human immunodeficiency virus [HIV] infection) or a lymphoid neoplasm (lymphoma or Hodgkin's disease); such a finding justifies examination for (or inquiry about) lymphoid enlargement at distant sites, such as the axilla, inguinal region, and spleen, to confirm the generalized nature of the process. A successful outcome to cancer treatment is dependent on early detection and treatment, and hence the need for rapid follow-up investigation whenever unexplained lymph node enlargement is detected during examination of the neck. Enlargement of supraclavicular and cervical nodes may occur from lymphatic spread of tumor from the thorax, breast, and arm as well as from tumors of the oral cavity and nasopharynx. Conditions to be considered in a patient with cervical lymph node enlargement include acute bacterial, viral, and rickettsial infections of the head and neck (eg, acute abscesses, infectious mononucleosis, cat-scratch disease, and mucocutaneous lymph node syndrome); chronic bacterial infections, such as syphilis and tuberculosis; leukemia, lymphoma, metastatic carcinoma, collagen disease, and allergic reactions (especially serum sickness); and sarcoidosis.

CRANIAL NERVE FUNCTION

In examining patients with oral sensory or motor complaints, it is important to know if there is any objective evidence of abnormality of cranial nerve function that might relate to the patient's oral symptoms. A definitive answer to this question usually comes from specific testing of cranial nerve function as part of a general physical examination carried out by either the patient's physician, an internist, or a neurologist. When the results of a neurologist's examination are not readily available, a cranial nerve examination carried out by the dentist may help direct diagnostic efforts in the interim. The following schema (summarized in Table 2-7) is provided with such circumstances in mind and not as a substitute for a thorough neurologic examination carried out by a skilled specialist. On the other hand, dentists and oral surgeons in hospitals are often responsible for the admitting history and physical examination of their patients. In view of the focus of dentistry, it is logical that the physical examination carried out by a dentist should be complete as far as the head and neck are concerned and should include an assessment of cranial nerve function. The dentist's professional training and experience give him or her a specialized knowledge of the range of normal oral function, providing a level of accuracy usually not available to one less experienced in the examination of the mouth. For these reasons, instruction and experience in the evaluation of cranial nerve function, particularly as it relates to the oral cavity (eg, cranial nerves V, VII, IX, and XII), are fully justified as part of a dentist's education.

The routine cranial nerve examination is carried out systematically according to the sequence of nerves (from I to XII). Each examiner will develop a personal routine, but it should always be standardized so that the results of repeated examinations will be comparable. In addition to the standard evaluation described here, there are a number of other techniques of special interest in particular clinical situations.

Cranial Nerve I (Olfactory Nerve). Olfactory nerve function is traditionally tested by closing one of the patient's nostrils with a finger and asking if the patient can smell a strongly scented volatile substance such as coffee or lemon extract. The test is then repeated for the other nostril. The patient should sniff strongly to draw the volatile molecules well into the nose. This procedure tests for olfactory nerve function only when the nasal airway is patent to the olfactory receptors and when the substance being tested does not produce a response solely on the basis of chemical irritation of nonspecific somatic sensory receptors in the nasal mucosa. Such responses are due to stimulation of branches of the trigeminal nerve. For this reason, substances such as ammonia, perfumes (because of alcoholic content), and onions, although strongly scented, cannot be used to test for olfactory function. A compact "scratch-and-sniff" test (suitable for clinical use) that uses 50 different microencapsulated olfactory stimulants (the University of Pennsylvania Smell Identification Test [UP-SIT], Sensonics, Inc., Haddon Heights, N.J.) has been developed by the University of Pennsylvania Clinical Smell

TABLE 2-7   Summary of Cranial Nerve Examinations

Cranial Nerve	Function	Usual Complaint	Test of Function	Physical Findings
I (olfactory)	Smell	None, or loss of "taste" if bilateral	Sense of smell*	No response to olfactory stimuli
II (optic)	Vision	Loss of vision	Visual acuity; visual fields of each eye	Decreased visual acuity, or loss of visual field
III (oculomotor)	Eye movement; pupillary construction	Double vision	Pupil and eye movement	Failure to move eye in field of motion of muscle; pupillary abnormalities
IV (trochlear)	Eye movement	Double vision, especially on down and medial gaze	Ability to move eye down and in	Negligible†
V (trigeminal)	Facial, nasal, and oral sensation; jaw movement	Numbness; paresthesia	Pinprick sensation on face; corneal reflex; masseter muscle contraction	Decreased pin and absent corneal reflex; weakness of masticatory muscles
VI (abducens)	Eye movement	Double vision on lateral gaze	Move eyes laterally	Failure of eye to abduct
VII (facial)	Facial movement	Lack of facial movement, eye closure; dysarthria	Facial contraction; smiling	Asymmetry of facial contraction
VIII (auditory and vestibular)	Hearing; balance	Hearing loss; tinnitus; vertigo	Hearing test; nystagmus; balance	Decreased hearing; nystagmus; ataxia
IX (glossopharyngeal)	Palatal movement	Trouble swallowing	Elevation of palate	Asymmetric palate
X (vagus)	Palatal movement; vocal cords	Hoarseness; trouble swallowing	Elevation of palate; vocal cords	Asymmetric palate; "brassy" voice
XI (spinal accessory)	Turns neck	None	Contraction of sternocleidomastoid and trapezius	Paralysis of sternocleidomastoid muscle
XII (hypoglossal)	Moves tongue	Dysarthria	Extrusion of tongue	Wasting and fasciculation or deviation of tongue

Adapted from Balciunas BA, Siegel MA. A clinical approach to the diagnosis of facial pain. Dent Clin North Am 1992;36:987–1000.

*Each nostril tested individually.

†May be difficult to detect anything if the third nerve is intact.

and Taste Research Center, for more accurate and comprehensive testing of olfactory function.

Cranial Nerve II (Optic Nerve).   Optic nerve function is tested by the investigation of visual acuity and the visual fields. In addition, clinicians who are trained in the use of the ophthalmoscope can use this instrument to examine the ocular fundus directly for lesions. Visual acuity is tested with the familiar wall chart, but it can also be evaluated by asking the patient to read print of various sizes in a book or newspaper held at various distances from the patient's eyes.

Gross defects in the field of vision can be detected by having the patient indicate how close to the midline a pencil held in the observer's hand must be brought before it can be seen. For this test (known as the confrontation test), hold the pencil 2 to 3 feet to one side of the patient's face while the patient covers the other eye. Move the pencil in turn along the main axes of the field of vision until the patient can see it.

Cranial Nerves III, IV, and VI (Ocular Nerves).   The three ocular nerves are concerned with the pupillary reflex (III), accommodations (III), and eye movements (III, IV, and VI). These nerves are tested simultaneously by examining the size, outline, and reaction of each pupil to light and dark and to accommodation for near and far vision. Conjugate eye movements, individual eye movements, and convergent vision (all

under the control of bilateral extraocular eye muscles) are tested by having the patient follow the path of a pencil held both at a distance and close up as it traverses right to left and up and down.

Cranial Nerve V (Trigeminal Nerve).   The trigeminal nerve is tested for both motor and sensory function. The small motor branch of this nerve supplies the muscles of mastication, and the strength of these muscles is used as a measure of the intactness of their motor supply. The force of contraction and muscle bulk (motor loss leads to laxity and muscle atrophy) of the masseter and temporal muscles are noted by external palpation of these muscles bilaterally while the patient clenches. Lateral movement of the jaw against the examiner's finger is one test of pterygoid function. Weakness of the temporalis, masseter, and pterygoid muscles may also manifest itself by deviation of the jaw when the patient opens the mouth. (Disorders of the temporomandibular joint may produce similar signs, however, with the instability of the jaw to passive displacement at the temporomandibular joint resulting in easy subluxation of the joint.)

Another useful indicator of the motor power of the masticatory muscles is their ability to carry out voluntary displacement of the jaw against the imposed resistance of the examiner's hand, tested as follows: place the thumb on the lower molar table, with fingers externally about the body and ramus; the patient moves the jaw forward, sideways, and upward, with his or her head steadied by your other hand.

Abnormalities of the jaw jerk may indicate muscular weakness or an abnormality of the proprioceptive reflex arc controlling jaw movements. Press your index finger downward and posteriorly above the mental eminence, and lightly strike the finger with a percussion hammer or with one or two fingers of the other hand. In normal subjects, a single reflex response can usually be discerned by palpation. The principle is the same as that of the more familiar knee jerk test.

Sensory function of the trigeminal nerve should logically be tested for all three divisions (ophthalmic, maxillary, and mandibular), but testing is often focused on the corneal reflex to touch (ophthalmic division), with rather cursory testing of touch and pinprick sensation on the facial skin and often with no testing of the intraoral mucosa. The dentist's interest in orofacial problems will often require more detailed evaluation of intraoral sensitivity and skin sensitivity for the lower half of the face; however, a complete evaluation of all sensory modalities subserved by branches of cranial nerve V—pain, touch, temperature, two-point discrimination, and taste (ie, gustatory fibers of cranial nerve VII traveling with the lingual branch of cranial nerve V)—is rarely possible and is usually attempted only as part of a thorough research investigation.

The following instruments, many of which can be adapted for the testing of trigeminal sensory function, are available as aids in sensory evaluation:

1. Graded Frey's hairs (a series of fine hairs or nylon fibers calibrated according to the force required to bend the filament when it is placed against skin, mucosa, or tooth)
2. Two-point esthesiometers, often designed with a pistol grip to facilitate the placement of the points of the instrument on the oral mucosa (similar testing can be carried out with a simple caliper)
3. Calibrated thermal devices for the application of hot and cold
4. Discs of various grades of sandpaper for the evaluation of textural differences
5. Stereognostic forms for the evaluation of oral stereotactic ability
6. Two-dimensional maps of the oral mucosa on which sensory response about a lesion or area of paresthesia can be accurately recorded.
7. Taste testing

Abnormalities in any of these various modalities of trigeminal sensory function may be taken as evidence of an abnormality of the affected branch of cranial nerve V and provide additional evidence of the diagnosis of neuropathy that may be suggested by the patient's subjective report of paresthesia, numbness, or other unusual sensations.

Cranial Nerve VII (Facial Nerve). The facial nerve is tested for abnormalities of motor function involving the "mimetic" muscles of facial expression and also for gustatory disorders.

A gustatory salivary reflex involves facial nerve gustatory stimuli and increased salivary function, and affections of the chorda tympani may be associated with failure of the salivary flow to increase following the application of lemon juice or citric acid to the affected side of the mouth.

Motor function of cranial nerve VII is tested by observing facial muscle function in response to requests to wrinkle the forehead, frown, close the eyelids tightly, wink, open the mouth, retract the mouth, blow out the cheeks, pucker the lips, "screw up" the nose, whistle, and speak. Close observation and comparison of the right and left sides may be necessary to detect minor degrees of facial paralysis in some patients; in other patients, the defect will be obvious and disfiguring.

Cranial Nerve VIII (Acoustic Nerve). Acoustic nerve function includes both cochlear (hearing) and vestibular (balance) components, which are physiologically distinct and which are tested separately. Hearing may be tested at three levels of sophistication in the following ways:

1. By observing the patient's ability to hear (a) normal speech and a whisper or (b) the ticking of a watch held at varying distances from each ear
2. By holding one or more tuning forks near each ear, on the mastoid process, and on the forehead (allowing separation of nerve and conduction deafness as well as identification of unilateral defects)
3. By audiometric testing (the most precise method)

Simple tests for vestibular function include the past-pointing test and assessment for the eye movements that are characteristic of nystagmus when the patient is asked to look to one side and then upward (nystagmus will cause a fast jerk to the direction indicated, followed by a slow return to the midline, with or without rotary movements of the eyeball). More elaborate studies of vestibular function involve tests for the occurrence of past-pointing, nystagmus, and vertigo and nausea when cold water or a blast of cold air is injected into the external auditory canal of the upright patient.

Cranial Nerve IX (Glossopharyngeal Nerve). The glossopharyngeal nerve provides taste fibers to the posterior aspect of the tongue, somatic sensory fibers to the same area of the tongue as well as to the pharynx and soft palate (tested along with sensory function of cranial nerve X, below), and motor fibers to the stylopharyngeus muscle, which plays only a minor role in palatal function. Thus, any accurate testing of cranial nerve IX motor function is impossible.

Cranial Nerve X (Vagus Nerve). The vagus nerve is the chief motor nerve of the pharynx and larynx; it also provides sensory fibers to the pharyngeal and faucial mucous membrane. Routine testing is carried out by observation of pharyngeal movements (eg, symmetric elevation of the soft palate and shortening of the uvula when the patient says "ah") and the pharyngeal (gag) reflex (ie, contraction of the palate and faucial muscles in response to the examiner's touching the mucosa of the posterior pharynx). The gag reflex may be temporarily eliminated with a topical analgesic spray so that the soft palate and pharynx can be palpated manually for masses and muscular tonus. Since the major clinical problem associated with cranial nerve X dysfunction is dysphagia, a more detailed evaluation of this nerve's function can include the careful observation of swallowing. The laryngeal component of the vagus nerve is studied by inspection of laryngeal function with indirect laryngoscopy (using a headlamp and a dental mirror, with the patient's tongue extended) and by various vocal tests of phonation. Pulse and respiratory rates are measures of the visceral component of the vagus nerve although a variety of other factors also affect these rates.

Cranial Nerve XI (Accessory Nerve). The spinal accessory nerve is tested through its motor supply to the trapezius and sternomastoid muscles. For the trapezius, ask the patient to shrug his or her shoulders against the resistance of your hands; for the sternomastoid, have the patient turn and flex the head against the same resistance.

Cranial Nerve XII (Hypoglossal Nerve). The hypoglossal nerve provides the motor supply to the tongue; hypoglossal paralysis causes deviation of the tongue when the patient extrudes it. Atrophy of the tongue's musculature may be noted on oral examination, and its muscular tonus can be ascertained by the force with which the patient can push the tongue against either cheek or by evaluation of the tongue jerk. Dyskinesia (such as may occur in parkinsonism and amyotrophic lateral sclerosis) is observed on the dorsal surface of the tongue, particularly when the tongue comes to the resting position after vigorous or forceful activity. Crenation of the margin of the tongue caused by forceful and persistent molding of the organ against irregular lingual surfaces of the dental arch is frequently seen in neurologically normal patients and is difficult to evaluate as a sign of lingual atrophy. More often than not, crenation is the result of muscle tension that may also be manifest in other parts of the body or that may accompany severe malocclusion. Occasionally, it may be due to true macroglossia.

SUPPLEMENTARY EXAMINATION PROCEDURES

With the information obtained from the history and routine physical examination, a diagnosis can usually be made, or the information can at least provide the clinician with direction for subsequent diagnostic procedures. Additional questioning of the patient or more specialized examination procedures may still be needed to confirm a diagnosis or distinguish between several possible diagnoses. Examples of more specialized physical examination procedures are the charting of dental restorations, caries, and periodontal defects; dental pulp vitality testing; detailed evaluation of salivary gland function (see Chapter 9, Salivary Gland Disease); and assessments of occlusion, masticatory muscles, and temporomandibular joint function (see Chapter 10, Temporomandibular Disorders). Radiography of the teeth and jaws, computer-assisted scanning (computed

tomography [CT]), and magnetic resonance imaging (MRI) of the temporomandibular joint, salivary glands, and other soft-tissue structures of the head and neck (see Chapter X) can provide visible evidence of suspected physical abnormalities, and a variety of laboratory aids to diagnosis (such as serology, biopsy, and blood chemistry, hematologic, and microbiologic procedures) can be used to confirm a suspected diagnosis or to identify a systemic abnormality contributing to the patient's signs and symptoms.

LABORATORY STUDIES

It is important to realize the limitations of any laboratory test. There are no tests that can detect "health"; rather, laboratory tests are used to discriminate between the presence or absence of disease or are used as a predictor of disease. The frequency with which a test indicates the presence of a disease is called sensitivity; specificity is the frequency with which a test indicates the absence of the disease.[47] A test that identifies a disease every time has a sensitivity of 100% whereas a test that identifies the absence of disease every time has a specificity of 100%. Consequently, a test with a sensitivity of 98% has a 2% false-negative rate, and a test with a specificity of 98% has a 2% false-positive rate. The significance of choosing a test with a particular sensitivity or specificity usually corresponds with the outcome of the test result. For instance, it is highly desirable to use an HIV test with a high sensitivity to minimize false-negative results because individuals who believe they are HIV-negative may continue to transmit the disease and may not seek medical care. However, sensitivity improves at the expense of specificity, and vice versa.

Another important aspect of a test is its efficacy, or predictive value. Predictive value is defined as the value of positive results indicating the presence of a disease (positive predictive value) or the value of negative results indicating the absence of a disease (negative predictive value). These predictive values are dependent on the prevalence of the particular condition in the population, as well as on the sensitivity and specificity of the test.

Even normal values in tests used to screen asymptomatic populations for disease fall within two standard deviations of the mean. Consequently, a single test will produce an abnormal result 5% of the time. For a "panel" of tests the percentage of abnormal results increases significantly. Thus, for any decision (or even diagnosis) based on any laboratory test, many different criteria need to be considered.

Laboratory studies are an extension of the physical examination; tissue, blood, urine, or other specimens are obtained from the patient and are subjected to microscopic, biochemical, microbiologic, or immunologic examination. A laboratory test alone rarely establishes the nature of an oral lesion, but when interpreted in conjunction with information obtained from the history and the physical examination, the results of laboratory tests will frequently establish or confirm a diagnostic impression. Specimens obtained directly from the oral cavity (eg, scrapings of oral mucosal cells, tissue biopsy specimens, and swabs of exudates), as well as the specimens more commonly submitted to the clinical diagnostic laboratory (eg, blood), may provide information that is of value in the diagnosis of oral lesions such as candidiasis, pulpal and periodontal abscesses, pharyngitis, and lesions of the oral mucosa and jaw bones.

Lesions of the oral cavity may also be complicated by coexistent systemic disease or may be the direct result of such disease. Many of the laboratory studies needed in dental practice are those that are widely used in medicine. The systemic disease suspected by the dentist may often be of greater significance to the patient's health than the presenting oral lesion may be. By investigating a problem of this type, the dentist is, in effect, investigating a medical problem. It has been argued that the patient in whom systemic disease is suspected should be referred to a physician without further tests being ordered by the dentist. This procedure is clearly the correct one under some circumstances, and professional judgment is required. However, in many situations, laboratory studies made by the dentist prior to medical referral are appropriate and may be necessary to identify the nature of the patient's problem or to assess the severity of an underlying medical condition.

Diseases affecting the oral cavity often exhibit features peculiar to this region, and a dentist trained in the management of diseases of the oral cavity may be better equipped to select appropriate laboratory tests and evaluate their results than is a physician with no specific knowledge of the region.

A diagnostic problem can be solved by referral only when the patient accepts the referral. If a lesion is minor or if the patient is unwilling to admit that the lesion may be of systemic origin, then she or he may reject the dentist's advice, delay in following up the referral, or even seek treatment elsewhere. Failure to follow up a referral may sometimes stem from the patient's belief that the dentist is straying beyond his or her area of competence but is more often the result of anxiety created by the dentist's suggesting that the patient may have an undiagnosed medical problem. Referral to a physician is possible only when confidence is firmly established between dentist and patient. Patients who seem unwilling to accept referral to a physician often agree to a screening laboratory test (eg, blood sugar, hematocrit) carried out through the dentist's office. When the results of such tests are positive, they strengthen the dentist's recommendation and often achieve the desired referral.

Screening diagnostic clinical and laboratory procedures, such as blood pressure measurement, complete blood count, blood chemistry screening, throat culture for infections with beta-hemolytic streptococci, and detection of antibodies to hepatitis viruses and HIV, have also been used for epidemiologic purposes in dentistry.[48–51] Except in limited situations, however, the cost of standard screening tests such as a complete blood count or blood sugar determination has discouraged their routine use in dental offices and clinics, even though the detection of elevated blood pressure has become customary.

The results of screening tests of this type (and, in fact, the majority of studies carried out by dentists for the detection of systemic diseases) do not themselves constitute a diagnosis. For example, a dentist who finds glucose in the blood of a patient should not tell the patient that he or she has diabetes but should inform the patient that the results of the test indicate an abnormality and should then advise the patient to seek medical consultation. Reports of abnormal results for any of the tests should be sent directly to the patient's physician, and the diagnosis of diabetes, hypertension, or other disease should be made by the physician on the basis of physical examination, history, and (possibly) further laboratory tests. The management of any systemic problem detected is also the prerogative of the physician, and the dentist should not consider prescribing medication or other treatment for systemic disease detected in this way, even though he might be required to provide local care for the oral manifestations. The physician may decide that in the latent stage of the disease, only surveillance and advice to the patient are required.

The success of all screening for systemic disease, whether carried out by the public health authorities or by dentists, depends on the availability of physicians who are willing to accept such referrals. When ordering or carrying out a laboratory test for the detection of systemic disease, always consider what can practically be done with the results of the test. Laboratory testing without follow-up is not only futile but can lead to serious anxiety in the patient.

SPECIALIZED EXAMINATION OF OTHER ORGAN SYSTEMS

The compact anatomy of the head and neck and the close relationship between oral function and the contiguous nasal, otic, laryngopharyngeal, gastrointestinal, and ocular structures often require that evaluation of an oral problem be combined with evaluation of one or more of these related organ systems. For detailed evaluation of these extraoral systems, the dentist should request that the patient consult the appropriate medical specialist, who is informed of the reason for the consultation. The usefulness of this consultation will usually depend on the dentist's knowledge of the interaction of the oral cavity with adjacent organ systems, as well as the dentist's ability to recognize symptoms and signs of disease in the extraoral regions of the head and neck. Superficial inspection of these extraoral tissues is therefore a logical part of the dentist's examination for the causes of certain oral problems.

Disorders of the temporomandibular joint, referred pain, oropharyngeal and skin cancer screening, dysgeusia, salivary gland disease, postsurgical oropharyngeal and oronasal defects, and various congenital syndromes affecting the head and neck are all conditions that are frequently brought to the dentist's attention and that require the dentist to look beyond the oral cavity when examining the head and neck. The details of special examinations of the ears, nose, eyes, pharynx, larynx, and facial musculature and integument are beyond the scope of this chapter; the reader is advised to consult texts that describe the physical examination of these organs and to obtain training in the use of the headlamp, the otoscope, and the ophthalmoscope, as well as in techniques such as indirect laryngoscopy and the inspection of the nasal cavity. Knowledge of disease processes that affect these organ systems is also a prerequisite.

The dentist's initial evaluations of extraoral tissues neither infringe on the rights of other medical specialists nor reduce their professional activities. These evaluations can contribute significantly to the collaboration of dentist and physician in the management of many oral problems. More important, information gathered during these examinations will provide invaluable diagnostic information that is necessary to ensure a proper referral to a medical specialist. Provided the patient's permission is obtained before these nonsurgical procedures are carried out, there seems to be no legal bar to the dentist's examining these extraoral organ systems. *However, the dentist may be prohibited by law from specifically diagnosing and treating extraoral problems.* In all cases in which there is any concern about the presence of disease in any of these extraoral organ systems, referral and treatment for the patient must be sought from the appropriate medical service. The dentist needs to clearly indicate the preliminary nature of the examination of extraoral tissues and that the area of legal diagnostic competency is restricted to the oral cavity by recording and describing the results of the extraoral examination as impressions and not as diagnosis. Moreover, attempts at making an appropriate referral to a physician when systemic disease is suspected should also be recorded.

▼ ESTABLISHING THE DIAGNOSIS

In some circumstances, the diagnosis (ie, an explanation for the patient's symptoms and identification of other significant disease process) may be self-evident. When clinical data are more complex, the diagnosis may be established by

1. reviewing the patient's history and physical, radiographic, and laboratory examination data;
2. listing those items that either clearly indicate an abnormality or that suggest the possibility of a significant health problem requiring further evaluation;
3. grouping these items into primary versus secondary symptoms, acute versus chronic problems, and high versus low priority for treatment; and
4. categorizing and labeling these grouped items according to a standardized system for the classification of disease.

The rapidity and accuracy with which a diagnosis or set of diagnoses can be achieved depends on the history and examination data that have been collected and on the clinician's knowledge and ability to match these clinical data with a conceptual representation of one or more disease processes. In general, experienced clinicians have an extensive knowledge of human physiology and disease etiology, as well as recollections of past clinical experiences, and this enables them to establish the correct diagnosis fairly rapidly. Such "mental models" of disease syndromes also increase the efficiency with which experienced clinicians gather and evaluate clinical data and focus supplemental questioning and testing at all stages of the diagnostic process.

For effective treatment as well as for health insurance and medicolegal reasons, it is important that a diagnosis (or diagnostic summary) is entered into the patient's record after the detailed history and physical, radiographic, and laboratory examination data. The patient (or a responsible family member or guardian) should also be informed of the diagnosis. When more than one health problem is identified, the diagnosis for the primary complaint (ie, the stated problem for which the patient sought medical or dental advice) is usually listed first, followed by subsidiary diagnoses of concurrent problems. Previously diagnosed conditions that remain as actual or potential problems are also included, with the qualification "by history," "previously diagnosed," or "treated" to indicate their status. Problems that were identified but not clearly diagnosed during the current evaluation can also be listed with the comment "to be ruled out." Because oral medicine is concerned with regional problems that may or may not be modified by concurrent systemic disease, it is common for the list of diagnoses to include both oral lesions and systemic problems of actual or potential significance in the etiology or management of the oral lesion. Items in the medical history that do not relate to the current problem and that are not of major health significance usually are not included in the diagnostic summary. For example, a diagnosis might read as follows:

> (i) Alveolar abscess, lower left first molar; (ii) Rampant dental caries secondary to radiation-induced salivary hypofunction; (iii) Carcinoma of tonsillar fossa, by history, excised and treated with 6.5 Gy 2 years ago; (iv) Cirrhosis and prolonged bleeding time, by history; (v) Hyperglycemia, R/O (rule out) diabetes.

A definite diagnosis cannot always be made, despite a careful review of all history, clinical, and laboratory data. In such cases, a descriptive term (rather than a formal diagnosis) may be used for the patient's symptoms or lesion, with the added word "idiopathic," "unexplained," or (in the case of symptoms without apparent physical abnormality) "functional" or "symptomatic." The clinician must decide what terminology to use in conversing with the patient and whether to clearly identify this diagnosis as "undetermined." Irrespective of that decision, it is important to recognize the equivocal nature of the patient's problem and to schedule additional evaluation, by referral to another consultant, additional testing, or placement of the patient on recall for follow-up studies.

Unfortunately, there is no generally accepted system for identifying and classifying diseases, and diagnoses are often written with concerns related to third-party reimbursement and to medicolegal and local peer review as well as for the purpose of accurate description and communication of the patient's disease status.[52] Most practitioners probably follow the systems of disease classification and nomenclature that they were taught during their training since these usually serve as the framework for the mental models of disease syndromes on which they base their diagnoses.

Some standardization of diagnoses has been achieved in the United States as a result of the introduction (in the 1980s) of the diagnosis-related group (DRG) system as an obligatory cost-containment measure for the reimbursement of hospitals for inpatient care[52–56] and the more recent requirement that all requests for Medicare reimbursement for both inpatient and outpatient care include a diagnosis coded according to the lists contained in the International Classification of Diseases, 9th Revision, Clinical Modification (ICD-9-CM) codes, prepared under the auspices of the World Health Organization.[57–60] The DRG system[53,54] consists of 470 categories derived from multivariate analysis of data from a million hospitalized patients, including age, the patient's International Classification of Diseases (ICD) diagnosis, surgical procedures, intrahospital complications, and length of hospital stay. Although scientifically derived, the DRG system is designed for fiscal use rather than as a system for the accurate classification of disease. It also emphasizes procedures rather than diseases and has a number of serious flaws in its classification and coding system.[52] The ICD system, by contrast, was developed from attempts at establishing an internationally accepted list of causes of death and has undergone numerous revisions in the past 150 years, related to the various emphases placed on clinical, anatomic, biochemical, and perceived etiologic classification of disease at different times and different locations. There is still no official set of operational criteria for assigning the various diagnoses included in the ICD (even though many specialities[61–64] have attempted to match ICD codes with well-defined criteria for the differentiation of diseases affecting a given organ system), and codes are probably assigned in fairly arbitrary fashion in many circumstances. In addition, the categories for symptoms, lesions, and procedures applicable to disease of the oral cavity are limited and often outdated. Medicare and other third-party reimbursers are usually concerned only with diagnoses of those conditions that were actively diagnosed or treated at a given visit; concurrent problems not specifically addressed at that visit are omitted from the reimbursement diagnosis, even if they are of major health significance. The clinician, therefore, must address a number of concerns in formulating a diagnosis, selecting appropriate language for recording diagnoses on the chart and documenting requests for third-party reimbursement.

Patients must also be informed of their diagnoses as well as the results of the various examinations and tests carried out, they correlate with the patient's signs and symptoms and they clearly establish that a particular diagnostic concern has not been confirmed. Because patients' anxieties frequently emphasize the possibility of a potentially serious diagnosis, it is important to point out (when the facts allow) that the biopsy specimen revealed no evidence of a malignant growth, the blood test revealed no abnormality, and that no evidence of diseases such as diabetes, anemia, leukemia, or cancer was found. Equally important is the necessity to explain to the patient the nature, significance, and treatment of any lesion or disease that has been clearly diagnosed.

▼ FORMULATING A PLAN OF TREATMENT AND ASSESSING MEDICAL RISK

Plan of Treatment

The diagnostic procedures (history, physical examination, and imaging and laboratory studies) outlined in the preceding pages are designed to assist the dentist in establishing a plan of treatment directed at those disease processes that have been identified as responsible for the patient's symptoms. A plan of treatment of this type, which is directed at the causes of the patient's symptoms rather than at the symptoms themselves, is often referred to as rational, scientific, or definitive (in contrast to symptomatic, which denotes a treatment plan directed at the relief of symptoms, irrespective of their causes).

Like the diagnostic summary, the plan of treatment should be entered in the patient's record and explained to the patient in detail (procedure, chances for cure [prognosis], complications and side effects, and required time and expense). As initially formulated, the plan of treatment usually lists recommended procedures for the control of current disease as well as preventive measures designed to limit the recurrence or progression of the disease process over time. For medicolegal reasons, the treatment that is most likely to eradicate the disease and preserve as much function as possible (ie, the ideal treatment) is usually entered in the chart, even if the clinician realizes that compromises may be necessary to obtain the patient's consent to treatment. It is also unreasonable for the clinician to prejudge a patient's decision as to how much time, energy, and expense should be expended on treating the patient's disease or how much discomfort and pain the patient is willing to tolerate in achieving a cure.

The plan of treatment may be itemized according to the components of the diagnostic summary and is usually written prominently in the record to serve as a guide for the scheduling of further treatment visits. If the plan is complex or if there are reasonable treatment alternatives, a copy should also be given to the patient to allow consideration of the various implications of the plan of treatment he or she has been asked to agree to. Modifications of the ideal plan of treatment, agreed on by patient and clinician, should also be entered in the chart, together with a signed disclaimer from the patient if the modified plan of treatment is likely to be significantly less effective or unlikely to eradicate a major health problem.

Medical Risk Assessment

The diagnostic procedures described above are also designed to help the dentist (1) recognize significant deviations from normal general health status that may affect dental treatment, (2) make informed judgments on the risk of dental procedures, and (3) identify the need for medical consultation to provide assistance in diagnosing or treating systemic disease that may be an etiologic factor in oral disease or that is likely to be worsened by the proposed dental treatment. The end point of the diagnostic process is thus twofold, and an evaluation of any special risks posed by a patient's compromised medical status under the circumstances of the planned anesthetic, diagnostic, or medical or surgical treatment procedures must also be entered in the chart, usually as an addendum to the plan of treatment. This process of medical risk assessment is the responsibility of all clinicians prior to any anesthetic, diagnostic, or therapeutic procedure and applies to outpatient as well as inpatient situations.

A routine of initial history taking and physical examination is essential for all dental patients because even the apparently healthy patient may on evaluation be found to have history or examination findings of sufficient significance to cause the dentist to re-evaluate the plan of treatment, modify a medication, or even defer a particular treatment until additional diagnostic data are available. To respect the familiar medical axiom *primum non nocere* (first, do no harm), all procedures carried out on a patient and all prescriptions given to a patient should be preceded by the dentist's conscious consideration of the risk of the particular procedure. Medical risk assessment, by establishing a formal summary in the chart of the specific risks that are likely to occur in treating a particular patient, ensures that continuous self-evaluation will be carried out by the clinician.

A decision for or against dental treatment for a medically complex patient is traditionally arrived at by the dentist's requesting the patient's physician to "clear the patient for dental care." Unfortunately, in many cases, the physician is provided with little information about the nature of the proposed dental treatment and may have little (other than personal experience with dental care) on which to judge the stress likely to be associated with the proposed dental treatment. The response of a given patient to specific dental treatment situations may also be unpredictable, particularly when the patient has a number of disease processes and is maintained on a variety of medications. In addition, the practitioner identified by the patient as his or her physician may not have adequate or complete data from previous evaluations, data necessary to make an informed judgment on the patient's likely response to dental care. All too frequently, the dentist receives the brief comment "OK for dental care," which suggests that clearances are often given casually and subjectively rather than being based on objective physiologic data.

More important, the practice of having the patient "cleared" for dental care confuses the issue of responsibility for untoward events occurring during dental treatment. Although the dentist often must rely on the physician or a consultant for expert diagnostic information and for an opinion about the advisability of dental treatment or the need for special precautions, *the dentist retains the primary responsibility for the procedures actually carried out and for the immediate management of any untoward complications*. The dentist is most familiar with the procedures he or she is carrying out, as well as with their likely complications, but the dentist must also be able to assess patients for medical or other problems that are likely to set the stage for the development of complications. Thus, physicians can only advise on what type of modifications are necessary to treat a patient, but the treating dentist is ultimately responsible for the safety of the patient.

A number of guides have been developed to facilitate efficient and accurate preoperative assessment of medical risk.[65–67] The majority of these guides were developed for the assessment of risks associated with general anesthesia or major surgery and focus on mortality as the dependent variable; guides for the assessment of hazards associated with dental or oral surgical procedures performed under local or regional anesthesia usually take the same approach. Of these, the most commonly used are the American Society of Anesthesiologists (ASA) Physical Scoring System[68] (illustrated, in a form modified for dental use, in Table 2-8) and Goldman's Cardiac Risk Index[69] (Table 2-9). Although scores such as these are commonly included in the preoperative evaluation of patients admitted to hospitals for dental surgery, they use relatively broad risk categories, and their applicability to both inpatient and outpatient dental procedures is limited. The validity of preanesthetic risk assessment has also been questioned by several authors in light of data suggesting that the "demonstrable competence" of the anesthetist can also be a significant factor in anesthetic outcome.[70]

Medical Referral (Consultation) Procedure

Patients for whom a dentist may need to obtain medical consultation include (1) the patient with known medical problems who is scheduled for either inpatient or outpatient dental treatment, (2) the patient in whom abnormalities are detected dur-

---

TABLE 2-8   American Society of Anesthesiologists Physical Scoring System for Dental Treatment and Anesthesia

ASA Classification	Dental and Anesthesia Considerations
Physical status 1: patient without systemic disease; normal patient	Routine dental therapy, without modification
Physical status 2: patient with mild systemic disease	Routine dental therapy, with possible treatment limitations or special considerations*
Physical status 3: patient with severe systemic disease that limits activity but is not incapacitating	Dental therapy when significant complications can be anticipated and should be addressed
Physical status 4: patient with incapacitating systemic disease that is a constant threat to life	Emergency dental therapy only, preferably in close cooperation with patient's physician

Reproduced with permission from Keats AS.[68]

ASA = American Society of Anesthesiologists.

*Examples: timing and duration of therapy, interventions to reduce stress, and prophylactic medications.

TABLE 2-9 Computation of Cardiac Risk Index

Criterion	Points*
History	
Age > 70 years	5
MI in previous 6 months	10
Physical examination	
S3 gallop or JVD	11
Important VAS	3
Electrocardiography	
Rhythm other than sinus or PAC on last preoperative ECG	7
> 5 PVCs per minute documented at any time before operation	7
General status	
PO_2 < 60 mm Hg or PCO_2 > 50 mm Hg, K < 3.0 mEq/L or HCO_3 < 20 mEq/L, BUN > 50 mg/dL or CR > 3.0 mg/dL, abnormal SGOT, signs of chronic liver disease, or patient bedridden from noncardiac causes	3
Operation type	
Intraperitoneal, intrathoracic, or aortic operation	3
Emergency operation	4

Adapted from Feneck R. Cardiovascular function and the safety of anesthesia. In: Taylor TH, Major E, editors. Hazards and complications of anesthesia. New York: Churchill Livingstone; 1987.

MI = myocardial infarction; JVD = jugular venous distension; VAS = vascular aortic stenosis; PAC = premature atrial contraction; ECG = electrocardiogram; PVCs = premature ventricular contractions; PO_2 = partial pressure of oxygen; PCO_2 = partial pressure of carbon dioxide; K = potassium; HCO_3 = bicarbonate; BUN = blood urea nitrogen; CR = creatinine; SGOT = serum glutamic oxaloacetic transaminase.

*Total possible points = 53.

ing history taking or on physical examination or laboratory study, and (3) the patient who has a high risk for the development of particular medical problems.[71,72]

When there is need for a specific consultation, the consultant should be selected for appropriateness to the particular problem, and the problem and the specific questions to be answered should be clearly transmitted to the consultant in writing. Adequate details of the planned dental procedure, with an assessment of time, stress to the patient, and expected period of post-treatment disability, should be given, as well as details of the particular symptom, sign, or laboratory abnormality that occasioned the consultation. The written request should be brief and should specify the particular items of information needed from the consultant. Requests for "medical clearance" rarely produce a response other than "OK for dental treatment" and should be avoided.

Medical risk assessment of patients before dental treatment offers the opportunity for greatly improving dental services for patients with compromised health. It does require considerably more clinical training and understanding of the natural history and clinical features of systemic disease processes than have been customarily taught in undergraduate dental education programs; however, a partial solution to this problem has been achieved through undergraduate assignments in hospital dentistry and (most important) through hospital-based dental general-practice oral medicine and oral

surgery residency programs. It is hoped that revisions in dental undergraduate curricula will recognize this need and provide greater emphasis on both the pathophysiology of systemic disease and the practical clinical evaluation and management of medically compromised patients in the dental student's program.

Modification of Dental Care for Medically Complex Patients

Dental care causes changes to the patient's homeostasis. The results of the microbiologic, physical, and psychological stimuli caused by dental care may be altered by underlying medical conditions. Therefore, modifications necessary for providing safe and appropriate dental care are often determined by underlying medical conditions. A risk assessment needs to be performed to evaluate and determine what modifications should be implemented before, during, and after dental treatment. Different modifications may be necessary at each stage of treatment. For example, antibiotic prophylaxis or steroid replacement may be necessary before treatment,[73–75] or it may not be possible to place the patient in a supine position during dental procedures, or specific hemostatic agents may need to be employed after extractions.

In this book, many different medical conditions are discussed, and protocols for the modification of dental care are suggested. However, it is the responsibility of the oral health care provider to obtain all the pertinent information that may have an impact on the patient's care.

Before initiating dental care, the risk to the patient must be assessed. It is helpful to focus on the following three questions (which will change according to severity of the underlying disease or condition):

1. What is the likelihood that the patient will experience an adverse event due to dental treatment?
2. What is the nature and severity of the potential adverse event?
3. What is the most appropriate setting in which to treat the patient?

Each of these questions can be subdivided into smaller entities, which will facilitate the assessment of the patient.

The four major concerns that must be addressed when assessing the likelihood of the patient to experience an adverse event are (1) possible impaired hemostasis, (2) possible susceptibility to infections, (3) drug actions and drug interactions, and (4) the patient's ability to withstand the stress of the dental procedure.

The adverse event may be (1) minor and effectively dealt with at "chairside" (minor complications and adverse events are anticipated) or (2) major, in which case austere interventions may be necessary (major complications and adverse events are anticipated).

Finally, based on the type and severity of the medical condition, the likelihood of the patient's experiencing an adverse event and the severity of that event will determine the most appropriate setting for the dental care. The patient can be treated as one of the following:

1. Outpatient in a general dental office
2. Outpatient in a dental office with more extended resources for resuscitation
3. Patient in a short procedure unit in a hospital
4. Inpatient in an operating room

Most medically complex patients can be safely treated when the factors mentioned above have been addressed.

Summary

The following sample evaluation should summarize all pertinent information given in the above text.

A 45-year-old Caucasian female presents for evaluation of a swelling in her lower lip. The swelling has been present for 1 month.

Her past medical history is remarkable for several anginal attacks during the past 4 years. The angina is being treated with nitroglycerins only when necessary. Patient is not taking any daily medications. No history of any other cardiovascular disease. No chest pains for the past 6 months. ROS findings are noncontributory.

Examination reveals a 2 mm × 2 mm hard nonmovable pea-shaped lesion 10 mm medial to the right lip commisure and 5 mm inferior to the vermilion border. The lesion is consistent with a traumatic injury of a minor salivary gland.

Patient has been advised that the lesion may resolve by itself or the she can have it surgically removed with local anesthesia.

Any dental treatment of this patient needs to address her cardiovascular condition.

▼ MONITORING AND EVALUATING UNDERLYING MEDICAL CONDITIONS

Several major medical conditions can be monitored by oral health care personnel. Signs and symptoms of systemic conditions, the types of medications taken, and the patient's compliance with medications can reveal how well a patient's underlying medical condition is being controlled. Signs of medical conditions are elicited by physical examination, which includes measurements of blood pressure and pulse, or laboratory or other diagnostic evaluations. Symptoms are elicited through a review of systems, whereby subjective symptoms that may indicate changes in a patient's medical status are ascertained. A list of the patient's present medications, changes of medications, and daily doses and a record of the patient's compliance with medications usually provide a good indicator of how a medical condition is being managed. The combined information on signs, symptoms, and medications is ultimately used to determine the level of control and status of the patient's medical condition.

▼ ORAL MEDICINE CONSULTATIONS

Both custom and health insurance reimbursement systems recognize the need of individual practitioners to request the assistance of a colleague who may have more experience with the treatment of a particular clinical problem or who has received advanced training in a medical or dental specialty pertinent to the patient's problem. However, this practice of specialist consultation is usually limited to defined problems, with the expectation that the patient will return to the referring primary care clinician once the nature of the problem has been identified (diagnostic consultation) and appropriate treatment has been prescribed or performed (consultation for diagnosis and treatment). In general, referrals for oral medicine consultation cover the following:

1. Diagnosis and nonsurgical treatment of a variety of orofacial problems, including oral mucosal disease, temporomandibular and myofascial dysfunction, chronic jaw and facial pain, dental anomalies and jaw bone lesions, salivary hypofunction and other salivary gland disorders, and disorders of oral sensation, such as dysgeusia, dysesthesia, and glossodynia
2. Dental treatment of patients with medical problems that affect the oral cavity or for whom modification of standard dental treatment is required, to avoid adverse effects
3. Opinion on the management of dental disease that does not respond to standard treatment, such as rampant dental caries and such as periodontal disease in which there is a likelihood that systemic disease is an etiologic cofactor

In response to a consultation request, the diagnostic procedures outlined in this chapter are followed, with the referral problem listed as the chief complaint and with supplementary questioning (ie, HPI) directed to the exact nature, mode of development, prior diagnostic evaluation/treatment, and associated symptomatology of the primary complaint. A thorough examination of the head, neck, and oral cavity is essential and should be fully documented, and the systems review should include a thorough exploration of any associated symptoms. When pertinent, existing laboratory, radiographic, and medical records should be reviewed and documented in the consultation record, and any additional testing or specialized examinations should be ordered.

A comprehensive consultation always includes a written report of the consultant's examination, usually preceded by a history of the problem under investigation and any items from the medical or dental history that may be pertinent to the problem. A formal diagnostic summary follows, together with the consultant's opinion on appropriate treatment and management of the problem. Any other previously unrecognized abnormalities or significant health problem should also be drawn to the attention of the referring clinician. When a biopsy or some initial treatment is required before a definitive diagnosis is possible and when the terms of the consultation request are not clear, a discussion of the initial findings with the referring clinician is often appropriate before proceeding. Likewise, the consultant usually discusses the details of his report with the patient unless the referring dentist specifies otherwise. In community practice, patients are sometimes referred for consultation by telephone or are simply directed to arrange an appointment with a consultant and acquaint him or her with the details of the problem at that time; a written report is still necessary to clearly identify the consultant's recommendations, which otherwise may not be transmitted accurately by the patient.

In hospital practice, the consultant is always advisory to the patient's attending dentist or physician, and the recommendations listed at the end of the consultation report are not implemented unless specifically authorized by the attending physician, even though the consultation report becomes a part of the patient's official hospital record. For some oral lesions and mucosal abnormalities, a brief history and examination of the lesion will readily identify the problem, and only a short written report is required; this accelerated procedure is referred to as a limited consultation.

▼ THE DENTAL/MEDICAL RECORD: ORGANIZATION, CONFIDENTIALITY, AND INFORMED CONSENT

The patient's record is customarily organized according to the components of the history, physical examination, diagnostic summary, plan of treatment, and medical risk assessment described in the preceding pages. Test results (diagnostic laboratory tests, radiographic examinations, and consultation and biopsy reports) are filed after this, followed by dated progress notes recorded in sequence. Separate sheets for (1) a summary of the medications prescribed for or dispensed to the patient, (2) a description of surgical procedures, (3) the anesthetic record, and (4) a list of the patient's problems and their proposed and actual treatment are also incorporated into the record. This pattern of organization of the patient's record may be modified according to local custom and to varying approaches to patient evaluation and diagnostic methodology taught in different institutions.

Organization

In recent years, educators have explored a number of methods[76] for organizing and categorizing clinical data, with the aim of maximizing the matching of the clinical data with the "mental models" of disease syndromes referred to earlier in this chapter. The problem-oriented record and the condition diagram are two such approaches; both use unique methods for establishing a diagnosis and also involve a reorganization of the clinical record.

PROBLEM-ORIENTED RECORD

The problem-oriented record (POR)[77,78] focuses on problems requiring treatment rather than on traditional diagnoses. It stresses the importance of complete and accurate collecting of clinical data, with the emphasis on recording abnormal findings, rather than on compiling the extensive lists of normal and abnormal data that are characteristic of more traditional methods (consisting of narration, checklists, questionnaires, and analysis summaries). Problems can

be subjective (symptoms), objective (abnormal clinical signs), or otherwise clinically significant (eg, psychosocial) and need not be described in prescribed diagnostic categories. Once the patient's problems have been identified, priorities are established for further diagnostic evaluation or treatment of each problem. These decisions (or assessments) are based on likely causes for each problem, risk analysis of the problem's severity, cost and benefit to the patient as a result of correcting the problem, and the patient's stated desires. The plan of treatment is formulated as a list of possible solutions for each problem. As more information is obtained, the problem list can be updated, and problems can be combined and even reformulated into recognized disease categories. The POR is helpful in organizing a set of complex clinical data about an individual patient, maintaining an up-to-date record of both acute and chronic problems, ensuring that all of the patient's problems are addressed, and ensuring that preventive as well as active therapy is provided. It is also adaptable to computerized patient-tracking programs. However, without any scientifically based or accepted nomenclature and operational criteria for the formulation of the problem list, data cannot be compared across patients or clinicians.[52]

Despite these shortcomings, two features of the POR have received wide acceptance and are often incorporated into more traditionally organized records—the collection of data and the generation of a problem list. In dentistry, the value of the POR has been documented in orthodontics and hospital dentistry but otherwise appears to have attracted little attention in dental education.

The value of a problem list for individual patient care is generally acknowledged,[79,80] and it is considered a necessary component of the hospital record in institutions accredited by the Joint Commission on Accreditation of Healthcare Organizations.

The four components of a problem—subjective, objective, assessment, and plan (SOAP)—are widely taught as the SOAP mnemonic[81] for organizing progress notes or summarizing an outpatient encounter. The components of the SOAP mnemonic are as follows:

S Subjective: the patient's complaint, symptoms, and medical history (a brief review)
O Objective: the clinical examination, including a brief generalized examination, as previously described, and then a focused evaluation of the chief complaint or the area of the procedure to be undertaken
A Assessment: the diagnosis (or differential diagnosis) for the specific problem being addressed
P Plan: the treatment either recommended or performed

The SOAP note is a useful tool for organizing progress notes in the patient record for routine office procedures and follow-up appointments. It is also quite useful in a hospital record when a limited oral medicine consultation must be documented. An example of each type of SOAP note is shown below.

Example 1: Routine Office Procedure.

S: This 21-year-old female presented for routine extraction of the maxillary right first molar. As found by history, the tooth "broke in half" while the patient was chewing ice. The patient had been in pain since the tooth fractured 24 hours ago. The discomfort was sharp, constant, and was exacerbated with cold and mastication. Past medical history was unremarkable. The patient was taking no medication and had not been seriously ill or hospitalized since her last visit 6 months ago.

O: The patient was afebrile, and her blood pressure (BP) and pulse were normal (BP = 110/70 RASit [right arm sitting]; pulse = 72 reg [regular rhythm]). There was no swelling or adenopathy. The maxillary right first molar was vertically fractured through the central fossa and progressed into the furcation.

A: Irreversible pulpitis, vertical fracture, nonrestorable.

P: Extraction, using a local anesthetic of 1.8 cc of 3% carbocaine infiltration. The tooth was extracted with forceps without incident. The patient tolerated the procedure well; advised to take acetaminophen as necessary for discomfort. Postoperative instructions were given. The patient will return in 7 days for follow-up.

Example 2: Follow-Up Appointment.

S: The patient returned 1 week after routine extraction of the maxillary right first molar. The patient reported uneventful healing and was "surprised" at how well she felt.

O: No palpation tenderness or suggestion of bleeding or infection. Mucosal color at the extraction site was normal.

A: Healing normally.

P: The patient is to be scheduled to discuss prosthetic replacement of this tooth.

Example 3: Limited Oral Medicine Consultation.

S: A 55-year-old male who is an inpatient for reconstructive knee surgery, due to a skiing accident. The patient has had a recent onset of oral ulceration; he has also complained of gastrointestinal distress. There is no previous history of similar oral ulceration or gastrointestinal disease. The patient is in ASA class I and is not presently taking any medication except for ibuprofen (800 mg) given as an analgesic postsurgically.

O: Classic aphthalike ulcerations of the buccal and labial mucosae and lateral tongue borders. The largest lesion is 0.6 cm in diameter. The total number of lesions is six.

A: Erythema multiforme secondary to ibuprofen therapy.

P: Recommend that attending physician discontinue the use of ibuprofen and substitute acetaminophen, as necessary for analgesia.

CONDITION DIAGRAM

The condition diagram (CD)[82] uses a standardized approach to categorizing and diagramming the clinical data, formulating a differential diagnosis, prevention factors, and interventions (treatment or further diagnostic procedures). It relies heavily on graphic or non-narrative categorization of clinical data and provides students with a concise strategy for summarizing the "universe of the patient's problems" at a given time. Although currently used in only a limited number of institutions, the graphic method of conceptualizing a patient's problems is supported by both educational theory and by its proven success with medical students.

▼ CONFIDENTIALITY OF PATIENT RECORDS

Patients provide dentists and physicians with confidential dental, medical, and psychosocial information on the understanding that this information may be necessary for effective diagnosis and treatment and that the information will remain confidential and will be not released to other individuals without the patient's specific permission. This information may also be entered into the patient's record and shared with other clinical personnel involved in the patient's treatment unless the patient specifically requests otherwise. Patients are willing to share such information with their dentists and physicians only to the extent that the patient believes that this contract is being honored.

There are also specific circumstances in which the confidentiality of clinical information is protected by law and may be released to authorized individuals only after compliance with legally defined requirements for informed consent (eg, psychiatric records, and confidential HIV-related information). Conversely, some medical information that is considered to be of public health significance is a matter of public record when reported to the local health authorities (eg, clinical or laboratory confirmation of reportable infectious diseases such as syphilis, hepatitis, or acquired immunodeficiency syndrome [AIDS]). Courts also have the power to subpoena medical and dental records under defined circumstances, and records of patients participating in clinical research trials may be subject to inspection by a pharmaceutical sponsor or an appropriate drug regulatory authority. Dentists are generally authorized to obtain and record information about a patient to the extent that the information may be pertinent to the diagnosis of oral disease and its effective treatment. The copying of a patient's record for use in clinical seminars, case presentations,[83] and scientific presentations is a common and acceptable practice, provided that the patient is not identifiable in any way.

Conversations about patients, discussion with a colleague about a patient's personal problems and correspondence about a patient should be limited to those occasions when information essential to the patient's treatment has to be transmitted. Lecturers and writers who use clinical cases to illustrate a topic should avoid mention of any item by which a patient might be identified and should omit confidential information. Conversations about patients, however casual, should never be held where they could possibly be overheard by unauthorized individuals, and discussion of patients with nonclinical colleagues, friends, family, and others should always be kept to a minimum and should never include confidential patient information.

▼ INFORMED CONSENT

Prior consent of the patient is needed for all diagnostic and treatment procedures, with the exception of those considered necessary for treatment of a life-threatening emergency in a comatose patient.[84–86] In dentistry, such consent is more often implied than formally obtained although written consent is generally considered necessary for all surgical procedures (however minor), for the administration of general anesthetics, and for the majority of clinical research procedures.

Consent of the patient is often required before clinical records are transmitted to another dental office or institution. Many communities also have specific laws that discourage discrimination against individuals infected with HIV[87] by requiring specific written consent from the patient before any HIV-related testing can be carried out and before any HIV-related information can be released to insurance companies, other practitioners, family members, and fellow workers. Dentists treating patients whom they believe may be infected with HIV must therefore be cognizant of local law and custom when they request HIV-related information from a patient's physician, and they must establish procedures in their own offices to protect this information from unauthorized release. In response to requests for the release of psychiatric records or HIV-related information, hospital medical record departments commonly supply the practitioner with the necessary additional forms for the patient to sign before the records are released. Psychiatric information that is released is usually restricted to the patient's diagnoses and medications.

▼ REFERENCES

1. US Department of Health and Human Services, Office of Disease Prevention and Health Promotion. Developing objectives for healthy people 2010. Washington (DC): US Government Printing office. 1998 Sept.
2. US Bureau of the Census. Population projections of the United States by age, sex, race and Hispanic origin: 1995 to 2050. Washington (DC): US Government Printing Office; 1996. Current Population Reports, Series P25-1130.
3. Centers for Disease Control and Prevention. Total tooth loss among persons aged ≥ 65 years. Selected states, 1995–1997. Morb Mortal Wkly Rep 1999; 48:206–10.
4. US Department of Health and Human Services. Oral health in America: a report of the Surgeon General. Rockville (MD): US Department of Health and Human Services, National Institute of Dental and Craniofacial Research, National Institutes of Health; 2000.
5. McAlister FA, Straus SE, Sackett DL. Why we need large, simple studies of the clinical examination: the problem and a proposed solution. Lancet 1999;354:1721.
6. Brodman K, Erdmann AJ, Lorge I, Wolff HG. The Cornell Medical Index. An adjunct to medical interview. JAMA 1949;140:530.
7. Ramsey PG, Curtis JR, Paauw DS, et al. History-taking and preventive medicine skills among primary care physicians: an assessment using standardized patients. Am J Med 1998;104:152.
8. Schechter GP, Blank LL, Godwin HA Jr, et al. Refocusing on history-taking skills during internal medicine training. Am J Med 1996;101:210.
9. Guggenheimer J, Orchard TJ, Moore PA, et al. Reliability of self-reported heart murmur history: possible use of antibiotic use in dentistry. J Am Dent Assoc 1998;129:861.
10. McDaniel TF, Miller D, Jones R, Davis M. Assessing patient willingness to reveal health history information. J Am Dent Assoc 1995;126:375.
11. Lebenbom-Mansour MH, Oesterle JR, Ownby DR, et al. The incidence of latex sensitivity in ambulatory surgical patients: a correlation of historical factors with positive serum immunoglobin E levels. Anesth Analg 1997;85:44.
12. Hamann CP, Turjanmaa K, Rietschel R, et al. Natural latex rubber hypersensitivity: incidence and prevalence of type 1 allergy in the dental professional. J Am Dent Assoc 1998;129:43.
13. Spina AM, Levine HJ. Latex allergy: a review for the dental professional. Oral Surg Oral Med Oral Pathol Oral Radiol Endod 1999;87:5.
14. Safadi GS, Safadi TJ, Terezhalmy GT, et al. Latex hypersensitivity: its prevalence among dental professionals. J Am Dent Assoc 1996;127:83.
15. Rees TD. Drugs and oral disorders. Periodontol 2000 1998; 18:21–36.
16. Physician's desk reference. 54th ed. Montvale (NJ): Medical Economics Co.; 2000.
17. PDR for nonprescription drugs and dietary supplements. Montvale (NJ): Medical Economics Co.; 2000.
18. Wynn RL, Meiller TF, Crossley HL. Drug information handbook for dentistry. 6th ed. Cleveland: Lexi-Comp, 2000.
19. 1996 Physicians' GenRx. The complete drug reference. 7th ed. Smithtown (NY): Data Pharmaceutica Inc.; 1996.
20. Reynolds JEF. Martindale: the extra pharmacopoeia. 31st ed. London: The Pharmaceutical Press, 1998.
21. Facts and comparison. St. Louis (MO): A. Wolters Kluwer Co.; 2000.
22. Fishman DL. Computerized clinical information system—CCIS from Micromedex. Database 1992;15:58.
23. Leggatt V, Mackay J, Yates JR. Evaluation of questionnaire on cancer family history in identifying patients at increased genetic risk in general practice. BMJ 1999;319:757–8.
24. Aldred MJ, Bartold PM. Genetic disorders of the gingivae and periodontium. Periodontology 2000 1998;18:7.
25. Bolan BJ, Wollan PC, Silverstein MD. Review of systems, physical examination, and routine tests for case-finding in ambulatory patients. Am J Med Sci 1995;309:194.
26. Verdon ME, Siemens K. Yield of review of systems in a self-administered questionnaire. J Am Board Fam Pract 1997;10:20.
27. Orient JM. Sapira's art & science of bedside diagnosis. 3rd ed. Philadelphia: Lippincott Williams & Wilkins, 2000.
28. Schneiderman H, Peixoto AJ. Bedside diagnosis: an annotated bibliography of literature on physical examination and interviewing. 3rd ed. Philadelphia: American College of Physicians; 1997.
29. Bickley LS, Hoekelman RA. Bates' guide to physical examination and history taking. 7th ed. Philadelphia: Lippincott Williams & Wilkins; 1998.
30. Libb JW, Murray J, Thurstin H, Alarcon RD. Concordance of the MCMI-II, the MMPI, and Axis I discharge diagnosis in psychiatric in patients. J Pers Assess 1992;58:580.
31. Greenberger NJ, Hinthorn DR. History taking and physical examination: essentials and clinical correlates. St. Louis: Mosby Year Book, 1993.

32. Darowski A, Najim Z, Weinberg JR, Guz A. Normal rectal, auditory canal, sublingual and axillary temperatures in elderly afebrile patients in a warm environment. Age Ageing 1991; 20:113–19.

33. Darowski A, Najim Z, Weinberg JR, Guz A. The increase in body temperature of elderly patients in the first twenty-four hours following admission to hospital. Age Ageing 1991; 20:107–12.

34. Darowski A, Najim Z, Weinberg JR, Guz A. The febrile response to mild infections in elderly hospital in-patients. Age Aging 1991;20:193–8.

35. Poiset M, Johnson R, Nakamura R. Pulse rate and oxygen saturation in children during routine dental procedures. ASDC J Dent Child 1990;57:279.

36. Gortzak RA, Abraham-Inpijn L. Blood pressure measurements during dental check ups representative of 26-hour registration. Oral Surg Oral Med Oral Pathol 1990;70:730–3.

37. Gortzak RA, Abraham-Inpijn L, Oosting J. Blood pressure response to dental check up: a continuous, non-invasive registration. Gen Dent 1991;39:339–42.

38. Glick M. New guidelines for prevention, detection, evaluation and treatment of high blood pressure. J Am Dent Assoc 1998;129;1588.

39. Berman CL, Van Stewart A, Ramazzotto LT, Davis FD. High blood pressure detection: a new public health measure for the dental profession. J Am Dent Assoc 1976;92:116.

40. Renson CE. The dental patient with hypertension. Dent Update 1990;17:223–5.

41. The sixth report of the Joint National Committee on prevention, detection, evaluation, and treatment of high blood pressure. Arch Intern Med 1997;157:2413–46.

42. Prisant LM, Alpert BS, Robbins CB, et al. American National Standard for nonautomated sphygmomanometers: summary report. Am J Hypertens 1995;8:210.

43. Nesselroad JM, Flacco VA, Phillips DM, Kruse J. Accuracy of automated finger blood pressure devices. Fam Med 1996; 28:189.

44. Bates B , Kirkendall WM, Burton AC, et al. Recommendations for human blood pressure determination by sphygmomanometers. Circulation 1967;36:980.

45. Westesson PL. Physical diagnosis continues to be the gold standard. Cranio 1999;17:3–4.

46. Yellowitz JA. The oral cancer examination. In: Ord RA, Blanchaerd R, editors. Oral cancer: the dentist's role in diagnosis, management, rehabilitation and prevention. Carol Stream (IL): Quintessence, 1999.

47. Saah AJ, Hoover DR. "Sensitivity" and "specificity" reconsidered: the meaning of these terms in analytical and diagnostic settings. Ann Intern Med 1997;126:91.

48. Gortzak RA, Abraham-Inpijn L, ter Horst G, Peters G. High blood pressure screening in the dental office: a survey among Dutch dentists. Gen Dent 1993;41:246.

49. Glick M. Know thy hepatitis: A through TT. J Calif Dent Assoc 1999;27:376–85.

50. Patton LL, Shugars DC. Immunologic and viral markers of HIV-1 disease progression: implications for dentistry. J Am Dent Assoc 1999;130:1313.

51. Atkinson JC, O'Connell A, Aframian D. Oral manifestations of primary immunological diseases. J Am Dent Assoc 2000; 131:345.

52. Feinstein AR. ICD, POR, and DRG. Unsolved scientific problems in the nosology of clinical medicine. Arch Intern Med 1988;148:2269.

53. Fetter RB, Shin Y, Freeman JL, et al. Case-mix definition by diagnosis-related groups. Med Care 1980;18 Suppl 2:1.

54. Vladeck BC. Medicare hospital payment by diagnosis-related groups. Ann Intern Med 1984;100:576.

55. Mullin RL. Diagnosis-related groups and severity. JAMA 1985;254:1208.

56. Kahn KL, Rubenstein LV, Draper D, et al. The effects of the DRG-based prospective payment system on quality of care for hospitalized Medicare patients. An introduction to the series. JAMA 1990;264:1953–5.

57. ICD.9.CM. 1993. International classification of diseases. 9th revision. Clinical modification. 4th ed. Salt Lake City: Med-Index Publications, 1993.

58. Pennsylvania Blue Shield. Diagnosis code monitoring. Medicare report. Camp Hill (PA): Pennsylvania Blue Shield Corporate Affairs Division, 1991.

59. Code it right. Methods for proper reimbursement. Salt Lake City: Med-Index Publications, 1991.

60. McMahon LJ Jr, Smits HL. Can Medicare prospective payment survive the ICD-9-CM disease classification system? Ann Intern Med 1986;104:562.

61. World Health Organization. Application of the International Classification of Diseases to dentistry and stomatology, ICD-DA. 3rd ed. Geneva, Switzerland: World Health Organization, 1995.

62. American Psychiatric Association. Diagnostic and statistical manual of mental disorders. Revised (DSM-IV-TR). 4th ed. Washington (DC): American Psychiatric Association, 1994.

63. Levitsky S. Using ICD-9-CM and CPT in the nineties [editorial]. Ann Thorac Surg 1990;50:519.

64. Rothwell DJ. Systematized nomenclature of medicine (SNOMED). Microglossary for surgical pathology. Skokie (IL): College of American Pathologists; 1980.

65. Rose LF, Roizen MF. Preoperative evaluation of patients for dental surgery. In: Dionne RA, Laskin DM, editors. Anesthesia and sedation in the dental office. New York: Elsevier, 1986. p. 67.

66. DeRossi SS, Glick M. Dentistry in the operating room. Compend Contin Educ Dent 1997;18:614–6, 618–24.

67. Brown DL. Anesthesia risk: a historical perspective. Introduction. In: Brown DL, editor. Risk and outcomes in anesthesia. Philadelphia: J.B. Lippincott; 1988.

68. Keats AS. The ASA classification of physical status: a recapitulation. Anesthesiology 1978;49:233.

69. Goldman L, Caldera DL, Nussbaum SR, et al. Multifactorial index of cardiac risk in noncardiac surgical procedures. New Engl J Med 1977;297:845–50.

70. Slogoff S, Keats AS. Does perioperative myocardial ischemia lead to postoperative myocardial infarction? Anesthesiology 1988;62:107.

71. CAN's professional liability risk management. Information for dentists. Referrals. Pa Dent J 1990;57(6):6.

72. American Dental Association Council on Dental Practice. General guidelines for referring dental patients to specialists and other settings for care. Chicago: American Dental Association, 1991.

73. Dajani AS, Taubert KA, Wilson W, et al. Prevention of bacterial endocarditis: recommendations by the American Heart Association. J Am Dent Assoc 1997;128:1142.

74. American Dental Association, American Academy of Orthopaedic Surgeons. Advisory statement: antibiotic prophylaxis for dental patients with total joint replacements. J Am Dent Assoc 1997;128:1004.

75. De Rossi SS, Glick M. Lupus erythematosus: considerations for dentistry. J Am Dent Assoc 1998;129:330.

76. Sheagren JN, Zweifler A, Woolliscroft JO. The present medical database needs reorganization. It's time for a change! Arch Intern Med 1990;150:2014.

77. Weed LL. Medical records, medical education and patient care; the problem-oriented record as a basic tool. Cleveland: Press of Case Western Reserve, 1969.

78. Hershey SE, Bayleran ED. Problem-oriented orthodontic record. J Clin Orthod 1986;20:106–10.

79. Donaldson MS, Povar GT. Improving the master problem list: a case study in changing clinician behavior. QRB Qual Rev Bull 1985;11:327–33.

80. Papa RP. An emergency medicine clinical problem-solving system. Ann Emerg Med 1985;14:660.

81. Exstrom S. Gollner ML. There is more than one use of SOAP. Nurs Manage 1990;21(10):12.

82. Russell IK, Hendricson WD, Harris GD, Gobut DV. A comparison of two methods for facilitating clinical data integration by medical students. Acad Med 1990;65:333.

83. Kroenke K. The case presentation: stumbling blocks and stepping stones. Am J Med 1985;79:605.

84. Widdop FT. On informed consent in dentistry. Aust Dent Assoc News Bull 1991;Feb:35.

85. Schafler NL. Medical malpractice. Handling dental cases. 2nd ed. Colorado Springs (CO): Shepard's/McGraw-Hill Inc.; 1991.

86. Seear J, Walters L. Law and ethics in dentistry. 3rd ed. Boston: Wright/Butterworth-Heinemann Ltd.; 1991.

87. Burris S. Dental discrimination against the HIV-infected: empirical data, law and public policy. Yale J Regul 1996;13:1.

3

Maxillofacial Imaging

Sharon L. Brooks, DDS, MS

The role of imaging in oral medicine varies greatly with the type of problem being evaluated. Certain problems, such as pain in the orofacial region, frequently require imaging to determine the origin of the pain. For other conditions, however, such as soft-tissue lesions of the oral mucosa, imaging offers no new diagnostic information.

The variety of imaging techniques available to the clinician has grown in number and in degree of sophistication over the years. While this means that there is an imaging procedure that will provide the information desired by the clinician, it also means that choosing the best technique is not necessarily an easy process.

This chapter first explores the underlying principles the clinician should consider when deciding whether imaging is appropriate for the case in question and then discusses the imaging techniques that are available in dental offices and in referral imaging centers. Examples of specific imaging protocols are then described, followed by a discussion of risk-benefit analysis of imaging in oral medicine.

▼ SELECTION CRITERIA

The decision to order diagnostic imaging as part of the evaluation of an orofacial complaint should be based on the principle of selection criteria. Selection criteria are those historical and/or clinical findings that suggest a need for imaging to provide additional information so that a correct diagnosis and an appropriate management plan can be determined. The use of selection criteria requires the clinician to obtain a history, perform a clinical examination, and then determine both the type of additional information required (if any) and the best technique for obtaining this information. The emphasis is on the acquisition of new information that affects the outcome, not just the routine application of a diagnostic modality.

There are many reasons for requesting imaging information, including the determination of the nature of a condition, the confirmation of a clinical diagnosis, the evaluation of the extent of a lesion, and the monitoring of the progression or regression of a lesion over time. Each of these may require a different imaging strategy.

Over the years, there have been some attempts to offer guidance to the clinician in the selection of the most appropriate imaging protocol. In 1986, the Food and Drug Administration convened a panel of experts to develop guidelines for selecting appropriate radiologic examinations for new and recall dental patients, both those who present for routine examination without complaints and those with specific signs or symptoms of disease.[1] These guidelines have been approved by the American Dental Association and all dental specialty organizations. A convenient chart of these recommendations can be obtained from Eastman Kodak Company, Rochester, New York (pamphlet No. N-80A).

Guidance for imaging of the temporomandibular joint (TMJ)[2] and dental implant preoperative site assessment[3] has been developed in the form of position papers published by the American Academy of Oral and Maxillofacial Radiology. That group has also produced a document describing parameters of care for a variety of imaging tasks.[4]

Whether or not there are published guidelines, it is incumbent upon the individual clinician to use diagnostic imaging wisely. This means determining specifically what information is needed, deciding whether imaging is the best way to obtain this information, and (if so) selecting the most appropriate technique, after considering the information needed, the radiation dose and cost, the availability of the technique, and the expertise needed to interpret the study.

▼ IMAGING MODALITIES AVAILABLE IN DENTAL OFFICES AND CLINICS

Intraoral and Panoramic Radiography

There are a number of imaging modalities that are readily available to the clinician for evaluating patients' conditions. Virtually every dental office has the equipment to perform intraoral radiography, and many offices also have panoramic x-ray machines. These two types of radiographic equipment will provide the majority of images needed for evaluating patients' orofacial complaints.

Clinicians who treat patients who have oral medical problems should be able to make a variety of occlusal radiographs in addition to standard periapical and bite-wing radiographs. Occlusal radiographs may be valuable for detecting sialoliths in the submandibular duct, localizing lesions or foreign bodies (by providing a view at right angles to that of the periapical radiograph), and evaluating the buccal and lingual cortex of the mandible for perforation, erosion, or expansion. The advantage of intraoral radiography is the fine detail provided in its visualization of the teeth and supporting bone.

Panoramic radiography demonstrates a wide view of the maxilla and mandible as well as surrounding structures, including the neck, TMJ, zygomatic arches, maxillary sinuses and nasal cavity, and orbits although it does so with less sharpness and detail than are seen in intraoral views (Figure 3-1).

Comparison of right and left sides is easier with a panoramic projection, and this view provides an excellent initial view of the osseous structures of the TMJ and of the integrity of the sinus floor. Additional views targeting these tissues can be obtained later if needed.

Some panoramic x-ray machines also have the capability of providing a variety of skull projections, including lateral, oblique lateral, posteroanterior, anteroposterior, and submentovertex views. Typically, these are done with a cephalometric attachment to the machine. Although these views are relatively easy to take and can provide valuable information in certain circumstances, they demonstrate complex anatomy and should be interpreted by someone with experience in the field, preferably an oral and maxillofacial radiologist.

Digital Imaging

While most intraoral radiography is still performed with film as the recording medium, the use of digital imaging techniques is rapidly increasing. Although it is possible to produce a digital image by scanning a film radiograph, that technique does not provide any of the advantages of speed and radiation dose reduction that are available when digital images are acquired directly.

There are two major techniques for acquiring digital images: (1) a single-step wired system using a charge-coupled device (CCD) or complementary metal oxide semiconductor (CMOS) sensor and (2) a two-step wireless system using a photostimulable storage phosphor (PSP) plate (Figure 3-2). The CCD or CMOS sensor is a device that transforms the energy from ionizing radiation into an electrical signal that is displayed as an image on a computer monitor within a few seconds. The sensor is housed in a rigid plastic case that is attached to the computer by a long cord. The sensor is placed in the mouth, the computer is activated, and the exposure is made. Once the image appears on the screen (generally within a few seconds) (Figure 3-3), a number of different software

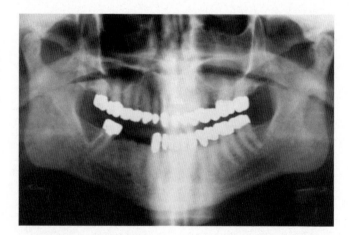

FIGURE 3-1   Panoramic radiograph of a 75-year-old man with a history of discomfort in the left TMJ region. Note the large osteophyte on the left mandibular condyle. The left maxillary sinus is also radiopaque due to chronic sinusitis. The cervical spine is visible as a radiopaque shadow in the anterior because the patient could not extend his neck as a result of severe osteoarthritis.

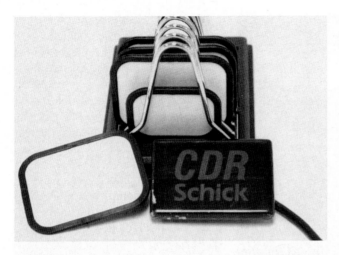

FIGURE 3-2 Digital imaging sensors. Left, photostimulable storage phosphor (Digora, Soredex/Orion, Helsinki, Finland); right, charge-coupled device (CCD) sensor (CDR [Computed Dental Radiography], Schick Technologies, Long Island City, N.Y.).

"enhancements" can be applied although some studies have shown the unenhanced images to have higher diagnostic capabilities than the enhanced ones, most likely due to processing done before the image appears on the screen.[5]

With the PSP technique, the imaging plate (sensor) is thinner and more flexible and is not attached to the computer. After the exposure is made, a plate is inserted into a machine that scans it with a laser, converting the latent image into a visual image on the computer screen. This process takes from 30 s to 2.5 min, depending on the system. The sensor plate must then be discharged before reuse.

Both CCD and PSP digital imaging systems are available for both intraoral and panoramic radiography. They use a standard x-ray machine but replace the film or standard panoramic cassette with a digital sensor. Even though digital systems do not have higher diagnostic capabilities than their film-based counterparts do for the detection of dental caries,[6] periodontal disease,[7] and periapical lesions,[8] there are a number of other advantages to using digital imaging, including reduced radiation exposure, reduced time of image acquisition, the ability to transmit images electronically, and the ability to be used with a number of image analysis tools.

Once the image is in the computer, a number of procedures can be done, depending on the software available. In addition to the standard contrast and brightness enhancements, there is a measurement tool that can be used to determine the dimensions of a lesion. Specialized software is available for digital subtraction, a method of evaluating changes in radiographs over time. Ideally, "before" and "after" radiographs should be identical other than for the area of interest (although algorithms are being developed that can take similar [although not necessarily identical] images and mathematically "warp" them so that the geometry is the same). The two images are then registered, and the gray levels of the same pixels of both images are compared. Typically, increasing mineral (tooth or

bone gain) is portrayed as white, and decreasing mineral is shown as black (Figure 3-4). One commercially available program uses red and green to portray bone loss and gain, respectively. Digital subtraction can be useful for evaluating changes in bone height and/or density in periodontitis and for judging the degree of healing and remineralization of periapical lesions after endodontic therapy. Theoretically, any lesion (including bony cysts or tumors) with the potential of change over time can be studied by the subtraction technique, given a method for standardizing the images.

This need for standardization means that the decision to use digital subtraction must be made at the time of the initial imaging so that follow-up images can be made with the same technique since there is a limit to the amount of geometric image correction that can be done. In addition, a step wedge or other device must be incorporated into the imaging system to allow for correction of differences in density and contrast between radiographs, which would affect the subtraction outcome. Because of the difficulty in standardizing panoramic imaging, digital subtraction is currently more feasible for evaluating changes in lesions small enough to be visualized on intraoral views.

Other software is available for the evaluation of other aspects of the digital images, including software for histogram analysis and for a variety of pattern analyses of the trabecular bone.[9] Although these are currently considered research tools, they may have clinical application in the future.

All of the analyses described above can be done on any type of digital image, whether acquired by CCD or PSP or scanned from a film image.

Some interesting new clinical applications of digital imaging will soon be available. With tuned-aperture computed tomography (TACT®), a series of digital images is acquired at slightly varying angles; the computer then reconstructs the

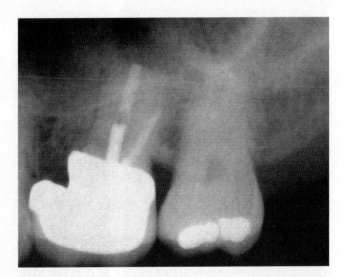

FIGURE 3-3 Periapical radiograph made with a charge-coupled device (CCD) type of direct digital imaging system. The mesial root of the first molar was amputated 10 years previously due to a vertical fracture. Note the letter "E" in the corner of the image, indicating that the image has been exported from the program used to acquire it initially.

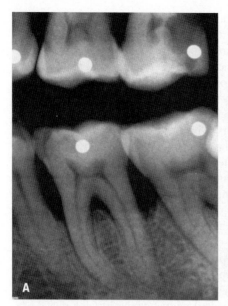
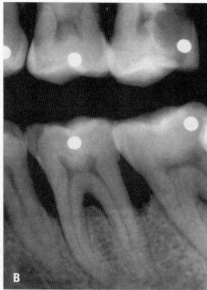
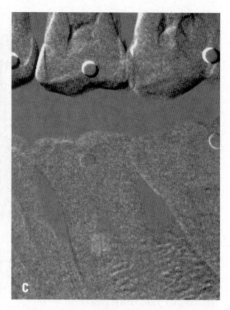

FIGURE 3-4   Digital subtraction images of a periodontal furcation defect. **A,** Reference radiograph showing a defect in the furcation of the mandibular first molar. **B,** Follow-up radiograph after placement of 2 mg of crushed bone in soft wax in the defect. The bone "graft" is undetectable. **C,** Subtracted and contrast-enhanced combination of reference and follow-up images. The bone "graft" is visible as a square white area in the furcation. (Courtesy of Dr. Onanong Chai-U-Domn, University of North Carolina School of Dentistry, Chapel Hill, N.C.)

resultant data to provide information about depth. The image can be manipulated to bring various layers into focus, thus permitting determination of depths of lesions and relationships between structures[10] (Figure 3-5).

Another computer reconstruction technique under development uses a Scanora panoramic x-ray machine (Soredex/ Orion Co., Helsinki, Finland) and a special image intensifier to produce three-dimensional data of a cylindrical volume of tissue. The data can be reconstructed to provide an image at any angle through the volume, providing a high-resolution computed tomography (CT) scan at a radiation dose a fraction of that required by conventional CT.[11] The developers have dubbed this technique "ortho-cubic CT" and expect to make it available soon (Figure 3-6).

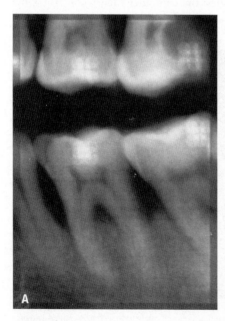
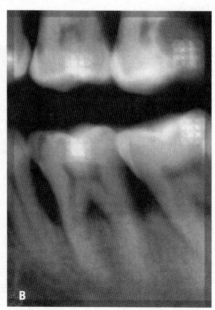
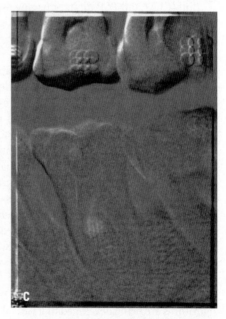

FIGURE 3-5   Tuned-aperture computed tomography (TACT®) images of the same periodontal defect shown in Figure 3-4.   **A,** Reference image with the TACT® slice centered on the buccolingual location of bone apposition. **B,** Follow-up image in the same plane, after placement of 2 mg of crushed bone. **C,** Contrast-enhanced images after subtraction of the two TACT® slices. The bone mass is clearly visible in the furcation as a white area. (Courtesy of Dr. Onanong Chai-U-Domn, University of North Carolina School of Dentistry, Chapel Hill, N.C.)

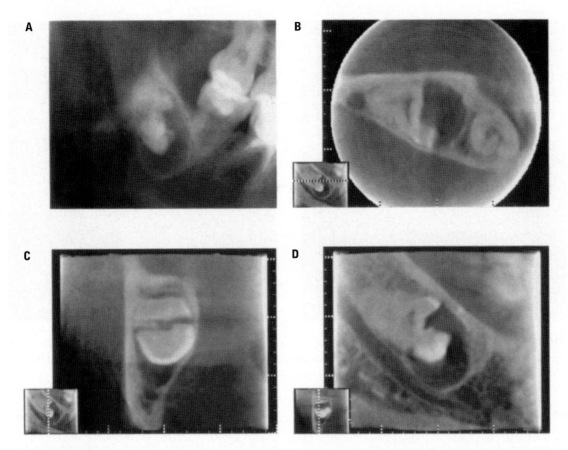

FIGURE 3-6 Dentigerous cyst in the mandibular third molar region. **A,** Portion of a panoramic radiograph. **B,** Horizontal ortho–computed tomography (CT) image. **C,** Ortho-CT image perpendicular to dental arch. **D,** Ortho-CT image parallel to dental arch. (Courtesy of Drs. Koji Hashimoto and Yoshinori Arai, Nihon University School of Dentistry, Tokyo, Japan)

Conventional Tomography

Plain (or conventional) tomography is a radiographic technique that has been available for many years, generally in institutions such as dental schools or hospitals, due to the size and expense of the equipment. However, tomographic capability has been added to some sophisticated computer-controlled panoramic x-ray machines, making tomography potentially more readily available in dental offices and clinics.

In conventional tomography, an image is made of a thin layer of tissue; tissues that are superficial and deep to the desired region blur out due to movement of the x-ray tube and film. Some machines use a relatively simple linear movement of the tube, which can unfortunately produce streaking artifacts. More complex tube movements (such as spiral and hypocycloidal movements) can blur out undesired tissues more completely, thus making the area of interest more prominent.

In the past, the primary use of tomography in dentistry has been for detailed evaluation of the osseous structures of the TMJ (Figure 3-7, A). However, some of the newer machines will also produce cross-sectional images of the jaws (see Figure 3-7, B). While these are excellent for the assessment of the bone prior to the placement of dental implants, they also can be used whenever a cross-sectional view of the jaws would be

helpful, such as when determining the relationship between a lesion and the apex of the tooth or when evaluating the integrity of the buccal or lingual cortical bone.

For the evaluation of large or complex lesions such as facial fractures or tumors, conventional tomography has generally been superceded by CT or magnetic resonance imaging because of the clarity of the images, the lack of blurring from other structures, and the ability to produce images in multiple planes. However, plain tomography may still be of value in imaging lesions confined to the jaw bones.

▼ IMAGING MODALITIES AVAILABLE IN HOSPITALS AND RADIOLOGY CLINICS

While the standard imaging modalities that are available in dental offices will suffice for many of the cases being evaluated in oral medicine, there are situations in which it is appropriate to refer the patient to a hospital or other facility for a specialized imaging procedure.

The decision of which type of imaging to request depends on the question to be answered. Is there a need for information on hard tissue, soft tissue, or both? Is the disease process

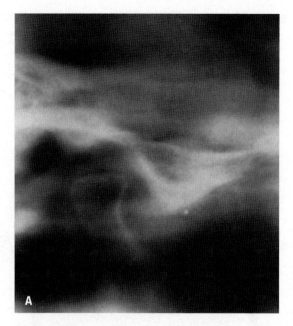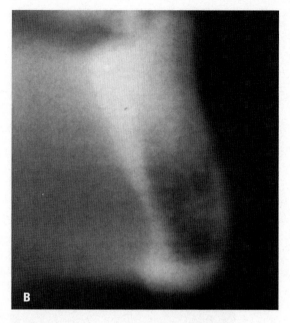

FIGURE 3-7   A, Linear tomogram of a temporomandibular joint exhibiting severe flattening of the condyle with sclerosis of the superior surface. **B,** Cross-sectional linear tomogram of the mandible, made for preoperative site assessment for dental implants.

apparently localized or widespread? Is functional information needed in addition to or in place of anatomic information? How much anatomic detail is necessary? Is three-dimensional reconstruction of the image contemplated?

The rest of this section discusses the imaging modalities that are available in most imaging centers today.

Computed Tomography

Computed tomography (CT) permits the imaging of thin slices of tissue in a wide variety of planes. Most CT is done in the axial plane, and many CT scans also provide coronal views; sagittal slices are less commonly used. During CT scanning, the x-ray source and detectors move around the desired region of the body while the patient lies on a table. Modern generations of CT scanners use a spiral motion of the gantry to produce the x-ray data that are then reconstructed by computer. The operator selects the region of the anatomy and the thickness of the slices of tissue to be scanned, along with the kilovolt and milliampere settings. Slice thickness is usually 10 mm through the body and brain and 5 mm through the head and neck, unless three-dimensional reconstruction is anticipated. In such cases, the slice thickness is 1.0 to 1.5 mm in order to provide adequate data.

CT scans are usually evaluated on computer monitors although they may also be printed on radiographic film. The contrast and brightness of the image may be adjusted as necessary although the images are usually viewed in two modes: bone windowing and soft-tissue windowing. In bone windowing, the contrast is set so that osseous structures are visible in maximal detail. With soft-tissue windowing, the bone looks uniformly white, but various types of soft tissues can be distinguished (Figure 3-8). Viewing the images in these different formats does not require rescanning the patient.

There are many advantages to CT of the head and neck region compared to imaging this area by plain films or conventional tomography. Thin slices of tissue can be viewed in multiple planes without superimposition by adjacent structures or the blurring out of other layers. Fine detail of osseous and other calcified structures can be obtained. Various soft tissues can be differentiated by their attenuation of the x-ray beam. Fascial planes between muscle groups can be identified, as can lymph nodes and blood vessels. Three-dimensional images that may make it easier to visualize certain abnormalities can be produced, and some software programs will color certain structures (such as tumors) to simplify visualization of the lesion. Three-dimensional models can also be milled out of plastic, based on data from CT scans. Cross-sectional images can also be reconstructed from axial CT scans, producing, for example, views of the mandible for use in preoperative assessments for implant placement.

The major disadvantages of CT relate to the relatively high cost and high radiation dose of this examination compared to those of plain-film radiography. In addition, resolution of fine structures of the head and neck may be less than optimal although the newly developed super-high-resolution ortho-CT described above is attempting to address these problems. Careful attention must also be paid to the imaging plane through the jaws if the patient has metallic restorations; these restorations produce streak artifacts that may obscure portions of the anatomy (Figure 3-9).

CT is typically used in dentistry to evaluate (1) the extent of lesions suspected or detected with other radiographic techniques, (2) the degree of maxillofacial involvement in cases of trauma, (3) the integrity and condition of the paranasal sinuses, and (4) the quality and quantity of bone in proposed dental

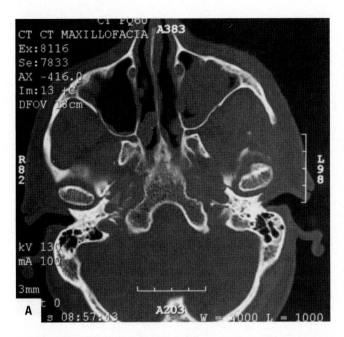 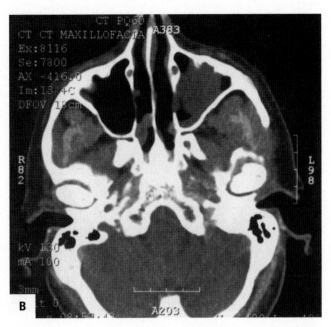

FIGURE 3-8 **A,** Bone window computed tomography (CT) scan of the same patient as in Figure 3-1. The left condyle exhibits alterations in size, shape, and degree of sclerosis, with an osteophyte in the anterior lateral aspect. Soft-tissue densities can be seen in the maxillary and ethmoid sinuses, consistent with chronic sinusitis and mucous retention cyst on the left. **B,** Soft-tissue window CT scan in the same imaging plane.

implant sites, particularly when there are multiple sites or when there has been bone grafting. CT is rarely indicated for evaluation of the TMJ since the osseous structures can be visualized adequately with less expensive techniques such as conventional tomography or panoramic radiography,[2] and disk displacement and other joint soft-tissue information can be better obtained with magnetic resonance imaging. CT may be of value in complex TMJ situations, such as in cases of suspected anky-

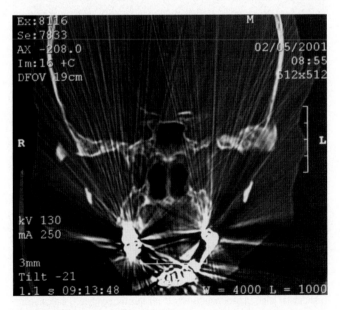

FIGURE 3-9 Streak artifact on a computed tomography (CT) scan as a result of metallic dental restorations in the imaging plane.

losis or severe joint destruction or when there is a history of polytetrafluoroethylene or silicon-sheeting TMJ implants.

Magnetic Resonance Imaging

Magnetic resonance imaging (MRI) uses electrical and magnetic fields and radiofrequency (RF) pulses, rather than ionizing radiation, to produce an image. The patient is placed within a large circular magnet that causes the hydrogen protons of the body to be aligned with the magnetic field. At this point, energy in the form of RF pulses is added to the system, and the equilibrium is destabilized, with the protons altering their orientation and magnetic moment. After the RF pulse is removed, the protons gradually return to equilibrium, giving up the excess energy in the form of a radio signal that can be detected and converted to a visible image. This return to equilibrium is called relaxation, and the time that it takes is dependent on tissue type. "T1 relaxation" describes the release of energy from the proton to its immediate environment, and "T2 relaxation" designates the interaction between adjacent protons. This whole sequence of applying RF pulses and then picking up the returning signal later is repeated many times in forming the image.

By manipulating the time of repetition (TR) of the pulses and the time of signal detection (time of echo [TE]), the various tissues can be highlighted, allowing the determination of tissue characteristics. For example, when both TR and TE are short (eg, 500 ms/20 ms), the image contrast is due primarily to differences in T1 relaxation times (ie, T1-weighted image) (Figure 3-10, A). Fat produces a bright signal whereas fluids and muscle produce an intermediate signal. If the parameters are adjusted so that both TR and TE are long (2,000 ms/80 ms—a T2-weighted image), fluids become bright and fat

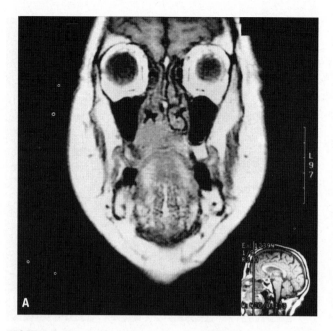 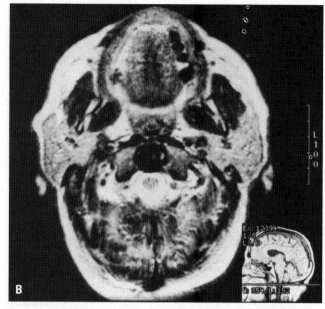

FIGURE 3-10 **A,** T1-weighted (time of repetition [TR]/time of echo [TE] = 500 ms/11 ms) magnetic resonance imaging (MRI) scan in a patient with squamous cell carcinoma of the maxillary sinus and nasal cavity on the right side, coronal plane. **B,** T2-weighted (TR/TE = 5,901 ms/90 ms) MRI scan in the same patient, axial view. The carcinoma has invaded the right alveolar ridge and palate.

becomes darker (see Figure 3-10, B). By running a variety of different sequences, significant information about tissue character can be obtained. The addition of an intravenous contrast agent (gadolinium-diethylenetriamine pentaacetic acid [DTPA]) allows even more tissue differentiation because certain tumors enhance (ie, produce a brighter signal) in a characteristic way due to increased blood flow.

Similarly to CT, MRI produces images of thin slices of tissue in a wide variety of planes, including oblique angles. Quasi-dynamic motion studies can also be performed, as can three-dimensional reconstruction.

MRI is used primarily for evaluating soft tissues because bone always produces a low signal (black) due to a relative paucity of hydrogen protons. While some information about osseous tissue can be obtained (particularly about alterations in the bone marrow), detailed study of bone is usually reserved for CT. Due to signals emanating from flowing blood, MRI can also be used to evaluate blood vessels, with differentiation between arteries and veins possible. Three-dimensional magnetic resonance (MR) angiography can rival conventional angiography in detail but without the need for the injection of a contrast medium.

Although MRI was first introduced clinically for the evaluation of the brain, it is now used throughout the body, not only for soft tissue but also for the assessment of joints since ligaments (both intact and torn), menisci, surface cartilage, bone marrow abnormalities, and synovial membrane proliferation can all be studied with MRI.

In dentistry, the primary uses of MRI have been the evaluation of various pathologic lesions (such as tumors) and the assessment of the TMJ. A number of cadaver and clinical studies have demonstrated that MRI can accurately depict the location, morphology, and function of the articular disk, thus

allowing the diagnosis of internal derangement to be made or confirmed[12] (Figure 3-11). Information on joint effusion and pannus formation can also be obtained, and some osseous changes can also be evaluated.[13,14] Recent reports have also described the correlation of MR appearance with histology in cases of bone marrow edema or necrosis.[15]

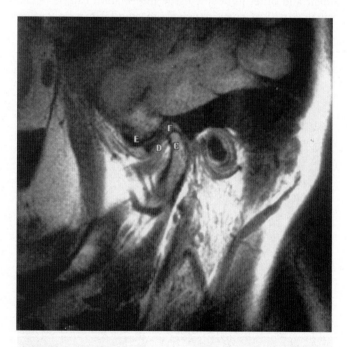

FIGURE 3-11 Magnetic resonance imaging (MRI) scan of the temporomandibular joint, closed-mouth view. C indictes the condyle, D indicates the disk, E marks the articular eminence, and F marks the articular fossa. The disk is anteriorly displaced.

The typical MRI examination of the TMJ consists of both closed- and open-mouth views in an oblique sagittal plane, with the sections oriented perpendicular to the long axis of the condyle. Some institutions also routinely obtain images in the coronal plane for easier identification of a lateral or medial displacement of the disk.

The sagittal images are used to evaluate disk position with respect to the head of the condyle. The disk is considered to be in a normal location when the posterior band is superior to the condyle (the so-called twelve-o'clock position) when the mouth is closed, but there is not complete agreement about how far the disk must be from twelve o'clock before anterior displacement is diagnosed.[16] Because there can also be a rotational component to the disk displacement, all slices through the joint should be evaluated, not just the ones that show the disk most clearly. In the open-mouth views, the disk can be seen to be interposed between the condyle and articular eminence (normal or reducing) or to remain anterior to the condyle (nonreducing).

MRI has many advantages over other imaging techniques, including the capability of imaging soft tissue in virtually any plane. It also uses no ionizing radiation and is thus generally considered safe although there are limits on the magnitude of the magnetic field used and although animal studies have shown teratogenicity resulting from MRI in pregnant mice.[17]

The major disadvantage of MRI is its cost, which is typically more than $1,000 per examination. Not only are the equipment, physical facility, and supplies (such as cryogens for the supercooled magnet) costly, the procedure also requires specially trained technologists and radiologists.

MRI is contraindicated for certain patients, including those with demand-type cardiac pacemakers, due to interference by the electrical and magnetic fields. Patients with ferromagnetic metallic objects in strategic places (such as aneurysm clips in the brain and metallic fragments in the eye) also should not be placed in the magnet. Most machines have weight and girth limits for patients because of the size of the bore of the magnet. Some patients feel claustrophobic inside the magnet and may need to be sedated for the procedure. Because of the length of time for each scan in the series (typically several minutes), patients who cannot remain motionless are not good candidates for MRI.

Ultrasonography

Ultrasonography (US) uses the reflection of sound waves to provide information about tissues and their interfaces with other tissues. This is a noninvasive and relatively inexpensive technique for imaging superficial tissues in "real time." The operator applies a probe over the area of interest and receives information immediately on the computer monitor. In regard to the head and neck region, there has been a great deal of recent interest in the imaging of salivary glands (Figure 3-12). Several researchers have studied the ultrasonographic features of a variety of tumors and other conditions in the parotid gland, in an attempt to make a diagnosis before biopsy as the surgical management of these tumors may vary.[18] Others have

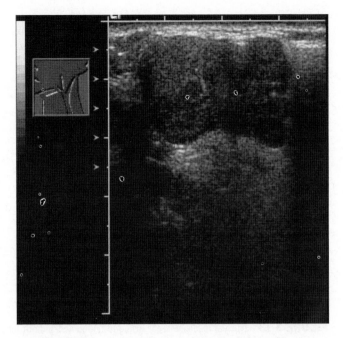

FIGURE 3-12 Ultrasonography of a pleomorphic adenoma of the pole of the parotid gland, showing a lobular shape, homogeneous internal echoes, and enhanced posterior echoes. (Courtesy of Dr. Mayumi Shimizu, Kyushu University Faculty of Dentistry, Fukuoka, Japan)

looked at the heterogeneity of sonic echo production within the parenchyma of parotid glands affected by a variety of inflammatory or autoimmune conditions.[19]

Efforts are being made to categorize lymph nodes in the neck as metastatic, reactive, or normal in patients with head and neck neoplasms.[20] Evaluation of stenosis of carotid arteries is also usually done with US.

US has been used to assess some joints in the body for evidence of inflammation, tears in ligaments and tendons, and other abnormalities. Unfortunately, US does not appear to be useful for determining internal derangement of the TMJ at this time[21] although work is continuing in this area.

Nuclear Medicine

In radionuclide imaging (nuclear medicine, scintigraphy), a substance labeled with a radioactive isotope is injected intravenously. Depending on the specific material used, the substance will be taken up preferentially by the thyroid (technetium [Tc] 99m–labeled iodine), salivary glands (Tc 99m pertechnetate), or bone (Tc 99m methylene diphosphonate [MDP]). Gallium 67 citrate is also sometimes used to assess infections and inflammation in bone. At various times after radionuclide injection, a gamma camera is used to count the radioactivity in the various organs and tissues of the body and to display the results visually. High concentrations of the isotope show up as "hot spots" and generally indicate high metabolic activity (Figure 3-13). Nuclear-medicine scans are used to assess conditions that may be widespread, such as metastasis to bone or other tissues or such as fibrous dysplasia in an active phase. Unfortunately, areas of dental periapical and peri-

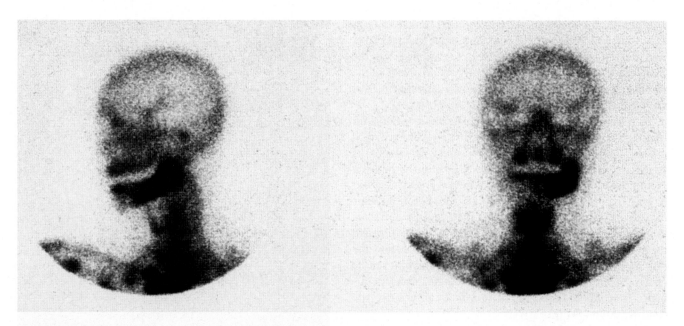

FIGURE 3-13 Nuclear medicine scans (using technetium 99m methylene diphosphonate) of a patient with osteomyelitis in the left mandible (frontal and lateral views). (Courtesy of Dr. Soon-Chul Choi, Seoul National University College of Dentistry, Seoul, Korea)

odontal inflammation also take up the tracer, presenting as hot spots in the jaws, and must be differentiated from other pathologic conditions.

A variation of bone scintigraphy that can be used to localize and quantify bone activity is single-photon emission computed tomography (SPECT). In this technique, the gamma rays given off by the Tc 99m MDP are detected by a rotating gamma camera, and the data are processed by computer to provide cross-sectional images that can later be reconstructed as images in other planes. Volumetric measurements may also be obtained to quantify the distribution of radioactivity in the tissue, allowing better assessment of tissue function.[22] A recent study demonstrated the use of SPECT in the evaluation of osseointegration in dental implants.[23] However, in another study, both the sensitivity and specificity of SPECT were low for the detection of painful sites in patients with idiopathic jaw pain.[24]

Contrast-Enhanced Radiography

Radiography with the use of contrast agents is still performed in some facilities, but its usage has decreased significantly with the evolution of advanced imaging techniques. The major contrast-enhanced examinations used in dentistry are arthrography and sialography.

In arthrography of the TMJ, radiopaque material is injected into the lower (and sometimes also the upper) joint space under fluoroscopic guidance. Once the dye is in place, fluoroscopic recordings of the joint in motion may be made in order to assess the shape, location, and function of the articular disk.[25] Radiography or tomography may also be performed afterwards (Figure 3-14). Arthrography is invasive and technically difficult and has been replaced by MRI in most institutions.

In sialography, contrast medium is injected into the major duct of the salivary gland of interest. The distribution of the

ductal system, along with any patterns such as narrowing or dilation of ducts or such as contrast extravasation or retention, can provide helpful information regarding the inflammatory, obstructive, or neoplastic condition affecting the gland[26,27] (Figure 3-15). In many institutions, CT, MRI, or US is used more often than sialography to evaluate the salivary glands.

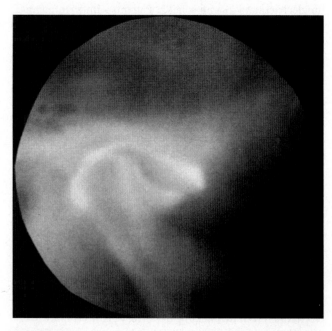

FIGURE 3-14 Arthrogram of the temporomandibular joint. Radiopaque contrast material was injected into both upper and lower joint spaces. The disk is anteriorly displaced. (Courtesy of Dr. L. George Upton, University of Michigan School of Dentistry, Ann Arbor, Mich.)

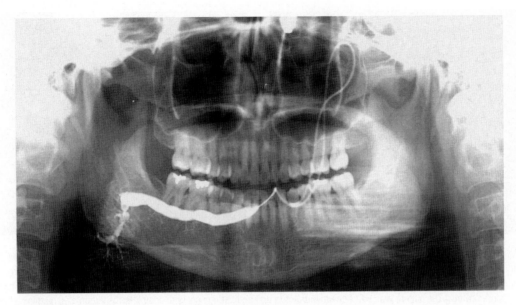

FIGURE 3-15 Sialography, using panoramic radiography, of the submandibular gland. The patient has chronic obstruction of the gland due to a radiolucent sialolith. (Courtesy of Dr. Soon-Chul Choi, Seoul National University College of Dentistry, Seoul, Korea)

▼ IMAGING PROTOCOLS

Orofacial Pain

In deciding whether to use imaging during the assessment of a patient with orofacial pain, the clinician must first obtain enough information from the history and clinical examination to determine the nature and probable cause of the problem and to decide whether imaging will provide any benefits in the diagnosis and management of the patient. In many cases, it may be necessary to rule out the teeth as a source of the pain. Select intraoral and/or panoramic radiography combined with the clinical examination can generally help in this situation.

If the patient's symptoms are suggestive of temporomandibular disorder (TMD), a thorough clinical examination may provide enough information to establish a diagnosis and to select a management strategy without imaging, even though it has been shown that clinical examination alone will not detect all cases of internal derangement.[28]

When there appears to be a bony component to the temporomandibular problem or if the patient is refractory to conservative treatment, it may be useful to obtain information on the condition of the osseous structures of the joints.[2] A number of techniques can be used to confirm or rule out a variety of developmental, inflammatory, degenerative, traumatic, or neoplastic processes. Panoramic radiography provides a good overview of both joints as well as the rest of the maxillofacial complex. Although only gross structural abnormalities will be visualized with this type of radiography, this degree of detail may be adequate in many cases to determine the presence or absence of bony changes.[29] If more detail is necessary to make the diagnosis or prognosis, conventional tomography should be performed, generally in oblique sagittal views, corrected for condylar angle, in both open- and closed-mouth positions.[30] Coronal or frontal tomography complements the lateral view by providing images at 90° to the first view. While some studies show that TMJ tomography provides additional information not anticipated clinically,[31] others show mixed results as to the effect of the findings on the management of the patient.[32,33]

If an internal derangement is suspected and if patient management depends on confirmation or rejection of this diagnosis, the position and function of the articular disk can be determined by either MRI or arthrography. In most institutions, MRI is the preferred examination because it is noninvasive and can provide information about the disk as well as other soft-tissue and bony structures.

There are other causes besides TMD for pain in the head region. Panoramic radiography may be helpful in the initial evaluation of the maxillary sinus if that structure is thought to be the origin of the facial pain. The floor of the sinus is well visualized, and discontinuity of the bony margins, thickening of the mucous membrane, partial or total opacification of the antrum, and the presence of mucous retention cysts can be noted on the resultant radiograph (Figure 3-16). A full imaging evaluation of the paranasal sinuses usually requires CT although a series of plain films may be made at some institutions.

If a central lesion is suspected of being the cause of the pain, an evaluation of the skull by CT or MRI is in order. The choice of the specific imaging examination depends on the presumptive diagnosis and should be determined in conjunction with the treating clinician and the radiologist.

Disease Entities Affecting Salivary Glands

There are a number of disease entities that can affect the salivary glands: these entities include obstructive, inflammatory,

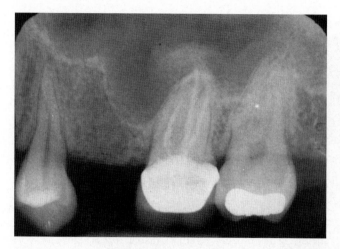
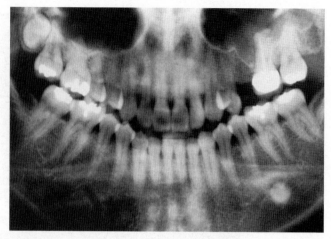

FIGURE 3-16 **A,** Periapical radiograph of a 29-year-old woman who presented with a throbbing toothache in the maxillary left. Endodontic treatment on the first molar had been completed 10 years earlier. The second premolar was extracted due to similar symptoms 1 year before. There is a thickening of the mucous membrane above the molars and a general cloudiness of the maxillary sinus. **B,** Panoramic radiograph taken the same day. The unilateral clouding of the sinus is more obvious. The patient was treated with antibiotics and antihistamines, with complete resolution of symptoms within 24 hours. The round radiopaque lesion in the mandible was not investigated at the initial appointment, and the patient did not return for further treatment.

autoimmune, and neoplastic processes. In addition, swellings or enlargements in the region of the major salivary glands can arise in structures outside the glands, including lymph nodes, cysts, nonsalivary neoplasms, and muscle hypertrophy. Imaging may be of value in differentiating between various diseases and in staging the degree of tissue destruction.

Plain films are frequently helpful when an obstructive disease is suspected, although about 20% of the sialoliths in the submandibular gland and 40% of the sialoliths in the parotid gland are not well calcified and will thus appear radiolucent on radiographs.[34] Occlusal radiography can be used to demonstrate submandibular sialoliths, with a standard topographic or cross-sectional view and with the beam entering under the chin and striking the film at 90° (Figure 3-17). In the posterior

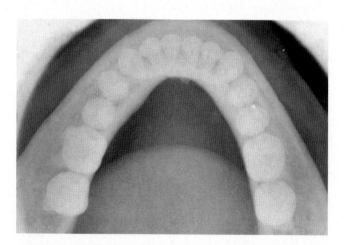

FIGURE 3-17 Mandibular cross-sectional occlusal radiograph demonstrating a tubular radiopaque object just lingual to the left premolars in the floor of the mouth. The sialolith, which had been causing periodic obstruction of the submandibular gland for 4 years, was surgically removed, and the duct orifice was repositioned.

region, a more oblique angle may be needed to visualize the stone, projecting it forward onto the film. In general, a reduced exposure time is needed because the stone is less calcified than bone or teeth. Periapical radiography in the buccal vestibule may demonstrate a sialolith in the parotid duct. Various extraoral views may also be needed to visualize a stone, depending on its location.

Sialography, in which a radiopaque contrast medium is instilled into the duct of a salivary gland prior to imaging, permits a thorough evaluation of the ductal system of the major glands. It can demonstrate the branching pattern as well as the number and size of the ducts. Radiolucent sialoliths that are not visible on plain films can be seen as voids in the contrast medium. Sialography is indicated primarily for the evaluation of chronic inflammatory diseases and ductal pathosis, but other imaging techniques are preferred for the investigation of space-occupying masses.

Tumors in the salivary glands or surrounding areas may be investigated by a variety of techniques, including CT, MRI, and US. The selection of specific examinations should be made in consultation with a radiologist. In many institutions, CT is the procedure of choice for evaluating the salivary glands and particularly the extent of a mass since glandular tissue usually can be readily distinguished from surrounding fat and muscle. MRI, however, may better delineate the internal structure of the tumor and demonstrate extension into adjacent tissues. Ultrasonography has typically been used to differentiate solid lesions from cystic lesions in the salivary glands, but recent studies have begun to look more closely at the ultrasonographic features of various salivary tumors in an effort to aid the differential diagnosis by using a noninvasive and relatively inexpensive technique.[18,19]

For many years, sialography has been considered the "gold standard" for evaluating the salivary component of autoimmune diseases such as Sjögren's syndrome.[26] The presence of punctate (< 1 mm) or globular (1 to 2 mm) collections of contrast medium (sialectasis) may be seen throughout the glands, progressing over time into larger pools of extraductal contrast material that may signal more advanced gland destruction.

Recently, there has been increased interest in the use of US to examine the glands in patients with Sjögren's syndrome, primarily in respect to the degree of homogeneity of the parenchyma.[19] While its diagnostic accuracy is not as high as that of sialography, particularly in the early stages of the disease, US may be useful in those cases in which sialography cannot be done. It has also been suggested that US could be done first, followed by sialography only in those cases that yield abnormal or equivocal ultrasonographic results.[20]

Scintigraphy with Tc 99m pertechnetate can be used to evaluate the function of all of the salivary glands simultaneously. However, there is disagreement over how useful this technique is in determining the cause of xerostomic states. One recent study concluded that scintigraphy was not useful in determining which patients would respond to pilocarpine after radiotherapy-induced salivary dysfunction.[35]

Jaw Lesions

The imaging evaluation of jaw lesions may range from a combination of intraoral and panoramic radiography to CT, MRI, US, and/or scintigraphy, depending on the size, location, margins, and behavior of the lesion. For small well-defined lesions occurring in the jaws, standard dental radiography may be adequate to characterize the lesion and permitting the development of a differential diagnosis prior to confirmation by biopsy.

However, if the jaw lesion is large, causes jaw expansion, has indistinct or irregular margins, or appears to be a tumor originating in soft tissues, additional information is usually needed either before or after biopsy, to determine the extent of the lesion and its relationship to adjacent tissues. If the lesion is malignant, evaluation for metastasis is necessary. Although CT is frequently used to examine the lymph nodes of the neck, recent reports have suggested that US can reliably distinguish metastatic nodes from reactive and normal nodes.[36] In some cases, CT and MRI may be of more value in planning the treatment than in making the diagnosis since appropriate treatment is predicated on knowing the full extent of the lesion, including any invasion of adjacent structures (Figure 3-18).

▼ BENEFITS AND RISKS

In determining whether to order a particular type of imaging, the clinician first must decide what information is needed and whether diagnostic imaging can provide it. If the answer is yes, the next step is to determine the best imaging technique for the situation. It is possible that several techniques could provide the desired data. For example, an expansile lesion in the mandible may be viewed with panoramic radiography, perhaps supplemented with an occlusal view. However, it could also be visualized with plain-film radiography (at various

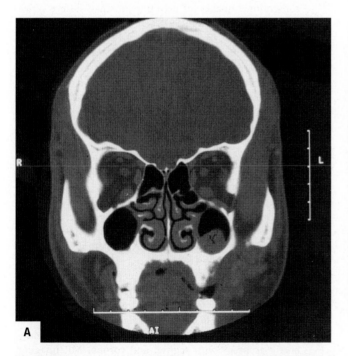 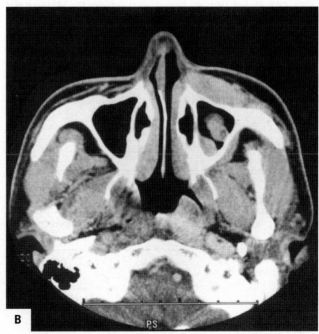

FIGURE 3-18 Computed tomography scans of a patient with adenocystic carcinoma arising in the maxillary sinus. The clinical presentation was advanced periodontitis, a nonhealing sinus track in the maxillary anterior where a tooth had exfoliated, and slight facial swelling. **A,** Coronal view, bone window. A soft-tissue mass is seen in the left maxillary sinus. There is also erosion of bone on the buccal surface of the left maxillary alveolar ridge. **B,** Axial view, soft-tissue window. A soft-tissue mass can be seen under the skin anterior to the left maxillary sinus. A mass within the sinus can be seen as well. There was extensive involvement by this tumor throughout the entire head.

angles), CT, MRI, or a combination of techniques. How much information is necessary? If a lesion is contained and well defined, panoramic radiography alone may be adequate. However, if a lesion is large and poorly defined, the information on lesion extension and effects on adjacent structures may be critical to the management of the patient, and CT may be almost mandatory. On the other hand, if the results of the CT or MRI studies will not affect the diagnosis or management of the case, the procedure could be considered superfluous and a waste of time, money, and radiation risk.

All imaging techniques, with the exception of US and perhaps MRI, carry some type of radiobiologic risk. Current practice is to convert the absorbed dose from the radiation to an effective dose, which is a quantity weighted for radiation type and dose and for radiosensitivity of the tissues. This practice allows expression of a dose to a limited portion of the body equivalent, in terms of detriment, to a smaller dose to the entire body, thus allowing comparison between radiographic techniques. Reported average effective doses for several imaging examinations of the head and neck, along with days of equivalent natural exposure, are listed in Table 3-1.

The cost of imaging procedures varies significantly. Intraoral and panoramic radiography is the least expensive; an examination typically costs less than $75.00 (US). Plain films of the skull may be obtained for about $135.00 (US) each in a hospital radiology facility. A typical ultrasound examination of the neck costs about $250.00 (US). CT scans of the maxillofacial region are in the range of $850.00 to $1,000.00 (US) and cost more if there is three-dimensional reconstruction of the image whereas MRI scans usually cost more than $1,200.00 (US). (All stated fees are based on the fees at a Midwestern teaching hospital in the year 2000.) The majority of advanced imaging procedures will be billed to medical insurance rather than to dental insurance. The regulations of the patient's health care insurer must be followed if payment is not to be denied. For example, in a health maintenance organization (HMO), CT or MRI may need to be ordered by the patient's primary care physician for payment to be authorized.

A prudent principle to follow when ordering an imaging study is to select the technique that has the lowest cost and radiation dose but that is still capable of providing the needed information. Consultation with an oral and maxillofacial radiologist can help the clinician select the best study for the particular situation.

▼ REFERENCES

1. US Department of Health and Human Services. The selection of patients for x-ray examinations: dental radiographic examinations. DHHS Publication FDA 88-8273. Rockville (MD): US Department of Health and Human Services; 1987.
2. Brooks SL, Brand JW, Gibbs SJ, et al. Imaging of the temporomandibular joint. A position paper of the American Academy of Oral and Maxillofacial Radiology. Oral Surg Oral Med Oral Pathol Oral Radiol Endod 1997;83:609–18.
3. Tyndall DA, Brooks SL, editors. Selection criteria for dental implant site imaging: a position paper of the American Academy of Oral and Maxillofacial Radiology. Oral Surg Oral Med Oral Pathol Oral Radiol Endod 2000;89:630–7.
4. White SC, Heslop EW, Hollender LG, et al. Parameters of radiologic care. An official report of the American Academy of Oral and Maxillofacial Radiology. Oral Surg Oral Med Oral Pathol Oral Radiol Endod 2001; 91:498–511.
5. Tyndall DA, Ludlow JB, Platin E, Nair M. A comparison of Kodak Ektaspeed Plus film and the Siemens Sidexis digital imaging system for caries detection using receiver operating characteristic analysis. Oral Surg Oral Med Oral Pathol Oral Radiol Endod 1998;85:113–8.
6. White SC, Yoon DC. Comparative performance of digital and conventional images for detecting proximal surface caries. Dentomaxillofac Radiol 1997;26:32–8.
7. Nair MK, Ludlow JB, Tyndall DA, et al. Periodontitis detection efficacy of film and digital images. Oral Surg Oral Med Oral Pathol Oral Radiol Endod 1998;85:608–12.
8. Paurazas SB, Geist JR, Pink FE, et al. Comparison of diagnostic accuracy of digital imaging by using CCD and CMOS-APS sensors with E-speed film in the detection of periapical bony lesions. Oral Surg Oral Med Oral Pathol Oral Radiol Endod 2000;89:356–62.
9. White SC, Rudolph DJ. Alterations of the trabecular pattern of the jaws in patients with osteoporosis. Oral Surg Oral Med Oral Pathol Oral Radiol Endod 1999;88:628–35.
10. Webber RL, Messura JK. An in vivo comparison of diagnostic information obtained from tuned-aperture computed tomography and conventional digital radiographic imaging modalities. Oral Surg Oral Med Oral Pathol Oral Radiol Endod 1999; 88:239–47.
11. Terakado M, Hashimoto K, Arai Y, et al. Diagnostic imaging with newly developed ortho cubic super-high resolution computed tomography (Ortho-CT). Oral Surg Oral Med Oral Pathol Oral Radiol Endod 2000;89:509–18.
12. Tasaki MM, Westesson P-L. Temporomandibular joint: diagnostic accuracy with sagittal and coronal MR imaging. Radiology 1993;186:723–9.
13. Westesson P-L, Brooks SL. Temporomandibular joint: relationship between MR evidence of effusion and the presence of pain and disk displacement. AJR Am J Roentgenol 1992;159:559–63.

TABLE 3-1 Effective Dose and Equivalent Natural Exposure from Diagnostic Radiographic Examinations of the Head and Neck

Survey	Effective Dose (E) (μSv)	Equivalent Natural Exposure (d)
Full-mouth intraoral survey		
Round collimation, D-speed film	150	18.8
Rectangular collimation, E-speed film	33	4.1
Panoramic radiography	26	3.3
Computed tomography		
Maxilla	104–1,202	13.0–150.3
Mandible	761–3,324	95.1–415.5
Skull	220	27.5

Adapted from Frederiksen NL. Health physics. In: White SC, Pharoah MJ. Oral radiology: principles and interpretation. 4th ed. St. Louis: Mosby; 2000. p. 49.

14. Smith HJ, Larheim TA, Aspestrand F. Rheumatic and non-rheumatic disease in the temporomandibular joint: gadolinium-enhanced MR imaging. Radiology 1992;185:229–34.

15. Larheim TA, Westesson PL, Hicks DG, et al. Osteonecrosis of the temporomandibular joint: correlation of magnetic resonance imaging and histology. J Oral Maxillofac Surg 1999;57:888–98.

16. Orsini MG, Kuboki T, Terada S, et al. Diagnostic value of 4 criteria to interpret temporomandibular joint normal disk position on magnetic resonance imaging. Oral Surg Oral Med Oral Pathol Oral Radiol Endod 1998;86:489–97.

17. Tyndall DA, Sulik KK. Effects of magnetic resonance imaging on eye development in the C57BL/6J mouse. Teratology 1991;43:263–75.

18. Shimizu M, Ussmüller J, Hartwein J, et al. Statistical study for sonographic differential diagnosis of tumorous lesions in the parotid gland. Oral Surg Oral Med Oral Pathol Oral Radiol Endod 1999;88:226–33.

19. Shimizu M, Ussmüller J, Hartwein J, Donath K. A comparative study of sonographic-histopathologic findings of tumorous lesions in the parotid gland. Oral Surg Oral Med Oral Pathol Oral Radiol Endod 1999;88:723–37.

20. Yoshiura K, Yuasa K, Tabata O, et al. Reliability of ultrasonography and sialography in the diagnosis of Sjögren's syndrome. Oral Surg Oral Med Oral Pathol Oral Radiol Endod 1997;83:400–7.

21. Emshoff R, Bertram S, Rudisch A, Gassner R. The diagnostic value of ultrasonography to determine the temporomandibular disk position. Oral Surg Oral Med Oral Pathol Oral Radiol Endod 1997;84:688–96.

22. Ell PJ, Khan O. Emission computerized tomography: clinical applications. Semin Nucl Med 1981;11:50-60.

23. Khan O, Archibald A, Thomson E, Maharaj P. The role of quantitative single photon emission computerized tomography (SPECT) in the osseous integration process of dental implants. Oral Surg Oral Med Oral Pathol Oral Radiol Endod 2000;90:228–32.

24. DeNucci DJ, Chen CC, Sobiski C, Meehan S. The use of SPECT bone scans to evaluate patients with idiopathic jaw pain. Oral Surg Oral Med Oral Pathol Oral Radiol Endod 2000;90:750–7.

25. Westesson P-L, Bronstein SL. Temporomandibular joint: comparison of single- and double-contrast arthrography. Radiology 1987;164:65–70.

26. Whaley K, Blair S, Low PS, et al. Sialographic abnormalities in Sjögren's syndrome, rheumatoid arthritis, and other arthritides and connective tissue diseases: a clinical and radiological investigation using hydrostatic sialography. Clin Radiol 1972;23:474–82.

27. O'Hara AE. Sialography: past, present and future. CRC Crit Rev Clin Radiol Nucl Med 1973;15:87–139.

28. Paesani D, Westesson P-L, Hatala MP, et al. Accuracy of clinical diagnosis for TMJ internal derangement and arthrosis. Oral Surg Oral Med Oral Pathol 1992;73:360–3.

29. Habets LL, Bezuur JN, Jimenez Lopez V, Hansson TL. The OPG: an aid in TMJ diagnosis. III. A comparison between lateral tomography and dental rotational panoramic radiography (orthopantomography). J Oral Rehabil 1989;16:401–6.

30. Eckerdal O, Lundberg M. The structural situation in temporomandibular joints: a comparison between conventional oblique transcranial radiography, tomography, and histologic sections. Dentomaxillofac Radiol 1979;8:42–9.

31. Pullinger AG, White SC. Efficacy of TMJ radiographs in terms of expected versus actual findings. Oral Surg Oral Med Oral Pathol Oral Radiol Endod 1995;79:367–74.

32. White SC, Pullinger AG. Impact of TMJ radiographs on clinician decision making. Oral Surg Oral Med Oral Pathol Oral Radiol Endod 1995;79:375–81.

33. Callender KI, Brooks SL. The usefulness of tomography in the evaluation of patients with temporomandibular disorders: a retrospective clinical study. Oral Surg Oral Med Oral Pathol Oral Radiol Endod 1996;81:710–9.

34. Rubin P, Holt JF. Secretory sialography in diseases of the major salivary glands. AJR Am J Roentgenol 1957;77:575–98.

35. Cooper RA, Cowan RA, Owens SE, et al. Does salivary gland scintigraphy predict response to pilocarpine in patients with post-radiotherapy xerostomia. Eur J Nucl Med 1999;26:220–5.

36. Sato N, Kawabe R, Fujita K, Omura S. Differential diagnosis of cervical lymphadenopathy with intranodal color Doppler flow signals in patients with oral squamous cell carcinoma. Oral Surg Oral Med Oral Pathol Oral Radiol Endod 1998;86:482–8.

4

ULCERATIVE, VESICULAR, AND BULLOUS LESIONS

MARTIN S. GREENBERG, DDS

▼ THE PATIENT WITH ACUTE MULTIPLE LESIONS
Herpesvirus Infections
Primary Herpes Simplex Virus Infections
Coxsackievirus Infections
Varicella-Zoster Virus Infection
Erythema Multiforme
Contact Allergic Stomatitis
Oral Ulcers Secondary to Cancer Chemotherapy
Acute Necrotizing Ulcerative Gingivitis

▼ THE PATIENT WITH RECURRING ORAL ULCERS
Recurrent Aphthous Stomatitis
Behçet's Syndrome
Recurrent Herpes Simplex Virus Infection

▼ THE PATIENT WITH CHRONIC MULTIPLE LESIONS
Pemphigus
Subepithelial Bullous Dermatoses
Herpes Simplex Virus Infection in Immunosuppressed Patients

▼ THE PATIENT WITH SINGLE ULCERS
Histoplasmosis
Blastomycosis
Mucormycosis

A clinician attempting to diagnose an ulcerative or vesiculobullous disease of the mouth is confronted with the fact that many diseases have a similar clinical appearance. The oral mucosa is thin, causing vesicles and bullae to break rapidly into ulcers, and ulcers are easily traumatized from teeth and food, and they become secondarily infected by the oral flora. These factors may cause lesions that have a characteristic appearance on the skin to have a nonspecific appearance on the oral mucosa.

Mucosal disorders may occasionally be correctly diagnosed from a brief history and rapid clinical examination, but this approach is most often insufficient and leads to incorrect diagnosis and improper treatment. The history taking is frequently underemphasized, but, when correctly performed, it gives as much information as does the clinical examination. A detailed history of the present illness is of particular importance when attempting to diagnose oral mucosal lesions. A complete review of systems should be obtained for each patient, including questions regarding the presence of skin, eye, genital, and rectal lesions. Questions should also be included regarding symptoms of diseases associated with oral lesions; that is, each patient should be asked about the presence of symptoms such as joint pains, muscle weakness, dyspnea, diplopia, and chest pains. The clinical examination should include a thorough inspection of the exposed skin surfaces; the diagnosis of oral lesions requires knowledge of basic dermatology because many disorders occurring on the oral mucosa also affect the skin. Dermatologic lesions are classified according to their clinical appearance and include the following basic lesions:

1. Macules. Well-circumscribed, flat lesions that are noticeable because of their change from normal skin color. They may be red due to the presence of vascular lesions or inflammation, or pigmented due to the presence of melanin, hemosiderin, and drugs.

2. Papules. Solid lesions raised above the skin surface that are smaller than 1 cm in diameter. Papules may be seen in a wide variety of diseases including erythema multiforme simplex, rubella, lupus erythematosus, and sarcoidosis.

3. Plaques. Solid raised lesions that are over 1 cm in diameter; they are large papules.

4. Nodules. These lesions are present deep in the dermis, and the epidermis can be easily moved over them.

5. Vesicles. Elevated blisters containing clear fluid that are under 1 cm in diameter.

6. Bullae. Elevated blisterlike lesions containing clear fluid that are over 1 cm in diameter.

7. Erosions. Moist red lesions often caused by the rupture of vesicles or bullae as well as trauma.

8. Pustules. Raised lesions containing purulent material.

9. Ulcers. A defect in the epithelium; it is a well-circumscribed depressed lesion over which the epidermal layer has been lost.

10. Purpura. Reddish to purple flat lesions caused by blood from vessels leaking into the subcutaneous tissue. Classified by size as petechiae or ecchymoses, these lesions do not blanch when pressed.

11. Petechiae. Purpuric lesions 1 to 2 mm in diameter. Larger purpuric lesions are called ecchymoses.

A detailed history of the present illness is essential in making the diagnosis of oral mucosal disease. Three pieces of information that should be obtained early in the history will help the clinician rapidly categorize a patient's disease and simplify the diagnosis: length of time the lesions have been present (acute or chronic lesions), past history of similar lesions (primary or recurrent disease), and number of lesions present (single or multiple). In this chapter, the diseases are grouped according to the information just described. This information serves as an excellent starting point for the student who is just learning to diagnose these disorders, as well as the experienced clinician who is aware of the potential diagnostic pitfalls.

The first section of this chapter describes acute multiple lesions that tend to occur only once, the second portion of the chapter covers recurring oral mucosal syndromes, and the third portion presents the patient with chronic multiple lesions. The final section describes diseases that present as chronic single lesions. It is hoped that classifying the disorders in this way will help the clinician avoid the common diagnostic problem of confusing viral infections with recurring oral syndromes, such as recurrent aphthous stomatitis, or disorders that present as chronic progressive disease, such as pemphigus and pemphoid.

▼ THE PATIENT WITH ACUTE MULTIPLE LESIONS

The major diseases that cause acute multiple oral lesions include viral stomatitis, allergic reactions (particularly erythema multiforme and contact allergic stomatitis), and lesions caused by cancer chemotherapy or blood dyscrasias.

Herpesvirus Infections

There are 80 known herpesviruses, and eight of them are known to cause infection in humans: herpes simplex virus (HSV) 1 and 2, varicella-zoster virus, *Cytomegalovirus*, Epstein-Barr virus, and human herpesvirus 6 (HHV6). All herpesviruses contain a deoxyribonucleic acid (DNA) nucleus and can remain latent in host neural cells, thereby evading the host immune response.[1] HHV6, a herpesvirus discovered in 1986, has been shown by seroprevalence studies to infect over 80% of the population by adult life. Two variants, HHV6A and HHV6B have been identified. The virus is commonly isolated from saliva and causes roseola infantum (exanthema subitum), a common childhood illness that is characterized by fever and a rash. The virus also is a cause of a mononucleosis-like syndrome in older children and adults. In immunocompromised patients, HHV6 can cause interstitial pneumonitis and bone marrow suppression.[2] HHV7, which is commonly isolated from saliva, is presently not associated with a specific disease, whereas HHV8 has been closely associated with Kaposi's sarcoma in human immunodeficiency virus (HIV)–infected patients. There is also evidence linking HHV8 to forms of lymphoma and Castleman's disease.

HSV1, HSV2, and varicella-zoster are viruses that are known to cause oral mucosal disease. *Cytomegalovirus* is an occasional cause of oral ulceration in immunosuppressed patients, and it is suspected as a cause of salivary gland disease in HIV-infected patients.[3]

The herpes simplex virus is composed of four layers: an inner core of linear double-stranded DNA, a protein capsid, a tegument, and a lipid envelope containing glycoproteins that is derived from the nuclear membrane of host cells. The two major types, HSV1 and 2, can be distinguished serologically or by restriction endonuclease analysis of the nuclear DNA. Classically, HSV1 causes a majority of cases of oral and pharyngeal infection, meningoencephalitis, and dermatitis above the waist; HSV2 is implicated in most genital infections. Although this distinction applies to a majority of cases, changing sexual habits are making that distinction less important. Both types can cause primary or recurrent infection of either the oral or the genital area, and both may cause recurrent disease at either site.[1] Primary infection may also occur concurrently in both oral and genital sites from either HSV1 or HSV2,[4] although HSV1 recurs more frequently in the oral region and HSV2 more frequently in the genital region.[5,6]

Humans are the only natural reservoir of HSV infection, and spread occurs by direct intimate contact with lesions or secretions from an asymptomatic carrier. This latter method of spread of HSV is common; between 2 and 9% of asymptomatic individuals shed HSV in saliva or genital secretions.[7–9]

Latency, a characteristic of all herpesviruses, occurs when the virus is transported from mucosal or cutaneous nerve endings by neurons to ganglia where the HSV viral genome remains present in a nonreplicating state.[10] During the latent phase, herpes DNA is detectable, but viral proteins are not produced.[11] Reactivation of the latent virus occurs when HSV switches to a replicative state; this can occur as a result of a number of factors including peripheral tissue injury from trauma or sunburn, fever, or immunosuppression.[12]

The concept that HSV is a possible cause of Bell's palsy was initially suggested in 1972,[13] but recent evidence using genetic and molecular techniques has demonstrated that reactivation of HSV is the most common cause of this disorder.[14,15]

There is evidence linking HSV to carcinogenesis.[16] Epidemiologic studies have demonstrated an increased incidence of HSV2 serum antibodies or positive HSV2 cultures in patients with cervical carcinoma. Animal studies on hamster cheek pouches show an enhanced development of invasive squamous cell carcinoma when HSV1 infection is combined with topical snuff.[17]

Primary Herpes Simplex Virus Infections

There are approximately 600,000 new cases of primary HSV infections per year in the United States. Primary HSV infection occurs in patients who do not have immunity resulting from previous contact with the virus. HSV is contracted after intimate contact with an individual who has active HSV primary or recurrent lesions. Primary HSV may also be spread by asymptomatic shedders with HSV present in salivary secretions. The majority of oral HSV infections is caused by HSV1, but primary oral HSV2 infections may also occur chiefly as a result of oral-genital contact.[11] Infection of the fingers (herpetic whitlows) of health professionals may occur during treatment of infected patients. Dentists may experience primary lesions of the fingers from contact with lesions of the mouth or saliva of patients who are asymptomatic carriers of HSV, although the incidence of this disorder should be minimal if gloves are worn (Figure 4-1).[18] Use of gloves should also prevent the spread of HSV from the fingers of health care workers infected with herpetic whitlows to patients.

Primary HSV infection of the newborn was previously believed to be caused by direct contact with vaginal HSV lesions during birth, but it has now been established that a majority of mothers giving birth to children with primary HSV are asymptomatic carriers without lesions.[19] These infections of the newborn result in viremia and disseminated infection of the brain, liver, adrenals, and lungs.[20]

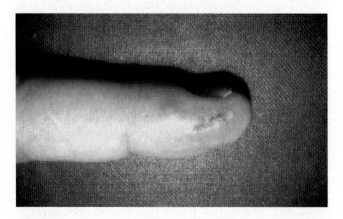

FIGURE 4-1   Primary herpetic whitlow on the finger of a dentist.

Newborns of mothers with antibody titers are protected by placentally transferred antibodies during the first 6 months of life. After 6 months of age, the incidence of primary HSV1 infection increases. The incidence of primary HSV1 infection reaches a peak between 2 and 3 years of age. Incidence of primary HSV2 infection does not increase until the age when sexual activity begins. Studies of neutralizing and complement-fixing antibodies to HSV have shown a continual rise in the percentage of patients who have had contact with the virus until 60 years of age, demonstrating that although the primary infection with HSV1 is chiefly a disease of infants and children, new cases continue to appear during adult life. This is consistent with the many reports of adults with primary herpetic gingivostomatitis.

The incidence of primary herpes infection has been shown to vary according to socioeconomic group. In lower socioeconomic groups, 70 to 80% of the population have detectable antibodies to HSV by the second decade of life, indicating prior HSV infection, whereas, in a group of middle class individuals, only 20 to 40% of the patients in the same age group have evidence of contact with HSV.[21,22]

A significant percentage of cases of primary herpes are subclinical, although the apparently low incidence of a history of classic primary herpetic gingivostomatitis is also influenced by the young age of patients who develop the infection, by the improper diagnosis of some cases, and by the cases of primary herpetic pharyngitis that cannot be clinically distinguished from other causes of viral pharyngitis.

CLINICAL MANIFESTATIONS OF PRIMARY ORAL HERPES

The patient usually presents to the clinician with full-blown oral and systemic disease, but a history of the mode of onset is helpful in differentiating lesions of primary HSV infection from other acute multiple lesions of the oral mucosa. The incubation period is most commonly 5 to 7 days but may range from 2 to 12 days.

Patients with primary oral herpes have a history of generalized prodromal symptoms that precede the local lesions by 1 or 2 days. This information is helpful in differentiating this viral infection from allergic stomatitis or erythema multiforme, in which local lesions and systemic symptoms appear together. These generalized symptoms include fever, headache, malaise, nausea, and vomiting. A negative past history of recurrent herpes labialis and a positive history of direct intimate contact with a patient with primary or recurrent herpes are also helpful in making the diagnosis.

Approximately 1 or 2 days after the prodromal symptoms occur, small vesicles appear on the oral mucosa; these are thin-walled vesicles surrounded by an inflammatory base (Figure 4-2). The vesicles quickly rupture, leaving shallow round discrete ulcers. The lesions occur on all portions of the mucosa. As the disease progresses, several lesions may coalesce, forming larger irregular lesions.

An important diagnostic criterion in this disease is the appearance of generalized acute marginal gingivitis. The entire gingiva is edematous and inflamed (Figures 4-3, A and

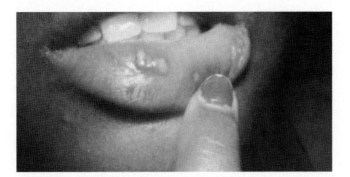

FIGURE 4-2   A 12-year-old female with primary herpetic gingivostomatis causing discrete vesicles and ulcers surrounded by inflammation.

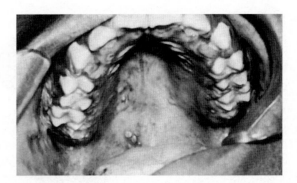

FIGURE 4-4   Primary herpes infection in a 17-year-old male. Note the unruptured palatal vesicles and intense marginal gingivitis.

B, and 4-4). Several small gingival ulcers are often present. Examination of the posterior pharynx reveals inflammation, and the submandibular and cervical lymph nodes are characteristically enlarged and tender. On occasion, primary HSV may cause lesions of the labial and facial skin without intraoral lesions.

Primary HSV in otherwise healthy children is a self-limiting disease. The fever ordinarily disappears within 3 or 4 days, and the lesions begin healing in a week to 10 days, although HSV may continue to be present in the saliva for up to a month after the onset of disease.

LABORATORY DIAGNOSIS

The diagnosis of primary herpetic gingivostomatitis is straightforward when patients present with a typical clinical picture of generalized symptoms followed by an eruption of oral vesicles, round shallow symmetric oral ulcers, and acute marginal gingivitis. Laboratory tests are rarely required in these cases. Other patients, especially adults, may have a less typical clinical picture, making the diagnosis more difficult. This is especially important when distinguishing primary herpes from erythema multiforme since proper therapy differs significantly.

The following laboratory tests are helpful in the diagnosis of a primary herpes infection.

Cytology.   For cytology, a fresh vesicle can be opened and a scraping made from the base of the lesion and placed on a microscope slide. The slide may be stained with Giemsa, Wright's, or Papanicolaou's stain and searched for multinucleated giant cells (Figure 4-5), syncytium, and ballooning degeneration of the nucleus. Fluorescent staining of cytology smears has been shown to be more sensitive (83%) compared with routine cytology (54%); it is the cytologic test of choice, when available.[23]

HSV Isolation.   Isolation and neutralization of a virus in tissue culture is the most positive method of identification and has a specificity and sensitivity of 100%.[23] A clinician must remember that isolation of HSV from oral lesions does not necessarily mean that HSV caused the lesions. Patients who have lesions from other causes may also be asymptomatic shedders of HSV.

Antibody Titers.   Conclusive evidence of a primary HSV infection includes testing for complement-fixing or neutralizing antibody in acute and convalescent sera. However, it is rarely necessary in routine clinical situations and is often not helpful since the results are not available until the infection is gone. In special circumstances, such as immunocompromised

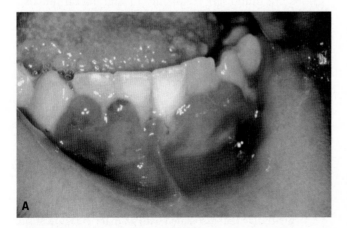

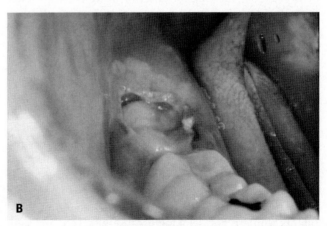

FIGURE 4-3   Acute marginal gingivitis characteristic of primary HSV infection. **A,** mandibular anterior gingiva; **B,** vesicles and inflammation around mandibular molars.

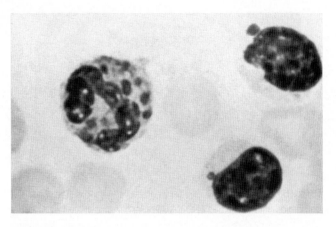

FIGURE 4-5 Cytology smear stained with Giemsa, demonstrating multinucleated giant cells.

patients, an acute serum specimen should be obtained within 3 or 4 days of the onset of symptoms. The absence of detectable antibodies plus the isolation of HSV from lesions is compatible with the presence of a primary HSV infection. Antibody to HSV will begin to appear in a week and reach a peak in 3 weeks. A convalescent serum can confirm the diagnosis of primary HSV infection by demonstrating at least a fourfold rise in anti-HSV antibody. If anti-HSV antibody titers are similar in both the acute and convalescent sera, then the lesions from which HSV was isolated were recurrent lesions.

TREATMENT

A significant advance in the management of herpes simplex infections was the discovery of acyclovir, which has no effect on normal cells but inhibits DNA replication in HSV-infected cells.[24] Acyclovir has been shown to be effective in the treatment of primary oral HSV in children when therapy was started in the first 72 hours. Acyclovir significantly decreased days of fever, pain, lesions, and viral shedding.[25] Newer anti-herpes drugs are now available, including valacyclovir and famciclovir. The advantage of the newer drugs is increased bioavailability, allowing for effective treatment with fewer doses.[26] Milder cases can be managed with supportive care only. The use of antiviral drugs in the management of recurrent disease or in immunocompromised patients is discussed later in this chapter in sections on recurrent and chronic HSV.

Routine supportive measures include aspirin or acetaminophen for fever and fluids to maintain proper hydration and electrolyte balance. If the patient has difficulty eating and drinking, a topical anesthetic may be administered prior to meals. Dyclonine hydrochloride 0.5% has been shown to be an excellent topical anesthetic for the oral mucosa. If this medication is not available, a solution of diphenhydramine hydrochloride 5 mg/mL mixed with an equal amount of milk of magnesia also has satisfactory topical anesthetic properties. Infants who are not drinking because of severe oral pain should be referred to a pediatrician for maintenance of proper fluid and electrolyte balance.

Antibiotics are of no help in the treatment of primary herpes infection, and use of corticosteroids is contraindicated. Future therapy may include prevention of the infection with use of a genetically disabled HSV vaccine.

Coxsackievirus Infections

Coxsackieviruses are ribonucleic acid (RNA) enteroviruses and are named for the town in upper New York State where they were first discovered. Coxsackieviruses have been separated into two groups, A and B. There are 24 known types of coxsackievirus group A and 6 types of coxsackievirus group B. These viruses cause hepatitis, meningitis, myocarditis, pericarditis, and acute respiratory disease. Three clinical types of infection of the oral region that have been described are usually caused by group A coxsackieviruses: herpangina, hand-foot-and-mouth disease, and acute lymphonodular pharyngitis. Types of coxsackievirus A have also been described as causing a rare mumpslike form of parotitis.

HERPANGINA

Coxsackievirus A4 has been shown to cause a majority of cases of herpangina, but types A1 to A10 as well as types A16 to A22 have also been implicated. Because many antigenic strains of coxsackievirus exist, herpangina may be seen more than once in the same patient. Unlike herpes simplex infections, which occur at a constant rate, herpangina frequently occurs in epidemics that have their highest incidence from June to October. The majority of cases affect young children ages 3 through 10, but infection of adolescents and adults is not uncommon.

Clinical Manifestations. After a 2- to 10-day incubation period, the infection begins with generalized symptoms of fever, chills, and anorexia. The fever and other symptoms are generally milder than those experienced with primary HSV infection. The patient complains of sore throat, dysphagia, and occasionally sore mouth. Lesions start as punctate macules, which quickly evolve into papules and vesicles involving the posterior pharynx, tonsils, faucial pillars, and soft palate. Lesions are found less frequently on the buccal mucosa, tongue, and hard palate (Figure 4-6). Within 24 to 48 hours, the vesicles rupture, forming small 1 to 2 mm ulcers. The disease is usually mild and heals without treatment in 1 week.

Herpangina may be clinically distinguished from primary HSV infection by several criteria:

1. Herpangina occurs in epidemics; HSV infections do not.
2. Herpangina tends to be milder than HSV infection.
3. Lesions of herpangina occur on the pharynx and posterior portions of the oral mucosa, whereas HSV primarily affects the anterior portion of the mouth.
4. Herpangina does not cause a generalized acute gingivitis like that associated with primary HSV infection.
5. Lesions of herpangina tend to be smaller than those of HSV.

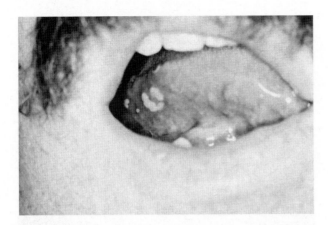

FIGURE 4-6   A cluster of vesicles on the tongue in a patient with herpangina. The patient had lesions of the posterior pharyngeal wall and tonsils, but there was no gingivitis. Coxsackievirus A4 was isolated in tissue culture.

Laboratory Studies.   A smear taken from the base of a fresh vesicle and stained with Giemsa will not show ballooning degeneration or multinucleated giant cells. This helps to distinguish herpangina from herpes simplex and herpes zoster, which do show these changes.

Treatment.   Herpangina is a self-limiting disease, and treatment is supportive, including proper hydration and topical anesthesia when eating or swallowing is difficult. Specific antiviral therapy is not available.

ACUTE LYMPHONODULAR PHARYNGITIS

This is a variant of herpangina caused by coxsackievirus A10. The distribution of the lesions is the same as in herpangina, but yellow-white nodules appear that do not progress to vesicles or ulcers. The disease is self-limiting, and only supportive care is indicated.

HAND-FOOT-AND-MOUTH DISEASE

Hand-foot-and-mouth disease is caused by infection with coxsackievirus A16 in a majority of cases, although instances have been described in which A5, A7, A9, A10, B2, or B5 or enterovirus 71 has been isolated. The disease is characterized by low-grade fever, oral vesicles and ulcers, and nonpruritic macules, papules, and vesicles, particularly on the extensor surfaces of the hands and feet. The oral lesions are more extensive than are those described for herpangina, and lesions of the hard palate, tongue, and buccal mucosa are common. Severe cases with central nervous system involvement, myocarditis, and pulmonary edema have been reported in epidemics caused by enterovirus 71.[27]

Adler and colleagues[28] studied 20 cases of hand-foot-and-mouth disease. The patients ranged in age from 8 months to 33 years, with 75% of cases occurring below 4 years of age. The clinical manifestations lasted 3 to 7 days. The most common complaint of the 20 patients was a sore mouth, and, clinically, all 20 patients had lesions involving the oral mucosa. Because of the frequent oral involvement, dentists are more likely to see

patients with this disease than with herpangina, and they should remember to examine the hands and feet for maculopapular and vesicular lesions when patients present with an acute stomatitis and fever. Treatment is supportive.

Varicella-Zoster Virus Infection

Varicella zoster (VZV) is a herpesvirus, and, like other herpesviruses, it causes both primary and recurrent infection and remains latent in neurons present in sensory ganglia.[29] VZV is responsible for two major clinical infections of humans: chickenpox (varicella) and shingles (herpes zoster [HZ]). Chickenpox is a generalized primary infection that occurs the first time an individual contacts the virus. This is analogous to the acute herpetic gingivostomatitis of herpes simplex virus. After the primary disease is healed, VZV becomes latent in the dorsal root ganglia of spinal nerves or extramedullary ganglia of cranial nerves. A child without prior contact with VZV can develop chickenpox after contact with an individual with HZ.

In 3 to 5 of every 1,000 individuals, VZV becomes reactivated, causing lesions of localized herpes zoster. The incidence of HZ increases with age or immunosuppression.[30] Patients who are immunocompromised due to HIV disease, cancer chemotherapy, immunosuppressive drug therapy, or hematologic malignancy have an increased susceptibility to severe and potentially fatal HZ. These HZ infections may be deep-seated and disseminated, causing pneumonia, meningoencephalitis, and hepatitis; however, otherwise normal patients who develop HZ do not have a significant incidence of underlying malignancy.

CLINICAL MANIFESTATIONS

General Findings.   Chickenpox is a childhood disease characterized by mild systemic symptoms and a generalized intensely pruritic eruption of maculopapular lesions that rapidly develop into vesicles on an erythematous base. Oral vesicles that rapidly change to ulcers may be seen, but the oral lesions are not an important symptomatic, diagnostic, or management problem.

HZ commonly has a prodromal period of 2 to 4 days, when shooting pain, paresthesia, burning, and tenderness appear along the course of the affected nerve. Unilateral vesicles on an erythematous base then appear in clusters, chiefly along the course of the nerve, giving the characteristic clinical picture of single dermatome involvement. Some lesions spread by viremia occur outside the dermatome. The vesicles turn to scabs in 1 week, and healing takes place in 2 to 3 weeks. The nerves most commonly affected with HZ are C3, T5, L1, L2, and the first division of the trigeminal nerve.

When the full clinical picture of HZ is present with pain and unilateral vesicles, the diagnosis is not difficult. Diagnostic problems arise during the prodromal period, when pain is present without lesions. Unnecessary surgery has been performed because of the diagnosis of acute appendicitis, cholecystitis, or dental pulpitis.[31] A more difficult diagnostic problem is pain caused by VZ virus without lesions developing along the course of the nerve (zoster sine herpete; zoster sine eruptione). Diagnosis in these cases is based on clinical symptoms and serologic evidence of a rising antibody titer.

HZ may also occasionally affect motor nerves. HZ of the sacral region may cause paralysis of the bladder. The extremities and diaphragm have also been paralyzed during episodes of HZ.

The most common complication of HZ is postherpetic neuralgia, which is defined as pain remaining for over a month after the mucocutaneous lesions have healed, although some clinicians do not use the term postherpetic neuralgia unless the pain has lasted for at least 3 months after the healing of the lesions. The overall incidence of postherpetic neuralgia is 12 to 14%, but the risk increases significantly after the age of 60 years, most likely due to the decline in cell-mediated immunity.[32–34] Immunosuppression does not increase the risk of postherpetic neuralgia.[35]

Oral Findings. Herpes zoster involves one of the divisions of the trigeminal nerve in 18 to 20% of cases, but the ophthalmic branch is affected several times more frequently than are the second or third divisions. HZ of the first division can lead to blindness secondary to corneal scarring and should be managed by an ophthalmologist. Facial and intraoral lesions are characteristic of HZ involving the second and third divisions of the trigeminal nerve.

Each individual oral lesion of HZ resembles lesions seen in herpes simplex infections. The diagnosis is based on a history of pain and the unilateral nature and segmental distribution of the lesions (Figures 4-7 and 4-8). When the clinical appearance is typical and vesicles are present, oral HZ can be distinguished clinically from other acute multiple lesions of the mouth, which are bilateral and are not preceded or accom-

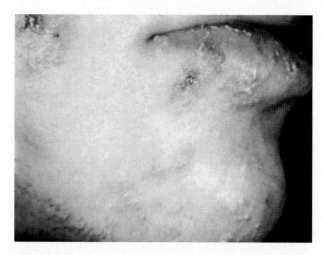

FIGURE 4-8 Herpes zoster of the third division of fifth nerve, right side.

panied by pain along the course of one trigeminal nerve branch[36] (Figure 4-9).

HZ has been associated with dental anomalies and severe scarring of the facial skin when trigeminal HZ occurs during tooth formation. Pulpal necrosis and internal root resorption have also been related to HZ.[37] In immunocompromised patients, large chronic HZ lesions have been described that have led to necrosis of underlying bone and exfoliation of teeth.[38]

HZ of the geniculate ganglion, Ramsay Hunt syndrome, is a rare form of the disease characterized by Bell's palsy, unilateral vesicles of the external ear, and vesicles of the oral mucosa.

Because oral lesions occurring without facial lesions are rare, isolated oral HZ can be misdiagnosed, particularly when erythema, edema, and nonspecific ulceration are seen without the presence of intact vesicles. In these cases, a cytology smear or viral culture is often necessary for diagnosis. An incorrect diagnosis can be made when prodromal pain is present prior to the appearance of the characteristic lesions. During this period, endodontic therapy, extractions, or other surgery may be performed unnecessarily. Similar problems occur in zoster sine eruptione.

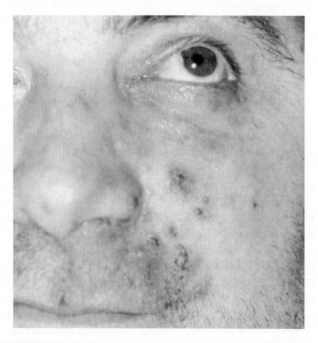

FIGURE 4-7 Facial lesions of herpes zoster involving the second division of trigeminal nerve.

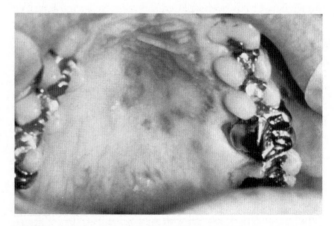

FIGURE 4-9 Unilateral palatal lesions of herpes zoster of the second division of trigeminal nerve.

LABORATORY FINDINGS

Cytology is a rapid method of evaluation that can be used in cases in which the diagnosis is uncertain. Fluorescent-antibody stained smears using fluorescein conjugated monoclonal antibodies is more reliable than is routine cytology and is positive in over 80% of cases. The most accurate method of diagnosis is viral isolation in tissue culture, but this test is more expensive and the results take days rather than hours. Demonstration of a rising antibody titer is rarely necessary for diagnosis except in cases of zoster sine eruptione, when it is the only means of confirming suspected cases.

TREATMENT

Management should be directed toward shortening the course of the disease, preventing postherpetic neuralgia in patients over 50 years of age, and preventing dissemination in immunocompromised patients. Acyclovir or the newer anti-herpes drugs valacyclovir or famciclovir accelerate healing and reduce acute pain, but they do not reduce the incidence of postherpetic neuralgia.[35] The newer drugs have greater bioavailability and are more effective in the treatment of HZ.[39]

The use of systemic corticosteroids to prevent postherpetic neuralgia in patients over 50 years of age is controversial; a recent review of the data indicated a reduction of pain and disability during the first 2 weeks but no effect on the incidence or severity of post-herpetic neuralgia.[33,34] Some clinicians advocate the use of a combination of intralesional steroids and local anesthetics to decrease healing time and prevent postherpetic neuralgia, but a controlled study of this therapy has not been performed.

Effective therapy for postherpetic neuralgia includes application of capsaicin, a substance extracted from hot chili peppers.[40] Topical capsaicin is safe but must be used for a prolonged period to be effective and may cause a burning sensation of the skin. When topical capsaicin therapy is ineffective, use of a tricyclic antidepressant or gabapentin is indicated.[41] Chemical or surgical neurolysis may be necessary in refractory cases (see Chapter 11, Orofacial Pain).

Erythema Multiforme

Erythema multiforme (EM) is an acute inflammatory disease of the skin and mucous membranes that causes a variety of skin lesions—hence the name "multiforme." The oral lesions, typically inflammation accompanied by rapidly rupturing vesicles and bullae, are often an important component of the clinical picture and are occasionally the only component. Erythema multiforme may occur once or recur, and it should be considered in the diagnosis of multiple acute oral ulcers whether or not there is a history of similar lesions. There is also a rare chronic form of EM. EM has several clinical presentations: a milder self-limiting form and severe life-threatening forms that may present as either Stevens-Johnson syndrome or toxic epidermal necrolysis (TEN).

ETIOLOGY

EM is an immune-mediated disease that may be initiated either by deposition of immune complexes in the superficial microvasculature of skin and mucosa, or cell-mediated immunity. Kazmierowski and Wuepper studied specimens of lesions less than 24 hours old from 17 patients with EM; 13 of the 17 had deposition of immunoglobulin (Ig) M and complement (C) 3 in the superficial vessels.[42] Other health care workers have detected elevated levels of immune complexes and decreased complement in fluid samples taken from vesicles.

Although the histopathology is not specific, two major histologic patterns have been described: an epidermal pattern characterized by lichenoid vasculitis and intraepidermal vesicles, and a dermal pattern characterized by lymphocytic vasculitis and subepidermal vesiculation.[43]

The most common triggers for episodes of EM are herpes simplex virus and drug reactions. The drugs most frequently associated with EM reactions are oxycam nonsteroidal anti-inflammatory drugs (NSAIDs); sulfonamides; anticonvulsants such as carbamazepine, phenobarbital, and phenytoin; trimethoprim-sulfonamide combinations, allopurinol, and penicillin.[44] A majority of the severe cases of Stevens-Johnson syndrome or TEN are caused by drug reactions.

The relationship of HSV to episodes of EM has been known for over 50 years, but improved diagnostic techniques, including polymerase chain reaction (PCR) and in situ hybridization have demonstrated that herpes-associated EM is a common form of the disease, accounting for at least 20 to 40% of the cases of single episodes of EM and approximately 80% of recurrent EM[45] (Figures 4-10 and 4-11). Herpes antigens have been demonstrated in the skin and immunocomplexes obtained from patients with EM. Many investigators now believe that the major cause of EM is a cellular immune response to HSV antigens deposited in keratinocytes of the skin and mucosa.[46] The tendency to develop mucous membrane lesions during episodes of herpes-associated EM appears to be genetically determined and related to specific human leukocyte antigen (HLA) types.[47] Oral mucosal lesions were detected in 8 of 12 children with HSV-associated EM.[48] Other triggers for EM include progesterone, *Mycoplasma* benign and malignant tumors, radiotherapy, Crohn's disease, sarcoidosis, histoplasmosis, and infectious mononucleosis.[49–51]

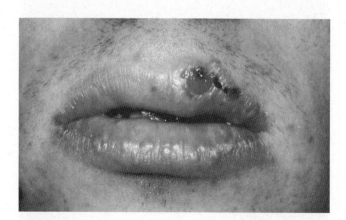

FIGURE 4-10 Early vesicular lesions in a patient who develops erythema multiforme after each episode of recurrent herpes labialis.

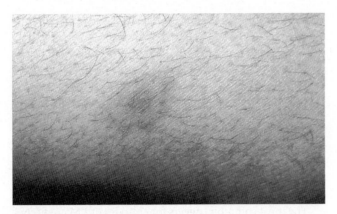

FIGURE 4-11   Target lesion on the arm of the patient with erythema multiforme shown in Figure 4-10.

Many cases of EM continue to have no obvious detectable cause after extensive testing for underlying systemic disease and allergy and are labeled idiopathic.

CLINICAL MANIFESTATIONS

General Findings.   EM is seen most frequently in children and young adults and is rare after age 50 years. It has an acute or even an explosive onset; generalized symptoms such as fever and malaise appear in severe cases. A patient may be asymptomatic and in less than 24 hours have extensive lesions of the skin and mucosa. EM simplex is a self-limiting form of the disease and is characterized by macules and papules 0.5 to 2 cm in diameter, appearing in a symmetric distribution.

The most common cutaneous areas involved are the hands, feet, and extensor surfaces of the elbows and knees. The face and neck are commonly involved, but only severe cases affect the trunk. Typical skin lesions of EM may be nonspecific macules, papules, and vesicles. More typical skin lesions contain petechiae in the center of the lesion. The pathognomonic lesion is the target or iris lesion, which consists of a central bulla or pale clearing area surrounded by edema and bands of erythema (Figure 4-12).

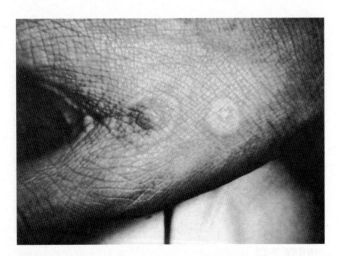

FIGURE 4-12   Target lesions in a patient with erythema multiforme.

The more severe vesiculobullous forms of the disease, Stevens-Johnson syndrome and TEN, have a significant mortality rate.[52] EM is classified as Stevens-Johnson syndrome when the generalized vesicles and bullae involve the skin, mouth, eyes, and genitals[53] (Figure 4-13).

The most severe form of the disease is TEN, (tone epidermal neurolysis), which is usually secondary to a drug reaction and results in sloughing of skin and mucosa in large sheets. Morbidity, which occurs in 30 to 40% of patients, results from secondary infection, fluid and electrolyte imbalance, or involvement of the lung, liver, or kidneys.[54] Patients with this form of the disease are most successfully managed in burn centers, where necrotic skin is removed under general anesthesia and healing takes place under sheets of porcine xenografts.

Oral Findings.   Oral lesions commonly appear along with skin lesions in approximately 70% of EM patients[55] (Figure 4-14). In some cases, oral lesions are the predominant or single site of disease. When the oral lesions predominate and no target lesions are present on the skin, EM must be differentiated from other causes of acute multiple ulcers, especially primary herpes simplex infection. This distinction is important because corticosteroids may be the treatment of choice in EM, but they are specifically contraindicated in primary herpes simplex infections. When there are no skin lesions and the oral lesions are mild, diagnosis may be difficult and is usually made by exclusion of other diseases. Cytologic smears and virus isolation may be done to eliminate the possibility of primary herpes infection. Biopsy may be performed when acute pemphigus is suspected. The histologic picture of oral EM is not considered specific, but the finding of a perivascular lymphocytic infiltrate and epithelial edema and hyperplasia is considered suggestive of EM.

The diagnosis is made on the basis of the total clinical picture, including the rapid onset of lesions. The oral lesions start as bullae on an erythematous base, but intact bullae are rarely seen by the clinician because they break rapidly into irregular ulcers. Viral lesions are small, round, symmetric, and shallow, but EM lesions are larger, irregular, deeper, and often bleed. Lesions may occur anywhere on the oral mucosa with EM, but involvement of the lips is especially prominent, and gingival involvement is rare. This is an important criterion for distinguishing EM from primary herpes simplex infection, in which generalized gingival involvement is characteristic.

In full-blown clinical cases, the lips are extensively eroded, and large portions of the oral mucosa are denuded of epithelium. The patient cannot eat or even swallow and drools blood-tinged saliva. Within 2 or 3 days the labial lesions begin to crust. Healing occurs within 2 weeks in a majority of cases, but, in some severe cases, extensive disease may continue for several weeks.

TREATMENT

Mild cases of oral EM may be treated with supportive measures only, including topical anesthetic mouthwashes and a soft or liquid diet. Moderate to severe oral EM may be treated with a

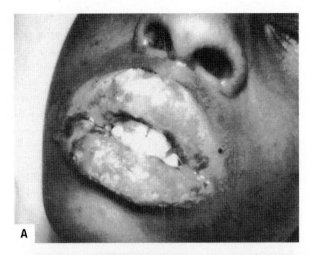

A

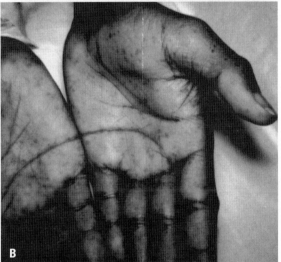

B

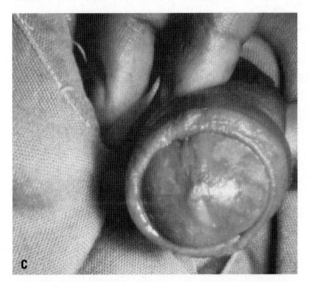

FIGURE 4-13 Labial **(A)**, skin **(B)**, and penile **(C)** lesions in a 17-year-old male with Stevens-Johnson form of erythema multiforme. The lesions began to arise less than 12 hours before the pictures were taken.

C

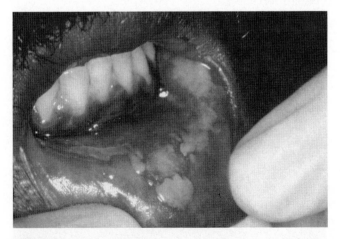

FIGURE 4-14 Intraoral lesions of erythema multiforme in an 18-year-old male.

short course of systemic corticosteroids in patients without significant contraindications to their use. Systemic corticosteroids should only be used by clinicians familiar with the side effects, and, in each case, potential benefits should be carefully weighed against potential risks. Young children treated with systemic steroids for EM appear to have a higher rate of complications than do adults, particularly gastrointestinal bleeding and secondary infections. Adults treated with short-term systemic steroids have a low rate of complications and a shorter course of EM.[56] The protein-wasting and adrenal-suppressive effects of systemic steroids are not significant when used short-term, and the clinical course of the disease may be shortened. An initial dose of 30 mg/d to 50 mg/d of prednisone or methylprednisolone for several days, which is then tapered, is helpful in shortening the healing time of EM, particularly when therapy is started early in the course of the disease. It should be noted that the efficacy of this treatment has not been proven by controlled clinical trials and is controversial.

Patients with severe cases of recurrent EM have been treated with dapsone, azathioprine, levamisole, or thalidomide. EM triggered by progesterone, also referred to as autoimmune progesterone dermatitis and stomatitis, has been treated successfully with tamoxifen. In resistant cases, oophorectomy has been necessary to cure the disorder.[57] Antiherpes drugs such as acyclovir or valacyclovir can be effective in preventing susceptible patients from developing herpes-associated EM, if the drug is administered at the onset of the recurrent HSV lesion. Prophylactic use of antiherpes drugs is effective in preventing frequent recurrent episodes of HSV-associated EM.[56,58] Systemic steroids are recommended for management of Stevens-Johnson syndrome and are considered life saving in severe cases.[59,60]

Contact Allergic Stomatitis

Contact allergy results from a delayed hypersensitivity reaction that occurs when antigens of low molecular weight penetrate the skin or mucosa of susceptible individuals. These antigens combine with epithelial-derived proteins to form haptens that bind to Langerhans' cells in the epithelium. The Langerhans' cells migrate to the regional lymph nodes and present the antigen to T lymphocytes, which become sensitized and undergo clonal expansion. After re-exposure to the antigen, sensitized individuals develop an inflammatory reaction confined to the site of contact. Since the reaction resulting from contact allergy appears as nonspecific inflammation, contact dermatitis or stomatitis may be difficult to distinguish from chronic physical irritation. The incidence of contact stomatitis is unknown, but it is believed to be significantly less common than contact dermatitis for the following reasons:

1. Saliva quickly dilutes potential antigens and physically washes them away and digests them before they can penetrate the oral mucosa.
2. Since the oral mucosa is more vascular than the skin, potential antigens that do penetrate the mucosa are rapidly removed before an allergic reaction can be established.
3. The oral mucosa has less keratin than does the skin, decreasing the possibility that haptens will be formed.

Contact stomatitis may result from contact with dental materials, oral hygiene products, or foods. Common causes of contact oral reactions are cinnamon or peppermint, which are frequently used flavoring agents in food, candy, and chewing gum, as well as oral hygiene products such as toothpaste, mouthwash and dental floss[61] (Figure 4-15).

Dental materials that have been reported to cause cases of contact allergic stomatitis include mercury in amalgam, gold in crowns, free monomer in acrylic, and nickel in orthodontic wire.[62–64] Pyrophosphates and zinc citrate, which are components of tartar control toothpaste, cause superficial peeling of the mucosa in some users, but this reaction is believed to be caused by physical irritation rather than an allergic reaction.[65]

CLINICAL MANIFESTATIONS

The clinical signs and symptoms of contact oral allergy are nonspecific and are frequently difficult to distinguish from physical irritation. The reaction occurs only at the site of contact and includes a burning sensation or soreness accompanied by erythema, and occasionally the formation of vesicles and ulcers. Burning sensations without the presence of lesions is not a result of contact allergy, and obtaining allergy tests for patients with burning mouth syndrome with normal-appearing mucosa is not indicated.

Lesions that appear lichenoid both clinically and histologically may also be a result of contact allergy when the lichenoid lesion is in direct contact with the potential allergen. These lesions occur most frequently as a result of mercury in amalgam, and appear on the buccal mucosa and lateral border of the tongue in direct contact with the restoration. These lesions disappear when the amalgam is removed. It should be emphasized that there is no evidence that generalized lesions of oral lichen planus not in direct contact with restorations heal when amalgam restorations are removed.

Another oral manifestation of contact allergy is plasma cell gingivitis, which is characterized by generalized erythema and edema of the attached gingiva, occasionally accompanied by cheilitis and glossitis[66] (Figure 4-16). The histopathology is described as sheets of plasma cells that replace normal connective tissue. Some cases have been related to an allergen present in toothpaste, chewing gum, or candy, whereas other cases remain of unknown etiology even after extensive allergy testing. Plasma cell gingivitis must be distinguished from neoplastic plasma cell diseases such as plasmacytoma or multiple myeloma.

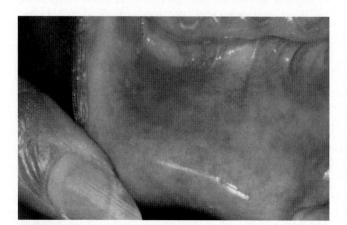

FIGURE 4-15 Contact allergy of the labial mucosa, due to peppermint.

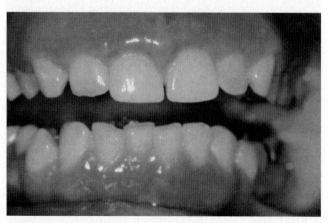

FIGURE 4-16 Plasma cell gingivitis of unknown etiology.

DIAGNOSIS

Contact allergy is most accurately diagnosed by the use of a patch test.[67] This test is performed by placing the suspected allergens in small aluminum disks, called Finn chambers, which are taped onto hairless portions of the skin. The disks remain in place for 48 hours. A positive response to a contact allergen is identified by inflammation at the site of the test, which is graded on a scale of 0 to 3. Patch tests should be performed by clinicians trained and experienced in using the test, so the results are interpreted accurately.

TREATMENT

Management of oral contact allergy depends on the severity of the lesions. In mild cases, removal of the allergen suffices. In more severe symptomatic cases, application of a topical corticosteroid is helpful to speed healing of painful lesions.

Oral Ulcers Secondary to Cancer Chemotherapy

Chemotherapeutic drugs are frequently used to effect remission of both solid tumors, hematologic malignancies, and bone marrow transplantation. Similar drugs are used for patients with bone marrow transplants. One of the common side effects of the anticancer drugs is multiple oral ulcers. Dentists who practice in hospitals where these drugs are used extensively may see oral ulcers secondary to such drug therapy more frequently than any other lesion described in this chapter.[68,69]

Anticancer drugs may cause oral ulcers directly or indirectly. Drugs that cause stomatitis indirectly depress the bone marrow and immune response, leading to bacterial, viral, or fungal infections of the oral mucosa. Others, such as methotrexate, cause oral ulcers via direct effect on the replication and growth of oral epithelial cells by interfering with nucleic acid and protein synthesis, leading to thinning and ulceration of the oral mucosa.

A recent publication by Sonis describes a new hypothesis that explains the severe stomatitis observed in patients receiving cytotoxic drugs for stem cell transplantation.[70] It is noted that an inflammatory reaction precedes ulceration and that anti-inflammatory drugs may be useful in minimizing bone marrow–related ulceration.

Details of the diagnosis and management of these lesions are discussed in Chapters 19, Transplantation Medicine, and 16, Hematologic Disease.

Acute Necrotizing Ulcerative Gingivitis

Acute necrotizing ulcerative gingivitis (ANUG) is an endogenous oral infection that is characterized by necrosis of the gingiva. Occasionally, ulcers of the oral mucosa also occur in patients with hematologic disease or severe nutritional deficiencies (see Chapter 16).

ANUG became known notoriously as "trench mouth" during World War I because of its prevalence in the combat trenches, and it was incorrectly considered a highly contagious disease. Since then, studies have shown that the disease is accompanied by an overgrowth of organisms prevalent in normal oral flora and is not transmissible. The organisms most frequently mentioned as working symbiotically to cause the lesions are the fusiform bacillus and spirochetes.

Plaque samples taken from ANUG patients demonstrate a constant anaerobic flora of *Treponema* spp, *Selenomonas* spp, *Fusobacterium* spp, and *Bacteroides intermedius*.[71] The tissue destruction is thought to be caused by endotoxins that act either directly on the tissues or indirectly by triggering immunologic and inflammatory reactions.

Classic ANUG in patients without an underlying medical disorder is found most often in those between the ages of 16 and 30 years, and it is associated with three major factors:

1. Poor oral hygiene with pre-existing marginal gingivitis or faulty dental restorations
2. Smoking
3. Emotional stress

Systemic disorders associated with ANUG are diseases affecting neutrophils (such as leukemia or aplastic anemia), marked malnutrition, and HIV infection. Malnutrition-associated cases are reported from emergent countries where the untreated disease may progress to noma, a large necrotic ulcer extending from the oral mucosa through the facial soft tissues.

The prevalence of the disease was reported by Giddon and colleagues,[72] who studied the prevalence of ANUG in 12,500 students served by the Harvard University Dental Health Service. About 0.9% of the total sample developed ANUG during the period of study. A 4% prevalence in those students who made use of the dental clinic was observed. Members of the junior class were most often affected. A relation to stress was noted by an increased frequency during examination and vacation periods. Studies of military trainees or college students demonstrated a prevalence of 5 to 7%.

There are three forms of periodontal diseases observed in patients with acquired immunodeficiency syndrome (AIDS): linear gingival erythema (LGE), necrotizing ulcerative gingivitis (NUG), and necrotizing ulcerative periodontitis (NUP).

LGE is an intense red band involving the marginal gingiva that does not resolve with standard oral hygiene procedures. Some cases are believed to be caused by candidal overgrowth, and these cases resolve with antifungal therapy. NUG and NUP are clinically similar to ANUG; the term "NUG" is used when the disease involves only the gingiva, and "NUP" involves a loss of periodontal attachment.[73,74] There is evidence that, in patients with AIDS, the host response in the gingival crevice is altered. Levels of proinflammatory cytokines such as interleukin-1 β are increased in the gingival crevice of patients with human immunodeficiency virus (HIV), which alters the regulation of neutrophils. This alteration in neutrophil function may explain the increase in NUP-related organisms including fusobacteria and *Candida*, which results in the rapid necrosis of gingival tissues.[75]

A fulminating form of ulcerative stomatitis related to ANUG is noma (cancrum oris), which predominantly affects children in sub-Saharan Africa. This disease is characterized by extensive necrosis that begins on the gingiva and then progresses from the mouth through the cheek to the facial skin, causing extensive disfigurement (Figure 4-17). The major risk factors associated with noma include malnutrition, poor oral hygiene, and concomitant infectious diseases such as measles.[76] Living in close proximity to livestock is also believed to play a role, and *Fusobacterium necrophorum*, a pathogen associated with disease in livestock, has been isolated from over 85% of noma lesions.[77] The mortality rate without appropriate therapy exceeds 70%.

CLINICAL MANIFESTATIONS

The onset of acute forms of ANUG is usually sudden, with pain, tenderness, profuse salivation, a peculiar metallic taste, and spontaneous bleeding from the gingival tissues. The patient commonly experiences a loss of the sense of taste and a diminished pleasure from smoking. The teeth are frequently thought to be slightly extruded, sensitive to pressure, or to have a "woody sensation." At times they are slightly movable. The signs noted most frequently are gingival bleeding and blunting of the interdental papillae (Figure 4-18).

The typical lesions of ANUG consist of necrotic punched-out ulcerations, developing most commonly on the interdental papillae and the marginal gingivae. These ulcerations can be observed most easily on the interdental papillae, but ulceration may develop on the cheeks, the lips, and the tongue, where these tissues come in contact with the gingival lesions or following trauma. Ulcerations also may be found on the palate and in the pharyngeal area (Figure 4-19). When the lesions have spread beyond the gingivae, blood dyscrasias and immunodeficiency should be ruled out by ordering appropriate laboratory tests, depending upon associated signs and symptoms.

The ulcerative lesions may progress to involve the alveolar process, with sequestration of the teeth and bone. When gingival hemorrhage is a prominent symptom, the teeth may become superficially stained a brown color, and the mouth odor is extremely offensive.

The tonsils should always be examined since these organs may be affected. The regional lymph nodes usually are slightly

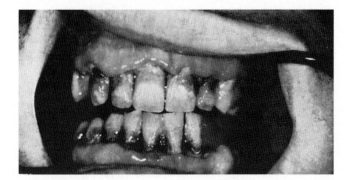

FIGURE 4-18 Extensive necrosis of the interdental papillae, and marginal and attached gingivae caused by acute necrotizing ulcerative gingivitis.

enlarged, but occasionally the lymphadenopathy may be marked, particularly in children.

The constitutional symptoms in primary ANUG are usually of minor significance when compared with the severity of the oral lesions. Significant temperature elevation is unusual, even in severe cases, and, when it exists, other accompanying or underlying diseases should be ruled out, particularly blood dyscrasias and AIDS. HIV-infected patients with NUG have rapidly progressing necrosis and ulceration first involving the gingiva alone, and then NUP with the periodontal attachment and involved alveolar bone. The ulcerated areas may be localized or generalized and often are very painful. In severe cases, the underlying bone is denuded and may become sequestrated, and the necrosis may spread from the gingiva to other oral tissues.

TREATMENT

The therapy of ANUG uncomplicated by other oral lesions or systemic disease is local débridement. At the initial visit, the gingivae should be débrided with both irrigation and periodontal curettage. The extent of the débridement depends on the soreness of the gingivae. The clinician should remember that the more quickly the local factors are removed, the faster is the resolution of the lesions. Special care should be taken by the clinician to débride the area just below the marginal gin-

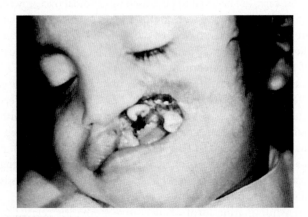

FIGURE 4-17 Cancrum oris or noma. (Courtesy of Dr. Gustavo Berger, Guatemala City, Guatemala).

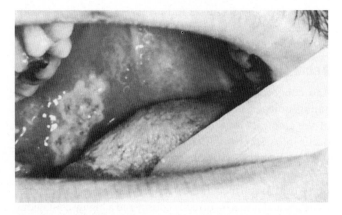

FIGURE 4-19 Palatal ulceration in a 21-year-old male with fusospirochetal stomatitis, which began as a necrotizing lesion of a pericoronal flap.

givae. Complete débridement may not be possible on the first visit because of soreness. The patient must return, even though the pain and other symptoms have disappeared, to remove all remaining local factors.

Treatment of ANUG is not finished until there has been a complete gingival curettage and root planing, including removal of overhanging margins and other predisposing local factors. After the first visit, careful home care instruction must be given to the patient regarding vigorous rinsing and gentle brushing with a soft brush. Patients should be made aware of the significance of such factors as poor oral hygiene, smoking, and stress.

Antibiotics are usually not necessary for routine cases of ANUG confined to the marginal and interdental gingivae. These cases can be successfully treated with local débridement, irrigation, curettage, and home care instruction including hydrogen peroxide (approximately 1.5 to 2% in water) mouth rinses three times a day and chlorhexidine 12% rinses. Antibiotics should be prescribed for patients with extensive gingival involvement, lymphadenopathy, or other systemic signs, and in cases in which mucosa other than the gingivae is involved. Metronidazole and penicillin are the drugs of choice in patients with no history of sensitivity to these drugs. Patients whose lesions have extended from the gingivae to the buccal mucosa, tongue, palate, or pharynx should be placed on antibiotics and should have appropriate studies to rule out blood dyscrasias or AIDS. After the disease is resolved, the patient should return for a complete periodontal evaluation. Periodontal treatment should be instituted as necessary. The patient must be made aware that, unless the local etiologic factors of the disease are removed, ANUG may return or become chronic and lead to periodontal disease.

▼ THE PATIENT WITH RECURRING ORAL ULCERS

Recurring oral ulcers are among the most common problems seen by clinicians who manage diseases of the oral mucosa. There are several diseases that should be included in the differential diagnosis of a patient who presents with a history of recurring ulcers of the mouth, including recurrent aphthous stomatitis (RAS), Behçet's syndrome, recurrent HSV infection, recurrent erythema multiforme, and cyclic neutropenia.

Recurrent Aphthous Stomatitis

RAS is a disorder characterized by recurring ulcers confined to the oral mucosa in patients with no other signs of disease. Many specialists and investigators in oral medicine no longer consider RAS to be a single disease but, rather, several pathologic states with similar clinical manifestations. Immunologic disorders, hematologic deficiencies, and allergic or psychological abnormalities have all been implicated in cases of RAS.

RAS affects approximately 20% of the general population, but when specific ethnic or socioeconomic groups are studied, the incidence ranges from 5 to 50%.[78] RAS is classified according to clinical characteristics: minor ulcers, major ulcers (Sutton's disease, periadenitis mucosa necrotica recurrens),

and herpetiform ulcers. Minor ulcers, which comprise over 80% of RAS cases, are less than 1 cm in diameter and heal without scars. Major ulcers, are over 1 cm in diameter and take longer to heal and often scar. Herpetiform ulcers are considered a distinct clinical entity that manifests as recurrent crops of dozens of small ulcers throughout the oral mucosa.

ETIOLOGY

It was once assumed that RAS was a form of recurrent HSV infection, and there are still clinicians who mistakenly call RAS "herpes." Many studies done during the past 40 years have confirmed that RAS is not caused by HSV.[79,80] This distinction is particularly important at a time when there is specific effective antiviral therapy available for HSV that is useless for RAS. "Herpes" is an anxiety-producing word, suggesting a sexually transmitted disease among many laypersons, and its use should be avoided when it does not apply. There continue to be investigations studying the relationship of RAS to other herpesviruses such as varicella-zoster virus or *Cytomegalovirus,* but the results of these studies continue to be inconclusive.[81,82]

The current concept is that RAS is a clinical syndrome with several possible causes. The major factors identified include heredity, hematologic deficiencies, and immunologic abnormalities.[83,84] The best documented factor is heredity.[85] Miller and colleagues studied 1,303 children from 530 families and demonstrated an increased susceptibility to RAS among children of RAS-positive parents.[86] A study by Ship and associates showed that patients with RAS-positive parents had a 90% chance of developing RAS, whereas patients with no RAS-positive parents had a 20% chance of developing the lesions.[85] Further evidence for the inherited nature of this disorder results from studies in which genetically specific HLAs have been identified in patients with RAS, particularly in certain ethnic groups.[87,88]

Hematologic deficiency, particularly of serum iron, folate, or vitamin B_{12}, appears to be an etiologic factor in a subset of patients with RAS.[84] The size of the subset is controversial, but most estimates range from 5 to 15%. A study by Rogers and Hutton reported clinical improvement in 75% of patients with RAS when a specific hematologic deficiency was detected and corrected with specific replacement therapy.[89] Some cases of nutritional deficiency, such as celiac disease, are reported to be secondary to malabsorption syndrome.[90]

Most of the research into the etiology of RAS centers on immunologic abnormalities. Early work suggested either an autoimmune disorder or hypersensitivity to oral organisms such as *Streptococcus sanguis.*[91] Investigations using more sophisticated immune assays have not supported the early work and suggest a role of lymphocytotoxicity,[92] antibody-dependent cell-mediated cytotoxicity, and defects in lymphocyte cell subpopulations.[93–95] Burnett and Wray showed that sera and monocytes induced significantly more cytolysis in patients with RAS than in control patients.[96] Thomas and colleagues showed that T lymphocytes from patients with RAS had increased cytotoxicity to oral epithelial cells.[92] Work by Pedersen and colleagues and other studies demonstrated an alteration in CD4:CD8 lymphocyte ratio, or a dysfunction of the mucocutaneous cytokine network.[97–99] Further work is needed to determine if these are specific or nonspecific responses.

Other factors that have been suggested as being etiologic in RAS include trauma, psychological stress, anxiety, and allergy to foods.[100] It is well documented that cessation of smoking increases the frequency and severity of RAS.[101] In cases of refractory disease, Hay and Reade reported the benefit of an elimination diet in some patients with suspected or proven allergy to foods such as milk, cheese, wheat, and flour.[102]

A detergent present in toothpaste, sodium lauryl sulfate (SLS), was suspected as an etiologic factor in RAS development,[103] but a recent double-blind crossover study showed that use of an SLS-free toothpaste had no significant effect on ulcer development.[104]

CLINICAL MANIFESTATIONS

The first episodes of RAS most frequently begin during the second decade of life and may be precipitated by minor trauma, menstruation, upper respiratory infections, or contact with certain foods. The lesions are confined to the oral mucosa and begin with prodromal burning any time from 2 to 48 hours before an ulcer appears. During this initial period, a localized area of erythema develops. Within hours, a small white papule forms, ulcerates, and gradually enlarges over the next 48 to 72 hours. The individual lesions are round, symmetric, and shallow (similar to viral ulcers), but no tissue tags are present from ruptured vesicles (this helps to distinguish RAS from disease with irregular ulcers such as EM, pemphigus, and pemphigoid). Multiple lesions are often present, but the number, size, and frequency of them vary considerably (Figure 4-20). The buccal and labial mucosae are most commonly involved. Lesions are less common on the heavily keratinized palate or gingiva. In mild RAS, the lesions reach a size of 0.3 to 1.0 cm and begin healing within a week. Healing without scarring is usually complete in 10 to 14 days.

Most patients with RAS have between two and six lesions at each episode and experience several episodes a year. The disease is an annoyance for the majority of patients with mild RAS, but

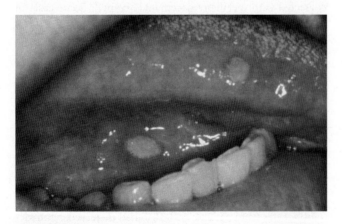

FIGURE 4-20   Recurrent aphthous stomatitis of the tongue and floor of the mouth.

it can be disabling for patients with severe frequent lesions, especially those classified as major aphthous ulcers. Patients with major ulcers develop deep lesions that are larger than 1 cm in diameter and may reach 5 cm (Figure 4-21, A and B). Large portions of the oral mucosa may be covered with large deep ulcers that can become confluent. The lesions are extremely painful and interfere with speech and eating. Many of these patients continually go from one clinician to another, looking for a "cure." The lesions may last for months and sometimes be misdiagnosed as squamous cell carcinoma, chronic granulomatous disease, or pemphigoid. The lesions heal slowly and leave scars that may result in decreased mobility of the uvula and tongue and destruction of portions of the oral mucosa. The least common variant of RAS is the herpetiform type, which tends to occur in adults. The patient presents with small punctate ulcers scattered over large portions of the oral mucosa.

DIAGNOSIS

RAS is the most common cause of recurring oral ulcers and is essentially diagnosed by exclusion of other diseases. A detailed history and examination by a knowledgeable clinician should distinguish RAS from primary acute lesions such as viral stomatitis or from chronic multiple lesions such as pemphigoid, as well as from other possible causes of recurring ulcers, such as connective tissue disease, drug reactions, and dermatologic disorders. The history should emphasize symptoms of blood dyscrasias, systemic complaints, and associated skin, eye, genital, or rectal lesions. Laboratory investigation should be used when ulcers worsen or begin past the age of 25 years. Biopsies are only indicated when it is necessary to exclude other diseases, particularly granulomatous diseases such as Crohn's disease or sarcoidosis.

Patients with severe minor aphthae or major aphthous ulcers should have known associated factors investigated, including connective-tissue diseases and abnormal levels of serum iron, folate, vitamin B_{12}, and ferritin (Figure 4-22). Patients with abnormalities in these values should be referred to an internist to rule out malabsorption syndromes and to initiate proper replacement therapy. The clinician may also choose to have food allergy or gluten sensitivity investigated in severe cases resistant to other forms of treatment.[102] HIV-infected patients, particularly those with CD4 counts below 100/mm³, may develop major aphthous ulcers (Figure 4-23).

TREATMENT

Medication prescribed should relate to the severity of the disease. In mild cases with two or three small lesions, use of a protective emollient such as Orabase (Bristol-Myers Squibb, Princeton, NJ) or Zilactin (Zila Pharmaceutions, Phoenix, AZ) is all that is necessary. Pain relief of minor lesions can be obtained with use of a topical anesthetic agent or topical diclofenac, an NSAID frequently used topically after eye surgery.[105] In more severe cases, the use of a high-potency topical steroid preparation, such as fluocinonide, betamethasone or clobetasol, placed directly on the lesion shortens healing time and reduces the size of the ulcers. The effectiveness of the topical steroid is partially based upon good instruction and

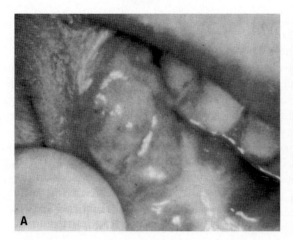
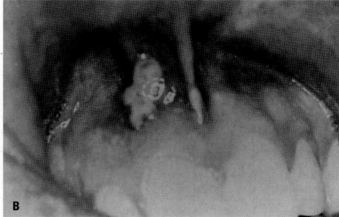

FIGURE 4-21 Major aphthous ulcers of the labial mucosa **(A)** and alveolar mucosa **(B)**.

patient compliance regarding proper use. The gel can be carefully applied directly to the lesion after meals and at bedtime two to three times a day, or mixed with an adhesive such as Orabase prior to application. Larger lesions can be treated by placing a gauze sponge containing the topical steroid on the ulcer and leaving it in place for 15 to 30 minutes to allow for longer contact of the medication. Other topical preparations that have been shown to decrease the healing time of RAS lesions include amlexanox paste and topical tetracycline, which can be used either as a mouth rinse or applied on gauze sponges. Intralesional steroids can be used to treat large indolent major RAS lesions. It should be emphasized that no available topical therapy decreases the onset of new lesions. In patients with major aphthae or severe cases of multiple minor aphthae not responsive to topical therapy, use of systemic therapy should be considered. Drugs that have been reported to reduce the number of ulcers in selected cases of major aphthae include colchicine, pentoxifylline, dapsone, short bursts of systemic steroids, and thalidomide.[106–108] Each of these drugs has the potential for side effects, and the clinician must weigh the

potential benefits versus the risks. Thalidomide has been shown to reduce both the incidence and severity of major RAS in both HIV-positive and HIV-negative patients, but this drug must be used with extreme caution in women during childbearing years owing to the potential for severe life-threatening and deforming birth defects.[109] All clinicians prescribing thalidomide in the United States must be registered in the STEPS (System for Thalidomide Education and Prescribing Safety) program, and patients receiving the drug must be thoroughly counseled regarding effective birth control methods that must be used whenever thalidomide is prescribed. For example, two methods of birth control must be used, and the patient must have a pregnancy test monthly. Other side effects of thalidomide include peripheral neuropathy, gastrointestinal complaints, and drowsiness.

Behçet's Syndrome

Behçet's syndrome, described by the Turkish dermatologist Hulûsi Behçet, was classically described as a triad of symptoms including recurring oral ulcers, recurring genital ulcers, and

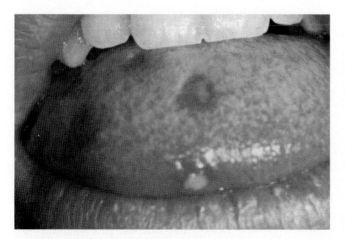

FIGURE 4-22 A 42-year-old woman with a recent increase in severity of recurrent aphthous ulcers. An iron deficiency was detected, and the ulcers resolved when this deficiency was corrected.

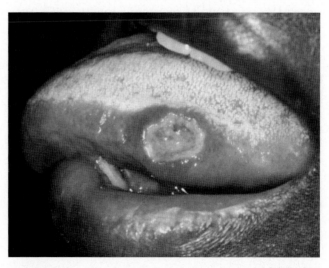

FIGURE 4-23 Major aphthous ulcer in an HIV-infected patient.

eye lesions. The concept of the disease has changed from a triad of signs and symptoms to a multisystem disorder.[110] The highest incidence of Behçet's syndrome has been reported in eastern Asia, where 1 in 10,000 is affected, and the eastern Mediterranean, where it is a leading cause of blindness in young men; however, cases have been reported worldwide, including in North America, where it is estimated that 1 in 500,000 persons is affected. The highest incidence of Behçet's syndrome is in young adults, but cases of Behçet's syndrome in children are being reported with increasing frequency.[111]

ETIOLOGY

Behçet's syndrome is caused by immunocomplexes that lead to vasculitis of small and medium-sized blood vessels and inflammation of epithelium caused by immunocompetent T lymphocytes and plasma cells.[112,113] Increased neutrophil activity has also been noted.[114] There is a genetic component to the disease, with a strong association with HLA-B51. Studies of the immune abnormalities associated with Behçet's syndrome have included findings described above for patients with RAS. This has led some investigators to believe that Behçet's syndrome and RAS are both manifestations of a similar disorder of the immune response.

CLINICAL MANIFESTATIONS

The most common single site of involvement of Behçet's syndrome is the oral mucosa. Recurring oral ulcers appear in over 90% of patients; these lesions cannot be distinguished from RAS (Figure 4-24). Some patients experience mild recurring oral lesions; others have the deep large scarring lesions characteristic of major RAS. These lesions may appear anywhere on the oral or pharyngeal mucosa. The genital area is the second most common site of involvement and involves ulcers of the scrotum and penis in males and ulcers of the labia in females. The eye lesions consist of uveitis, retinal infiltrates, edema and vascular occlusion, optic atrophy, conjunctivitis, and keratitis.

Generalized involvement occurs in over half of patients with Behçet's syndrome. Skin lesions are common and usually manifest as large pustular lesions. These lesions may be precipitated by trauma, and it is common for patients with Behçet's syndrome to have a cutaneous hyper-reactivity to intracuta-

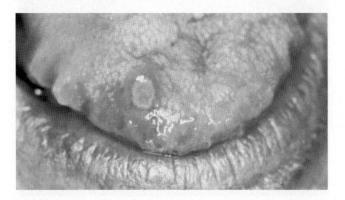

FIGURE 4-24 Aphthous-like lesion in a patient with Behçet's syndrome.

neous injection or a needlestick (pathergy). Positive pathergy is defined as an inflammatory reaction forming within 24 hours of a needle puncture, scratch, or saline injection.

Arthritis occurs in greater than 50% of patients and most frequently affects the knees and ankles.[115] The affected joint may be red and swollen as in rheumatoid arthritis, but involvement of small joints of the hand does not occur, and permanent disability does not result.

In some patients, central nervous system involvement is the most distressing component of the disease. This may include brainstem syndrome, involvement of the cranial nerves, or neurologic degeneration resembling multiple sclerosis that can be visualized by magnetic resonance imaging of the brain. Other reported signs of Behçet's syndrome include thrombophlebitis, intestinal ulceration, venous thrombosis, and renal and pulmonary disease. Involvement of large vessels is life threatening because of the risk of arterial occlusion or aneurysms.

Behçet's syndrome in children, which most frequently presents between the ages of 9 and 10 years, has similar manifestations as does the adult form of the disease, but oral ulcers are a more common presenting sign in children, and uveitis is less common.[116] Oral lesions are the presenting symptom in over 95% of children with Behçet's syndrome. A variant of Behçet's syndrome, MAGIC syndrome, has been described. It is characterized by Mouth And Genital ulcers with Inflammed Cartilage.[117]

DIAGNOSIS

Because the signs and symptoms of Behçet's syndrome overlap with those of several other diseases, particularly the connective-tissue diseases, it has been difficult to develop criteria that meet with universal agreement. Five different sets of diagnostic criteria have been in use during the past 20 years. In 1990, an international study group reviewed data from 914 patients from seven countries.[118] A new set of diagnostic criteria was developed that includes recurrent oral ulceration occurring at least three times in one 12-month period plus two of the following four manifestations:

1. Recurrent genital ulceration
2. Eye lesions including uveitis or retinal vasculitis
3. Skin lesions including erythema nodosum, pseudofolliculitis, papulopustular lesions, or acneiform nodules in postadolescent patients not receiving corticosteroids
4. A positive pathergy test

TREATMENT

The management of Behçet's syndrome depends on the severity and the sites of involvement. Patients with sight-threatening eye involvement or central nervous system lesions require more aggressive therapy with drugs with a higher potential for serious side effects.[119] Azathioprine combined with prednisone has been shown to reduce ocular disease as well as oral and genital involvement.[120] Pentoxifylline, which has fewer side effects than do immunosuppressive drugs or systemic steroids, has also been reported to be effective in decreasing disease activity, particularly eye involvement.[121] Cyclosporine or colchicine in combination with corticosteroids has also been shown to be useful in severe disease.[122,123] Colchicine[124] and thalidomide[125] have been shown to be useful in mucocutaneous and gastrointestinal manifestations. Systemic corticosteroids remain a mainstay of treatment and are particularly useful in rapidly controlling the disease until immunosuppressive agents begin to work. Plasmapheresis has also been used successfully in emergencies.

Oral mucosal lesions not adequately controlled by systemic therapy may be treated with topical or intralesional steroids in regimens described in the section on RAS.

Recurrent Herpes Simplex Virus Infection

Recurrent herpes infection of the mouth (recurrent herpes labialis [RHL]; recurrent intraoral herpes simplex infection [RIH]) occurs in patients who have experienced a previous herpes simplex infection and who have serum-antibody protection against another exogenous primary infection. In otherwise healthy individuals, the recurrent infection is confined to a localized portion of the skin or mucous membranes. Recurrent herpes is not a re-infection but a reactivation of virus that remains latent in nerve tissue between episodes in a nonreplicating state.[126,127] Herpes simplex has been cultured from the trigeminal ganglion of human cadavers, and recurrent herpes lesions commonly appear after surgery involving the ganglion.[128,129] Recurrent herpes may also be activated by trauma to the lips, fever, sunburn, immunosuppression, and menstruation.[130] The virus travels down the nerve trunk to infect epithelial cells, spreading from cell to cell to cause a lesion.

The published evidence demonstrating that RAS is not caused by herpesvirus induced many to believe that recurrent herpes infection of the oral region occurred only on the lips and not on the oral mucosa; this has been shown to be false. RAS and herpes lesions can both exist intraorally and are two separate and distinct disease processes.[131–133]

All patients who experience primary herpes infection do not experience recurrent herpes. The number of patients with a history of primary genital infection with HSV1 who subsequently experience recurrent HSV infections is approximately 15%.[134] The recurrence rate for oral HSV1 infections is estimated to be between 20 and 40%.

Studies have suggested several mechanisms for reactivation of latent HSV, including low serum IgA,[135] decreased cell-mediated immunity, decreased salivary antiherpes activity,[136] and depression of ADCC (antibody-dependent cell-mediated cytotoxicity)[137] and interleukin-2 caused by prostaglandin release in the skin.

Individuals with T-lymphocyte deficiencies owing to AIDS or transplant or cancer chemotherapy may develop large chronic lesions[138] (see "Herpes Simplex Virus Infection in Immunosuppressed Patients," below) or, rarely, disseminated HSV infection.

CLINICAL MANIFESTATIONS

RHL, the common cold sore or fever blister, may be precipitated by fever, menstruation, ultraviolet light, and perhaps emotional stress. The lesions are preceded by a prodromal period of tingling or burning. This is accompanied by edema at the site of the lesion, followed by formation of a cluster of small vesicles (Figure 4-25). Each vesicle is 1 to 3 mm in diameter, with the size of the cluster ranging from 1 to 2 cm. Occasionally, the lesions may be several centimeters in diameter, causing discomfort and disfigurement. These larger lesions are more common in immunosuppressed individuals. The frequency of recurrences varies.

RIH lesions in otherwise normal patients are similar in appearance to RHL lesions, but the vesicles break rapidly to form ulcers. The lesions are typically a cluster of small vesicles or ulcers, 1 to 2 mm in diameter, clustered on a small portion of the heavily keratinized mucosa of the gingiva, palate, and alveolar ridges, although RIH lesions can occasionally involve other mucosal surfaces[139] (Figure 4-26). In contrast, lesions of RAS tend to be larger, to spread over a larger area of mucosa, and to have a predilection for the less heavily keratinized buccal mucosa, labial mucosa, or floor of the mouth.[131]

DIAGNOSIS

If laboratory tests are desired, RIH can be distinguished from RAS by cytology smears taken from the base of a fresh lesion. Smears from herpetic lesions show cells with ballooning degeneration and multinucleated giant cells; those from RAS lesions do not. For more accurate results, cytology smears may also be tested for HSV using fluorescein-labeled HSV antigen. Viral cultures also are used to distinguish herpes simplex from other viral lesions, particularly varicella-zoster infections.

TREATMENT

Recurrent herpes infections of the lips and mouth are seldom more than a temporary annoyance in otherwise normal individuals and should be treated symptomatically. Patients who experience frequent, large, painful, or disfiguring lesions may request professional consultation. The clinician should first attempt to minimize obvious triggers. Some recurrences can be eliminated by the wearing of sunblock during intense sun exposure.

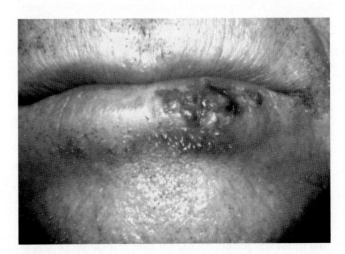

FIGURE 4-25 Crusted lesions of recurrent herpes labialis.

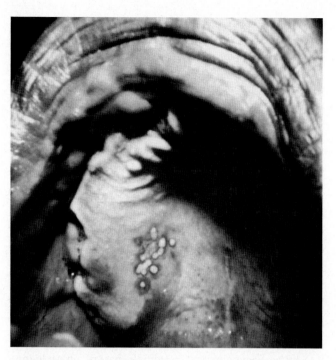

FIGURE 4-26 Typical lesions of recurrent intraoral herpes simplex virus infection in patients with normal immunity are clusters of small vesicles and ulcers on the heavily keratinized oral mucosa.

Drugs are available that suppress the formation and shorten the healing time of new recurrent lesions. Acyclovir, the original antiherpes drug, has been shown to be both safe and effective. The newer antiviral drugs such as valacyclovir, a prodrug of acyclovir, and famciclovir, a prodrug of penciclovir, have greater bioavailability than does acyclovir, but they do not eliminate established latent HSV. However, in the mouse model, famciclovir appeared to decrease the rate of HSV latency.[140,141] The clinical importance of this finding in human HSV infection is not known. The effectiveness of these antiherpes drugs to prevent recurrences of genital HSV has been studied extensively. Acyclovir 400 mg twice daily, valacyclovir 250 mg twice daily, and famciclovir 250 mg were each highly effective in preventing genital recurrences.[142,143] The use of antiherpes nucleoside analogues to prevent and treat RHL in otherwise normal individuals is controversial. Systemic therapy should not be used to treat occasional or trivial RHL in otherwise healthy individuals, but episodic use to prevent lesions in susceptible patients before high-risk activities such as skiing at high altitudes or before undergoing procedures such as dermabrasion or surgery involving the trigeminal nerve is justifiable. Some clinicians advocate the use of suppressive antiherpes therapy for the small percentage of RHL patients who experience frequent deforming episodes of RHL. Acyclovir 400 mg twice daily has been shown to reduce the frequency and severity of RHL in this group of patients.[144] Both acyclovir and penciclovir are available in topical formulations, but use of these preparations shortens the healing time of RHL by less than 2 days.

▼ THE PATIENT WITH CHRONIC MULTIPLE LESIONS

Patients with chronic multiple lesions are frequently misdiagnosed for weeks to months since their lesions may be confused with recurring oral mucosal disorders. The clinician can avoid misdiagnosis by carefully questioning the patient on the initial visit regarding the natural history of the lesions. In recurring disorders such as severe aphthous stomatitis, the patient may experience continual ulceration of the oral mucosa, but individual lesions heal and new ones form. In the category of disease described in this section, the same lesions are present for weeks to months. The major diseases in this group are pemphigus vulgaris, pemphigus vegetans, bullous pemphigoid, mucous membrane pemphigoid, linear IgA disease, and erosive lichen planus. Herpes simplex infections may cause chronic lesions in patients immunocompromised by cancer chemotherapy, immunosuppressive drugs, or HIV infection.

Pemphigus

Pemphigus is a potentially life-threatening disease that causes blisters and erosions of the skin and mucous membranes. These epithelial lesions are a result of autoantibodies that react with desmosomal glycoproteins that are present on the cell surface of the keratinocyte. The immune reaction against these glycoproteins causes a loss of cell-to-cell adhesion, resulting in the formation of intraepithelial bullae.[145,146] There are 0.5 to 3.2 cases reported each year per 100,000 population, with the highest incidence occurring in the fifth and sixth decades of life, although rare cases have been reported in children and the elderly.[147] Pemphigus occurs more frequently in the Jewish population, particularly among Ashkenazi Jews, in whom studies have shown a strong association with major histocompatibility complex (MHC) class II alleles HLA-DR4 and DQW3. Familial pemphigus has also been reported.

The major variants of pemphigus are pemphigus vulgaris (PV), pemphigus vegetans, pemphigus foliaceus, pemphigus erythematosus, paraneoplastic pemphigus (PNPP), and drug-related pemphigus. Pemphigus vegetans is a variant of pemphigus vulgaris, and pemphigus erythematosus is a variant of pemphigus foliaceus. Each form of this disease has antibodies directed against different target cell surface antigens, resulting in a lesion forming in different layer of the epithelium. In pemphigus foliaceus, the blister occurs in the superficial granular cell layer, whereas, in pemphigus vulgaris, the lesion is deeper, just above the basal cell layer. Mucosal involvement is not a feature of the foliaceus and erythematous forms of the disease.

PEMPHIGUS VULGARIS

PV is the most common form of pemphigus, accounting for over 80% of cases. The underlying mechanism responsible for causing the intraepithelial lesion of PV is the binding of IgG autoantibodies to desmoglein 3, a transmembrane glycoprotein adhesion molecule present on desmosomes. The presence of desmoglein 1 autoantibodies is a characteristic of pemphigus foliaceus, but these antibodies are also detected in patients with long-standing PV. Evidence for the relationship of the IgG autoantibodies to PV lesion formation includes studies demonstrating the formation of blisters on the skin of mice after passive transfer of IgG from patients with PV.[148] The mechanism by which antidesmoglein antibodies cause the loss of cell-to-cell adhesion is controversial. Some investigators believe that binding of the PV antibody activates proteases, whereas more recent evidence supports the theory that the PV antibodies directly block the adhesion function of the desmogleins.[146,149,150]

The separation of cells, called acantholysis, takes place in the lower layers of the stratum spinosum (Figure 4-27). Electron microscopic observations show the earliest epithelial changes as a loss of intercellular cement substance; this is followed by a widening of intercellular spaces, destruction of desmosomes, and finally cellular degeneration. This progressive acantholysis results in the classic suprabasilar bulla, which involves increasingly greater areas of epithelium, resulting in loss of large areas of skin and mucosa.

Pemphigus has been reported coexisting with other autoimmune diseases, particularly myasthenia gravis.[147] Patients with thymoma also have a higher incidence of pemphigus. Several cases of pemphigus have been reported in patients with multiple autoimmune disorders or those with neoplasms such as lymphoma. Death occurs most frequently in elderly patients and in patients requiring high doses of corticosteroids who develop infections and bacterial septicemia, most notably from *Staphylococcus aureus*.[151,152]

Clinical Manifestations. The classical lesion of pemphigus is a thin-walled bulla arising on otherwise normal skin or mucosa. The bulla rapidly breaks but continues to extend peripherally, eventually leaving large areas denuded of skin (Figure 4-28). A characteristic sign of the disease may be obtained by application of pressure to an intact bulla. In patients with PV, the bulla enlarges by extension to an apparently normal surface. Another characteristic sign of the disease is that pressure to an appar-

ently normal area results in the formation of a new lesion. This phenomenon, called the Nikolsky sign, results from the upper layer of the skin pulling away from the basal layer. The Nikolsky sign is most frequently associated with pemphigus but may also occur in epidermolysis bullosa.

Some patients with pemphigus develop acute fulminating disease, but, in most cases, the disease develops more slowly, usually taking months to develop to its fullest extent.

Oral Manifestations. Eighty to ninety percent of patients with pemphigus vulgaris develop oral lesions sometime during the course of the disease, and, in 60% of cases, the oral lesions are the first sign.[153] The oral lesions may begin as the classic bulla on a noninflamed base; more frequently, the clinician sees shallow irregular ulcers because the bullae rapidly break. A thin layer of epithelium peels away in an irregular pattern, leaving a denuded base. The edges of the lesion continue to extend peripherally over a period of weeks until they involve large portions of the oral mucosa. Most commonly the lesions start on the buccal mucosa, often in areas of trauma along the occlusal plane. The palate and gingiva are other common sites of involvement.[154]

It is common for the oral lesions to be present up to 4 months before the skin lesions appear. If treatment is instituted during this time, the disease is easier to control, and the chance for an early remission of the disorder is enhanced. Frequently, however, the initial diagnosis is missed, and the lesions are misdiagnosed as herpes infection or candidiasis. Zegarelli and Zegarelli studied 26 cases of intraoral PV. The average time from onset of the disease to diagnosis was 6.8 months.[155] They also noted that several patients had coexisting candidiasis, which sometimes masked the typical clinical picture of the pemphigus lesions. There is also a subgroup of pemphigus patients whose disease remains confined to the oral mucosa. These patients often have negative results on direct immunofluorescence (DIF).

If a proper history is taken, the clinician should be able to distinguish the lesions of pemphigus from those caused by acute viral infections or erythema multiforme because of the acute nature of the latter diseases. It is also important for the clinician to distinguish pemphigus lesions from those in the RAS category. RAS lesions may be severe, but individual lesions heal and recur. In pemphigus, the same lesions continue to extend peripherally over a period of weeks to months. Lesions of pemphigus are not round and symmetric like RAS lesions but are shallow and irregular and often have detached epithelium at the periphery (see Figure 4-27). In early stages of the disease, the sliding away of the oral epithelium resembles skin peeling after a severe sunburn. In some cases, the lesions may start on the gingiva and be called desquamative gingivitis. It should be remembered that desquamative gingivitis is not a diagnosis in itself; these lesions must be biopsied to rule out the possibility of PV as well as bullous pemphigoid, mucous membrane pemphigoid, and erosive lichen planus.

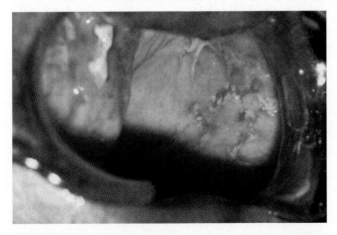

FIGURE 4-27 Histologic picture of pemphigus vulgaris. The bulla is intraepithelial because of acantholysis (×32 original magnification). (Courtesy of Margaret Wood, MD)

Laboratory Tests. PV is diagnosed by biopsy. Biopsies are best done on intact vesicles and bullae less than 24 hours old; however, because these lesions are rare on the oral mucosa, the

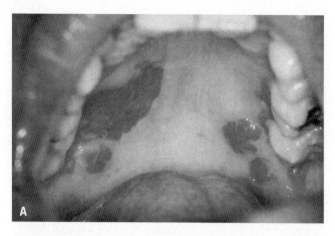 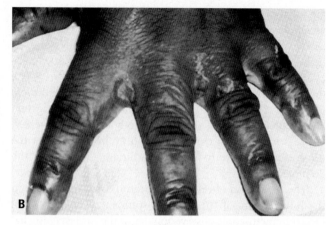

FIGURE 4-28   A, Shallow irregular erosions on the buccal mucosa and ventral surface of the tongue caused by pemphigus. **B,** Bullae between the fingers of the same patient.

biopsy specimen should be taken from the advancing edge of the lesion, where areas of characteristic suprabasilar acantholysis may be observed by the pathologist. Specimens taken from the center of a denuded area are nonspecific histologically as well as clinically. Sometimes several biopsies are necessary before the correct diagnosis can be made. If the patient shows a positive Nikolsky sign, pressure can be placed on the mucosa to produce a new lesion; biopsy may be done on this fresh lesion.

A second biopsy, to be studied by DIF, should be performed whenever pemphigus is included in the differential diagnosis. This study is best performed on a biopsy specimen that is obtained from clinically normal-appearing perilesional mucosa or skin. In this technique for DIF, fluorescein-labeled antihuman immunoglobulins are placed over the patient's tissue specimen. In cases of PV, the technique will detect antibodies, usually IgG and complement, bound to the surface of the keratinocytes.

Indirect immunofluorescent antibody tests have been described that are helpful in distinguishing pemphigus from pemphigoid and other chronic oral lesions and in following the progress of patients treated for pemphigus. In this technique, serum from a patient with bullous disease is placed over a prepared slide of an epidermal structure (usually monkey esophagus). The slide is then overlaid with fluorescein-tagged antihuman gamma globulin. Patients with pemphigus vulgaris have antikeratinocyte antibodies against intercellular substances that show up under a fluorescent microscope. The titer of the antibody has been directly related to the level of clinical disease. An ELISA (enzyme-linked immunosorbent assay) has been developed that can detect desmoglein 1 and 3 in serum samples of patients with PV. These laboratory tests should provide a new tool for the accurate diagnosis of PV and may also prove useful in monitoring the progress of the disease.[156,157]

Treatment.   An important aspect of patient management is early diagnosis, when lower doses of medication can be used for shorter periods of time to control the disease. The mainstay of treatment remains high doses of systemic corticosteroids, usually given in dosages of 1 to 2 mg/kg/d. When steroids must be used for long periods of time, adjuvants such as azathioprine or cyclophosphamide are added to the regimen to reduce the complications of long-term corticosteroid therapy. Prednisone is used initially to bring the disease under control, and, once this is achieved, the dose of prednisone is decreased to the lowest possible maintenance levels. Patients with only oral involvement also may need lower doses of prednisone for shorter periods of time, so the clinician should weigh the potential benefits of adding adjuvant therapy against the risks of additional complications such as blood dyscrasias, hepatitis, and an increased risk of malignancy later in life. There is no one accepted treatment for pemphigus confined to the mouth, but one 5-year follow-up study of the treatment of oral pemphigus showed no additional benefit of adding cyclophosphamide or cyclosporine to prednisone versus prednisone alone, and it showed a higher rate of complications in the group taking the immunosuppressive drug.[158] Most studies of pemphigus of the skin show a decreased mortality rate when adjuvant therapy is given along with prednisone.[159] One new immunosuppressive drug, mycophenolate, has been effective when managing patients resistant to other adjuvants.[160] The need for systemic steroids may be lowered further in cases of oral pemphigus by combining topical with systemic steroid therapy, either by allowing the prednisone tablets to dissolve slowly in the mouth before swallowing or by using potent topical steroid creams. Other therapies that have been reported as beneficial are parenteral gold therapy, dapsone, tetracycline, and plasmapheresis.[161] Plasmapheresis is particularly useful in patients refractory to corticosteroids. A therapy described by Rook and colleagues involves administration of 8-methoxypsoralen followed by exposure of peripheral blood to ultraviolet radiation.[162]

PARANEOPLASTIC PEMPHIGUS

PNPP is a severe variant of pemphigus that is associated with an underlying neoplasm—most frequently non-Hodgkin's lymphoma, chronic lymphocytic leukemia, or thymoma.

Castleman's disease and Waldenströms macroglobulinemia are also associated with cases of PNPP. Patients with this form of pemphigus develop severe blistering and erosions of the mucous membranes and skin. Treatment of this disease is difficult, and most patients die from the effects of the underlying tumor, respiratory failure due to acantholysis of respiratory epithelium, or the severe lesions that do not respond to the therapy successful in managing other forms of pemphigus.[163,164]

Histopathology of lesions of PNPP includes inflammation at the dermal-epidermal junction and keratinocyte necrosis in addition to the characteristic acantholysis seen in PV. The results of direct and indirect immunofluorescence also differ from those in PV. DIF shows deposition of IgG and complement along the basement membrane as well as on the keratinocyte surface. Indirect immunofluorescence demonstrates antibodies that not only bind to epithelium but to liver, heart, and bladder tissue as well.

PEMPHIGUS VEGETANS

Pemphigus vegetans, which accounts for 1 to 2% of pemphigus cases, is a relatively benign variant of pemphigus vulgaris because the patient demonstrates the ability to heal the denuded areas. Two forms of pemphigus vegetans are recognized: the Neumann type and the Hallopeau type. The Neumann type is more common, and the early lesions are similar to those seen in pemphigus vulgaris, with large bullae and denuded areas. These areas attempt healing by developing vegetations of hyperplastic granulation tissue. In the Hallopeau type, which is less aggressive, pustules, not bullae, are the initial lesions. These pustules are followed by verrucous hyperkeratotic vegetations.

Biopsy results of the early lesions of pemphigus vegetans show suprabasilar acantholysis.[165] In older lesions, hyperkeratosis and pseudoepitheliomatous hyperplasia become prominent. Immunofluorescent study shows changes identical to those seen in PV.

Oral Manifestations. Oral lesions are common in both forms of pemphigus vegetans and may be the initial sign of disease.[166] Gingival lesions may be lace-like ulcers with a purulent surface on a red base or have a granular or cobblestone appearance (Figure 4-29). Oral lesions that are associated with inflammatory bowel disease and resemble pemphigus vegetans both clinically and histologically are referred to by some authors as pyostomatitis vegetans.[167]

Treatment. Treatment is the same as that for PV.

Subepithelial Bullous Dermatoses

Subepithelial bullous dermatoses are a group of mucocutaneous autoimmune blistering diseases that are characterized by a lesion in the basement membrane zone. The diseases in this group include bullous pemphigoid (BP), mucous membrane (cicatricial) pemphigoid (MMP), linear IgA disease (LAD), chronic bullous dermatosis of childhood (CBDC), and erosive

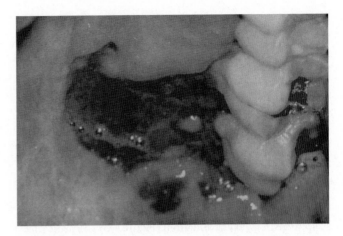

FIGURE 4-29 Chronic palatal lesions of pemphigus vegetans.

and bullous lichen planus. There is significant overlap among these diseases, and the diagnosis often depends on whether the disease is categorized by clinical manifestations combined with routine histopathology or the newer techniques of molecular biology. Recent research into pathologic mechanisms is defining the specific antigens in the basement membrane complex involved in triggering the autoantibody response.

BULLOUS PEMPHIGOID

BP, which is the most common of the subepithelial blistering diseases, occurs chiefly in adults over the age of 60 years; it is self-limited and may last from a few months to 5 years. BP may be a cause of death in older debilitated individuals.[168] BP has occasionally been reported in conjunction with other diseases, particularly multiple sclerosis and malignancy, or drug therapy, particularly diuretics.[169] In pemphigoid, the initial defect is not intraepithelial as in PV, but it is subepithelial in the lamina lucida region of the basement membrane[170] (Figure 4-30). There is no acantholysis, but the split in the basement membrane is accompanied by an inflammatory infiltrate that is characteristically rich in eosinophils.

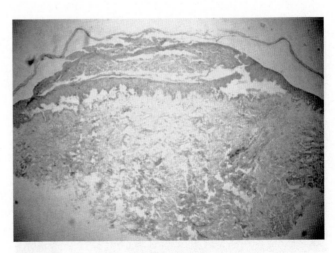

FIGURE 4-30 Histologic picture of bullous pemphigoid. The bulla is subepithelial.(Courtesy of Margaret Wood, MD)

Direct immunofluorescent study of a biopsy specimen demonstrates deposition of IgG bound to the basement membrane. Indirect immunoflourescent study of serum obtained from patients with BP demonstrates IgG antibodies bound to the epidermal side of salt-split skin onto antigens that have been named BP antigens 1 and 2. This latter test is particularly useful in distinguishing BP from another subepithelial bullous disease, epidermolysis bullosa aquisita, which has IgG antibodies localized to the dermal side of the salt-split skin.

Clinical Manifestations.   The characteristic skin lesion of BP is a blister on an inflamed base that chiefly involves the scalp, arms, legs, axilla, and groin (Figure 4-31). Pruritic macules and papules may also be a presenting sign. The disease is self-limiting but can last for months to years without therapy. Patients with BP may experience one episode or recurrent bouts of lesions. Unlike pemphigus, BP is rarely life threatening since the bullae do not continue to extend at the periphery to form large denuded areas, although death from sepsis or cardiovascular disease secondary to long-term steroid use has been reported to be high in groups of sick elderly patients.[171]

Oral Manifestations.   Oral involvement is common in BP. Lever reported 33 patients with bullous pemphigoid. Oral lesions were present in 11.[172] In 3 of the cases, the oral lesions preceded the skin lesions, most frequently on the buccal mucosa. Venning and colleagues reported oral lesions in 50% (18 of 36) of BP patients studied.[170]

The oral lesions of pemphigoid are smaller, form more slowly, and are less painful than those seen in pemphigus vulgaris, and the extensive labial involvement seen in pemphigus is not present. Desquamative gingivitis has also been reported as a manifestation of BP. The gingival lesions consist of generalized edema, inflammation, and desquamation with localized areas of discrete vesicle formation. The oral lesions are clinically and histologically indistinguishable from oral lesions of mucous membrane pemphigoid, but early remission of BP is more common.

Treatment.   Patients with localized lesions of BP may be treated with high-potency topical steroids,[168] whereas patients with severe disease require use of systemic corticosteroids alone or combined with immunosuppressive drugs such as azathioprine, cyclophosphamide, or mycophenolate. Patients with moderate levels of disease may avoid use of systemic steroids by use of dapsone or a combination of tetracycline and nicotinamide.

MUCOUS MEMBRANE PEMPHIGOID (CICATRICIAL PEMPHIGOID)

MMP is a chronic autoimmune subepithelial disease that primarily affects the mucous membranes of patients over the age of 50 years, resulting in mucosal ulceration and subsequent scarring. The primary lesion of MMP occurs when autoantibodies directed against proteins in the basement membrane zone, acting with complement (C3) and neutrophils, cause a subepithelial split and subsequent vesicle formation (Figure 4-32). The antigens associated with MMP are most frequently present in the lamina lucida portion of the basement membrane, but recent research has demonstrated that the identical antigen is not involved in all cases, and the lamina densa may be the primary site of involvement in some cases. The circulating autoantibodies are not the same in all cases, and subsets of MMP have been identified by the technique of immunofluorescent staining of skin that has been split at the basement membrane zone with the use of sodium chloride.[173] The majority of cases of MMP demonstrate IgG directed against antigens on the epidermal side of the salt-split skin, which have been identified as BP 180 (also called type XVII collagen); however, cases of MMP have also been identified where the antigen is present on the dermal side of the split. This latter antigen has been identified as epiligrin (laminin 5), an adhesion molecule that is a component of the anchoring filaments of the basement membrane.[174,175]

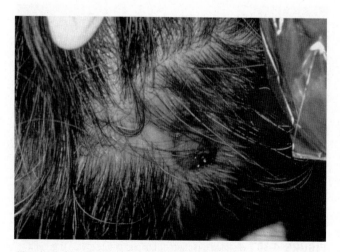

Figure 4-31   Bullous pemphigoid lesion of the scalp.

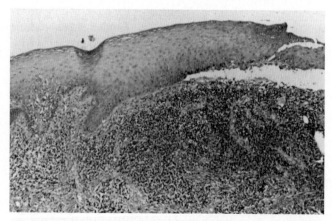

FIGURE 4-32   Histopathology of mucous membrane pemphigoid, demonstrating subepithelial separation at the basement membrane.

Clinical Manifestations. The subepithelial lesions of MMP may involve any mucosal surface, but they most frequently involve the oral mucosa. The conjunctiva is the second most common site of involvement and can lead to scarring and adhesions developing between the bulbar and palpebral conjunctiva called symblepharon (Figure 4-33, A and B). Corneal damage is common, and progressive scarring leads to blindness in close to 15% of patients. Lesions may also affect the genital mucosa, causing pain and sexual dysfunction. Laryngeal involvement causes pain, hoarseness, and difficulty breathing, whereas esophageal involvement may cause dysphagia, which can lead to debilitation and death in severe cases. Skin lesions, usually of the head and neck region, are present in 20 to 30% of patients.

Oral Manifestations. Oral lesions occur in over 90% of patients with MMP. Desquamative gingivitis is the most common manifestation and may be the only manifestation of the disease (Figure 4-34). Since these desquamative lesions resemble the lesions of erosive lichen planus and pemphigus, all cases of desquamative gingivitis should be biopsied and studied with both routine histology and direct immunofluorescence to determine the correct diagnosis. Lesions may present as intact vesicles of the gingival or other mucosal surfaces, but more frequently they appear as nonspecific-appearing erosions (Figure 4-35). The erosions typically spread more slowly than pemphigus lesions and are more self-limiting.

Diagnosis. Patients with MMP included in the differential diagnosis must have a biopsy done for both routine and direct immunofluorescent study. Routine histopathology shows subbasilar cleavage. Using the direct immunofluorescent technique (see "Laboratory Tests" under "Pemphigus Vulgaris" for description), biopsy specimens taken from MMP patients demonstrate positive fluorescence for immunoglobulin and complement in the basement membrane zone in 50 to 80% of patients. Splitting the biopsy specimen at the basement membrane zone with 1 M NaCl prior to direct immunofluorescence increases the sensitivity of the test. The direct immunofluorescent technique is excellent for distinguishing MMP from pemphigus, and specimens obtained show immunoglobulin and complement deposition in the intercellular substance of the prickle cell layer of the epithelium. Only 10% of MMP patients demonstrate positive indirect immunofluorescence for circulating antibasement membrane-zone antibodies; however, use of salt-split skin as a substrate increases the sensitivity of this test.

Treatment. Management of MMP depends on the severity of symptoms. When the lesions are confined to the oral mucosa, systemic corticosteroids will suppress their formation, but the clinician must weigh the benefits against the hazards from side effects of the drug.[176] Unlike pemphigus, MMP is not a fatal disease, and long-term use of steroids for this purpose must be carefully evaluated, particularly because most cases are chronic, most patients are elderly, and treatment is required for a long period of time.

Patients with mild oral disease should be treated with topical and intralesional steroids. Desquamative gingivitis can often be managed with topical steroids in a soft dental splint that covers the gingiva, although the clinician using topical steroids over large areas of mucosa must closely monitor the patient for side effects such as candidiasis and effects of systemic absorption. When topical or intralesional therapy is not successful, dapsone therapy may be attempted. Rogers and Mehregan have developed a protocol for use of dapsone in patients with MMP.[177] The effectiveness of this protocol for the management of MMP was recently confirmed by Ciarrocca and Greenberg.[178] Since dapsone causes hemolysis and methemoglobinemia, glucose-6-phosphate dehydrogenase deficiency must be ruled out, and the patient's hemoglobin must be closely monitored. Methemoglobinemia can be reduced with the use of cimetidine and vitamin E.[151] Another rare side effect of dapsone is dapsone hypersensitivity syndrome, an idiosyncratic disorder characterized by fever, lymphadenopathy, skin eruptions, and occasional liver involvement. Patients resistant to dapsone should be treated with a combination of systemic corticosteroids and immunosuppressive drugs,[152] particularly when there is risk of blindness from conjunctival involvement,

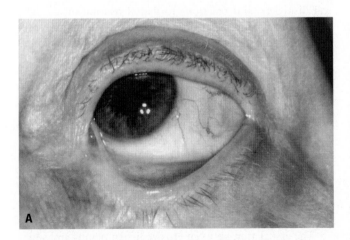
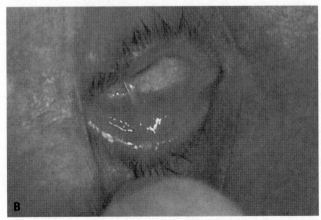

FIGURE 4-33 Mucous membrane pemphigoid; early **(A)** and advanced **(B)** cicatricial pemphigoid of the conjunctiva with symblepharon formation.

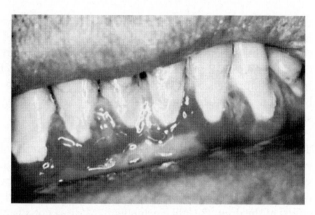

FIGURE 4-34 Chronic desquamative gingival lesions of mucous membrane pemphigoid.

or significant laryngeal or esophageal damage. Reports suggest that tetracycline and nicotinamide may also be helpful in controlling the lesions of MMP.[179,180]

LINEAR IgA DISEASE

LAD is characterized by the deposition of IgA rather than IgG at the basement membrane zone, and the clinical manifestations may resemble either dermatitis herpetiformis or pemphigoid. The cause of the majority of cases is unknown, but a minority of cases have been drug induced.[181] As in MMP, the antigens associated with LAD are heterogeneous and may be found in either the lamina lucida or lamina densa portions of the basement membrane.[182,183]

The skin lesions of LAD may resemble those observed in patients with dermatitis herpetiformis, which are characterized by pruritic papules and blisters at sites of trauma such as the knees and elbows. Other patients have bullous skin lesions similar to those seen in patients with bullous pemphigoid.

Oral lesions are common in LAD and may be seen in up to 70% of patients. These lesions are clinically indistinguishable from the oral lesions of MMP, with blisters and erosions of the mucosa frequently accompanied by desquamative gingivitis.

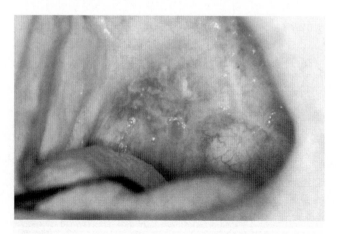

FIGURE 4-35 Mucous membrane pemphigoid causing scarring of the soft palate.

The oral lesions of LAD may be managed with the use of topical steroids, but dapsone is effective therapy for more severe cases. Resistant cases may require systemic corticosteroids.

CHRONIC BULLOUS DISEASE OF CHILDHOOD

CBDC is another blistering disorder, which chiefly affects children below the age of 5 years. It is characterized by the deposition of IgA antibodies in the basement membrane zone,[184] which are detected by direct immunofluorescence on the epidermal side of salt-split skin or mucosa. The onset of the disease may be precipitated by an upper respiratory infection or drug therapy.[185] The characteristic lesion of CBDC is a cluster of vesicles and bullae on an inflamed base. The genital region is involved; conjunctival, rectal, and oral lesions may also be present. Oral mucosal involvement is present in up to 50% of cases, and the oral lesions are similar to those observed in patients with MMP.

Diagnosis is made by biopsy demonstrating a subepithelial lesion on routine histology and by deposition of IgA in the basement membrane zone on direct immunofluorescence. Indirect immunofluorescence demonstrates circulating IgA in 80% of cases.[186] This disease is self-limiting, and the lesions characteristically heal within 2 years. As with LAD, the lesions are responsive to sulfapyridine or dapsone therapy. Corticosteroids may be required for severe cases.

EROSIVE LICHEN PLANUS

The majority of cases of lichen planus present as white lesions (discussed in detail in Chapter 5). An erosive and bullous form of this disease presents as chronic multiple oral mucosal ulcers. Erosive and bullous lesions of lichen planus occur in the severe form of the disease when extensive degeneration of the basal layer of epithelium causes a separation of the epithelium from the underlying connective tissue.[187,188] In some cases, the lesions start as vesicles or bullae—this has been classified as "bullous lichen planus"; in a majority of cases, the disease is characterized by ulcers and is called "erosive lichen planus." Both of these disorders are variations of the same process and should be considered together. The erosive form of lichen planus has been associated with drug therapy, underlying medical disorders, and reactions to dental restorations.[189] The drugs most commonly associated with severe lichenoid reactions include NSAIDs, hydrochlorothiazide, penicillamine, and angiotensin-converting enzyme inhibitors. The most frequently reported underlying disease associated with oral lichenoid reactions is chronic hepatitis caused by hepatitis C, particularly in Japan and the Mediterranean region.[190,191] Contact allergic reactions to flavoring agents such as cinnamon and peppermint and to dental materials such as mercury in amalgam may also result in lichenoid reactions of the oral mucosa.[192,193] Lichen planus lesions suspected of being caused by contact allergy should be in direct contact with the suspected allergen. Graft-versus-host disease due to bone marrow transplantation also causes oral lichenoid lesions.[194]

The association between erosive lichen planus and squamous cell carcinoma remains controversial. There have been many case reports of carcinoma developing in areas of lichen planus.[195–198] A case by Massa and colleagues shows histologic progression from lichen planus, lichen planus with epithelial atypia, and frank squamous cell carcinoma.[199] Reviews of large numbers of patients with lichen planus by Silverman and colleagues and Murti and associates show an association between the two diseases of between 0.4 and 1.2%.[200,201] Affected patients were frequently tobacco users; this leads to speculation that lichen planus is a cofactor in malignant transformation.

Clinical Manifestations.   Erosive lichen planus is characterized by the presence of vesicles, bullae, or irregular shallow ulcers of the oral mucosa[187] (Figures 4-36 and 4-37). The lesions are usually present for weeks to months and thus can be distinguished from those of aphthous stomatitis, which form and heal in a period of 10 days to 2 weeks. A significant number of cases of erosive lichen planus present with a picture of desquamative gingivitis[202] (Figure 4-38). It is important to remember that desquamative gingivitis is not a disease entity but a sign of disease that can be caused by erosive lichen planus, pemphigus vulgaris, or cicatricial pemphigoid. Desquamative gingivitis caused by lichen planus may be accompanied by characteristic Wickham's striae, simplifying the diagnosis, or they may be present without other lesions.

Diagnosis.   A diagnosis of erosive lichen planus should be suspected when erosive or bullous lesions are accompanied by typical lichenoid white lesions. Biopsy is necessary for definitive diagnosis. Biopsy of the erosive lesions shows hydropic degeneration of the basal layer of epithelium. This can help to distinguish it from mucous membrane pemphigoid, which is also a subepithelial lesion but which shows an intact basal layer, or from pemphigus vulgaris, in which acantholysis is demonstrated. Direct immunofluorescence should be performed on biopsy specimens when pemphigus, pemphigoid, or discoid lupus erythematosus is included in the differential diagnosis.

Management.   Patients with severe lichen planus should have drug therapy and underlying disease ruled out as possible causes. The bullous and erosive forms of lichen planus can be

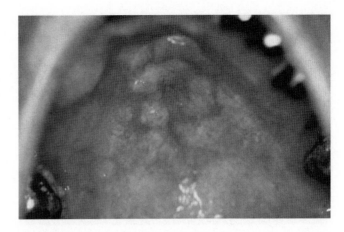

FIGURE 4-37   Palatal lesions of erosive lichen planus.

distressingly painful. The treatment of choice is topical corticosteroids (Figure 4-39). Intralesional steroids can be used for indolent lesions, and, in cases of severe exacerbation, systemic steroids may be considered for short periods of time. Cyclosporine rinses may be effective for patients with severe erosions resistant to topical steroids, although the expense may be a limiting factor.[203,204] Tacrolimus, another immunosuppressive drug, has recently been marketed in a topical form and has been reported useful in the management of oral erosive lichen planus. Systemic etretinate, dapsone, or photochemotherapy have also been reported to be effective in severe resistant cases.[205–207] Because patients with oral lichen planus appear to be in a higher risk group for development of squamous cell carcinoma, it is prudent to periodically evaluate all patients with erosive and bullous forms of lichen planus for the presence of suspicious lesions requiring biopsy (Figure 4-40).

Herpes Simplex Virus Infection in Immunosuppressed Patients

Immunosuppressed patients may develop an aggressive or chronic form of herpes infection; therefore, herpes simplex infection should be included in the differential diagnosis when immunosuppressed patients develop chronic oral

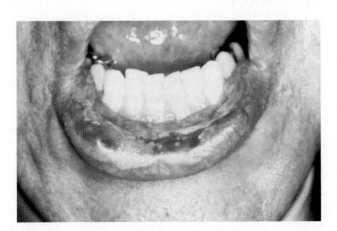

FIGURE 4-36   Erosive lichen planus of the labial mucosa.

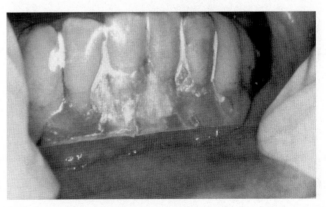

FIGURE 4-38   Desquamative gingival lesions in a patient with erosive lichen planus.

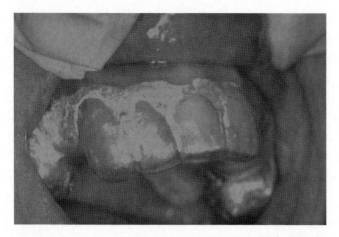

FIGURE 4-39   Soft medication splint used to treat desquamative gingivitis secondary to erosive lichen planus.

ulcers. The chronic form of herpes is a variation of recurrent herpes simplex infection rather than a primary infection.[208,209] AIDS patients, transplant patients taking immunosuppressed drug therapy, patients on high doses of corticosteroids, and patients with leukemia, lymphoma, or other disorders that alter the T-lymphocyte response are those most susceptible to aggressive HSV lesions.

Lesions appear on the skin or the mucosa of the mouth, rectal, or genital area. They begin as an ordinary recurrent herpes infection but remain for weeks to months and develop into large ulcers up to several centimeters in diameter (Figure 4-42). Chronic herpes simplex infection has been reported with both type 1 and type 2 herpesviruses. This disease causes significant local morbidity and occasional dissemination.

ORAL MANIFESTATIONS

Lesions of chronic or aggressive recurrent HSV may occur on the lips or intraoral mucosa. Schneidman and colleagues[210] reviewed 18 cases of chronic herpes infection; 7 cases occurred in renal transplant patients, and 8 occurred in patients with

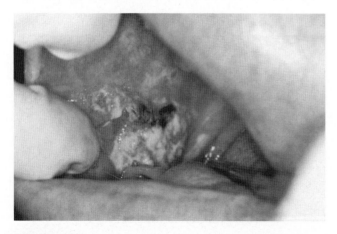

FIGURE 4-40   Squamous cell carcinoma forming on the buccal mucosa of a patient with erosive lichen planus.

hematologic malignancies. Fourteen of the 18 patients had oral or perioral lesions. Greenberg and colleagues studied 98 immunosuppressed patients: 68 renal transplant patients and 30 acute leukemic patients receiving chemotherapy.[209] Fifty percent of the leukemic patients and 15% of the transplant patients developed aggressive or chronic recurrent HSV. HSV was the most common cause of oral lesions in both groups, producing lesions that were previously thought to be due to the toxic effects of chemotherapy or bacterial infection. The oral lesions may be small, round, symmetric, and associated with recurrent herpes infection, or they may be large and deep and often confused with lesions of other diseases (see Figure 4-41, A and B) The lesions last from weeks to months and may reach several centimeters in diameter. The larger lesions often have raised white borders composed of small vesicles (Figure 4-42).

DIAGNOSIS

HSV must be ruled out whenever oral mucosal vesicles or ulcers occur in immunosuppressed or myelosuppressed patients. Both a cytology for staining with fluorescent HSV antibody and a viral culture should be obtained. If these lesions occur in a patient without an obvious known cause, they should be thoroughly evaluated for an immunologic deficiency disease.

TREATMENT

Immunosuppressed patients with HSV infection respond well to acyclovir administered orally or intravenously.[21] Occasional cases of acyclovir-resistant HSV have been reported in AIDS patients. Foscarnet has been effective therapy for these patients.[211]

▼ THE PATIENT WITH SINGLE ULCERS

The most common cause of single ulcers on the oral mucosa is trauma. Trauma may be caused by teeth, food, dental appliances, dental treatment, heat, chemicals, or electricity (Figure 4–43). The diagnosis is usually not complicated and is based on the history and physical findings. The most important differentiation is to distinguish trauma from squamous cell carcinoma. The dentist must examine all single ulcers for significant healing in 1 week; if healing is not evident in this time, a biopsy should be done to rule out cancer. (Cancer of the mouth is discussed in detail in Chapter 8.)

Infections that may cause a chronic oral ulcer include the deep mycoses histoplasmosis, blastomycosis, mucormycosis, aspergillosis, cryptococcosis, and coccidioidomycosis as well as a chronic herpes simplex infection. Syphilis, another infection that may cause a single oral ulcer in the primary and tertiary stages, is described in Chapter 20.

The deep mycoses were rare causes of oral lesions prior to HIV infection and immunosuppressive drug therapy. The dentist must consider this group of diseases in the differential diagnosis whenever isolated ulcerative lesions develop in known or suspected immunosuppressed patients. Biopsy of

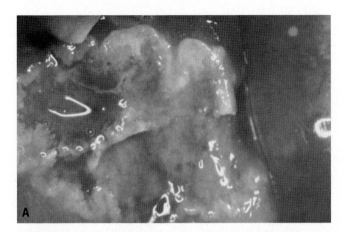
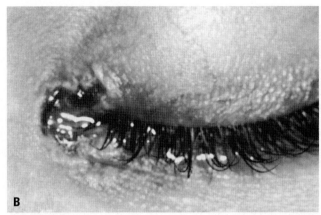

FIGURE 4-41 **A,** This large ulcer of the buccal mucosa was caused by a chronic herpes simplex infection in a kidney transplant patient receiving immunosuppressive drug therapy. **B,** A herpetic ulcer near the eye of the same patient.

suspected tissue, accompanied by a request for appropriate stains, is necessary for early diagnosis (Figure 4-44). Deep mycoses in immunosuppressed patients are discussed in greater detail in Chapters 16 and 18.

Histoplasmosis

Histoplasmosis is caused by the fungus *Histoplasma capsulatum*, a dimorphic fungus that grows in the yeast form in infected tissue. Infection results from inhaling dust contaminated with droppings, particularly from infected birds or bats. An African form of this infection is caused by a larger yeast, which is considered a variant of *H. capsulatum* and is called *H. duboisii*.

Histoplasmosis is the most common systemic fungal infection in the United States; in endemic areas such as the Mississippi and Ohio River valleys, serologic evidence of previous infection may be found in 75 to 80% of the population. In most cases, particularly in otherwise normal children, primary infection is mild, manifesting as a self-limiting pulmonary disease that heals to leave fibrosis and calcification similar to tuberculosis. In a small percentage of cases, progressive disease results in cavitation of the lung and dissemination of the organism to the liver, spleen, adrenal glands, and meninges. Patients with the disseminated form of the disease may develop anemia and leukopenia secondary to bone marrow involvement. Immunosuppressed or myelosuppressed patients are more likely to develop the severe disseminated form of the disease. During the past decade, most reported cases of oral lesions of histoplasmosis have been reported in HIV-infected individuals who live in or have visited endemic areas.

ORAL MANIFESTATIONS

Oral involvement is usually secondary to pulmonary involvement and occurs in a significant percentage of patients with disseminated histoplasmosis. Oral mucosal lesions may appear as a papule, a nodule, an ulcer, or a vegetation. If a single lesion is left untreated, it progresses from a firm papule to a nodule, which ulcerates and slowly enlarges. The cervical lymph nodes are enlarged and firm. The clinical appearance of the lesions, as well as the accompanying lymphadenopathy, often resembles that of squamous cell carcinoma, other chronic fungal infections, or even Hodgkin's disease.

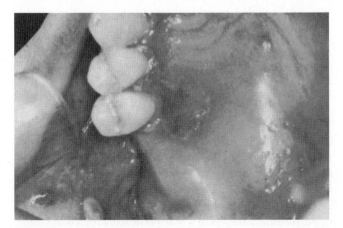

FIGURE 4-42 Chronic herpes simplex infection of the palate in a patient taking chemotherapy for acute leukemia.

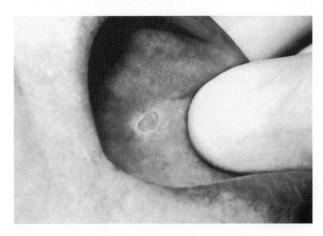

FIGURE 4-43 Traumatic ulcer of the buccal mucosa secondary to cheek biting.

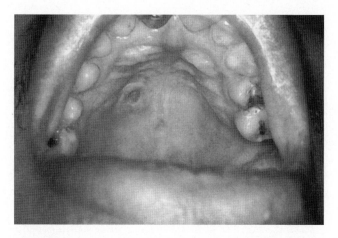

FIGURE 4-44   Palatal ulcer can be the initial sign of *Cryptococcus* in an AIDS patient.

Cases of oral histoplasmosis have been reported as the initial sign of HIV infection. The most common oral lesion of histoplasmosis in patients with HIV is an ulcer with an indurated border, which is most commonly seen on the gingiva, palate, or tongue.[212] These oral histoplasmosis lesions in patients with HIV may occur alone or as part of a disseminated infection.[213,214]

DIAGNOSIS

Definitive diagnosis of histoplasmosis is made by a culture of infected tissues or exudates on Sabouraud's dextrose agar or other appropriate media. Biopsy of infected tissue shows small oval yeasts within macrophages and reticuloendothelial cells as well as chronic granulomas, epithelioid cells, giant cells, and occasionally caseation necrosis. Skin tests and serology are not definitive because of significant numbers of false-negative and false-positive reactions.

TREATMENT

Mild to moderate cases of histoplasmosis can be treated with ketoconazole or itraconazole for 6 to 12 months. Immunosuppressed patients or patients with severe disease require intravenous amphotericin B for up to 10 weeks.

Blastomycosis

Blastomycosis is a fungal infection caused by *Blastomyces dermatitidis*. This dimorphic organism can grow in either a yeast or as a mycelial form. The organism is found as a normal inhabitant of soil; therefore, the highest incidence of this infection is found in agricultural workers, particularly in the middle Atlantic and southeastern portions of the United States. This geographic distribution of the infection has led to the designation by some as "North American blastomycosis." Infection by the same organism, however, has also been found in Mexico and Central and South Americas.

Infection with *Blastomyces* begins in a vast majority of cases by inhalation; this causes a primary pulmonary infection. Although an acute self-limiting form of the disease exists, the infection commonly follows a chronic course beginning with mild symptoms such as malaise, low-grade fever, and mild cough. If the infection goes untreated, the symptoms worsen to include shortness of breath, weight loss, and production of blood-tinged sputum. Infection of the skin, mucosa, and bone may also occur, resulting from metastatic spread of organisms from the pulmonary lesions through the lymphatic system. The skin and mucosal lesions start as subcutaneous nodules and progress to well-circumscribed indurated ulcers.

ORAL MANIFESTATIONS

Oral lesions are rarely the primary site of infection. When oral lesions have been reported as a first sign of blastomycosis, they have occurred in patients with mild pulmonary symptoms that have been overlooked by the patient or physician. Most cases of oral involvement demonstrate concomitant pulmonary lesions on chest radiographs.

The most common appearance of the oral lesions of blastomycosis is a nonspecific painless verrucous ulcer with indurated borders, often mistaken for squamous cell carcinoma. Occasionally, this mistake is perpetuated by an inexperienced histopathologist who confuses the characteristic pseudoepitheliomatous hyperplasia with malignant changes.

Other oral lesions that have been reported include hard nodules and radiolucent jaw lesions. Page and colleagues reported two cases of painless oral mucosal ulcers as the first sign of blastomycosis; in both cases, a careful history taking revealed mild respiratory symptoms.[215] Bell and colleagues reported 7 cases of oral lesions occurring in patients with blastomycosis; 4 presented as chronic oral ulcers and 3 as radiolucent bone lesions.[216] Chest radiographs showed concomitant pulmonary involvement in all cases.

Dentists should include the diagnosis of blastomycosis in the differential diagnosis of a chronic oral ulcer. The diagnosis cannot be made on clinical grounds alone. The index of suspicion should increase when a chronic painless oral ulcer appears in an agricultural worker or when the review of systems reveals pulmonary symptoms. Diagnosis is made on the basis of biopsy and on culturing the organism from tissue.[217] The histologic appearance shows pseudoepitheliomatous hyperplasia with a heavy infiltrate of chronic inflammatory cells and microabscesses.

TREATMENT

Treatment for blastomycosis is similar to that described for histoplasmosis.

Mucormycosis

Mucormycosis (phycomycosis) is caused by an infection with a saprophytic fungus that normally occurs in soil or as a mold on decaying food. The fungus is nonpathogenic for healthy individuals and can be cultured regularly from the human nose, throat, and oral cavity. (The organism represents an opportunistic rather than a true pathogen.) Infection occurs in individuals with decreased host resistance, such as those with poorly controlled diabetes or hematologic malignancies, or those undergoing cancer chemotherapy or immunosuppressive drug therapy.[218,219] In the debilitated patient, mucormycosis may appear as a pulmonary, gastrointestinal, disseminated, or rhinocerebral infection.

The rhinomaxillary form of the disease, a subdivision of the rhinocerebral form, begins with the inhalation of the fungus by a susceptible individual. The fungus invades arteries and causes damage secondary to thrombosis and ischemia. The fungus may spread from the oral and nasal region to the brain, causing death in a high percentage of cases. Symptoms include nasal discharge caused by necrosis of the nasal turbinates, ptosis, proptosis secondary to invasion of the orbit, fever, swelling of the cheek, and paresthesia of the face.

ORAL MANIFESTATIONS

The most common oral sign of mucormycosis is ulceration of the palate, which results from necrosis due to invasion of a palatal vessel.[218,220] The lesion is characteristically large and deep, causing denudation of underlying bone (Figure 4-45). Ulcers from mucormycosis have also been reported on the gingiva, lip, and alveolar ridge. The initial manifestation of the disease may be confused with dental pain or bacterial maxillary sinusitis caused by invasion of the maxillary sinus. The clinician must include mucormycosis in the differential diagnosis of large oral ulcers occurring in patients debilitated from diabetes, chemotherapy, or immunosuppressive drug therapy.

Early diagnosis is essential if the patient is to be cured of this infection. Negative cultures do not rule out mucormycosis because the fungus is frequently difficult to culture from infected tissue; instead, a biopsy must be performed when mucormycosis is suspected. The histopathologic specimen shows necrosis and nonseptate hyphae, which are best demonstrated by a periodic acid–Schiff stain.

TREATMENT

When diagnosed early, mucormycosis may be cured by a combination of surgical débridement of the infected area and systemic administration of amphotericin B for up to 3 months. Proper management of the underlying disorder is an important aspect affecting the final outcome of treatment. All patients given amphotericin B must be closely observed for renal toxicity by repeated measurements of the blood urea nitrogen and creatinine.

▼ REFERENCES

1. Scully C. Orofacial herpes simplex virus infections. Current concepts in the epidemiology, pathogenesis and treatment. Oral Surg 1989;68:701–10.
2. Levy JA. Three new human herpesviruses (HHV-6, 7 and 8). Lancet 1997;349:558–62.
3. Greenberg MS, Glick M, Nghiem L, et al. Relationship of cytomegalovirus to salivary gland dysfunction in HIV-infected patients. Oral Surg Oral Med Oral Pathol Oral Radiol Endod 1997;83:334–9.
4. Embil JA, Manuel R, McFarlane S. Concurrent oral and genital infection with an identical strain of herpes simplex type I. Sex Transm Dis 1981;8:70–2.
5. Fife KH, Schmidt O, Remington M, Corely L. Primary and recurrent concomitant genital infection with herpes simplex virus types 1 and 2. J Infect Dis 1983;147:163.
6. Christenson B, Bottinger M, Svenson A, Jeansson S. A 15 year surveillance study of antibodies to herpes simplex types 1 and 2 in a cohort of young girls. J Infect 1992;25:147.
7. Scott DA, Coulter WA, Lamey PJ. Oral shedding of herpes simplex virus type 1: a review. J Oral Pathol Med 1997;26:441–7.
8. Wheeler CE. The herpes simplex problem. J Am Acad Dermatol 1988;18:163–8.
9. Wald A. Herpes. Transmission and viral shedding. Dermatol Clin 1998;16:795–7.
10. Roizman B, Sears AE. An inquiry into the mechanisms of herpes simplex virus latency. Ann Rev Microbiol 1987;41:543–57.
11. Riley LE. Herpes simplex virus. Semin Perinatol 1998;22:284–92.
12. Miller CS, Danaher RJ, Jacob RJ. Molecular aspects of herpes simplex virus I latency, reactivation, and recurrence. Crit Rev Oral Biol Med 1998;9:541–62.
13. McCormick DD. Herpes simplex virus as cause of Bell's palsy. Lancet 1972;1:937–9.
14. Murakami S, Mizobuchi M, Nakashiro Y, et al. Bell's palsy and herpes simplex virus. Ann Intern Med 1996;124:27–30.
15. Rodriguez AS, Martin Oterino JA, Ruiz VA. Arch Intern Med 1998;158:1577–78.
16. Rapp F, Duff R. Transformation of hamster embryo fibroblasts by herpes simplex viruses type 1 and type 2. Cancer Res 1973;33:1527.
17. Scully C. Herpes simplex virus (HSV). In: Millard HD, Mason DK, editor. 1988 World Workshop on Oral Medicine. Yearbook Medical Publishers, 1988. Ann Arbor, MI. p. 160.
18. Brightman VJ, Guggenheimer JG. Herpetic paronychia—primary herpes simplex infection of the finger. J Am Dent Assoc 1970;80:112.
19. Stone KM, Brooks CA, Guinan ME, Alexander ER. National surveillance for neonatal herpes simplex infections. Sex Transm Dis 1989;16:152–6.
20. Nahmias AJ. Disseminated herpes simplex virus infections. N Engl J Med 1970;282:684.
21. Whitley RJ, Kimberlin DW, Roizman B. Herpes simplex viruses. Clin Infect Dis 1998;26:541–53.

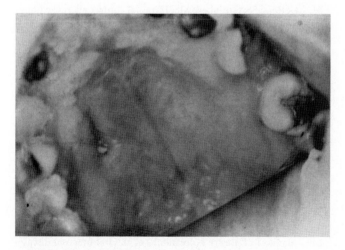

FIGURE 4-45 Mucormycosis of the palate in a kidney transplant patient taking immunosuppressive drugs (azathioprine and prednisone).

22. Greenberg MS, Brightman VJ, Ship II. Clinical and laboratory differentiation of recurrent intraoral herpes simplex infections following fever. J Dent Res 1969;48:435.

23. Bagg J, Mannings A, Munso J, Walker DM. Rapid diagnosis of oral herpes simplex or zoster virus infections by immunofluorescence: comparison with Tzanck cell preparations and viral culture. Br Dent J 1989;167:235.

24. Penna JJ, Eskinazi DP. Treatment of oro-facial herpes simplex infections with acyclovir: a review. Oral Surg 1988;65:689.

25. Amir J, Harel L, Smetana Z, Varsano I. Treatment of herpes simplex gingivostomatitis with acyclovir in children: a randomized double blind placebo controlled study. J Pediatr 1998;132:185.

26. Balfour HH. Antiviral drugs. N Engl J Med 1999;340:1255–68.

27. Ho M, Chen ER, Hsu KH, et al. An epidemic of enterovirus 71 infection in Taiwan. N Engl J Med 1999;341:929.

28. Adler L, Epidemiologic investigation of hand-foot-and-mouth disease. Am J Dis Child 1970;120:309.

29. Dueland AN. Latency and reactivation of varicella zoster virus infections. Scand J Infect Dis 1996;100:46–50.

30. Morgan R, King D. Shingles: a review of diagnosis and management. Hosp Med 1998;59:770–6.

31. Lopes MA, de Souza Filho FJ, Jorge J Jr, de Almeida OP. Herpes zoster infection as a differential diagnosis of acute pulpitis. J Endod 1998;24:143–4.

32. Petursson G, Helgason S, Gudmundsson S, Sigurdsson JA. Herpes zoster in children and adolescents. Pediatr Infect Dis J 1998;17:905–8.

33. MacFarlane LL, Simmons MM, Hunter MH. The use of corticosteroids in the management of herpes zoster. J Am Board Fam Pract 1998;11:224–8.

34. Kost RG, Straus SE. Postherpetic neuralgia—pathogenesis, treatment, and prevention. N Engl J Med 1996;335:32–42.

35. Kost RG, Straus SE. Postherpetic neuralgia: predicting and preventing risk. Arch Intern Med 1997;157:1166–7.

36. McKenzie CD, Gobetti JP. Diagnosis and treatment of orofacial herpes zoster: report of cases. J Am Dent Assoc 1990;120:679.

37. Solomon CS, Coffiner MO, Chalfin HE. Herpes zoster revisited: implicated in root resorption. J Endod 1986;12:210.

38. Schwartz O, Kvorning SA. Tooth exfoliation, osteonecrosis of the jaw and neuralgia following herpes zoster of the trigeminal nerve. Int J Oral Surg 1982;11:364.

39. Wood MJ, Shukla S, Fiddian PA, Crooks RJ. Treatment of acute herpes zoster: effect of early (< 48 h) versus late (48–72 h) therapy with acyclovir and valacyclovir on prolonged pain. J Infect Dis 1998;178 Suppl 1:S81–4.

40. Menke JJ, Heins JR. Treatment of postherpetic neuralgia. J Am Pharm Assoc 1999;39:217–21.

41. Robotham M, Harden N, Stacey B, et al. Gabapentin for the treatment of postherpetic neuralgia: a randomized controlled trial. J Am Med Assoc 1998;280:1837–42.

42. Kazmierowski JA, Wuepper KD. Erythema multiforme: immune complex vasculitis of the superficial cutaneous microvasculature. J Invest Dermatol 1978;71:366.

43. Reed RJ. Erythema multiforme: a clinical syndrome and a histologic complex. Am J Dermatopathol 1985;7:143.

44. Roujeau J-C, Kelly JP, Naldi L, et al. Medication use and the risk of Stevens-Johnson syndrome or toxic epidermal necrolysis. N Engl J Med 1995;333:1600–7.

45. Huff JC. Erythema multiforme and latent herpes simplex infection. Semin Dermatol 1992;11:207–10.

46. Aurelian L, Kokuba H, Burnett JW. Understanding the pathogenesis of HSV-associated erythema multiforme. Dermatology 1998;197:219–22.

47. Malo A, Kampgen E, Wank R. Recurrent herpes simplex virus induced erythema multiforme: different HLA-DQB1 alleles associate with severe mucous membrane versus skin attacks. Scand J Immunol 1998;47:408–11.

48. Weston WL, Morelli JG. Herpes simplex virus–associated erythema multiforme in prepubertal children. Arch Pediatr Adolesc Med 1997;151:1014–6.

49. Wojnarowska F Progesterone induced erythema multiforme. J R Soc Med 1985;78:407.

50. Kroonen LM. Erythema multiforme: case report and discussion. J Am Board Fam Pract 1998;11:63–5.

51. Chan HL, Stern RS, Arndt KA, et al. The incidence of erythema multiforme, Stevens-Johnson syndrome and toxic epidermal necrolysis. A population based study with particular reference to reactions caused by drugs among outpatients. Arch Dermatol 1990;126:43.

52. Stevens AM, Johnson FC. A new eruptive fever associated with stomatitis and ophthalmia. Am J Dis Child 1922;24:526.

53. Lever WF. My concept of erythema multiforme. Am J Dermatolpathol 1985;7:141.

54. Patterson R, Dykewicz MS, Gonzales A, et al. Erythema multiforme and Stevens-Johnson syndrome. Descriptive and therapeutic controversy. Chest 1990;98:331.

55. Pisanty S, Tzukert A, Sheskin J. Erythema multiforme: a clinical study on ninety patients. Ann Dent 1986;45:23.

56. Fine JD. Drug therapy: management of acquired bullous skin diseases. N Engl J Med 1995;333:1475–84.

57. Rodenas JM, Herranz MT, Tercedor J. Autoimmune progesterone dermatitis: treatment with oophorectomy. Br J Dermatol 1998;139:508–11.

58. Tatnall FM, Schofield JK, Leight IM. A double-blind, placebo-controlled trial of continuous acyclovir therapy in recurrent erythema multiforme. Br J Dermatol 1995;132:267–70.

59. Patterson R, Miller M, Kaplan M, et al. Effectiveness of early therapy with corticosteroids in Stevens-Johnson syndrome: experience with 41 cases and a hypothesis regarding pathogenesis. Ann Allergy 1994;73:27–34.

60. Cheriyan S, Patterson R, Greenberger PA, et al. The outcome of Stevens-Johnson syndrome treated with corticosteroids. Allergy Proc 1995;16:151–5.

61. DeRossi SS, Greenberg MS. Intraoral contact allergy: a literature review and case reports. J Am Dent Assoc 1998;129:1435.

62. Pang BK, Freeman S. Oral lichenoid lesions caused by allergy to mercury in amalgam fillings. Contact Dermatitis 1995;33:423–7.

63. Marcusson JA. Contact allergies to nickel sulfate, gold sodium thiosulfate and palladium chloride in patients claiming side-effects from dental alloy components. Contact Dermatitis 1996;34:320–3.

64. Rasanen L, Laimo K, Laine J, et al. Contact allergy to gold in dental patients. Br J Dermatol 1996;134:673–7.

65. Kowitz G, Jacobson J, Meng Z, Lucatorto F. The effects of tartar-control toothpaste on the oral soft tissue. Oral Surg Oral Med Oral Pathol 1990;70:529–36.

66. Sollecito TP, Greenberg MS. Plasma cell gingivitis: a report of two cases. Oral Surg Oral Med Oral Pathol Oral Radiol Endod 1992;73:690.

67. Alanko K, Kanerva L, Jolanki R, et al. Oral mucosal diseases investigated by patch testing with a dental screening series. Contact Dermatitis 1996;34:263–7.

68. Dreizen S, Bodey GP, Rodriquez V. Oral complications of cancer chemotherapy. Postgrad Med 1975;58:75.

69. Dreizen S, McCredie KB, Keating MJ. Chemotherapy induced oral mucositis in adult leukemia. Postgrad Med 1981;69:103.

70. Sonis ST. Mucositis as a biological process: a new hypothesis for the development of chemotherapy induced stomatotoxicity. Oral Oncol 1998;34:39.

71. Loesche WJ, Syed SA, Laughon BE, Stoll J. The bacteriology of acute necrotizing ulcerative gingivitis. J Periodontol 1982;53:223.

72. Giddon DB, Zackin SJ, Goldhaber P. Acute necrotizing ulcerative gingivitis in college students. J Am Dent Assoc 1964;68:381.

73. Winkler JR, Grassi M, Murray PA. Clinical description and etiology of HIV-associated periodontal diseases. In: Robertson PB, Greenspan JS, editors. Perspectives on oral manifestations of AIDS. Proceedings of First International Symposium on Oral Manifestations of AIDS. Littleton (MA): PSG Publishing Company; 1988. p. 49.

74. Holmstrup P, Westergaard J. HIV infection and periodontal disease. Periodontol 2000 1998;18:37.

75. Lamster IB, Grbic JT, Mitchell-Lewis DA, et al. New concepts regarding the pathogenesis of periodontal disease in HIV infection. Ann Periodontol 1998;3:62.

76. Enwonwu CO, Falker WA, Idigbe EO, Savage KO. Noma (cancrum oris) questions and answers. Oral Dis 1999;5:144.

77. Falker WA, Enwonwa CO, Idigbe EO. Microbiological understandings and mysteries of noma. Oral Dis 1999;5:150.

78. Roger RS. Recurrent aphthous stomatitis: clinical characteristics and associated systemic disorders. Semin Cutan Med Surg 1997;16:278–83.

79. Ship II, Ashe WK, Scherp HW. Recurrent "fever blister" and "canker sore" tests for herpes simplex and other viruses with mammalian cell cultures. Arch Oral Biol 1961;3:117.

80. Lennette EH, Magoffin RL. Virologic and immunologic aspects of major oral ulcerations. J Am Dent Assoc 1973;87:1055.

81. Peterson A, Hornsieth A. Recurrent aphthous ulceration: possible clinical manifestations of varicella zoster in cytomegalovirus infection. J Oral Pathol Med 1993;22:64–8.

82. Ghodratnama F, Riggio MP, Wray D. Search for human herpesvirus 6, human cytomegalovirus and varicella zoster virus DNA in current aphthous stomatitis tissue. J Oral Pathol Med 1997;26:192–7.

83. Scully C, Porter S. Recurrent aphthous stomatitis current concepts of etiology, pathogenesis and management. J Oral Pathol Med 1989;18:21.

84. Challacombe SJ, Barkhan P, Lehner T. Hematologic features and differentiation of recurrent oral ulcerations. Br J Oral Surg 1977;15:37.

85. Ship JJ. Epidemiologic aspects of recurrent aphthous ulcerations. Oral Surg 1972;33:400.

86. Miller MF, Garfunkel AA, Ram CA, Ship II. The inheritance of recurrent aphthous stomatitis observations on susceptibility. Oral Surg 1980;49:409.

87. Savage NW, Seymour AJ, Kruger BJ. Expression of class I and class II major histocompatibility complex antigens on epithelial cells in recurrent aphthous stomatitis. J Oral Pathol 1986;15:191.

88. Eversole LR. Immunopathogenesis of oral lichen planus and recurrent aphthous stomatitis. Semin Cutan Med Surg 1997;16:284–94.

89. Rogers RS, Hutton KP. Screening for haematinic deficiencies in patients with recurrent aphthous stomatitis. Aust J Dermatol 1986;27:98.

90. Ferguson MM, Wray D, Carmichael HA, et al. Coeliac disease associated with recurrent aphthae. Gut 1980;21:223.

91. Donatsky O, Bendixen G. In vitro demonstration of cellular hypersensitivity to Strep 2A in recurrent aphthous stomatitis by means of the leukocyte migration test. Acta Allergol 1972;27:137.

92. Thomas DW, Bagg J, Walker DM. Characterization of the effector cells responsible for the in vitro cytotoxicity of blood leucocytes from aphthous ulcer patients for oral epithelial cells. Gut 1990;31:294.

93. Hoover CI, Olson JA, Greenspan JA. Humoral responses and cross-reactivity to viridians streptococci in recurrent aphthous ulceration. J Dent Res 1986;65:1101.

94. Savage NW, Seymour GJ, Kruger BJ. T-lymphocyte subset changes in recurrent aphthous stomatitis. Oral Surg 1985;60:175.

95. Greenspan JL, Gadol N, Olson JA, et al. Lymphocyte function in recurrent aphthous ulceration. J Oral Pathol 1985;14:592.

96. Burnett PR, Wray D. Tyler effects of serum and mononuclear leukocytes on oral epithelial cells in recurrent aphthous stomatitis. Clin Immunol Immunopathol 1985;34:197.

97. Pedersen A, Klausen B, Hougen HP, Stenvang JP. T-lymphocyte subsets in recurrent aphthous ulceration. J Oral Pathol Med 1989;18:59.

98. Galliani EA, Infantolino D, Tarantello M, et al. Recurrent aphthous stomatitis: which role for viruses, food and dental materials? Ann Ital Med Int 1998;13:152–6.

99. Buno IJ, Huff JC, Weston WL, et al. Elevated levels of interferon gamma, tumor necrosis factor alpha, interleukins 2, 4, 5, but not interleukin 10, are present in recurrent aphthous stomatitis. Arch Dermatol 1998;134:827–31.

100. Rennu JS, Reade PC, Hay KD, Scully C. Recurrent aphthous stomatitis. Br Dent J 1985;159:361.

101. Axell T, Henricsson V. Association between recurrent aphthous ulcers and tobacco habits. Scand J Dent Res 1985;93:239.

102. Hay KD, Reade PC. The use of elimination diet in the treatment of recurrent aphthous ulceration in the oral cavity. Oral Surg 1984;57:504.

103. Chahine L, Sempson N, Wagoner C. The effect of sodium lauryl sulfate on recurrent aphthous ulcers: a clinical study. Comp Continu Educ Dent 1997;18:1238–40.

104. Healy CM, Paterson M, Joyston-Bechal S, et al. The effect of sodium lauryl sulfate-free dentifrice on patients with recurrent oral ulceration. Oral Dis 1999;5:39–43.

105. Saxen MA, Ambrosius WT, Rehemtula al-KF, Eckert GJ. Sustained relief of oral aphthous ulcer pain from topical diclofenac in hyaluronan: a randomized, double-blind clinical trial. Oral Surg Oral Med Oral Pathol Oral Radiol Endod 1997;84:356–61.

106. Wahba-Yahav AV. Pentoxifylline in intractable recurrent aphthous stomatitis: an open trial. J AM Acad Dermatol 1995;33:680.

107. Katz J, Langeritz P, Shemer J. Prevention of RAS with colchicines: an open trial. J Am Acad Dermatol 1994;31:459–61.

108. Tananis R, DeRossi S, Sollecito TP, Greenberg MS. Management of recurrent aphthous stomatitis with colchicine and pentoxifylline. Oral Surg Oral Med Oral Pathol Oral Radiol Endod 2000;89:449.

109. Jacobson JM, Greenspan J, Spritzler N, et al. Thalidomide for the treatment of oral aphthous ulcers in patients with human immunodeficiency virus infection. N Engl J Med 1997;336:1487–93.

110. O'Duffy JD. Behçet's syndrome. N Engl J Med 1990;322:326.

111. Kone-Paut I, Yurdakul S, Bahabri SA, et al. Clinical features of Behçet's disease in children: an international collaborative study of 86 cases. J Pediatr 1998;132:721–5.

112. Matsumoto T, Vekusa T, Fukuda Y. Vasculo-Behçet's disease; a pathologic study of eight cases. Hum Pathol 1991;22:45.

113. O'Duffy JD. Vasculitis in Behçet's disease. Rheum Dis Clin North Am 1990;16:423.

114. Yasui K, Ohta K, Kobayashi M, et al. Successful treatment of Behçet disease with pentoxifylline. Ann Intern Med 1996;124:891–3.

115. Benamour S, Zeroual B, Alaoui FZ. Joint manifestation in Behçet's disease: a review of 340 cases. Rev Rhum 1998;65:299-307.

116. Krause I, Uziel Y, Guedj D, et al. Mode of presentation and multisystem involvement in Behçet's disease: the influence of sex and age of disease onset. J Rheumatol 1998;25:1566–9.

117. Imai H, Motegi M, Mizuki N, et al. Mouth and genital ulcers with inflamed cartilage (MAGIC syndrome): a case report and literature review. Am J Med Sci 1997;314:330–2.

118. International Study Group. Criteria for diagnosis of Behçet's disease. Lancet 1990;335:1078.

119. Bang D. Treatment of Behçet's disease. Yonsei Med J 1997;38:401–10.

120. Yazici H, Yurdakul S, Hamuryudan V. Behçet's syndrome. Curr Opin Rhematol 1999;1:53–7.

121. Arici, M, Kiraz S, Ertenli I. Treatment of Behçet disease with pentoxifylline. Ann Intern Med 1997;126:493–4.

122. Masuda K, Nakajima A, Urayama A. Double-masked trial of cyclosporine versus colchicine and long term open study of cyclosporine in Behçet's disease. Lancet 1989;1:1093.

123. O'Duffy JD, Robertson DM, Goldstein NP. Chlorambucil in the treatment of uveitis and meningoencephalitis of Behçet's disease. Am J Med 1984;76:75.

124. Muzulu SI, Walton S, Keczkes K. Colchicine therapy in Behçet's syndrome. A report of five cases. Clin Exp Dermatol 1989;14:298.

125. Eisenbud L, Horowitz I, Kay B. Recurrent aphthous stomatitis of the Behçet's type: successful treatment with thalidomide. Oral Surg 1987;64:289.

126. Blyth WA, Hill TJ. Establishment, maintenance and control of herpes simplex virus (HSV-1) latency. In: Rouse BT, Lopez C, editors. Immunobiology of herpes simplex virus infection. Boca Raton: CRC Press; 1984. p. 9.

127. Roizman B, Sears AE. An inquiry into the mechanism of herpes simplex virus latency. Ann Rev Microbiol 1987;41:543.

128. Croen KD, Ostrove JM, Dragovic MD, et al. Latent herpes simplex virus in human trigeminal ganglia: detection of an immediate early gene "antisense" transcript by in situ hybridization. N Engl J Med 1987;317:1427.

129. Carton CA, Kilbourne ED. Activation of latent herpes simplex by trigeminal sensory-root section. N Engl J Med 1952;246:172.

130. Halford WP, Gebhardt BM, Carr DJ. Mechanisms of herpes simplex virus type 1 reactivation. J Virol 1996;70:5051–60.

131. Greenberg MS, Brightman VJ, Ship II. Clinical and laboratory differentiation of recurrent intra-oral herpes simplex virus infections following fever. J Dent Res 1969;48:435.

132. Griffin JW. Recurrent intraoral herpes simplex virus infection. Oral Surg 1965;19:209.

133. Weathers DR, Griffin JW. Intraoral ulcerations of recurrent herpes simplex and recurrent aphthae—two distinct clinical entities. J Am Dent Assoc 1970;81:81.

134. Reeves WC, Corey L, Adams HG. Risk of recurrence after first episodes of genital herpes: relation of HSV type and antibody response. N Engl J Med 1981;305:315.

135. Greenberg MS, Brightman VJ. Serum immunoglobulins in patients with recurrent intraoral herpes simplex infections. J Dent Res 1971;50:781.

136. Heineman HS, Greenberg MS. Cell protective effect of human saliva specific for herpes simplex virus. Arch Oral Biol 1980;25:257–61.

137. Greenberg MS, Friedman H, Cohen SG, et al. A comparative study of herpes simplex infections in renal transplant and leukemic patients. J Infect Dis 1987;156:280.

138. Greenberg MS, Cohen SG, Boosz B, Friedman H. Oral herpes simplex infections in patients with leukemia. J Am Dent Assoc 1987;114:483.

139. Eisen D. The clinical characteristics of intraoral herpes simplex virus infection in 52 immunocompetent patients. Oral Surg Oral Med Oral Pathol Oral Radiol Endod 1998;86:432-7.

140. Thackray AM, Field HJ. Famciclovir and valacyclovir differ in the prevention of herpes simplex virus type 1 latency in mice: a quantitative study. Antimicrob Agents Chemother 1998;42:1555–62.

141. Thackray AM, Field HJ. Differential effects of famciclovir and valacyclovir on the pathogenesis of herpes simplex virus in a murine infection model including reactivation from latency. J Infect Dis 1996;173:291–9.

142. Reitano M, Tyring S, Lang W, et al. Valacyclovir for the suppression of recurrent genital herpes simplex virus infection: a large-scale dosage range-finding study. International Valacyclovir HSV Study Group. J Infect Dis 1998;178:603–10.

143. Diaz-Mitoma E, Sibbald RG, Shafran SD, et al. Oral famciclovir for the suppression of recurrent genital herpes: a randomized controlled trial. Collaborative Famciclovir Genital Herpes Research Group. JAMA 1998;280:887–92.

144. Rooney JF, Straus SE, Mannix ML, et al. Oral acyclovir to suppress frequently recurrent herpes labialis: a double-blind, placebo-controlled trial. Ann Intern Med 1993;118:268–72.

145. Amagai M, Koch PJ, Nishikawa T, Stanley JR. Pemphigus vulgaris antigen (desmoglein 3) is localized in the lower epidermis, the site of blister formation in patients. J Invest Dermatol 1996;106:351–5.

146. Mahoney MG, Wang Z, Rothenberger K, et al. Explanations for the clinical and microscopic localization of lesions in pemphigus foliaceus and vulgaris. J Clin Invest 1999;103:461–8.

147. Williams DM. Vesiculobullous mucocutaneous disease: pemphigus vulgaris. J Oral Pathol Med 1989;18:544.

148. Anhalt GJ, Labib RS, Voorhees JJ, et al. Induction of pemphigus in neonatal mice by passive transfer of IgG from patients with the disease. N Engl J Med 1982;506:1189–96.

149. Jensen PJ, Baird J, Morioka S, et al. Epidermal plasminogen activation is abnormal in cutaneous lesions. J Invest Dermatol 1988;90:777.

150. Stanley JR. Cell adhesion molecules as targets of autoantibodies in pemphigus and pemphigoid, bullous diseases due to defective epidermal cell adhesion. Adv Immunol 1993;53:291–325.

151. Coleman MD. Dapsone: modes of action, toxicity and possible strategies for increasing patient tolerance. Br J Dermatol 1993;129:507–13.

152. Anhalt GJ. Pemphigoid: bullous and cicatricial. Dermatol Clin 1990;8:701.

153. Gilmore HK. Early detection of pemphigus vulgaris. Oral Surg 1978;46:641.

154. Lamey PJ, Rees TD, Binnie WH, et al. Oral presentation of pemphigus vulgaris and its response to systemic steroid therapy. Oral Surg 1992;74:54.

155. Zegarelli DJ, Zegarelli EV. Intraoral pemphigus vulgaris. Oral Surg 1977;44:384.

156. Lenz P, Amagai M, Volc-Platzer B, et al. Desmoglein 3-ELISA: a pemphigus vulgaris–specific diagnostic tool. Arch Dermatol 1999;135:143–148.

157. Nishikawa T. Desmoglein ELISAs: a novel diagnostic test for pemphigus. Arch Dermatol 1999;135:195–6.

158. Chrysommlis F, Ioannides D, Teknetzis A, et al. Treatment of oral pemphigus vulgaris. Int J Dermatol 1994;33:803–7.

159. Stanley JR. Therapy of pemphigus vulgaris. Arch Dermatol 1999;135:76–7.

160. Enk AH. Mycophenolate is effective in the treatment pemphigus vulgaris. Arch Dermatol 1999;135:54–6.

161. Calebotta A, Saenz AM, Gonzalez F, et al. Pemphigus vulgaris: benefits of tetracycline as adjuvant therapy in a series of thirteen patients. Int J Dermatol 1999;38:217–21.

162. Rook AH, Jegasothy BV, Heald P, et al. Extracorporeal photochemotherapy for drug-resistant pemphigus vulgaris. Ann Intern Med 1990;112:303.

163. Nousari HC, Deterding R, Wojtczak KH, et al. The mechanism of respiratory failure in paraneoplastic pemphigus. N Engl J Med 1999;340:1406–10.

164. Anhalt GJ. Paraneoplastic pemphigus. Adv Dermatol 1997;12:77–96.

165. Virgils A, Trombelli L, Calura G. Sudden vegetation of the mouth. Pemphigus vegetans of the mouth (Hallopeau type). Arch Dermatol 1992;128:398.

166. Iwata M, Watanabe S, Tamaki K. Pemphigus vegetans presenting as scrotal tongue. J Dermatol 1989;16:159.

167. Thornhill MH, Zakrzewska JM, Gilkes JJ. Pyostomatitis vegetans. Report of three cases and review of the literature. J Oral Pathol Med 1992;21:128.

168. Korman NJ. Bullous pemphigoid: the latest in diagnosis, prognosis and therapy. Arch Dermatol 1998;134:1137–41.

169. Bastuji-Garin S, Joly P, Picard-Dahan C, et al. Drugs associated with bullous pemphigoid: a case-control study. Arch Dermatol 1996;132:272–6.

170. Venning VA, Frith PA, Bron AJ, et al. Mucosal involvement in bullous and cicatricial pemphigoid. A clinical and immunopathological study. Br J Dermatol 1988;118:7.

171. Roujeau JC, Lok C, Bastuji-Garin S, et al. High risk of death in elderly patients with extensive bullous pemphigoid. Arch Dermatol 1998;134:465.

172. Lever WF. Pemphigus and pemphigoid. J Am Acad Dermatol 1979;1:2.

173. Chan LS, Hammerberg C, Cooper KD. Cicatricial pemphigoid. Identification of two distinct sets of epidermal antigens by IgA and IgG class circulating autoantibodies. Arch Dermatol 1990;126:1466.

174. Albritton JI, Nousari HC, Anhalt GJ. Antiepiligrin (laminin-5) cicatricial pemphigoid. Br J Dermatol 1997;137:992–6.

175. Nousari HC, Rencic A, Hsu R, et al. Anti-epiligrin cicatricial pemphigoid with antibodies against the gamma2 subunit of laminin 5. Arch Dermatol 1999;135:173–6.

176. Lamey PJ, Rees TD, Binnie WH, Rankin KV. Mucous membrane pemphigoid. Treatment experience at two institutions. Oral Surg 1992;74:50.

177. Rogers RS, Mehregan DA. Dapsone therapy of cicatricial pemphigoid. Semin Dermatol 1988;7:201.

178. Ciarrocca KN, Greenberg MS. A retrospective study of the management of oral mucous membrane pemphigoid with dapsone. Oral Surg Oral Med Oral Pathol Oral Radiol Endod 1999;88:159–63.

179. Berk MA, Lorincz AL. The treatment of bullous pemphigoid with tetracycline and nicotinamide. Arch Dermatol 1986;122:670.

180. Korman NJ, Eyra RW, Zone J, Stanley JR. Drug-induced pemphigus. J Invest Dermatol 1991;96:273.

181. Wakelin SH, Allen J, Zhou S, Wojnarowska F. Drug-induced linear IgA disease with antibodies to collagen vii. Br J Dermatol 1998;138:310.

182. Zhou S, Ferguson DJ, Allen J, Wojnarowska F. The localization of target antigens and autoantibodies is variable. Br J Dermatol 1998;139:591.

183. Dabelsteen E. Molecular biological aspects of acquired bullous diseases. Crit Rev Oral Biol Med 1998;9:162.

184. Marsden RA. Linear IgA disease of childhood. In: Wojnarowska F, Briggaman RA, editors. Management of blistering diseases. New York: Chapman & Hall; 1990. p. 119–26.

185. Lear JT, Smith AG. Multiple blisters in a young boy. Arch Dermatol 1998;134:625.

186. Marsden RA, Mckee PH, Bhogal B, et al. A study of chronic bullous disease of childhood and comparison with dermatitis herpetiformis and bullous pemphigoid occurring in childhood. Clin Exp Dermatol 1980;5:159.

187. Greenspan JS, Yeoman CM, Harding SM. Oral lichen planus. Br Dent J 1978;144:83.

188. Walsh LJ, Savage NW, Ishii T, Seymour GJ. Immunopathogenesis of oral lichen planus. J Oral Pathol Med 1990;19:389.

189. Bolewska J, Hansen HJ, Holmstrup P, et al. Oral mucosal lesions related to silver amalgam restorations. Oral Surg 1990;70:55.

190. Carrozzo M, Gandolpho S, Carbone M, et al. Hepatitis C virus infection in Italian patients with oral lichen planus: a prospective case controlled study. J Oral Pathol Med 1997;26:36.

191. Bagan JV, Ramon C, Gonzalez L, et al. Preliminary investigation of the association of oral lichen planus and hepatitis C. Oral Surg Oral Med Oral Pathol Oral Radiol Endod 1998;85:532.

192. DeRossi S, Greenberg MS. Intraoral contact allergy: a literature review and case reports. J Am Dent Assoc 1998;129:1435.

193. Yiannias JA, el Azhary RA, Hand JH, et al. Relevant contact sensitivities in patients with the diagnosis of oral lichen planus. J Am Acad of Dermatol 2000;42:177.

194. Schubert MM, Sullivan KM. Recognition, incidence and management of oral graft-versus-host disease. N C I Monogr 1990;9:135.

195. Fowler CB, Rees TD, Smith BR. Squamous cell carcinoma on the dorsum of the tongue arising in a longstanding lesion of erosive lichen planus. J Am Dent Assoc 1987;15:707.

196. Katz RW, Brahim JS, Travis WD. Oral squamous cell carcinoma arising in a patient with longstanding lichen planus: a case report. Oral Surg 1990;70:282.

197. Lind PO, Koppang HS, Eigil AAS. Malignant transformation in oral lichen planus. Int J Oral Surg 1985;14:509.

198. Kaplan B, Barnes L. Oral lichen planus and squamous carcinoma: case report and update of the literature. Arch Otolaryngol 1985;111:543.

199. Massa MC, Greancy V, Kron T, Armin A. Malignant transformation of oral lichen planus: case report and review of the literature. Cutis 1990;45:45.

200. Silverman S, Gorsky M, Lozada-Nur F. A prospective follow-up study of 570 patients with oral lichen planus: persistence, remission and malignant association. Oral Surg 1985;60:30.

201. Murti PR, Daftary DK, Bhonsle RR, et al. Malignant potential of oral lichen planus: observations in 722 patients from India. J Oral Pathol 1986;15:71.

202. Jungell P. Oral lichen planus. A review. Int J Oral Maxillofac Surg 1991;20:129.

203. Eisen D, Ellis CN, Duell EA, et al. Effect of topical cyclosporine rinse on oral lichen planus. A double blind analysis. N Engl J Med 1990;323:290.

204. Jungell P, Malmstrom M. Cyclosporin A mouthwash in the treatment of oral lichen planus. Int J Oral Maxillofac Surg 1996;25:60.

205. Gorsky M, Raviv M. Efficacy of etretinate (Tigason) in symptomatic oral lichen planus. Oral Surg 1992;73:52.

206. Lundquist G, Forsgren H, Gajecki M, et al. Photochemotherapy of oral lichen planus. A controlled study. Oral Surg Oral Med Oral Pathol Oral Radiol Endod 1995;79:554

207. McCreary CE, McCartan BE. Clinical management of oral lichen planus. Br J Oral Maxillofac Surg 1999;37:338.

208. Greenberg MS, Cohen SG, Boosz B, Friedman H. Oral herpes simplex infections in patients with leukemia. J Am Dent Assoc 1987;114:483.

209. Greenberg MS, Friedman H, Cohen SG, et al. A comparative study of herpes simplex infections in renal transplant and leukemic patients. J Infect Dis 1987;156:280.

210. Schneidman DW, Barr RJ, Graham JH. Chronic cutaneous herpes simplex. JAMA 1979;241:542.

211. MacPhail LA, Greenspan D, Schiodt M, et al. Acyclovir-resistant Foscarnet-sensitive oral herpes simplex type 2 lesion in a patient with AIDS. Oral Surg 1989;67:427.

212. Economopoulou P, Laskaris G, Kittas C. Oral histoplasmosis as an indicator of HIV infection. Oral Surg Oral Med Oral Pathol Oral Radiol Endod 1998;86:203.

213. Warnakulasuriya KAAS, Harrison JD, Johnson NW, et al. Localized oral histoplasmosis associated with HIV infection. J Oral Pathol Med 1997;26:294.

214. Chinn H, Chernoff DN, Migliorati CA, et al. Oral histoplasmosis in HIV infected patients: a report of two cases. Oral Surg Oral Med Oral Pathol Oral Radiol Endod 1995;79:710.

215. Page LR, Drummond JF, Daniels HT, et al. Blastomycosis with oral lesions. Oral Surg 1979;47:157.

216. Bell WA, Gamble GE, Garrington GE. North American blastomycosis with oral lesions. Oral Surg 1969;28:914.

217. Rose HD, Gingrass DJ. Localized oral blastomycosis mimicking actinomycosis. Oral Surg 1982;54:12.

218. Cohen SG, Greenberg MS. Rhinomaxillary mucormycosis in a kidney transplant patient. Oral Surg 1980;50:33.

219. Salisbury PL, Caloss R, Cruz JM, et al. Mucormycosis of the mandible after dental extractions in a patient with acute myelogenous leukemia. Oral Surg Oral Med Oral Pathol Oral Radiol Endod 1997;83:340.

220. Jones AC, Bentsen TY, Freedman PD. Mucormycosis of the oral cavity. Oral Surg 1993;75:455.

5

RED AND WHITE LESIONS OF THE ORAL MUCOSA

INDRANEEL BHATTACHARYYA, DDS, MSD
DONALD M. COHEN, DMD, MS, MBA
SOL SILVERMAN JR., DDS, MS

Any condition that increases the thickness of the epithelium causes it to appear white by increasing the distance to the vascular bed. Lesions most often appear white because of a thickening of the keratin layer, or hyperkeratosis. Other common causes of a white appearance include acanthosis (a thickening of the spinous cell layer), an increase in the amount of edema fluid in the epithelium (ie, leukoedema), and reduced vascularity in the underlying lamina propria. Surface ulcerations covered by a fibrin cap can also appear white, as would collapsed bullae. (These latter two types of lesions are covered in Chapter 4, "Ulcerative, Vesicular, and Bullous Lesions.")

▼ HEREDITARY WHITE LESIONS

Leukoedema

Leukoedema is a common mucosal alteration that represents a variation of the normal condition rather than a true pathologic change.[1,2] It has been reported in up to 90% of black adults and up to 50% of black teenagers.[3,4] The incidence in white persons in different studies is highly variable (10 to 90%).[3] This difference can be attributed to the darker coloration of the mucosa in black persons, rendering the alteration more visible.[5,6] Similar edematous changes have been reported in other mucosal surfaces, such as the vagina and larynx.[5]

FEATURES

The most frequent site of leukoedema is the buccal mucosa bilaterally, and it may be seen rarely on the labial mucosa, soft palate, and floor of the mouth. It usually has a faint, white, diffuse, and filmy appearance, with numerous surface folds resulting in wrinkling of the mucosa (Figure 5-1). It cannot be scraped off, and it disappears or fades upon stretching the mucosa. Microscopic examination reveals thickening of the epithelium, with significant intracellular edema of the stratum spinosum. The surface of the epithelium may demonstrate a thickened layer of parakeratin.

TREATMENT

No treatment is indicated for leukoedema since it is a variation of the normal condition. No malignant change has been reported.[2]

White Sponge Nevus

White sponge nevus (WSN) is a rare autosomal dominant disorder with a high degree of penetrance and variable expressivity; it predominantly affects noncornified stratified squamous epithelium.[7] The disease usually involves the oral mucosa and (less frequently) the mucous membranes of the nose, esophagus, genitalia, and rectum.[7,8] The lesions of WSN may be present at birth or may first manifest or become more intense at puberty. Genetic analyses of families with WSN have identified a missense mutation in one allele of keratin 13 that leads to proline substitution for leucine within the keratin gene cluster on chromosome 17.[9,10] A new study, using sequence analysis, has reported a glutamine insertion localized in the helix initiation motif of the 1A alpha helical domain of Keratin 4 gene.[9]

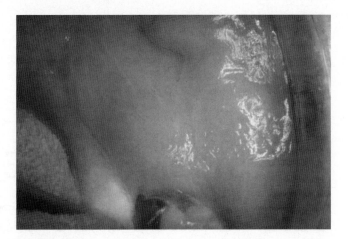

FIGURE 5-1   Leukoedema with a faint white diffuse filmy appearance and mild wrinkling of the mucosa.

FEATURES

White sponge nevus presents as bilateral symmetric white, soft, "spongy," or velvety thick plaques of the buccal mucosa. However, other sites in the oral cavity may be involved, including the ventral tongue, floor of the mouth, labial mucosa, soft palate, and alveolar mucosa. The condition is usually asymptomatic and does not exhibit tendencies toward malignant change. The characteristic histopathologic features are epithelial thickening, parakeratosis, a peculiar perinuclear condensation of the cytoplasm, and vacuolization of the suprabasal layer of keratinocytes. Electron microscopy of exfoliated cells shows numerous cellular granules composed of disordered aggregates of tonofilaments.[7,8]

DIFFERENTIAL DIAGNOSIS

The lesions of WSN may be grossly similar to those of other hereditary mucosal syndromes such as hereditary benign intraepithelial dyskeratosis or pachyonychia congenita, infections such as candidiasis, traumatic lesions seen in cheek chewing, and chemical burns or preneoplastic/neoplastic processes.[7] This differential diagnosis is best resolved in many cases by incisional biopsy specimens interpreted in the context of the clinical history and physical findings.[8]

TREATMENT

No treatment is indicated for this benign and asymptomatic condition. Patients may require palliative treatment if the condition is symptomatic. One study has reported some relief of symptoms with a tetracycline rinse.[11]

Hereditary Benign Intraepithelial Dyskeratosis

Hereditary benign intraepithelial dyskeratosis (HBID), also known as Witkop's disease, is a rare autosomal dominant disorder characterized by oral lesions and bilateral limbal conjunctival plaques.[12,13] This condition is noted specifically in a triracial isolate of white, Native American, and African American people and their descendants in Halifax county, North Carolina. It exhibits a high degree of penetrance.[12]

FEATURES

The oral lesions are similar to those of WSN, with thick, corrugated, asymptomatic, white "spongy" plaques involving the buccal and labial mucosa. Other intraoral sites include the floor of the mouth, the lateral tongue, the gingiva, and the palate. The oral lesions are generally detected in the first year of life and gradually increase in intensity until the teens. The most significant aspect of HBID involves the bulbar conjunctiva, where thick, gelatinous, foamy, and opaque plaques form adjacent to the cornea. The ocular lesions manifest very early in life (usually within the first year). Some patients exhibit chronic relapsing ocular irritation and photophobia. The plaques may exhibit seasonal prominence, with many patients reporting more-pronounced lesions in the spring and regression during the summer months. A few cases of blindness due to corneal vascularization following HBID have been reported.[12] The histopathologic features of HBID are characteristic, and the epithelium exhibits marked parakeratin production with thickening of the stratum spinosum and the presence of numerous dyskeratotic cells. Ultrastructural findings in patients with HBID reveal the the presence of numerous vesicular bodies in immature dyskeratotic cells, densely packed tonofilaments within the cytoplasm of these cells, and the disappearance of cellular bridging in mature dyskeratotic cells.[14]

TREATMENT

Since HBID is a benign condition, no treatment is required for the oral lesions. For evaluation and treatment of the ocular lesions, the patient should be referred to an ophthalmologist.[12]

Dyskeratosis Congenita

Dyskeratosis congenita, a recessively inherited genodermatosis, is unusual due to the high incidence of oral cancer in young affected adults.[15] It is a rare X-linked disorder characterized by a series of oral changes that lead eventually to an atrophic leukoplakic oral mucosa, with the tongue and cheek most severely affected.[15] The oral changes occur in association with severely dystrophic nails and a prominent reticulated hyperpigmentation of the skin of the face, neck, and chest.[15] Many cases also exhibit hematologic changes including pancytopenia, hypersplenism, and an aplastic or Fanconi's anemia (ie, an anemia associated with an inherited inability to repair deoxyribonucleic acid [DNA] defects, leading to a high frequency of leukemia and lymphoma).[16,17]

The oral lesions commence before the age of 10 years as crops of vesicles with associated patches of white ulcerated necrotic mucosa often infected with *Candida*. Erythroplakic changes and nail dystrophy follow, with leukoplakic lesions and carcinoma supervening on the oral lesions in early adulthood.[15]

▼ REACTIVE AND INFLAMMATORY WHITE LESIONS

Linea Alba (White Line)

As the name implies, linea alba is a horizontal streak on the buccal mucosa at the level of the occlusal plane extending from the commissure to the posterior teeth. It is a very common finding and is most likely associated with pressure, frictional irritation, or sucking trauma from the facial surfaces of the teeth. This alteration was present in about 13% of the population in one study.[18–20]

CLINICAL FEATURES

Linea alba is usually present bilaterally and may be pronounced in some individuals. It is more prominent in individuals with reduced overjet of the posterior teeth. It is often scalloped and restricted to dentulous areas.[18]

TREATMENT

No treatment is indicated for patients with linea alba. The white streak may disappear spontaneously in some people.[18,19]

Frictional (Traumatic) Keratosis

CLINICAL FEATURES

Frictional (traumatic) keratosis is defined as a white plaque with a rough and frayed surface that is clearly related to an identifiable source of mechanical irritation and that will usually resolve on elimination of the irritant. These lesions may occasionally mimic dysplastic leukoplakia; therefore, careful examination and sometimes a biopsy are required to rule out any atypical changes.[20,21] Histologically, such lesions show varying degrees of hyperkeratosis and acanthosis.[22] Prevalence rates as high as 5.5% have been reported.[21] Such lesions are similar to calluses on the skin. Traumatic keratosis has never been shown to undergo malignant transformation.[23] Lesions belonging to this category of keratosis include linea alba and cheek, lip, and tongue chewing. Frictional keratosis is frequently associated with rough or maladjusted dentures (Figure 5-2) and with sharp cusps and edges of broken teeth.[20]

TREATMENT

Upon removal of the offending agent, the lesion should resolve within 2 weeks. Biopsies should be performed on lesions that do not heal to rule out a dysplastic lesion.

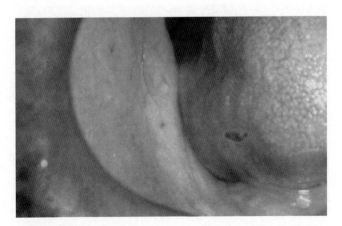

FIGURE 5-2 Leukoplakic-appearing area of frictional keratosis from an ill-fitting denture.

Cheek Chewing

White lesions of the oral tissues may result from chronic irritation due to repeated sucking, nibbling, or chewing.[24–29] These insults result in the traumatized area becoming thickened, scarred, and paler than the surrounding tissues. Cheek chewing is most commonly seen in people who are under stress or in psychological situations in which cheek and lip biting become habitual. Most patients with this condition are somewhat aware of their habit but do not associate it with their lesions. The white lesions of cheek chewing may sometimes be confused with other dermatologic disorders involving the oral mucosa, which can lead to misdiagnosis.[30] Chronic chewing of the labial mucosa (morsicatio labiorum) and the lateral border of the tongue (morsicatio linguarum) may be seen with cheek chewing or may cause isolated lesions. Prevalence rates ranging from 0.12 to 0.5% have been reported in Scandinavian populations, compared with a prevalence rate of 4.6% for South African school children in mental health treatment facilities; these rates support the role of stress and anxiety in the etiology of this condition.[26–28]

TYPICAL FEATURES

The lesions are most frequently found bilaterally on the posterior buccal mucosa along the plane of occlusion. They may be seen in combination with traumatic lesions on the lips or tongue. Patients often complain of roughness or small tags of tissue that they actually tear free from the surface. This produces a distinctive frayed clinical presentation (Figure 5-3). The lesions are poorly outlined whitish patches that may be intermixed with areas of erythema or ulceration. The occurrence is twice as prevalent in females and three times more common after the age of 35 years.

The histopathologic picture is distinctive and includes hyperparakeratosis and acanthosis. The keratin surface is usually shaggy and ragged with numerous projections of keratin that demonstrate adherent bacterial colonies. When the lesion is seen on the lateral tongue, the clinical and histomorphologic features mimic those of oral hairy leukoplakia.[29]

TREATMENT AND PROGNOSIS

Since the lesions result from an unconscious and/or nervous habit, no treatment is indicated. However, for those desiring treatment and unable to stop the chewing habit, a plastic occlusal night guard may be fabricated. Isolated tongue involvement requires further investigation to rule out oral hairy leukoplakia especially when appropriate risk factors for infection with human immunodeficiency virus (HIV) are present. Differential diagnosis also includes WSN, chemical burns, and candidiasis.

Chemical Injuries of the Oral Mucosa

Transient nonkeratotic white lesions of the oral mucosa are often a result of chemical injuries caused by a variety of agents that are caustic when retained in the mouth for long periods of time, such as aspirin, silver nitrate, formocresol, sodium hypochlorite, paraformaldehyde, dental cavity varnishes, acid-etching materials, and hydrogen peroxide.[31–42] The white lesions are attributable to the formation of a superficial pseudomembrane composed of a necrotic surface tissue and an inflammatory exudate.

SPECIFIC CAUSATIVE AGENTS

Aspirin Burn. Acetylsalicylic acid (aspirin) is a common source of burns of the oral cavity.[43–45] Usually, the tissue is damaged when aspirin is held in the mucobuccal fold area for prolonged periods of time for the relief of common dental pain (Figure 5-4).

Silver Nitrate. Silver nitrate is commonly used by health care practitioners as a chemical cautery agent for the treatment of aphthous ulcers.[46] It brings about almost instantaneous relief of symptoms by burning the nerve endings at the site of the ulcer. However, silver nitrate often destroys tissue around the immediate area of application and may result in delayed healing or (rarely) severe necrosis at the application site (Figure 5-5).[46] Its use should be discouraged.

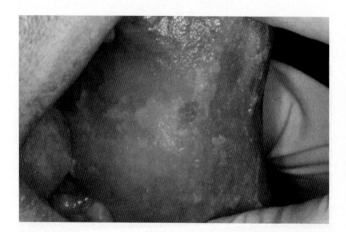

FIGURE 5-3 Morsicatio buccarum represented by a frayed macerated irregular leukoplakic area in the cheek.

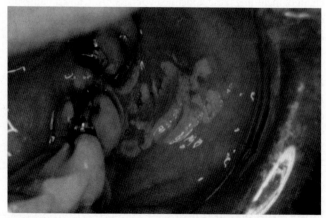

FIGURE 5-4 Aspirin burn, creating a pseudomembranous necrotic white area.

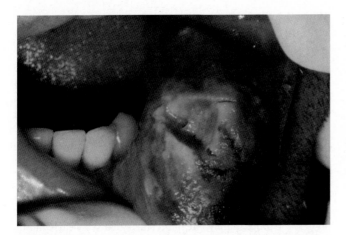

FIGURE 5-5 Extensive tissue necrosis caused by injudicious use of silver nitrate.

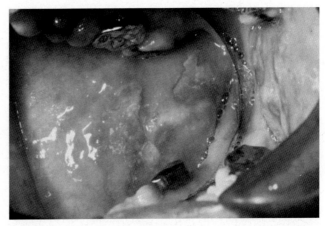

FIGURE 5-7 Severe ulceration and sloughing of mucosa, caused by use of a cinnamon-containing dentifrice.

Hydrogen Peroxide. Hydrogen peroxide is often used as an intraoral rinse for the prevention of periodontal disease. At concentrations of ≥ 3%, hydrogen peroxide is associated with epithelial necrosis.[40]

Sodium Hypochlorite. Sodium hypochlorite, or dental bleach, is commonly used as a root canal irrigant and may cause serious ulcerations due to accidental contact with oral soft tissues.[32]

Dentifrices and Mouthwashes. Several cases of oral injuries and ulcerations due to the misuse of commercially available mouthwashes and dentifrices have been reported (Figure 5-6).[31,33,42,47] An unusual sensitivity reaction with severe ulcerations and sloughing of the mucosa has been reported to have been caused by a cinnamon-flavored dentifrice (Figure 5-7). However, these lesions probably represent a sensitivity or allergic reaction to the cinnamon aldehyde in the toothpaste.[47] This reaction can appear to be very similar to the reactions caused by other chemical agents such as aspirin and hydrogen

peroxide. Caustic burns of the lips, mouth, and tongue have been seen in patients who use mouthwashes containing alcohol and chlorhexidine.[33,42] A case of an unusual chemical burn, confined to the masticatory mucosa and produced by abusive ingestion of fresh fruit and by the concomitant excessive use of mouthwash, has also been reported.[42]

TYPICAL FEATURES

The lesions are usually located on the mucobuccal fold area and gingiva. The injured area is irregular in shape, white, covered with a pseudomembrane, and very painful. The area of involvement may be extensive. When contact with the tissue is brief, a superficial white and wrinkled appearance without resultant necrosis is usually seen. Long-term contact (usually with aspirin, sodium hypochlorite, phenol, paraformaldehyde, etc) can cause severer damage and sloughing of the necrotic mucosa. The unattached nonkeratinized tissue is more commonly affected than the attached mucosa.

TREATMENT AND PROGNOSIS

The best treatment of chemical burns of the oral cavity is prevention. Children especially should be supervised while taking aspirin tablets, to prevent prolonged retention of the agent in the oral cavity.[31,41,45] The proper use of a rubber dam during endodontic procedures reduces the risk of iatrogenic chemical burns. Most superficial burns heal within 1 or 2 weeks. A protective emollient agent such as a film of methyl cellulose may provide relief.[37,45] However, deep-tissue burns and necrosis may require careful débridement of the surface, followed by antibiotic coverage. In case of ingestion of caustic chemicals or accidental exposure to severely corrosive agents, extensive scarring that may require surgery and/or prosthetic rehabilitation may occur.[48]

Actinic Keratosis (Cheilitis)

Actinic (or solar) keratosis is a premalignant epithelial lesion that is directly related to long-term sun exposure.[49] These lesions are classically found on the vermilion border of the

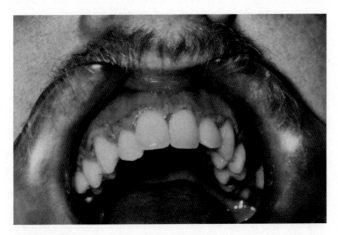

FIGURE 5-6 Diffuse slough of marginal gingivae due to misuse of commercial mouthwash.

lower lip as well as on other sun-exposed areas of the skin. A small percentage of these lesions will transform into squamous cell carcinoma.[50] Biopsies should be performed on lesions that repeatedly ulcerate, crust over, or show a thickened white area. These lesions are commonly found in individuals with extensive sun exposure, such as those with outdoor occupations and/or fair complexions.[49]

TYPICAL FEATURES

Actinic keratosis may be seen on the skin of the forehead, cheeks, ears, and forearms. On the lip, it appears as a white plaque, oval to linear in shape, usually measuring < 1 cm in size (Figure 5-8). The surface may be crusted and rough to the touch. Histopathologically, the surface epithelium appears atrophic, with a basophilic homogenous amorphous alteration of the collagen (solar elastosis) in the lamina propria. Varying degrees of atypical features such as increased nucleocytoplasmic ratios, loss of cellular polarity and orientation, and nuclear and cellular atypia are found within the epithelium. A mild lymphocytic infiltrate may also be noted in the lamina propria.[49]

TREATMENT AND PROGNOSIS

The mainstay of treatment of actinic keratosis is surgery. Chemotherapeutic agents such as topical 5-fluorouracil have been used with some success.[50] However, follow-up biopsies in individuals who were treated with 5-fluorouracil showed that the dysplastic changes persist in clinically healthy-appearing epithelium. Patients treated with nonsurgical methods therefore require long-term follow-up. About 10% of these lesions will undergo malignant transformation.[51]

Smokeless Tobacco–Induced Keratosis

Chewing tobacco is an important established risk factor for the development of oral carcinoma in the United States.[52] Habitually chewing tobacco leaves or dipping snuff results in the development of a well-recognized white mucosal lesion in the area of tobacco contact, called smokeless tobacco keratosis, snuff dipper's keratosis, or tobacco pouch keratosis.[53]

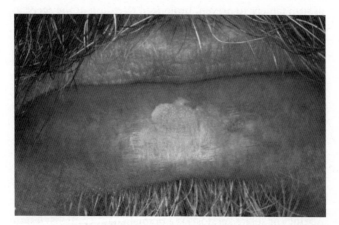

FIGURE 5-8 Distinctive raised white plaque, representing actinic cheilitis.

While these lesions are accepted as precancerous, they are significantly different from true leukoplakia and have a much lower risk of malignant transformation.[54]

This habit was once almost universal in the United States and is very common among certain other populations, most notably in Sweden, India, and Southeast Asia.[52,55–60] Smokeless tobacco use among white males in the United States has shown a recent resurgence.[60–62] The estimated proportion of adult men in the United States who regularly use "spit" tobacco ranges from 6 to 20%.[58,63] This range is attributed to significant geographic, cultural, and gender variations in chewing habits.[54] The cumulative incidence for smokeless tobacco use was highest for non-Hispanic white males.[54] Unfortunately, the habit starts relatively early in life, usually between the ages of 9 and 15 years, and is rarely begun after 20 years of age. Recent epidemiologic data indicate that over five million Americans use smokeless tobacco and that more than 750,000 of these users are adolescents. It is estimated that each year in the United States, approximately 800,000 young people between the ages of 11 and 19 years experiment with smokeless tobacco and that about 300,000 become regular users.[55–59,63]

Smokeless tobacco contains several known carcinogens, including N-nitrosonornicotine (NNN), and these have been proven to cause mucosal alterations.[64] In addition to its established role as a carcinogen, chewing tobacco may be a risk factor in the development of root surface caries and, to a lesser extent, coronal caries. This may be due to its high sugar content and its association with increased amounts of gingival recession.[58] The duration of exposure is very important in the production of mucosal damage. Leukoplakia has been reported to develop with the habitual use of as little as three cans of snuff per week for longer than 3 years.[53] Although all forms of smokeless tobacco may result in mucosal alterations, snuff (a finely powdered tobacco) appears to be much more likely to cause such changes than is chewing tobacco.[53,59]

Smokeless tobacco is not consistently associated with increased rates of oral cancer.[54] Approximately 20% of all adult Swedish males use moist snuff, yet it has not been possible to detect any significant increase in the incidence of cancer of the oral cavity or pharynx in Sweden. By international standards, the prevalence of oral cancer is low in Sweden.[52] This has been attributed to variations in the composition of snuff, in particular, the amount of fermented or cured tobacco in the mixture. The carcinogen NNN is present in much lower concentrations in Swedish snuff, probably because of a lack of fermentation of the tobacco. Also, the high level of snuff use might decrease the amount of cigarette smoking and therefore lead to a lesser prevalence of oral cancer.[52,54]

TYPICAL FEATURES

Numerous alterations are found in habitual users of smokeless tobacco. Most changes associated with the use of smokeless tobacco are seen in the area contacting the tobacco. The most common area of involvement is the anterior mandibular vestibule, followed by the posterior vestibule.[53] The surface of the mucosa

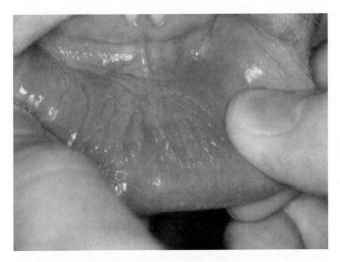

FIGURE 5-9 Snuff pouch with a white wrinkled mucosal surface.

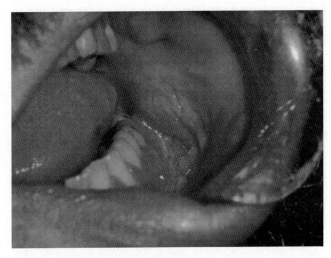

FIGURE 5-11 White leathery nodular tobacco pouch. These thickened areas are more worrisome for malignant transformation.

appears white and is granular or wrinkled (Figure 5-9); in some cases, a folded character may be seen (tobacco pouch keratosis). Commonly noted is a characteristic area of gingival recession with periodontal-tissue destruction in the immediate area of contact (Figure 5-10). This recession involves the facial aspect of the tooth or teeth and is related to the amount and duration of tobacco use. The mucosa appears gray or gray-white and almost translucent. Since the tobacco is not in the mouth during examination, the usually stretched mucosa appears fissured or rippled, and a "pouch" is usually present. This white tobacco pouch may become leathery or nodular in long-term heavy users (Figure 5-11). Rarely, an erythroplakic component may be seen. The lesion is usually asymptomatic and is discovered on routine examination. Microscopically, the epithelium is hyperkeratotic and thickened. A characteristic vacuolization or edema may be seen in the keratin layer and in the superficial epithelium. Frank dysplasia is uncommon in tobacco pouch keratosis.[62]

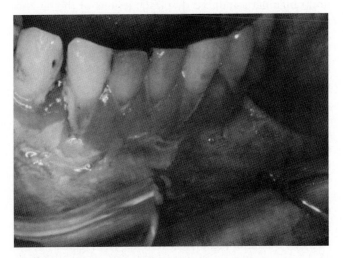

FIGURE 5-10 Snuff pouch showing extensive periodontal tissue destruction and a thickened area of leukoplakia. (Courtesy of Dr. Robert Howell, West Virginia University, School of Dentistry)

TREATMENT AND PROGNOSIS

Cessation of use almost always leads to a normal mucosal appearance within 1 to 2 weeks.[54,64,65] Biopsy specimens should be obtained from lesions that remain after 1 month. Biopsy is particularly indicated for those lesions that appear clinically atypical and that include such features as surface ulceration, erythroplakia, intense whiteness, or a verrucoid or papillary surface.[53,62,64] The risk of malignant transformation is increased fourfold for chronic smokeless tobacco users.[66]

Nicotine Stomatitis

Nicotine stomatitis (stomatitis nicotina palati, smoker's palate) refers to a specific white lesion that develops on the hard and soft palate in heavy cigarette, pipe, and cigar smokers. The lesions are restricted to areas that are exposed to a relatively concentrated amount of hot smoke during inhalation. Areas covered by a denture are usually not involved. The lesion has become less common since pipe smoking has lost popularity. Although it is associated closely with tobacco smoking, the lesion is not considered to be premalignant.[67–69] Interestingly, nicotine stomatitis also develops in individuals with a long history of drinking extremely hot beverages.[70] This suggests that heat, rather than toxic chemicals in tobacco smoke, is the primary cause. Prevalence rates as high as 1.0 to 2.5% have been reported in populations of different cultures.[69–72] "Reverse smoking" (ie, placing the burning end of the cigarette in the oral cavity), seen in South American and Asian populations, produces significantly more pronounced palatal alterations that may be erythroleukoplakic and that are definitely considered premalignant.[73]

TYPICAL FEATURES

This condition is most often found in older males with a history of heavy long-term cigar, pipe, or cigarette smoking. Due to the chronic insult, the palatal mucosa becomes diffusely gray or white (Figure 5-12, A). Numerous slightly elevated papules with punctate red centers that represent inflamed and metaplastically altered minor salivary gland ducts are noted.

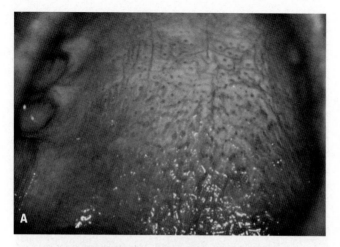

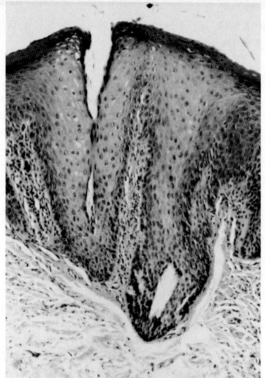

FIGURE 5-12   A, Nicotine stomatitis with diffuse white change in the palatal mucosa, along with elevated papules with red centers. **B,** Histologic appearance of nicotine stomatitis, showing hyperkeratosis and acanthosis with squamous metaplasia of the dilated salivary duct. (Hematoxylin and eosin, ×40 original magnification)

Microscopically, the surface epithelium exhibits hyperkeratosis and acanthosis with squamous metaplasia and hyperplasia of the salivary ducts as they approach the surface (see Figure 5-12, B). The subjacent connective tissue and minor salivary glands exhibit a mild to moderate scattered chronic inflammation. No atypical or dysplastic changes are usually identified.[72]

TREATMENT AND PROGNOSIS

Nicotine stomatitis is completely reversible once the habit is discontinued. The severity of inflammation is proportional to the duration and amount of smoking.[72] The lesions usually resolve within 2 weeks of cessation of smoking. Biopsy of nicotine stomatitis is rarely indicated except to reassure the patient. However, a biopsy should be performed on any white lesion of the palatal mucosa that persists after 1 month of discontinuation of smoking habit.

Sanguinaria-Induced Leukoplakia

Sanguinaria extract, a mixture of benzophenanthridine alkaloids derived from the common bloodroot plant (*Sanguinaria canadensis*), has been used in oral rinses and toothpaste products since 1982. The most widely used product with Sanguinaria, Viadent, has been shown, through extensive clinical trials, to be effective against plaque buildup and gingivitis.[74,75] Importantly, sanguinaria extract has also been shown to be carcinogenic in many studies.[76,77] In 1999, Damm and associates[78] reported an increased prevalence of leukoplakia of the maxillary vestibule in patients who used sanguinaria-based products on a routine basis. They conducted a retrospective review of 88 patients with leukoplakia of the maxillary vestibule and found that 84.1% of the patients reported having used Viadent. The prevalence of Viadent use was only 3% among randomly selected adults in their study. Eversole and colleagues[79] compared and contrasted biomarkers and ploidy data from maxillary gingival leukoplakias associated with dentifrices and mouth rinses containing sanguinaria with those from other forms of benign and premalignant mucosal keratosis. They used computerized image analysis and biomarker immunohistochemical assays to assess ploidy, DNA content, and p53 and proliferating cell nuclear antigen immunoreactivity of nuclei in tissue from these groups. A significantly higher (fourfold) DNA content and higher numbers of cells with hyperploid nuclei were found in the group with sanguinaria-associated keratoses. Although this group did not harbor significant numbers of p53-expressing nuclei, a significant elevation in nuclei labeled with proliferating cell nuclear antigen was noted. The authors concluded that sanguinaria-associated keratoses show marker and image analysis profiles similar to those of non-sanguinaria-induced dysplastic lesions of the lip and mucosa.[79] Hence, preparations containing sanguinaria should be avoided until the risk for malignant transformation is determined.[80] This recommendation is further supported by the lack of regression in some Viadent-induced leukoplakias months after the cessation of Viadent use.

TYPICAL FEATURES

Most patients are adults in the fourth to ninth decades of life. In the study by Damm and colleagues, the range of Viadent use before the development of lesions was 6 months to 12 years, with a mean of 4.4 years.[78] Typically, patients present with a white, velvety, wrinkled or corrugated patch of leukoplakia in the maxillary vestibule, involving both the attached gingiva and vestibular mucosa (Figure 5-13, A). The lesions may also be seen in the anterior mandibular vestibule (see Figure 5-13, B). The area is usually very distinct and sharply demarcated from the surrounding tissue. The lesions are localized to these areas since the anterior portions of the maxillary and mandibular

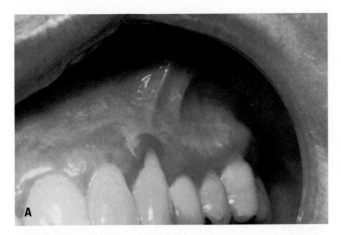

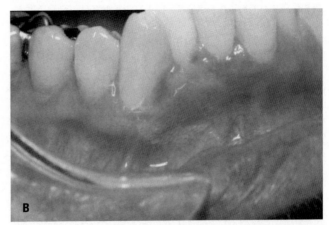

FIGURE 5-13   A, Typical white corrugated leukoplakia in the maxillary vestibule, associated with sanguinaria use. **B,** Mandibular vestibular lesion in the same patient.

vestibule exhibit prolonged retention of the product due to the greater distance from the major salivary ducts. Histopathologically, all biopsy specimens demonstrate significant surface keratosis with a verrucoid pattern. Minimal atypical changes (including basilar hyperplasia, nuclear hyperchromatism, and increased nucleocytoplasmic ratios) limited to the lower one-third of the epithelium are noted in most specimens. More significant atypical changes have also been reported.[78]

TREATMENT

No appropriate treatment has been established for sanguinaria-induced leukoplakia. However, an initial biopsy is mandatory. If a histopathologic diagnosis of dysplasia is rendered, the condition should be treated in a fashion similar to the treatment of other potentially premalignant processes. The less severe changes should be managed according to clinical judgment, depending on the extent and duration of the lesion. In all cases, complete discontinuation of Sanguinaria-containing products and cessation of any other harmful habits such as tobacco or alcohol use is mandatory. All patients should be given careful clinical follow-up, with a biopsy of any recurrent or worsening lesion(s).

▼ INFECTIOUS WHITE LESIONS AND WHITE AND RED LESIONS

Oral Hairy Leukoplakia

Oral hairy leukoplakia is a corrugated white lesion that usually occurs on the lateral or ventral surfaces of the tongue in patients with severe immunodeficiency.[81,82] The most common disease associated with oral hairy leukoplakia is HIV infection.[82] Oral hairy leukoplakia is reported in about 25% of adults with HIV infection but is not as common in HIV-infected children. Its prevalence reaches as high as 80% in patients with acquired immunodeficiency syndrome (AIDS).[83] Epstein-Barr virus (EBV) is implicated as the causative agent in oral hairy leukoplakia.[84–86] A positive correlation with decreasing cluster designation 4 (CD4) cell counts has been

established in HIV-positive patients. The presence of this lesion has been associated with the subsequent development of AIDS in a large percentage of HIV positive patients.[83] Hairy leukoplakia has also occasionally been reported in patients with other immunosuppressive conditions, such as patients undergoing organ transplantation and patients undergoing prolonged steroid therapy.[87–89] Rare cases may occur in immunocompetent persons after topical steroid therapy.[90,91]

TYPICAL FEATURES

Oral hairy leukoplakia most commonly involves the lateral border of the tongue but may extend to the ventral or dorsal surfaces. Lesions on the tongue are usually corrugated and may have a shaggy or frayed appearance, mimicking lesions caused by tongue chewing (Figure 5-14). Oral hairy leukoplakia may also present as a plaquelike lesion and is often bilateral. Histopathologic examination of the epithelium reveals severe hyperparakeratosis with an irregular surface, acanthosis with superficial edema, and numerous koilocytic cells (virally affected

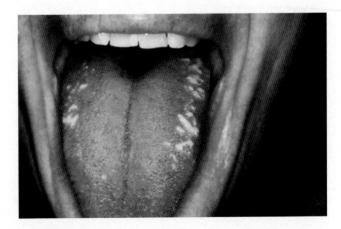

FIGURE 5-14   Bilateral linear leukoplakic lesions on the dorsolateral tongue, suggestive of oral hairy leukoplakia. (Courtesy of Dr. Parnell Taylor, Riverton, Wyoming)

"balloon" cells) in the spinous layer. The characteristic microscopic feature is the presence of homogeneous viral nuclear inclusions with a residual rim of normal chromatin.[92–94] The definitive diagnosis can be established by demonstrating the presence of EBV through in situ hybridization, electron microscopy, or polymerase chain reaction (PCR).[85,86]

DIFFERENTIAL DIAGNOSIS

It is important to differentiate this lesion from other clinically similar entities such as hyperplastic candidiasis, idiopathic leukoplakia, leukoplakia induced by tongue chewing, tobacco-associated leukoplakia, lichen planus, lupus erythematosus, WSN, and verrucous leukoplakia. Since oral hairy leukoplakia is considered to be highly predictive of the development of AIDS, differentiation from other lesions is critical.[95]

TREATMENT AND PROGNOSIS

No treatment is indicated. The condition usually disappears when antiviral medications such as zidovudine, acyclovir, or gancyclovir are used in the treatment of the HIV infection and its complicating viral infections.[81] Topical application of podophyllin resin or tretinoin has led to short-term resolution of the lesions, but relapse is often seen.[81] The probability of patients developing AIDS was found to be 48% at 16 months and as high as 83% at 31 months after the initial diagnosis of oral hairy leukoplakia.[83]

TABLE 5-1 Classification of Oral Candidiasis

Acute

    Pseudomembranous

    Atrophic (erythematous)

        Antibiotic stomatitis

Chronic

    Atrophic

        Denture sore mouth

        Angular cheilitis

        Median rhomboid glossitis

    Hypertrophic/hyperplastic

        Candidal leukoplakia

        Papillary hyperplasia of the palate (see denture sore mouth)

        Median rhomboid glossitis (nodular)

    Multifocal

Mucocutaneous

    Syndrome associated

        Familial +/– endocrine candidiasis syndrome

        Myositis (thymoma associated)

    Localized

    Generalized (diffuse)

Immunocompromise (HIV) associated

HIV = human immunodeficiency virus.

Candidiasis

"Candidiasis" refers to a multiplicity of diseases caused by a yeastlike fungus, *Candida*, and is the most common oral fungal infection in humans. The various diseases are classified in Table 5-1 according to onset and duration (acute or chronic); clinical features, including color (erythematous/atrophic); location (median rhomboid glossitis, denture stomatitis, multifocal candidiasis, and angular cheilitis); the presence of skin lesions as well as oral lesions (mucocutaneous); and association with an immunocompromised host (HIV associated). Other clinical features include a hyperplastic or hypertrophic appearance (papillary hyperplasia of the palate, candidal leukoplakia, and hyperplastic median rhomboid glossitis). *Candida* is predominantly an opportunistic infectious agent that is poorly equipped to invade and destroy tissue. The role of *Candida* as opportunistic invader versus etiologic agent in patients with oral white lesions has not been clearly established. However, the demonstration of the catalytic role of some *Candida* strains in endogenous cellular nitrosamine production,[96] the statistically significant association of certain strains with dysplastic red and white lesions (speckled leukoplakia),[97,98] and the hyperplastic effects on epithelium of *Candida* in vitro,[99] indicate that *Candida* may be a carcinogen or promoting agent, rather than only an innocuous opportunistic infectious entity.

ACUTE PSEUDOMEMBRANOUS CANDIDIASIS (THRUSH)

Clinical Features.   Thrush is the prototype of the oral infections caused by *Candida*. It is a superficial infection of the outer layers of the epithelium, and it results in the formation of patchy white plaques or flecks on the mucosal surface (Figure 5-15, A). Removal of the plaques by gentle rubbing or scraping usually reveals an area of erythema or even shallow ulceration. Because of their prevalence, characteristic appearance, and ease of removal, the lesions of thrush are easily recognized, and a diagnosis of thrush is frequently made on the basis of the appearance of the lesion. A smear demonstrating a yeast or myelin is helpful when the diagnosis is uncertain.

Thrush is seen in children and in adults of all ages whenever the number of *Candida* organisms in the oral cavity increases significantly. When *Candida* is reduced or eliminated by the administration of antifungal agents, the lesions of thrush rapidly disappear. Transient episodes of thrush may occur as isolated phenomena, with lesions that disappear spontaneously with minimal or no treatment. These episodes are usually unrelated to any recognized predisposing factor and are common in neonates and young children. Alternatively, the lesions may promptly recur following treatment, suggesting the persistence of a predisposing factor, as is often seen in adult patients with candidiasis.

The typical lesions in infants are described as soft white adherent patches on the oral mucosa. The intraoral lesions are generally painless and can be removed with little difficulty. In the adult, inflammation, erythema, and painful eroded areas are more often associated with this disease, and the typical

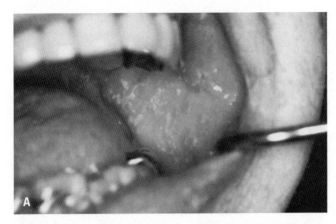
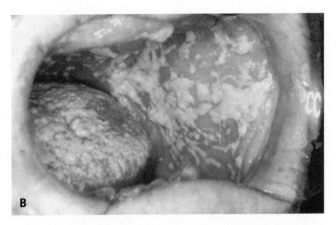

FIGURE 5-15   A, Patchy white plaque and flecks that rubbed off represent thrush. The patient complained of a burning mouth. **B,** More-extensive pseudomembranous lesions associated with an erythematous base in an adult with severe thrush. (Courtesy of Dr. T.J. Johnson, University of Nebraska Medical Center, College of Dentistry)

pearly white plaquelike lesions are relatively inconspicuous at times. Any mucosal surface may be involved, and erythematous or white areas often develop beneath partial or complete dentures. The lesions may involve the entire oral mucosa (see Figure 5-15, B) or may involve relatively localized areas where normal cleansing mechanisms are poor.

A prodromal symptom of a rapid onset of a bad taste and the loss of taste discrimination is described by some adults. A burning sensation of the mouth and throat may also precede the appearance of the white pseudomembranous lesions. Symptoms of this type in a patient receiving broad-spectrum antibiotics are strongly suggestive of thrush or other forms of oral candidiasis. Patients with immunodeficiencies, such as those suffering from AIDS or hematologic malignancies, are also especially susceptible to this form of candidiasis.

The differential diagnosis of thrush includes food debris, habitual cheek biting, and rarely, a genetically determined epithelial abnormality such as white sponge nevus.

Causative Organism and Frequency.   The yeastlike fungus that causes thrush and other manifestations of candidiasis occurs in both yeast and mycelial forms in the oral cavity. The organism grows by a budding of the yeast cells to form germ tubes and individual hyphal elements, which undergo limited peripheral branching to form a pseudomycelium. These phenomena can be demonstrated in smears and tissue sections and form the basis for confirmatory laboratory diagnostic tests for candidiasis.

Candida species are normal inhabitants of the oral flora of many individuals, but are present in the mouth of the healthy carrier in a low concentration of 200 to 500 cells per milliliter of saliva.[100,101] At this concentration, the organism cannot usually be identified by direct microscopic examination of smears from the oral mucosa, and its presence can be demonstrated only by inoculation onto a selective medium such as Sabouraud agar. Saliva samples give a carrier rate of 20 to 30% for healthy young adults whereas imprint cultures, which sample colonized sites rather than detached cells and organisms in

the mixed saliva, give a figure as high as 44%.[102] Imprint cultures suggest that the papillae of the posterior oral surface of the tongue are the primary colonization site in the oral cavity of healthy dentate carriers and that other areas are contaminated or secondarily colonized from this site.

The asymptomatic carrier state is affected by a number of known factors, including the immune status of the host, the strain of *Candida*, the local oral environment, smoking, prior use of antibiotics, and the general health of the host. The carrier state is more prevalent in diabetic individuals, and the density of *Candida* at various oral sites is also increased in persons with diabetes. As reported by Guggenheimer and colleagues, diabetic patients with clinical features of candidiasis were more likely to have a longer duration of insulin-dependent diabetes mellitus (IDDM), to have poorer glycemic control, and to experience the complications of nephropathy and retinopathy.[103] The wearing of removable prosthetic appliances is also associated with higher asymptomatic carrier prevalence rates. Importantly, simple measures to improve the oral health of the patient will reduce the rate of *Candida* colonization of the oral mucosa and denture.[104]

Because *Candida* spp are normal oral inhabitants, thrush and other forms of oral candidiasis may be classified as specific endogenous infections. A variety of species of *Candida* have been isolated from carriers and from patients with candidiasis. *Candida albicans, Candida tropicalis,* and *Candida glabrata* account for over 80% of medical isolates; *Candida parapsilopsis, Candida guilliermondii, Candida krusei,* and *Candida pseudotropicalis* are also recognized as pathogens. Candidiasis in HIV-positive patients is often associated with a shift in species, from *Candida albicans* to *Candida glabrata* and *Candida krusei.*[105] The particular species involved with a given oral infection is generally not thought to be of any significance, but *Candida albicans* is most commonly found in thrush, and several subtypes of this species have been implicated as cocarcinogens in speckled leukoplakia.[96,97] Severity and refractoriness of *Candida* infection to treatment possibly depend more on the site of involvement and on predisposing factors than on properties of the infecting species. While certain phenotypic characteristics such as tissue invasion may give strains of *Candida* a competitive advantage in the oral cavity, it is the host's immunocompetence that ultimately determines whether clearance, colonization, or candidiasis occurs.[106] Like other microorganisms involved in endogenous infections, *Candida* spp are of low virulence, are not usually considered contagious, and are involved in mucosal infection only where there is a definite local or systemic predisposition to their enhanced reproduction and invasion.

Predisposing Factors.   The following predisposing factors for oral candidiasis have been defined by clinical observation:

1. Marked changes in oral microbial flora (due to the use of antibiotics [especially broad-spectrum antibiotics], excessive use of antibacterial mouth rinses, or xerostomia).
2. Chronic local irritants (dentures and orthodontic appliances)
3. Administration of corticosteroids (aerosolized inhalant and topical agents are more likely to cause candidiasis than systemic administration)
4. Poor oral hygiene
5. Pregnancy
6. Immunologic deficiency
   — congenital or childhood (chronic familial mucocutaneous candidiasis ± endocrine candidiasis syndrome [hypoparathyroidism, hypoadrenocorticism], and immunologic immaturity of infancy)
   — acquired or adult (diabetes, leukemia, lymphomas, and AIDS)
   — iatrogenic (from cancer chemotherapy, bone marrow transplantation, and head and neck radiation)
7. Malabsorption and malnutrition

So important are these predisposing factors in the etiology of this infection that it is extremely rare to find a case of oral candidiasis in which one or more of these factors cannot be identified. A diagnosis of thrush should always be followed by a search for a possible undiagnosed medical disorder, a review of the patient's medications, and a search for some locally acting predisposing factor such as a denture.

Xerostomia and chronic local irritants may alter the oral mucous membranes, predisposing them to colonization and invasion. Shifts in the bacterial flora often accompany these situations and provide an opportunity for *Candida* spp to increase. Radiation to the head and neck also affects the oral mucous membranes and produces xerostomia. In Sjögren's syndrome, sarcoidosis, and other diseases of the salivary glands, xerostomia often develops gradually and is tolerated by the patient until superinfection with *Candida* develops. The mucosal lesions, pain, and associated symptoms of thrush then cause the patient to seek medical or dental care.

Knowledge of the ecology and epidemiology of *Candida* in the human mouth has increased substantially in recent years, particularly in regard to the attachment of the organism to oral mucosal surfaces.[107,108] *Candida* colonization and infection depend on the initial ability of the organism to adhere to host surfaces. In immunocompromised hosts, adhesion varies significantly among species of *Candida*.[109] Also, the quality of the epithelial cells in immunocompromised (HIV-positive) patients, including the cells' receptivity to *Candida*, may play a role in increasing the oral concentration of yeast.[110]

Histologic Features.   Microscopic examination of the lesions of thrush reveals a localized superficial inflammatory reaction, with hyperparakeratosis and ulceration of the surface. The ulcer is covered with a fibrinoid exudate, in which are found large numbers of yeast and pseudohyphae. The fungi rarely penetrate below this superficial layer. This pseudomembrane imparts the characteristic white-flecked appearance to the mucosal lesions. Thrush is correctly described as an acute pseudomembranous candidiasis.

ACUTE ATROPHIC CANDIDIASIS

Acute atrophic candidiasis presents as a red patch of atrophic or erythematous raw and painful mucosa, with minimal evidence of the white pseudomembranous lesions observed in thrush. Antibiotic sore mouth, a common form of atrophic candidiasis, should be suspected in a patient who develops symptoms of oral burning, bad taste, or sore throat during or after therapy with broad-spectrum antibiotics. Patients with chronic iron deficiency anemia may also develop atrophic candidiasis (Figure 5-16).

CHRONIC ATROPHIC CANDIDIASIS

Chronic atrophic candidiasis includes denture stomatitis (denture sore mouth), angular cheilitis, and median rhomboid glossitis.

Denture Stomatitis (Denture Sore Mouth).   Denture stomatitis is a common form of oral candidiasis[111] that manifests as a diffuse inflammation of the maxillary denture-bearing areas and that is often (15 to 65% of cases) associated with angular cheilitis.

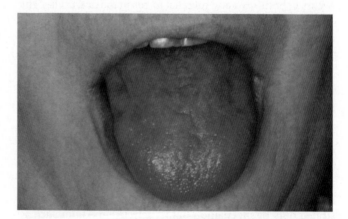

FIGURE 5-16   A patient with a history of chronic iron deficiency anemia developed red, raw, and painful areas of the mucosa, diagnosed as acute atrophic candidiasis.

At least 70% of individuals with clinical signs of denture stomatitis exhibit fungal growth, and this condition most likely results from yeast colonization of the oral mucosa, combined with bacterial colonization.[112] *Candida* spp act as an endogenous infecting agent on tissue predisposed by chronic trauma to microbial invasion.[113] Lesions of chronic atrophic candidiasis have also been frequently reported in HIV-positive and AIDS patients.[113]

Three progressive clinical stages of denture sore mouth have been described.[114,115] The first stage consists of numerous palatal petechiae (Figure 5-17, A). The second stage displays a more diffuse erythema involving most (if not all) of the denture-covered mucosa (see Figure 5-17, B and C). The third stage includes the development of tissue granulation or nodularity (papillary hyperplasia) (see Figure 5-17, D), commonly involving the central areas of the hard palate and alveolar ridges.

Antifungal treatment will modify the bright red appearance of denture sore mouth and papillary hyperplasia specifically but will not resolve the basic papillomatous lesion, especially if the lesions have been present for more than 1 year. Antifungal therapy and cessation of denture wearing usually is advisable before surgical excision since elimination of the mucosal inflammation often reduces the amount of tissue that needs to be excised.

Yeast attached to the denture plays an important etiologic role in chronic atrophic candidiasis.[116] The attachment of yeast to the patient's appliances is increased by mucus and serum and decreased by the presence of salivary pellicle, suggesting an explanation for the severity of candidiasis in xerostomic patients. Rinsing the appliance with a dilute (10%) solution of household bleach, soaking it in boric acid, or applying nystatin cream before inserting the denture will eliminate the yeast. Disinfection of the appliance is an important part of the treatment of denture sore mouth. Soft liners in dentures provide a porous surface and an opportunity for additional mechanical locking of plaque and yeast to the appliance. In general, soft liners are considered to be an additional hazard for patients who are susceptible to oral candidiasis.

Denture sore mouth is rarely found under a mandibular denture. One possible explanation for this is that the negative pressure that forms under the maxillary denture excludes salivary antibody from this region, and yeast may reproduce, undisturbed, in the space between the denture and mucosa. The closer adaptation of the maxillary denture and palate may also bring the large number of yeasts adhering to the denture surface into contact with the mucosa.

Angular Cheilitis. Angular cheilitis is the term used for an infection involving the lip commissures (Figure 5-18). The majority of cases are *Candida* associated and respond

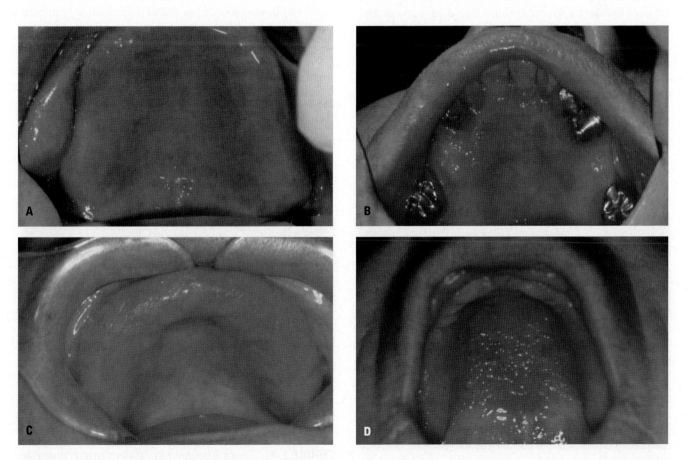

FIGURE 5-17 Three progressive stages of denture sore mouth. **A,** Numerous palatal petechiae in a patient with an ill-fitting denture. **B** and **C,** More diffuse erythema is seen under a partial denture (**B**) and a full upper denture (**C**). **D,** This patient has developed a granular nodular overgrowth of the palate (papillary hyperplasia) secondary to a candidal infection and an ill-fitting denture. (Courtesy of Dr. Robert Howell, West Virginia University, School of Dentistry)

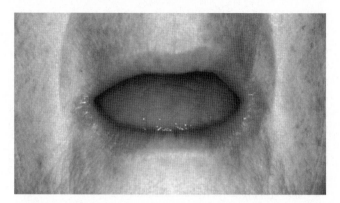

FIGURE 5-18   Candidal infection of the lip commissures (angular cheilitis).

promptly to antifungal therapy. There is frequently a coexistent denture stomatitis, and angular cheilitis is uncommon in patients with a natural dentition. Other possible etiologic cofactors include reduced vertical dimension; a nutritional deficiency (iron deficiency anemia and vitamin B or folic acid deficiency) sometimes referred to as perlèche; and (more rarely) diabetes, neutropenia, and AIDS, as well as co-infection with *Staphylococcus* and beta-hemolytic *Streptococcus*. More-extensive desquamative lesions affecting the full width of the lip and sometimes extending to the adjacent skin are associated with habitual lip sucking and chronic *Candida* infection.

Median Rhomboid Glossitis.   Erythematous patches of atrophic papillae located in the central area of the dorsum of the tongue are considered a form of chronic atrophic candidiasis (Figure 5-19). When these lesions become more nodular, the condition is referred to as hyperplastic median rhomboid glossitis. These lesions were originally thought to be developmental in nature but are now considered to be a manifestation of chronic candidiasis.

CHRONIC HYPERPLASTIC CANDIDIASIS

Chronic hyperplastic candidiasis (CHC) includes a variety of clinically recognized conditions in which mycelial invasion of the deeper layers of the mucosa and skin occurs, causing a proliferative response of host tissue (Figure 5-20).[117]

Candidal leukoplakia is considered a chronic form of oral candidiasis in which firm white leathery plaques are detected on the cheeks, lips, palate, and tongue (Figure 5-21). The differentiation of candidal leukoplakia from other forms of leukoplakia is based on finding periodic acid–Schiff (PAS)–positive hyphae in leukoplakic lesions. CHC also occurs as part of chronic mucocutaneous candidiasis, often with identifiable predisposing immunologic or endocrine abnormalities. These patients develop similar lesions around the nails and other skin sites or alternatively develop only isolated oral lesions. CHC also occurs on the dorsum of the tongue and may resemble median rhomboid glossitis (Figure 5-22).

Approximately 10% of oral leukoplakias satisfy the clinical and histologic criteria for CHC.[118] Epithelial dysplasia occurs four to five times more frequently in candidal (speckled) leukoplakia than in leukoplakia in general[119] and has been reported in as many as 50% of cases of candidal (speckled) leukoplakia in some series.[120] *Candida* is known to cause epithelial proliferation, and this high number of cases of dysplasia may be exaggerated because of the induction of inflammatory or atypical (reactive) changes in the epithelium (ie, changes that do not constitute actual dysplasia). However, dysplastic and carcinomatous changes are more common in speckled leukoplakia than in homogeneous leukoplakia.[121]

CHRONIC MULTIFOCAL CANDIDIASIS

Patients may present with multiple areas of chronic atrophic candidiasis. These are most often seen in immunocompromised individuals or in patients with predisposing factors such as ill-fitting dentures. The changes frequently affect the dor-

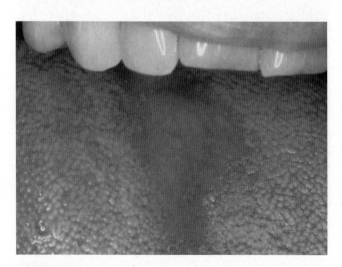

FIGURE 5-19   A patient with a long-standing atrophic (red) area in the midline of the tongue, just anterior to the circumvallate papillae. This was diagnosed as median rhomboid glossitis.

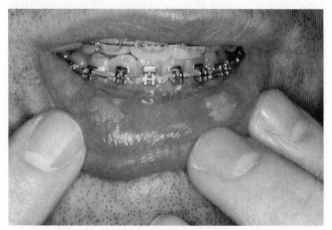

FIGURE 5-20   Chronic hyperplastic candidiasis presenting as multiple wartlike growths on the patient's lower lip. A biopsy specimen revealed a pseudoepitheliomatous hyperplasia with numerous pseudohyphae in the keratin layer.

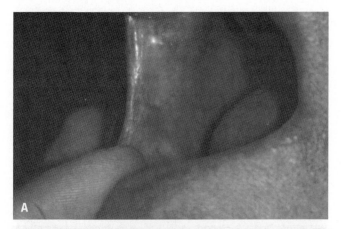

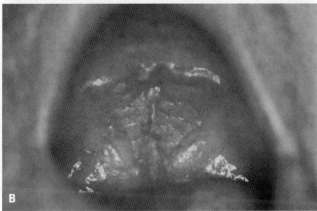

FIGURE 5-21 **A,** Candidal leukoplakia, a chronic form of candidiasis in which firm red white plaques form, most often in the cheeks. **B,** Occasionally, the plaques develop in the palate opposite a tongue lesion (kissing lesions). (Courtesy of Dr. Robert Howell, West Virginia University, School of Dentistry)

sum of the tongue and midline of the hard palate (kissing lesions), commissure area (angular cheilitis), and denture-bearing mucosal surfaces (Figure 5-23). Smoking may also play an important role in immunocompetent patients.

CHRONIC MUCOCUTANEOUS CANDIDIASIS

Persistent infection with *Candida* usually occurs as a result of a defect in cell-mediated immunity or may be associated with iron deficiency. Hyperplastic mucocutaneous lesions, localized granulomas, and adherent white plaques on affected mucous membranes are the prominent lesions that identify chronic mucocutaneous candidiasis (CMC) (Figure 5-24). In many cases, persistent and significant predisposing factors can be identified. Two categories of CMC have been described: (1) syndrome-associated CMC and (2) localized and diffuse CMC. Syndrome-associated CMC is further categorized as either familial or chronic. The familial form, candidiasis endocrinopathy syndrome (CES), is a rare autosomal recessive disorder characterized by an onset of CMC during infancy or early childhood, associated with the appearance of hypoparathyroidism, hypoadrenocorticism, and other endocrine anomalies.[122] Patients develop persistent oral candidiasis and hyperplastic

infections of the nail folds at an early age. Some patients also have low serum iron and iron-binding capacity. The other syndrome-associated form is chronic candidiasis associated with thymoma, which appears with other autoimmune abnormalities such as myasthenia gravis, polymyositis, bullous lichen planus,[123] and hypogammaglobulinemia.

Localized CMC is a variant associated with chronic oral candidiasis and lesions of the skin and nails. Lesions usually begin within the first two decades of life. The diffuse variant is characterized by randomly occurring cases of severe mucocutaneous candidiasis with widespread skin involvement and development of *Candida* granulomas. It is often associated with other opportunistic fungal and bacterial infections. A majority of patients are iron deficient.

Both oral and cutaneous lesions of CMC can be controlled by the continuous use of systemic antifungal drugs; once treatment is discontinued, however, the lesions rapidly reappear.

IMMUNOCOMPROMISED (HIV)-ASSOCIATED CANDIDIASIS

Oral candidiasis is the most frequent opportunistic infection associated with immunocompromised individuals.[124] The role of weakened specific immune defense mechanisms is apparent from the fact that patients who are on immunosuppressive drug regimens[125] or who have HIV infection,[126] cancer, or hematologic malignancies have an increased susceptibility to oral candidiasis. This supports an important role for T lymphocytes in immunity to *Candida*, especially in regard to chronic candidiasis. Host factors affecting the adherence of *Candida* to mucosal cells (such as salivary ABO antigens),[127] as well as variation in the virulence and invasiveness of the fungal organism, also play a role.

The possible importance of local immunoglobulin A (IgA) as a first line of protection against acute candidiasis has been emphasized.[124–129] Salivary IgA (but not immunoglobulin G [IgG]) affects the adherence of *Candida* to buccal epithelial cells,[130] and levels of *Candida*-specific IgA are elevated in the saliva of healthy patients with chronic oral candidiasis. In HIV-infected patients who develop oral candidiasis, the level of salivary anti-*Candida* IgG is increased while serum and

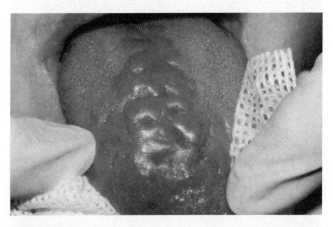

FIGURE 5-22 Chronic hyperplastic candidiasis occurs on the dorsum of the tongue as a mammilated form of median rhomboid glossitis.

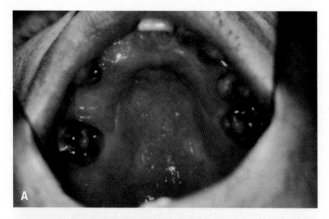

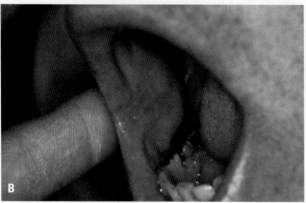

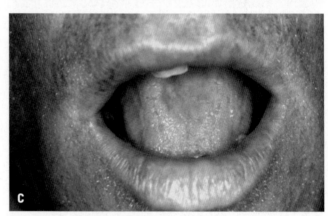

FIGURE 5-23   A, B, and **C,** Chronic multifocal candidiasis presents with multiple areas of chronic atrophic candidiasis, usually involving the palate (midline and under a denture) (**A**), the commissures (**B**), and the dorsum of the tongue (**C**). The tongue lesion is almost healed after 14 days of nystatin therapy. The patient had poor oral hygiene and was a heavy smoker but was not immunocompromised.

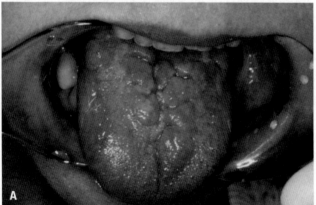

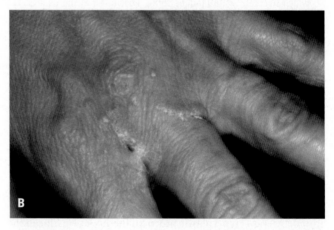

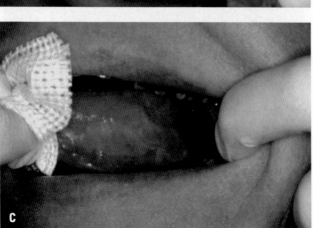

FIGURE 5-24   Chronic mucocutaneous candidiasis manifests as hyperplastic mucocutaneous lesions including granulomas and nodules. **A,** Localized granulomas and nodules on the tongue. **B,** The same condition, affecting the skin. **C,** Adherent white plaques that represent speckled leukoplakia.

salivary IgA decrease, despite an increased antigenic load.[130] This helps explain the strong association between candidiasis and HIV positivity, especially in those who are about to develop full-blown AIDS.[131]

TREATMENT OF ORAL CANDIDIASIS

A variety of topical and systemically administered medications are now available to supplement the older polyene antifungal antibiotics nystatin and amphotericin B. An imidazole derivative (clotrimazole) is available for topical use. Systemic therapy includes the use of any one of these three: ketoconazole, itraconazole, and fluconazole. Fluconazole and amphotericin B may be used intravenously for the treatment of the resistant lesions of CMC and systemic candidiasis.

The majority of acute oral *Candida* infections respond rapidly to topical nystatin and will not recur, provided that the predisposing factors have also been eliminated. Seven to 21 days' use of a nystatin rinse three to four times daily is usually adequate although some resistant cases may require a second course of treatment. Nystatin in cream form may also be applied directly to the denture or to the corners of the mouth. Patients for whom predisposing factors such as xerostomia and immunodeficiency cannot be eliminated may need either continuous or repeated treatment to prevent recurrences. Clotrimazole troches can also be used for treatment of oral lesions. The consumption of yogurt two to three times per week and improved oral hygiene can also help, especially if underlying predisposing factors cannot be eliminated.

Better patient compliance and more effective treatment of both acute and chronic candidiasis can usually be attained by a once-daily dose of 200 mg of ketoconazole, 100 mg of fluconazole,[132] or itraconazole oral suspension (100 to 200 mg/d) for 2 weeks. When these medications are used for this short period, side effects such as increased liver enzymes, abdominal pain, and pruritus are rare. Vaginal candidiasis responds to ketoconazole and fluconazole even more rapidly than does oral candidiasis, and the likelihood of re-infection is reduced by the control of *Candida* at various sites. Fluconazole is more effective than ketoconazole, but its frequent use can lead to the development of resistance to the drug. Fluconazole therapy for oral candidiasis associated with HIV infection often results in the development of resistance to fluconazole. Itraconazole can be substituted for fluconazole in resistant patients, but fluconazole is still the mainstay of therapy for HIV-associated candidiasis.[105] Fluconazole interacts with a number of other medications and must be prescribed with care for patients who are using anticoagulants, phenytoin, cyclosporine, and oral hypoglycemic agents. The simultaneous administration of ketoconazole (or the related antifungal itraconazole) and cisapride or antihistamines (terfenadine and astemizole) is associated occasionally with ventricular arrhythmias and other serious cardiovascular events.

Mucous Patches

A superficial grayish area of mucosal necrosis is seen in secondary syphilis; this lesion is termed a "mucous patch."[133] Secondary syphilis usually develops within 6 weeks after the primary lesion and is characterized by diffuse maculopapular eruptions of the skin and mucous membranes. On the skin, these lesions may present as macules or papules.[133,134] In the oral cavity, the lesions are usually multiple painless grayish-white plaques overlying an ulcerated necrotic surface. The lesions occur on the tongue, gingiva, palate, and buccal mucosa.[134,135] Associated systemic signs and symptoms (including fever, sore throat, general malaise, and headache) may also be present. The mucous patches of the secondary stage of syphilis resolve within a few weeks but are highly infective because they contain large numbers of spirochetes.

Parulis

A parulis, or gumboil, is a localized accumulation of pus located with the gingival tissues (Figure 5-25). It originates from either an acute periapical abscess or an occluded periodontal pocket. The cortical bone is destroyed by the inflammatory process, and the gumboil often appears as a yellowish white bump on the gingiva. The lesion is usually painful, and pain relief occurs when the "boil" ruptures or drains spontaneously. To permanently resolve this problem, the nonvital tooth or periodontal abscess must be treated.

▼ IDIOPATHIC "TRUE" LEUKOPLAKIA

Leukoplakia is a white oral precancerous lesion with a recognizable risk for malignant transformation. In 1972, the World Health Organization (WHO) defined a precancerous lesion as a "morphologically altered tissue in which cancer is more likely to occur than in its apparently normal counterpart."[136] The most commonly encountered and accepted precancerous lesions in the oral cavity are leukoplakia and erythroplakia. Leukoplakia is currently defined as "a white patch or plaque that cannot be characterized clinically or pathologically as any other disease" (WHO, 1978).[136–138] This definition has no histologic connotation and is used strictly as a clinical description. The risk of malignant transformation varies according to the histologic and clinical presentation, but the total lifetime risk of malignant transformation is estimated to be 4 to 6%.[139–144]

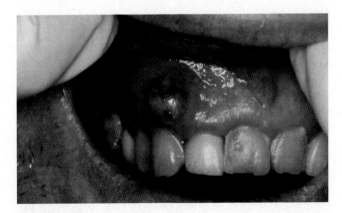

FIGURE 5-25 The elevated white nodule above the maxillary right canine is a parulis, or gumboil.

Etiology

A number of locally acting etiologic agents, including tobacco, alcohol, candidiasis, electrogalvanic reactions, and (possibly) herpes simplex and papillomaviruses, have been implicated as causative factors for leukoplakia. True leukoplakia is most often related to tobacco usage;[136] more than 80% of patients with leukoplakia are smokers. The development of leukoplakia in smokers also depends on dose and on duration of use, as shown by heavier smokers' having a more frequent incidence of lesions than light smokers. Cessation of smoking often results in partial to total resolution of leukoplakic lesions. Smokeless tobacco is also a well-established etiologic factor for the development of leukoplakia; however, the malignant transformation potential of smokeless tobacco–induced lesions is much lower than that of smoking-induced lesions.[54]

Alcohol consumption alone is not associated with an increased risk of developing leukoplakia, but alcohol is thought to serve as a promoter that exhibits a strong synergistic effect with tobacco, relative to the development of leukoplakia and oral cancer.[52]

In addition to tobacco, several other etiologic agents are associated with leukoplakia. Sunlight (specifically, ultraviolet radiation) is well known to be an etiologic factor for the formation of leukoplakia of the vermilion border of the lower lip.[43] *Candida albicans* is frequently found in histologic sections of leukoplakia and is consistently (60% of cases) identified in nodular leukoplakias but rarely (3%) in homogeneous leukoplakias. The terms "candidal leukoplakia" and "hyperplastic candidiasis" have been used to describe such lesions.[117,120] Whether *Candida* constitutes a cofactor either for excess production of keratin or for dysplastic or malignant transformation is unknown[145] (see previous section on candidiasis). Human papillomavirus (HPV), particularly subtypes HPV-16 and HPV-18, have been identified in some oral leukoplakias. The role of this virus remains questionable, but there is evidence that HPV-16 may be associated with an increased risk of malignant transformation.[146] Of interest, there is some evidence that oral leukoplakia in nonsmokers has a greater risk for malignant transformation than oral leukoplakia in smokers.[147]

Clinical Features

The incidence of leukoplakia varies by geographic location and patients' associated habits. For example, in locations where smokeless tobacco is frequently used, leukoplakia appears with a higher prevalence.[64] Leukoplakia is more frequently found in men, can occur on any mucosal surface, and infrequently causes discomfort or pain (Figure 5-26). Leukoplakia usually occurs in adults older than 50 years of age. Prevalence increases rapidly with age, especially for males, and 8% of men older than 70 years of age are affected. Approximately 70% of oral leukoplakia lesions are found on the buccal mucosa, vermilion border of the lower lip, and gingiva. They are less common on the palate, maxillary mucosa, retromolar area, floor of the mouth, and tongue. However, lesions of the tongue and the floor of the mouth account for more than 90% of cases that show dysplasia or carcinoma.[140]

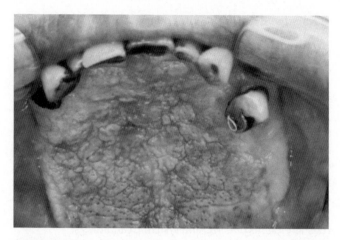

FIGURE 5-26   Hyperkeratosis of the palate in a heavy pipe smoker appears as an area of leukoplakia.

Subtypes

Many varieties of leukoplakia have been identified.

"Homogeneous leukoplakia" (or "thick leukoplakia") refers to a usually well-defined white patch, localized or extensive, that is slightly elevated and that has a fissured, wrinkled, or corrugated surface (Figure 5-27). On palpation, these lesions may feel leathery to "dry, or cracked mud-like."[140]

Nodular (speckled) leukoplakia is granular or nonhomogeneous. The name refers to a mixed red-and-white lesion in which keratotic white nodules or patches are distributed over an atrophic erythematous background (Figure 5-28). This type of leukoplakia is associated with a higher malignant transformation rate, with up to two-thirds of the cases in some series showing epithelial dysplasia or carcinoma.[139,140]

"Verrucous leukoplakia" or "verruciform leukoplakia" is a term used to describe the presence of thick white lesions with papillary surfaces in the oral cavity (Figure 5-29). These lesions are usually heavily keratinized and are most often seen in older adults in the sixth to eighth decades of life. Some of these lesions may exhibit an exophytic growth pattern.[137]

Proliferative verrucous leukoplakia (PVL) was first described in 1985.[147] The lesions of this special type of leukoplakia have been described as extensive papillary or verrucoid white plaques that tend to slowly involve multiple mucosal sites in the oral cavity and to inexorably transform into squamous cell carcinomas over a period of many years (Figure 5-30).[147,148] PVL has a very high risk for transformation to dysplasia, squamous cell carcinoma[148] or verrucous carcinoma (Figure 5-31). Verrucous carcinoma is almost always a slow growing and well-differentiated lesion that seldom metastasizes.

Histopathologic Features

The most important and conclusive method of diagnosing leukoplakic lesions is microscopic examination of an adequate biopsy specimen.[149] Benign forms of leukoplakia are characterized by variable patterns of hyperkeratosis and chronic inflammation. The association between the biochemical process of hyperkeratosis and malignant transformation remains an enigma.

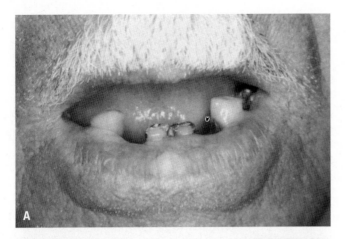

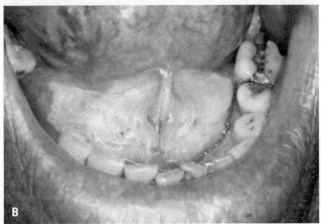

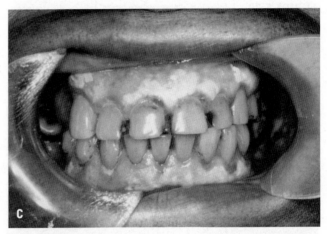

FIGURE 5-27 Homogeneous leukoplakia as it appears at different sites: **A,** the lower lip; **B,** the floor of mouth; and **C,** the gingiva.

However, the increased risk for malignant transformation and thus "premalignant designation" is documented in Table 5–2.[143]

Waldron and Shafer, in a landmark study of over 3,000 cases of leukoplakia, found that 80% of the lesions represented benign hyperkeratosis (ortho- or parakeratin) with or without a thickened spinous layer (acanthosis).[140] About 17% of the cases were epithelial dysplasias or carcinomas in situ. The dysplastic changes typically begin in the basal and parabasal zones of the epithelium. The higher the extent of epithelial involvement, the higher the grade of dysplasia. Dysplastic alterations of the epithelium are characterized by enlarged and hyperchromatic nuclei, cellular and nuclear pleomorphism, premature keratinization of individual cells, an increased nucleocytoplasmic ratio, increased and abnormal mitotic activity, and a generalized loss of cellular polarity and orientation (Figure 5-32). When the entire thickness of the epithelium is involved ("top-to-bottom" change), the term "carcinoma in situ" (CIS) is used. There is no invasion seen in CIS. Only 3% of the leukoplakic lesions examined had evolved into invasive squamous cell carcinomas.[140]

Diagnosis and Management

A diagnosis of leukoplakia is made when adequate clinical and histologic examination fails to reveal an alternative diagnosis and when characteristic histopathologic findings for leukoplakia are present. Important clinical criteria include location,

appearance, known irritants, and clinical course. Many white lesions can mimic leukoplakia clinically and should be ruled out before a diagnosis of leukoplakia is made. These include lichen planus, lesions caused by cheek biting, frictional keratosis, smokeless tobacco–induced keratosis, nicotinic stomatitis, leukoedema, and white sponge nevus.[140,141]

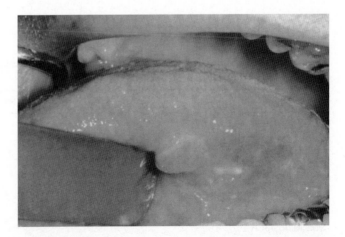

FIGURE 5-28 Nodular or speckled leukoplakia appears as a red velvety plaque with associated white spots or papules on the lateral border of the tongue. The nodular ulcerated area anterior to the red plaque is a spindle cell squamous cell carcinoma.

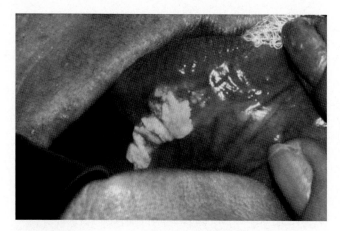

FIGURE 5-29 Thick white plaque on the lateral border of tongue represents verrucous leukoplakia. The small ulcerated lesion anterior to the white bumpy lesion is a squamous cell carcinoma (proven by biopsy). (Courtesy of Dr. Gregg A. Peterson, Grand Island, Nebr.)

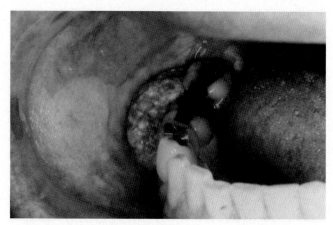

FIGURE 5-31 Buccal leukoplakia and an adjacent verrucous carcinoma.

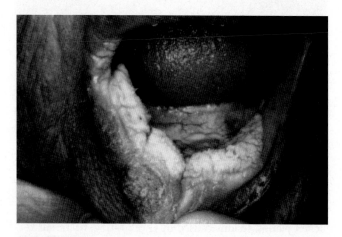

FIGURE 5-30 Proliferative verrucous leukoplakia of the floor of the mouth and of the lip. In this form of leukoplakia, the risk for malignant transformation is very high.

If a leukoplakic lesion disappears spontaneously or through the elimination of an irritant, no further testing is indicated.[150] For the persistent lesion, however, the definitive diagnosis is established by tissue biopsy. Adjunctive methods such as vital staining with toluidine blue and cytobrush techniques are helpful in accelerating the biopsy and/or selecting the most appropriate spot at which to perform the biopsy.

Toluidine blue staining uses a 1% aqueous solution of the dye that is decolorized with 1% acetic acid. The dye binds to dysplastic and malignant epithelial cells with a high degree of accuracy.[151] The cytobrush technique uses a brush with firm bristles that obtain individual cells from the full thickness of the stratified squamous epithelium; this technique is significantly more accurate than other cytologic techniques used in the oral cavity.[152] It must be remembered that staining and cytobrush techniques are adjuncts and not substitutes for an incisional biopsy. When a biopsy has been performed and the lesion has not been subsequently removed, another biopsy is recommended if and when changes in signs or symptoms occur.

TABLE 5–2 Malignant Transformation in Oral Leukoplakia

Investigator (Country)	Year	No. of Patients	Malignancies (%)	Yr Observed (Avg)
Silverman (India)	1976	4,762	0.13	2
Gupta (India [Bhavnagar])	1980	360	0.30	1–10 (7)
Gupta (India [Ernakulam])	1980	410	2.20	1–10 (7)
Roed-Petersen (Denmark)	1971	331	3.60	>1
Einhorn (Sweden)	1967	782	4.00	1–20
Pindborg (Denmark)	1968	248	4.40	1–9
Kramer (England)	1969	187	4.80	1–16
Banoczy (Hungary)	1977	670	5.90	1–30 (9.8)
Silverman (USA)	1968	117	6.00	1–11 (3.5)
Schepman (Netherlands)	1998	166	12.00	5–17 (2.7)
Silverman (USA)	1984	257	17.50	1–39 (7.2)

Reproduced with permission from Schepman KP et al.[143]

Avg = average.

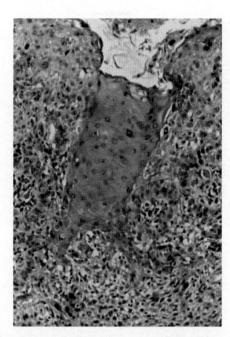

FIGURE 5-32 Epithelium showing full-thickness change (ie, carcinoma in situ) and central area of severe dysplasia. Dysplastic cells have enlarged hyperchromatic nuclei, cellular and nuclear pleomorphism, an increased nucleocytoplasmic ratio, and (most importantly) a generalized loss of cellular polarity and orientation. Note central pink (cytoplasm-rich) area of "normal" epithelium. (Hematoxylin and eosin, ×65 original magnification)

Definitive treatment involves surgical excision although cryosurgery and laser ablation are often preferred because of their precision and rapid healing.[153–155] Total excision is aggressively recommended when microscopic dysplasia is identified, particularly if the dysplasia is classified as severe or moderate. Most leukoplakias incur a low risk for malignant transformation. Following attempts at removal, recurrences appear when either the margins of excision are inadequate or the causative factor or habit is continued. In any event, such patients must be observed periodically because of the risk of eventual malignancy.

The use of antioxidant nutrients and vitamins have not been reproducibly effective in management. Programs have included single and combination dosages of vitamins A, C, and E; beta carotene; analogues of vitamin A; and diets that are high in antioxidants and cell growth suppressor proteins (fruits and vegetables).[156–158]

Prognosis

After surgical removal, long-term monitoring of the lesion site is important since recurrences are frequent and because additional leukoplakias may develop.[159,160] In one recent series of these lesions, the recurrence rate after 3.9 years was 20%.[143] Smaller benign lesions that do not demonstrate dysplasia should be excised since the chance of malignant transformation is 4 to 6%.[140] For larger lesions with no evidence of dysplasia on biopsy, there is a choice between removal of the remaining lesion and follow-up evaluation, with or without local medication.

Repeated follow-up visits and biopsies are essential, particularly when the complete elimination of irritants is not likely to be achieved. In such cases, total removal is strongly advisable. Follow-up studies have demonstrated that carcinomatous transformation usually occurs 2 to 4 years after the onset of leukoplakia but that it may occur within months or after decades.[159]

Each clinical appearance or phase of leukoplakia has a different potential for malignant transformation. Speckled leukoplakia carries the highest average transformation potential, followed by verrucous leukoplakia; homogeneous leukoplakia carries the lowest risk. For dysplastic leukoplakia, the clinician must consider the histologic grade when planning treatment and follow-up. In general, the greater the degree of dysplasia, the greater the potential for malignant change. In addition, multiple factors play a role in determining the optimum management procedure. These factors include the persistence of the lesion over many years, the development of leukoplakia in a nonsmoker, and the lesion's occurrence on high-risk areas such as the floor of the mouth, the soft palate, the oropharynx, or the ventral surface of the tongue.

▼ BOWEN'S DISEASE

Bowen's disease is a localized intraepidermal squamous cell carcinoma of the skin that may progress into invasive carcinoma over many years. Bowen's disease also occurs on the male and female genital mucosae and (rarely) in the oral mucosa as an erythroplakic, leukoplakic, or papillomatous lesion.[161]

Bowen's disease occurs most commonly on the skin, as a result of arsenic ingestion. It grows slowly as an enlarging erythematous patch, with little to suggest a malignant process. The histologic picture is very characteristic, with the epithelium exhibiting a significant loss of cellular polarity and orientation, increased and abnormal mitoses, multiple highly atypical hyperchromatic nuclei, and cellular pleomorphism. Individual cell keratinization at different levels of the epithelium is seen. Lesions of this type are often associated with visceral cancer.[161,162]

Because of the clinical and histologic similarity between Bowen's disease and erythroplakia (both of which can be characterized as red patches of the mucous membrane that histologically contain severely dysplastic epithelium or intraepithelial carcinoma), the question has been raised as to whether they are the same disorder.[162] Current opinion, based on the comparison of oral erythroplakias with the oral lesions of Bowen's disease, holds that they are separate disorders.[162]

A nodular, benign, and virus-associated epithelial dysplasia with a histologic picture resembling Bowen's disease (bowenoid papulosis) occurs on the genital mucosa of sexually active young adults and has been reported on multiple oral mucosal surfaces on rare occasions.[163]

▼ ERYTHROPLAKIA

Erythroplakia has been defined as a "bright red velvety plaque or patch which cannot be characterized clinically or pathologically as being due to any other condition."[164] The word is an adaptation of the French term "erythroplasie de Queyrat,"[171] which describes a similar-appearing lesion of the glans penis with a comparable premalignant tendency. Although red lesions of the oral mucosa have been noted for many years, the use of the term "erythroplakia" in this context has been common for only about 25 years.[165,166] Erythroplakic lesions are easily overlooked, and the true prevalence of the condition is unknown. Erythroplakia is far less common than leukoplakia in most histopathologic series, but this reflects the fact that leukoplakias are more likely to have biopsies performed on them and emphasizes the lack of appreciation of the clinical significance of erythroplakia[140,167] since it has been proposed that most erythroplakic lesions are precursors of oral squamous cell carcinoma.[168] A number of studies have shown that the majority of erythroplakias (particularly those located under the tongue, on the floor of the mouth, and on the soft palate and anterior tonsillar pillars) exhibit a high frequency of premalignant and malignant changes.[169,170]

Although the etiology of erythroplakia is uncertain, most cases of erythroplakia are associated with heavy smoking, with or without concomitant alcohol abuse.[136,171]

Clinical Features

Several clinical variants of erythroplakia have been described, but there is no generally accepted classification. Shear[172] described "homogeneous erythroplakia, erythroplakia interspersed with patches of leukoplakia, and granular or speckled erythroplakia"; most authors consider this last category to be identical to speckled leukoplakia (Figure 5-33). Many of these lesions are irregular in outline, and some contain islands of normal mucosa within areas of erythroplakia, a phenomenon that has been attributed to the coalescence of a number of precancerous foci.

Erythroplakia occurs predominantly in older men, in the sixth and seventh decades of life.

Erythroplakias are more commonly seen on the floor of the mouth, the ventral tongue, the soft palate, and the tonsillar fauces, all prime areas for the development of carcinoma. Multiple lesions may be present. These lesions are commonly described as erythematous plaques with a soft velvety texture. Almost all of the lesions are asymptomatic and therefore unlikely to be drawn to the dentist's attention by the patient.[165,166,169]

Histopathologic Features

Different studies have demonstrated that 80 to 90% of cases of erythroplakia are histopathologically severe epithelial dysplasia, carcinoma in situ, or invasive carcinoma. In one study, none of the cases of erythroplakia was histologically found to represent benign keratosis.[140,172]

Differential Diagnosis

In view of the clinical significance of erythroplakia, its differentiation from other red inflammatory lesions of the oral mucosa is critical. Clinically similar lesions may include ery-

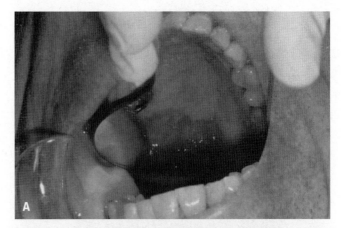
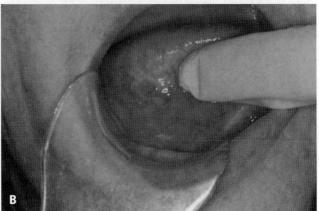

FIGURE 5-33   Clinical variations of erythroplakia. **A,** Homogeneous erythroplakia consisting of a bright red well-demarcated velvety patch seen here in the posterior hard palate/soft palate area. **B,** Homogeneous erythroplakia as a mixed area of leukoplakia and erythroplakia, called speckled leukoplakia, seen in the floor of the mouth and on the lateral border of the tongue.

thematous candidiasis, areas of mechanical irritation, denture stomatitis, vascular lesions, and a variety of nonspecific inflammatory lesions.[169] Because localized areas of redness are not uncommon in the oral cavity, areas of erythroplakia are likely to be disregarded by the examiner, and they are often falsely determined to be a transient inflammatory response to local irritation. Differentiation of erythroplakia from benign inflammatory lesions of the oral mucosa can be enhanced by the use of a 1% solution of toluidine blue, applied topically with a swab or as an oral rinse. Although this technique was previously found to have limited usefulness in the evaluation of keratotic lesions, prospective studies of the specificity of toluidine blue staining of areas of early carcinoma contained in erythroplakic and mixed leukoplakic-erythroplakic lesions reported excellent results, with false-negative (underdiagnosis) and false-positive (overdiagnosis) rates of well below 10%.[151]

Treatment and Prognosis

The treatment of erythroplakia should follow the same principles outlined for that of leukoplakia (see section on management of leukoplakia, above). Observation for 1 to 2 weeks following the elimination of suspected irritants is acceptable, but prompt biopsy at that time is mandatory for lesions that persist. The toluidine blue vital staining procedure may be redone following the period of elimination of suspected irritants. Lesions that stain on this second application frequently show extensive dysplasia or early carcinoma. Epithelial dysplasia or carcinoma in situ warrants complete removal of the lesion. Actual invasive carcinoma must be treated promptly according to guidelines for the treatment of cancer. Most asymptomatic malignant erythroplakic lesions are small; 84% are ≤ 2 cm in diameter, and 42% are ≤ 1 cm.[165–167] However, since recurrence and multifocal involvement is common, long-term follow-up is mandatory.

▼ ORAL LICHEN PLANUS

Oral lichen planus (OLP) is a common chronic immunologic inflammatory mucocutaneous disorder that varies in appearance from keratotic (reticular or plaquelike) to erythematous and ulcerative. About 28% of patients who have OLP also have skin lesions.[173–175] The skin lesions are flat violaceous papules with a fine scaling on the surface. Unlike oral lesions, skin lesions are usually self-limiting, lasting only 1 year or less. The lack of sound epidemiologic studies and the variations in signs as well as symptoms make estimates of prevalence difficult.

Etiology and Diagnosis

The etiology of lichen planus involves a cell-mediated immunologically induced degeneration of the basal cell layer of the epithelium. Lichen planus is one variety of a broader range of disorders of which an immunologically induced lichenoid lesion is the common denominator.[176–178] Thus, there are many clinical and histologic similarities between lichen planus and lichenoid dermatoses and stomatitides associated with drugs, some autoimmune disorders, and graft-versus-host reactions.[179,180] Although lichen planus may manifest as a particularly well-defined and characteristic lesion, the differential diagnosis for less specific lesions is extensive. Speculated cofactors in causation, such as stress, diabetes, hepatitis C, trauma, and hypersensitivity to drugs and metals, have varying degrees of support, with the last three having the most convincing evidence.[174,175,181,182] At the very least, some of these factors may add to the risk of developing OLP in susceptible patients.

As stated above, in "true" OLP a specific causative factor cannot be identified. However, clinical and microscopic changes that are consistent with OLP will often occur in response to a variety of agents (eg, drugs, chemicals, metals, and foods).[174,183,184] When these manifestations take place, they are referred to as "lichenoid" reactions. When the offending agent or antigen is removed, the signs and symptoms are reversed; examples in reported cases include reactions to dental restorations, mouth rinses, antibiotics, gold injections for arthritis, and immunocompromised status such as graft-versus-host disease.[174,176,183] These reactions are not to be confused with other hypersensitivity reactions such as urticaria or erythema multiforme, which differ both clinically and microscopically.

These often confusing clinical variations (Figure 5-34) mandate a thorough clinical work-up and histologic examination to rule out possible dysplasia and carcinoma. This requires not only an initial biopsy but also follow-up biopsies when changes in signs and symptoms occur.

(Because some lesions of oral lichen planus are erosive and others are bullous, this disorder is also discussed in Chapter 4. The emphasis in this chapter is on the white non-erosive non-bullous forms of lichen planus.)

Clinical Features

In general, studies of patients with OLP reveal that there is no evident genetic bias or uniform etiologic factor. The mean age of onset is the fifth decade of life, and there is clearly a female predominance. Although OLP may occur at any oral mucosal site, the buccal mucosa is the most common site. OLP may be associated with pain or discomfort, which interferes with function and with quality of life. Approximately 1% of the population may have cutaneous lichen planus. The prevalence rate of OLP ranges between 0.1 and 2.2%.[27,30,173,174] The skin lesions of lichen planus have been classically described as purple, pruritic, and polygonal papules.

OLP is classified as reticular (lacelike keratotic mucosal configurations), atrophic (keratotic changes combined with mucosal erythema), or erosive (pseudomembrane-covered ulcerations combined with keratosis and erythema) and bullous (vesiculobullous presentation combined with reticular or erosive patterns).[181,185] Apart from the erosive and bullous forms of the disorder, reticular OLP is quite frequently an indolent and painless lesion that is usually asymptomatic before it is identified during a routine oral examination. The clinical features of the lesions in a given patient often vary with time, as does their extent and the area of erosion of the atrophic mucosa.[181]

The reticular form consists of (a) slightly elevated fine whitish lines (Wickham's striae) that produce either a lacelike pattern or a patern of fine radiating lines or (b) annular lesions. This is the most common and most readily recognized form of lichen planus. Most patients with lichen planus at some time exhibit some reticular areas. The most common sites include the buccal mucosa (often bilaterally), followed by the tongue; lips, gingivae, the floor of the mouth, and the palate are less frequently involved. Whitish elevated lesions, or papules, usually measuring 0.5 to 1.0 mm in diameter, may be seen on the well-keratinized areas of the oral mucosa. However, even large plaquelike lesions may occur on the cheek, tongue, and gingivae, and these are difficult to distinguish from leukoplakia.

Bullous lichen planus (see Chapter 4) is rare and may sometimes resemble a form of linear IgA disease.[186] Atrophic lichen planus presents as inflamed areas of the oral mucosa covered by thinned red-appearing epithelium. Erosive lesions probably develop as a complication of the atrophic process when the thin epithelium is abraded or ulcerated. These lesions are invariably symptomatic, with symptoms that range from mild burning to severe pain.

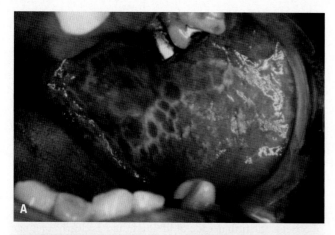

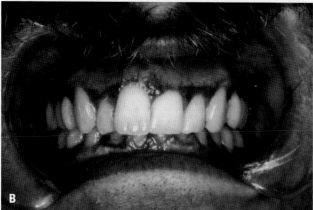

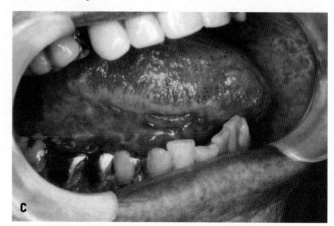

FIGURE 5-34   Forms of lichen planus. **A,** Reticular lichen planus of the buccal mucosa. **B,** Atrophic lichen planus of the gingiva. **C,** Erosive lichen planus of the tongue.

Papular, plaquelike, atrophic, and erosive lesions are very frequently accompanied by reticular lesions, a search for which is an essential part of the clinical evaluation in suspected cases of lichen planus. Characteristically, the affected areas of the oral mucosa are not bound down or rendered inelastic by lichen planus, and the keratotic white lines cannot be eliminated by either stretching the mucosa or rubbing its surface. Reticular papular lesions are generally asymptomatic; atrophic, erosive, and bullous forms are generally associated with pain.

Atrophic or erosive lichen planus involving the gingivae results in desquamative gingivitis (see Figure 5-34, B), a condition characterized by bright red edematous patches that involve the full width of the attached gingivae. Lichen planus must be distinguished histologically from other diseases that cause desquamative gingivitis, such as mucous membrane pemphigoid and pemphigus. Lichen planus has occasionally been described in association with autoimmune diseases.[174,177,187]

Histopathologic Features

Three features are considered essential for the histopathologic diagnosis of lichen planus: (1) areas of hyperparakeratosis or hyperorthokeratosis, often with a thickening of the granular cell layer and a saw-toothed appearance to the rete pegs; (2) "liquefaction degeneration," or necrosis of the basal cell layer, which is often replaced by an eosinophilic band; and (3) a

dense subepithelial band of lymphocytes (Figure 5-35). Isolated epithelial cells, shrunken with eosinophilic cytoplasm and one or more pyknotic nuclear fragments (Civatte bodies), are often scattered within the epithelium and superficial lamina propria. These represent cells that have undergone apoptosis. The linear sub-basilar lymphocytic infiltration is composed largely of T cells. Immunohistochemical studies have confirmed that the T4/T8 ratio of the lymphocytes in the epithelium and lamina propria in lichenoid lesions is higher than in either normal or leukoplakic mucosa, thus providing an additional feature for distinguishing leukoplakia from a lichenoid reaction.[177]

Immunofluorescent Studies

Immunofluorescent studies of biopsy specimens from lesions of lichen planus reveal a number of features that are not seen in hematoxylin-eosin (H&E)–stained sections and that both reflect the mode of development of these lesions and aid in distinguishing lichen planus from a number of other dermatoses. Direct immunofluorescence demonstrates a shaggy band of fibrinogen in the basement membrane zone in 90 to 100% of cases.[187–189] Patients also may have multiple mainly IgM-staining cytoid bodies, usually located in the dermal papilla or in the peribasalar area. These cytoid bodies are considered to be highly suggestive of lichen planus if they are present in large numbers or grouped in clusters.[189]

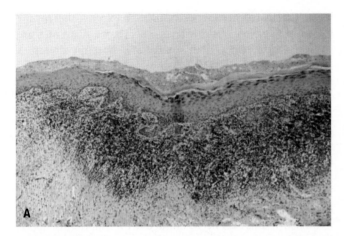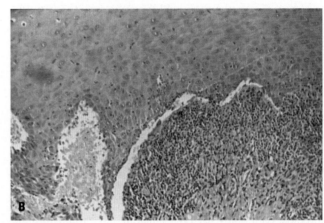

FIGURE 5-35   A, The essential microscopic features of lichen planus include hyperkeratosis, epithelial atrophy, and a dense subepithelial band of lymphocytes. (Hematoxylin and eosin, ×40 original magnification) **B,** Also characteristic of lichen planus are saw-toothed rete ridges, liquefactive degeneration or necrosis of the basal cell layer, and separation of the epithelium from the lamina propria. (Hematoxylin and eosin, ×65 original magnification)

Differential Diagnosis

Differential diagnosis of lichen planus must consider the range of other lichenoid lesions (eg, drug-induced lesions, contact mercury hypersensitivity, erythema multiforme, lupus erythematosus, and graft-versus-host reaction), as well as leukoplakia, squamous cell carcinoma, mucous membrane pemphigoid, and candidiasis.[173,175,180] A detailed history of the clinical appearance and distribution of the lesions is very helpful.

Although it does not always provide an unequivocal diagnosis, a biopsy should be carried out before treatment of the lesions, because of the tendency for corticosteroids to confuse the diagnosis. Asymptomatic reticular lichen planus is often left untreated, and biopsy is not usually performed. Biopsy of papular and plaquelike OLP should be performed to rule out dysplastic changes and leukoplakia. Biopsy is usually performed on the erosive and bullous forms, partly because they are symptomatic (and thus brought to the clinician's attention) and partly to differentiate them from other vesiculobullous disorders.[181]

Clinical Course and Prognosis

The lesions of OLP appear, regress, and re-appear in a somewhat unpredictable fashion. Andreasen[190] calculated that 41% of reticular lesions healed spontaneously whereas 12% of atrophic lesions, 7% of plaquelike lesions, and 0% of erosive lesions healed without treatment. Silverman and Griffith[191] reported that when observed longer than 1 year, approximately 10% of a group of patients with predominantly erosive lesions had remissions. In a more recent, larger, and prospective study, Thorn and associates [181] reported that papular and ulcerative (erosive) changes were short-term lesions whereas atrophic and plaquelike changes were characterized by many remissions and newly developing lesions. Thorn and co-workers demonstrated that long-term topical steroid and antimycotic therapy had no apparent effect on the course of the disease. Numerous reports have related lichenoid lesions to a contact sensitivity to mercury and, less often, gold and food flavorings.

Removal of amalgam fillings in mercury-sensitive individuals who have contact-related lesions has almost always led to the complete resolution of the disease or at least to significant improvement.[176,183]

It must be stressed that lichenoid lesions that are caused by a contact allergy to dental materials such as amalgam occur only directly opposite the restoration. In patients with lichen planus, the general removal of amalgam fillings that are not directly opposite a lesion is not justified.

The status of OLP as a premalignant condition has been debated for many years. Numerous publications have described the clinical and histopathologic follow-up of lesions (in some cases, over many decades).[191–198] The occurrence of squamous cell carcinoma in most series ranges from 0.4 to 2.0% per 5-year observation period.[195] The most recent and extensive study reported a rate of 1.5% for patients observed over 7.5 years.[198] These rates are similar to those quoted for malignant change in leukoplakia and represent some 50 times the rate for the general population. OLP fulfills the criteria for a "premalignant" condition and was so designated at the 1984 International Seminar on Oral Leukoplakia and Associated Lesions Related to Tobacco Habits.[136] Although malignant transformation is reported to be more likely in erosive lesions, possibly due to the exposure of deeper layers of the epithelium to oral environmental carcinogens, there appears to be no consistent clue to the identity of those lesions that are likely to become malignant. Several investigators have described a lesion (referred to as oral lichenoid dysplasia) on the basis of a defined histopathologic picture and have postulated that this lesion is an independent precancerous lesion that mimics lichen planus and represents the true precursor of malignant change in lichen planus.[199,200] There is no general agreement on the grading of lichen planus, either clinically or histopathologically. Therefore, continued surveillance, repeated biopsy, and (where possible) eradication of erosive lesions and those lesions demonstrating dysplastic changes remain the safest course. Most cases of squamous cell carcinoma arising in an area of lichen planus are found on the tongue.[185,192–194] However, those cases of lichen planus exhibiting dysplastic changes are reportedly more prevalent on the buccal mucosa.[199,200]

Treatment

There is no known cure for OLP; therefore, the management of symptoms guides therapeutic approaches. Corticosteroids have been the most predictable and successful medications for controlling signs and symptoms. Topical and/or systemic corticosteroids are prescribed electively for each patient after orientation to OLP and by patient choice.[178,179,185,201–203]

Topical medications include high-potency corticosteroids, the most commonly used of which are 0.05% fluocinonide (Lidex) and 0.05% clobetasol (Temovate).[202,203] These are frequently prescribed as pastes or as gels. The topical forms are applied daily to meet each patient's needs. Topical steroids can be applied to the lesions with cotton swabs or (especially on the buccal mucosa) with gauze pads impregnated with steroid. In addition, extensive erosive lesions of OLP on the gingiva (desquamative gingivitis) may be treated effectively by using occlusive splints as carriers for the topical steroid. Long-term studies show no adverse systemic side effects with topical steroids, but occlusive therapy with high-potency steroids does cause systemic absorption, and patients should be carefully monitored and treated with the minimal amount of medication required to manage each individual.[204] *Candida* overgrowth with clinical thrush may develop, requiring concomitant topical or systemic antifungal therapy. Some studies have shown that the use of an antibacterial rinse such as chlorhexidine before steroid application helps prevent fungal overgrowth.

Systemic steroids are rarely indicated for brief treatment of severe exacerbations or for short periods of treatment of recalcitrant cases that fail to respond to topical steroids.[201] Systemic administration of prednisone tablets may be done with dosages varying between 40 and 80 mg daily for less than 10 days without tapering. The time and dosage regimens are determined individually, based on the patient's medical status, severity of disease, and previous treatment responses. End points and stabilization of treatment are determined by each patient since symptoms are managed only to individual satisfaction or acceptance. Consultation with the patient's primary care physician is important when underlying medical problems are present.[204]

Retinoids are also useful, usually in conjunction with topical corticosteroids as adjunctive therapy for OLP.[205,206] Systemic and topically administered beta all-*trans* retinoic acid, vitamin A acid, systemic etretinate, and systemic and topical isotretinoin are all effective, and topical application of a retinoid cream or gel will eliminate reticular and plaquelike lesions in many patients. However, following withdrawal of the medication, the majority of lesions recur. Topical retinoids are usually favored over systemic retinoids since the latter may be associated with adverse effects such as liver dysfunction, cheilitis, and teratogenicity.[205,206] A new systemically administered retinoid, temarotene, is reported to be an effective therapy for OLP and to be free of side effects other than a slight increase in liver enzymes.[207] Other topical and systemic therapies reported to be useful, such as dapsone, doxycycline, and antimalarials, require additional research.[185]

Topical application of cyclosporine appears to be helpful in managing recalcitrant cases of OLP. Although this has been confirmed in double-blind trials, the cost of cyclosporine solution, its hydrophobicity and unpleasant taste, and the yet unanswered questions regarding the drug's ability to promote viral reproduction and malignant change in epithelial cells have limited its use except for patients with extensive and otherwise intractable oral lesions.[184,208–210]

When lesions have been confined to the mucosa just opposite amalgam restorations and when patients have been positive for patch tests to mercury or other metals, complete removal of the amalgam restorations has been curative in most patients.[211–213] Surgical excision is usually not indicated for the treatment of OLP except in cases where concomitant dysplasia has been identified.[199]

▼ LICHENOID REACTIONS

Lichenoid reactions and lichen planus exhibit similar histopathologic features.[174] Lichenoid reactions were differentiated from lichen planus on the basis of (1) their association with the administration of a drug, contact with a metal, the use of a food flavoring, or systemic disease and (2) their resolution when the drug or other factor was eliminated or when the disease was treated.[174,212] Clinically, lichenoid lesions may exhibit the classic appearance of lichen planus, but atypical presentations are seen, and some of the dermatologic lesions included in this category show little clinical lichenification.[174]

Table 5-3 lists some of the disorders that are currently proposed as lichenoid reactions.[214]

Drug-Induced Lichenoid Reactions

Drug-induced lichenoid eruptions include those lesions that are usually described in the dental literature under the topic of lichenoid reactions (ie, oral mucosal lesions that have the clinical and histopathologic characteristics of lichen planus, that are associated with the administration of a drug, and that resolve following the withdrawal of the drug).[174,216]

A drug history can be one of the most important aspects of the assessment of a patient with an oral or oral-and-skin

TABLE 5-3   Diseases Exhibiting Lichenoid Tissue Reaction[18,22,169,214,215]

Site of Reaction	Disease
Skin and oral mucosa	Lichen planus, lupus erythematosus, erythema multiforme, lichenoid and fixed drug eruptions, secondary syphilis, graft-versus-host disease

Reproduced with permission from Weedon D.[214]

lichenoid reaction. Clinically, there is often little to distinguish drug-induced lichenoid reactions from lichen planus. However, lichenoid lesions that include the lip and lichenoid lesions that are symmetric in distribution and that also involve the skin are more likely to be drug related.[214] Histopathologically, lichenoid drug eruptions may show a deep as well as superficial perivascular lymphocytic infiltrate rather than the classic bandlike infiltrate of lichen planus, and eosinophils, plasma cells, and neutrophils may also be present in the infiltrate.

Drug-induced lichenoid reactions may resolve promptly when the offending drug is eliminated. However, many lesions take months to clear; in the case of a reaction to gold salts, 1 or 2 years may be required before complete resolution. Gold therapy, nonsteroidal anti-inflammatory drugs (NSAIDs), diuretics, other antihypertensives, and oral hypoglycemic agents of the sulfonylurea type are all important causes of lichenoid reactions (Table 5-4; Figure 5-36).[216–224] (Because more drugs are being added to it on a continual basis, this list should by no means be considered complete.)

Surveys of medication use among patients with various oral keratoses, including lichen planus, have found the use of antihypertensive drugs to be more common among lichen planus patients.[219] The use of NSAIDs was 10 times more frequent among those with erosive lichen planus.[216,218,222] Penicillamine is associated with many adverse reactions, including lichenoid reactions, pemphigus-like lesions, lupoid reactions and stomatitis, and altered taste and smell functions.[220,223] A number of the drugs that have been associated with lichenoid reactions may also produce lesions of discoid lupus erythematosus (lupoid reactions).[216]

Graft-versus-Host Disease

Graft-versus-host disease (GVHD)[225–240] is a complex multisystem immunologic phenomenon characterized by the interaction of immunocompetent cells from one individual (the donor) to a host (the recipient) who is not only immunodeficient but who also possesses transplantation isoantigens foreign to the graft and capable of stimulating it.[226] Reactions of this type occur in up to 70% of patients who undergo allogenic bone marrow transplantation, usually for treatment of refractory acute leukemia. There may be both acute (< 100 days after bone marrow transplantation) and chronic (after day 100, post transplantation) forms of the condition. The pathogenesis is probably related to an antigen-dependent proliferation of transplanted donor T-cell lymphocytes that are genetically disparate from the recipient's own tissues and that give rise to a generation of effector cells that react with and destroy recipient tissues. Of these, the epidermal (skin and mucous membrane) lesions are often most helpful clinically in establishing a diagnosis.[227]

CLINICAL FEATURES

The epidermal lesions of acute GVHD range from a mild rash to diffuse severe sloughing. This may include toxic epidermal necrolysis (Lyell's disease), a type of erythema multiforme in

TABLE 5-4 Drugs and Materials Implicated in Oral Lichenoid Reactions

Category	Drugs or Materials
Antimicrobials	Dapsone
	Ketoconazole
	Para-aminosalicylic acid
	Sodium aminosalicylate
	Streptomycin
	Sulfamethoxazole
	Tetracycline
Antiparasitics	Antimony compounds (stibophen, stibocaptate)
	Organic arsenicals
	Chloroquine
	Pyrimethamine
	Quinacrine
Antihypertensives	ACE inhibitors
	Chlorothiazide
	Hydrochlorothiazide
	Labetalol
	Mercurial diuretics
	Methyldopa
	Practolol
Antiarthritics	Aurothioglucose
	Colloidal gold (Europe only)
	Gold sodium thiomalate, thiosulfate
Anxiolytics	Lorazepam
NSAIDs	Fenclofenac
	Ibuprofen
	Naproxen
	Phenylbutazone
Oral hypoglycemic agents	Chlorpropamide
	Tolazamide
	Tolbutamide
Uricosuric agents	Allopurinol
Miscellaneous drugs	Iodides
	Penicillamine
	Quinidine sulfate
Chemicals; dental restorative materials	Substituted paraphenylenediamines used in color film developers; dental casting alloys and amalgam restorations

Adapted from Firth NA, Reade PD;[216] Hay KD et al;[217] Mason C et al;[218] McCartan BE, McCreary CE;[219] Cohen DM et al;[220] Potts AJC et al;[221] Robertson WD, Wray D;[222] Seehafer JR et al;[223] Regezi JA, Sciubba JJ;[224] Bez C et al.[225]

ACE = angiotensin-converting enzyme; NSAIDs = nonsteroidal anti-inflammatory drugs.

which large flaccid bullae develop with detachment of the epidermis in large sheets, leaving a scalded skin appearance.[226,228] Oral mucosal lesions occur in only about one-third of cases and are only a minor component of this problem.[229]

Chronic GVHD is associated with lichenoid lesions that affect both skin and mucous membranes. Oral lesions occur in

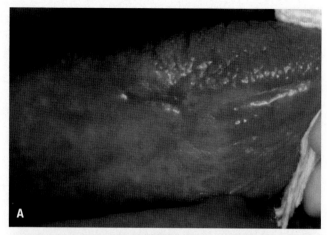

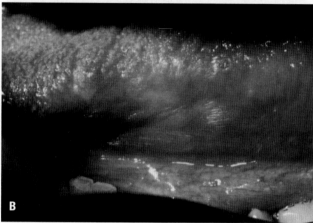

FIGURE 5-36 Lichenoid drug reaction. **A,** This patient had an 8-year history of a painful red-white plaque on the lateral border of the tongue. The plaque appears somewhat lichenoid, with radiating white lines. The patient was on a β-blocker for hypertension for 9 years and had these lesions continuously for 8 years. **B,** Within 1 month of discontinuing the medication, the patient's lesions completely disappeared.

80% of cases of chronic GVHD; salivary and lacrimal gland epithelium may also be involved.[230–233] In some cases, the intraoral lichenoid lesions are extensive and involve the cheeks, tongue, lips, and gingivae. In most patients with oral GVHD, a fine reticular network of white striae that resembles OLP is seen. Patients may often complain of a burning sensation of the oral mucosa. Xerostomia is a common complaint due to the involvement of the salivary glands. The development of a pyogenic granuloma on the tongue has been described as a component of chronic GVHD.[234,235]

The mouth is an early indicator of a variety of reactions and infections associated with transplantation-related complications. The majority of these infections are opportunistic *Candida* infections although infections with other agents (such as gram-negative anaerobic bacilli and *Aspergillus*) have also been described.[236] The differential diagnosis of oral lesions that develop in patients some months after bone marrow transplantation thus includes candidiasis and other opportunistic infections, toxic reactions to chemotherapeutic drugs that are

often used concomitantly, unusual viral infections (herpesvirus, *Cytomegalovirus*), and lichenoid drug eruptions.[226,230–232,237,238] Because of the potential involvement of salivary glands in chronic GVHD, biopsy of minor salivary glands is a useful diagnostic procedure in some cases.[227] The histopathologic features of chronic GVHD may resemble those of OLP.

TREATMENT AND PROGNOSIS

The principle basis for management of GVHD is prevention by careful histocompatibility matching and judicious use of immunosuppressive drugs. In some cases, topical corticosteroids and palliative medications may facilitate the healing of the ulcerations. Ultraviolet A irradiation therapy with oral psoralen has also been shown to be effective in treating resistant lesions.[229,239]

Topical azathioprine suspension has been used as an oral rinse and then swallowed, thereby maintaining the previously prescribed systemic dose of azathioprine. This resulted in improvement in cases of oral GVHD that was resistant to other approaches to management. Topical azathioprine may provide additional therapy in the management of immunologically-mediated oral mucosal disease.[240]

Clinicians evaluating cases of lichen planus should rule out the possibility of oral lichenoid reactions. Lichenoid drug reactions manifesting in the oral cavity have received some attention, and oral lichenoid GVHD has been well described, but it is likely that oral lichen planus as currently diagnosed also represents a heterogeneous group of lesions that require more specific identification and customized focused treatment.

▼ LUPUS ERYTHEMATOSUS (SYSTEMIC AND DISCOID)

Clinical Features, Diagnosis, and Treatment

Systemic lupus erythematosus (SLE) is a prototypical example of an immunologically mediated inflammatory condition that causes multiorgan damage. (SLE is discussed in more detail in Chapter 18, under "Connective Tissue Diseases"; the brief description here emphasizes its clinical manifestations on the oral mucosa.)

The oral lesions of systemic lupus are generally similar to those of discoid lupus (see below) and are most prevalent on the buccal mucosa, followed by the gingival tissues, the vermilion border of the lip, and the palate, in decreasing order of frequency. The lesions are frequently symptomatic, especially if the patient ingests hot or spicy foods, and often consist of one or more of the following components: erythema, surface ulceration, keratotic plaques, and white striae or papules (Figure 5-37). These lesions frequently appear lichenoid although they may be nonspecific and resemble leukoplakia, vesiculobullous disease, or even a granulomatous lesion (Figure 5-38). They typically respond well to topical or systemic steroids. Clobetasol (a potent topical steroid) placed under an occlusive tray is very effective for temporary relief of these lesions.[241] Long-term remission of these lesions obviously depends on treatment of the underlying systemic disease.

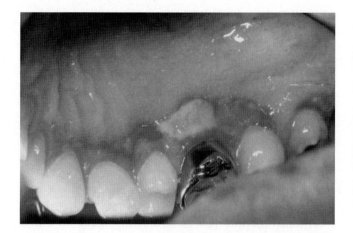

FIGURE 5-37 Symptomatic gingival lesion of systemic lupus erythematosus. The lesion is composed of the characteristic elements of a lupus reaction, including areas of erythema, ulceration, and hyperkeratosis (leukoplakia).

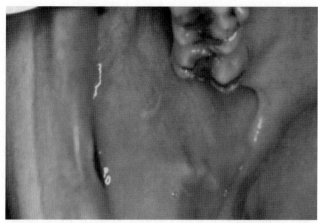

FIGURE 5-38 Lupus lesions frequently appear lichenoid but may be nonspecific and resemble leukoplakia.

Discoid lupus erythematosus (DLE) is a relatively common disease and occurs predominantly in females in the third or fourth decade of life.[242] DLE can present in both localized and disseminated forms and is also called chronic cutaneous lupus (CCL). DLE is confined to the skin and oral mucous membranes and has a better prognosis than SLE.[20] Typical cutaneous lesions appear as red and somewhat scaly patches that favor sun-exposed areas such as the face, chest, back, and extremities. These lesions characteristically expand by peripheral extension and are usually disk-shaped. The oral lesions can occur in the absence of skin lesions, but there is a strong association between the two. As the lesions expand peripherally, there is central atrophy, scar formation, and occasional loss of surface pigmentation. Lesions often heal in one area only to occur in a different area later.

The oral mucosal lesions of DLE frequently resemble reticular or erosive lichen planus. The primary locations for these lesions include the buccal mucosa, palate, tongue, and vermilion border of the lips. Unlike lichen planus, the distribution of DLE lesions is usually asymmetric, and the peripheral striae are much more subtle (Figure 5-39). The lesions may be atrophic, erythematous, and/or ulcerated and are often painful. Hyperkeratotic lichen planus–like plaques are probably twice as common in patients with CCL as compared to patients with SLE.[243,244] The oral lesions of DLE are markedly variable and can also simulate leukoplakia. Therefore, the diagnosis must be based not only on the clinical appearance of the lesions but also on the coexistence of skin lesions and on the results of both histologic examination and direct immunofluorescence testing. Despite their similar clinical features, lichen planus and lupus erythematosus yield markedly different immunofluorescent findings. Some authors [245] believe that the histology of oral lupus erythematosus is characteristic enough to provide a definitive diagnosis at the level of light microscopy, but most feel that the diagnostic standard must involve direct immunofluorescence. Importantly, lesions

with clinical and immunofluorescent features of both lichen planus and lupus erythematosus have also been described (overlap syndrome).[244]

Histopathologic Features

The histopathologic changes of oral lupus consist of hyperorthokeratosis with keratotic plugs, atrophy of the rete ridges, and (most especially) liquefactive degeneration of the basal cell layer. Edema of the superficial lamina propria is also quite prominent. Most of the time, lupus patients lack the bandlike leukocytic inflammatory infiltrate seen in patients with lichen planus. Immediately subjacent to the surface epithelium is a band of PAS-positive material, and frequently there is a pronounced vasculitis in both superficial and deep connective tissue. Another important finding in lupus is that direct immunofluorescence testing of lesional tissue shows the deposition of various immunoglobulins and C3 in a granular band

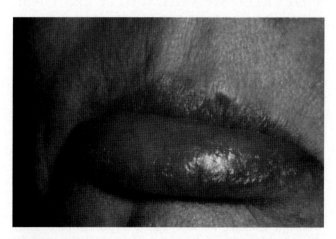

FIGURE 5-39 Lupus lesions are common on the lip. Unlike lichen planus, lupus lesions are usually asymmetric in distribution, and the peripheral striae are much more subtle.

involving the basement membrane zone. Importantly, direct immunofluorescent testing of uninvolved skin in a case of SLE will show a similar deposition of immunoglobulins and/or complement. This is called the positive lupus band test, and discoid lesions will not show this result.

Malignant Potential, Importance, and Scope of Oral Lesions

The precancerous potential of intraoral discoid lupus is controversial. Basal cell and (more commonly) squamous cell carcinomas have been reported to develop in healing scars of discoid lupus. However, this malignant change may have been caused by the radiation and ultraviolet light used in the treatment of lupus in the early twentieth century. The development of squamous cell carcinoma has been described in lesions of discoid lupus involving the vermilion border of the lip, and actinic radiation may play an important adjunct role in this.

Oral ulcers are one of the defining features of lupus erythematosus. The frequency of oral lesions in all forms of lupus combined varies from 5 to > 50%. Importantly, oral ulcers are found in SLE patients who have a higher level of disease activity as measured by the system lupus activity measure.[246] One study of 446 SLE patients showed that the extent of oral mucosal involvement was 40 to 54%, with the higher figure occurring in more severely involved patients.[247] The validity of these percentages, however, may be in question. In a recent survey of international centers devoted to the treatment of lupus, there was an extremely low level of agreement on the incidence of oral manifestations of this disease.[246,248]

An increase in the frequency of generalized periodontal disease has been reported with SLE.[249] However, most studies have found that there is either a decrease in periodontal probing depth in lupus or no change in periodontal status.[250,251] In fact, recent evidence suggests that the tendency of periodontitis to be more severe or progressive in some patients with collagen vascular diseases is a consequence of xerostomia and not a result of the primary disease.[250]

▼ DEVELOPMENTAL WHITE LESIONS: ECTOPIC LYMPHOID TISSUE

Cystic ectopic lymphoid tissue (oral lymphoepithelial cyst) may be found in several locations in the oral cavity. The most common locations are the posterior lateral border of the tongue (where the lymphoid tissue is called the lingual tonsil) and the floor of the mouth and ventral surface of the tongue. These lesions can also occur in the soft palate. Lymphoid tissue is normally present in the oral cavity as a ring of tonsillar tissue located in the pharynx and tongue, called Waldeyer's ring. This ring of tonsillar tissue includes the lingual, pharyngeal, and palatine tonsils. Connections between the overlying surface epithelium and the tonsillar tissue can often be seen in histologic sections. These so-called crypts can be become plugged with keratin and form lymphoepithelial cysts.[252–254] These are keratin-filled cysts within the accessory lymphoid tissue; they usually appear as reddish yellow or white submucosal dome-shaped nodules. In the absence of cystic obstruction, these lymphoid aggregates can become enlarged due to allergy or other inflammatory conditions and can appear as hyperplastic nodules.[255] These are particularly common in the oropharynx, soft palate, and faucial tonsillar area. These lesions can often be diagnosed by clinical features alone. Occasionally, they may become large enough to require a biopsy. Especially in the soft palate area, they can cause some irritation and itching, which will necessitate their removal as well.

▼ FORDYCE'S GRANULES

Fordyce's granules are ectopic sebaceous glands or sebaceous choristomas (normal tissue in an abnormal location) within the oral mucosa. Normally, sebaceous glands are seen within the dermal adnexa, in association with hair follicles; however, Fordyce's granules do not exhibit any association with hair structures in the oral cavity. This condition is seen in approximately 80 to 90% of the population.[256,257]

Features

Fordyce's granules present as multiple yellowish white or white papules. They are often seen in aggregates or in confluent collections, most commonly on the buccal mucosa (Figure 5-40, A) and vermilion border of the upper lip. Occasionally, these may be seen on the retromolar pad area and the anterior tonsillar pillars. Men usually exhibit more Fordyce's granules than women exhibit. The granules tend to appear during puberty and increase in number with age. Fordyce's granules are completely asymptomatic and are often discovered on routine examination. Histologically, they are identical to normal sebaceous glands found in the dermis (see Figure 5-40, B).

Treatment

Usually no treatment is indicated, and since the clinical appearance is virtually diagnostic, no biopsy is usually required. Fordyce's granules on the vermilion border of the upper lip may require surgical removal for esthetic reasons. Rare cases of pseudocysts and sebaceous cell hyperplasia and adenoma have been reported.[258–262]

▼ GINGIVAL AND PALATAL CYSTS OF THE NEWBORN AND ADULT

Features in the Newborn

Gingival cysts of the newborn are often multiple sessile dome-shaped lesions measuring about 2 to 3 mm in diameter. They are chalk white and present predominantly on the maxillary anterior alveolar ridge just lingual to the crest. Those in the posterior region of the jaw are found directly on the crest of the ridge occlusal to the crowns of the molar teeth (Figure 5-41). These lesions are usually seen in newborn or very young infants and disappear shortly after birth; they are thought to originate from remnants of the dental lamina. These cysts tend

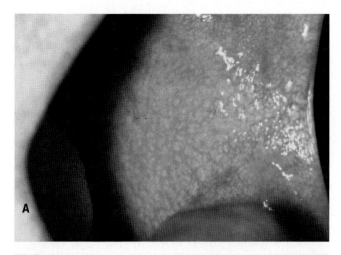

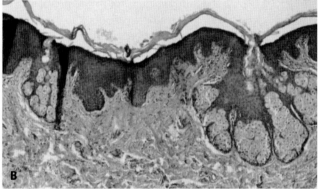

FIGURE 5-40 A, Fordyce's granules, appearing as multiple yellowish white papules and often seen as aggregates in the buccal mucosa. **B,** Photomicrograph of Fordyce's granules, which microscopically are identical to normal sebaceous glands. (Hematoxylin and eosin, ×20 original magnification)

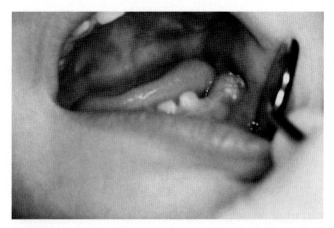

FIGURE 5-41   Gingival cysts of the newborn in a 2-year-old with retained teeth. These cysts appear as clusters of pearly white papules on the crest of the ridge in the mandibular molar area.

to rupture and disappear spontaneously. The eponyms "Epstein's pearls" and "Bohn's nodules" have both been used to describe odontogenic cysts of dental lamina origin, but these terms are not considered to be accurate. Epstein originally described keratin-filled nodules found along the mid-palatal region, probably derived from entrapped epithelium along the lines of fusion of the palatal processes. These are considered quite rare. Bohn's nodules are thought to be keratin-filled cysts scattered across the palate but most plentiful along the junction of the hard palate and soft palate and are thought to be derived from palatal salivary glands. Bohn's nodules probably relate to what are presently called gingival cysts of the newborn. Krisover reported finding 65 examples of gingival cysts in 17 infants.[242] The incidence in Japanese infants was almost 90%, an incidence considered significantly higher than that seen in black or white newborns.[263] Palatal cysts of the newborn occasionally persist into adult life and appear as peripheral odontogenic keratocysts.

Features in the Adult

Gingival cysts of the adult are thought to arise from dental lamina rests or from entrapment of surface epithelium.[264,265] They are most common in the canine and premolar area of the mandible and maxillary lateral incisor area and usually occur during the fifth and sixth decades of life. They have a very strong resemblance to lateral periodontal cysts, and there is a strong correlation between these two types of lesions. Patients have had lateral periodontal cysts subsequent to the development of a gingival cyst,[266] and lateral periodontal cysts are thought to be the intrabony counterpart of the gingival cyst. Gingival cysts usually appear as sessile painless growths involving the interdental area of the attached gingiva. These lesions often appear to be white or yellow white to blue and measure about 0.5 to 1 cm in diameter. They occasionally cause some superficial destruction of the underlying bone. A definite radiolucency is thought to represent a lateral periodontal cyst.[267–272]

▼ MISCELLANEOUS LESIONS

Geographic Tongue

Geographic tongue (erythema migrans, benign migratory glossitis, erythema areata migrans, stomatitis areata migrans) is a common benign condition affecting primarily the dorsal surface of the tongue. Its incidence varies from slightly over 2% in the US population to 11 to 16% in other populations. The condition is usually asymptomatic, but in one study of patients who experienced burning in the mouth, the burning was associated with geographic tongue in 24% of the patients. Tongue lesions are occasionally associated with similar-appearing ectopic lesions on the palate, buccal mucosa, or gingiva (Figure 5-42); this is called erythema circinata migrans or ectopic geographic tongue. Both conditions feature annular, circinate, or serpiginous lesions of the tongue with slightly depressed atrophic centers (devoid of filiform papillae) and raised white borders[15] (Figure 5-43).

ASSOCIATION WITH PSORIASIS

There may be an association between certain types of psoriasis (especially pustular psoriasis) and geographic tongue.[273]

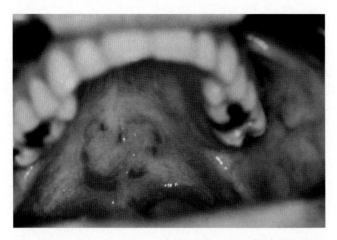

FIGURE 5-42 Ectopic geographic tongue involving the palate. Note the circinate configuration and strong resemblance to classic geographic tongue.

However, there is controversy over whether the psoriasis patients who manifest geographic tongue actually have intraoral psoriasis. A report of two patients with concurrent pustular psoriasis and mucosal lesions having the characteristic picture of geographic tongue seems to support this hypothesis.[273] Both skin lesions and oral lesions responded positively and in a parallel manner to systemic retinoid treatment, and both had identical histopathologic features. Further support for this association is seen in report of an unusual case of mucositis with features of psoriasis.[274] In that case, a patient had skin psoriasis including crusted lesions of the upper lip and diffuse erythematous lesions of the labial and buccal mucosa and denture-bearing palatal mucosa. Classic geographic tongue and ectopic geographic tongue were also seen. Importantly, all the lesions had multiple pustules. These references seem to suggest an association between geographic tongue and psoriasis in some cases. Furthermore, both psori-

asis and benign migratory glossitis are associated with human leukocyte antigen (HLA)-Cw6 and HLA-DR5.[275,276] Also, stomatitis areata migrans was found in 5.4% of patients with psoriasis and in 1% of control patients whereas benign migratory glossitis was found in 10.3% of patients with psoriasis and in 2.5% of control patients.[277] This association between these disorders gives supporting evidence that geographic tongue may be a manifestation of psoriasis.[277] However, another study found that 10% of psoriasis patients had oral lesions histologically suggestive of psoriasis but that only 1% had classic geographic tongue.[278]

OTHER ASSOCIATED CONDITIONS

Ectopic geographic tongue is frequently associated with similar tongue lesions. This is especially true in patients with atopy.[279] There is a significant increase in the prevalence of ectopic geographic tongue in atopic patients who have intrinsic asthma and rhinitis versus patients with negative skin test reactions to various antigens.[224] Also, patients with geographic tongue have a significantly greater personal or family history of asthma, eczema, and hay fever, when compared to control populations.[279] Benign migratory glossitis is seen with a fourfold increase in frequency in patients with juvenile diabetes, possibly due to an increased frequency of elevated amounts of the HLA-B15 tissue type.[280] Importantly, this tissue type also has a higher prevalence in atopic individuals.

Geographic tongue has also been seen with increased frequency in patients with pernicious anemia (this often appears as an erythematous form of geographic tongue) (Figure 5-44) and in pregnant patients, in whom it is possibly associated with folic acid deficiency or hormonal fluctuations. Association with the latter condition is supported by one report in which the severity of geographic tongue appeared to vary with hormonal levels.[280] Lesions that are histologically indistinguishable from those of geographic tongue can also be seen in Reiter's syndrome. The development of geographic tongue has also been associated with the administration of lithium carbonate.[281]

Hairy Tongue (Black Hairy Tongue)

"Hairy tongue" is a clinical term describing an abnormal coating on the dorsal surface of the tongue. The incidence of this condition ranges from 0.5% in the United States to 12.8% among Israeli male geriatric patients and 57% among imprisoned Greek drug addicts.[282–284] Hairy tongue results from the defective desquamation of cells that make up the secondary filiform papilla. This buildup of keratin results in the formation of highly elongated hairs, which is the hallmark of this entity.[285] The cause of black hairy tongue is unknown; however, there are several initiating or contributing factors. These include tobacco (heavy smoking) and psychotropic agents.[286–288] Other predisposing factors include broad-spectrum antibiotics such as penicillin and the use of systemic steroids.[224] The use of oxidizing mouthwashes or antacids and the overgrowth of fungal or bacterial organisms have also been associated with this condition. Radiation therapy for head and neck malignancies is

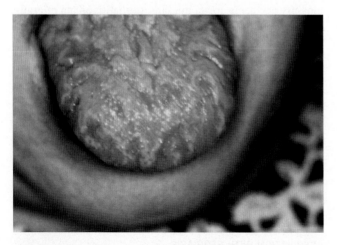

FIGURE 5-43 Florid geographic tongue in a pregnant woman. Note classic lesions containing red areas with atrophic filiform papillae and white circinate borders.

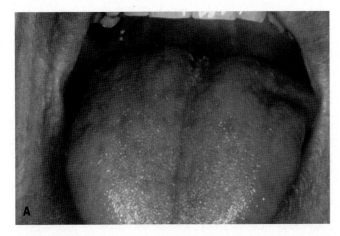
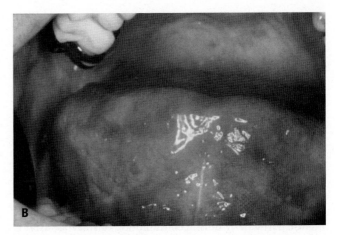

FIGURE 5-44 Red geographic tongue seen in patients with pernicious anemia. **A,** Typical red lesions involving the dorsum. **B,** Typical red lesions involving the ventral tongue.

considered a major factor as well. Importantly, poor oral hygiene can exacerbate this condition. The common etiologic factor for all of these influences may be the alteration of the oral flora by the overgrowth of yeast and chromogenic bacteria.[283] (See Chapters 4 and 7 for a more thorough discussion of this entity and its treatment.)

Hairy tongue usually involves the anterior two-thirds of the dorsum of the tongue, with a predilection for the midline just anterior to the circumvallate papillae. The patient presents with elongated filiform papillae and lack of desquamation of the papillae. The tongue therefore appears thickened and matted. Depending on the diet and the type of organisms present, the lesions may appear to range from yellow to brown to black or tan and white. Although the lesions are usually asymptomatic, the papillae may cause a gag reflex or a tickle in the throat if they become especially elongated (Figure 5-45). They may also result in halitosis or an abnormal taste. A biopsy is usually unnecessary. Treatment consists of eliminating the predisposing factors

if any are present. Cessation of smoking or discontinuation of oxygenating mouthwashes or antibiotics will often result in resolution. Improvement in oral hygiene is also important, especially brushing or scraping of tongue, in addition to other good oral hygiene practices. Podophyllin resin (a keratolytic agent) has been used in treatment, but there are some questions about its safety. However, a 1% solution of podophyllin resin is available for the treatment of hairy tongue. The efficacy of tooth brushing can be enhanced by a prior application of a 40% solution of urea. Topical tretinoin has recently been tried as treatment of this entity.[289,290]

Oral Submucous Fibrosis

Oral submucous fibrosis (OSF) is a slowly progressive chronic fibrotic disease of the oral cavity and oropharynx, characterized by fibroelastic change and inflammation of the mucosa, leading to a progressive inability to open the mouth, swallow, or speak.[291,292] These reactions may be the result of either direct stimulation from exogenous antigens like *Areca* alkaloids or changes in tissue antigenicity that may lead to an autoimmune response. It occurs almost exclusively in inhabitants of Southeast Asia, especially the Indian subcontinent.[292–295] The inflammatory response releases cytokines and growth factors that promote fibrosis by inducing the proliferation of fibroblasts, up-regulating collagen synthesis and down-regulating collagenase production.[292,296]

ETIOLOGY

Even though the etiopathology is incompletely understood, several factors are believed to contribute to the development of OSF, including general nutritional and vitamin deficiencies and hypersensitivity to certain dietary constituents such as chili peppers, chewing tobacco, etc.[293] However, the primary factor is the habitual use of betel and its constituents, which include the nut of the areca palm (*Areca catechu*), the leaf of the betel pepper (*Piper betle*), and lime (calcium hydroxide). Approximately 200 million persons chew betel regularly throughout the western

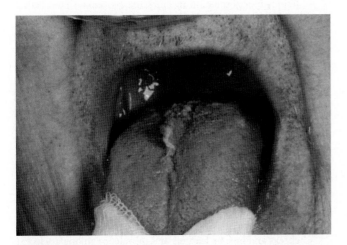

FIGURE 5-45 Elongated papillae in a patient with black hairy tongue. Such papillae can sometimes cause gagging and irritation of the palate.

Pacific basin and south Asia.[291,292,294,295,297] Only three drugs (nicotine, ethanol, and caffeine) are consumed more widely than betel. When betel is chewed, it produces mild psychoactive and cholinergic effects. Betel use is also associated with oral leukoplakia and squamous cell carcinoma.[294] OSF is regarded as a premalignant condition, and many cases of oral cancer have been found coexisting with submucous fibrosis.[298–300] Cases of submucous fibrosis have been reported in many Western countries, especially in individuals who have immigrated from the Indian subcontinent.[301,302]

CLINICAL FEATURES

The disease first presents with a burning sensation of the mouth, particularly during consumption of spicy foods. It is often accompanied by the formation of vesicles or ulcerations and by excessive salivation or xerostomia and altered taste sensations. Gradually, patients develop a stiffening of the mucosa, with a dramatic reduction in mouth opening and with difficulty in swallowing and speaking. The mucosa appears blanched and opaque with the appearance of fibrotic bands that can easily be palpated. The bands usually involve the buccal mucosa, soft palate, posterior pharynx, lips, and tongue. OSF usually affects young individuals in the second and third decades of life but may occur at any age. Histologic examination reveals severely atrophic epithelium with complete loss of rete ridges. Varying degrees of epithelial atypia may be present. The underlying lamina propria exhibits severe hyalinization, with homogenization of collagen. Cellular elements and blood vessels are greatly reduced.[292,303]

TREATMENT AND PROGNOSIS

OSF is very resistant to treatment. Many treatment regimens have been proposed to alleviate the signs and symptoms, without much success. Submucosal injected steroids and hyaluronidase, oral iron preparations, and topical vitamin A and steroids are some of the agents that have been used.[304] All of these therapies are essentially palliative. In severe cases, surgical intervention is the only treatment, but the fibrous bands and other symptoms often recur within a few months to a few years.[305] The use of an oral stent as an adjunct to surgery to prevent relapse has also been studied.[306] OSF is considered to be a premalignant condition. In a 17-year follow-up study in India, oral cancer developed in 7.6% of patients with submucous fibrosis. The malignant transformation rate for submucous fibrosis was 4 to 13%.[298–300]

▼ REFERENCES

1. Martin JL. Leukoedema: a review of the literature. J Natl Med Assoc 1992;84(11):938–40.
2. Durocher RT, Thalman R, Fiore-Donno G. Leukoedema of the oral mucosa. J Am Dent Assoc 1972;85:1105–9.
3. Martin JL, Crump EP. Leukoedema of the buccal mucosa in Negro children and youth. Oral Surg Oral Med Oral Pathol 1972;34:49–58.
4. Martin JL. Leukoedema: an epidemiological study in white and African Americans. J Tenn Dent Assoc 1997;77(1):18–21.
5. Van Wyk CW. An investigation into the association between leukoedema and smoking. J Oral Pathol 1985;4:491–9.
6. Axell T, Henricsson V. Leukoedema — an epidemiologic study with special reference to the influence of tobacco habits. Community Dent Oral Epidemiol 1981;9(3):142–6.
7. Jorgenson RJ, Levin S. White sponge nevus. Arch Dermatol 1981;117(2):73–6.
8. Morris R, Gansler TS, Rudisill MT, Neville B. White sponge nevus. Diagnosis by light microscopic and ultrastructural cytology. Acta Cytol 1988;32(3):357–61.
9. Terrinoni A, Candi E, Oddi S, et al. A glutamine insertion in the 1A alpha helical domain of the keratin 4 gene in a familial case of white sponge nevus. J Invest Dermatol 2000; 114(2):388–91.
10. Richard G, De Laurenzi V, Didona B, et al. Keratin 13 point mutation underlies the hereditary mucosal epithelial disorder white sponge nevus. Nat Genet 1995;11(4):453–5.
11. Lim J, Ng SK. Oral tetracycline rinse improves symptoms of white sponge nevus. J Am Acad Dermatol 1992;26(6):1003–5.
12. Shields CL, Shields JA, Eagle RC Jr. Hereditary benign intraepithelial dyskeratosis. Arch Ophthalmol 1987;105(3):422–3.
13. McLean IW, Riddle PJ, Schruggs JH, Jones DB. Hereditary benign intraepithelial dyskeratosis. A report of two cases from Texas. Ophthalmology 1981;88(2):164–8.
14. Sadeghi EM, Witkop CJ. Ultrastructural study of hereditary benign intraepithelial dyskeratosis. Oral Surg Oral Med Oral Pathol 1977;44(4):567–77.
15. Lynch MA, editor. Burkett's oral medicine: diagnosis and treatment. 9th ed. Lippincott-Raven, 1997. p. 60–73, 99, 258–60.
16. Dodd JH, Devereux S, Sarkany I. Dyskeratosis congenita with pancytopenia. Clin Exp Dermatol 1984;10:73.
17. Kalb RE, Grossman ME, Hutt C. Avascular necrosis of bone in dyskeratosis congenital. Am J Med 1986;80:511.
18. Wood NK, Goaz PW. White lesions of the oral mucosa. In: Wood NK, Goaz PW, editors. Differential diagnosis of oral lesions. 5th ed. St. Louis: Mosby, 1997. p. 96, 98.
19. Neville BW, Damm DD, Allen CM, Bouquot JE. Oral and maxillofacial pathology. Philadelphia: W. B. Saunders Company; 1995. p. 211, 280–8, 580.
20. Kashani HG, Mackenzie IC, Kerber PE. Cytology of linea alba using a filter imprint technique. Clin Prev Dent 1980;2:21–4.
21. Kovac-Kovacic M, Skaleric U. The prevalence of oral mucosal lesions in a population in Ljubljana, Slovenia. J Oral Pathol Med 2000;29(7):331–5.
22. Axell T. Occurrence of leukoplakia and some other oral white lesions among 20,333 adult Swedish people. Community Dent Oral Epidemiol 1987;15(1):46–51.
23. Shafer WG, Waldron CA. A clinical histopathologic study of oral leukoplakia. Surg Gynecol Obstet 1961;112:411.
24. Glass LF, Maize JC. Morsicatio buccarum et labiorum (excessive cheek and lip biting). Am J Dermatopathol 1991;13(3):271–4.
25. Schiodt M, Larsen V, Bessermann M. Oral findings in glassblowers. Community Dent Oral Epidemiol 1980;8(4):195–200.
26. Sewerin I. A clinical and epidemiologic study morsicatio buccarum-labiorum. Scand J Dent Res 1971;79(2):73–80.
27. Bouquot JE. Common oral lesions found during a mass screening examination. J Am Dent Assoc 1986;112(1):50–7.
28. Van Wyk CW, Staz J, Farman AG. The chewing lesion of the cheeks and lips: its features and prevalence among a selected group of adolescents. J Dent 1977;5(3):193–9.
29. Hjorting-Hansen E, Holst E. Morsicatio mucosae oris and suc-

tio mucosae oris. An analysis of oral mucosal changes due to biting and sucking habits. Scand J Dent Res 1970;78(6):492–9.

30. Bouquot JE, Gorlin RJ. Leukoplakia, lichen planus, and other oral keratoses in 23,616 white Americans over the age of 35 years. Oral Surg Oral Med Oral Pathol 1986;61(4):373–81.

31. Muhlendahl KE, Oberdisse U, Krienke EG. Local injuries by accidental ingestion of corrosive substances by children. Arch Toxicol 1978;39(4):299–314.

32. Gatot A, Arbelle J, Leiberman A, Yanai-Inbar I. Effects of sodium hypochlorite on soft tissues after its inadvertent injection beyond the root apex. J Endod 1991;17(11):573–4.

33. Moghadam BK, Gier R, Thurlow T. Extensive oral mucosal ulcerations caused by misuse of a commercial mouthwash. Cutis 1999;64(2):131–4.

34. Isenberg SR, Hier LA, Chauvin PJ. Chemical burns of the oral mucosa: report of a case. J Can Dent Assoc 1996;62(3):262–4.

35. Murdoch-Kinch CA, Mallatt ME, Miles DA. Oral mucosal injury caused by denture cleanser tablets: a case report. Oral Surg Oral Med Oral Pathol 1995;80(6):756–8.

36. Spiller HA, Quadrani-Kushner DA, Cleveland P. A five year evaluation of acute exposures to phenol disinfectant (26%). J Toxicol Clin Toxicol 1993;31(2):307–13.

37. Baruchin AM, Lustig JP, Nahlieli O, Neder A. Burns of the oral mucosa. Report of 6 cases. J Craniomaxillofac Surg 1991; 19(2):94–6.

38. Murrin JR, Abrams H, Barkmeier WW. Chemical burn of oral tissue caused by dental cavity varnish. Report of a case. Ill Dent J 1978;47(10):580–1.

39. Fanibunda KB. Adverse response to endodontic material containing paraformaldehyde. Br Dent J 1984;157(7):231–5.

40. Rees TD, Orth CF. Oral ulcerations with use of hydrogen peroxide. J Periodontol 1986;57(11):689–92.

41. Mucklow ES. Accidental feeding of a dilute antiseptic solution (chlorhexidine 0.05% with cetrimide 1%) to five babies. Hum Toxicol 1988;7(6):567–9.

42. Touyz LZ, Hille JJ. A fruit-mouthwash chemical burn. Report of a case. Oral Surg Oral Med Oral Pathol 1984;58(3):290–2.

43. Kawashima Z, Flagg RH, Cox DE. Aspirin-induced oral lesion: report of case. J Am Dent Assoc 1975;91(1):130–1.

44. Glick GL, Chaffee RB Jr, Salkin LM, Vandersall DC. Oral mucosal chemical lesions associated with acetyl salicylic acid. Two case reports. N Y State Dent J 1974;40(8):475–8.

45. Maron FS. Mucosal burn resulting from chewable aspirin: report of case. J Am Dent Assoc 1989;119(2):279–80.

46. Frost DE, Barkmeier WW, Abrams H. Aphthous ulcer—a treatment complication. Report of a case. Oral Surg Oral Med Oral Pathol 1978;45(6):863–9.

47. Lamey PJ, Lewis MA, Rees TD, et al. Sensitivity reaction to the cinnamonaldehyde component of toothpaste. Br Dent J 1990;10;168(3):115–8.

48. Seals RR Jr, Cain JR. Prosthetic treatment for chemical burns of the oral cavity. J Prosthet Dent 1985;53(5):688–91.

49. Gupta PC, Mehta FS, Daftary DK, et al. Incidence rates of oral cancer and natural history of oral precancerous lesions in a 10-year follow–up study of Indian villagers. Community Dent Oral Epidemiol 1980;8(6):283–333.

50. Douglass CW, Gammon MD. Reassessing the epidemiology of lip cancer. Oral Surg Oral Med Oral Pathol 1984;57(6):631–42.

51. Warnock GR, Fuller RP Jr, Pelleu GB Jr . Evaluation of 5-fluorouracil in the treatment of actinic keratosis of the lip. Oral Surg Oral Med Oral Pathol 1981;52(5):501–5.

52. Lewin F, Norell SE, Johansson H, et al. Smoking tobacco, oral snuff, and alcohol in the etiology of squamous cell carcinoma of the head and neck: a population-based case-referent study in Sweden. Cancer 1998;82(7):1367–75.

53. Hirsch JM, Heyden G, Thilander HJ. A clinical, histomorphological and histochemical study on snuff-induced lesions of varying severity. J Oral Pathol 1982;11(5):387–98.

54. Bouquot JE, Meckstroth RL. Oral cancer in a tobacco-chewing US population—no apparent increased incidence or mortality. Oral Surg Oral Med Oral Pathol 1998;86(6):697–706.

55. Rigotti NA, Lee JE, Wechsler H. US college students' use of tobacco products: results of a national survey. JAMA 2000; 284(6):699–705.

56. Walsh MM, Ellison J, Hilton JF, et al. Spit (smokeless) tobacco use by high school baseball athletes in California. Tob Control 2000;9 Suppl;2:1132–9.

57. Horn KA, Gao X, Dino GA, Kamal-Bahl S. Determinants of youth tobacco use in West Virginia: a comparison of smoking and smokeless tobacco use. Am J Drug Alcohol Abuse 2000;26(1):125–38.

58. Tomar SL, Winn DM. Chewing tobacco use and dental caries among U.S. men. J Am Dent Assoc 1999;130(11):1601–10.

59. Smith SS, Fiore MC. The epidemiology of tobacco use, dependence, and cessation in the United States. Prim Care 1999;26(3):433–61.

60. Wasnik KS, Ughade SN, Zodpey SP, Ingole DL. Tobacco consumption practices and risk of oro-pharyngeal cancer: a case-control study in Central India. Southeast Asian J Trop Med Public Health 1998;29(4):827–34.

61. Tomar SL, Giovino GA. Incidence and predictors of smokeless tobacco use among US youth. Am J Public Health 1998; 88(1):20–6.

62. Daniels TE, Hansen LS, Greenspan JS, et al. Histopathology of smokeless tobacco lesions in professional baseball players. Associations with different types of tobacco. Oral Surg Oral Med Oral Pathol 1992;73(6):720–5.

63. From the Centers for Disease Control and Prevention. State-specific prevalence among adults of current cigarette smoking and smokeless tobacco use and per capita tax-paid sales of cigarettes—United States, 1997. JAMA 1999;281(1):29–30.

64. Everett SA, Husten CG, Warren CW, et al. Trends in tobacco use among high school students in the United States, 1991–1995. J Sch Health 1998;68(4):137–40.

65. Martin GC, Brown JP, Eifler CW, Houston GD. Oral leukoplakia status six weeks after cessation of smokeless tobacco use. J Am Dent Assoc 1999;130(7):945–54.

66. Nilsson R. A qualitative and quantitative risk assessment of snuff dipping. Regul Toxicol Pharmacol 1998;28(1):1–16.

67. Mirbod SM, Ahing SI. Tobacco-associated lesions of the oral cavity: part I. Nonmalignant lesions. J Can Dent Assoc 2000;66(5):252–6.

68. Mani NJ. Tobacco smoking and associated oral lesions. Ann Dent 1984;43(1):6–14.

69. Dayal PK, Mani NJ, Bhargava K, Malaowalla AM. Prevalence of oral leukoplakia and nicotine stomatitis in smokers. A clinical study in textile mill workers. Indian J Cancer 1974; 11(3):272–9.

70. Rossie KM, Guggenheimer J. Thermally induced 'nicotine' stomatitis. A case report. Oral Surg Oral Med Oral Pathol 1990;70(5):597–9.

71. Mani NJ. Preliminary report on prevalence of oral cancer and

precancerous lesions among dental patients in Saudi Arabia. Community Dent Oral Epidemiol 1985;13(4):247–8.

72. Van Wyk CW. Nicotinic stomatitis of the palate: a clinico-histological study. J Dent Assoc S Afr 1967;22(4):106–11.

73. Pindborg JJ, Mehta FS, Gupta PC, et al. Reverse smoking in Andhra Pradesh, India: a study of palatal lesions among 10,169 villagers. Br J Cancer 1971;25(1):10–20.

74. Mandel ID. Antimicrobial mouthrinses: overview and update. J Am Dent Assoc 1994;125 Suppl 2:2S–10S.

75. Kopczyk RA, Abrams H, Brown AT, et al. Clinical and microbiological effects of a sanguinaria-containing mouthrinse and dentifrice with and without fluoride during 6 months of use. J Periodontol 1991;62(10):617–22.

76. Hakim SA. Sanguinarine—a carcinogenic contaminant in Indian edible oils. Indian J Cancer 1968;5(2):183–97.

77. Sen A, Ray A, Maiti M. Thermodynamics of the interactions of sanguinarine with DNA: influence of ionic strength and base composition. Biophys Chem 1996;7:59(1–2):155–70.

78. Damm DD, Curran A, White DK, Drummond JF. Leukoplakia of the maxillary vestibule—an association with Viadent? Oral Surg Oral Med Oral Pathol 1999;87(1):61–6.

79. Eversole LR, Eversole GM, Kopcik J. Sanguinaria-associated oral leukoplakia: comparison with other benign and dysplastic leukoplakic lesions. Oral Surg Oral Med Oral Pathol 2000;89(4):455–64.

80. Allen CM. Viadent-related leukoplakia—the tip of the iceberg? Oral Surg Oral Med Oral Pathol 1999;87(4):393–4.

81. Reichart PA, Langford A, Gelderblom HR, et al. Oral hairy leukoplakia: observations in 95 cases and review of the literature. J Oral Pathol Med 1989;18(7):410–5.

82. Greenspan D, Greenspan JS. Oral manifestations of human immunodeficiency virus infection. Dent Clin North Am 1993;37(1):21–32.

83. Greenspan D, Greenspan JS, Hearst NG, et al. Relation of oral hairy leukoplakia to infection with the human immunodeficiency virus and the risk of developing AIDS. J Infect Dis 1987;155(3):475–81.

84. Felix DH, Jalal H, Cubie HA, et al. Detection of Epstein-Barr virus and human papillomavirus type 16 DNA in hairy leukoplakia by in situ hybridisation and the polymerase chain reaction. J Oral Pathol Med 1993;22(6):277–81.

85. Mabruk MJ, Flint SR, Toner M, et al. Detection of Epstein-Barr virus DNA in tongue tissues from AIDS autopsies without clinical evidence of oral hairy leukoplakia. J Oral Pathol Med 1995;24(3):109–12.

86. Mabruk MJ, Flint SR, Toner M, et al. In situ hybridization and the polymerase chain reaction (PCR) in the analysis of biopsies and exfoliative cytology specimens for definitive diagnosis of oral hairy leukoplakia (OHL). J Oral Pathol Med 1994;23(7):302–8.

87. Syrjanen S, Laine P, Niemela M, Happonen RP. Oral hairy leukoplakia is not a specific sign of HIV-infection but related to immunosuppression in general. J Oral Pathol Med 1989;18(1):28–31.

88. King GN, Healy CM, Glover MT, et al. Prevalence and risk factors associated with leukoplakia, hairy leukoplakia, erythematous candidiasis, and gingival hyperplasia in renal transplant recipients. Oral Surg Oral Med Oral Pathol 1994;78(6):718–26.

89. Schiodt M, Norgaard T, Greenspan JS. Oral hairy leukoplakia in an HIV-negative woman with Behcet's syndrome. Oral Surg Oral Med Oral Pathol 1995;79(1):53–6.

90. Lozada-Nur F, Robinson J, Regezi JA. Oral hairy leukoplakia in

nonimmunosuppressed patients. Report of four cases. Oral Surg Oral Med Oral Pathol 1994;78(5):599–602.

91. Eisenberg E, Krutchkoff D, Yamase H. Incidental oral hairy leukoplakia in immunocompetent persons. A report of two cases. Oral Surg Oral Med Oral Pathol 1992;74(3):332–3.

92. Epstein JB, Fatahzadeh M, Matisic J, Anderson G. Exfoliative cytology and electron microscopy in the diagnosis of hairy leukoplakia. Oral Surg Oral Med Oral Pathol 1995;79(5):564–9.

93. Kratochvil FJ, Riordan GP, Auclair PL, et al. Diagnosis of oral hairy leukoplakia by ultrastructural examination of exfoliative cytologic specimens. Oral Surg Oral Med Oral Pathol 1990;70(5):613–8.

94. Mabruk MJ, Flint SR, Coleman DC, et al. A rapid microwave-in situ hybridization method for the definitive diagnosis of oral hairy leukoplakia: comparison with immunohistochemistry. J Oral Pathol Med 1996;25(4):170–6.

95. Green TL, Greenspan JS, Greenspan D, De Souza YG. Oral lesions mimicking hairy leukoplakia: a diagnostic dilemma. Oral Surg Oral Med Oral Pathol 1989;67(4):422–6.

96. Krogh P, Hald B, Holmstrup P. Possible mycological etiology of oral mucosal cancer: catalytic potential of infecting Candida albicans and other yeasts in production of N-nitrosobenzyl-methylamine. Carcinogenesis 1987;8:1543.

97. Krogh P, Holmstrup P, Vedtofte P, Pindborg JJ. Yeast organisms associated with human oral leukoplakia. Acta Derm Venerol Suppl (Stockh) 1986;121:51–5.

98. Barrett AW, Kingsmill UT, Speight PM. The frequency of fungal infection of oral mucosal lesions. Oral Dis 1998;4(1):26–31.

99. Cawson RA. Leukoplakia and oral cancer. Proc R Soc Med 1969;62:610.

100. Kozinn PJ, Taschdjian CL, Wiener H. Incidence and pathogenesis of neonatal candidiasis. Pediatrics 1958;21:421.

101. Epstein JB, Pearsall NN, Truelove EL. Quantitative relationships between Candida albicans in saliva and the clinical status of human subjects. J Clin Microbiol 1980;12:475.

102. Santarpia RP, Pollock JJ, Renner RP, Spiechowitz E. An in vivo replica method for site-specific detection of Candida albicans on the denture surface in denture stomatitis patients: correlation with clinical disease. J Prosthet Dent 1990;63:437.

103. Guggenheimer J, Moore PA, Rossie, K, et al. Insulin-dependent diabetes mellitus and oral soft tissue pathologies: II Prevalence and characteristics of Candida and candidal lesions. Oral Surg Oral Med Oral Pathol 2000;89(5):570-6.

104. Bud FZ, Jorgensen E, Mojon P, et al. Effects of an oral health program on the occurrence of oral candidiasis in a long-term care facility. Community Dent Oral Epidemiol 2000;28(2):141–9.

105. Reichart PA. [Infections of the oral mucosa II. Bacteria, mycotic and viral infections.] Mund Kiefer Gesichtschir 1999;3(6):298–308.

106. Cannon RD, Holmes AR, Mason AB, Monk BC. Oral Candida: clearance, colonization or candidiasis. J Dent Res 1995; 74(5):1152–61.

107. Olsen I. Oral adhesion of yeasts. Acta Odontol Scand 1990;48:45.

108. Darwazeh AMG, Lamey PJ, Samaranayake LP, et al. The relationship between colonization, secretor status and in vitro adhesion of Candida albicans to buccal epithelial cells from diabetics. J Med Microbiol 1990;33:43.

109. Fernanado PH, Panagoda GJ, and Samaranayake LE. The relationship between the acid and alkaline phosphatase activity and the adherence of clinical isolates of Candida parapsiposis to human buccal epithelial cells. APMIS 1999;107(11):1034–42.

110. Tsang CS, Samaranayake LE. Factors affecting the adherence of *Candida albicans* to human buccal epithelial cells in human immunodeficiency virus infection. Br J Dermatol 1999; 141(5):852–8.

111. Kulak Y, Arikan A, Kazazoglu E. Existence of *Candida albicans* and microorganisms in denture stomatitis patients. J Oral Rehabil 1997;24(10):780–90.

112. McMullan-Vogel CG, Jude HD, Ollert MW, Vogel CW. Serotype distribution and secretory proteinase activity of *Candida albicans* isolated from the oral mucosa of patients with denture stomatitis. Oral Microbiol Immunol 1999;14(3):183–9.

113. Reichart PA, Geldesblom HR, Becker J, Kuntz A. AIDS and the oral cavity. The HIV infection, virology, aetiology, immunology, precautions and clinical observations in 100 patients. Int J Oral Maxillofac Surg 1987;16:129.

114. Newton AV. Denture sore mouth. Br Dent J 1962;112:357.

115. Bergendahl T, Issacson G. Effect of nystatin in the treatment of denture stomatitis. Scand J Dent Res 1980;88:446.

116. Davenport J. The oral distribution of *Candida* in denture stomatitis. Br Dent J 1970;129:151.

117. Cawson RA, Lehner T. Chronic hyperplastic candidiasis-candidal leukoplakia. Br J Dermatol 1968;80:9.

118. Burkhardt A, Seifert G. Morphologische klassification den oralen leukoplakien. Dtsch Med Wochenschr 1977;102:223–9.

119. Pindborg JJ. Oral cancer and precancer. Bristol, UK: John Wright and Sons, 1980.

120. Walker DM, Arendorf TM. Candidal leukoplakia, chronic multifocal candidiasis and median rhomboid glossitis. In: Samaranayake LP, MacFarlane TW. Oral candidosis. Boston: Wright/Butterworth Scientific; 1990.

121. Banoczy J. Oral leukoplakias. The Hague: Martinus Nijhoff; 1982.

122. Porter SR, Scully C. Chronic mucocutaneous candidosis and related syndromes. In: Samaranayake LP, MacFarlane TW. Oral candidosis. Boston: Wright/Butterworth Scientific; 1990.

123. Rothberg MS, Eisenbud L, Griboff S. Chronic mucocutaneous candidiasis-thymoma syndrome. A case report. Oral Surg Oral Med Oral Pathol 1989;68:411.

124. Dongari-Bagtzoglou A, Wen K, Lamster IB. *Candida albicans* triggers interleukin-6 and interleukin-8 responses by oral fibroblasts in vitro. Oral Microbiol Immunol 1999;14(6):364–70.

125. Harvey RL, Myers JP. Nosocomial fungemia in a large community hospital. Arch Intern Med 1987;147:2117.

126. Klein RS, Harris CA, Small CB, et al. Oral candidiasis in high-risk patients as the initial manifestation of the acquired immunodeficiency syndrome. N Engl J Med 1984;311:354.

127. Blackwell CC, Aly FZM, James VS, et al. Blood group, secretor status and oral carriage of yeasts among patients with diabetes mellitus. Diabetes Res 1989;12:101.

128. Challacombe SJ. Immunology of oral candidosis. In: Samaranayake LP, MacFarlane TW. Oral candidosis. Boston: Wright/Butterworth Scientific; 1990.

129. Wray D, Felix DH, Cumming CG. Alteration of humoral responses to *Candida* in HIV infection. Br Dent J 1990;168:326.

130. Epstein JB, Kimura LH, Menard TW, et al. Effects of specific antibodies on the interaction between the fungus *Candida albicans* and human oral mucosa. Arch Oral Biol 1982;27:469.

131. Klein R, Harris C, Small C, et al. Oral candidiasis in high-risk patients as the initial manifestation of the acquired immunodeficiency syndrome. N Engl J Med 1984;311:354–8.

132. Hay RJ. Overview of studies of fluconazole in oropharyngeal candidiasis. Rev Infect Dis 1990;12 Suppl:334.

133. Meyer I, Shklar G. The oral manifestations of acquired syphilis. A study of eighty-one cases. Oral Surg Oral Med Oral Pathol 1967;23(1):45–57.

134. Wong PN. Secondary syphilis with extensive oral manifestations. Aust Dent J 1985;30(1):22–4.

135. Mani NJ. Secondary syphilis initially diagnosed from oral lesions. Report of three cases. Oral Surg Oral Med Oral Pathol 1984;58(1):47–50.

136. Axell T, Pindborg JJ, Smith CJ, van der Waal I. Oral white lesions with special reference to precancerous and tobacco-related lesions: conclusions of an international symposium held in Uppsala, Sweden, May 18–21 1994. International Collaborative Group on Oral White Lesions. J Oral Pathol Med 1996;25(2):49–54.

137. Bouquot JE. Reviewing oral leukoplakia: clinical concepts for the 1990s. J Am Dent Assoc 1991;122(7):80–2.

138. Payne TF. Why are white lesions white? Observations on keratin. Oral Surg Oral Med Oral Pathol 1975;40(5):652–8.

139. Banoczy J. Follow-up studies in oral leukoplakia. J Maxillofac Surg 1977;5(1):69–75.

140. Waldron CA, Shafer WG. Leukoplakia revisited. A clinicopathologic study of 3256 oral leukoplakias. Cancer 1975;36(4):1386–92.

141. Silverman S Jr, Gorsky M, Kaugars GE. Leukoplakia, dysplasia, and malignant transformation. Oral Surg Oral Med Oral Pathol 1996;82:117.

142. Silverman S Jr, Gorsky M, Lozada F. Oral leukoplakia and malignant transformation. A follow-up study of 257 patients. Cancer 1984;53:563–8.

143. Schepman KP, van der Meij EH, Smeele LE, et al. Malignant transformation of oral leukoplakia: a follow-up study of a hospital based population of 166 patients with oral leukoplakia from the Netherlands. Oral Oncol 1998;34:270–5.

144. Lumerman H, Freedman P, Kerpel S. Oral epithelial dysplasia and the development of invasive squamous carcinoma. Oral Surg Oral Med Oral Pathol 1995;79:321–9.

145. Field EA, Field JK, Martin MV. Does *Candida* have a role in oral epithelial neoplasia? J Med Vet Mycol 1989;27(5):277–94.

146. Sugerman PB, Shillitoe EJ. The high risk human papillomaviruses and oral cancer: evidence for and against a causal relationship. Oral Dis 1997;3:130–47.

147. Hansen LS, Olson JA, Silverman S Jr. Proliferative verrucous leukoplakia. A long-term study of thirty patients. Oral Surg Oral Med Oral Pathol 1985;60(3):285–98.

148. Silverman S Jr, Gorsky M. Proliferative verrucous leukoplakia: a follow-up study of 54 cases. Oral Surg Oral Med Oral Pathol Oral Radiol Endod 1997;84:154–7.

149. Abbey LM, Kaugars GE, Gunsolley JC, et al. Intraexaminer and interexaminer reliability in the diagnosis of oral epithelial dysplasia. Oral Surg Oral Med Oral Pathol 1995;80:188–91.

150. Mashberg A, Samit A. Early diagnosis of asymptomatic oral and oropharyngeal squamous cancers. CA Cancer J Clin 1995;45:328–51.

151. Warnakulasuriya KAAS, Johnson NW. Sensitivity and specificity of OraScan toluidine blue mouthrinse in the detection of oral cancer and precancer. J Oral Pathol Med 1996;25:97–103.

152. Sciubba JJ. Improving detection of precancerous and cancerous oral lesions. Computer-assisted analysis of the oral brush biopsy. J Am Dent Assoc 1999;130:1445–57.

153. Silverman S Jr. Diagnosis and management of leukoplakia and premalignant lesions. Atlas Oral Maxillofac Surg Clin North Am 1998;10:13–23.

154. Al-Drouby HA. Oral leukoplakia and cryotherapy. Br Dent J 1983;155(4):124–5.

155. Horch HH, Gerlach KL, Schaefer HE. CO2 laser surgery of oral premalignant lesions. Int J Oral Maxillofac Surg 1986;15(1):19–24.

156. Kaugars GE, Silverman S Jr, Lovas JL, et al. A review of the use of antioxident supplements in the treatment of human oral leukoplakia. Oral Surg Oral Med Oral Pathol 1996;81:5–14.

157. Krebs-Smith SM. Progress in improving diet to reduce cancer risk. Cancer 1998;83:1425–32.

158. Enwonwu CO, Meeks VI. Bionutrition and oral cancer in humans. Crit Rev Oral Biol Med 1995;6(1):5–17.

159. Pindborg JJ, Daftary DK, Mehta FS. A follow-up study of sixty-one oral dysplastic precancerous lesions in Indian villagers. Oral Surg Oral Med Oral Pathol 1977;43(3):383–90.

160. Schepman KP, van der Meij EH, Smeele LE, van der Waal I. Concomitant leukoplakia in patients with oral squamous cell carcinoma. Oral Dis 1999;5:206–9.

161. Gorlin RJ. Bowen's disease of the mucous membrane of the mouth. A review of the literature and a presentation of six cases. Oral Surg Oral Med Oral Pathol 1950;3:35.

162. Daley T, Birek C, Wysocki GP. Oral bowenoid lesions: differential diagnosis and pathogenetic insights. Oral Surg Oral Med Oral Pathol Oral Radiol Endod 2000;90(4):466–73.

163. Kratochvil FJ, Cioffi GA, Auclair PL, Rathburn WA. Virus-associated dysplasia (bowenoid papulosis?) of the oral cavity. Oral Surg Oral Med Oral Pathol 1989;68:312.

164. Brightman VJ. Red and white lesions of the oral mucosa. In: Lynch MA, Brightman VJ, Greenberg MS, editors. Burket's oral medicine. 9th ed. Philadelphia: J.B. Lippincott; 1997.

165. Crissman JD, Visscher DW, Sakr W. Premalignant lesions of the upper aerodigestive tract: pathologic classification. J Cell Biochem Suppl 1993;17F:49–56.

166. Hashibe M, Mathew B, Kuruvilla B, et al. Chewing tobacco, alcohol, and the risk of erythroplakia. Cancer Epidemiol Biomarkers Prev 2000;9(7):639–45.

167. Kramer IR, Lucas RB, Pindborg JJ, Sobin LH. Definition of leukoplakia and related lesions: an aid to studies on oral pre-cancer. Oral Surg Oral Med Oral Pathol 1978;46(4):518–39.

168. Mashberg A, Garfinkel L. Early diagnosis of oral cancer: the erythroplastic lesion in high risk sites. CA Cancer J Clin 1978;28(5):297–303.

169. Mashberg A, Samit A. Early diagnosis of asymptomatic oral and oropharyngeal squamous cancers. CA Cancer J Clin 1995;45(6):328–51.

170. Seoane J, Varela-Centelles PI, Diz Dios P, et al. Experimental intervention study about recognition of erythroplakia by undergraduate dental students. Int Dent J 1999;49(5):275–8.

171. Shafer WG, Waldron CA. Erythroplakia of the oral cavity. Cancer 1975;36(3):1021–8.

172. Shear M. Erythroplakia of the mouth. Int Dent J 1972;22(4):460–73.

173. Zegarelli DJ, Sabbagh E. Relative incidence of intraoral pemphigus vulgaris, mucous membrane pemphigoid and lichen planus. Ann Dent 1989;48(1):5–7.

174. Black MM. Lichen planus and lichenoid eruptions. In: Rook A, Wilkinson DS, Ebling FJG, et al, editors. Textbook of dermatology. 4th ed, Boston: Blackwell; 1986.

175. Conklin RJ, Blasberg B. Oral lichen planus. Dermatol Clin 1987;5(4):663–73.

176. Scully C, El-Kom M. Lichen planus: review and update on pathogenesis. J Oral Pathol 1985;14(6):431–58.

177. Porter SR, Kirby A, Olsen I, et al. Immunologic aspects of dermal and oral lichen planus. Oral Surg Oral Med Oral Pathol Oral Radiol Endod 1997;83:858–63.

178. Vincent SD, Fotos PG, Baker KA, et al. Oral lichen planus: the clinical, historical and therapeutic features of 100 cases. Oral Surg Oral Med Oral Pathol 1990;70:165–71.

179. Silverman S Jr, Gorsky M, Lozada-Nur F, Gionnotti K. A prospective study of findings and management in 214 patients with oral lichen planus. Oral Surg Oral Med Oral Pathol 1991;72:665–70.

180. McClatchy KD, Silverman S Jr, Hansen LS. Studies on oral lichen planus III: clinical and histologic correlations in 213 patients. Oral Surg Oral Med Oral Pathol 1975;39:122–7.

181. Thorn JJ, Holmstrup P, Rindum J, Pindborg JJ. Course of various clinical forms of oral lichen planus: a prospective follow-up study of 611 patients. J Oral Pathol 1988;17(5):213–8.

182. Allen CM, Beck FM, Rossie KM, Kaul TJ. Relation of stress and anxiety to oral lichen planus. Oral Surg Oral Med Oral Pathol 1986;61(1):44–6.

183. Yiannias JA, el-Azhary RA, Hand JH, et al. Relevant contact sensitivities in patients with the diagnosis of oral lichen planus. J Am Acad Dermatol 2000;42:177–82.

184. Palestine AG, Nussenblat RB, Chan C-C, et al. Side effects of systemic cyclosporine in patients not undergoing transplantation. Am J Med 1984;77(4):652–6.

185. Silverman S Jr, Bahl S. Oral lichen planus update: clinical characteristics, treatment responses, and malignant transformation. Am J Dent 1997;10:259-63.

186. Cohen DM, Bhattacharyya I, Zunt SL, Tomich CE. Linear IgA disease histopathologically and clinically masquerading as lichen planus. Oral Surg Oral Med Oral Pathol 1999;88(2):196–201.

187. Boisnic S, Frances C, Branchet MC, et al. Immunohistochemical study of oral lesions of lichen planus: diagnostic and pathophysiologic aspects. Oral Surg Oral Med Oral Pathol 1990;70(4):462–5.

188. Laskaris G, Sklavounou A, Angelopoulos A. Direct immunofluorescence in oral lichen planus. Oral Surg Oral Med Oral Pathol 1982;53(5):483–7.

189. Rinaggio J, Neiders ME, Aguirre A, Kumar V. Using immunofluorescence in the diagnosis of chronic ulcerative lesions of the oral mucosa. Compend Contin Educ Dent 1999;20(10):943–50.

190. Andreasen JO. Oral lichen planus. 1. A clinical evaluation of 115 cases. Oral Surg Oral Med Oral Pathol 1968;25(1):31–42.

191. Silverman S Jr, Griffith M. Studies on oral lichen planus II. Follow-up on 200 patients: clinical characteristics and associated malignancy. Oral Surg Oral Med Oral Pathol 1974;37(5):705–10.

192. Silverman S Jr, Gorsky M, Lozada-Nur F. A prospective follow-up study of 570 patients with oral lichen planus: persistence, remission, and malignant association. Oral Surg Oral Med Oral Pathol 1985;60:30–4.

193. Krutchkoff DK, Cutler L, Laskowski S. Oral lichen planus: the evidence regarding potential malignant transformation. Oral Surg Oral Med Oral Pathol 1978;7(1):1–7.

194. Murti PR, Daftary DK, Bhousi RB, et al. Malignant potential of lichen planus: observations in 722 patients from India. J Oral Pathol 1986;15(2):71–7.

195. van der Meij EH, Schepman KP, Smeele LE, et al. A review of the recent literature regarding malignant transformation

of oral lichen planus. Oral Surg Oral Med Oral Pathol 1999;88(3):307–10.

196. Cohen DM, Bhattacharyya I, Zunt SL, Tomich CE. Linear IgA disease histopathologically and clinically masquerading as lichen planus. Oral Surg Oral Med Pathol 1999;88:196-201.

197. Eisenberg E, Krutchkoff DJ. Lichenoid lesions of oral mucosa. Diagnostic criteria and their importance in the alleged relationship to oral cancer. Oral Surg Oral Med Oral Pathol 1992;73(6):699–704.

198. Hietanen J, Paasonen MR, Kuhlefelt M, Malmstrom M. A retrospective study of oral lichen planus patients with concurrent or subsequent development of malignancy. Oral Oncol 1999;35(3):278–82.

199. Krutchkoff DJ, Eisenberg E. Lichenoid dysplasia: a distinct histopathologic entity. Oral Surg Oral Med Oral Pathol 1985;60(3):308–15.

200. Lovas JGI, Harsanyi BB, El Generdy AK. Oral lichenoid dysplasia: a clinicopathologic analysis. Oral Surg Oral Med Oral Pathol 1989;68(1):57–63.

201. Silverman S Jr, Lozada-Nur F, Migliorati C. Clinical efficacy of prednisone in the treatment of patients with oral inflammatory ulcerative diseases: a study of 55 patients. Oral Surg Oral Med Oral Pathol 1985;59:360–3.

202. Lozada-Nur F, Silverman S Jr. Topically applied fluocinonide in an adhesive base in the treatment of oral vesiculoerosive diseases. Arch Dermatol 1980;116(8):898–901.

203. Lozada-Nur F, Huang MZ. Open preliminary clinical trial of clobetasol proprionate ointment in adhesive paste for treatment of chronic vesiculoerosive disease. Oral Surg Oral Med Oral Pathol 1991;71:283–7.

204. Plemons JM, Rees TD, Zachariah NY. Absorption of a topical steroid and evaluation of adrenal suppression in patients with erosive lichen planus. Oral Surg Oral Med Oral Pathol 1990;69(6):688–93.

205. Giustina TA, Stewart JCB, Ellis CN, et al. Topical application of isotretinoin gel improves oral lichen planus. A double-blind study. Arch Dermatol 1986;122(5):534–6.

206. Camisa C, Allen CM. Treatment of oral erosive lichen planus with systemic isotretinoin. Oral Surg Oral Med Oral Pathol 1986;62(4):393–6.

207. Bollag W, Ott F. Treatment of oral lichen planus with temarotene. Lancet 1989;21;2(8669):974.

208. Eisen D, Ellis CN, Duell EA, et al. Effect of topical cyclosporine rinse on oral lichen planus: a double-blind analysis. N Engl J Med 1990;323(5):290–4.

209. Frances C, Boisnic S, Etiennes C, Szpirglas H. Effect of the local topical application of cyclosporine A on chronic erosive lichen planus of the oral cavity. Dermatologia 1988;177(3):194–5.

210. Balato N, DeRosa S, Bordone F, et al. Dermatological application of cyclosporine A. Arch Dermatol 1989;125(10):1430–1.

211. Koch P, Bahmer FA. Oral lesions and symptoms related to metals used in dental restorations: a clinical, allergological, and histologic study. J Am Acad Dermatol 1999;41(3 Pt 1):422–30.

212. Finne KAJ, Goransson K, Winckler L. Oral lichen planus and contact allergy to mercury. Int J Oral Surg 1982;11(4):236–9.

213. Eversole LK, Ringer M. The role of dental restorative metal in the pathogenesis of oral lichen planus. Oral Surg Oral Med Oral Pathol 1984;57(4):383–7.

214. Weedon D. The lichenoid tissue reaction. Int J Dermatol 1982;21:203.

215. Brook PM, Day RO. Nonsteroidal anti-inflammatory drugs—differences and similarities. N Engl J Med 1991;324:1716.

216. Firth NA, Reade PD. Angiotensin-converting enzyme inhibitors implicated in oral mucosal lichenoid reactions. Oral Surg Oral Med Oral Pathol 1989;67(1):41–4.

217. Hay KD, Mullen HK, Reade PC. D-penicillamine-induced mucocutaneous lesions with features of pemphigus. Oral Surg Oral Med Oral Pathol 1978;45:385.

218. Mason C, Grisius R, McKean T. Stomatitis medicamentosa associated with gold therapy for rheumatoid arthritis. US Navy Med 1978;69(1):23–5.

219. McCartan BE, McCreary CE. Oral lichenoid drug eruptions. Oral Dis 1997;3(2):58–63.

220. Cohen DM, Bhattacharyya I, Lydiatt WM. Recalcitrant oral ulcers caused by calcium channel blockers: diagnosis and treatment considerations. J Am Dent Assoc 1999; 130(11):1611–8.

221. Potts AJC, Hamburger J, Scully C. The medication of patients with oral lichen planus and the association of nonsteroidal anti-inflammatory drugs with erosive lesions. Oral Surg Oral Med Oral Pathol 1987;64(5):541–3.

222. Robertson WD, Wray D. Ingestion of medication among patients with oral keratoses including lichen planus. Oral Surg Oral Med Oral Pathol 1992;74(2):183–5.

223. Seehafer JR, Rogers RS, Fleming R, et al. Lichen planus-like lesions caused by penicillamine in primary biliary cirrhosis. Arch Dermatol 1981;117(3):140–2.

224. Regezi JA, Sciubba JJ. Oral pathology: clinical pathologic correlations. 3rd ed. Philadelphia: WB Saunders; 1999. p. 99–101,104.

225. Bez C, Lodi G, Sardella A, et al. Oral lichenoid lesions after thalidomide treatment. Dermatology 1999;199(2):195.

226. Woo SB, Lee SJ, Schubert MM. Graft-vs.-host disease. Crit Rev Oral Biol Med 1997;8(2):201–16.

227. Sale GE, Shulman HM, Schubert MM, et al. Oral and ophthalmic pathology of graft versus host disease in man: predictive value of the lip biopsy. Hum Pathol 1981; 12(11):1022–30.

228. Peck GL, Herzig GP, Elias PM. Toxic epidermal necrolysis in a patient with graft-vs-host reaction. Arch Dermatol 1972;105(4):561–9.

229. Schubert MM, Sullivan KR, Truelove EL. Head and neck complications of bone marrow transplantation. In: Petersen DE, Elias EG, Sonis ST, editors. Head and neck management of the cancer patient. Boston: Martinus Nijhoff; 1986. p. 401.

230. Nakamura S, Hiroki A, Shinohara M, et al. Oral involvement in chronic graft-versus-host disease after allogeneic bone marrow transplantation. Oral Surg Oral Med Oral Pathol 1996;82(5):556–63.

231. Schubert MM, Sullivan KM. Recognition, incidence, and management of oral graft-versus-host disease. NCI Monogr 1990;9:135–43.

232. Rodu B, Gockerman JP. Oral manifestations of the chronic graft-vs-host reaction. JAMA 1983;249(4):504–7.

233. Nagler R, Marmary Y, Krausz Y, et al. Major salivary gland dysfunction in human acute and chronic graft-versus-host disease (GVHD). Bone Marrow Transplant 1996;17(2):219–24.

234. Kanda Y, Arai C, Chizuka A, et al. Pyogenic granuloma of the tongue early after allogeneic bone marrow transplantation for multiple myeloma. Leuk Lymphoma 2000;37(3–4):445–9.

235. Lee L, Miller PA, Maxymiw WG, et al. Intraoral pyogenic granuloma after allogeneic bone marrow transplant. Report of three cases. Oral Surg Oral Med Oral Pathol 1994;78(5):607–10.

236. Schubert MM, Sullivan KM, Morton TH, et al. Oral manifestations of chronic graft-vs-host disease. Arch Intern Med 1984;144(8):1591–5.

237. Majorana A, Schubert MM, Porta F, et al. Oral complications of pediatric hematopoietic cell transplantation: diagnosis and management. Support Care Cancer 2000;8(5):353–65.

238. Lloid ME, Schubert MM, Myerson D, et al. *Cytomegalovirus* infection of the tongue following marrow transplantation. Bone Marrow Transplant 1994;14(1):99–104.

239. Redding SW, Callander NS, Haveman CW, Leonard DL. Treatment of oral chronic graft-versus-host disease with PUVA therapy: case report and literature review. Oral Surg Oral Med Oral Pathol 1998;86(2):183–7.

240. Epstein JB, Nantel S, Sheoltch SM. Topical azathioprine in the combined treatment of chronic oral graft-versus-host disease. Bone Marrow Transplant 2000;25(6):683–7.

241. Brown RS, Flaitz CM, Hays GL, Trejo PM. The diagnosis and treatment of discoid lupus erythematosus with oral manifestations only. A case report. Compendium 1994;15(6): 724,726–8,730.

242. Shafer WG, Hine MK, Levi BM. A textbook of oral pathology. 4th ed. Philadelphia: W.B. Saunders; 1983. p. 269, 842.

243. Burge SM, Frith PA, Juniper RP, Wojnarowski F. Mucosal involvement and systemic and chronic cutaneous lupus erythematosus. Br J Dermatol 1989;121(6):727–41.

244. Rossi A, Euzzauto MT. Association of lichen planus and discoid lupus erythematosus: the clinical and histolopathologic study of two cases. G Ital Dermatol Venereol 1990;125(12):583–91.

245. Karjalinen TK, Tomich CE. Pathologic study of oral mucosal lupus erythematosus. Oral Surg 1989;67(5):547–54.

246. Parodi A, Mussone C, Cacciapuoti M, et al. Measuring the activity of disease in patients with cutaneous lupus erythematosus. Br J Dermatol 2000;142(3):457–60.

247. Meyer U, Kleinheinz J, Gaubitz M, et al. [Oral manifestations in patients with systemic lupus erythematosus.] Mund Kiefer Gesichtschir 1997;1(2):90–4.

248. Vitali C, Doria A, Tincani A, et al. International survey on management of patients with SLE. I. General data on the participating centers and the results of a questionnaire regarding mucotaneous involvement. Clin Exp Rheumatol 1996;14 Suppl 16:S1722.

249. Nagler RM, Wilber M, Ben-Arieh Y, et al. Generalized periodontal involvement in a younger patient with systemic lupus erythematosus. Lupus 1999:8(9):770–2.

250. Gonzales TS, Coleman CG. Periodontal manifestations of collagen vascular disorders. Periodontol 2000 1999;Oct 21:94–105.

251. Mutlu S, Richards A, Maddison P, Scully C. Gingival and periodontal health in systemic lupus erythematosus. Community Dent Oral Epidemiol 1993;21(3):158–61.

252. Bhaskar SN. Lymphoepithelial cysts of the oral cavity. Oral Surg 1996;21:120.

253. Buchner A, Hansen LS. Lymphoepithelial cysts of the oral cavity. Oral Surg 1980;50:441.

254. Giunta J, Cataldo E. Lymphoepithelial cysts of the oral mucosa. Oral Surg 1973;35:77.

255. Mogi K. Ectopic tonsillar tissue in the muscoa of the floor of the mouth simulating a benign tumor. Case report. Aust Dent J 1991;36(6):456–8.

256. Sewerin I, Praetorius F. Keratin-filled pseudocysts of ducts of sebaceous glands in the vermillion border of the lip. J Oral Pathol 1974;3(6):279–83.

257. Halperin V, Kolas S, Jefferis KR, et al. The occurrence of Fordyce spots, benign migratory glossitis, median rhomboid glossitis and fissured tongue in 2,478 dental patients. Oral Surg Oral Med Oral Pathol 1953;6:1072.

258. Sewerin I. The sebaceous glands in the vermillion border of the lips and in the oral mucosa of man. Acta Odonto Scand Suppl 1975;33:1.

259. Daley TD. Intraoral sebaceous hyperplasia. Diagnostic criteria. Oral Surg Oral Med Oral Pathol 1993;75(3):343–7.

260. Batsakis JG, el-Naggar AK. Sebaceous lesions of salivary glands and oral cavity. Ann Otol Rhinol Laryngol 1990;99(5 Pt 1):416–8.

261. Lipani C, Woytash JJ, Greene GW Jr. Sebaceous adenoma of the oral cavity. J Oral Maxillofac Surg 1983;41(1):56–60.

262. Orlian AI, Salman L, Reddi T, et al. Sebaceous adenoma of the oral mucosa. J Oral Med;1987;42(1):38–9.

263. Chehade A, Daley TD, Wysocki GP, Miller AS. Peripheral odontogenic keratocyst. Oral Surg Oral Med Oral Pathol 1994;77(5):494–7.

264. Shear M. Developmental odontogenic cyst. An update. J Oral Pathol Med 1994;23(1):1–11.

265. Ikemura K, Kakinoki Y, Inshio K, Suenaga Y. Cysts of the oral mucosa in newborns: a clinical observation. J UOEH 1983;1(52):163–8.

266. Tolson GE, Czuszak A, Billman MA, Lewis DM. Report of a lateral periodontal cyst and gingival cyst occurring in the same patient. J Periodontal 1996;67(5):541–4.

267. Buchner A, Hansen LS. The histomorphologic spectrum of the gingival cyst in the adult. Oral Surg Oral Med Oral Pathol 1979;48:532–9.

268. Catalvo E, Berkman MB. Cysts of the oral mucosa in newborns. Am J Dis Child 1968;116:44.

269. Fromm A. Epstein's pearls, Bowen's nodules and inclusion cyst of the oral cavity. J Dent Child 1967;34:275–87.

270. Maher WP, Swindle PF. Etiology and vascularization of dental lamina cysts. Oral Surg Oral Med Oral Pathol 1970;29:590–7.

271. Reeve CM, Levy BP. Gingival cysts: a review of the literature and report of four cases. Periodontics 1968;6:115–7.

272. Wysocki GP, Brannon RB, Gardner DG, Sapp P. Histogenesis of the lateral periodontal cyst and the gingival cyst of the adult. Oral Surg Oral Med Oral Pathol 1980;50:327–34.

273. Casper U, Seiffert K, Dippel E, Zouboulis CC. [Exfoliatio areata lingua et mucosae oris: a mucous membrane manifestation of psoriasis pustulosa?] Hautarzt 1998;49(11):850–4.

274. Younai FS, Phelan JA. Oral mucositis with features of psoriasis: report of a case and review of the literature. Oral Surg Oral Med Oral Pathol 1997;84(1):61–70.

275. Gonzaga HF, Torres EA, Alchorne MM, Gerbase-Delima M. Both psoriasis and benign migratory glossitis are associated with HLA-CW6. Br J Dermatol 1996;135(3):368–70.

276. Feneli A, Papanicolaou S, Papanicolaou M, Laskaris G. Histocomaptibility of antigens and geographic tongue. Oral Surg Oral Med Oral Pathol 1993(76):476–9.

277. Morris LF, Phillips CM, Binnie WH, et al. Oral lesions and patients with psoriasis: a controlled study. Cutis 1992; 49(5):339–44.

278. Hietanen J, Salo OP, Kanerva L, Juvakoski T. Study of the oral mucosa in 200 consecutive patients with psoriasis. Scan J Dent Res 1984;92(4)50–4.

279. Marks R, Simons MJ. Geographic tongue: a manifestation of atopy. Br J Dermatol 1979;101(2):159–62.

280. Waltimo J. The geographic tongue during a year of oral contraceptive cycles. Br Dent J 1991;171(3–4):94–6.

281. Patki AH. Geographic tongue developing in a patient on lithium carbonate therapy. Int J Dermatol 1992;31(5):368–9.

282. Kaplin I, Moskona D. A clinical survey of oral soft tissue lesions in institutionalized geriatric patients in Israel. Gerodontology 1990,9(2):59–62.

283. Suzuki N, Seiko K, Shiota T, et al. Fundamental and clinical studies of long-acting amoxicillin granules in oral and maxillofacial surgery infections. Jpn J Antibiot 1983;36(2):452–63.

284. Donta AN, Lampadakis J, Pilalitos P, Spyropoulos ND. [Findings from the clinical examination of the oral cavity of 100 drug addicts.] Hell Stomatol Chron 1989;33(2):101–5.

285. Manabe M, Lim HW, Winzer M, Loomis CA. Architectural organization of the filiform papilla in normal and black hairy tongue epithelium: dissection of differentiation pathways in a complex human epithelium according to their keratin expression. Arch Dermatol 1999;135(2):177–81.

286. Mirbod SM, Ahing SI. Tobacco-associated lesions of the oral cavity: part I nonmalignant lesions. J Can Dent Assoc 2000; 66(5):252–6.

287. Heymann WR. Psychotropic agent-induced black hairy tongue. Cutis 2000;66(1):25–6.

288. Andersson G, Vala EK, Curval M. The influence of cigarette consumption and smoking machine yields of tar and nicotine on the nicotine uptake and oral mucosal lesions in smokers. J Oral Pathol Med 1997;26(3):117–23.

289. Langtry JA, Car MM, Steele MC, Ivy FA. Topical tretinoin: a new treatment for black hairy tongue (lingua villosa nigra). Clin Exp Dermatol 1992;17(3):163–4.

290. McGregor JM, Hay RJ. Oral retinoids to treat black hairy tongue. Clin Exp Dermatol 1993;18(3):291.

291. Zain RB, Ikeda N, Gupta PC, et al. Oral mucosal lesions associated with betel quid, areca nut and tobacco chewing habits: consensus from a workshop held in Kuala Lumpur, Malaysia, November 25–27, 1996. J Oral Pathol Med 1999;28:1–4.

292. Rajendran R. Oral submucous fibrosis: etiology, pathogenesis, and future research. Bull World Health Organ 1994; 72(6):985–96.

293. Gupta PC, Hebert JR, Bhonsle RB, et al. Dietary factors in oral leukoplakia and submucous fibrosis in a population-based case control study in Gujarat, India. Oral Dis 1998;4(3):200–6.

294. Norton SA. Betel: consumption and consequences. J Am Acad Dermatol 1998;38(1):81–8.

295. Sinor PN, Gupta PC, Murti PR, et al. A case-control study of oral submucous fibrosis with special reference to the etiologic role of areca nut. J Oral Pathol Med 1990;19(2):94–8.

296. Haque MF, Harris M, Meghji S, Barrett AW. Immunolocalization of cytokines and growth factors in oral submucous fibrosis. Cytokine 1998;10(9):713–9.

297. Shah N, Sharma PP. Role of chewing and smoking habits in the etiology of oral submucous fibrosis (OSF): a case-control study. J Oral Pathol Med 1999;28(1):1–4.

298. Pindborg JJ, Murti PR, Bhonsle RB, et al. Oral submucous fibrosis as a precancerous condition. Scand J Dent Res 1984;92(3):224–9.

299. Murti PR, Bhonsle RB, Pindborg JJ, et al. Malignant transformation rate in oral submucous fibrosis over a 17-year period. Community Dent Oral Epidemiol 1985;13(6):340–1.

300. Pindborg JJ, Mehta FS, Daftary DK. Incidence of oral cancer among 30,000 villagers in India in a 7-year follow-up study of oral precancerous lesions. Community Dent Oral Epidemiol 1975;3(2):86–8.

301. VanWyk CW. Oral submucous fibrosis. The South African experience. Indian J Dent Res 1997;8(2):39–45.

302. Oliver AJ, Radden BG. Oral submucous fibrosis. Case report and review of the literature. Aust Dent J 1992; 37(1):31–4.

303. Haque MF, Harris M, Meghji S, Speight PM. An immunohistochemical study of oral submucous fibrosis. J Oral Pathol Med 1997;26(2):75–82.

304. Borle RM, Borle SR . Management of oral submucous fibrosis: a conservative approach. J Oral Maxillofac Surg 1991;49(8):788–91.

305. Khanna JN, Andrade NN. Oral submucous fibrosis: a new concept in surgical management. Report of 100 cases. Int J Oral Maxillofac Surg 1995;24(6):433–9.

306. Le PV, Gornitsky M, Domanowski G. Oral stent as treatment adjunct for oral submucous fibrosis. Oral Surg Oral Med Oral Pathol 1996;81(2):148–50.

6

PIGMENTED LESIONS OF THE ORAL MUCOSA

LEWIS R. EVERSOLE, DDS, MSD

In the course of disease, the mucosal tissues can assume a variety of discolorations. Disease processes can culminate in the formation of pseudomembranes, in increased keratinization (white lesions), or in increased vascularization (red lesions). Blue, brown, and black discolorations constitute the pigmented lesions of the oral mucosa, and such color changes can be attributed to the deposition of either endogenous or exogenous pigments. Although there are many biochemical substances and metabolic products that are pigmented, only a few become deposited in the oral soft tissues although some accumulate in developing dentin during odontogenesis (eg, bilirubin pigment, porphyrins, and hemosiderin).

The endogenous pigmentation of the oral mucous membrane is most often explained by the presence of hemoglobin, hemosiderin, and melanin (Table 6-1). Hemoglobin imparts a red or blue appearance to the mucosa and represents pigmentation associated with vascular lesions; the coloration is rendered by circulating erythrocytes coursing through patent vessels. In contrast, hemosiderin appears brown and is deposited as a consequence of blood extravasation, which may occur as a consequence of trauma or a defect in hemostatic mechanisms. Hemochromatosis (generalized hemosiderin tissue deposition) may occur as a result of a variety of pathologic states.

Melanin is the pigment derivative of tyrosine and is synthesized in melanocytes, which subsequently transfer the melanin granules into adjacent basal cells to protect against the damaging effects of actinic irradiation. An increase in melanin pigment occurs when melanocytes oversynthesize or overpopulate. Overproduction (basilar melanosis) may be caused by a variety of mechanisms, including increased sun exposure, drugs, the pituitary adrenocorticotropic hormone (ACTH), and genetic factors (in association with certain syndromes). Melanocyte overpopulation occurs in benign nevi and in malignant melanomas.

TABLE 6-1 Endogenous Pigmentation in Oral Mucosal Disease

Pigment	Color	Disease Process
Hemoglobin	Blue, red, purple	Varix, hemangioma, Kaposi's sarcoma, angiosarcoma, hereditary hemorrhagic telangiectasia
Hemosiderin	Brown	Ecchymosis, petechia, thrombosed varix, hemorrhagic mucocele, hemochromatosis
Melanin	Brown, black or gray	Melanotic macule, nevus, melanoma, basilar melanosis with incontinence

The distribution of these various pigments in the oral mucosa is quite variable, ranging from a focal macule to broad diffuse tumefactions. The specific coloration, tint, location, multiplicity, size, and configuration of the pigmented lesion(s) are of diagnostic importance.

Exogenous pigments are usually traumatically deposited directly into the submucosa. However, some may be ingested, absorbed, and distributed hematogenously, to be precipitated in connective tissues, particularly in areas subject to chronic inflammation, such as the gingiva (Table 6-2). In the past, various metallic compounds were used medicinally, but currently, this therapy is rarely prescribed. For that reason, lesions attributable to heavy-metal therapy are no longer seen, with the exception of lesions caused by gold, which is still used systemically to treat arthritis. Lastly, exogenous pigment may be generated by chromogenic bacteria that colonize the keratinized surface of the tongue (hairy tongue).

In this chapter, the differential diagnosis of oral pigmentation is organized according to color, configuration, and distribution (Table 6-3).

▼ BLUE/PURPLE VASCULAR LESIONS

Hemangioma

Vascular lesions presenting as proliferations of vascular channels are tumorlike hamartomas when they arise in childhood; in adults (particularly elderly persons), benign vascular proliferations are generally varicosities. The hemangiomas of childhood are found on the skin, in the scalp, and within the connective tissue of mucous membranes. Approximately 85% of childhood-onset hemangiomas spontaneously regress after puberty.[1,2]

TABLE 6-2 Exogenous Pigmentation of Oral Mucosa

Source	Color	Disease Process
Silver amalgam	Gray, black	Tattoo, iatrogenic trauma
Graphite	Gray, black	Tattoo, trauma
Lead, mercury, bismuth	Gray	Ingestion of paint or medicinals
Chromogenic bacteria	Black, brown, green	Superficial colonization

Depending on the depth of the vascular proliferation within the oral submucosa, the lesion may harbor vessels close to the overlying epithelium and appear reddish blue or, if a little deeper in the connective tissue, a deep blue. Angiomatous lesions occurring within muscle (so-called intramuscular hemangiomas) may fail to show any surface discoloration. Whereas most hemangiomas are raised and nodular, some may be flat, macular, and diffuse, particularly on the facial skin, where they are referred to as port-wine stains. The port-wine hemangioma of facial skin may concomitantly involve the oral mucosa, where the angioma may continue in macular fashion or become tumefactive. Thus, the clinical appearance of benign vascular hamartomas can be quite variable, ranging from a flat reddish blue macule to a nodular blue tumefaction.

Most oral hemangiomas are located on the tongue, where they are multinodular and bluish red. The multinodularity is racemose and diffuse. Tongue angiomas frequently extend deeply between the intrinsic muscles of the tongue. The lip mucosa is another common site for hemangiomas in children; these tumors are usually localized, blue, and raised. The aforementioned port-wine stain involves the facial skin and is flat and magenta in color. When there is a concurrent history of seizures, the condition represents encephalotrigeminal angiomatosis (Sturge-Weber syndrome). Vascular lesions occur in the brain as well as on the facial skin; skull radiography may disclose vessel wall calcifications that yield bilamellar radiopaque tracks referred to as "tram line" calcifications.

Hemodynamics in angiomas are perturbed, and stasis with thrombosis is commonly encountered. Most patent vascular lesions will blanch under pressure; indeed, placing a microscope glass slide over the pigmented area and adding pressure will often demonstrate this feature dramatically. Conversely, when intraluminal clots form, they become palpable and the lesion will usually not blanch. Thrombi in angiomas may eventually calcify, and such lesions will feel hard on palpation. The calcified nodules, or phleboliths, may be radiographically evident.

Microscopically, a hemangioma may comprise numerous large dilated vascular channels lined by endothelial cells without a muscular coat; such lesions are referred to as cavernous hemangiomas. Rarely, cavernous hemangiomas may show a media muscularis. Cellular- or capillary-type hemangiomas show significant endothelial proliferation, and the vascular lumina are very small. Both types may occur only in the subepithelial connective tissue or may extend deeply between muscle fibers (so-called intramuscular hemangiomas). This biologic feature is of clinical importance since intramuscular lesions may extend quite deeply and are more difficult to manage if treatment is required for functional or esthetic reasons.

Since many hemangiomas spontaneously involute during teenage years, treatment may be withheld in children. Patients who require treatment can undergo conventional surgery, laser surgery, or cryosurgery. Larger lesions that extend into muscles are more difficult to eradicate surgically, and sclerosing agents such as 1% sodium tetradecyl sulfate may be administered by intralesional injection. These agents result in postoperative pain, and the patient must be managed with a

TABLE 6-3   Clinical Classification of Oral Pigmentations

| Color | Solitary | | Multifocal |
	Focal	Diffuse	
Blue/Purple	Varix Hemangioma	Hemangioma	Kaposi's sarcoma Hereditary hemorrhagic telangiectasia
Brown	Melanotic macule Nevus Melanoma	Ecchymosis Melanoma Drug-induced pigmentation Hairy tongue	Physiologic pigment Neurofibromatosis Hemochromatosis Lichen planus Addison's disease Drug-induced pigmentation Peutz-Jeghers syndrome Petechia
Gray/Black	Amalgam tattoo Graphite tattoo Nevus Melanoma	Amalgam tattoo Melanoma Hairy tongue	Heavy-metal ingestion pigmentation

moderate-level analgesic such as oxycodone or aspirin with codeine. Cutaneous port-wine stains can be treated by subcutaneous tattooing or by argon laser (see also Chapter 5, "Red and White Lesions of the Oral Mucosa").

Varix

Pathologic dilatations of veins or venules are varices or varicosities, and the chief site of such involvement in the oral tissues is the ventral tongue.[3–5] Varicosities become progressively prominent with age; thus, lingual varicosities are encountered in elderly individuals. Lingual varicosities appear as tortuous serpentine blue, red, and purple elevations that course over the ventrolateral surface of the tongue, with extension anteriorly. Even though they may be quite striking in some patients, they represent a degenerative change in the adventitia of the venous wall and are of no clinical consequence. They are painless and are not subject to rupture and hemorrhage.

A focal dilatation of a vein or group of venules is known as a varix (Figure 6-1). These lesions also tend to occur in elderly persons and are primarily located on the lower lip, appearing as a focal raised pigmentation. They may be blue, red, or purple, and the surface mucosa is often lobulated or nodular. Whereas some can be blanched, others are not, due to the formation of intravascular thrombi. The varix resembles the hemangioma both clinically and histologically, yet it is distinguished by two features: (1) the patient's age at its onset and (2) its etiology. As previously mentioned, a hemangioma is usually congenital and has a tendency to spontaneously regress whereas a varix arises in older individuals and, once formed, does not regress. Alternatively, a varix has a finite growth potential; once a varix has formed, further enlargement is uncommon. Whereas hemangiomas are vascular hamartomas of unknown etiology, the varix represents a venous dilatation that may evolve from trauma such as lip or cheek biting. The traumatic event probably damages and weakens the vascular wall and culminates in dilation.

Microscopically, varices resemble cavernous hemangiomas. They may be represented by a single dilated vascular channel lined by endothelial cells lacking a muscular coat, or they may comprise numerous tortuous channels. Most show intraluminal thrombosis, and the thrombi show evidence of organization and canalization.

Varices of the lips and buccal mucosa may be unsightly and may interfere with mastication. The lesion can be excised or removed by other surgical methods, including electrosurgery and cryosurgery. Intralesional 1% sodium tetradecyl sulfate injection is effective as well, yet it is usually more painful than simple excision. This sclerosing agent should be injected directly into the lumina with a tuberculin syringe (depositing .05 to 0.15 mL/cm^3).

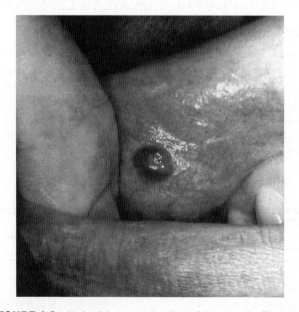

FIGURE 6-1   Varix of the mucosal surface of the upper lip. The lesion appears as a blue nodule.

Angiosarcoma

Malignant vascular neoplasms, distinct from Kaposi's sarcoma, are not related to human immunodeficiency virus (HIV) and can arise anywhere in the body. Although the oral cavity is an extremely rare site for such tumors, those that occur will (if superficial) appear red, blue, or purple. They are rapidly proliferative and therefore present as nodular tumors. Angiosarcomas can arise from blood or lymph vessel endothelial cells or from pericytic cells of the vasculature. They have a poor prognosis and are treated by radical excision.

Kaposi's Sarcoma

A tumor of putative vascular origin, Kaposi's sarcoma (KS)[6,7] was rarely encountered in the oral cavity prior to 1983. The classic form generally appeared in two distinct clinical settings: (1) elderly men (in the oral mucosa and on the skin of the lower extremities) and (2) children in equatorial Africa (in lymph nodes). The former is the classic form as originally described by Moritz Kaposi and is an indolent tumor with slowly progressive growth. Although classified as a malignancy, classic Kaposi's sarcoma does not show a great tendency for metastasis and probably has never caused the death of a patient. The oral and cutaneous tumors are considered to be of multifocal origin rather than metastases from a distant primary tumor. The oral tumors are red, blue, and purple, and the hard palate is the favored site; the skin tumors tend to localize in the dorsal aspect of the feet and great toe. The African form is characterized by lymph node enlargement and can progressively involve many node groups, being an aggressive and potentially lethal disease. Since it does not present with oral lesions, this form of KS is not discussed further.

After 1983, oral KS became much more prevalent, being the most common neoplastic process to accompany HIV infection. Indeed, the mere presence of KS lesions in HIV-seropositive subjects constitutes a diagnostic sign for acquired immunodeficiency syndrome (AIDS). The cutaneous lesions begin as red macules and enlarge to become blue, purple, and ultimately brown nodular tumefactions. The lower extremity shows no predilection over other cutaneous sites, and lesions may appear on the arms, face, scalp, or trunk. The oral lesions continue to show a predilection for the posterior hard palate, and they also begin as flat red macules of variable size and irregular configuration (Figure 6-2). Although they may appear as a focal lesion, typical oral KS lesions are multifocal, with numerous isolated and coalescing plaques. Eventually, these lesions increase in size to become nodular growths, and some will involve the entire palate, protruding below the plane of occlusion. The facial gingiva is the second most-favored oral site; in the early stages, the differential diagnosis includes pyogenic granuloma and giant cell granuloma. It is uncommon for AIDS-associated KS to arise in the buccal mucosa, tongue, and lips.

Laboratory studies have disclosed that the cell population is not transplantable into athymic nude mice as with most malignant tumors; rather, the human neoplastic cells secrete a variety of cytokines that induce KS lesions of mouse origin in

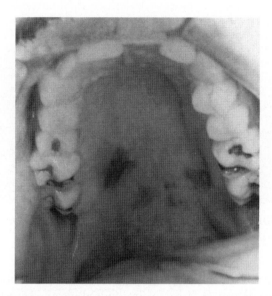

FIGURE 6-2 Multifocal reddish purple macules of the posterior palate, representing early-stage Kaposi's sarcoma in an HIV-seropositive patient.

the transplant recipient animals. Thus, even in the context of HIV infection, KS should be considered a low-grade sarcoma.

Microscopically, KS lesions show proliferating spindle cells with mild pleomorphism associated with plump endothelial cells oriented about small lumina. Typically, extravasation of erythrocytes is a prominent feature, and hemosiderin granules are commonly encountered. The more hemosiderin present, the browner the tumor will appear clinically. Overall, the pattern of growth in larger lesions is multinodular.

The early plaque or macular stage lesions are painless and do not require treatment. Nodular lesions may become unsightly and interfere with mastication; in this situation, therapy may be desirable. Surgical excision is not usually attended by severe hemorrhage, but electrocautery is recommended, either as a primary form of surgery or as a coagulative hemostatic adjunct to conventional excision. Intralesional injection of 1% sodium tetradecyl sulfate will result in necrosis of the tumefactions; however it is painful, and the patient should be prescribed a moderate-strength analgesic. Intralesional 1% vinblastine sulfate is also beneficial; because it is not a sclerosing agent, it is not associated with significant postinjection pain. Multiple biweekly injections of vinblastine can be given to eradicate the tumors.

Hereditary Hemorrhagic Telangiectasia

Characterized by multiple round or oval purple papules measuring less than 0.5 cm in diameter, hereditary hemorrhagic telangiectasia (HHT) is a genetically transmitted disease, inherited as an autosomal dominant trait[8,9] (Figure 6-3). The lesions represent multiple microaneurysms, owing to a weakening defect in the adventitial coat of venules. The lesions are so distinct as to be pathognomonic. There may be more than 100 such purple papules on the vermilion and mucosal surfaces of the lips as well as on the tongue and buccal mucosa. The facial skin and neck are also involved. Examination of the

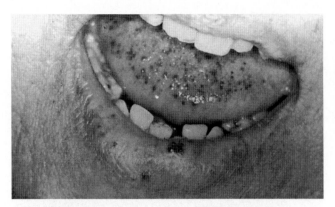

FIGURE 6-3 Multiple small purple papules of hereditary hemorrhagic telangiectasia.

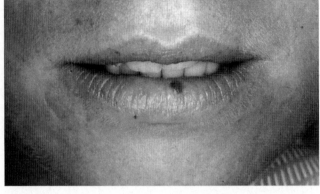

FIGURE 6-4 Ephelis of the lower lip, appearing as a brown macule.

nasal mucosa will reveal similar lesions, and a past history of epistaxis may be a complaint. Indeed, deaths have been reported in HHT attributable to epistaxis. The lesions may be seen during infancy but are usually more prominent in adults.

Although the differential diagnosis should include petechial hemorrhages with an attending platelet disorder, petechiae are macular rather than papular and (as foci of erythrocyte extravasation with breakdown to hemosiderin) red or brown rather than purple. Furthermore, HHT is genetic and should have been noticed in other family members. If any doubt exists, platelet studies can be ordered to rule out a blood dyscrasia.

Microscopically, HHT shows numerous dilated vascular channels with some degree of erythrocyte extravasation around the dilated vessels.

There is no treatment for the disease. If the patient would like to have the telangiectatic areas removed for cosmetic reasons, the papules can be cauterized by electrocautery in a staged series of procedures using local anesthesia.

▼ BROWN MELANOTIC LESIONS

Ephelis and Oral Melanotic Macule

The common cutaneous freckle, or ephelis,[10,11] represents an increase in melanin pigment synthesis by basal-layer melanocytes, without an increase in the number of melanocytes. On the skin, this increased melanogenesis can be attributed to actinic exposure. Ephelides can therefore be encountered on the vermilion border of the lips, with the lower lip being the favored site since it tends to receive more solar exposure than the upper lip (Figure 6-4). The lesion is macular and ranges from being quite small to over a centimeter in diameter. Some patients report a prior episode of trauma to the area. Lip ephelides are asymptomatic and occur equally in men and women. They are rarely seen in children.

The intraoral counterpart to the ephelis is the oral melanotic macule.[10,11] These lesions are oval or irregular in outline, are brown or even black, and tend to occur on the gingiva, palate, and buccal mucosa. Once they reach a certain size, they do not tend to enlarge further (Figure 6-5). The differential diagnosis includes nevus, early superficial spreading melanoma,

amalgam tattoo, and focal ecchymosis. If such pigmented lesions are present after a 2-week period, hemosiderin pigment associated with ecchymosis can be ruled out, and a biopsy specimen should be obtained to secure a definitive diagnosis.

Microscopically, a normal epithelial layer is seen, and the basal cells contain numerous melanin pigment granules without proliferation of melanocytes. Melanin incontinence into the submucosa is commonly encountered. Rarely, melanin-containing dendritic cells are seen to extend high into a thickened spinous layer. Lesions of this nature are diagnosed as melanoacanthoma.

The oral melanotic macule is innocuous, does not represent a melanocytic proliferation, and does not predispose to melanoma. Once it is removed, no further surgery is required.

Nevocellular Nevus and Blue Nevus

Unlike ephelides and melanotic macules, which result from an increase in melanin pigment synthesis, nevi are due to benign proliferations of melanocytes.[12,13] There are two major types, based on histology, and these two types tend to show differences clinically as well, particularly in tint and

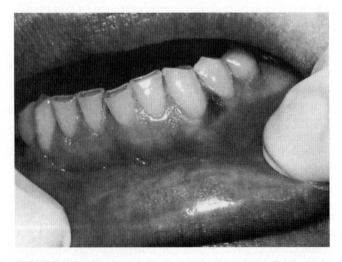

FIGURE 6-5 Oral focal melanotic macule of the gingiva. This lesion is the oral counterpart of the ephelis.

coloration. Nevocellular nevi arise from basal-layer melanocytes early in life. In the evolutionary stages, the nevus cells maintain their localization to the basal layer, residing at the junction of the epithelium and the basement membrane and underlying connective tissue. Since proliferation is minimal, these nevi are macular and are classified as junctional nevi. In general, they are flat and brown and have a regular round or oval outline. With time, the melanocytes form clusters at the epitheliomesenchymal junction and begin to proliferate down into the connective tissue although they do not invade vessels or lymphatics. Such nevi assume a dome-shaped appearance (since more cells have accumulated) and are referred to as compound nevi. In late puberty, the melanocytes (now known as nevus cells) in compound nevi lose their continuity with the surface epithelium, and the cells become localized to the deeper connective tissues. They are then termed intradermal nevi when on skin and intramucosal nevi when in the mouth. On the skin, they are elevated brown nodules that often have hair protruding from them. Thus, in adults, junctional nevi should not exist. When a nevus shows microscopic evidence of junctional activity, premelanomatous change should be suspected.

The second type of nevus, not derived from basal-layer melanocytes, is the blue nevus. The blue nevus is blue on the skin because the melanocytic cells reside deep in the connective tissue and because the overlying vessels dampen the brown coloration of melanin, yielding a blue tint. The melanocytes of a blue nevus differ morphologically from those of a nevocellular nevus by being more spindle shaped while containing significant amounts of pigment. Such cells are neuroectodermally derived yet are believed to represent cells that failed to reach the epithelium. A rare cellular form of blue nevus also exists, and neither the ordinary nor the cellular form has the potential to become a melanoma.

In the oral mucosa, both nevocellular and blue nevi tend to be brown and may be macular or nodular (Figure 6-6). They may be seen at any age and are found most frequently on the palate and gingiva but may also be encountered in the buccal mucosa and on the lips. Once they reach a given size, their growth ceases, and the lesions remain static. Biopsy is necessary for diagnostic confirmation since the clinical diagnosis includes many other focal pigmentations, such as melanotic macule, melanoma, and amalgam tattoo. Simple excision is the treatment of choice.

Malignant Melanoma

On the facial skin, the malar region is a common site for melanoma[14,15] because this area of the face is subject to significant solar exposure. In fact, cutaneous melanoma is most common among white populations that live in sunbelt regions of the world. Facial cutaneous melanomas may appear macular or nodular, and the coloration can be quite varied, ranging from brown to black to blue, with zones of depigmentation. An important difference is that unlike common nevi that exhibit smooth outlines, melanomas show jagged irregular margins. These lesions are more common among elderly

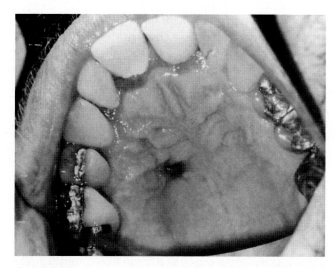

FIGURE 6-6 Nevocellular nevus of the palate. The nevus is raised and gray brown.

patients and show a male predilection. The term "lentigo maligna melanoma" or "Hutchinson's freckle" has been applied to these facial skin lesions that exhibit atypical melanocytic hyperplasia or melanoma in situ. The melanocytic tumor cells spread laterally and therefore superficially; this pattern has been referred to as a radial growth phase. These lesions have a good prognosis if they are detected and treated before the appearance of nodular lesions, which indicates invasion into the deeper connective tissue (ie, a vertical growth phase). The level of invasion is determined by the Breslow method, by which millimeter depths of invasion are measured (depth correlating with prognosis).

Mucosal melanomas are extremely rare. Their prevalence appears to be higher among Japanese people than among other populations. Melanomas arising in the oral mucosa tend to occur on the anterior labial gingiva and the anterior aspect of the hard palate. In the early stages, oral melanomas are macular brown and black plaques with an irregular outline. They may be focal or diffuse and mosaic, and the differential diagnosis should include nevi, melanotic macules, and amalgam tattoo. Any pigmented oral lesion with an irregular margin or with a history of growth should be suspect, and a biopsy of it should be performed without delay. Eventually, melanomas become more diffuse, nodular, and tumefactive, with foci of hyper- and hypopigmentation.

Microscopically, oral mucosal melanomas (like cutaneous melanomas) may exhibit a radial or a vertical pattern of growth. The radial or superficial spreading pattern is seen in macular lesions; clusters and theques of nevus cells showing nuclear atypia and hyperchromatism proliferate within the basal cell junctional region of the epithelium, and many of the neoplastic cells invade the overlying epithelium as well as the submucosa. Once vertical growth into the connective tissue progresses, the lesions can become clinically tumefactive. The vertical growth phase connotes a poor prognosis because of the likelihood of lymphatic and hematogenous metastasis, and grading systems are based on the quantitation of vertical penetration of the submucosa. The Breslow classification has not been applied to oral melanomas, principally because they are generally quite advanced and invasive when biopsy specimens are initially obtained.

Excision with wide margins is the treatment of choice; once nodularity has evolved, however, the lesion has probably already metastasized. Computed tomography and magnetic resonance imaging studies should be undertaken to explore regional metastases to the submandibular and cervical lymph nodes. A variety of chemo- and immunotherapeutic strategies can be used once metastases have been identified.

Drug-Induced Melanosis

A variety of drugs can induce oral mucosal pigmentation.[16–18] These pigmentations can be large yet localized, usually to the hard palate, or they can be multifocal, throughout the mouth. In either case, the lesions are flat and without any evidence of nodularity or swelling. The chief drugs implicated are the quinoline, hydroxyquinoline, and amodiaquine antimalarials. These medications have also been used in the treatment of autoimmune diseases. Minocycline, used in the treatment of acne, can also produce oral pigmentation. The pigment is not confined to oral mucosa and is also encountered in the nail bed and on the skin. Last, oral contraceptives and pregnancy are occasionally associated with hyperpigmentation of the facial skin, particularly in the periorbital and perioral regions (Figure 6-7). This condition is referred to as melasma or chloasma. Endocrine disease should be excluded by appropriate laboratory studies when oral or facial nonphysiologic melanosis is encountered.

The cause is unknown, and the pigment may remain for quite some time after withdrawal of the incriminated drug. Microscopically, basilar melanosis without melanocytic proliferation is observed, and melanin incontinence is commonly seen.

Physiologic Pigmentation

Black people, Asians, and dark-skinned Caucasians frequently show diffuse melanosis of the facial gingiva.[19,20] In addition, the lingual gingiva and tongue may exhibit multiple, diffuse, and reticulated brown macules. Although other causes of hyperpigmentation are possible, racial pigmentation, representing basilar melanosis, evolves in childhood and usually does not arise de novo in the adult. Therefore, any multifocal or diffuse pigmentation of recent onset should be investigated further to rule out endocrinopathic disease.

Café au Lait Pigmentation

In neurofibromatosis, an autosomal dominant inherited disease, both nodular and diffuse pendulous neurofibromas occur on the skin and (rarely) in the oral cavity. A concomitant finding is the presence of "café au lait" pigmentation.[21,22] As the term implies, these lesions have the color of coffee with cream and vary from small ephelis-like macules to broad diffuse lesions. They tend to appear in late childhood and can be multiple; many overlie the neurofibromatous swellings on the skin.

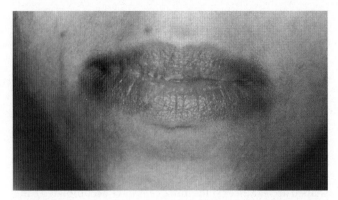

FIGURE 6-7   Perioral melanosis (melasma) in a young woman taking birth control pills.

Rarely, oral pigmentation is encountered. Importantly, the patient will manifest cutaneous signs as the predominant feature of the disease.

Microscopically, café au lait spots represent basilar melanosis without melanocyte proliferation.

Smoker's Melanosis

Diffuse macular melanosis of the buccal mucosa, lateral tongue, palate, and floor of the mouth is occasionally seen among cigarette smokers[23,24] (Figure 6-8). Although no cause-and-effect relationship has been proven and although most smokers (even heavy smokers) usually fail to show such changes, those who do are said to exhibit smoker's melanosis. Thus, it is probable that in certain individuals, melanogenesis is stimulated by tobacco smoke products. Indeed, among dark-skinned individuals who normally exhibit physiologic

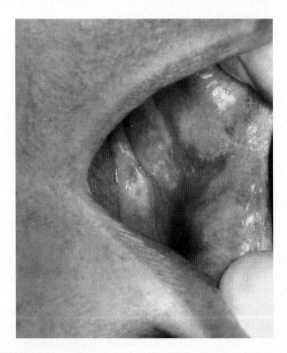

FIGURE 6-8   Diffuse melanosis of the buccal mucosa in a cigarette smoker (smoker's melanosis).

pigmentation, studies have disclosed that tobacco use stimulates an increase in oral pigmentation. The lesions are brown, flat, and irregular; some are even geographic or maplike in configuration. Histologically, basilar melanosis with melanin incontinence is observed, and the lesions have no premalignant potential.

Pigmented Lichen Planus

Lichen planus (discussed in detail in Chapter 5) is a disease that generally presents as a white lesion, with variants showing red and desquamative lesions. Rarely, erosive lichen planus can be associated with diffuse melanosis. In such instances, the classic lesions of lichen planus remain recognizable, usually in the buccal mucosa and vestibule.[25] Reticulated white patches, with or without a red erosive component, overlie or are flanked by diffuse brown macular foci (Figure 6-9). This increase in melanogenesis may be stimulated by the infiltrate into the basal layer of T lymphocytes that contribute to basal cell degeneration. Histologically, the usual features of lichen planus are observed, along with basilar melanosis and melanin incontinence.

Endocrinopathic Pigmentation

Bronzing of the skin and patchy melanosis of the oral mucosa are signs of Addison's disease and pituitary-based Cushing's syndrome.[26] In both of these endocrine disorders, the cause of hyperpigmentation is oversecretion of ACTH, a hormone with melanocyte-stimulating properties. In Addison's disease, adrenocortical insufficiency evolves as a consequence of granulomatous infection of the cortex or autoimmune cortical destruction. As steroid hormones decrease, the feedback loop is stimulated with excess secretion of ACTH by the neurohypophysis. With a decrease in mineralocorticoids and glucocorticoids, the patient develops hypotension and hypoglycemia, respectively.

In Cushing's syndrome, adrenocortical hyperactivity is observed, and if such activity is caused by a cortical secretory adenoma or cortical hyperplasia of adrenal origin, ACTH secretion will be shut down. Alternatively, if the hypercorticism is the consequence of a pituitary ACTH-secreting tumor that secondarily induces an adrenal hypersecretion, then melanocyte-stimulating effects may evolve. Patients with Cushing's syndrome may be hypertensive and hyperglycemic and may show facial edema ("moon face").

In both cases, the skin may appear tanned, and the gingiva, palate, and buccal mucosa may be blotchy. These changes in pigmentation are due to an accumulation of melanin granules as a consequence of increased hormone-dependent melanogenesis. Endocrinopathic disease should be suspected whenever oral melanotic pigmentation is accompanied by cutaneous bronzing. Serum steroid and ACTH determinations will aid the diagnosis, and the pigment will disappear once appropriate therapy for the endocrine problem is initiated.

HIV Oral Melanosis

HIV-seropositive patients with opportunistic infections may have adrenocortical involvement by a variety of parasites,

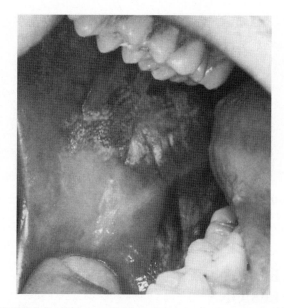

FIGURE 6-9 White speckled foci, plaques, and striae, seen overlying diffuse brown melanosis in pigmented lichen planus.

which manifests signs and symptoms of Addison's disease.[27–29] Such patients undergo progressive hyperpigmentation of the skin, nails, and mucous membranes. In actuality, most HIV-seropositive patients presenting with diffuse multifocal macular brown pigmentations of the buccal mucosa show no features of adrenocortical disease. The oral pigmentation cannot be attributed to medications in this population because cases have been recorded in individuals who have not received any medications that could be so implicated. Thus, the etiology remains undetermined. As mentioned, the pigmentation resembles most of the other diffuse macular pigmentations discussed so far; the buccal mucosa is the most frequently affected site, but the gingiva, palate, and tongue may also be involved.

Like all diffuse melanoses, HIV-associated pigmentation is microscopically characterized by basilar melanin pigment, with incontinence into the underlying submucosa.

Peutz-Jeghers Syndrome

In Peutz-Jeghers syndrome (discussed more fully in Chapter 7), oral pigmentation is distinctive and is usually pathognomonic.[30,31] Multiple focal melanotic brown macules are concentrated about the lips while the remaining facial skin is less strikingly involved. The macules appear as freckles or ephelides, usually measuring < 0.5 cm in diameter (Figure 6-10). Similar lesions may occur on the anterior tongue, buccal mucosa, and mucosal surface of the lips. Ephelides are also seen on the fingers and hands.

Lesions on the perioral areas are essentially pathognomonic although in individuals who have diffuse cutaneous ephelides (such as red-haired light-complected individuals), an erroneous diagnosis could be made.

Histologically, these lesions show basilar melanogenesis without melanocytic proliferation.

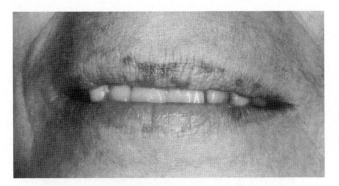

FIGURE 6-10 Multiple labial brown melanotic ephelides, characteristic of Peutz-Jeghers syndrome.

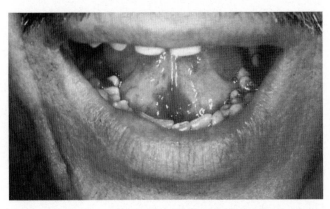

FIGURE 6-11 Ecchymosis in the floor of the mouth, secondary to trauma.

▼ BROWN HEME-ASSOCIATED LESIONS

Ecchymosis

Traumatic ecchymosis[32,33] is common on the lips and face yet is uncommon in the oral mucosa. Immediately following the traumatic event, erythrocyte extravasation into the submucosa will appear as a bright red macule or as a swelling if a hematoma forms. The lesion will assume a brown coloration within a few days, after the hemoglobin is degraded to hemosiderin (Figure 6-11). The differential diagnosis must include other focal pigmented lesions. If the patient recalls an episode of trauma, however, the lesion should be observed for 2 weeks, by which time it should have resolved if it represents a focus of ecchymosis.

When multiple brown macules or swellings are observed and ecchymosis is included in the differential diagnosis, a hemorrhagic diathesis should be considered. Certainly, patients taking anticoagulant drugs may present with oral ecchymosis, particularly on the cheek or tongue, either of which can be traumatized while chewing. Coagulopathic ecchymosis of the skin and oral mucosa may also be encountered in hereditary coagulopathic disorders and in chronic liver failure. A coagulation panel including prothrombin time and partial thromboplastin time should be ordered in instances of unprovoked ecchymoses to explore defects in the extrinsic and intrinsic pathways, respectively. The clotting time will also be prolonged.

Petechia

Capillary hemorrhages will appear red initially and turn brown in a few days once the extravasated red cells have lysed and have been degraded to hemosiderin. Petechiae secondary to platelet deficiencies or aggregation disorders are usually not limited to the oral mucosa but occur concomitantly on skin.[33] Autoimmune or idiopathic thrombocytopenic purpura (ITP), HIV-related ITP, disorders of platelet aggregation, aspirin toxicity, myelophthistic lesions, and myelosuppressive chemotherapy all will lead to purpura, with petechiae being the major lesions. Alternatively, most oral petechiae are not associated with thrombocytopenia or thrombocytopathia; rather, they are usually confined to the soft palate, where 10 to 30 petechial lesions may be seen and can be attributed to suction. Excessive suction of the soft palate against the posterior tongue is self-inflicted by many patients who have a pruritic palate at the onset of a viral or an allergic pharyngitis; they simply "click" their palate. Palatal petechiae can also appear following fellatio. When traumatic or suction petechiae are suspected, the patient should be instructed to cease whatever activity may be contributing to the presence of the lesions. By 2 weeks, the lesions should have disappeared. Failure to do so should arouse suspicion of a hemorrhagic diathesis, and a platelet count and platelet aggregation studies must be ordered.

Hemochromatosis

The deposition of hemosiderin pigment in multiple organs and tissues occurs in a primary heritable disease with a prominent male predilection or may evolve secondary to a variety of diseases and conditions, including chronic anemia, porphyria, cirrhosis, postcaval shunt for portal hypertension, and excess intake of iron.[34,35] The oral mucosal lesions of hemochromatosis are brown to gray diffuse macules that tend to occur in the palate and gingiva. Although these pigmentations are predominantly the result of iron deposition in the submucosa, basilar melanosis is also observed microscopically and may be the result of a secondary addisonian complication, whereby hemosiderin deposition within the adrenal cortex may lead to hypocorticism and ACTH hypersecretion.

When hemochromatosis is suspected, an oral biopsy may be helpful in the diagnosis. The tissue can be stained for iron by using Prussian blue; iron levels will be elevated in the serum if hemochromatosis is present. Since the condition can be the consequence of a variety of disease states, medical referral is recommended.

▼ GRAY/BLACK PIGMENTATIONS

Amalgam Tattoo

By far, the most common source of solitary or focal pigmentation in the oral mucosa is the amalgam tattoo.[36] The lesions are macular and bluish gray or even black and are usually seen in the buccal mucosa, gingiva, or palate (Figure 6-12). Importantly, they are found in the vicinity of teeth with large amalgam restorations or crowned teeth that probably had amalgams removed when the teeth were being prepared for the fabrication of the crown. Such lesions are the consequence of an iatrogenic mishap whereby the dentist's bur, loaded with small amalgam particles that accumulate during the removal of amalgam, accidently veers into the adjacent mucosa and traumatically introduces the metal flecks. The metallic particles are quite fine, but in some instances (when large enough), they are identifiable on radiographs of the area. Amalgam fragments can also be deposited in oral tissue during multiple tooth extractions. Metal particles may fall unnoticed into extraction sockets, and during the healing phase, the amalgam becomes entombed within the connective tissue while re-epithelialization occurs. In these instances, radiography almost always demonstrates the presence of the metal.

Microscopically, amalgam tattoos show a fine brown granular stippling of reticulum fibers, particularly around vessel walls, and in many instances, large chunks of black metallic particles can be seen. A giant cell reaction is uncommon; however, a mononuclear inflammatory cell infiltrate is often noted.

Since amalgam tattoos are innocuous, their removal is not required, particularly when they can be documented radiographically. Alternatively, biopsy is recommended when a gray pigmented lesion suddenly appears or when such a lesion arises distant from any restored teeth; the differential diagnosis must include nevi and melanoma in such instances.

Graphite Tattoo

Graphite tattoos tend to occur on the palate and represent traumatic implantation from a lead pencil.[37] The lesions are usually macular, focal, and gray or black. Since the traumatic event usually occurred in the classroom during grade school,

many patients may not recall the injury. Microscopically, graphite resembles amalgam in tissue although special stains can segregate the two.

Hairy Tongue

Hairy tongue is a relatively common condition of unknown etiology.[38,39] The lesion involves the dorsum, particularly the middle and posterior one-third. Rarely are children affected. The papillae are elongated, sometimes markedly so, and have the appearance of hairs. The hyperplastic papillae then become pigmented by the colonization of chromogenic bacteria, which can impart a variety of colors ranging from green to brown to black. Various foods, particularly coffee and tea, probably contribute to the diffuse coloration.

Microscopically, the filiform papillae are extremely elongated and hyperplastic with keratosis. External colonization of the papillae by basophilic microbial colonies is a prominent feature. Otherwise, there are no pathologic findings in the remaining epithelium or in the connective tissue. The condition is so classic in its clinical presentation that biopsy is not required, and a clinical diagnosis is appropriate.

Treatment consists of having the patient brush the tongue and avoid tea and coffee for a few weeks. Since the cause is undetermined, the condition can recur.

Pigmentation Related to Heavy-Metal Ingestion

Many years ago, a variety of metallic compounds were used medicinally, but such medicaments are either no longer or rarely still in use. Ingestion of heavy metals or metal salts can be an occupational hazard since many metals are used in industry and in paints. Lead, mercury, and bismuth have all been shown to be deposited in oral tissue if ingested in sufficient quantities or over a long course of time.[40,41] These ingested pigments tend to extravasate from vessels in foci of increased capillary permeability such as inflamed tissues. Thus, in the oral cavity, the pigmentation is usually found along the free marginal gingiva, where it dramatically outlines the gingival cuff, resembling eyeliner. This metallic line has a gray to black appearance. The heavy metals may be associated with systemic symptoms of toxicity, including behavioral changes, neurologic disorders, and intestinal pain. This condition is now rarely seen.

▼ SUMMARY

Oral pigmentations may be focal, diffuse, or multifocal. They may be blue, purple, brown, gray, or black. They may be flat or tumefactive. Importantly, some are harbingers of internal disease; some are localized harmless accumulations of melanin, hemosiderin, or exogenous metal; and some can be highly lethal. The differential diagnosis can be lengthy, particularly when the pigmentation is macular and diffuse or multifocal. Although biopsy is a helpful aid to diagnosis for localized lesions, the more diffuse lesions will require a thorough history and laboratory studies in order to arrive at a definitive diagnosis.

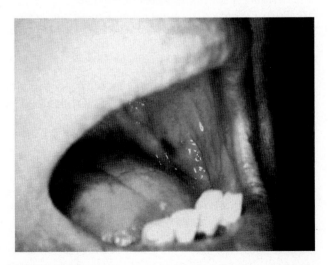

FIGURE 6-12 Amalgam tattoo of the buccal mucosa. The lesion appears gray black.

▼ REFERENCES

1. Watson WL, McCarthy WE. Blood and lymph vessel tumors: a report of 1,056 cases. Surg Gynecol Obstet 1970;71:569.

2. Royle HR, Lapp R, Ferrara ED. The Sturge-Weber syndrome. Oral Surg Oral Med Oral Pathol 1979;71:569.

3. Weathers DR, Fine RM. Thrombosed varix of the oral cavity. Arch Dermatol 1971;104:1971.

4. Shklar G, Meyer I. Vascular tumors of the mouth and jaws. Oral Surg Oral Med Oral Pathol 1965;19:335.

5. Minkow B, Laufer D, Gutman JD. Treatment of oral hemangiomas with local sclerosing agents. Int J Oral Maxillofac Surg 1979;8:18.

6. Eversole LR, Leider AS, Jacobsen PL, Shaber EP. Oral Kaposi's sarcoma associated with acquired immunodeficiency syndrome among homosexual males. J Am Dent Assoc 1983;107:248.

7. Silverman S Jr. AIDS update: oral findings, diagnosis and precautions. J Am Dent Assoc 1987;115:559.

8. Everett FG, Hahn CR. Hereditary hemorrhagic telangiectasia with gingival lesions: review and case reports. J Periodontol 1976;47:295.

9. Austin GB, Quart AM, Novak B. Hereditary hemorrhagic telangiectasia with oral manifestations: report of peridontal treatment in two cases. Oral Surg Oral Med Oral Pathol 1981;51:245.

10. Buchner A, Hansen LS. Melanotic macule of the oral mucosa: a clinicopathologic study of 105 cases. Oral Surg Oral Med Oral Pathol 1979;48:244.

11. Kaugars GE, Heise AP, Riley WT, et al. Oral melanotic macules. A review of 353 cases. Oral Surg Oral Med Oral Pathol 1993;76:59–61.

12. Buchner A, Hansen LS. Pigmented nevi of the oral mucosa: a clinicopathologic study of 32 new cases and review of 75 cases from the literature. Oral Surg Oral Med Oral Pathol 1979;48:131.

13. Buchner A, Leider AS, Merrell PW, Carpenter WM. Melanocytic nevi of the oral mucosa: a clinicopathologic study of 130 cases from northern California. J Oral Pathol Med 1990;19:197-201.

14. Nandapalan V, Roland NJ, Helliwell TR, et al. Mucosal melanoma of the head and neck. Clin Otolaryngol 1998;23:107–16.

15. Doval DC, Rao CR, Saitha KS, et al. Magliant melanoma of the oral cavity: report of 14 cases from a regional cancer centre. Eur J Surg Oncol 1996;22:245–9.

16. Eisen D, Hakim MD. Minocycline-induced pigmentation. Incidence, prevention and management. Drug Saf 1998;18:431–40.

17. Manor A, Sperling I, Buchner A. Gingival pigmentation associated with antimalarial drugs. Isr J Dent Med 1981;25:13.

18. Birek C, Main JHP. Two cases of oral pigmentation associated with quinidine therapy. Oral Surg Oral Med Oral Pathol 1989;66:59.

19. Moghadam BK, Gier RE. Melanin pigmentation disorders of the skin and oral mucosa. Compendium 1991;12:14,16–20.

20. Dummett CO. Oral pigmentation—physiologic and pathologic. N Y State Dent J 1959;25:407.

21. O'Driscoll PM. The oral manifestations of multiple neurofibromatosis. Br J Oral Maxillofac Surg 1965;3:22.

22. White AK, Smith RJ, Bigler CR, et al. Head and neck manifestations of neurofibromatosis. Laryngoscope 1986;96:732.

23. Kleinegger CL, Hammond HL, Finkelstein MW. Oral mucosal hyperpigmentation secondary to antimalarial drug therapy. Oral Surg Oral Med Oral Pathol Oral Radiol Endod 2000;90:189–94.

24. Hedin CA, Axell T. Oral melanin pigmentation in 467 Thai and Malaysian people with special emphasis on smoker's melanosis. J Oral Pathol Med 1991;20:8.

25. Murti PR, Bhousle RB, Daftary DK, Mehta FS. Oral lichen planus associated with pigmentation. J Oral Pathol Med 1979;34:23.

26. Lamey PJ, Carmichael F, Scully C. Oral pigmentation, Addison's disease and the results of screening for adrenocortical insufficiency. Br Dent J 1985;158:297.

27. Esposito R. Hyperpigmentation of skin in patients with AIDS. BMJ 1987;294:840.

28. Chermosky ME, Finley VK. Yellow nail syndrome in patients with acquired immunodeficiency disease. J Am Acad Dermatol 1985;13:731.

29. Ficarra G, Shillitoe EJ, Adler-Storthz K, et al. Oral melanotic macules in patients infected with human immunodeficiency virus. Oral Surg Oral Med Oral Pathol 1990;70:748–55.

30. Kitagawa S, Townsend BL, Hebert AA. Peutz-Jeghers syndrome. Dermatol Clin 1995;13:127–33.

31. Lucky AW. Pigmentary abnormalities in genetic disorders. Dermatol Clin 1988;6:193.

32. Linenberg WBP. Idiopathic thrombocytopenic purpura. Oral Surg Oral Med Oral Pathol 1964;17:22.

33. Damm DD, White DK, Brinker DM. Variations in palatal erythema secondary to fellatio. Oral Surg Oral Med Oral Pathol 1981;52:417.

34. Frantzis TG, Sheridan PJ, Reeve CM, Young LL. Oral manifestations of hemochromatosis. Report of a case. Oral Surg Oral Med Oral Pathol 1972;33:186.

35. Dean DH, Hiramoto RN. Submandibular salivary gland involvement in hemochromatosis. J Oral Med 1984;39:197–8.

36. Buchner A, Hansen LS. Amalgam pigmentation (amalgam tattoo) of the oral mucosa. A clinicopathologic study of 268 cases. Oral Surg Oral Med Oral Pathol 1980;49:139.

37. Peters E, Gardner DF. A method of distinguishing between amalgam and graphite in tissue. Oral Surg Oral Med Oral Pathol 1986;62:73.

38. Farman AG. Hairy tongue (lingua villosa). J Oral Med 1977;32:85–91.

39. Svejda J, Skach M, Plackova A. Hairlike variations of filiform papillae in the human tongue. Oral Surg Oral Med Oral Pathol 1977;43:97.

40. Bruggenkate CM, Cordozo EL, Maaskant P, van der Waal I. Lead poisoning with pigmentation of the oral mucosa. Oral Surg Oral Med Oral Pathol 1975;39:747.

41. Gordon NC, Brown S, Khosla VM, Hansen LS. Lead poisoning: a comprehensive review and report of a case. Oral Surg Oral Med Oral Pathol 1977;47:500.

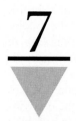

7

BENIGN TUMORS OF THE ORAL CAVITY

LEWIS R. EVERSOLE, DDS, MSD

▼ NORMAL STRUCTURAL VARIANTS

▼ INFLAMMATORY (REACTIVE) HYPERPLASIAS
Fibrous Inflammatory Hyperplasias and Traumatic Fibromas
Pyogenic Granuloma, Pregnancy Epulis, and Peripheral Ossifying Fibroma
Giant Cell Granuloma (Peripheral and Central)
Pseudosarcomatous Fasciitis (Nodular Fasciitis) and Proliferative Myositis
Pseudoepitheliomatous Hyperplasia
Benign Lymphoid Hyperplasia

▼ HAMARTOMAS
Hemangioma and Angiomatous Syndromes
Lymphangioma
Glomus Tumor and Other Vascular Endothelial Growths
Granular Cell Tumor and Granular Cell Epulis
Nerve Sheath Tumors and Traumatic Neuroma
Melanotic Neuroectodermal Tumor of Infancy
Fibrous Dysplasia of Bone and Albright's Syndrome
Other Benign Fibro-Osseous Lesions
Teratomas and Dermoid Cysts

▼ CYSTS OF THE JAW AND BENIGN ODONTOGENIC TUMORS
Cysts of the Jaw
Benign Odontogenic Tumors

▼ BENIGN "VIRUS-INDUCED" TUMORS (ORAL SQUAMOUS PAPILLOMAS AND WARTS)

▼ SYNDROMES WITH BENIGN ORAL NEOPLASTIC OR HAMARTOMATOUS COMPONENTS
Von Recklinghausen's Neurofibromatosis
Gardner's Syndrome
Peutz-Jeghers Syndrome
Nevoid Basal Cell Carcinoma Syndrome
Multiple Endocrine Neoplasia Type III (Multiple Mucosal Neuroma Syndrome)
Tuberous Sclerosis
Acanthosis Nigricans
Albright's Syndrome
Paget's Disease of Bone (Osteitis Deformans)
Cowden's Syndrome
Xanthomas
Langerhans Cell (Eosinophilic) Histiocytosis
Amyloidosis

▼ ACUTE AND GRANULOMATOUS INFLAMMATIONS
Cervicofacial Actinomycosis
Cat-Scratch Disease
Hansen's Disease (Leprosy)
Orofacial Granulomatosis

▼ GINGIVAL ENLARGEMENTS
Inflammatory Gingival Enlargement
Fibrotic Gingival Enlargement
Phenytoin-Induced Gingival Hyperplasia
Gingival Hyperplasia Induced by Cyclosporin A and Calcium Channel Blockers
Syndromes Associated with Diffuse Gingival Enlargement

This chapter is concerned with the clinical features, diagnosis, and management of localized nonmalignant growths of the oral cavity. A variety of lesions of miscellaneous etiologies are discussed, many of which are not true neoplasms. Tissue enlargements attributable to irritation or injury represent a hyperplastic reaction and are collectively grouped as "reactive proliferations."

If left untreated, some of the lesions discussed in this chapter will lead to extensive tissue destruction and deformity whereas others will interfere with mastication and will become secondarily infected following masticatory trauma. Regardless, the major clinical consideration in the management of all of these tumors is to identify their benign nature and to distinguish them from potentially life-threatening malignant lesions. Since this decision usually can be made with certainty only by microscopic examination of excised tissue, biopsy is generally an essential step.[1]

▼ NORMAL STRUCTURAL VARIANTS

Structural variations of the jaw bones and overlying oral soft tissues are sometimes mistakenly identified as tumors, but they are usually easily recognized as within the range of normal variation for the oral cavity; biopsy in these cases is rarely indicated. Examples of such structural variants are ectopic lymphoid nodules,[2] or "oral tonsils" (small and slightly reddish nodular elevations of a localized area of the oral mucosa as distinct from the pharyngeal mucosa); tori; a pronounced retromolar pad remaining after the extraction of the last molar teeth; localized nodular connective-tissue thickening of the attached gingiva; the papilla associated with the opening of Stensen's duct; a circumvallate dorsum of the tongue; and sublingual varicosities in older individuals.

Localized nodular enlargements of the cortical bone of the palate (torus palatinus) and jaws (torus mandibularis) occur frequently[3] and are considered to be normal structural variants that are analagous to the spurs encountered on other bones (eg, on the malleoli of the tibia and fibula) (Figure 7-1). The lack of obvious irritants for most tori and the negligible growth of most tori after an initial slow but steady period of development also suggest that they are usually neither inflammatory hyperplasias nor neoplasms. Histologically, tori consist of layers of dense cortical bone-covered periosteum and an overlying layer of thin epithelium, with minimal rete peg development.

Tori may pose a mechanical problem in the construction of dentures; they are frequently traumatized as a result of their prominent position and thin epithelial covering, and the resulting ulcers are slow to heal. Rarely, tori on the palate or lingual mandibular ridge may become sufficiently large to interfere with eating and speaking. Unless a torus is exceptionally large, its surgical removal (when dictated by mechanical concerns or by a patient's anxiety) is not a major procedure, provided that splints or stents are fabricated beforehand to provide a protective dressing during healing.

Similar nodular growths or exostoses arise on the buccal aspect of the maxillary and mandibular alveolae and must be differentiated from bony hyperplasia secondary to a chronic periapical abscess. Nodular bony enlargements of the alveolus also can occur in fibrous dysplasia and in Paget's disease, in which they represent superficial evidence of a more generalized bony dysplasia.

The mylohyoid ridge, located just lingual to the third molars, may be traumatized, resulting in ulceration of the overlying mucosa. This focus of ulceration is painful and can be subject to infection, leading to osteomyelitis. Perhaps the most common insult to this area is intubation for general anesthesia.

Biopsy specimens from oral and perioral tissues, like those from any regional tissue, may contain normal structures that are unique to that area, but such structures have occasionally been mistakenly identified as an abnormality or even as a malignancy. For example, the organ of Chievitz (a group of epithelial cell nests typically located adjacent to the temporal fossa and the long buccal nerve) has in a number of cases been incorrectly diagnosed as a perineuronal invasion of cells from an oral carcinoma,[4] leading to a second and unnecessarily wider surgical excision. In similar fashion, pseudoepitheliomatous hyperplasia, an exuberant but common benign proliferation of the oral epithelium, has been overdiagnosed as invasive carcinoma.

▼ INFLAMMATORY (REACTIVE) HYPERPLASIAS

The term "inflammatory hyperplasia" is used to describe a large range of commonly occurring nodular growths of the oral mucosa that histologically represent inflamed fibrous and granulation tissue. The size of these reactive hyperplastic masses may be greater or lesser, depending on the degree to which one or more of the components of the inflammatory reaction and healing response are exaggerated in the particular lesion. Some are predominantly epithelial overgrowths with only scanty connective-tissue stroma; others are fibromatous with a thin epithelial covering and may exhibit either angiomatous, desmoplastic (collagenous), or fibroblastic features. In many lesions, different sections may reveal examples of each of these histologic patterns. Like scar tissue, some inflammatory hyperplasias appear to mature and become less vascular (paler and less friable) and more collagenous (firmer and smaller) with time. Others appear to have a high proliferative ability for exophytic growth until they are excised.

This variability of histologic appearance is reflected in the wide range of clinical characteristics that inflammatory hyperplasias show and in the clinical names many of them have acquired that suggest a specific etiology or natural history. Names such as "fibroma" and "papilloma" are therefore often used to describe these lesions even though there is no evidence to suggest a neoplastic etiology. The major etiologic factor for these lesions is generally assumed to be chronic trauma (such as that produced by ill-fitting dentures, calculus, overhanging dental restorations, acute or chronic tissue injury from biting, and fractured teeth), and chronic irritants can be convincingly demonstrated in many cases (eg, palatal papillary hyper-

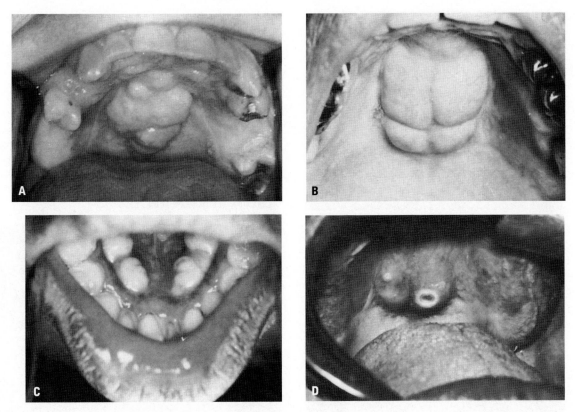

FIGURE 7-1 **A** and **B,** Torus palatinus. **C,** Torus mandibularis. Both are common localized nodular enlargements of the cortical bone of the palate and jaws, usually considered to be normal structural variants of these bones. **D,** Ulcer resulting from trauma. Such ulcers are often slow to heal because of the dense and relatively avascular bone in these lesions and their susceptibility to recurrent trauma.

plasia associated with aged maxillary dentures). With some of these lesions, (eg, pregnancy epulis and the central giant cell tumor associated with hyperparathyroidism), the levels of circulating hormones also undoubtedly play a role. The majority of lesions occur on the surface of the oral mucous membrane, where irritants are quite common. Two deeper lesions (pseudosarcomatous fasciitis and giant cell reparative granuloma of bone) are also classified as inflammatory hyperplasias, on the basis of their histologic structure and clinical behavior.

As surface outgrowths of the oral mucous membrane, most inflammatory hyperplasias are subject to continual masticatory trauma and frequently are ulcerated and hemorrhagic. Dilated blood vessels, acute and chronic inflammatory exudates, and localized abscesses are additional reasons for the swollen, distended, and red to purple inflamed appearance of some inflammatory hyperplasias. Epithelial hyperplasia frequently produces a lesion with a textured surface or an area of mucosa resembling carpet pile. Erosion of the underlying cortical bone rarely occurs with inflammatory hyperplasia of the oral mucosa; when it is noted, there should be a strong suspicion that an aggressive process or even malignancy is involved, and a section of the affected bone should be included with the biopsy specimen.

Unless otherwise specified in the following description of lesions of this type, excisional biopsy is indicated except when the procedure would produce marked deformity; in such a case, incisional biopsy is mandatory. If the chronic irritant is eliminated when the lesion is excised, the majority of inflammatory hyperplasias will not recur. This confirms the benign nature of these lesions (as would be expected from their histologic structure).

The following are examples of inflammatory hyperplasias: fibrous inflammatory hyperplasias (clinical fibroma, epulis fissuratum, and pulp polyp); palatal papillary hyperplasia; pyogenic granuloma; pregnancy epulis; giant cell granuloma (giant cell epulis and central giant cell tumor of the jaw); pseudosarcomatous fasciitis; proliferative myositis; and pseudoepitheliomatous hyperplasia.

Fibrous Inflammatory Hyperplasias and Traumatic Fibromas

FIBROMA, EPULIS FISSURATUM, AND PULP POLYP

Fibrous inflammatory hyperplasias may occur as either pedunculated or sessile (broad-based) growths on any surface of the oral mucous membrane (Figure 7-2). They are called fibromas if they are sessile, firm, and covered by thin squamous epithelium. On the gingiva, a similar lesion is often referred to as an epulis[5,6] (Figure 7-3). The majority remain small, and lesions that are > 1 cm in diameter are rare. An exception to this rule occurs with a lesion that is associated with the periphery of ill-fitting dentures,[7] the so-called epulis fissuratum, in which the

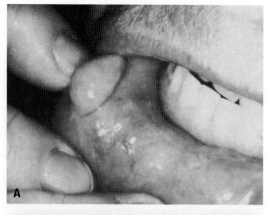

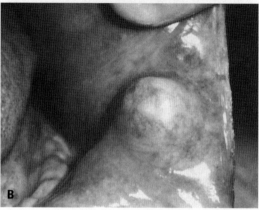

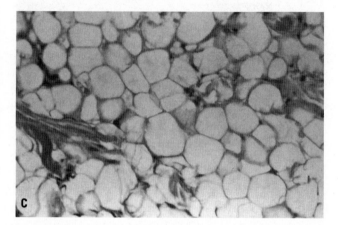

FIGURE 7-2 A, Pedunculated fibrous inflammatory hyperplasia of the cheek, possibly associated with dental trauma. **B** and **C,** On biopsy, a comparable soft nodular swelling of the lip proved to be a small benign growth made up of mature fat cells (lipoma). (**B** and **C** courtesy of Gary Cohen, DMD, Philadelphia, Pa.)

growth is often split by the edge of the denture, one part of the lesion lying under the denture and the other part lying between the lip or cheek and the outer denture surface. This lesion may extend the full length of one side of the denture. Many such hyperplastic growths will become less edematous and inflamed following the removal of the associated chronic irritant, but they rarely resolve entirely. In the preparation of the mouth to

receive dentures, these lesions are excised to prevent further irritation and to ensure a soft-tissue seal for the denture periphery. Pulp polyps represent an analogous condition (chronic hyperplastic pulpitis) involving the pulpal connective tissue, which proliferates through a large pulpal exposure and fills the cavity in the tooth with a mushroom-shaped polyp that is connected by a stalk to the pulp chamber. Masticatory

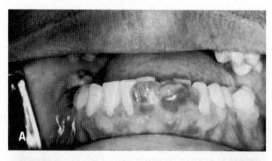

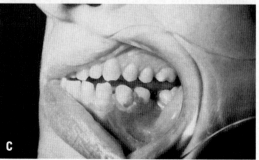

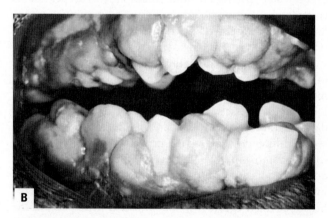

FIGURE 7-3 Three examples of inflammatory hyperplasia affecting the gingiva. **A,** A fibrous epulis associated with calculus. **B,** Generalized hyperplasia of the gingivae as a result of local irritants in a brain-damaged child maintained on phenytoin (Dilantin). **C,** A pregnancy epulis in an otherwise healthy dental arch; oral hygiene was excellent and the epulis was associated with a "food pack" area that developed after loss of the mandibular first molar. The lesion resolved after delivery.

pressure usually leads to keratinization of the epithelial covering of these lesions. Characteristically, pulp polyps (like granulation tissue) contain few sensory nerve fibers and are remarkably insensitive. The crowns of teeth affected by pulp polyps are usually so badly destroyed by caries that endodontic treatment is not considered; however, when restorative considerations do not preclude it, root canal therapy can be satisfactorily completed on these teeth after the extirpation of the polyp and remaining pulp tissue.

The differential diagnosis of fibrous inflammatory hyperplasia[8] should include consideration of the possibility that the lesion is a true papilloma (a cauliflower-like mass made up of multiple fingerlike projections of stratified squamous epithelium with a central core of vascular connective tissue) or a small verrucous carcinoma. Multiple oral papillomatous lesions also may be virus-induced warts (see "Benign 'Virus-Induced' Tumors") or one feature of a syndrome with more serious manifestations in other organs (eg, acanthosis nigricans or ichthyosis hystrix). On the dorsal surface of the tongue, nodular lesions may represent scars, neurofibroma, and granular cell tumor as well as fibrous inflammatory hyperplasia. Both pedunculated and broad-based nodules on the pharyngeal surface of the tongue are usually lymphoid nodules or cystic dilatations of mucous gland ducts (see Figure 7-3, C). Condyloma latum, one of the characteristic oral lesions of secondary syphilis, has been reported to involve the intraoral mucosa.[9]

Fibrous inflammatory hyperplasias have no malignant potential, and recurrences following excision are almost always a result of the failure to eliminate the particular form of chronic irritation involved. The occasional report of squamous cell carcinoma arising in an area of chronic denture irritation, however, underlines the fact that no oral growth, even those associated with an obvious chronic irritant, can be assumed to be benign until proven so by histologic study. Thus, whenever possible, all fibrous inflammatory hyperplasias of the oral cavity should be treated by local excision, with microscopic examination of the excised tissue.

PALATAL PAPILLARY HYPERPLASIA

Palatal papillary hyperplasia (denture papillomatosis) is a common lesion with a characteristic clinical appearance that develops on the hard palate in response to chronic denture irritation in approximately 3 to 4% of denture wearers.[7,10] Full dentures in which relief areas or "suction chambers" are cut in the palatal seating surface appear to be the strongest stimuli, but the lesion is also seen under partial dentures, and occasional case reports have described the lesion in patients who have never worn dentures.

The palatal lesion is usually associated with some degree of denture sore mouth (stomatitis) due to chronic candidal infection, which influences the appearance of the papillary hyperplasia. When complicated by candidal infection, the lesion may be red to scarlet, and the swollen and tightly packed projections resemble the surface of an overripe berry. Such lesions are friable, often bleed with minimal trauma, and may be covered with a thin whitish exudate. When the candidal infection is eliminated, either by removing the denture or by topical administration of an antifungal agent, the papillary lesion becomes little different in color from the rest of the palate and consists of more or less tightly packed nodular projections. If tiny, the nodular projections simply give a feltlike texture to that portion of the palate, and the lesion may even pass unnoticed unless it is stroked with an instrument or disturbed by a jet of air.

The microscopic appearance of these lesions is little different from that of "papillomas" elsewhere in the mouth although the degree of branching and polypoid proliferation that develop on the epithelial surface occluded by the denture is often quite surprising. Low-power examination of these lesions demonstrates their exophytic nature, and neither epithelial invasion of the submucosa nor resorption of the palatine bone occurs, even under large or long-standing lesions. Despite their sometimes bizarre clinical appearance, these lesions have almost no neoplastic potential, a finding that is borne out by the absence of atypia and cellular dysplasia in biopsy specimens.

If the alveolar ridges are surgically prepared for new dentures,[11] papillary hyperplasia lesions are usually excised or removed (by electrocautery, cryosurgery, or laser surgery), and the old denture or a palatal splint is used to maintain a postoperative surgical dressing over the denuded area.

If florid papillomatosis of the palate occurs or persists in the absence of dentures, the differential diagnosis should also consider several granulomatous diseases that may manifest intraorally in this fashion (eg, infectious granulomas, Cowden disease, and verrucous carcinoma), particularly when the papillary lesions are white and extend beyond the palatal vault and onto the alveolar mucosa.

Pyogenic Granuloma, Pregnancy Epulis, and Peripheral Ossifying Fibroma

Pyogenic granuloma is a pedunculated hemorrhagic nodule that occurs most frequently on the gingiva and that has a strong tendency to recur after simple excision[12] (Figure 7-4). Chronic irritation as a causative factor for these lesions may sometimes be hard to identify, but the fact that they are usually located close to the gingival margin suggests that calculus,

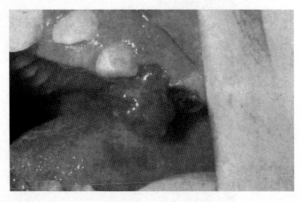

FIGURE 7-4 Pyogenic granuloma arising from the socket of an exfoliated upper first deciduous molar. (Courtesy of J.E. Bouquot, Morgantown, W.Va.)

food materials, and overhanging margins of dental restorations are important irritants that should be eliminated when the lesion is excised. Their friable, hemorrhagic, and frequently ulcerated appearance correlates with their histologic structure. They are comprised of proliferating endothelial tissue, much of which is canalized into a rich vascular network with minimal collagenous support. Polymorphs, as well as chronic inflammatory cells, are consistently present throughout the edematous stroma, with microabscess formation. Despite the common name for the lesion, a frank discharge of pus is not present; when such a discharge occurs, one is probably dealing with a fistula from an underlying periodontal or periapical abscess, the opening of which is often marked by a nodule of granulation tissue.

Identical lesions with the same histologic structure occur in association with the florid gingivitis and periodontitis that may complicate pregnancy.[13] Under these circumstances, the lesions are referred to as pregnancy epulis or pregnancy tumor (see Figure 7-3, C). The increased prevalence of pregnancy epulides toward the end of pregnancy (when levels of circulating estrogens are highest) and the tendency for these lesions to shrink after delivery (when there is a precipitous drop in circulating estrogens) indicate a definite role for these hormones in the etiology of the lesion.[14] Like pregnancy gingivitis, these lesions do not occur in mouths that are kept scrupulously free of even minor gingival irritation, and local irritation is clearly also an important etiologic factor. The relatively minor degree of chronic irritation that may be necessary to produce a pregnancy epulis is noteworthy.

Both pyogenic granulomas and pregnancy epulides may mature and become less vascular and more collagenous, gradually converting to fibrous epulides. Similar lesions also occur intraorally in extragingival locations. Histologically, differentiation from hemangioma is important.

A lesion that is closely related to pyogenic granulomas and peripheral giant cell granulomas (see below) is the peripheral ossifying fibroma. This lesion is found exclusively on the gingiva; it does not arise in other oral mucosal locations. Clinically, it varies from pale pink to cherry red and is typically located in the interdental papilla region. This reactive proliferation is so named because of the histologic evidence of calcifications and ossifications that are seen in the context of a hypercellular fibroblastic stroma. Like pyogenic granulomas, peripheral ossifying fibromas are commonly encountered among pregnant women.

The existence of these lesions indicates the need for a periodontal consultation, and treatment should include the elimination of subgingival irritants and gingival "pockets" throughout the mouth, as well as excision of the gingival growth. Small isolated pregnancy tumors occurring in a mouth that is otherwise in excellent gingival health may sometimes be observed for resolution following delivery, but the size of the lesion, episodes of hemorrhage or superimposed acute necrotizing ulcerative gingivitis, and the presence of a generalized pregnancy gingivitis usually dictate treatment during pregnancy. When possible, surgical and periodontal treatment should be completed during the second trimester, with continued surveillance of home care until after delivery.

Giant Cell Granuloma (Peripheral and Central)

Giant cell granuloma occurs either as a peripheral exophytic lesion on the gingiva (giant cell epulis, osteoclastoma, peripheral giant cell reparative granuloma) or as a centrally located lesion within the jaw,[15] skull, or facial bones[16] (Figures 7-5, A, and 7-6). It was first described (by Jaffe) as central giant cell reparative granuloma.[17] Both peripheral and central lesions are histologically similar and are considered to be examples of benign inflammatory hyperplasia in which cells with fibroblastic, osteoblastic, and osteoclastic potentials predominate. The

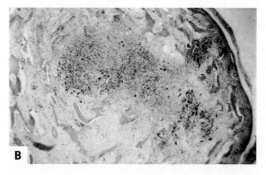

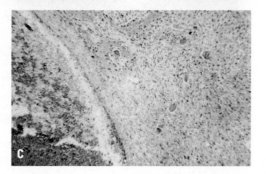

FIGURE 7-5 Giant cell reparative granuloma (peripheral giant cell tumor), an example of an inflammatory hyperplasia featuring osteoblastic and osteoclastic proliferation with a vascular stroma. The lesion in this patient was not associated with evidence of hyperparathyroidism. **A,** Clinical appearance of the lesion. **B** and **C,** Low- and higher-power views of stained sections from the lesion.

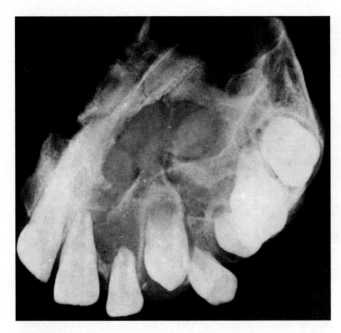

FIGURE 7-6 An active giant cell tumor. This radiograph is of a surgical specimen. (Courtesy of J.E. Hamner III, DDS, PhD, Washington, D.C.)

lesions are highly vascular; hemorrhage is a prominent clinical and histologic feature and also contributes a brown stain to the less common central lesions (Figure 7-7; see also Figure 7-5, B and C). True giant cell neoplasms, such as the giant cell tumor that occurs in the humerus and femur,[18] rarely occur in the jaw and usually occur only as a complication of Paget's disease (see "Paget's Disease of Bone," later in this chapter).

Peripheral giant cell granulomas are five times as common as the central lesions. Central lesions occur preferentially in the mandible, anterior to the first molar, and often cross the midline. Several large series of both peripheral and central giant cell granulomas have been reported in the literature.[19–22] The histologic structure of these lesions has been studied in detail,[23–25] as have their radiographic and computed tomo-

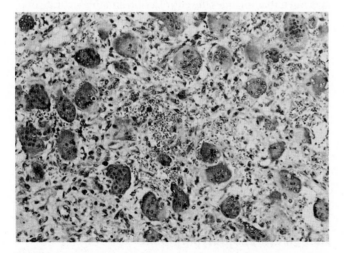

FIGURE 7-7 A benign giant cell tumor. (Hematoxylin and eosin, × 250 original magnification) (Courtesy of J.E. Hamner III, DDS, PhD, Washington, D.C.)

graphic appearances[26] (Figures 7-8 and 7-9; see also Figure 7-5, B and C, and Figures 7-6 and 7-7).

An important consideration in the management of these lesions is the necessity to search for evidence of hyperparathyroidism in all patients with histologically confirmed giant cell lesions of the jaw. There are documented examples of parathyroid lesions having been discovered as a result of blood and urine chemistry studies requested by a dentist following diagnosis of a giant cell lesion.[27] The frequency with which this is likely to happen is probably quite low since in most series of hyperparathyroidism,[28] lesions of the jaw have been among the last clinical manifestations of the disease to appear. Fewer than 10% of patients with hyperparathyroidism have radiographically visible cystic jaw lesions (see Figure 7-8) or even "loss of the lamina dura" (another effect of hyperparathyroidism, often used clinically to screen for the disease). Serum calcium, phosphorus, and alkaline phosphatase determinations should be requested prior to surgical removal of a jaw bone lesion that is radiographically compatible with a giant cell granuloma and immediately following the histologic diagnosis of central giant cell granuloma. Hyperparathyroidism may be primary, in which case there is a functional adenoma of the parathyroid glands, or secondary to renal disease, in which case renal osteodystrophy evolves as a consequence of tubular electrolyte retention abnormalities. In both cases, serum calcium is elevated, and phosphate is decreased. Parathormone levels are elevated.

In large lesions of the jaw bone, the chance that a biopsy specimen is not representative of the entire lesion is high, particularly since the pathologist is usually supplied with multiple small fragments curetted from the bony cavity rather than a solid specimen. In the interpretation of the results of the biopsy specimen analysis, consideration should always be given to the possibility that granulomatous giant cell–containing tissue may represent either a normal reparative response to some other bone lesion or an inflammatory hyperplasia.

The recurrence rate of central giant cell granulomas after initial conservative surgical therapy (curettage) is reported as 12 to 37%; repeat curettage usually prevents further recurrence.[15,19] On rare occasions, some giant cell lesions of the jaws behave more aggressively and may eventually require segmental jaw resection with a margin of normal tissue. Debate continues as to the validity of the histologic criteria that have been proposed to distinguish these more aggressive tumors,[15,24,25] and curettage with cryosurgery of the walls of the bony cavity is advised by some authors for any recurrent giant cell lesion. There is some evidence that the intralesional injection of steroids will cause the resolution of giant cell lesions of the jaws; however, a large controlled clinical series has yet to be reported.[29]

Pseudosarcomatous Fasciitis (Nodular Fasciitis) and Proliferative Myositis

Pseudosarcomatous fasciitis, a non-neoplastic connective-tissue proliferation, usually occurs on the trunk or extremities of young adults; it appears as a rapidly growing nodule that histologically imitates a malignant mesenchymal neoplasm but that clinically behaves benignly. Many cases have been origi-

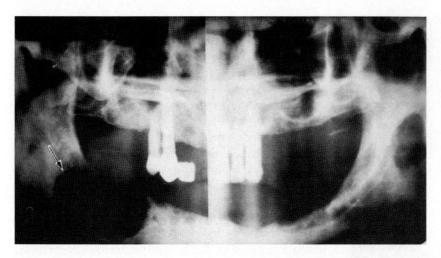

FIGURE 7-8 Panorex radiograph of a giant cell tumor (at the angle of the right mandible) that was associated with a parathyroid tumor (*arrow*). (Courtesy of J.E. Hamner III, DDS, PhD, Washington, D.C.)

nally mistaken as sarcomas due to the spindle cell nature and cellularity. Nodular fasciitis has distinctive microscopic features that allow for the diagnosis, and the predominant cell type is the myofibroblast. Similar lesions have been described intraorally and in the head and neck regions.[30,31]

Proliferative myositis[32] and focal myositis[33,34] are lesions of skeletal muscle that have similar clinical features that are identified on the basis of the histologic picture. Rare cases have been described in the tongue and in other neck and jaw muscles. Biologically, proliferative myositis is a reactive fibroblastic lesion that infiltrates around individual muscle fibers. Despite the nomenclature, these lesions are not inflamed histologically.

Pseudoepitheliomatous Hyperplasia

Pseudoepitheliomatous hyperplasia is a rather common exuberant oral epithelial response in which the rete pegs are extended deeply into the underlying connective tissue in an irregular fashion. Keratin pearl formation may be prominent, but other signs of cellular atypia characteristic of carcinoma

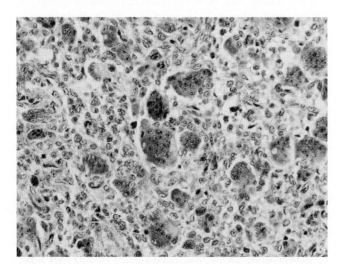

FIGURE 7-9 Histology of a giant cell tumor of the jaw bone. The tumor was associated with hyperparathyroidism. Compare with Figure 7-5, C, and Figure 7-7. (Hematoxylin and eosin, ×160 original magnification) (Courtesy of J.E. Hamner III, DDS, PhD, Washington, D.C.)

are absent. Neutrophilic infiltration about the elongated rete pegs is also prominent, in contrast to carcinoma. Sections may show isolated clumps of epithelial cells in the depth of the lesion, where the plane of sectioning cuts across long narrow rete pegs. However, true neoplastic invasion does not occur.

Clinically, lesions exhibiting pseudoepitheliomatous hyperplasia may be indistinguishable from epidermoid carcinoma, and if unnecessary surgery and radiation are to be avoided, the pathologist diagnosing the biopsy specimen must be familiar with the existence of this bizarre type of epithelial hyperplasia that is relatively common in the oral cavity. On occasion, experienced oral pathologists may be hesitant in deciding whether a particular lesion features this change or whether it is actually a carcinoma, despite the fact that morphometric analysis of the two lesions clearly differentiates them on the basis of size and shape of the squamous epithelial nuclei.[35]

Two oral lesions—granular cell tumor of the tongue and keratoacanthoma of the lip (both of which are described later in this chapter)—may exhibit pseudoepitheliomatous hyperplasia along the periphery of the lesion, and errors of diagnosis in which these lesions are wrongly identified as carcinoma are unfortunately not uncommon. The submission of a biopsy specimen that includes the entire lesion and the accurate documentation of the history and clinical appearance of the lesion can significantly help the pathologist recognize pseudoepitheliomatous hyperplasia. This change is also commonly seen in epulis fissuratum, in granulomatous inflammatory lesions attributable to tuberculosis or deep invasive fungi, in the gingival sulcus in cases of periodontitis (to a lesser degree), and (occasionally) in association with tumors such as malignant lymphoma. The pathogenesis of pseudoepitheliomatous hyperplasia has not been elucidated; the change may be related to the production of cellular growth factors by adjacent cells.[36]

Like other inflammatory hyperplasias, pseudoepitheliomatous hyperplasia is cured by local excision, provided that the chronic initiating irritant is also eliminated.

Benign Lymphoid Hyperplasia

Unencapsulated lymphoid aggregates that are normally present in the oral cavity (primarily on the soft palate, the foliate papillae on the posterolateral aspects of the tongue dorsum, and the anterior tonsillar pillar) can increase in size as a result of benign (reactive) processes as well as lymphoid neoplasms. In the absence of other evidence of lymphoid disease, diagnosis of intraoral swellings of this type may be difficult even when adequate biopsy specimens are obtained. The differential diagnosis of such swellings includes benign (follicular) lymphoid hyperplasia of the palate;[37,38] reactive hyperplasia of a buccal, facial, or submandibular lymph node, possibly associated with a chronic periapical or periodontal infection; viral infection (eg, Epstein-Barr virus) or a specific bacterial infection (eg, mycobacteria, Rochemela); and lymphoproliferative disease or lymphoma. Histologic criteria based on architectural, cytologic, and immunologic (leukocyte monoclonal antigen-antibody reactions) features of the lymphoid aggregate have been described in recent years.[38,39]

▼ HAMARTOMAS

Hamartomas are tumorlike malformations characterized by the presence of a cellular proliferation that is native to the part but that manifests growth cessation without potential for further growth.[40] On the one hand, hamartomas are to be distinguished from malformations such as extra digits, supernumerary teeth, and ectopic salivary gland tissue, in which excessive tissue is present in its usual histologic relationship. On the other hand, hamartomas are to be distinguished from true benign tumors that have a relatively unlimited capacity for expansive growth (which may continue after the exciting agent has ceased to operate).

Hamartomas are usually congenital and have their major period of growth when the rest of the body is growing. Once they have achieved their adult dimensions, they do not extend to involve more tissue and rarely increase in size unless trauma, thrombosis, or infection cause edema, inflammatory infiltration, and filling of new vascular channels. They are also to be distinguished from the excessive proliferation of reparative tissue described earlier in this chapter (see "Inflammatory [Reactive] Hyperplasias") and are usually easily separated histologically from such lesions. Hamartomas are found in many tissues of the body, and a tendency to such malformations is often hereditary. Individual oral hamartomas, therefore, often occur in association with other gross and microscopic developmental abnormalities that assist considerably in their diagnosis.

Hemangioma (both solitary and when found in association with other developmental anomalies in the various angiomatosis syndromes), lymphangioma, glomus tumor, nevi, granular cell tumor of the tongue and granular cell epulis, neuromas of the type III multiple endocrine neoplasia (MEN III) syndrome, fibrous dysplasia of bone, cherubism, various odontomas, some odontogenic tumors, and (possibly) the melanotic neuroectodermal tumor of infancy are all examples of hamartomatous development in the oral region. To a greater or lesser extent, these lesions all possess the characteristics of hamartomas. These variants aside, the treatment of hamartomas is essentially a cosmetic problem, and the complete removal of these lesions is often neither desirable nor possible. Neoplastic and malignant transformation are unusual in hamartomas although some have a greater tendency in this regard (eg, neurofibromas; see "Nerve Sheath Tumors and Traumatic Neuroma," below).

Teratomas (which are often thought of as malformations but which are actually neoplasms of developing tissues) are mentioned at the end of this section, in comparison with hamartomas (see "Teratomas and Dermoid Cysts," below).

Hemangioma and Angiomatous Syndromes

Hemangiomas are tumorlike malformations composed of seemingly disorganized masses of endothelium-lined vessels that are filled with blood and connected to the main blood vascular system.[41] They have been described in almost all locations in and about the oral cavity and face and may involve deep structures such as the jaw and facial bones, salivary glands, muscles,[42] and the temporomandibular joint, as well as the surface mucosa and skin. They may occur as isolated lesions in the oral cavity (Figure 7-10), as multiple lesions affecting different parts of the body, and in association with other developmental anomalies in the various angiomatous syndromes described below. They range from simple red patches (nevus flammeus, port-wine stain)[43] (Figure 7-11, A) or birthmarks (nongeneti-

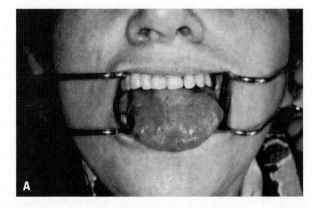
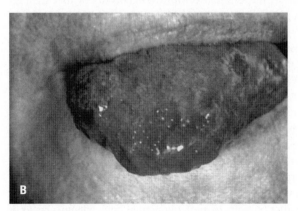

FIGURE 7-10 **A** and **B,** Bilateral hemangiomas of the tongue.

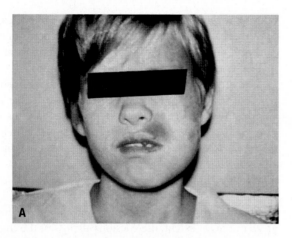 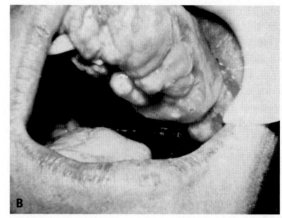

FIGURE 7-11   Encephalofacial angiomatosis (Sturge-Weber syndrome). **A,** Port-wine stain on a side of the face. **B,** Massive intraoral hemangioma of the maxilla. (Courtesy of E.P. Rossi, DDS, MS, Cleveland, Ohio)

cally transmitted embryologic mishaps),[44] which do not raise the mucosal or skin surface, to large fungating masses, which bury teeth and cause serious deformity and disfiguration. Small lesions may be clinically indistinguishable from pyogenic granulomas and superficial venous varicosities. Both cavernous and capillary types have been described; the former consists of relatively large blood-filled lakes, and the latter consists of masses of proliferating vessels of capillary dimension. In both cases, there is a simple endothelial lining to the vascular channels and little connective-tissue stroma. Such lesions characteristically bleed profusely when traumatized.

Many hemangiomas are evident at birth, and they frequently increase in size with general bodily growth. The filling of previously empty vascular channels also accounts for an increase in the size of these lesions, and such changes sometimes occur very rapidly following trauma. While such growth is to be distinguished from neoplasia, this distinction may not be easy to make clinically, and the clinician will quite reasonably sometimes be concerned that what is assumed to be a hamartomatous lesion may be developing a neoplastic tendency. Diascopy is the technique of applying pressure to a suspected vascular lesion to visualize the evacuation of coloration, a finding that supports the fact that patent blood-filled spaces constitute the lesion. If compression fails to evacuate the pigmentation, the lesion could be extravasated blood or some other type of intrinsic or extrinsic pigment that has been deposited in the tissues (see Chapter 6, "Pigmented Lesions of the Oral Mucosa").

When located on the surface of the skin or oral mucous membrane, hemangiomas are usually readily identified. Large lesions are warm and may even be pulsatile if associated with a large vessel. Hemangiomas of the tongue (see Figure 7-10) and gingiva are often covered by unusually rugose epithelium. Differentiation should be made from vascular inflammatory hyperplasias, sublingual varicosities (varicosities of the superficial veins on the ventral surface of the tongue that are common after 50 years of age), pigmented nevi, telangiectasias of various etiologies, and hematomas. Centrally located heman-

giomas[45] must be distinguished from the many osteolytic tumors and cystlike lesions that affect the jaws, as well as from both congenital and acquired arteriovenous aneurysms of the jaw. Care should be taken in excising or performing biopsies on hemangiomas, partly because of their tendency to uncontrolled hemorrhage and partly because of the difficulty of knowing the extent of the lesion, only a small part of which may be evident in the mouth.

Gingival hemangiomas may connect with similar lesions in the jawbone, and radiographic examination of the bone may not always reveal an abnormality of the trabecular architecture. Most such lesions are observed clinically as multilocular radiolucencies; therefore, when this radiographic pattern is observed, the lesion should be aspirated. Some central hemangiomas of bone represent arteriovenous malformations, and the blood coursing through them is under arterial pressure. A bright red aspirate is highly suggestive of central hemangioma and requires that imaging studies be instituted to confirm the clinical impression. Computed tomography, Doppler and conventional ultrasonography,[46] radionuclide-labeled red cell scintigraphic scanning,[47] and superselective microangiography[48] are used to define the extent of bony hemangiomas, and radiographic examination of the affected tissues may reveal not only bony defects but also phleboliths in the cheek that mark the location of abnormal vessels. Hemorrhage from centrally located hemangiomas of the jaw is especially difficult to control, and surgery on hemangiomas should be attempted only when provision has been made beforehand to control any untoward hemorrhage that may occur (typed and crossmatched blood, splints, and means of tying off branches of the external carotid artery). In general, electrocoagulation and cryosurgery cause less postoperative hemorrhage than incision with a scalpel causes.

The treatment of hemangiomas[49] continues to be a difficult problem fraught with the danger of uncontrollable hemorrhage. Conventional surgical techniques have been largely replaced by cryosurgery[50] and laser surgery,[51,52] often preceded by the injection of sclerosing solutions.[53,54] Also, intravascular embolization with plastic spheres[55,56] is now a commonly used and successful approach. Although radiation can be used to sclerose these lesions,[57] the risk of inducing neoplastic and other degenerative changes[58] later in life is very high, and its use is now generally contraindicated, particularly in children. Many of the reported cases of malignant change in hemangiomas undoubtedly are the results of radiation treatment. Intralesional injection of corticosteroids is sometimes a successful alternative to surgery for hemangiomas in infants.[59]

Hemangiomas of the skin and oral mucous membrane often coexist with similar lesions of the central nervous system and the meninges.[60,61] A variety of such angiomatous syndromes have been described, with eponyms applied to both complete and incomplete variants of each syndrome. Although the skin and oral lesions are the most deforming and disfiguring lesions, the central nervous system lesions are often associated with serious problems of epilepsy, hemiplegia, mental retardation, and retinal changes.

Sturge-Weber syndrome[59] (encephalofacial or encephalotrigeminal angiomatosis) is probably the most common of these malformations (see Figure 7-11). It is characterized by angiomatosis of the face (nevus flammeus), with a variable distribution sometimes matching the dermatomes of one or more trigeminal nerve divisions; leptomeningeal angiomas, particularly of the parietal and occipital lobes of the brain, with associated characteristic intracranial calcifications; contralateral hemiplegia; and one or more of the neurologic symptoms just mentioned. Oral changes occur in 40% of cases of this syndrome and may include massive growths of the gingiva and asymmetric jaw growth and tooth eruption sequence (due to differential blood flow to the affected area). Since many patients with this syndrome are treated for many years with phenytoin (Dilantin) as an anticonvulsant, a distinction needs to be made in these patients between gingival hypertrophy due to phenytoin and that due to angiomatous changes, particularly if gingivectomy is planned.[62,63] The intraoral lesions in this syndrome classically occur on the same side of the body as other angiomas in the patient, but the classic pattern is not always found in either the distribution or the expression of the various components of the syndrome. Fortunately, this serious malformation is not of hereditary origin (compare with Rendu-Osler-Weber syndrome[64] or hereditary hemorrhagic telangiectasia).

Other (rarer) angiomatous syndromes are Maffucci's syndrome[65,66] (multiple angioma of the skin and enchondromas of bone) and von Hippel-Lindau disease[67] (a familial syndrome involving hemangioblastomas in the retina and cerebellum, pancreatic and renal cysts, renal adenomas, hepatic hemangiomas, and multiple endocrine neoplasia)[68] (see pertinent section). Conditions such as Sturge-Weber syndrome and von Hippel-Lindau disease, which involve a visible congenitally acquired external lesion (ie, a birthmark or "phakos") and other systemic anomalies, are sometimes referred to as phakomatoses.

Many reviews and case reports[60,69,70] of both isolated oral hemangiomas and the various angiomatous syndromes are available and attest to the problems associated with treating these non-neoplastic lesions.

Lymphangioma

Lymphangioma is histologically and etiologically similar to hemangioma, except that the abnormal vessels are filled with a clear protein-rich fluid containing a few cells (lymph) rather than blood.[60,70–72] Lymphangiomas may occur alone or (more frequently) in association with hemangiomas or other anomalous blood vessels with which the lymphangiomatous vessels are anastomosed. The tongue is the most common oral location for this lesion. Together with hemangioma, lymphangioma is an important cause of congenital macroglossia.[73]

Lymphangiomas are frequently without a clear anatomic outline and present on clinical examination as soft masses that dissect tissue planes and turn out to be more extensive than anticipated. Large lymphangiomas spreading into and distending the neck are referred to as cystic hygromas.[74] Differential diagnoses of lymphangiomas of the tongue include hemangioma, congenital hypothyroidism, mongolism, amyloidosis, neurofibromatosis, various storage diseases (eg, Hurler's syndrome and glycogen storage disease), and primary muscular hypertrophy of the tongue, all of which may cause macroglossia. The differential diagnosis should also consider certain anomalies in the neck, including various inclusion cysts, cellulitis, and plunging ranula, which large angiomas of the neck may simulate. Abnormalities of the mucosa overlying a lymphangioma may give the appearance of a localized glossitis and may draw attention to the presence of a small lesion buried in the tongue. The typical clinical appearance of oral lymphangioma is that of a racemose surface. The problems of managing lymphangiomas are similar to those of managing hemangiomas.

In neonates, localized superficial cysts of the alveolar mucosa with a lymphangiomatous histologic picture are described as alveolar lymphangiomas.[71] Such lesions, which are more common in black neonates than in white neonates and which are probably often misidentified as eruption cysts or mucoceles, disappear spontaneously with chewing and with tooth eruption.

Glomus Tumor and Other Vascular Endothelial Growths

An unusual abnormality, glomus tumor[75] (glomangioma) develops as a small painful unencapsulated nodule as a result of hamartomatous proliferation of the modified smooth-muscle pericytic cells[76] found in the characteristic type of peripheral arteriovenous anastomosis known as the glomus. In addition to having a characteristic histology, these lesions also may secrete various catecholamines. The glomus tumor is rare in the mouth[76,77] but can occur in the pterygotemporotympanic region,[78,79] glomus jugulare, and skull base. Glomus tumors arising in the carotid and aortic bodies may produce neck masses; they are of a different cell derivation (ie, chemosensory) and are more appropriately referred to as chemodectomas or paragangliomas. Differentiation of the glomus tumor from other masses of proliferating vascular endothelial cells (hemangioendothelioma and hemangiopericytoma) requires special stains and considerable histopathologic diagnostic skills. Another important diagnostic feature that characterizes at least some glomus tumors is an autosomal dominant inheritance pattern. Because of the associated pain, glomus tumors tend to be removed while still quite small.

Granular Cell Tumor and Granular Cell Epulis

The granular cell tumor is an important oral hamartomatous lesion (1) because of its frequent occurrence as a nodule on the tongue and as its variant form on the gingiva (congenital epulis) (Figure 7-12) or other mucosal site; (2) because of the controversy as to its nature and cytologic structure; and (3) because of the overlying pseudoepitheliomatous hyperplasia that often leads to a misdiagnosis of squamous cell carcinoma and to unnecessary radical surgery.[75,78] Histologically, these lesions are composed of masses of large eosinophilic granular

cells interspersed with a collagenous stroma and covered with hyperplastic epithelium.

About one-third of oral granular cell tumors occur on the tongue; those occurring elsewhere in the mouth (ie, on the palate, gum, floor of mouth, buccal mucosa, and lips) and on the skin are similar in most of their clinical features and in their appearances on light and electron microscopy. Important distinctions between lingual and extralingual granular cell tumors are (in the latter) the absence of overlying pseudoepitheliomatous hyperplasia and a female sex predilection. The large granular cells have been variously identified as of muscle cell (Abrikosov's myocytes), histiocytic, Schwann cell, and mesenchymal origin. Immunocytochemical staining[80–82] reveals that nongingival lesions of this type are

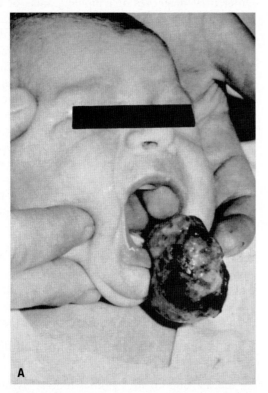

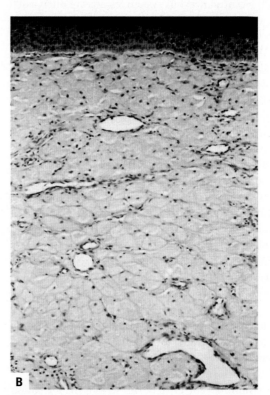

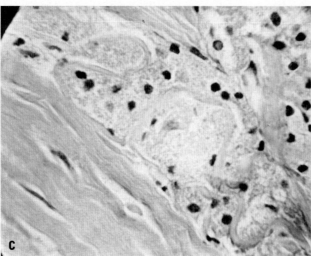

FIGURE 7-12 A, Congenital epulides arising from the upper and lower jaw of a 2-day-old infant. **B,** Section of one of these tumors; both showed identical histologic structure despite different clinical appearances. The lesions are composed of masses of granular eosinophilic cells characteristic of the granular cell–type of congenital epulis. (Reproduced with permission from Blair A, Edwards DM. Congenital epulis of the newborn. Oral Surg Oral Med Oral Pathol 1977;43:687) **C,** Similar cells from a granular cell myoblastoma presenting as a painless indurated mass in the anterior third of the tongue of a 49-year-old man. (Courtesy of E.P. Rossi, DDS, MS, Cleveland, Ohio)

immunologically reactive for S-100 protein and myelin but negative for myogenous and histiocytic markers and that they are probably derived from Schwann cells or their mesenchymal precursors.

Quite innocent-looking and often long-standing tongue nodules in biopsy specimens from adults may turn out to be granular cell tumors. Treatment of these oral lesions, both on the tongue and in extralingual locations, is by local excision. The differential diagnosis for congenital epulis includes other hamartomatous and hyperplastic oral mucosal lesions, odontogenic tumors, and ectopic tooth germs. Multiple and familially occurring oral granular cell tumors have been reported on several occasions. In contrast to the prevalence of the granular cell tumor, true neoplasms of the muscle of the body of the tongue (rhabdomyoma) are exceedingly rare and are positive for myogenous markers.[80]

Nerve Sheath Tumors and Traumatic Neuroma

The nerve sheath includes the Schwann cells, which surround individual axis cylinders; perineural fibroblasts, which form collagen networks between individual nerve fibers with their surrounding Schwann cells; and the epineurium, a sheath that envelops entire nerve trunks and that is composed of fibroblastic-type cells and collagen.[60,69,83,84] Most nerve sheath tumors are true neoplasms. The developmental abnormalities (ie, hamartomas and not neoplasms) of neurofibromatosis and traumatic neuroma arise from nerve sheath cells. Neurofibromas of the oral cavity are usually solitary;[85] a significant feature of neurofibroma is its tendency to be multiple and to be associated with a variety of other familial abnormalities in the syndrome of von Recklinghausen's neurofibromatosis, an inherited autosomal dominant condition in which there is also a tendency to develop sarcoma (see the later section, "Syndromes with Benign Oral Neoplastic or Hamartomatous Components"). Neurofibromatosis evolves as a consequence of a mutation in the *NF1* gene. Since 5% of patients with neurofibromatosis develop sarcoma,[86] recognition of an otherwise innocent-appearing nodule in the oral cavity as a neurofibroma can be an important diagnosis.

Histologically, neurofibromas are to be distinguished from neurilemomas (tumors of the nerve sheath, or schwannomas). Neurilemomas are encapsulated S-100 protein–positive tumors that show patterns of whorled connective-tissue elements interspersed with readily recognizable axons with or without a myelin sheath. Neurilemomas also exhibit a characteristic palisading of nuclei and other suggestions of a histologic organization referred to as an organoid structure; both features are usually absent from neurofibromas and neuromas.[87] Rarely, neurilemomas may occur in patients with neurofibromatosis. Oral lesions are usually asymptomatic and do not recur after local excision (Figure 7-13).

The term "traumatic neuroma" describes a localized exuberant growth of nerve and nerve sheath elements that develop after section or other local damage to a peripheral nerve.[88]

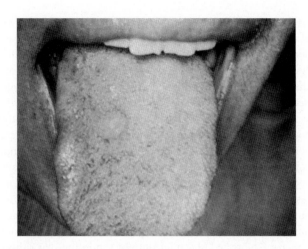

FIGURE 7-13 Asymptomatic neurofibroma of the tongue. This lesion was not associated with other evidence of neurofibromatosis.

Melanotic Neuroectodermal Tumor of Infancy

Melanotic neuroectodermal tumor of infancy has been classified both as a hamartoma and as a benign neoplasm, with recent authors favoring the latter etiology.[89,90] It is a rare tumor, occurring both orally and extraorally (usually in children under 6 months of age) and showing a characteristic biphasic histologic picture of melanin-containing epithelial cells lining slitlike spaces and small round cells resembling neuroblasts. Its origin is probably the neuroectoderm (the embryonic layer that contributes greatly to cranial and oral development) although its gnathic location has led some authors in the older literature to consider it to be of odontogenic origin and to use such synonyms as "melanotic ameloblastoma" and "pigmented epulis." Theories that assign its origin to ectopic retinal epithelium have produced the synonyms "retinal anlage tumor" and "melanotic progonoma." Recent immunohistochemical studies confirm that it is a tumor with "polyphenotypic expression of neural and epithelial markers, melanin production, and glial and rhabdomyoblastic differentiation."[89] The lesion usually protrudes into the mouth and may also involve underlying bone. The lesion does not necessarily appear pigmented clinically. It is rarely an aggressive lesion although aggressive behavior with recurrences after local excision have been described.[91] Findings on magnetic resonance imaging (MRI) have been recently described.[90]

Fibrous Dysplasia of Bone and Albright's Syndrome

Fibrous dysplasia of bone results from an abnormality in the development of bone-forming mesenchyme.[92–94] This is manifested by the replacement of spongy bone by a peculiar fibrous tissue, within which trabeculae or spherules of poorly calcified nonlamellar bone are formed by osseous metaplasia. Histologically, a given lesion may show a great variability of pattern, with some fields that are predominantly collagenous, some that are osteoid, and others that are fully ossified and calcified.

Radiographically, the lesion will usually present varying degrees of radiopacity and lucency; some areas will resemble compact bone, and others will be cystic areas. Surgical exploration of such cystic areas usually reveals either a soft fibrous tissue or (more characteristically) a tissue that is gritty on section or curettage. Because these lesions often develop to quite a large size with few symptoms other than a slowly developing asymmetry of the bone, they may exhibit a quite dramatic deformity and apparent bony destruction upon radiographic examination. Patients may have a small solitary focus (monostotic form) or may have many bones affected with multiple lesions (polyostotic form). Rare cases exist in which the lesions of fibrous dysplasia coexist with other developmental bony defects or with extraskeletal changes, notably a blotchy cutaneous hyperpigmentation and precocious puberty. The term "McCune-Albright syndrome" (or simply "Albright's syndrome") has been used to describe these more dramatic cases occurring in children (see "Syndromes with Benign Oral Neoplastic or Hamartomatous Components," below). Recently, the lesional tissues taken from patients with Albright's syndrome have revealed a mutation in the G protein of the internal signaling pathways. Solitary foci are far more common than multiple lesions, particularly in the jaw bone. Other than the greater variety of histologic patterns and sizes of lesions seen in the polyostotic form, there is no essential difference between the two lesions.[95]

The hamartomatous nature of the condition is exemplified by (1) the existence of congenital forms of the disease, (2) the association of fibrous dysplasia with other developmental bone problems in the same patient, (3) the frequency with which increasing size of the lesion correlates with periods of increased skeletal growth rate, (4) the association of endocrine abnormalities with bony lesions in patients with Albright's syndrome, and (5) the rarity of malignant transformation of these lesions (considering the frequency with which fibrous dysplasia is seen). Recent reviews have stressed that malignant transformation of these lesions probably occurs more frequently than is usually believed because small foci of fibrous dysplasia are often overlooked in the examination of a patient with a malignant bone lesion. In most cases, fibrous dysplasia can be safely handled as a benign developmental anomaly, and superficial recontouring of the lesion or curettage of a large cystic lesion remains appropriate management, provided that an adequate and representative bone biopsy specimen has been obtained.[96] Radiotherapy is contraindicated in the treatment of fibrous dysplasia. Radiotherapy administered in earlier decades of the twentieth century may have played a role in the rare cases of malignant transformation to fibrosarcoma or osteogenic sarcoma.

The extensive size and the nonuniform radiographic appearance of some lesions of fibrous dysplasia pose a problem to the surgeon who needs to obtain representative biopsy specimens with minimal disturbance of the lesion. Biopsy specimens of these lesions, as do other bone biopsy specimens, frequently reveal nothing more than superficial layers of reactive normal bone formation. Curettage of one of the cystic cavities usually provides material of more diagnostic value. At times, the hypercellularity, pleomorphism, and aggressiveness

of the fibrous tissue in these lesions will lead the pathologist to suspect a fibrosarcoma or an osteogenic sarcoma; consideration of both the clinical behavior and the histologic appearance of the lesion is needed to arrive at a diagnosis. Fibrous dysplasia has been described in association with giant cell reparative granuloma of bone, aneurysmal bone cyst, and a number of other fibro-osseous lesions, and the coexistence of different histologic pictures in one lesion or in one patient can provide added diagnostic difficulties.

The clinical problems associated with fibrous dysplasia of bone are related to the site and extent of involvement. Many small foci probably remain unrecognized throughout life. In the long bones, deformity and fractures are common complications that often lead to the initial diagnosis of the lesion. In the jaws and other parts of the craniofacial skeleton, involvement of adjacent structures such as the cranial sinuses, cranial nerves, and ocular contents can lead to serious complications in addition to cosmetic and functional problems. Intracranial lesions arising from the cranial bones may produce seizures and electroencephalographic changes. Extension into and occlusion of the maxillary and ethmoid sinuses and mastoid air spaces is common.[97] Proptosis, diplopia, and interference with jaw function also often prompt surgical intervention.

Computed tomography and technetium (Tc)-99m bone scans have proved to be of great help in the diagnosis of lesions of fibrous dysplasia.[98,99] Trimming and surface contouring of the affected bone, curettage of bony cavities, and packing with bone chips remain the recommended treatments. Surgical interventions before the patient has reached puberty may actually activate these fibro-osseous lesions and should be avoided except in cases of the more disfiguring lesions. Attempts at treating advanced cases of the polyostotic form with calcitonin[100] have not been greatly successful. There is laboratory evidence of increased bone turnover, increased alkaline phosphatase, and high urinary hydroxyproline levels with normal serum calcium and phosphate levels in large monostotic lesions of fibrous dysplasia and in the polyostotic form.

Opinions differ as to whether pain is a common feature of fibrous dysplasia. In the general skeleton, small lesions are undoubtedly often asymptomatic. Larger lesions associated with cortical fractures are painful and incapacitating and lead to extreme degrees of deformity in many cases. Pain is not a feature of craniofacial lesions. The extent of the deformity may be as great as that associated with untreated von Recklinghausen's disease of bone due to hyperparathyroidism, and in the early part of this century, fibrous dysplasia was often confused with this metabolic bone disorder.

Other Benign Fibro-Osseous Lesions

Before 1970, "fibrous dysplasia" was used as an all-inclusive term for both the monostotic and polyostotic forms of fibrous dysplasia described above and for a variety of other fibro-osseous lesions, notably ossifying fibroma, cementifying fibroma, and osteoblastoma[94] (Figure 7-14). Histologic studies often failed to establish definitive differences between these lesions, particularly in regard to the problems of the matura-

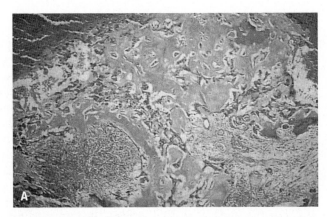

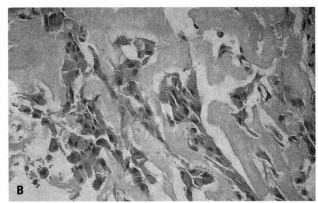

FIGURE 7-14 A, Low-power and **B,** high-power views of an aggressive osteoblastoma developing in association with a tooth socket. (Courtesy of D.R. Weathers, S. Mullër, Emory University, Atlanta, Ga.)

tion of the connective-tissue elements, the heterogeneity of large lesions, and inadequate biopsy specimens. The problem of separating these different lesions in the jaw bone is further compounded by the occurrence in the jaw of lesions with cemental as well as osseous differentiation (Figure 7-15) and the frequency of giant cell granulomas in this region. A number of papers that were published by oral pathologists during the late 1960s and early 1970s emphasized the variety of histologic appearances in fibro-osseous lesions that were derived from the periodontal membrane and distinguished them from similar lesions arising from medullary bone.[101–103]

The difficulty of differentiating tumors of periodontal membrane origin from tumors of medullary bone origin has long been recognized. Differentiation between the two is important because tumors of medullary bone origin usually behave in a more aggressive fashion even though they are essentially benign. The absolute proof of medullary bone origin in this group of tumors has not yet been shown, however. Benign fibro-osseous lesions of periodontal membrane origin are much more prevalent in the jaws than are fibro-osseous lesions of medullary bone origin. These latter lesions may be differentiated by clinical, radiographic, hematologic, and

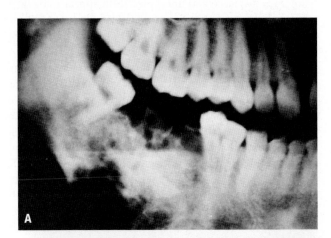

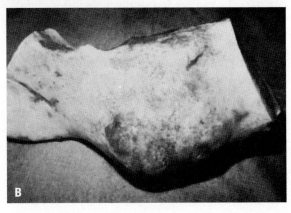

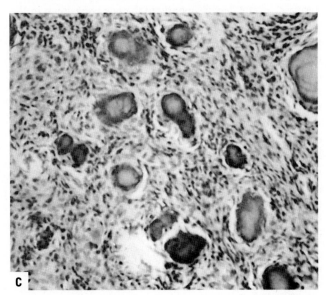

FIGURE 7-15 Large cemento-ossifying fibroma of the mandibular molar region in a 21-year-old black female with a 2-year history of localized enlargement of the body of the mandible associated with a dull throbbing pain and loosening of the teeth in this region. **A,** Radiographic examination revealed a large multilocular lesion extending from the third molar to the premolar area, with expansion of the bone. **C,** Histologic examination of the excised lesion revealed spherules of bone and cementum in a fibrous matrix. (Courtesy of T. Beckerman, DDS, Baltimore, Md.)

histopathologic considerations. (For additional information on this topic, the reader should consult the reviews by Hamner,[102] Waldron,[103] and Eversole.[104])

OSSIFYING FIBROMA

Differentiation of solitary lesions of ossifying fibroma and fibrous dysplasia can be quite difficult on histologic grounds alone, but the lesions generally can be distinguished if radiographic and clinical criteria are used together with an analysis of a biopsy specimen from the central part of the lesion. Fibrous dysplasia has a diffuse margin radiographically; ossifying fibroma is an expansile process with a clearly defined cortical margin (being a benign tumor). Fibrous dysplasia tends to favor the maxilla whereas ossifying fibroma occurs more often in the mandible. Both are slow growing and originate early in life, but fibrous dysplasia grows endosteally and follows the general structure of the affected bone, usually producing a thickening and irregular deformation of the bone. Ossifying fibroma, by contrast, grows into and fills cavities such as the nasal cavity and accessory sinuses and destroys surrounding bone as it enlarges. Management of the two benign lesions differs considerably. Fibrous dysplasia is treated by surface sculpting whereas ossifying fibromas are managed by surgical enucleation. Juvenile aggressive forms are seen and may require en bloc resection.

ANEURYSMAL BONE CYST, TRAUMATIC BONE CYST, AND STATIC BONE CYST

Aneurysmal bone cyst, unlike ossifying fibroma and fibrous dysplasia, occurs less frequently in the jaw bones than in the long bones and usually involves the mandible rather than the maxilla.[105,106] Eighty percent of aneurysmal bone cysts occur in patients younger than 30 years of age; both sexes are equally affected. Microscopically, curetted material from the cavity resembles giant cell reparative granuloma but has more prominent vascular spaces, with evidence of old and recent hemorrhages and thrombosis and hyalinization of some of the vascular spaces. Like giant cell granuloma, it has no epithelial lining despite the common use of the word "cyst" to describe it. Aneurysmal bone cyst is to be differentiated from two other pseudocysts of the jaw: the so-called traumatic bone cyst[107] (the name given to solitary and usually asymptomatic cavities that are found in the mandible, that are without any epithelial or other distinguishing lining and that contain only serum or are apparently empty), for which a traumatic etiology seems to be less convincingly established, and the submandibular salivary gland depression (static or latent bone cyst, or Stafne's cyst), located below the inferior mandibular canal just anterior to the angle of the mandible, where it presents as a well-delineated radiolucency that may contain salivary gland tissue.[108,109] A similar defect can be seen in the anterior mandible apical to the canine, where the sublingual gland resides, and is termed a sublingual salivary gland depression. For both the aneurysmal and traumatic bone cysts, a thorough curettage of the lesion and its walls and packing with bone chips result in the healing of the defect.

CHERUBISM

Cherubism is a rare disease of children that is characterized by bilateral painless mandibular (and often corresponding maxillary) swellings that cause fullness of the cheeks, firm protuberant intraoral alveolar masses, and missing or displaced teeth (Figure 7-16).[60,110,111] Submaxillary lymphadenopathy is an early and fairly constant feature that tends to subside after the age of 5 years and that usually has regressed by the age of 12 years. Maxillary involvement can often produce a slightly upward turning of the child's eyes, revealing an abnormal amount of sclera beneath them. It was the upward "looking toward heaven" cast of the eyes, combined with the characteristic facial chubbiness of these children, that prompted the term "cherubism."[112] Cherubism is inherited as a dominant gene, with a penetrance of nearly 100% in males and 50 to 75% in females; however, the exact cause of cherubism remains unknown, and other patterns of inheritance as well as the occurrence of cherubism in association with other syndromes have been described.[113–115] The clinical appearance may vary from barely discernible posterior swellings of a single jaw to a grotesque anterior and posterior expansion of both jaws, with concomitant difficulties in mastication, speech, swallowing, and respiration. Disease activity declines with advancing age.

Radiographically, the lesions are multiple well-defined multilocular radiolucencies in the mandible and maxilla. These rarefactions begin in the posterior alveolar region and ramus and can spread anteriorly. They are irregular in size and usually cause marked destruction of the alveolar bone. Numerous displaced and unerupted teeth appear to be floating in radiolucent spaces. Serum calcium and phosphorus are within normal limits, but the serum alkaline phosphatase level may be elevated.

Histologically, the jaw lesion can bear a close resemblance to benign giant cell granuloma. Other specimens have been described as being more mature, with a greater amount of fibrous tissue and collagen and fewer giant cells. The prominent eosinophilic perivascular cuffing material noted around capillaries in these lesions has been proved to be collagen; this finding is a distinctive histologic diagnostic feature (Figure 7-17).

The reported treatment of cherubism has varied considerably, and there are advocates for each of the following methods: no active treatment, extraction of teeth in the involved areas, surgical contouring of expanded lesions, and complete curettage. Long-term longitudinal clinical studies have disclosed that the childhood lesions give way to partial or complete resolution in the adult.

Teratomas and Dermoid Cysts

Teratomas are neoplasms that are composed of a mixture of tissues, more than one of which exhibits neoplastic proliferation.[116–118] They are congenitally acquired and are usually found in the ovary. Rare examples, either arising from the oral cavity or protruding into the oral cavity from the base of the skull, have been described in children. The finding of various organlike structures (ie, teeth, tissue, hair, and skin) in these tumors and their common location in the ovary may give the

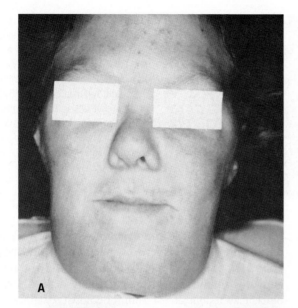

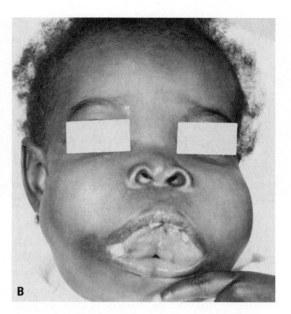

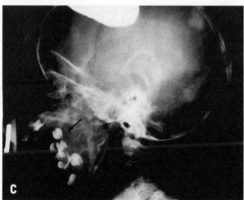

FIGURE 7-16 **A,** Cherubism in a 23-year-old female. (Courtesy of Sheldon Rovin, DDS, PhD, Philadelphia, Pa.) **B,** A severe case of cherubism in a 3-year-old female; **C,** Lateral head film depicts the radiographic features of cherubism. (Both courtesy of J.E. Hamner III, DDS, PhD, Washington, D.C.)

misleading impression that they are fetal malformations rather than neoplastic growths of developing tissue; the latter is the currently accepted understanding and clearly provides a more convincing explanation for oral teratomas than does the former. Teratomas that arise from the base of the skull often extend into the cranial cavity as well as the oral cavity, and

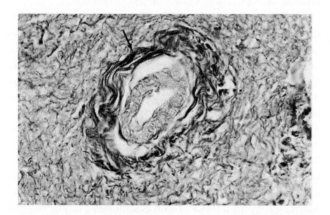

FIGURE 7-17   Histologic features of cherubism. Perivascular cuffing of collagen contributes the characteristic eosinophilic cuffing noted around capillaries in these lesions. (Courtesy of J.E. Hamner III, DDS, PhD, Washington, D.C.)

newborn infants with such lesions rarely survive. No single histologic picture is characteristic although the usual appearance of disorganized neoplastic tissues of various types readily identifies the lesion to the pathologist.

Some teratomas of the ovary are primarily cystic; these are often referred to as dermoid cysts because they may include epidermal tissue and even hair follicles. Dermoid cysts[118,119] of the oral cavity are most commonly encountered in the floor of the mouth although they may arise in other soft-tissue locations (Figures 7-18 and 7-19). These cysts also feature epidermal tissues and (even) hair follicles, sweat and sebaceous glands in the cyst wall, and keratin and sebum in the cyst cavity. Cysts that harbor tissues from all three germ layers are more correctly referred to as teratoid cysts.

▼ CYSTS OF THE JAWS AND BENIGN ODONTOGENIC TUMORS

Cysts of the Jaw

Cysts (ie, fluid-filled epithelial-lined cavities in the jaw bones and soft tissues of the face, floor of the mouth, and neck) may cause either intraoral or extraoral swellings that may clinically

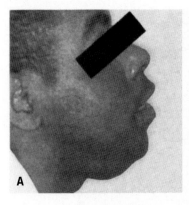 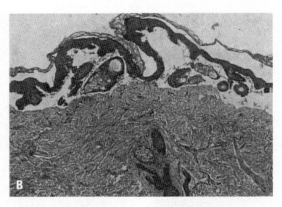

FIGURE 7-18 **A,** Dermoid (epidermoid) cyst of the floor of the mouth that developed in a young male adult as a mass in both the submental region and the floor of the mouth. **B,** The keratinized epithelial cyst lining with rudimentary hair follicles and sebaceous glands is apparent microscopically. (Courtesy of R.K. Wesley, University of Detroit-Mercy, Detroit, Mich. and R. Stampada, Sinai Hospital, Mich.)

resemble a benign tumor.[120–125] Unilocular and multilocular radiolucencies discovered in the jaw bones by radiographic examination must also be differentiated from solid growths in the jaw, a distinction that cannot always be made by inspecting the radiograph. However, the majority of cysts are small, do not distend surface tissues, and are often first recognized in routine dental radiographic examinations.[126] Others are discovered during investigation of a nonvital tooth or an acute dental abscess due to secondary infection of the cyst or by loosening of the teeth and by jaw fracture. Small isolated radiolucencies in the jaw bone that are not associated with a loss of pulp vitality are usually observed over several months for increase in size before surgical exploration. Radiolucencies that are suspected of being cysts or tumors and that are not associated with a necrotic tooth require biopsy.

Radiographic examination rarely provides a conclusive diagnosis as to the nature of a radiolucency in the jaw although it may be used to gauge the rate of growth of such lesions and to detect erosion of tooth roots and cortical destruction. These features are characteristic of aggressive benign lesions as well as malignant lesions. Contrary to traditional lore, there is no size range that separates periapical cysts from dental granulo-

mas, and microscopic examination of periapical lesions frequently reveals tiny cystic areas and areas of epithelial proliferation in what is clinically thought to be a granuloma. Similarly, caution must be used in diagnosing even large radiolucent jaw lesions as cysts simply because they appear "spherical" on the radiograph. The differential diagnosis of multiple radiolucencies in the jaw should include consideration of multiple myeloma, Langerhans cell histiocytosis, metastatic carcinoma, giant cell granuloma and hyperparathyroidism, multiple dental granulomas, periapical cysts, cemental dysplasia, ossifying fibroma, and fibrous dysplasia. Microscopic examination of the cyst wall provides the clear diagnosis that is important to the management of the lesion, and submission of all excised tissue (including fragments scraped from the wall of the jaw cyst and periapical tissues curetted at the time of dental extraction or apicoectomy) for histopathologic examination is strongly urged.

The treatment of choice for a cyst is local excision with complete removal of the cyst lining.[127] With larger lesions, the surgeon may decide to curet the lining through a relatively small window; removal of the lining can be expected to be incomplete, with recurrence a possibility. Alternatively, the lining of larger cysts may be sutured to the oral mucosa adjacent to the surgically created window, and the cyst may be "marsupialized." If such a lesion is kept patent by repeated irrigation, it will cease to expand, it will not become secondarily infected, and the defect in the jaw will gradually even out.

It is beyond the scope of this chapter to include detailed discussion of the clinical, radiographic, and histologic features of each of the different types of cysts that affect the jaws and adjacent oral tissues. The reader is referred to the more extensive coverage provided in most textbooks of oral pathology and oral radiology,[5,70,128] as well as to articles that review particular classes of cysts.[121–124,129–131]

The radiographic appearance of some odontogenic and non-odontogenic cysts is illustrated in Figures 7-20, 7-21, and 7-22. The 1971 World Health Organization (WHO) classification (also the 1992 revision)[122] of epithelial jaw cysts, which distinguishes cysts arising from the tooth germ tissues (odontogenic cysts) from those of non-odontogenic origin and also distinguishes cysts that represent an inflammatory process from those that arise "autonomously," remains the generally accepted classification. Minor revisions of this classification were pro-

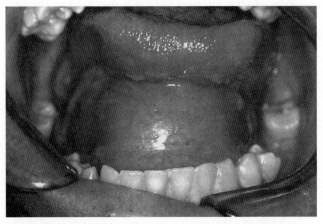

FIGURE 7-19 Dermoid (epidermoid) cyst on the floor of the mouth of a young male adult. The cyst developed as a mass in the floor of the mouth with upward displacement of the tongue (see Figure 7-18, A and B, for extraoral view and histopathology of cyst wall). (Courtesy of R.K. Wesley, University of Detroit, Detroit, Mich.)

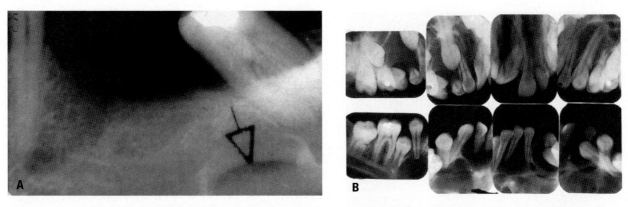

FIGURE 7-20   A, Pseudocyst ("Stafne's bone cyst") caused by developmental inclusion of salivary gland tissue within the body of the mandible. **B,** Multiple jaw cysts in a patient with nevoid basal cell carcinoma syndrome (see "Syndromes with Benign Oral Neoplastic or Hamartomatous Components," in this chapter). (Courtesy of Robert Beideman, Philadelphia, Pa.)

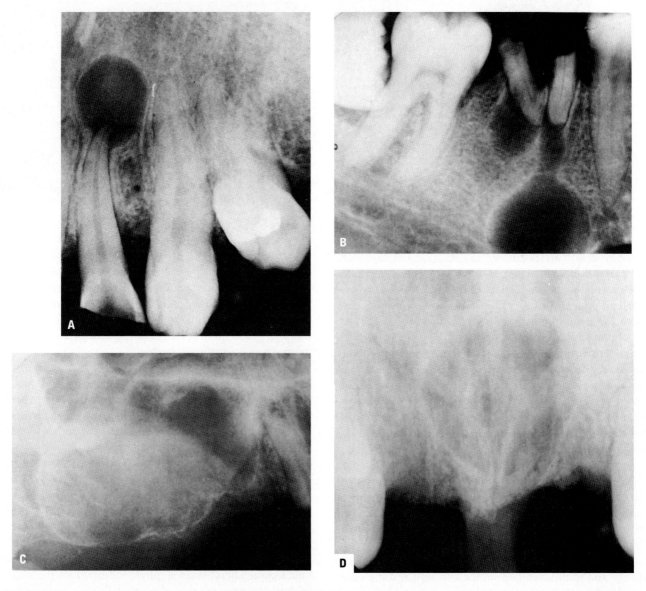

FIGURE 7-21   Radiographic appearance of several jaw cysts. **A** and **B,** Radicular (periapical) cysts, a result of pulp necrosis and infection. **C,** Mucous cyst of the maxillary sinus. **D,** Non-odontogenic fissural cyst in the midline of the anterior maxilla (note intact nasopalatine canal). (Courtesy of Robert Beideman, DMD, Philadelphia, Pa.)

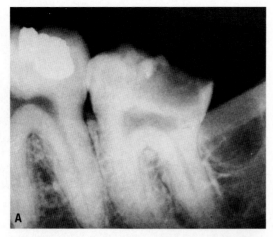

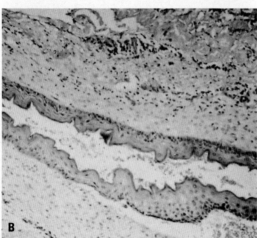

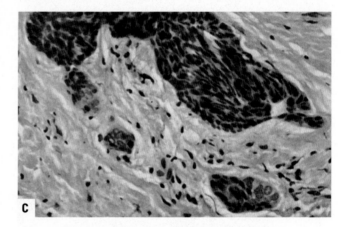

FIGURE 7-22 **A,** Asymptomatic odontogenic keratocyst in the mandibular third molar region, noted as an incidental finding in a periapical radiograph. **B** and **C,** Histologically, the cyst has a well-keratinized epithelial lining, with nests of cells of presumed odontogenic origin located in the surrounding connective tissue.

posed by Main[123] and Shear[120,124] in 1985. Main's revision of the WHO classification is presented in Table 7-1. Four types of cyst (follicular or dentigerous, nasopalatine, radicular, and keratocyst) constitute 95% of all epithelial jaw cysts and are frequently those that attain considerable size before they are recognized.

The follicular (or dentigerous) cyst arises from the reduced enamel epithelium of the dental follicle of an unerupted tooth, which may be part of the regular dentition or a supernumerary, and remains attached to the neck of the tooth, enclosing the crown within the cyst. Some unerupted teeth appear to be more susceptible than others to the development of such cysts (eg, third molars and canines). Studies with tooth germ isografts in the hamster cheek pouch and clinical observations suggest a correlation between cystic degeneration of the tooth follicle and enamel hypoplasia.[132] In addition to their potential for attaining large size, follicular cysts are noteworthy for their tendency to resorb the roots of adjacent teeth,[133] and for the occasional development of neoplastic changes such as plexiform ameloblastoma[134] and carcinoma[131,135] within an isolated segment of the cyst wall. This potential for neoplastic change and infiltration beyond the cyst wall and the occasional finding of other odontogenic tumors in association with a follicular cyst fully justify the need for histopathologic examination of all material derived from jaw cysts.

The eruption cyst is the soft-tissue analogue of the follicular cyst; it presents clinically as a bluish gray swelling of the mucosa over an erupting tooth and has been characterized as a "cyst arising within the oral mucosa by the separation of the follicle from around the anatomical crown of an erupting tooth."[123] Excision of a wedge of the mucosa to expose the tooth crown is usually adequate.

Radicular cysts (see Figure 7-21, A and B) derive from inflammatory proliferation and cystic degeneration of epithelial cell Malassez rests contained in periapical granulomatous tissue, usually secondary to pulp necrosis. When this change occurs in a granuloma that has not been eliminated by tooth extraction, the cyst is no longer associated with the apex of a tooth and is customarily referred to as a residual cyst. Radicular cysts are the most frequent type of jaw cyst and make up as much as 55% of jaw cysts in some series (once again, the difficulties of determining if a given radiolucency is a cyst, a granuloma, or some other lesion influence the validity of the estimates given for different series). There is a large body of literature devoted to elucidating the mechanism and cause of the epithelial proliferation, fluid accumulation, bone resorption, and expansion that underlie the development of radicular cysts.[123]

The odontogenic keratocyst (formerly, primordial cyst)[136,137] (Figures 7-23 and 7-24; see also Figure 7-20, B, and

TABLE 7-1 Proposed Revision of World Health Organization Jaw Cyst Classification

Developmental
    Odontogenic
        Odontogenic keratocyst (formerly, primordial cyst)
        Follicular cyst; eruption cyst
        Alveolar cyst of infants; gingival cyst of adults*
        Developmental lateral periodontal cyst[†]

    Nonodontogenic
        Midpalatal cyst of infants*
        Nasopalatine duct cyst
        Nasolabial cyst[‡]

Inflammatory
    Inflammatory follicular cyst[§]
    Radicular cyst
    Inflammatory lateral periodontal cyst

Adapted from Main DMG;[123] Kramer et al.[122]

* Minor cysts (< 5% of all jaw cysts) that develop from epithelial rests in gingival, alveolar, or midpalatal mucosa.

[†]Lateral follicular cysts that develop between vital maxillary lateral and cuspid teeth. Formerly referred to as globulomaxillary cysts, these are no longer believed to have a fissural origin (see Christ TF. The globulomaxillary cyst: an embryological misconception. Oral Surg Oral Med Oral Pathol 1970;30:515).

[‡]Rare cysts of uncertain origin developing in the nasolabial region.

[§]Arising from the spread of periapical inflammation from a nonvital deciduous tooth to the follicle of an underlying successor (see Shaw W, Smith M, Hill F. Inflammatory follicular cysts. ASDC J Dent Child 1980;47:97).

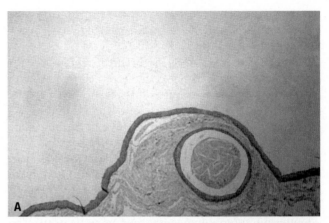
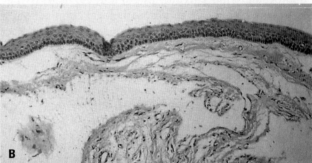

FIGURE 7-24 A and **B,** Histologic examinations of tissue excised from the patient illustrated in Figure 7-23 reveal a characteristic keratinizing squamous epithelial cyst lining and a "daughter" cyst. Differential diagnosis for cysts in this location includes the rare lateral periodontal (follicular) cyst, formerly referred to as globulomaxillary cyst (see Table 7-1). (Courtesy of D. Lovas, DDS, Halifax, N.S., Canada)

Figure 7-22), which arises from reduced enamel epithelium, dental lamina rests, and Malassez rests, are of considerable interest because of their tendency for recurrence after initial surgical intervention.[138] Keratocysts are characterized by keratinization and budding cyst lining. This cyst occurs as an isolated finding and in association with other basal cell cancers and various other lesions in nevoid basal cell carcinoma syndrome (see "Nevoid Basal Cell Carcinoma Syndrome," below).

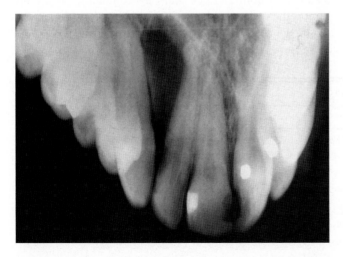

FIGURE 7-23 Radiograph of an odontogenic keratocyst located between the upper lateral incisor and cuspid teeth. (Courtesy of D. Lovas, DDS, Halifax, N.S., Canada)

The nasopalatine (incisive canal) cyst (see Figure 7-21, D) is derived from remnants of epithelium-lined vestigial oronasal duct tissue and possibly also from Jacobson's (vomeronasal) organ, which is said to account for the occasional finding of pigmented cells in the wall of these cysts. On the basis of radiographic surveys of dried skulls, the frequency of this cyst has been described as being as high as 1.8% although differences of opinion as to the maximum size the image of the incisive canal may attain without being considered cystic raise doubt as to the validity of this figure.[124] The surgical removal of a nasopalatine cyst commonly produces loss of sensation and paresthesia of the anterior palate supplied by the nasopalatine nerve; thus, unequivocal signs of cystic swelling in the canal are required before exploration of the area or excision of a suspected cyst is undertaken.

Cysts of the maxillary sinus (see Figure 7-21, C) were thought to arise from pseudostratified columnar respiratory-type epithelium rather than from the oral mucosa, but they are of interest because of the frequency (as high as 2.6% in one series)[139] with which they are recognized in panoramic dental radiographs, which demonstrate them more efficiently than the traditional Waters' projection.[140] In reality, most of these dome-shaped radiopacities of the sinus floor are nothing more than inflammatory polyps and are not true "retention" cysts. Cysts and odontogenic tumors arising in the maxilla, especially molar and premolar radicular cysts, may extend into the maxillary sinus but usually do so by expanding the floor of the sinus ahead of them.[141]

Cystic degeneration may also occur in benign odontogenic tumors, but the hamartomatous or neoplastic nature of odontogenic tumors requires that they be given special consideration (see following section). The misleading so-called cystic radiographic appearance of many odontogenic tumors (reflected in the synonym "multilocular cyst" for ameloblastoma), the majority of which develop within and expand the jaw, has also led to clinical confusion between the two classes of lesions.[124] Cystic degeneration is a common change in odontogenic tissue, and it is not surprising that odontogenic tumors frequently contain cystic areas. The importance of a thorough histopathologic examination of all curetted material is once again underlined by the fact that tumor tissue may be recognized in only a small section of a lesion, the bulk of which is represented by a relatively nonspecific odontogenic cyst.

Benign Odontogenic Tumors

With the exception of odontomas, odontogenic tumors are quite rare, probably constituting fewer than 1% of all jaw cysts and tumors.[75,123,142] Some, such as the ameloblastoma and the calcifying epithelial odontogenic (Pindborg) tumor, are undoubtedly neoplastic; others, such as the compound odontoma and periapical cemental dysplasia, are most likely hamartomas. Malignant variants of several odontogenic tumors also attest to the neoplastic nature of at least some odontogenic growths.[143] Although there have been many attempts at classifying odontogenic tumors, uncertainty concerning the cells of origin of many of these lesions, the bewildering array of histologic types of odontogenic tumors that result from inductive changes in the mesodermal component of these lesions, and their relative rarity all cause difficulty in the histopathologic diagnosis of some of these lesions.

For the majority of these lesions, the descriptions and illustrations included in the 1971 WHO classification of neoplasms and other tumors related to the odontogenic apparatus[121] remain unchanged although the categories of squamous odontogenic tumor and clear cell odontogenic carcinoma are generally included in more recent classifications. Subclassifications of epithelial, mesenchymal, and mixed epithelial and mesenchymal origin (Table 7-2) and subclassification of noninductive versus inductive[144] have also become common practice.

Of most significance to the clinician is the basis for the typing and classification of odontogenic tumors because the various designations are cause for bewilderment. These tumors are classified according to their emulation of the process of odontogenesis, their differentiation, and the tissues from which they are derived. Recall that the epithelial portion of the tooth germ arises as an invagination of the primative oral ectoderm into a linear strand of cells, the dental lamina. The tip of the lamina undergoes bulbous expansion to form the cap and bell stages of odontogenesis, with differentiation into the ameloblastic layer and the inner zone of stellate reticulum. During the differentiation of the odontogenic epithelium, the underlying connective tissues condense with cells recruited from the neural crest. This ectomesoderm transforms into the pulp, and those cells that lie in juxtaposition to the epithelium differentiate into odontoblasts. Once the crown morphology is outlined, dentinogenesis proceeds initially and is a requisite for subsequent amelogenesis. The cervical epithelial tissues then invaginate once again to outline the morphology of the roots as Hertwig's sheath. Surrounding periodontal connective tissues then form bone on the alveolus side of the process and form cementum on the tooth side.

These developmental stages are emulated in various odontogenic tumors. Those that derive strictly from epithelium do not show dentin formation since no ectomesoderm is a component of the neoplasm. Indeed, no enamel formation can be seen because dentin (the prerequisite for amelogenesis) is lacking. Conversely, the mixed odontogenic tumors.

CALCIFYING EPITHELIAL ODONTOGENIC CYST

Calcifying epithelial odontogenic cyst (CEOC) or Gorlin's cyst, occurs both as a cyst and (less commonly) as a solid tumor, the common characteristics being derivation from odontogenic epithelium, calcification, and so-called ghost

---

TABLE 7-2 Histopathologic Classification of Odontogenic Tumors

Ectodermal Origin	Mesodermal Origin	Mixed Ectodermal and Mesodermal Origin
Ameloblastoma	Odontogenic myxoma	Ameloblastic fibroma
Adenomatoid odontogenic tumor*	Central odontogenic fibroma	Ameloblastic fibro-odontoma
	Cementomas	Odontomas
	Periapical cemental dysplasia	Complex
Calcifying epithelial odontogenic tumor (Pindborg tumor)	Familial multiple gigantiform cementoma	Compound
Squamous odontogenic tumor	Cementifying fibroma	
Clear cell odontogenic tumor	Cementoblastoma	
Calcifying odontogenic cyst (Gorlin's cyst)†		

*Formerly called adenoameloblastoma.

†May occur as either a cyst or tumor.

cell keratinization (recently identified as coagulative necrosis of proliferated odontogenic epithelium)[145] (Figure 7-25). Both central and peripherally located lesions are described.[146] Calcifying odontogenic cysts or areas exhibiting these characteristic histologic changes are sometimes found in association with ameloblastomas or other odontogenic tumors, partially accounting for the variety of names under which this lesion has been described in the literature (Figure 7-26, F). Benign and malignant varieties are described, and the lesion mostly occurs in adolescents, appearing as a uni- or multilocular radiopacity enclosing calcified structures of variable size ("pepper-and-salt" appearance). Enucleation usually eliminates the lesion unless it is a component of another odontogenic tumor with a tendency to recur.

AMELOBLASTOMA

Without doubt, the best-known odontogenic tumor, the ameloblastoma, is often used as the norm by which other odontogenic tumors are judged.* Most tumor registries also list it as the most prevalent odontogenic tumor; but because these data are based on biopsy specimens of lesions and because well-differentiated and calcified lesions such as compound odontomas are often never removed, the data may not reflect the true frequency. However, the prevalence of ameloblastomas ensures that all pathologists have encountered them, and there is agreement among surgeons that ameloblastomas should be treated by block excision because of their tendency for local invasion. Thus, to describe a given odontogenic tumor as "more aggressive" or "less aggressive" than an ameloblastoma can be a useful means of communication in this rather uncertain field.[147–150]

In defining the ameloblastoma as the norm for odontogenic tumors, care must be given to the range of lesions accepted as ameloblastoma since several lesions of a quite different nature have been included under this diagnosis in past years. In particular, it is important that the melanotic neuroectodermal tumor of infancy (sometimes referred to as a melanotic ameloblastoma [see previous discussion]), the adenomatoid odontogenic tumor (formerly called adenoameloblastoma), and ameloblastic odontoma (odontoameloblastoma) are excluded from the category of ameloblastoma. Used in this restricted sense, ameloblastoma is a slow-growing benign neoplasm that has a strong tendency to local invasion and that can grow to be quite large without metastasizing (Figure 7-27). Rare examples of distant metastasis of an ameloblastoma in lungs or regional lymph nodes do exist.[143,151–153]

Ameloblastomas are rare in children; the greatest period of prevalence is in the age range of 20 to 50 years. The majority occur in the mandible, and over two-thirds occur in the molar-ramus area. Curettage of the unilocular or multilocular lesions (both radiographic appearances are characteristic) is often followed by local recurrence, and block excision of the lesion with a good margin of unaffected bone (or hemisection of the mandible, for a large lesion) is the treatment of choice and is rarely followed by recurrence.

Microscopically, all ameloblastomas show a fibrous stroma, with islands or masses of proliferating epithelium that always resembles the odontogenic epithelium of the enamel organ to some degree (ie, palisading of cells around proliferating nests of odontogenic epithelium in a pattern similar to ameloblasts). Follicular, plexiform, and acanthomatous histologic variants in which the appearances of basal cells, stellate reticulum (with varying degrees of cystic degeneration), and squamous metaplasia are reproduced

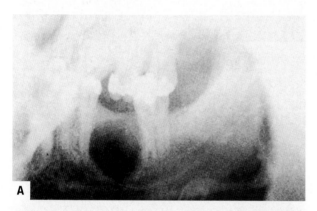

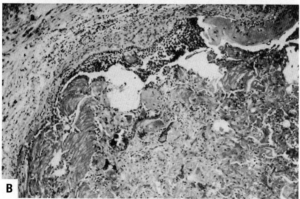

FIGURE 7-25 A, Asymptomatic lesion of the mandible of a 55-year-old male was discovered on routine radiographic examination. **B,** Histologic examination revealed a cystic lesion lined by a double-layered epithelium and containing larger eosinophilic masses of keratin and a calcified product resembling osteoid or dentinoid. The lesion was diagnosed as a cyst of odontogenic origin of the keratinizing and calcifying type (Gorlin's cyst). (Reproduced with permission from Gorlin RJ, Pindborg JJ, Clausen FJ, Vickers RA. The calcifying odontogenic cyst—a possible analogue of the cutaneous calcifying epithelioma of Malherbe. Oral Surg Oral Med Oral Pathol 1962;15:1235) (Courtesy of Charles E, Tomich, DDS, MD, Indianapolis, Ind.)

---

* Discussion of ameloblastoma under the heading of "Benign Odontogenic Tumors" may be questioned because the capacity for local invasion that this tumor can show certainly belies a "benign" character. Distant metastasis,[143] however, is quite rare, and the local invasion shown by this tumor probably differs biologically from that shown by squamous cell carcinoma, for example. Provided that the student fully recognizes the locally destructive tendency of this tumor and the need for block excision in its treatment, it is conveniently discussed at this point, because it provides a useful comparison with other rarer odontogenic tumors.

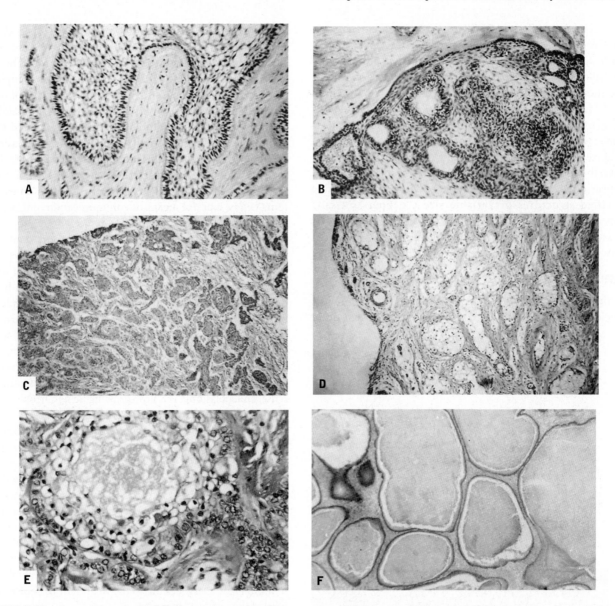

FIGURE 7-26   Some of the varied histologic appearances of ameloblastoma (hematoxylin and eosin sections). **A,** Follicular pattern. **B,** Cystic degeneration in an area of embryonal odontogenic epithelium. **C,** An area resembling basal cell carcinoma derived from odontogenic epithelium. **D,** Cystic degeneration of odontogenic follicles, giving an effect reminiscent of sebaceous cells (sebaceous cell variant). **E,** Detail of cystic degeneration of a follicle. **F,** Keratin-containing cysts lined by odontogenic epithelium, sometimes referred to as a keratoameloblastoma but more accurately as a keratinizing and calcifying odontogenic cyst (Gorlin's cyst; see also Figure 7-25).

have been described. These histologic variants show no correlation with either the clinical appearance of the lesion or its behavior, and different sections of the same tumor may show one or the other histologic variation (see Figure 7-26, A to E). There are only two significant subcategories of ameloblastoma; those that arise from the lining of an odontogenic cyst are called unicystic ameloblastomas, and those that are solid tumors are called solid or invasive ameloblastomas. The former tend to occur during teenage years; the latter tend to occur in midlife. The primary reason for distinguishing between these two variations of ameloblastoma is the difference in natural history and behavior. Fewer than 20% of unicystic ameloblastomas recur after curettage whereas over

75% of solid ameloblastomas will recur unless treated by resection. Attempts have been made to marsupialize unicystic tumors, yet this treatment eventuates in failure, with persistant and even progressive disease.

The distinction between an area of proliferating odontogenic epithelium in the wall of a dentigerous cyst and early ameloblastoma may be difficult to make (Figure 7-28), and studies of lectins and other cell markers on the proliferating epithelial cells have so far failed to identify those lesions that are most likely to develop into an ameloblastoma.[154] There is no clear origin for the ameloblastoma; the dentigerous cyst is only one possibility, but remnants of the dental lamina and the basal layer of the oral mucosal epithelium also are strong contenders.

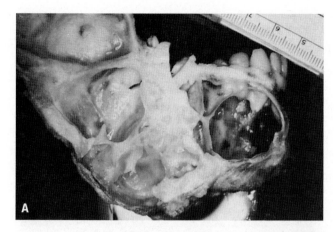

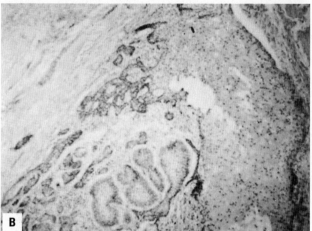

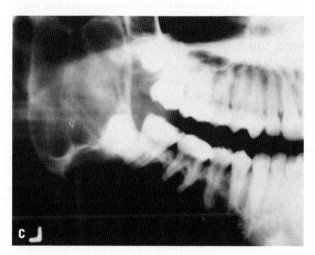

FIGURE 7-27 A, Gross appearance of a very large multilocular ameloblastoma that occupied and distended the entire mandible. **B,** Histologic appearance of the same lesion. **C,** Radiograph of an ameloblastoma of similar dimension.

However, there does seem to be good reason for repeated curettage or excision of the bony wall of a cyst in which such a change has been noted, especially in young patients.

There is no justification for the use of radiation therapy in the treatment of ameloblastomas; its use in past years has been associated with a considerable occurrence of radiation-induced sarcoma.[155]

ADENOMATOID ODONTOGENIC TUMOR

Adenomatoid odontogenic tumor (AOT) is a tumor of odontogenic epithelium with ductlike structures and with varying degrees of inductive change in the stroma.[156] It differs considerably from the ameloblastic norm and is usually now excluded from that category. By contrast with ameloblastoma, it reflects all of the characteristics of a hamartoma as a well-encapsulated lesion that rarely recurs even with conservative

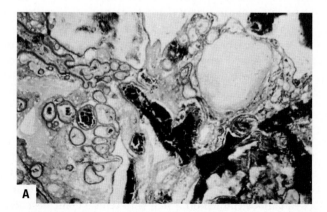

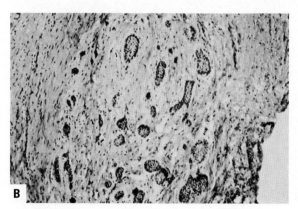

FIGURE 7-28 Proliferating islands of odontogenic epithelium are frequently seen in dental granulomas, as seen in **A,** and in cyst walls. The theory that these remnants of the dental lamina are one source of ameloblastomas is supported by the occasional finding of an ameloblastoma developing in the wall of a dentigerous cyst, as seen in **B.**

curettage. Recognition of its characteristic histology should prevent the need for block excision of the lesion. Clinically, it may be suspected because of its preference for the maxilla rather than the mandible and for anterior rather than posterior segments of the jaws. Often it presents as a cystic lesion that is not associated with a missing tooth and that is found (by biopsy specimen examination) to have several masses of tumor tissue in its wall. These mural nodules are composed of characteristic masses of ductlike structures lined with basal or columnar cells with peripherally placed nuclei. The "lumen" of some of these "ducts" is nonexistent, and that of others is dilated with an eosinophilic or fibrillar material, giving some suggestion of poorly formed stellate reticulum. Amorphous calcification may be apparent both microscopically and radiographically (Figure 7-29).

PINDBORG TUMOR (CALCIFYING EPITHELIAL ODONTOGENIC TUMOR)

The Pindborg tumor (Figure 7-30) resembles an ameloblastoma in that it is locally invasive and is commonly identified as a uni- or multilocular swelling in the molar-ramus region.[157,158] Histologically, it differs from ameloblastoma in being composed of masses of polyhedral epithelial cells with little stroma. The cells may be eosinophilic, exhibit intercellular bridges, and be quite pleomorphic, with multiple giant nuclei. In many ways, it appears microscopically like a potentially aggressive squamous cell carcinoma, with a predominance of cells resembling those of the stratum spinosum of oral epithelium, and many cases have undoubtedly been wrongly diagnosed as squamous cell carcinoma. The central location of the tumor in the jaw, often with expansion of the cortex (in contrast to the destructive lesion of carcinoma), and the areas of spotty calcification seen radiographically should alert the clinician to the possibility of a Pindborg tumor, but peripheral lesions are also occasionally reported.[159] Sections of such a tumor should be examined for the characteristic hyaline concentrically calcified globules of amyloid

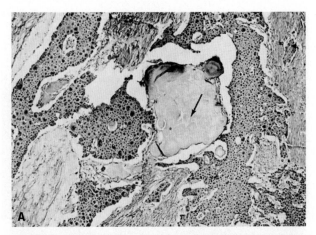

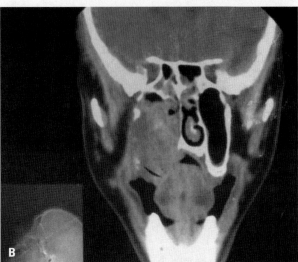

FIGURE 7-30 Calcifying epithelial odontogenic tumor (CEOT), or Pindborg tumor. **A,** Histology illustrates masses of polyhedral cells and calcified globules of amyloid (*arrow*). (Hematoxylin and eosin, × 65 original magnification) (Courtesy of J. E. Hamner III, DDS, PhD, Washington, D.C.) **B,** Magnetic resonance image of an unusual neoplastic CEOT arising in the maxilla and invading the maxillary sinus. (Courtesy of J. Fantasia, DDS, New Hyde Park, N.Y.)

within the masses of epithelioid cells that confirm the lesion as odontogenic in origin. Larger areas of calcification and dentin formation may also be found.

Treatment is by enucleation or local block excision; the recurrence rate is reported to be 20%. Exploration of regional nodes and follow-up radiation therapy (as might be used for squamous cell carcinoma) are quite unjustified for this odontogenic lesion.

OTHER EPITHELIAL ODONTOGENIC TUMORS

Two other relatively rare epithelial odontogenic tumors that have been recognized as separate entities in recent years are the squamous and clear cell odontogenic tumors. The squamous odontogenic tumor[160] is a lesion composed of multiple islands of squamous epithelium (often with central cystic degeneration) that arises in the alveolar process from proliferation of Malassez rests or gingival pseudoepitheliomatous hyperplasia. It occurs equally frequently in the maxilla or the mandible, and

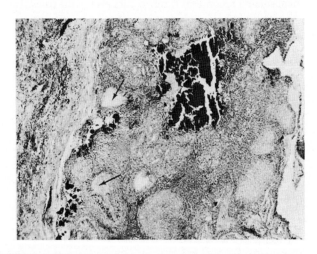

FIGURE 7-29 Adenomatoid odontogenic tumor with ductlike structures (*arrows*). (Hematoxylin and eosin, × 65 original magnification) (Courtesy of J. E. Hamner III, DDS, PhD, Washington, D.C.)

it may recur following enucleation; multiple lesions have been described. The clear cell odontogenic tumor,[161] previously considered a variant of ameloblastoma, is now considered to represent a malignant tumor. Histologic differentiation of this tumor from other oral and metastatic tumors (such as renal cell carcinoma) is important.

ODONTOGENIC TUMORS OF MESENCHYMAL ORIGIN

Odontogenic Myxoma and Central Odontogenic Fibroma.
Myxomas (tumors composed of very loose cellular connective tissue containing little collagen and large amounts of an inter-cellular substance that is rich in acid mucopolysaccharide) occur with some frequency in the jaw bones. Since similar lesions are rare in other bones and since some oral myxomas contain tiny epithelial remnants that resemble inactive odontogenic epithelium, tumors with this histologic appearance that occur in the jaw bone are referred to as odontogenic myxomas.[162] This lesion usually consists of rounded and angular cells lying in an abundant mucoid stroma that is reminiscent of dental pulp, with very scanty epithelial elements. It is a slow-growing but invasive tumor that sometimes reaches quite large dimensions and distends the jaw. Characteristically, it appears radiographically as a uni- or multilocular lesion ("soap bubble" effect) that may be indistinguishable from ameloblastoma, fibrous dysplasia, giant cell reparative granuloma, cherubism, and the jaw lesion of hyperparathyroidism (osteitis fibrosa cystica). Treatment is similar to that recommended for ameloblastoma although tooth root resorption in an area affected by a myxoma and recurrence after simple curettage may give the impression of a more aggressive lesion.

Central odontogenic fibroma[163,164] (a tumor composed of mature fibroblastic tissue with rare nests and strands of odontogenic epithelium) is an uncommon, slow-growing, and nonaggressive lesion. These tumors are generally small, yet they may cause root resorption, and many will underlie a distinct region of dimpling of the oral mucosa.

Cementomas. "Cementoma" is a nonspecific term often used to describe localized masses of radiopaque condensed areas of the alveolus adjacent to the roots of the teeth (see Figure 7-15).[102–104,121,165,166]

Periapical cementomas are often multiple and are distinguished from chronic periapical abscesses by their association with vital teeth.[167] There is good evidence that periapical cementomas are reactive lesions that pass through an osteolytic phase (in which they can be distinguished from periapical cysts and granulomas only by the retention of vitality in the tooth), through a stage in which one or more radiopaque zones appear within the radiolucent area, to a final stage of uniform radiopacity. "Periapical cemental dysplasia" (PACD)[168] is the accepted term for such lesions and emphasizes their benign hamartomatous nature (Figure 7-31). Provided that such lesions do not increase in size or otherwise exhibit atypical behavior, there seems to be no reason to remove them. Should caries or other pulpal disease warrant

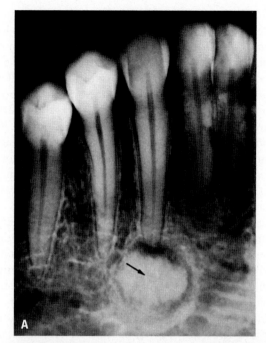

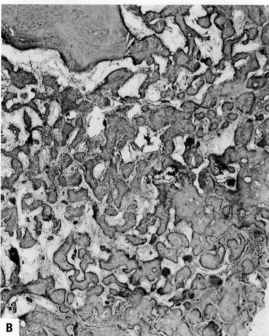

FIGURE 7-31 Periapical cementoma or cemental dysplasia. **A,** Radiographic appearance (*arrow*). **B,** Histologic appearance. (Courtesy of J.E. Hamner III, DDS, PhD, Washington, D.C.)

endodontic treatment of a tooth with associated PACD, apicoectomy with removal of the dense periapical lesion is desirable, if only to prevent complication of the postoperative evaluation of the success of the endodontic therapy.[169]

In addition to PACD, the WHO classification of odontogenic tumors distinguishes three other lesions with prominent and excessive cementum formation: familial multiple gigantiform cementoma,[170] cementifying fibroma,[171] and cementoblastoma.[172]

In regard to familial multiple gigantiform cementoma, females appear to be preferentially susceptible to both localized and widespread cementoma formation, in which both maxilla and mandible may be occupied by large globular and lobulated masses of dense acellular cementum. The differentiation of this condition from chronic sclerosing osteomyelitis, florid osseous dysplasia,[173] and ossifying fibroma is usually unproblematic since these tumors are huge, beginning in childhood years and progressively increasing in size into adult life (Figure 7-32). There is usually (but not invariably) a familial history, with variable penetrance in expressivity. Treatment is wide excision, followed by grafting and facial plastic surgery interventions.

Cementifying fibroma is merely a variant of ossifying fibroma and occurs in the mandible of older individuals. Radiographically, it passes through the stages that were described for periapical cemental dysplasia in younger patients. Histologically, it consists of cellular fibroblastic tissue containing rounded, heavily calcified, and basophilic masses of cementum, as opposed to ossifying fibroma, in which the hard tissue is represented by osseous trabeculae. Nevertheless, there are many tumors of this nature that elaborate both osseous and

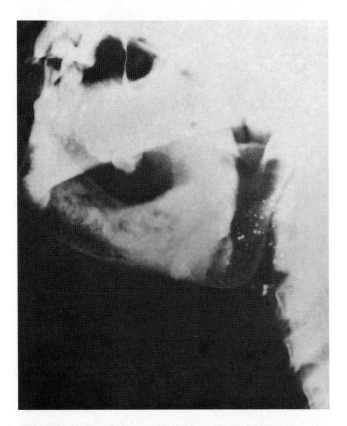

FIGURE 7-32 Radiographic appearance of chronic sclerosing osteomyelitis affecting the major portion of the body of the mandible. Clinical and histologic differentiation of this lesion from ossifying fibroma may be difficult, particularly if teeth have been extracted or surgery has been carried out adjacent to the area. (Reproduced with permission from Nichols C, Brightman VJ. Parotid calcifications and cementoma in a patient with Sjögren's syndrome and idiopathic thrombocytopenia. J Oral Pathol 1977;6:52)

cementicle trabeculae, and similar lesions are found in facial bones that do not bear teeth. Those lesions that are treated enucleate readily, and recurrence is uncommon.

Cementoblastoma (true cementoma) is a radiographically and histologically distinctive benign tumor that usually occurs around the root of a mandibular premolar or molar tooth. It is composed of layers of cemental tissue with prominent accretion lines; the inner layers are acellular, and the formative peripheral layers are uncalcified, allowing ready enucleation. Radiologically, the prominent linear calcifications provide a distinctive and unusual picture that may even suggest an osteosarcoma.

Focal osseous dysplasia and florid osseous dysplasia are benign fibro-osseous lesions that histologically resemble other "cementifying" lesions yet are self-limited non-neoplastic jaw lesions localized to tooth-bearing regions.[174] Radiologically, focal osseous dysplasia appears (usually in the mandible) as a localized small radiolucency with central calcifications. It is nonexpansile, and its etiology is unknown. Many such lesions are located in edentulous sites, and some may represent the residua of condensing osteitis, left behind after tooth extraction. Florid osseous dysplasia is typically seen in middle-aged black women but can occur in individuals of any race. This condition is characterized by multiple confluent "cotton wool" radiopacities with surrounding lucent regions that resemble traumatic bone cysts (vacant cavities in bone). Biopsy of these lesions may result in osteomyelitis, probably owing to the lack of vascularity in the dense bony regions. Both focal and florid osseous dysplasias show similar histologic features. There is a benign fibro-osseous lesion with foci of dense cortical bony structures.

ODONTOGENIC TUMORS OF MIXED EPITHELIAL AND MESENCHYMAL ORIGIN

Ameloblastic Fibroma and Fibro-odontoma. Odontogenic jaw tumors in which varying degrees of both dentin and enamel matrix (with or without calcification) occur are of two types. The ameloblastic fibroma is a child tumor that resembles an ameloblastoma radiologically and histologically (except that the stroma consists of pulp tissue rather than undifferentiated connective tissue) and that behaves less aggressively than an ameloblastoma (Figure 7-33). The other type comprises various odontomas such as ameloblastic fibro-odontoma and complex and compound odontomas.[175–177]

Calcification within an ameloblastoma does not occur unless there is reactive osteogenesis, as may occur in desmoplastic variants (Figure 7-34), and this feature can serve to distinguish ameloblastoma from both adenomatoid odontogenic tumor and ameloblastic fibro-odontoma or odontoameloblastoma. This latter lesion consists of ameloblastic tissue found in association with an abnormal mass of partially calcified dental tissues that histologically may contain enamel, dentin, osteodentin, bone, cementum, and pulp tissue as well as various developing stages of these tissues. This rare tumor should be treated the same way that a solid ameloblastoma is treated (generally by resection). In essense, it is an ameloblastoma arising in an odontoma.

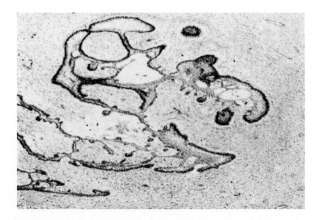

FIGURE 7-33 Ameloblastic fibroma, an odontogenic tumor of mixed epithelial and mesenchymal origin. Histologic examination reveals a pulp-like stroma enclosing a proliferating odontogenic epithelium. (Courtesy of Charles Halstead, DDS, PhD, Atlanta, Ga.)

Complex and Compound Odontomas. Complex and compound odontomas[177–179] are nonaggressive lesions that are more likely to be hamartomatous than neoplastic. They are often small and may remain undiscovered for many years until they are revealed by routine panoramic radiography or by a search for a missing permanent tooth. Their radiographic appearance is often characteristic, and if their presence does not interfere with orderly tooth eruption, they may safely be left undisturbed. Dentigerous cysts may form in association with these lesions, and this possibility may justify their removal and certainly justifies repeated radiographic examination for new cyst development every 2 to 3 years.

The term "complex odontoma" is used for lesions that contain mature calcified dental tissue that is poorly differentiated as to its exact identity as enamel, dentin, or cementum. Such lesions characteristically appear as dense radiopaque objects sometimes lying in a clear space or associated with a "cyst," but more often enclosed by a well-defined "lamina dura."

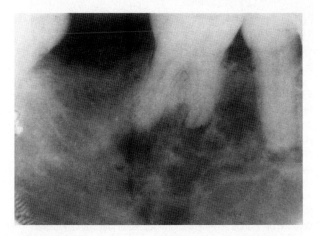

FIGURE 7-34 The "honeycomb" appearance of this ameloblastoma should not be confused with the partially calcified dental tissue found in association with ameloblastic tissue in some mixed odontogenic tumors. (Courtesy of Robert Beideman, Philadelphia, Pa.)

Compound odontomas contain calcified structures that grossly and radiographically resemble poorly formed and often small teeth in which enamel, dentin, and cementum can be distinguished. Remembering the common meanings of "complex" (complicated, hard to separate or analyze) and "compound" (a joining together of parts so as to form a whole) may help the student to distinguish these two types of odontoma, which are quite aptly described by these terms.

▼ BENIGN "VIRUS-INDUCED" TUMORS (ORAL SQUAMOUS PAPILLOMAS AND WARTS)

For many years, several benign oral epithelial growths that contain virus particles or viral antigens (warts, squamous papillomas and condyloma acuminata, focal epithelial hyperplasia, molluscum contagiosum, and keratoacanthoma) have been considered to be virus-induced neoplasms; leukoplakia, lichen planus, hairy leukoplakia, and squamous carcinoma have also been placed in this category by some authors.[180–183] More recently, molecular biologic techniques (eg, deoxyribonucleic acid [DNA] hybridization, restriction endonuclease analysis, the polymerase chain reaction,[184] which have proven to be more sensitive probes than electron microscopy or immunologic staining techniques that detect only virus or viral antigen) have revealed that viral DNA can be found in a number of oral mucosal lesions and that even normal oral mucosa may also harbor a limited number of viral strains, notably one that is related to human papillomavirus (HPV) subtype 16.[185] Although an extensive literature has documented the association of many of the 80 known strains of papillomavirus, herpes simplex virus, and Epstein-Barr virus with these lesions, the role of many of these viral strains remains unproven, and additional evidence is needed before particular viruses can be considered as etiologic agents.[180,183] For example, normal oral mucosa from as many as 40% of individuals, as well as 80% of leukoplakias and lichenoid lesions, contains the strain related to the HPV subtype 16. This HPV subtype is usually found only in genital carcinomas, and its presence in normal mucosa and in leukoplakia and lichenoid lesions suggests that some HPV subtypes at least may replicate in these tissues and are not necessarily causal. In contrast, HPV subtypes 1, 2, 4, 6, 11, 13, and 18, which are associated with various oral lesions, have not been detected in normal oral mucosa. Herpes simplex and Epstein-Barr viruses likewise have been detected in normal oral mucosa as well as in mucosal lesions.[186]

Although malignant transformation in these virus-associated lesions is quite unusual, the viral genomic material in oral mucosal cells can replicate, produce intact virus, and transform the host cell. The frequent development of unusual oral malignancies and of oral mucosal lesions that are associated with herpes simplex virus, Epstein-Barr virus, *Cytomegalovirus*, and papillomavirus in acquired immunodeficiency syndrome (AIDS) patients and in intentionally immunosuppressed patients also demonstrates that these oral viruses probably have clinical significance and that immunosuppressive medications (such as cyclosporine, corticosteroids, and azathioprine) should be administered with considerable caution, particularly if they must be used for extended periods of time.

Oral squamous papillomas and warts are proliferative epithelial lesions generally considered to be caused by HPV, with subtypes 6 and 11 being commonly implicated. Isolated reports of an association with subtypes 2 and 16 have not been confirmed.[181,182] Oral papillomas and warts (verrucae vulgaris) share many similarities. The term "verruca vulgaris" is usually applied when a crop of lesions develops, sometimes in association with similar skin lesions. Squamous papillomas usually occur in the third to the fifth decades, most commonly as isolated palatal lesions. When these lesions occur on the keratinized surface of the lips, alveolar gingivae, or palate, they are well keratinized and wartlike, often with a definite narrow pedicle (Figures 7-35 and 7-36). On the nonkeratinized mucosal surface, they may appear soft and redder and may be hard to differentiate from the lesions of fibrous hyperplasia described earlier. A rugose cauliflower-like exophytic lesion is more likely to be a papilloma than to be fibrous hyperplasia. Local excision of these lesions is desirable; electrocoagulation is the treatment of choice on the lips, where the lesions cause a cosmetic problem. Carbon dioxide laser treatment has also been described.[187]

Although these lesions are probably infectious, a history of direct contact with another infected person is unusual, except in the case of a multiple and often recurrent oral wart associated with sexual contact, referred to as condyloma acuminatum (see Chapter 22). HPV DNA sequences have also been described in condyloma acuminatum.[188]

Intraoral papillomatosis may be inherited in such rare conditions as ichthyosis hystrix, but other manifestations of this syndrome (a congenitally acquired deforming skin papillomatosis) serve to differentiate these lesions from other congenital conditions, such as Down syndrome, in which florid papillomatosis may also occur. The role of genetic predisposition in promoting HPV expression in these conditions has not yet been explored.

Focal epithelial hyperplasia[189] (Heck's disease), a condition characterized by numerous soft, well-circumscribed, flat, and sessile (ie, nonpapillomatous) papules that are distributed throughout the oral mucosa, is endemic in some Eskimo and Native American communities but is rare in white people. Examples among Puerto Ricans and (more recently) among black people suggest that further searches for this lesion may show it to be more widespread. Histologically, it is characterized by nondyskeratotic nodular acanthosis, which forms the basis of the papules, and a subepithelial lymphocytic infiltration. These lesions have been considered to be of viral origin for many years, initially on the basis of electron microscopic demonstration of *Papovavirus* particles[190] and (more recently) on the finding of DNA sequences for HPV subtypes 13 and 32,

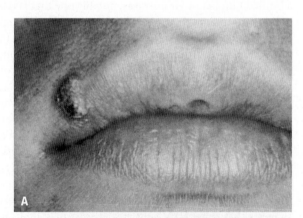

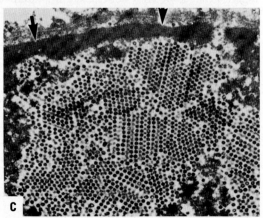

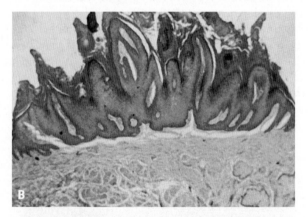

FIGURE 7-35 **A,** Viral warts (verruca vulgaris) on the keratinized skin surface of the upper lip of a 16-year-old male; the lesions were removed by electrocautery. **B,** Histologic section of one of the warts, showing exophytic epithelial hyperplasia and keratin-capped papillae. (Hematoxylin and eosin) **C,** Portion of a superficial cell nucleus from an intraoral lesion diagnosed histopathologically as verruca vulgaris. Note the numerous paracrystalline viral particles within the nucleus. The nuclear membrane is indicated by arrows. (×16,000 original magnification) (Reproduced with permission from Wysocki GC, Hardie J. Ultrastructural studies of intraoral verruca vulgaris. Oral Surg Oral Med Oral Pathol 1977;47:58)

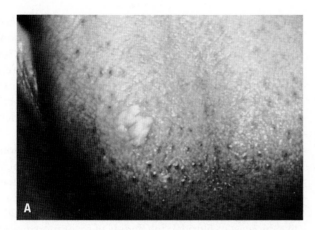 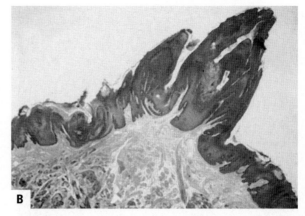

FIGURE 7-36 **A,** Inverted papilloma. A solitary exophytic and heavily keratinized wart on the dorsum of the tongue of a 22-year-old female. Before infiltration of anesthetic, the wart was inverted below the surface of tongue. **B,** Histologic appearance of the same papilloma.

which appear to be specific for this lesion and which are expressed only in those individuals who are genetically predisposed.[182,191] Once identified, the lesions require no treatment; malignant transformation does not occur.

Molluscum contagiosum,[192,193] a dermatologic infection acquired by direct skin contact and characterized by clusters of tiny firm nodules that can be curetted from the skin, is histologically composed of clumps of proliferating epithelial cells with prominent eosinophilic inclusion bodies. It is not a neoplasm, but it is included here as one of the spectra of oral epithelial proliferations that result from viral infection. Both intraoral and labial lesions of molluscum contagiosum have been reported.

Molluscum contagiosum is caused by a poxvirus that infects the skin, where the virus replicates in the stratum spinosum, producing the characteristic and pathognomonic Cowdry type A inclusion bodies that are commonly associated with poxvirus infections but apparently producing only a small number of complete viruses.[194] Cytotoxic T cells and delayed-type hypersensitivity are most likely the effective means of recovery from this infection, which explains the increased frequency and persistence of this infection in AIDS patients. Treatment usually involves the shelling out of the epithelial nodules with a curet.

Keratoacanthoma[195,196] is a localized lesion (usually found on sun-exposed skin, including the upper lip) whose rapid growth may be quite frightening, to the point where it is often mistakenly diagnosed as squamous or basal cell carcinoma (Figure 7-37). Like some carcinomas, these lesions appear fixed to the surrounding tissue, often grow rapidly, and are usually capped by thick keratin. Occasionally, the lesion matures, exfoliates, and heals spontaneously, but more frequently, block excision is carried out, and the diagnosis becomes apparent when the entire lesion is examined microscopically. Incisional biopsy specimens are almost always diagnosed as carcinoma since they lack the panoramic view of the entire lesion, which is of greatest help in differentiating it from carcinoma.

Epithelial tissue adjacent to the lesion is sharply demarcated from that of the lesion, which appears to lie in a cup-shaped depression. The proliferating epithelium constituting this amazing lesion consists of masses of reasonably well-differentiated squamous cells that often produce keratin pearls and show little cellular atypia. Viruslike inclusions have also been demonstrated in some specimens. Clumps of cells that appear to be separated along the base of the lesion and the accompanying chronic inflammatory exudate in this region presumably are the cause for the mistaken diagnosis of carcinoma, a diagnosis that seems, at the time, to be confirmed by the aggressive growth of the lesion. This fact and the lesion's usual location on the upper lip (where squamous cell carcinoma of actinic etiology is rare, compared with the lower lip) should remind the clinician to consider keratoacanthoma in the differential diagnosis. Intraoral lesions are rare.[197] Treatment of this lesion remains controversial; authors who believe that it is not clearly separable from squamous cell carcinoma advocate wide excision to prevent recurrence.[198]

▼ SYNDROMES WITH BENIGN ORAL NEOPLASTIC OR HAMARTOMATOUS COMPONENTS

The emphasis in this chapter has been on the accurate diagnosis of benign oral tumors by means of histopathologic examination, so that they may be clearly separated from malignant lesions and treated accordingly. The oral cavity and face can also provide evidence of malignancy elsewhere in the body, and clinicians need to be aware of a variety of oral signs that can serve as an index of internal malignancy, in much the same way that dermatologic conditions such as recurrent herpes zoster and erythema multiforme may occasionally signal the presence of an otherwise undetected lymphoma or carcinoma.

Of particular pertinence to this chapter are a group of conditions in which benign oral growths, which of themselves have no precancerous potential, are associated with a predisposition to a malignancy in another organ system. Such con-

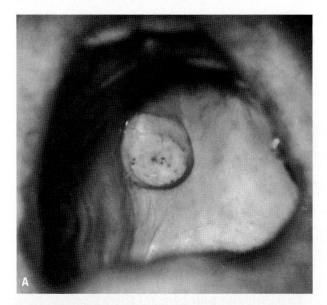

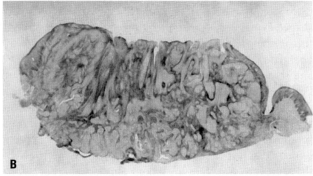

FIGURE 7-37 Keratoacanthoma on the hard palate of a 28-year-old white male cigarette smoker. **A,** The lesion is well circumscribed, abruptly elevated above the mucosal surface, and presents a roughened whitish surface. **B,** At low-power magnification, the histologic section shows the sharply circumscribed margin and the thinned surface epithelium that tends to "lip" the central cell mass. Epithelium at the margins of the lesion was well differentiated, with minimal pleomorphism and hyperchromatism. (Reproduced with permission from Scofield HH, Weining JT, Shukes RC. Solitary intraoral keratocanthoma. Oral Surg Oral Med Oral Pathol 1974;37:889.)

ditions, which are usually familial (often with autosomal dominant inheritance), are uncommon, but the very frequent association of a particular oral lesion in such families with the internal malignancy makes the recognition of these oral lesions very important.

Several authors have reviewed cancer syndromes that are associated with characteristic skin lesions.[199–202] Table 7-3 summarizes those syndromes that are associated with benign oral tumors. A brief discussion of these syndromes follows.

Von Recklinghausen's Neurofibromatosis

Two distinct varieties of this classic syndrome[69,203–205] ("elephant man" syndrome[206]) are now recognized: neurofibromatosis 1, which affects approximately 100,000 people in the United States and which is often associated with oral lesions;

and neurofibromatosis 2 (bilateral acoustic neurofibromatosis), which (1) is caused by a gene on a different chromosome, (2) is much less common, and (3) is less frequently associated with obvious peripheral neurofibromatosis or oral lesions even though it is often accompanied by other central nervous system tumors. Unidentified hormones or nerve growth factors are thought to contribute to tumor formation in both varieties of this syndrome.

Neurofibromatosis 1 is inherited as an autosomal dominant condition, but only half of the cases exhibit a familial history. The syndrome is characterized by the simultaneous occurrence, usually on the trunk, axilla, and pelvic area, of café au lait spots (light brown macules with a smooth outline "like the coast of Florida"; the finding of six or more macules ≥ 1.5 cm in diameter is diagnostic of neurofibromatosis),[†] axillary freckling (Crowe's sign), and a wide variety of nerve and nerve sheath tumors in both the central and peripheral nervous systems. The peripheral lesions are often indistinguishable from those described earlier in this chapter (see "Nerve Sheath Tumors and Traumatic Neuroma," above). The central lesions, because of their location within a bony cavity, often in association with various nerve roots, lead to neurologic symptoms, mental retardation, and vertebral anomalies. Large infiltrating lesions that occur both peripherally and centrally and that lead to severe deformity[206] are referred to as plexiform neuromas (Figure 7-38).

Malignant transformation of one or more neurofibromas occurs in about 5% of patients with this syndrome. Pheochromocytomas (tumors of the adrenal medulla and paraganglia) also may occur and produce hypertension by the secretion of excess catecholamines. Approximately 5% of patients with neurofibromatosis have well-developed oral lesions[207] and macroglossia (the tongue being the most common oral location for neurofibroma, both in this syndrome and in cases of solitary oral neurofibroma) (see Figure 7-13). This condition and the associated oral lesions are said to be more prevalent in patients in mental institutions. The lesions may be asymptomatic; about one-third are recognized on routine physical examination. The neurofibromatosis gene (NF1) has been cloned and is mutated in neurofibromatosis.

Gardner's Syndrome

Although rare, Gardner's syndrome is of importance because of the high frequency with which carcinomatous transformation occurs in the adenomatous intestinal (colonic and rectal) polyps that are characteristic of this condition.[208,209] Recognition of the multiple osteomas of the face and jaws and the accompanying skin cysts and tumors as phenotypic indicators of Gardner's syndrome fully justifies radiographic examination of the bowel and the resection of the polypoid tissue, even in young adults (Figure 7-39). Approximately 15

[†] Café au lait spots are also found in 10% of the normal population, especially in fair-skinned persons. Similar skin lesions with the same name occur in Albright's syndrome.

TABLE 7–3   Syndromes in which Benign Tumors and Other Mucosal Lesions of the Oral Cavity Are Associated with a Predisposition to Internal Malignancy

Syndrome	Oral Lesions	Other Skin Lesions	Associated Abnormalities	Associated Malignancies
Von Recklinghausen's neurofibromatosis	Intraoral neurofibromas (especially of tongue) leading to macroglossia Intrabony neurofibromas of jaws (rarely)	Multiple neurofibromas (especially trunk and extremities) Café au lait spots (especially trunk, axilla, pelvic area) Axillary freckles Giant nevi	CNS tumors (acoustic neuroma, meningioma, glioma, and plexiform neuroma) Bone cysts and hyperplasia associated with neuromas Mental retardation	Malignant neurilemmoma (5% of cases) Pheochromocytoma Astrocytoma and glioma
Gardner's syndrome	Multiple osteomas of cranial and facial skeleton (especially frontal bone, mandible, and maxilla) Compound odontomas and hypercementosis	Epidermoid and sebaceous cysts Desmoid tumors, lipomas, fibromas, and leiomyomas	Polyps of the colon and rectum	Adenocarcinoma of colon (very high incidence)
Peutz-Jeghers syndrome	Freckling and pigmentation of lips and oral mucosa	Similar lesions on fingers and toes	Intestinal polyposis (usually small intestine)	Gastric, duodenal, and colonic adenocarcinoma (low incidence)
Nevoid basal cell carcinoma syndrome	Multiple jaw cysts (simple and odontogenic keratocysts) Dilaceration of teeth adjacent to cysts Facial abnormalities (frontal bossing, sunken eyes, and wide nasal bridge; mild mandibular prognathism)	Epidermoid cysts Milia and calcium deposits	Rib and vertebral anomalies Short metacarpals Ovarian fibromas Calcification of ovarian fibromas and dura	Basal cell carcinoma of skin (often without sunlight exposure) Medulloblastoma Ameloblastoma and fibrosarcoma of jaws (low incidence)
Multiple mucosal neuroma syndrome (multiple endocrine neoplasia type III)	Neuromas of lips, tongue and buccal mucosa (oral cavity is most common site) Thick or "bumpy" lips Prognathism (infrequent)	Neuromas of eyelids and nasal laryngeal mucosa Abnormal triple response to intradermal histamine injections (no flare)	Parathyroid adenomas Hypertension	Medullary carcinoma of thyroid Pheochromocytoma
Tuberous sclerosis	Adenoma sebaceum Gingival lesions and enamel hypoplasia Cranial defects	Adenoma sebaceum	Epilepsy Mental retardation Hamartomas of brain, heart, and kidney	Astrocytoma and glioblastoma
Acanthosis nigricans	Perioral and oral mucosal papillomatosis with areas of black pigmentation	Similar lesions on neck, axilla, and groin	Absence of endocrine abnormalities, obesity, and family history	Gastric adenocarcinoma
Albright's syndrome	Solitary or multiple foci of fibrous dysplasia of jaw bones Oral pigmentation (rarely)	Café au lait spots	Polyostotic fibrous dysplasia and bony deformities (1% of cases) Precocious sexual development	Fibrosarcoma and osteogenic sarcoma developing in areas of fibrous dysplasia
Paget's disease of bone* (osteitis deformans)	Localized or generalized bony jaw growths Hypercementosis	—	Large head, curved back, and bowed legs deformity Raised serum alkaline phosphatase, usually with normal calcium and phosphorus levels	Osteogenic sarcoma, chondrosarcoma, fibrosarcoma, and giant cell tumor of bone developing in affected areas
Cowden's syndrome (multiple hamartoma and neoplasia syndrome)	Papillomatosis of lips, gingivae, palate, pharynx, and fauces Pebbly fissured tongue	Lichenoid and papillomatous lesions of perioral, perinasal, and periorbital areas, ear, and neck	Hamartomas of skin, gastrointestinal tract, breasts, and thyroid	A variety of neoplasms affecting principally the ovaries, colon, ear canal, and various soft and hard tissues

Continued

TABLE 7-3   Syndromes in which Benign Tumors and Other Mucosal Lesions of the Oral Cavity Are Associated with a Predisposition to Internal Malignancy (continued)

Syndrome	Oral Lesions	Other Skin Lesions	Associated Abnormalities	Associated Malignancies
Xanthomatosis	Pale yellow nodular subcutaneous deposits, especially on lips and cheeks	Similar deposits on skin, eyelids, and tendons	Abnormal and elevated serum triglycerides and cholesterol fractions, arteriosclerosis, hypertension, diabetes, and heart disease	Multiple myeloma
Langerhans cell (eosinophilic) granulomatosis*	Radiolucent jaw bone lesions, gingival swelling, "floating teeth"	Infiltrates on other mucous membrane and skin surfaces	Generalized lymphadenopathy, hepatomegaly, and splenomegaly; focal lesions in lung, thymus, and other organs	Malignant lymphomatous disease
Amyloidosis* (AL type)	Macroglossia, microscopic and gross waxy deposits in lips and submucosal tissues	Waxy papules or plaques clustered in axillae, anal, inguinal, facial, and neck regions	Similar deposits in heart, kidney, gastrointestinal tract, CNS, PNS, lung, endocrine glands, and joints	Multiple myeloma

AL = amyloid light chain; CNS = central nervous system; PNS =

*Oral lesions are only one part of a generalized neoplastic disease process.

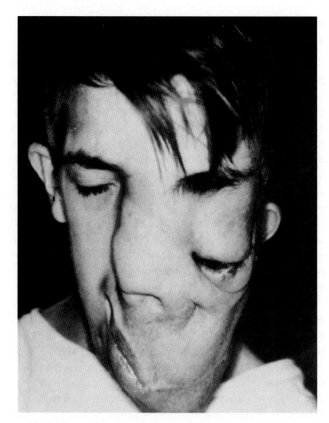

FIGURE 7-38 Gross facial deformity associated with neurofibromatosis in a 25-year-old male. (Courtesy of Robert M. Howell, DDS, MSD, Lincoln, Nebr.)

years may elapse between the development of the polyps and adenocarcinomatous change, but since this is a condition with autosomal dominant inheritance with marked penetrance, it is usual to examine (often by elective laparotomy) all family members who are beyond puberty. Several jaw bone and skin lesions have been described in families with genetic susceptibility to these conditions, including solitary and multiple osteomas, impacted teeth, odontomas, desmoid fibroma, and epidermoid cysts[209,210]

The adenomatous polyposis carcinoma (APC) gene is mutated, representing a tumor suppressor gene.[211]

Peutz-Jeghers Syndrome

True polyps of the gastrointestinal mucosa (ie, adenomatous tumors that frequently demonstrate malignant behavior with both local and lymphatic spread), are relatively rare except in the sigmoid colon and rectum.[60,212–214] In addition, a variety of polypoid lesions with very limited tendency to malignant change are found throughout the gastrointestinal tract. Many of these polypoid lesions are thought to be of inflammatory or hamartomatous origin[215] and are also occasionally associated with dermatologic or oral mucosal abnormalities. Peutz-Jeghers syndrome, in which perioral and lip freckling, patchy brown oral mucosal pigmentation, and freckling of the distal aspect of fingers and toes are associated with polypoid lesions that are mainly in the small intestine, is a well-known example of these inherited polypoid syndromes. The polypoid

lesions in this autosomal dominant condition generally behave as benign lesions although patients with carcinoma arising from adenomatous polyps have been reported.[211,216] Bleeding or intussusception are the most likely complications. The perioral freckling often fades as the affected individual matures, leaving oral mucosal pigmentation that may be indistinguishable from racial pigmentation or pigmentation associated with Addison's disease. Some members of affected families have the oral pigmentation but without any evidence of gastrointestinal polyposis.

Nevoid Basal Cell Carcinoma Syndrome

Nevoid basal cell carcinoma syndrome is inherited in a fashion similar to that by which Peutz-Jeghers syndrome is inherited, and thorough examination of all family members is justified when individuals present with characteristic jaw cysts,

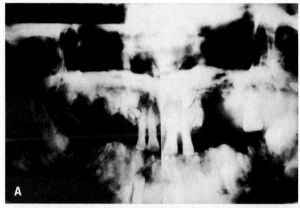

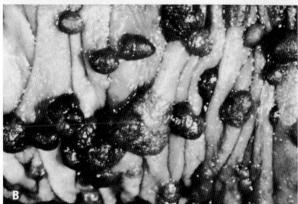

FIGURE 7-39 Gardner's syndrome in a 43-year-old black female with a history of multiple osteomas and odontomas of the jaws and multiple colonic polyps, one of which showed adenocarcinomatous change. Death occurred following the surgical removal of a large desmoid tumor of the abdominal wall. Additional findings at autopsy included an adrenal cortical adenoma, fibroadenoma of the breast, multiple leiomyomata of the uterus, multiple hamartomas of the kidney, and an exostosis above the left eyebrow. **A,** Panoramic radiograph of the jaws shows osteomas, odontomas, and multiple unerupted teeth. **B,** Multiple adenomatous polyps of the colonic mucosa. (Reproduced with permission from Archard HO. Biology and pathology of the oral mucosa. In: Fitzpatrick TB, editor. Dermatology in general medicine. New York: McGraw-Hill; 1971. p. 927)

facies (enlarged calvarium) and other bony abnormalities (calcification of the meninges and hypoplastic and bifid ribs), and skin lesions (basal cell carcinoma appearing as multiple pink or brown papules on the face, neck, and upper trunk).[217,218] Despite the syndrome's name, multiple basal cell carcinomas occur in only 50% of cases. In this condition, however, their multiple nature, appearance at an early age, and tendency to occur anywhere on the skin surface (often on areas covered by clothing) make early recognition and treatment difficult.

Many of the jaw cysts in affected individuals have a keratinized epithelial lining and may be filled with layers of desquamated squame. Such cysts are referred to as primordial or odontogenic keratocysts.[136–138,219,220] Considerable interest has been shown in cysts of this type in recent years because they frequently "bud" and produce daughter cysts, which may result in a recurrence of the cyst despite its removal and because a keratinizing cyst lining is more common in dentigerous cysts that have undergone carcinomatous change. Such cysts also occur without other evidence of this syndrome (see Figures 7-19, 7-20, and 7-21), and in the older literature, they were often mistakenly referred to as epidermal inclusion cysts of the jaws (ie, epidermoid or dermoid cysts, which also contain various epidermal appendages) or as primordial cysts, indicating an origin from a distal extension of the dental lamina. The finding of multiple odontogenic keratocysts, however, should always suggest the possibility of the syndrome and a search for its other features.

Pitting of the soles and palms (milia, local areas of undermaturation of the epithelial basal cells) is an obvious additional finding in about half of the individuals affected by the syndrome, and facies with ocular hypertelorism may be prominent. Continuous monitoring of these patients is advised, and any skin lesions that show signs of aggressiveness should be excised. Recurrences are reported to be rare, however.

There is no evidence that development of squamous cell carcinoma is a hazard associated with the odontogenic keratocysts in this syndrome, but occasional ameloblastoma and fibrosarcoma of the jaws have been reported. Although peripheral osseous curettage or ostectomy is sometimes recommended for odontogenic keratocysts to prevent recurrences,[221] the literature suggests that simple curettage or marsupialization of the cysts found in this syndrome is adequate treatment.[138,219,220]

The word "nevus," sometimes used in the name of this syndrome (eg, "basal cell nevus syndrome") and in certain other connotations (eg, "nevus flammeus" in Sturge-Weber syndrome, and "nevus unius lateris" for ichthyosis hystrix), refers to a genetically determined hamartoma or birthmark, not to a melanocytic nevus or mole. Nevoid basal cell carcinoma syndrome is inherited as an autosomal dominant condition with complete penetrance, and affected individuals have about a 50% chance of transmitting the condition. The *patched* gene, a component of the sonic hedgehog signaling pathway, is mutated. One mutation is germline; the other is acquired in lesional tissue. *Patched*, therefore, represents a tumor suppressor gene.

Multiple Endocrine Neoplasia Type III (Multiple Mucosal Neuroma Syndrome)

Multiple endocrine neoplasia types I to III (MEN I, II, and III) is a group of familial syndromes in which neoplastic change occurs in several endocrine glands in one individual.[‡] MEN I[222] involves lesions in some combination of pancreatic islets, adrenal cortex, and parathyroid and pituitary glands; it includes Zollinger-Ellison (or gastrinoma) syndrome, in which multiple primary gastrin-secreting adenomas or adenocarcinomas are located in the pancreas, duodenum, or even extra-abdominal sites such as the parathyroid gland. Stomach ulceration and hyperplasia of the pancreatic islets and parathyroid glands develop secondary to the excess gastrin release and account for the characteristic presenting symptoms. Between one-quarter and one-half of gastrinomas have other features of the MEN I syndrome, which is *not* associated with any skin or oral phakomatosis.

Likewise, MEN II,[223] which involves medullary carcinoma of the thyroid gland, pheochromocytoma of the adrenal medulla, and parathyroid hyperplasia or adenoma, is not associated with any phakomatosis. However, a subgroup of these patients exhibits multiple neuromas of the lips, tongue, and buccal, conjunctival, nasal, and pharyngeal mucosae, in association with their endocrine neoplasia (this is referred to as MEN III or multiple mucosal neuroma syndrome).[224,225] Since these neuromas may occasionally predate any overt endocrine neoplasia, the recognition of these oropharyngeal lesions as possible evidence of MEN III can lead to the early and sometimes successful treatment of the associated malignancies.[225]

Almost all individuals with MEN III have oral mucosal neuromas (Figure 7-40) that may be extensive enough to thicken the lip and produce a characteristic "bumpy" or "blubbery" lip appearance. In addition, these individuals may exhibit marfanoid habitus, café au lait spots, lentigines, and a history of diverticulosis or lower-bowel surgery.

Although there are complex interactions between the various involved endocrine organs in each of these three variant syndromes, the finding of multiple neoplastic endocrine involvement is thought to be due to a widespread predisposition to cancer in many tissues derived from neuroectoderm, rather than to endocrine interactions. Endocrine interaction is also evident in the occurrence of Cushing's syndrome, hyperinsulinism, hypertension, and hyperparathyroidism in some affected individuals. Various combinations of abnormalities are found in the relatives of affected individuals. The finding of oral mucosal neuromas in association with a family history of carcinoma of the thyroid or pheochromocytoma clearly indicates a need to search for other evidence of this syndrome.

---

‡ Endocrine abnormalities are also sometimes present in patients who have other inherited syndromes with neoplastic associations, such as neurofibromatosis 1, McCune-Albright syndrome, and von Hippel-Lindau syndrome. These conditions are usually excluded from the definition of multiple endocrine neoplasia.[68]

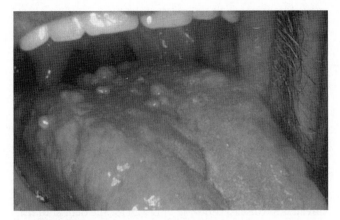

FIGURE 7-40 Multiple oral mucosal neuromas on the posterior third of the tongue of a patient with type III multiple endocrine neoplasia. (Courtesy of C. Dunlap, DDS, Kansas City, Mo.)

Tuberous Sclerosis

Tuberous sclerosis is an inherited disorder that is characterized by seizures and mental retardation associated with hamartomatous glial proliferations and neuronal deformity in the central nervous system.[226,227] Fine wartlike lesions (adenoma sebaceum) occur in a butterfly distribution over the cheeks and forehead, and histologically similar lesions (vascular fibromas) have been described intraorally.[228,229] Characteristic hypoplastic enamel defects (pitted enamel hypoplasia) occur in 70% of affected individuals and only rarely in unaffected relatives. Rhabdomyoma of the heart and other hamartomas of kidney, liver, adrenal glands, pancreas, and jaw[226] are described. The neoplastic transformation of the glial proliferations constitutes the "internal malignancy" of this syndrome.

Acanthosis Nigricans

The term "acanthosis nigricans" describes grayish brown thickened patches of skin, which are usually symmetrically distributed and which have a characteristic velvety papulosquamous texture. The axilla, base of neck, groin, and antecubital fossa are most commonly affected. A similar intraoral papillomatosis has also been described. Acanthosis nigricans is described in association with both benign and malignant systemic disease. Malignant acanthosis nigricans is often of sudden onset, is rapidly progressive, and is most commonly associated with gastric or other intra-abdominal adenocarcinomas (less commonly with lymphoma or squamous cell carcinoma). The skin change may precede the recognition of a malignancy and is considered to be an important diagnostic clue for possible internal malignancy. The skin pigmentation has been ascribed to the release of peptides from the tumor and usually fades following the tumor's removal. Apart from its rapidity of onset and progression, benign acanthosis nigricans is indistinguishable from the "malignant" variety. Idiopathic (obesity-associated), endocrine (associated with insulin-resistant diabetes, Addison's disease, or pituitary and pineal tumors), and drug-related (nicotinic acid, glucocorticoids, diethylstilbestrol) types of "benign" acanthosis nigricans are distinguishable.[60,201,230]

Albright's Syndrome

Polyostotic fibrous dysplasia with café au lait spots,[§] bony deformities, and precocious sexual development is referred to as McCune-Albright syndrome or Albright's syndrome (see "Fibrous Dysplasia of Bone and Albright's Syndrome," earlier in this chapter) and is an inherited form of fibrous dysplasia, usually with multiple bone involvement. Osteosarcoma develops in about 1% of patients with this syndrome. Since osteosarcoma also occasionally develops in patients with long-standing monostotic fibrous dysplasia (as the result of radiation therapy in some cases but even without such treatment in other cases) and in view of the greater volume of dysplastic bony tissue in which sarcoma can develop in polyostotic fibrous dysplasia, it is not known whether the lesion of Albright's syndrome is more predisposed to malignant transformation than the lesion of monostotic fibrous dysplasia. Polyostotic fibrous dysplasia may occur in the absence of the other components of the syndrome (ie, café au lait spots and precocious sexual development), and skeletal surveys are indicated for patients with large or multiple lesions of fibrous dysplasia of the jaws, even in the absence of skin pigmentation. The gene that is mutated in Albright's syndrome is an internal signaling G protein.

Paget's Disease of Bone (Osteitis Deformans)

Paget's disease of bone is by far the most common disease among those listed in Table 7-3, affecting about 3% of the population older than 45 years of age and about 6 to 7% of hospitalized patients. It is rare in patients younger than 40 years of age. The nature of this bone disease is unknown although evidence to suggest that it is a multicentric benign tumor of osteoclasts has been presented. No endocrine basis for the disease has been found, and the frequency with which malignant transformation occurs (in 1 to 2% of patients, especially those with multiple foci) and the heterogeneity of the osteoclasts in biopsy specimens from patients with Paget's disease suggest that the disease itself may be a benign (hormone-sensitive) neoplasm of bone cells.[231–233]

The possibility of an infective viral etiology for Paget's disease is suggested by the ultrastructural demonstration of intranuclear inclusions in the abnormal osteoclasts found in these patients, as well as in osteosarcoma cells in Paget's disease lesions that have undergone malignant transformation.[234] Similar inclusions have not been demonstrated in other human sarcomas or in osteoclasts in normal bone, fibrous dysplasia, or metabolic bone disorders such as hyperparathyroidism and rickets. However, similar inclusions have been reported in a giant cell tumor of bone.[235] These inclusions consisted of bundles of microfilaments with an electron-lucent

---

§ These lesions (compare with those of neurofibromatosis) are usually fewer than six in number although they are sometimes quite large and characteristically have an irregular ("coast of Maine") border. They are usually on the same side as bony lesions and may overlie them.

core and usually showed evidence of paracrystalline array. Similar inclusions are seen in cases of measles and in subacute sclerosing panencephalitis virus infections. Measles virus and respiratory syncytial (RS) virus antigens and ribonucleic acid (RNA)[236] have also been reported in osteoclasts from Paget's disease lesions, and it is possible that various *Paramyxovirus* infections modified by genetic or environmental factors are involved in the etiology of this multifocal neoplasm.

The bony lesions of Paget's disease produce characteristic deformities of the skull, jaw, back, pelvis, and legs and are readily recognized both clinically and radiologically. Irregular overgrowth of the jaw bones, especially the maxilla, may occur and may lead to the facial appearance described as "leontiasis ossea." A "ground-glass" change in the alveolar bones, which is often associated with loss of the lamina dura and root resorption, is sometimes apparent in dental radiographs made in the early (osteolytic) phase of the disease. Subsequently, the jaw bones and other affected bones are occupied by a dense sclerotic bony deposition that fixes the deformed skeleton in its characteristic shape and creates the diagnostic features of the calvarium (a "cotton wool" appearance between the widened bony tables of the skull), maxilla, maxillary sinuses, and elsewhere. Healing of dental extraction wounds in affected areas is poor, and excessive postsurgical bleeding from the highly vascular bone that is characteristic of this disease is a concern. The narrowing of skull foramina can cause ill-defined neuralgic pains. There is an increased incidence of both salivary and pulpal calculi. Jaw fractures do not usually occur (compare to Paget's disease of the long bones), but benign giant cell tumors and malignant sarcomatous transformation affect both the jaw bones and the long bones of these patients with some frequency. Multicentric sarcomas are not uncommon.

Although a few patients with Paget's disease have no symptoms, many suffer considerable pain and deformity. These problems, associated medical problems such as cardiac failure and hypercalcemia, and the high incidence of malignant transformation have encouraged the use of a variety of new treatments of this disease, many of which are still being tested.[232,234,237] The majority of these agents are designed to suppress some of the metabolic events by which bone cells remodel the calcified tissue and influence the exchange of mineral ions between bone and the circulating fluids. These agents include antibiotics (ie, intravenous mithramycin, an effective inhibitor of osteoclastic activity), hormones of human and animal origin (high-dose glucocorticoids and porcine, salmon, and human calcitonin administered subcutaneously or by nasal spray or suppository), salts such as the diphosphonate etidronate (which effectively reduces bone resorption), and cytotoxic agents like plicamycin and dactinomycin. A marked reduction in pain and some slowing in the progression of the disease have been attained with many of these agents.

Urinary levels of calcium and hydroxyproline (a measure of collagen metabolism) and serum alkaline phosphatase levels (a measure of osteoblastic activity) are useful for diagnosing Paget's disease and for monitoring bone resorption and deposition during treatment. Radiologic findings are also often diagnostic, and computed tomography and Tc-99m diphosphonate and gallium-67 bone scanning may be used to define the extent of bone involvement.

Usually not manifest until the patient's fifth decade, Paget's disease has a definite familial distribution, and susceptibility to this disease is probably inherited as an autosomal dominant condition, as are the majority of the syndromes listed in Table 7-3. It is clearly not in the same category of disease as the other listed syndromes, in which benign oral lesions may signal the presence of internal malignancy. The oral lesions in Paget's disease are simply the manifestation, in the jawbone, of a widespread bone disease; however, it is well for the dentist to realize that the patient with Paget's disease of the jaw bones has an increased chance of developing sarcoma both orally and wherever else the disease is manifested. In view of the rarity of a giant cell tumor in the jaws except as a complication of Paget's disease,[238] the finding of this lesion in a patient who is older than 40 years of age should raise the possibility of previously undiagnosed Paget's disease.

Cowden's Syndrome

Cowden's syndrome (multiple hamartoma and neoplasia syndrome) is characterized by the hamartomatous involvement of many organs, with a potential for neoplastic transformation.[201,239,240] It is inherited as an autosomal dominant character. Multiple papules on the lips and gingivae are often present, and papillomatosis (benign fibromatosis) of the buccal, palatal, faucial, and oropharyngeal mucosae often produces a "cobblestone" effect on these mucous membranes. The tongue is also pebbly, fissured, or scrotal. Multiple papillomatous nodules (histologically inverted follicular keratoses or trichilemmomas) are often present on the perioral, periorbital, and perinasal skin, and oropharyngeal mucosae often manifests a cobblestone effect on these mucous membranes. Multiple papillomatous nodules are often present also on the pinnae of the ears and neck, accompanied by lipomas, hemangiomas, neuromas, vitiligo, café au lait spots, and acromelanosis elsewhere on the skin. A variey of neoplastic changes occur in the organs exhibiting hamartomatous lesions, particularly an increased rate of breast and thyroid carcinoma and gastrointestinal malignancy.[214] Squamous cell carcinoma of the tongue and basal cell tumors of the perianal skin are also described.

Xanthomas

Xanthomas are localized deposits of lipoprotein that are usually found in the skin, subcutaneous tissue, or tendons.[201,241] They are of diverse origin; many are associated with vascular disease, and some are associated with internal malignancy. Similar nodules may occur intraorally and on the faces of individuals with a variety of disorders (lipidoses) characterized by an abnormal concentration of lipids in tissues or extracellular fluids. Many of these conditions are inherited, and some are secondary to diseases such as hypothyroidism, diabetes mellitus, obstructive liver diseases, and dysproteinemia (such as multiple myeloma). Isolated xanthomas sometimes occur in the absence of recognizable systemic abnormality, but they are almost certain to be a manifestation of a lipidosis when multiple lesions are found, and they are associated with similar lipid deposits elsewhere (in the skin, eyelids [xanthelasma], and cornea, and as nodules on the tendons). It is important that these lesions are recognized and that the patient is referred for plasma triglyceride, cholesterol, and lipoprotein measurement and medical consultation since several of the inherited lipidoses are associated with the early onset of severe coronary atherosclerosis and diabetes mellitus, which are likely to be fatal if not treated. A thorough description of the occurrence of oral and facial xanthomatosis in association with the various lipidoses does not appear to have been published although there are case reports of oral lesions of this type.[242–244] Many of the lipidoses are characterized in terms of the associated plasma lipoprotein abnormality. Xanthomatosis is manifest in types I to III and V hyperlipoproteinemias, and mucous membrane eruptions are frequent in types I and V (both of which exhibit hyperchylomicronemia). Xanthomas of the tendons, skin, and eyes and atheromatosis of the vascular endothelium are prominent features of types II and III (carbohydrate-induced) hyperlipoproteinemia, both of which carry a high risk of ischemic heart disease.

In Tangier disease, a familial high-density lipoprotein deficiency (a rare autosomal recessive condition) affects children, and adults exhibit startling orange or yellowish gray discolorations and a swelling of the tonsils, pharyngeal mucosa, and gingivae in association with hypocholestrolemia and the enlargement of other organs of the reticuloendothelial system (spleen, liver, and lymph nodes).[245] Xanthomas are also frequently associated with multiple myeloma,[246] leukemia, and some lymphomas, probably as a result of the dysproteinemia accompanying these malignancies.

Langerhans Cell (Eosinophilic) Histiocytosis

Osteolytic jaw lesions, xanthomas, and other oral soft-tissue swellings also occur in diseases that were previously referred to by the generic name of histiocytosis X but that have been renamed as Langerhans cell histiocytosis (LCH)[247,248] with the recognition that the key proliferative component in these lesions is the Langerhans' cell.[249] This group includes such variants as eosinophilic granuloma, Letterer-Siwe disease, and Hand-Schüller-Christian syndrome (triad of exophthalmos, diabetes insipidus, and destructive bone lesions). Widespread proliferation of tissue macrophages (formerly referred to as histiocytes)[250] and specialized bone marrow–derived Langerhans' cells characterize these diseases, which are often not benign. These eponyms have been respectively replaced with the following terms: acute disseminated LCH, chronic disseminated LCH, and chronic localized LCH.

Jaw bone lesions are relatively common in patients with Langerhans cell granulomatosis and may be the initial lesion detected. While the diagnosis must be established by examination of biopsy specimens, the presence of each of the following radiologic characteristics increases the likelihood that a given lesion is an example of Langerhans' cell proliferation:

a solitary intraosseous lesion, multiple "scooped-out" and sclerotic bone lesions with a well-defined periphery, periosteal new bone formation, and slight root resorption.[251] Small localized aggregates of Langerhans' cells that are occasionally noted in inflammatory periapical lesions are often interpreted as chronic localized Langerhans granulomatosis (incipient eosinophilic granuloma). Lesions of this type that have been followed clinically for as long as 10 years have remained localized, suggesting that local curettage may be adequate treatment of these microscopic lesions.[252] Jaw bone lesions that contain lipid-filled macrophages rather than Langerhans' cells are usually relegated to a category referred to as non-X histiocytosis and include such entities as xanthoma, xanthogranuloma, and benign fibrous histiocytoma.[253] Follow-up studies suggest that these lesions, although locally destructive in some cases, generally are benign, remain localized, and may occasionally heal spontaneously.

Amyloidosis

Deposits of the AL type of amyloid (see Chapter 16) frequently occur in the oral cavity, secondary to the proliferation of abnormal clones of plasma cells that characterizes multiple myeloma. These deposits are most common in the tongue and gingivae, and apart from the development of macroglossia (see Chapter 7), gross enlargement of oral tissues from this cause is unusual[254] although oral amyloidosis is generally included among the oral phakomatoses and has been the initial symptom of multiple myeloma on rare occasions.[255]

▼ ACUTE AND GRANULOMATOUS INFLAMMATIONS

Histopathologic examination of a biopsy specimen from a localized swelling of the jaws, tongue, lips, or oral mucosa occasionally reveals a chronic granulomatous inflammatory tissue response.[256] The etiology of such a lesion can be readily identified from the calculus, other foreign body, or specific microorganisms evident on microscopic examination of the tissue. When a foreign body, an infectious agent, or an associated systemic disease cannot be identified, the differential diagnosis can be extensive and includes sarcoidosis, tuberculosis and other mycobacterial infections, fungal infections (histoplasmosis, blastomycosis), actinomycosis, syphilis, leprosy (in endemic areas), Hodgkin's lymphoma, Crohn's disease, and Melkersson-Rosenthal and Meischer's syndromes. Tuberculosis, sarcoidosis, and cat-scratch fever are likely candidates if the swelling arises in a regional lymph node. Soft-tissue granulomas are usually small and are microscopically detectable only as focal collections of modified macrophages (epithelioid cells) and Langhans' cells or foreign-body-type giant cells with a peripheral rim of lymphocytes; fibroblasts, plasma cells, and neutrophils may also be present. Two classic types of granulomatous response are recognized:[257] (1) in tuberculosis, the granuloma or tubercle characteristically has a central area of amorphous granular debris (caseous necrosis) and usually contains acid-fast bacilli; (2) sarcoid granulomas are noncaseating and may exhibit asteroid bodies in the giant cells as well as concentric calcific concretions (Schaumann's bodies). Variations on either of these two patterns are seen in the other granulomas.[22] Actinomycosis, catscratch fever, leprosy, and Melkersson-Rosenthal and Meischer's syndromes are discussed below.

Cervicofacial Actinomycosis

Actinomycosis is an infectious disease caused by a slender gram-positive rod-shaped bacterium, *Actinomyces israelii*, that exhibits a number of simple funguslike characteristics, such as a tendency to grow as a mass of rounded bodies (clubs) and filaments in tissue (hence the term "ray fungus"), low virulence, and the property of eliciting suppuration, necrosis, and a chronic granulomatous tissue response.[258] Based on the shared feature of a granulomatous tissue response, actinomycosis, tuberculosis, and syphilis were once grouped as the "specific granulomatous diseases." However, these three infections have little in common as far as their natural histories, clinical features, or treatments are concerned, even though chronic pulmonary infection with *Actinomyces* occasionally can be clinically and radiographically confused with tuberculosis. Since *Actinomyces israelii* is an anaerobic or microaerophilic species, isolation of the organism in pure culture is difficult, and identification is often based on demonstration of the organisms as stained in tissue sections or as microcolonies (sulfur granules) in pus. The organism is included among the normal oral bacterial flora and is especially concentrated in dental plaque, calculus, carious lesions, and tonsillar crypts.[259] Almost all cervicofacial actinomycotic infections are endogenous in origin and occur when dental plaque, calculus, or gingival debris contaminates relatively deep wounds around the mouth. Although the classic lesions of cervicofacial actinomycosis are chronic low-grade persistent infections that may be difficult to eradicate, careful bacteriologic study of acute jaw and softtissue abscesses after surgical or other trauma has demonstrated that *Actinomyces israelii* may also be involved in acute and rapidly resolving suppurative lesions.[260,261] Microscopic examination of periapical tissues of nonvital and endodontically treated teeth may also occasionally reveal an isolated periapical actinomycotic granuloma, suggesting that this otherwise noninvasive organism can also be walled off and tolerated in the oral tissues for long periods of time without evidence of active disease.[262,263]

It is generally believed that pulmonary actinomycosis results from the aspiration of oral or tonsillar debris and that areas of localized atelectasis secondary to the obstruction of small air passages provide the necessary anaerobic conditions for the growth of *Actinomyces*. It is also possible that pulmonary actinomycosis may arise hematogenously, from an infected oral or cervicofacial focus. Ileocecal (intestinal) actinomycosis is the commonest other form of actinomycosis and usually arises following the rupture of an inflamed appendix, with the development of a mass in the right iliac fossa.[264] Pelvic actinomycosis has been recognized as an important complication of some intrauterine contraceptive devices (IUDs).[265] In immunocompromised individuals, spread via the bloodstream may occur from any of these primary foci of infection.

Approximately 60% of all actinomycotic infections occur in the cervicofacial area, and there is a history of tooth extraction or jaw fracture in about 15 to 20% of cases. It was once believed that the organism was implanted in the oral tissues by chewing wood splinters, blades, or stalks of grass and that the infection was more common in agricultural workers. More recent data fail to support this idea and have also cast doubt on *Actinomyces* as the universal etiologic agent for a cattle disease (referred to as "lumpy jaw") that was believed to be analogous to cervicofacial actinomycosis in man.

The submandibular region is the most frequent site of involvement in classic human cervicofacial actinomycosis, the disease usually having spread by direct tissue extension. There may be associated changes that are detectable at the portal of entry (such as a nonhealing tooth socket), exuberant granulation tissue, or periosteal thickening of the alveolus. On many occasions, however, the chronic infection spreads from the periapical region with minimal clinical signs until it is well established. Then, soft-tissue swelling or the development of a fistula causes the patient to seek treatment. The cheeks, the masseter region, and the parotid gland may also be involved. Extension to the skull and the meninges has occurred on rare occasions.

One of the characteristics of actinomycosis is the lack of immediate tissue reaction after implantation of the organism. It usually requires 6 weeks or longer for an actinomycotic swelling to break down and discharge pus. The multiple discharging sinuses that subsequently develop (Figure 7-41) and the sulfur granules that are often present in the pus are almost pathognomonic of the disease. The adjacent tissues usually have a hard, doughy consistency. The skin surrounding the discharging fistulae is purplish, and there may be small areas of hypertrophic granulation tissue. Acute pain is uncommon.

Primary actinomycosis of the tongue[266] (Figure 7-42) must be differentiated from neoplasms, tuberculous ulceration, syphilitic gumma, and other chronic infectious granulomatous diseases such as histoplasmosis. In actinomycosis of the tongue, there is usually a small deep-seated nodule[267] that is painless at first and causes little discomfort. The lesion gradually increases in size, and the overlying tissues soften and rupture. There may be temporary healing, after which the process is repeated, with the development of a more extensive lesion. Dysphagia is a prominent symptom in cases of extensive involvement.

Actinomycosis of the cervicofacial region may be confused with osteomyelitis. In osteomyelitis, pain is more severe, with greater destruction of bone and more rapidly developing suppuration. Radiologic studies aid in the diagnosis. Tuberculous adenitis and other causes of submandibular and cervical lymphadenopathy, such as cat-scratch disease, lymphogranuloma venereum, and Hodgkin's disease, should be considered. The presence of the boardlike induration found in actinomycosis

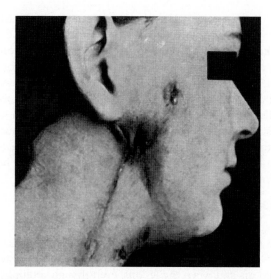

FIGURE 7-41 Multiple fistulae at the angle of the jaw and on the side of the face of a patient with chronic actinomycosis of the cervicofacial region. (Courtesy of the late Dr. Robert H. Ivy, Philadelphia, Pa.)

and the finding of acid-fast organisms on examination of the exudate help in making a diagnosis. A presumptive diagnosis can be made if "sulfur granules" are present and if gram-positive mycelia can be demonstrated. A positive diagnosis can be made only from anaerobic culture and isolation of *Actinomyces* from infected tissue or pus. As previously discussed, the opportunity for positive diagnosis in this disease is limited and will occur only when the clinician and the microbiologist collab-

orate to confirm a suspected actinomycotic infection or when the organism is demonstrated in tissue section. *Actinomyces* spp. have also been isolated from areas of osteomyelitis, and typical actinomycotic colonies are sometimes noted in excised sequestra, suggesting that this infection may play a role in osteoradionecrosis.[268]

Chronic cervicofacial actinomycosis is traditionally considered to be a difficult infection to eradicate, but more recent texts suggest that penicillin and tetracyclines are quite effective, particularly if high doses are used and continued for several weeks of treatment. At least four million units of penicillin should be given daily intramuscularly. Tetracyclines are administered at 500 mg every 6 hours. Preference is usually given to the use of tetracyclines for treatment of this infection to avoid the repeated intramuscular injections of penicillin. Iodides, sulfonamides, and radiation were all used at one time but no longer have any place in the treatment of these infections. Antifungal antibiotics do not affect the growth of actinomycetes. Surgical drainage of definable foci of infection may be needed and occasionally may be curative alone. Hyperbaric oxygenation is also used in eradicating chronic jaw bone infections.[269] The major problem associated with the treatment of actinomycosis is the development of allergic reactions to the prolonged high doses of antibiotics.

Asymptomatic periapical actinomycotic foci that are demonstrated in association with necrotic dental pulp tissue or endodontic treatment rarely result in progressive actinomycotic infection.[270,271] The apicoectomy procedure by which such foci are demonstrated is adequate treatment alone in most cases. The finding of the ray fungus in a periapical granuloma always raises the question of whether additional antibiotic treatment is needed. If antibiotics are given in this circumstance, a somewhat shorter period of administration (eg, 1 to 2 weeks) is probably adequate.[272]

Acute alveolar abscesses that are shown to be associated with *Actinomyces* infection have likewise usually resolved with the initial antibiotic treatment prior to recognition of *Actinomyces* as a possible causative agent.[260,261,273] Once again, increased doses of penicillin or tetracyclines may be given for an additional 1 to 2 weeks, but the need for this is not well established. The widespread use of penicillin and other antibiotics prophylactically after dental extractions, jaw fractures, and other orofacial trauma is considered to be responsible for a decreasing prevalence of cervicofacial actinomycosis over recent decades. Localized foci of actinomycotic infection have been reported following the intentional reimplantation of teeth,[274] and it is conceivable that localized actinomycotic lesions may become more frequent as dental implantology expands.

Cat-Scratch Disease

Localized lymphadenopathy of cervical lymph nodes because of an infectious agent that is indigenous to cats (clinically, there is often evidence of a recent infected cat scratch, bite, or other superficial injury on the hand or forearm of the patient) constitutes a specific infection that is referred to as cat-scratch disease or cat-scratch fever.[275–282] A variety of microorganisms

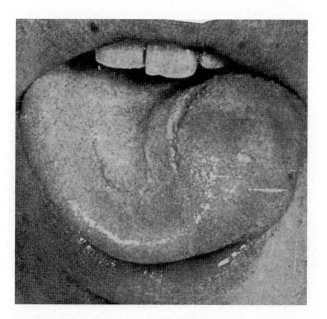

FIGURE 7-42 Actinomycotic nodule on the left lateral aspect of the dorsum of the tongue in a 27-year-old man. (Reproduced with permission from Dorph-Peterson L, Pindborg JJ. Actinomycosis of the tongue: report of a case. Oral Surg Oral Med Oral Pathol 1954;7:1178)

have been implicated in this disease; currently, a gram-negative partially cell wall–defective bacterium, *Rochalimaea hensele-lae*, appears to be the causative agent on the basis of cultural and seroepidemiologic studies of patients with lymphadenopathy of this type.[275,276] In most instances, the reactive lymphadenitis is restricted to one or more regional lymph nodes, in which case the differential diagnosis would include tuberculous adenitis, lymphadenitis from an abscessed tooth or infected tonsil, infectious mononucleosis, and even lymphoma. Less commonly, the reactive inflammation may spread beyond the lymph nodes and may produce a swelling that extends from the cervical region to the eye (Parinaud's syndrome),[278,279] frequently without significant systemic response. A biopsy specimen of the involved tissue may show a nonspecific reactive lymphadenitis or subsequent sarcoidlike granulomas that extend into perinodal tissue. Organisms similar to those cultured from lymph node aspirates can often be found in Warthin-Starry silver-stained sections of the nodes. However, the diagnosis is usually made on clinical grounds and occasionally by biopsy rather than by microbiologic or immunologic methods. Most infections are self-limited, and specific antibiotic treatment (eg, with cephalosporins) or treatment by incision and drainage is rarely indicated.[280,281]

Disseminated cat-scratch disease, which results in multiple liver abscesses, pleural effusion, and skin and mucosal lesions in addition to lymphadenopathy, is recognized as an indicator of opportunistic infection, signaling immunodeficiency in the patient who is infected with human immunodeficiency virus (HIV).[282]

Hansen's Disease (Leprosy)

Infection with *Mycobacterium leprae* remains endemic in many tropical countries.[283,284] A proportion of infected individuals develop characteristic lesions (primarily on the skin and extremities) that are referred to as tuberculoid, lepromatous, and borderline or reactional, depending on the stage of the infection. Tuberculoid leprosy appears clinically as macular lesions of the skin that on biopsy are found to overlie subepidermal tuberculoid granulomas containing small numbers of acid-fast bacilli. Patients with tuberculoid leprosy give positive delayed hypersensitivity responses (referred to as Fernandez or Mitsuda reactions) to intradermal injections of extracts of the organism (lepromin test) and are not considered infectious. By contrast, the patient with lepromatous leprosy[285] displays little evidence of immunity to the organism and develops multiple granulomatous masses (lepromas) affecting the face, nose, and ears (leonine facies) and the skin over the wrists, elbows, knees, and buttocks. Peripheral nerve tissue is also extensively involved, with both lepromatous nodules and apparently unaffected patches of skin often exhibiting hypoanesthesia or anesthesia. Histologically, lepromas consist of aggregates of lipid-rich foamy cells (lepra cells), with large numbers of acid-fast bacilli present and little evidence of the T-cell response that characterizes tuberculoid granulomas. Patients with lepromatous leprosy are infectious and usually have progressive disease requiring antimycobacterial therapy.

Borderline or reactional leprosy[286] represents an intermediate stage between the tuberculoid and lepromatous types.

The literature contains few descriptions of oral lesions in cases of tuberculoid leprosy. Lepromatous nodules of the tongue, palate, lips, and pharynx are reported more frequently, as reddish yellow or brown sessile or pedunculated mucosal nodules,[284] and destructive lesions of the palate and nasal bones can lead to deformities that are traditionally associated with this disease. Oral lesions have been reported in 20 to 60% of patients with Hansen's disease, the majority of these being lepromatous nodules.

Orofacial Granulomatosis

Sarcoidlike granulomatous lesions may be encountered anywhere in the oral cavity, head, and neck, and they may be multiple.[287,288] When there are no other manifestations of systemic sarcoidosis and when the lesions, even though multiple, are confined to the oral mucosa and facial skin, the appellation "orofacial granulomatosis" is applied. A biopsy performed on a persistent and usually painless diffuse swelling of one or both lips that is not associated with any identifiable allergic reaction (angioneurotic edema) or systemic disease occasionally will reveal the presence of noncaseating tuberculoid granulomas with Langhans' giant cells. If serial sectioning and special stains fail to reveal any foreign body or microorganism, the condition is often reported as cheilitis granulomatosa (Figure 7-43).

The terms "Miescher's syndrome" and "Melkersson-Rosenthal syndrome" may also be used clinically, the latter term usually being restricted to those cases that also exhibit facial paralysis and a folded or plicated tongue dorsum. The differential diagnosis in these circumstances also includes sarcoidosis (particularly if the lip lesions are associated with facial paralysis [Heerfordt's syndrome]) and Crohn's disease,[289] as well as the various infections known to be associated with tuberculoid reactions. Occasionally, similar granulomatous enlargements may involve the gingivae[290] (Figures 7-44, 7-45, and Figure 7-46). In the absence of any specific

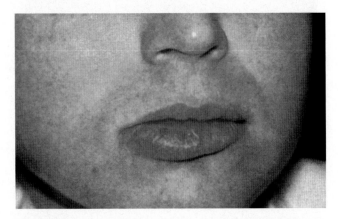

FIGURE 7-43 Cheilitis granulomatosa. A persistent swelling of the lip on biopsy revealed noncaseating tuberculoid-type granulomas with no evidence of any foreign body or microorganism. (Courtesy of D. Krutchkoff, DDS, PhD, Farmington, Conn.)

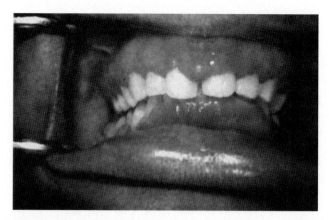

FIGURE 7-44 Marked gingival enlargement that developed in an adult with a history of Crohn's disease and that was not associated with use of phenytoin, cyclosporine, or calcium channel blockers. (Courtesy of Mark B. Snyder, Philadelphia, Pa.)

etiology, these lesions are usually treated with topical, intralesional,[291] and systemic corticosteroids, with surgical reduction of the lip when the persistent swelling is a cosmetic or functional problem.

▼ GINGIVAL ENLARGEMENTS

Gingival enlargement is usually caused by local conditions such as poor oral hygiene, food impaction, or mouth breathing. Systemic conditions such as hormonal changes, drug therapy, or tumor infiltrates may complicate the process or even set the stage for the development of unfavorable local conditions that lead to food impaction and difficulty with oral hygiene. Traditionally, a distinction was made between hypertrophy of the gingiva (an increase in the size of the cellular elements making up the gingiva) and hyperplasia (an actual increase in the number of the cellular elements). Both of these elements are usually present in inflammatory disease of the gingiva. In this section, the word "hyperplasia" is used simply to describe clinically evident gingival enlargement,

without reference to a particular histologic process underlying the change. When edema, vascular engorgement, and inflammatory cell infiltration predominate, gingival enlargement is referred to as inflammatory gingival hyperplasia. When the enlarged gingivae consist largely of dense fibrous tissue as a consequence of chronic inflammation or other causes, the condition is referred to as fibrotic gingival hyperplasia. The term "chronic hyperplastic gingivitis" is often used for either process.

Gingival enlargement may be associated with a wide variety of local and systemic factors. Enlargement is seen more consistently with some of these factors. Examples are local irritants; therapy with anticonvulsants, calcium channel blockers, and immunosuppressive medications; pregnancy and other hyperestrogenic states; monocytic leukemia; and clinical scurvy. A number of these are discussed elsewhere in this and other chapters (eg, congenital epulis and pregnancy epulis, phenytoin-induced hyperplasia, pyogenic granuloma, leukemic gingival enlargement, diabetic gingivitis, scurvy, and some of the congenital and inherited gingival enlargements).

Inflammatory Gingival Enlargement

In most instances, inflammatory gingival enlargement begins at an area of poor oral hygiene, food impaction, or other local irritation that can be readily controlled. However, the pseudopockets formed by gingival enlargement make the maintenance of good oral hygiene difficult, perpetuating a cycle of inflammation and fibrosis. The involved tissues are glossy, smooth, and odematous and bleed readily. A fetid odor may result from the decomposition of food debris and from the accumulation of bacteria in these inaccessible areas. Loss of interseptal bone and drifting of the teeth occur in long-standing cases of inflammatory enlargement. These changes are commonly referred to as gingivitis, or periodontal disease when the process involves the loss of gingival attachment and the subsequent loss of interproximal bone.[292,293]

Gingival inflammation affecting primarily the maxillary anterior region is observed in mouth breathers.[294] In some

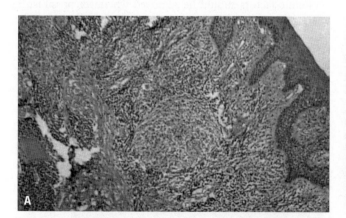
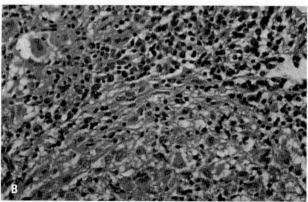

FIGURE 7-45 **A,** Low-power magnification of section of biopsied gingiva reveals grossly thickened submucosal tissue heavily infiltrated with round cells and containing focal granulomas. **B,** High-power magnification reveals noncaseating tuberculoid-type granulomas with giant cell formation. (Courtesy of Mark B. Snyder, Philadelphia, PA.).

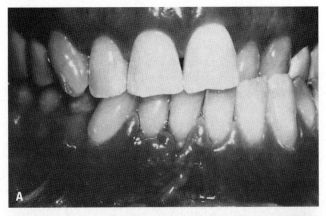

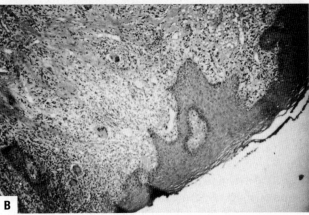

FIGURE 7-46 Inflammatory gingival enlargement associated with a noncaseating granulomatous tissue response. Such lesions have been described in patients diagnosed with Melkersson-Rosenthal syndrome and Crohn's disease and are often seen in association with granulomatous cheilitis and nodular enlargements of the tongue and other areas of the oral mucosa. **A,** Red shiny gingivae. **B,** Low-power micrograph of biopsy specimen of gingiva, showing granulomatous infiltrate with Langhans'-type giant cells. **C,** High-power micrograph of the same specimen.

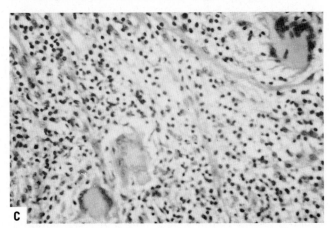

patients, abnormal facial development or malocclusion leads to a continued opening of the mouth, which predisposes these patients to this form of gingivitis. Varying degrees of gingival hyperplasia probably due to hormonal changes have been observed in association with the use of contraceptive pills.

The diagnosis of inflammatory gingival enlargement usually presents no difficulty. The edema of the tissues, their bright red or purplish red color, and their tendency to hemorrhage permits ready differentiation from fibrotic gingival enlargement. Although most gingival enlargements are inflammatory in nature, benign and malignant neoplasms of the gingivae also occur. A biopsy should be performed whenever the cause is unclear or whenever the lesion does not respond to local therapy (Figures 7-47 and 7-48).

Treatment of the inflammatory type of gingival enlargement consists of the establishment of excellent oral hygiene, the elimination of all local predisposing factors if possible, the elimination of any recognized systemic predisposing causes, and proper home care by the patient. In patients with extensive gingival hyperplasia,[295] the affected tissue must be removed surgically, and the remaining tissue must be properly contoured. All local irritative factors such as calculus, the margins of cervical cavities, or areas of food impaction should be corrected. Local treatment is often of value, even when gingival hyperplasia is associated with systemic disease. Although systemic factors should be removed whenever possible, the elimination of local irritative factors may be all that is necessary to obtain a reasonably satisfactory clinical result.

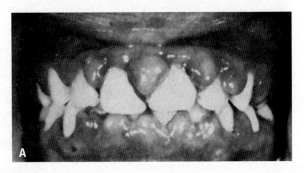

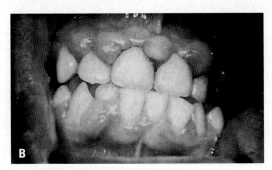

FIGURE 7-47 **A,** Inflammatory gingival enlargement with secondary ulceronecrotic gingivostomatitis. **B,** Fibrosis of the gingivae, secondary to long-standing periodontitis.

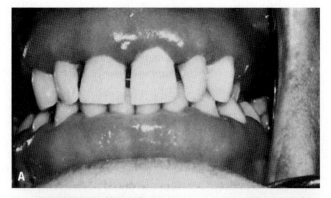

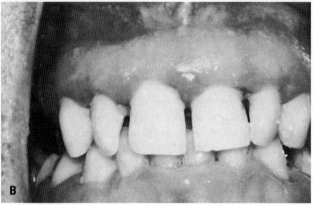

FIGURE 7-48 A, Inflammatory gingival enlargement ascribed to an ingredient formerly present in chewing gum. **B,** Partial regression of swelling after the discontinuation of gum chewing. **C,** Diffuse plasma cell infiltration characteristically associated with this type of reaction, which justifies the term "plasma cell gingivitis," sometimes used to describe this lesion. (Courtesy of C.C. Tomich, DDS, MSD, Indianapolis, Ind.)

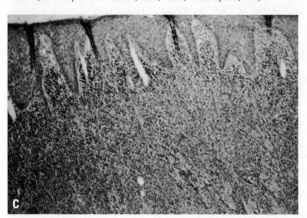

The successful treatment of gingival enlargement in mouth breathers depends mainly on the elimination of the habit. Referral to an otolaryngologist (to determine if there is some obstruction of the upper air passages, such as enlarged adenoids) or orthodontic treatment may be required to permit the normal closure of the lips during sleep. A protective ointment such as Vaseline or Orabase may be applied to the gums at night. The oral changes that are associated with blood dyscrasias are described in the sections devoted to that subject. Generalized gingival enlargement (Figure 7-49, A) is occasionally one of the earlier symptoms of these diseases.

Fibrotic Gingival Enlargement

Gingival lesions of the fibrotic type have a normal pink color, or they may be slightly paler than normal. The tissue is firm, hard, and fibrous in consistency (because of the increase in fibrous tissue) and does not bleed readily or pit on pressure. Typical examples of gingival fibrosis are found in the gingival enlargements associated with the administration of the immunosuppressant cyclosporine, several calcium channel blocking agents, or phenytoin (Dilantin) and its derivatives and in diffuse fibromatosis of the gingiva. A fibrotic gingival enlargement may develop in any patient with long-standing gingival hyperplasia.

Phenytoin-Induced Gingival Hyperplasia

Phenytoin-induced gingival hyperplasia[296–298] (see Figure 7-49, B) affects at least 40 to 50% of patients who use the drug for longer than 3 months. More severe effects may not develop until after several years of continued use. Evidence from animal studies, individual case reports, and clinical trials indicates that both the drug and local irritation from plaque and calculus or restorations and appliances are etiologic factors. If gingival irritation can be eliminated completely, gingival hyperplasia will be only minimal at most.[299] Continuous and obvious irritation, such as that associated with banded orthodontic appliances, is often associated with very severe hyperplasia. The pathogenesis of the gingival changes caused by phenytoin is still unknown; earlier suggestions that the gingival collagen is modified or that reduced serum and salivary immunoglobulin A (IgA) associated with the chronic use of phenytoin are the cause of the hyperplasia have not been confirmed. In fact, the available data still indicate that the mature fibrous-type phenytoin-induced gingival lesion represents neither hypertrophy, hyperplasia, nor fibrosis but is an example of the uncontrolled growth of a connective tissue of apparently normal cell and fiber composition.

The clinical appearance of phenytoin-induced gingival hyperplasia is characteristic although numerous variants are seen, depending on the location of the lesion, the particular irritant involved, and the extent of secondary inflammatory changes. The diagnosis is made from the history of chronic phenytoin use and the clinical appearance of the lesions; biopsy specimens and measurement of serum levels of phenytoin offer no additional diagnostic information. With very rare exceptions, the hyperplasia is restricted to the gingivae. After extraction of teeth and excision of the hyperplastic tissue, there is no recurrence.

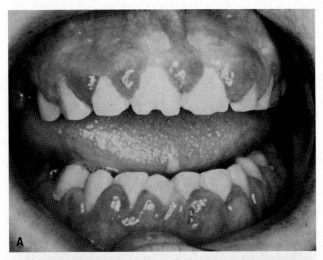

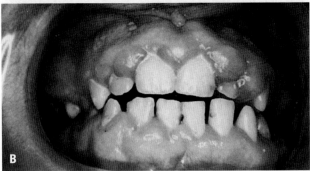

FIGURE 7-49   A, Generalized gingival enlargement in a patient with untreated monocytic leukemia. **B,** Fibrotic enlargement associated with the administration of phenytoin in a 17-year-old female.

Treatment of phenytoin-induced gingival hyperplasia[300] should emphasize the elimination of local gingival irritants, scrupulous oral hygiene, and interdental massage. Seizures can often be controlled by other nonhydantoin derivatives, and the physician, the patient, and the family may be willing to experiment with supervised alteration of the patient's anticonvulsive medications in order to reduce the hyperplasia.[301] In general, nonhydantoin derivatives are not associated with gingival hyperplasia although such an association has been described with primidone therapy.[302]

Menarche frequently brings a period of difficult management, partly because of the increased frequency of seizures that may occur at this time, partly because orthodontic treatment is usually begun about this time, and partly because of the patient's increased awareness of any orofacial cosmetic defects as adolescence progresses. Some authors advocate that phenytoin be routinely avoided in treating female adolescents, to exclude the possibility of both gingival hyperplasia and hirsutism. The epileptic patient's medication should at least always be reviewed before orthodontic treatment is begun.

Topically applied medications, including antiplaque agents such as chlorhexidine[303] have no effect on the gingival over-

growth although they provide effective plaque control and reduce gingivitis. Hyperplasia of any degree will not be resolved simply by removing local gingival irritants, and excision of hyperplastic gingivae, root planing, and the elimination of rough margins on restorations are usually necessary before adequate gingival hygiene and plaque control can be established. If gingivectomy is not followed by adequate home care and the use of interdental massage, hyperplasia will recur. A customized splint may be constructed to retain the periodontal dressing needed after gingivectomy, ligating it to anterior and posterior teeth to prevent the pack from being dislodged and aspirated during a convulsive seizure. The epileptic patient with brain damage and mental deficits often presents a difficult management problem, particularly if neither parents nor nurses can provide adequate toothbrushing and gingival hygiene. In such cases, the value of gingivectomy must be carefully considered; gingevectomy should be resorted to only when the overgrowth interferes with closure of the teeth or lips or is a source of severe halitosis or hemorrhage.

Other nonsurgical treatments proposed for phenytoin-induced gingival hyperplasia include topical antihistamines and corticosteroids (neither of which has been subjected to a controlled clinical trial) and topical and systemic treatment with folate. Phenytoin resembles folic acid structurally and may serve as a competitive inhibitor of folate metabolism. Folic acid deficiency (subnormal serum folate and macrocytosis) develops in 40 to 90% of patients treated with anticonvulsants, and defects in folic acid utilization have also been described in others who have apparently normal serum folic acid levels.[304] A controlled clinical trial of topical folate rinse (1 mg/mL) versus systemic folate (4 mg daily) in a small group of patients treated with phenytoin for a minimum of 3 months also showed some reduction in hyperplasia and mean periodontal probing depth, without any reduction in plaque or gingival indices.[305] Since the administration of folate supplements to patients who are receiving phenytoin anticonvulsant therapy appears not to increase the risk of seizures,[306] topical folate (which proved to be more effective than systemic folate in this trial) is a safe supplemental therapy for phenytoin-induced gingival hyperplasia. Phenytoin taken during pregnancy, with or without barbiturates, produces a two- to threefold increase in congenital anomalies. Affected offspring exhibit a variety of musculoskeletal growth defects, psychomotor retardation, and facial deformities, including ocular hypertelorism, depressed nasal bridge, hypertrichosis, and wide mouth. Although broad alveolar ridges have been reported in 30% of cases, gingival fibromatosis apparently does not occur with this route of administration.

Gingival Hyperplasia Induced by Cyclosporin A and Calcium Channel Blockers

For more than 40 years, phenytoin and its derivatives were the only drugs that were known to be associated with gingival hyperplasia.[298,307] In the last 10 years, however, two new classes of drugs, the immunosuppressant cyclosporine[308] and several calcium channel blockers[309–315] developed for treatment of hypertension and hypertensive cardiovascular disease, have been shown to have similar effects clinically, in experimental animals and in vitro.[316] In general, the changes that are produced by these new agents are very similar to changes that are associated with phenytoin therapy although differences in the latent period for the development of gingival changes have been described.‖ Two of the calcium channel blockers (oxodipine and nifedipine) also appear to cause hyperplasia of the labial mandibular gingiva rather than generalized gingival enlargement[314] although this phenomenon may reflect species and dose rather than specific drug effects. In comparison with phenytoin-induced gingival hyperplasia, hyperplasia caused by calcium channel blockers (both substituted dihydropyridines and verapamil) is probably of low incidence but is similarly dose dependent (with nifedipine, 48 mg/d produced gingival hyperplasia whereas 35 mg/d did not)[312] and positively correlated with oral hygiene and with the degree of gingival inflammation.[298] However, only limited epidemiologic investigations of drug-induced gingival hyperplasia other than those of phenytoin-induced changes have been reported.

Phenytoin, cyclosporin A, and the substituted dihydropyridines are chemically dissimilar compounds, and no common metabolic breakdown product that might serve as a common denominator has been identified. However, all three influence calcium/sodium (Ca^{++}/Na^+) flux, and this effect has been proposed as the common mechanism for development of the gingival hyperplasia associated with the three classes of drugs. Because folic acid is actively taken up at the cellular level by a Na^+-dependent transport mechanism, the effect of these three drugs on folic acid metabolism is being investigated. Two other findings associated with the gingival hyperplasia induced by these newer agents may provide new avenues for investigating the long-recognized but poorly understood phenomenon of drug-induced gingival overgrowth; these are

---

‖The following calcium channel blockers are associated with fibroblastic proliferation in vitro and gingival hyperplasia in man and experimental animals (specific data on unreferenced drugs are unavailable):[297]
1. Verapamil[309] (Calan, G.D. Searle & Co., Chicago, Ill.; Isoptin, Knoll Pharmaceuticals, Division BASF, K&F Corporation, Whippany, N.J.)
2. Substituted dihydropyridines currently marketed in the United States for treatment of hypertension, angina pectoris, cardiac arrhythmias, and other indications: diltiazem[310] (Cardiazem, Marion Merrell Dow Inc., Kansas City, Mo.), nicardipine (Cardene, Syntex Puerto Rico Inc., Humacao, Puerto Rico), nifedipine[311,312] (Procardia, Pfizer Inc., New York, N.Y.; Adalat, Miles Inc., West Haven, Conn.), nimodipine (Nimorop, Miles Inc.) (used for treatment of cerebrovascular spasm postsubarachnoid hemorrhage), bleomycin (Blenoxane, Bristol-Myers, Evansville, Ind.) (used for chemotherapy for brain tumors, multiple myeloma, and Hodgkin's and non-Hodgkin's lymphomas)
3. Other experimental substituted dihyropyridines, some currently marketed overseas: felodipine, isradipine, nisoldipine, nitrendipine (an analogue of nifedipine),[313] and oxodipine[314,315]

---

the production of gingival hyperplasia without inflammatory changes in rats treated with the experimental drug oxodipine[314] and the recognition of ultrastructural myofibroblastic modification of over 20% of the fibroblasts in human cyclosporine-induced hyperplastic gingiva.[317]

Syndromes Associated with Diffuse Gingival Enlargement

Diffuse or generalized fibromatosis, papillomatosis, or angiomatosis of the gingivae are less common forms of gingival hyperplasia and are congenital or inherited disorders in many cases (Figure 7-50) although diffuse enlargement of the gingivae can also be a response to widespread local irritants, with or without a systemic factor.[60,318–320] The enlargement may be present at birth or may become apparent only with the eruption of the deciduous or permanent dentitions. The following pathogenetic mechanisms are involved: hemangiomatous enlargement, infiltration of the gingival tissues by macrophages and other cells containing abnormal metabolic products, fibrotic reaction in gingivae overlying multiple impacted or grossly carious or hypoplastic teeth, and idiopathic fibrosis (possibly on a genetic basis). In many cases, the affected individuals have received phenytoin therapy to control the effects of associated central nervous system abnormalities and seizures. In such cases, it may be difficult to separate the basic gingival abnormality from a secondary phenytoin-induced hyperplasia.

If well developed, the dense and firm gingival tissue results in varying spacing of the teeth and in changes in profile and general facial appearance (Figure 7-51). The hyperplasia may be so excessive as to crowd the tongue, interfere with speech, cause difficulty in chewing food, and prevent normal closure of the lips. The surface of the hyperplastic tissue usually has a papillary or nodular appearance. Changes in the underlying alveolar bone are unusual in these patients unless progressive periodontitis develops as a complication of secondary plaque and calculus deposits.

Gingival fibromatosis can occur as a sporadic finding with or without associated physical or mental abnormalities; alter-

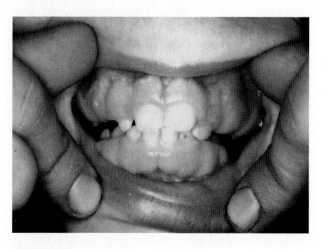

FIGURE 7-50   Familial gingival hyperplasia.

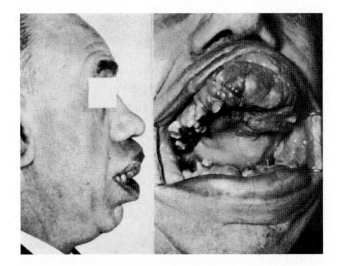

FIGURE 7-51   Profile and intraoral appearance of a 49-year-old male before all visible and easily accessible teeth were removed, after which he was able to appose his lips for the first time in his life. Gingivae had been resected several times before. The father, son, and daughter all suffered from hereditary gingivofibromatosis. (Reproduced with permission from Winstock D. Hereditary gingivofibromatosis. Br J Oral Surg 1964;2:61)

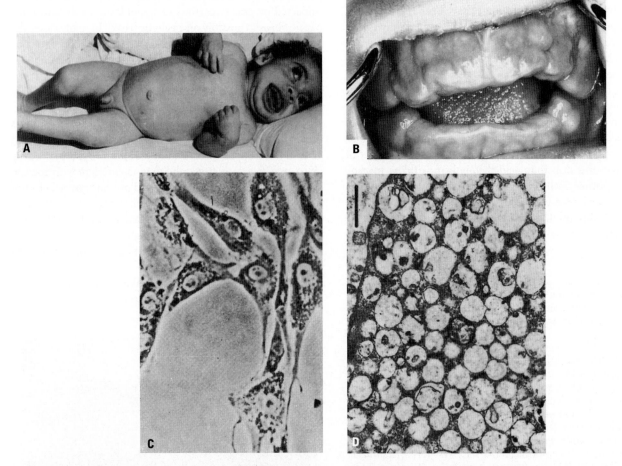

FIGURE 7-52   A, Pronounced gingival hyperplasia in this 12-month-old child is associated with mucolipidosis II (I-cell disease). (Reproduced with permission from Galili D et al.[335]) **B,** Hyperplasia, developed during the first year of life and before the eruption of deciduous dentition. This hyperplasia was noted in association with multiple developmental abnormalities, skeletal changes (similar to those of Hurler's syndrome) in the lower limbs and pelvis, unusual facies, and psychomotor retardation. The enlarged gingival tissue was firm and hard and obstructed mastication and closure of the mouth. (Reproduced with permission from Galili D et al[335]) **C,** Fibroblasts cultured from the skin biopsy specimen, showing numerous granular inclusions and the complete absence of lysosomal β-galactosidase activity. (Reproduced with permission from Terashima Y et al.[336]) **D,** Electron microscopic examination of gingival fibroblasts shows numerous membrane-limited empty vacuoles distending these cells. (Courtesy of Daniel Galili, DMD, Jerusalem, Israel) (Reproduced with permission from Mart JJ et al. Acta Neuropathol 1975;33:285)

TABLE 7-4 Syndromes Associated with Diffuse Gingival Enlargement (Gingival Fibromatosis, Papillomatosis, and Angiomatosis Syndromes)

Eponym* or Name of Syndrome	Characteristic Features	Associated Features	Reference
Autosomal dominant inheritance			
No eponym	Gingival fibromatosis with hypertrichosis, epilepsy, and mental retardation	Skeletal anomalies; commonest gingival fibromatosis syndrome	321, 322
Rutherford	Congenitally enlarged gingivae, delayed tooth eruption, "curtainlike" superior corneal opacities	Mental retardation, aggressive behavior, dentigerous cysts; only one kindred reported	323
Zimmerman-Laband	Gingival fibromatosis with defects of ears, nose, bones, nails, and terminal phalanges ("froglike" fingers and toes)	Hyperextensible joints, characteristic facies, hepatosplenomegaly	324, 325, 326
Cowden	Gingival papillomas as part of widespread oral, facial, and pharyngeal papillomatosis	Multiple hamartomas and neoplasms (see Table 7-3)	239, 240
No eponym	Familial gingival fibromatosis with progressive neurosensory hearing loss in young adults	Two extensive kindred reported	327
Tuberous sclerosis	Single or multiple fibromas of gingivae, oral mucosa, and skin (adenoma sebaceum), in association with other features of tuberous sclerosis	Epilepsy, mental retardation, and hamartomas of brain, heart, and kidney (see Table 7-3)	228, 229, 230
Gorlin-Goltz (focal dermal hypoplasia)	Gingival and other oral mucosal papillomatosis; lip and tooth defects	Poikiloderma, dermal fat herniation, adactyly and syndactyly; over 90% female	328, 329
Autosomal recessive inheritance			
Murray-Puretic-Drescher	Gingival fibromatosis with multiple juvenile PAS-positive hyaline fibromas of head ("turban tumors"), trunk, and extremities	Suppurative lesions of skin and mucosa, flexion contractures, mental retardation, elevated urinary hyaluronic acid and dermatan sulfate	330, 331, 332
Cross	Gingival and alveolar enlargement, microphthalmia cloudy corneas, hypopigmentation and athetosis	White hair, blond skin; melanocytes decreased with reduced tyrosine activity; mental retardation; very rare	333, 334
Ramon	Gingival fibromatosis, hypertrichosis, cherubism, mental retardation, and epilepsy; characteristic perivascular fibrosis in gingival biopsy specimens	Juvenile rheumatoid arthritis; gingival fibromatosis precedes cherubism	115
Lysosomal storage diseases†	Neonatal/childhood gingival enlargement (see Figure 7-46); widened alveolar ridges and/or widely spaced teeth	Specific enzymatic deficiencies; generalized visceromegaly (often with macroglossia) associated with lysosomal storage of intermediates (see Table 7-1)	60, 335, 336, 337
Sporadic or unknown pattern of inheritance			
No eponym	Gingival fibromatosis with or without bony involvement ("diffuse osteofibromatosis") and with no familial pattern or other associated findings	—	333, 339
No eponym	Gingival fibromatosis in a child with a new chromosome translocation	Hypertrichosis, facial anomalies, and sickle cell trait; single case reported	334
Sturge-Weber	Orofacial and meningeal angiomatosis with secondary mental deficiency, seizures, and hemiplegia; ipsilateral nevus flammeus and mild to severe gingival enlargement	Hyperplastic vascular gingivae blanch with pressure; bony hemangiomas and delayed tooth eruption	60, 63
Acanthosis nigricans (malignant variety)	Gingival papillomatosis associated with similar periorifacial, mucosal, and skin (pigmented) lesions	Gastric adenocarcinoma (see Table 7-3)	60, 201
Epidermal nevus (icthyosis hystrix lateris)	Cutaneous nevi that can extend to involve oral mucous membrane and gingiva, with localized warty papillomatosis	Mental deficiency, skeletal abnormalities, and hypoplastic teeth	338, 339

PAS = periodic acid–Schiff.

*A number of representative case reports are referenced in this table; see References 60 and 318 to 320 for additional citations.

†Hunter's (X-linked recessive), Hurler's, Morquio's, Maroteaux-Lamy, and Sly's syndromes; GM_1 gangliosidosis type I, aspartylglucosaminuria, mannosidosis, I-cell disease (see Figure 7-52), and sialic acid storage disease (sialuria).

natively, it may occur as part of a well-defined syndrome. Both autosomal dominant and autosomal recessive patterns of inheritance are recognized, as well as sporadic cases with no pedigree history. Genetic heterogeneity and variable expressivity also contribute to the difficulty encountered in assigning a diagnosis to familial gingival fibromatosis in specific clinical situations.[319] The treatment of gingival fibromatosis is often unsatisfactory. Gingivectomy is usually necessary although the tissue may regrow.

A list of the syndromes that are most consistently associated with diffuse gingival enlargement (Figure 7-52) is provided in Table 7-4.[321–339]

▼ REFERENCES

1. Bouquot JE, Gundlach KKH. Oral exophytic lesions in 23,616 white Americans over 35 years of age. Oral Surg Oral Med Oral Pathol 1986;62:284.

2. Knapp MJ. Oral tonsils: location, distribution, and histology, and pathology of oral tonsils. Oral Surg Oral Med Oral Pathol 1970;29:155–295.

3. King DR, King AC. Incidence of tori in three population groups. J Oral Med 1981;36:21.

4. Geist ET, Adams TO, Carr RF. The organ of Chievitz: its importance in the microscopic diagnosis of oral carcinoma. J Oral Med 1984;39:177.

5. MacLeod RI, Soames JV. Epulides: a clinicopathological study of a series of 200 consecutive lesions. Br Dent J 1987;163:51–3.

6. Daley TD, Wysocki GP, Wysocki PD, Wysocki DM. The major epulides: clinicopathological correlations. J Can Dent Assoc 1990;56:627.

7. Budtz-Jorgensen E. Oral mucosal lesions associated with the wearing of removable dentures. J Oral Pathol 1981;10:65.

8. Wood NK, Goaz PW. Oral exophytic lesions. In: Wood NK, Goaz PW. Differential diagnosis. 4th ed. St Louis: Mosby Year Book, 1991.

9. Manton SI, Egglestone SI, Alexander I, Scully C. Oral presentation of secondary syphilis. Br Dent J 1986;160:237.

10. Thwaites MS, Jeter TE, Ajagbe O. Inflammatory papillary hyperplasia: review of literature and case report involving a 10 year-old child. Quintessence Int 1990;21:133–8.

11. Rathofer SA, Gardner FM, Vermilyea SG. A comparison of healing and pain following excision of inflammatory papillary hyperplasia with electro-surgery and blade-loop knives in human patients. Oral Surg Oral Med Oral Pathol 1985;59:130.

12. Zain RB, Khoo SP, Yeo JF. Oral pyogenic granuloma (excluding pregnancy tumour)—a clinical analysis of 304 cases. Singapore Dent J 1995;20:8–10.

13. Daley TD, Nartley NI, Wysocki GP. Pregnancy tumor: an analysis. Oral Surg Oral Med Oral Pathol 1991;72:196.

14. Zachariasen RD. Ovarian hormones and oral health: pregnancy gingivitis. Compendium 1989;10:508.

15. Whitaker SB, Waldron CA. Central giant cell lesions of the jaws. A clinical, radiologic, and histopathologic study. Oral Surg Oral Med Oral Pathol 1993;75:199.

16. Ratner V, Dorfman HD. Giant-cell reparative granuloma of the hand and foot bones. Clin Orthop 1990;260:251.

17. Jaffe HL. Giant cell reparative granuloma, traumatic bone cyst, and fibrous (fibro-osseus) dysplasia of the jaw bones. Oral Surg Oral Med Oral Pathol 1953;6:159.

18. Hutter RVP, Worcester JN, Frances KC, et al. Benign and malignant giant cell tumors of bone. Cancer 1962;15:653.

19. Waldron CA, Shafer WG. The central giant cell reparative granuloma of the jaws: an analysis of 38 cases. Am J Clin Pathol 1966;45:437.

20. Giansanti JS, Waldron CA. Peripheral giant cell granuloma: review of 720 cases. Oral Surg Oral Med Oral Pathol 1969;277:787.

21. Eisenbud L, Stern M, Rothberg M, Sachs SA. Central giant cell granuloma of the jaws: experiences in the management of thirty-seven cases. J Oral Maxillofac Surg 1988;46:376.

22. Katsiteris N, Kakaranta-Angelopoulou E, Angelopoulou AP. Peripheral giant cell granuloma: clinicopathologic study of 224 new cases and review of 956 reported cases. Int J Oral Maxillofac Surg 1988;17:94.

23. Flaitz CM. Peripheral giant cell granuloma: a potentially aggressive lesion in children. Pediatr Dent 2000;22:232–3.

24. Abrams B, Shear M. A histological comparison of giant cells in the central giant cell granuloma of the jaws and the giant cell tumor of long bones. J Oral Pathol 1974;3:217.

25. Franklin CD, Craig GT, Smith CJ. Quantitative analysis of histological parameters in giant cell lesions of the jaws and long bones. Histopathology 1979;3:511.

26. Cohen MA, Hertzanu Y. Radiologic features including those seen with computed tomography of central giant cell granulomas of the jaws. Oral Surg Oral Med Oral Pathol 1988;65:255.

27. Macchia AF, Cassalia PT. Primary hyperparathyroidism: report of a case. J Am Dent Assoc 1970;81:1153.

28. Avioli LV. The diagnosis of primary hyperparathyroidism. Med Clin North Am 1968;52:451.

29. Khafif A, Krempl G, Medina JE. Treatment of giant cell granuloma of the maxilla with intralesional injection of steroids. Head Neck 2000;22:822–5.

30. Eversole LR, Christensen R, Ficarra G, et al. Nodular fasciitis and solitary fibrous tumor of the oral region: tumors of fibroblast heterogeneity. Oral Surg Oral Med Oral Pathol Oral Radiol Endod 1999;87:471–6.

31. Shimizu S, Hashimoto H, Enjoji M. Nodular fasciitis: an analysis of 250 patients. Pathology 1984;16:161.

32. Fujiwara K, Watanabe T, Katsuki T, et al. Proliferative myositis of the buccinator muscle: a case with immunohistochemical and electron microscopic analysis. Oral Surg Oral Med Oral Pathol 1987;63:597.

33. Azuma T, Komori A, Nagayama M. Focal myositis of the tongue. J Oral Maxillofac Surg 1987;45:953.

34. McLendon CI, Levine PA, Mills SE, Black WC. Squamous cell carcinoma masquerading as focal myositis of the tongue. Head Neck 1989;11:353.

35. van der Wal N, Baak JP, Schipper NW, van der Waal I. Morphometric study of pseudoepitheliomatous hyperplasia in giant cell tumors of the tongue. J Oral Pathol Med 1989;18:8–10.

36. Krasne DL, Warnke RA, Weiss LM. Malignant lymphoma presenting as pseudoepitheliomatous hyperplasia: a report of two cases. Am J Surg Pathol 1988;12:835.

37. Bradley G, Main JHP, Birt BD, From I. Benign lymphoid hyperplasia of the palate. J Oral Pathol 1987;16:18.

38. Napier SS, Newlands C. Benign lymphoid hyperplasia of the palate: report of two cases and immunohistochemical profile. J Oral Pathol Med 1990;19:221.

39. Wirt DP, Grogan TM, Jolley CS, et al. The immunoarchitecture of cutaneous pseudolymphoma. Hum Pathol 1985;16:492.

40. Willis RA. Hamartomas and hamartomatous syndromes. In: The borderland of embryology and pathology. London: Butterworth, 1962.

41. Stahl S, Hanilt S, Spira M. Hemangiomas, lymphangiomas and vascular malformations of the head and neck. Otolaryngol Clin North Am 1986;19:769.

42. Stofman GM, Reiter D, Feldman MD. Invasive intramuscular hemangiomas of the head and neck. Ear Nose Throat J 1989;68:612.

43. Ohtsuka H. Port-wine stain: distribution patterns on the face and neck. Ann Plastic Surg 1990;24:409.

44. Shanin R, Kohn G, Mctzker A. Nevus flammeus. Discordance in monozygotic twins. Am J Dis Child 1991;145:85.

45. Motamedi MH, Behnia H, Motamedi MR. Surgical technique for the treatment of high-flow arteriovenous malformations of the mandible. J Maxillofac Surg 2000;28(4):238–42.

46. Oates CP, Wilson AW, Ward-Booth RP, Williams FD. Combined use of Doppler and conventional ultrasound for the diagnosis of vascular and other lesions of the head and neck. Int J Oral Maxillofac Surg 1990;19:235.

47. Sloan GM, Bolton LL, Miller JH, et al. Radionuclide-labelled red blood cell imaging of vascular malformations in children. Ann Plastic Surg 1988;21:236.

48. Beltramello A, Benati A, Perini S, Maschio A. Interventional neuroangiography in neuropediatrics. Childs Nerv Syst 1989;5:87.

49. Bartlett JA, Riding KH, Salkeld LJ. Management of hemangiomas of the head and neck in children. J Otolaryngol 1988;17:11.

50. Gongloff RK. Treatment of intraoral hemangiomas with nitrous oxide cryosurgery. Oral Surg Oral Med Oral Pathol 1983;56:20.

51. Suen JY, Waner M. Treatment of oral cavity vascular malformations using the neodymium: YAG laser. Arch Otolaryngol Head Neck Surg 1989;115:1329.

52. Malm M, Jurell G, Glas JE. Argon laser treatment of port wine stain. Scand J Plast Reconstr Surg Hand Surg 1988;22:245.

53. Minkow B, Laufer D, Gutman D. Treatment of oral hemangiomas with local sclerosing agents. Int J Oral Surg 1979;8:18.

54. Fradis M, Podoskin L, Simon J, et al. Treatment of 7 cases of capillo-venous malformation localized to the head and neck with a fibrosing agent, Ethibloc, prior to surgery. J Laryngol Otol 1989;103:390.

55. Schwartz DN, Kellman RM, Cacayorin ED. Treatment of a lingual hemangioma by superselective embolization. Arch Otolaryngol Head Neck Surg 1986;112:96.

56. Hashimoto Y, Matsuhiro K, Nagaki M, Tanioka H. Therapeutic embolization for vascular lesions of the head and neck. Two cases. Int J Oral Maxillofac Surg 1989;18:47.

57. Furst CJ, Lundell M, Holm LE. Radiation therapy of hemangiomas, 1909–1959. A cohort based on 50 years of clinical practice at Radiumhemmet, Stockholm. Acta Oncol 1987;26:33.

58. Talmi Y, Valmanovitch M, Zohar Y. Thyroid carcinoma, cataract and hearing loss in a patient after irradiation for facial hemangioma. J Laryngol Otol 1988;102:91.

59. Sloan CM, Reinisch JF, Nichter LS, et al. Intralesional corticosteroid treatment for infantile hemangiomas. Plast Reconstr Surg 1989;83:459.

60. Gorlin RJ, Cohen MM, Jr. Levin LS. Syndromes of the head and neck. 3rd ed. New York: Oxford University Press; 1990.

61. Jellinger K. Vascular malformations of the central nervous system: a morphological overview. Neurosurg Rev 1986;9:177.

62. Hylton RP. Use of CO2 laser for gingivectomy in a patient with Sturge-Weber disease complicated by dilantin hyperplasia. J Oral Maxillofac Surg 1986;44:646.

63. Wilson S, Venzel JM, Miller R. Angiography, gingival hyperplasia and Sturge-Weber syndrome: report of case. ASDC J Dent Child 1986;53:283.

64. Flint SR, Keith O, Sully C. Hereditary hemorrhagic telangiectasia: family study and review. Oral Surg Oral Med Oral Pathol 1988;66:440.

65. Laskaris G, Skouteris C. Maffucci's syndrome: report of case with oral hemangiomas. Oral Surg Oral Med Oral Pathol 1984;57:263.

66. Wolf M, Engelberg S. Recurrent oral bleeding in Maffuci's syndrome: report of a case. J Oral Maxillofac Surg 1993;51:596.

67. Kounis NG, Karapanou E, Dimopoulos P. The von Hippel-Lindau syndrome: report of a case and review of the literature. Br J Clin Pract 1989;43:37.

68. Schimke RN. Multiple endocrine neoplasia: how many syndromes? Am J Med Genet 1990;37:375.

69. Caviness VS. Neurocutaneous syndromes and other developmental disorders of the central nervous system. In: Wilson JD, Braunwald E, Isselbacher KJ, et al, editors. Harrison's principles of internal medicine. 12th ed. New York: McGraw-Hill; 1991.

70. Gorlin RJ, Goldman HM. Thoma's oral pathology. 6th ed. St Louis: CV Mosby; 1970.

71. Levin LS, Jorgenson RJ, Jarvey BA. Lymphangiomas of the alveolar ridges in neonates. Pediatrics 1976;58:881.

72. Zacharides N, Koundouris I. Lymphangioma of the oral cavity: report of a case. J Oral Med 1984;39:33.

73. Dolan EA, Riski JE, Mason RM. Macroglossia: clinical considerations. Int J Orofacial Myology 1989;152:4.

74. Ricciardelli EJ, Richardson MA. Cervicofacial cystic hygroma. Patterns of recurrence and management of difficult cases. Arch Otolaryngol Head Neck Surg 1991;117:546.

75. Batsakis JG. Tumors of the head and neck. Clinical and pathological considerations. 2nd ed. Baltimore: Williams & Wilkins; 1979.

76. Moody GH, Myskow M, Musgrove C. Glomus tumor of the lip. A case report and immunohistochemical study. Oral Surg Oral Med Oral Pathol 1986;62:312.

77. Ficarra G, Merrell PW, Johnston WH, Hansen LS. Intraoral solitary glomus tumor (glomangioma): case report and literature review. Oral Surg Oral Med Oral Pathol 1986;62:306.

78. Griffin CJ. Glomus tumor in the bilaminar zone of the temporomandibular meniscus. Aust Dent J 1962;7:377.

79. Harvey JA, Walker F. Solid glomus tumor of the pterygoid fossa: a lesion mimicking an epithelial neoplasm of low-grade malignancy. Hum Pathol 1987;18:965.

80. Williams HK, Williams DM. Oral granular cell tumours: a histological and immunocytochemical study. J Oral Pathol Med 1997;26:164–9.

81. Stewart CM, Watson RE, Eversole LR, et al. Oral granular cell tumors: a clinicopathologic and immunocytochemical study. Oral Surg Oral Med Oral Pathol 1988;65:427.

82. Mittal KR, True LD. Origin of granules in giant cell tumors. Intracellular myelin formation with autodigestion. Arch Pathol Lab Med 1988;112:302.

83. Wright BA, Jackson D. Neural tumors of the oral cavity: a review of the spectrum of benign and malignant oral tumors of the oral cavity and jaws. Oral Surg Oral Med Oral Pathol 1980;49:509.

84. Zacharides N, Mezitis M, Vairaktaris E, et al. Benign neurogenic tumors of the oral cavity. Int J Oral Maxillofac Surg 1987;16:78.

85. Chrysomali E, Papanicolaou SI, Dekker NP, Regezi JA. Benign neural tumors of the oral cavity: a comparative immunohistochemical study. Oral Surg Oral Med Oral Pathol Oral Radiol Endod 1997;84(4):381–90.

86. Colmeneno C, Rivers T, Patron M, et al. Maxillofacial malignant peripheral nerve sheath tumors. J Craniomaxillofac Surg 1991;19:40.

87. Chavin PJ, Wysocki GP, Daley TD, Pringle GA. Palisaded encapsulated neuroma of oral mucosa. Oral Surg Oral Med Oral Pathol 1992;73:71.

88. Sist TC, Greene GW. Traumatic neuroma of the oral cavity: report of thirty-one new cases and review of the literature. Oral Surg Oral Med Oral Pathol 1981;51:394.

89. Pettinato G, Manivel JC, d'Amore ESG, et al. Melanotic neuroectodermal tumor of infancy. A reexamination of a histogenetic problem based on immunohistochemical, flow cytometric and ultrastructural study of 10 cases. Am J Surg Pathol 1991;15:233.

90. Bouckaert MM, Raubenheimer EJ. Gigantiform melanotic neuroectodermal tumor of infancy. Oral Surg Oral Med Oral Pathol Oral Radiol Endod 1998;86:569–72.

91. Stokry A, Briner J, Makek M. Malignant neuroectodermal tumor of infancy: a case report. Pediatr Pathol 1986;5:217.

92. Grabias SL, Campbell CJ. Fibrous dysplasia. Orthop Clin North Am 1977;8:771–83.

93. Mirra JM, Picci P, Gold RH. Bone tumors: clinical, radiologic and pathologic correlations. Philadelphia: Lea & Febiger; 1989.

94. Waldron CA. Fibro-osseous lesions of the jaws. J Oral Maxillofac Surg 1985;43:249.

95. Hall MB, Sclar AG, Gardner DF. Albright's syndrome with reactivation of fibrous dysplasia secondary to pituitary adenoma and further complicated by osteogenic sarcoma: report of a case. Oral Surg Oral Med Oral Pathol 1984;54:616.

96. Blomgren I, Lilja J, Lauritzen C, Magnusson B. Multiple craniofacial surgical interventions during 25 years of follow-up in a case of giant fibrous dysplasia. Case report. Scand J Plast Reconstr Surg 1986;20:327.

97. Williams HK, Mangham C, Speight PM. Juvenile ossifying fibroma. An analysis of eight cases and a comparison with other fibro-osseous lesions. J Oral Pathol Med 2000;29(1):13–8.

98. Higashi T, Iguchi M, Shimura A, Kruglik GD. Computed tomography and bone scintigraphy in polyostotic fibrous dysplasia. Report of a case. Oral Surg Oral Med Oral Pathol 1980;50:580.

99. Stuhler T, Brucker W, Kaiser G, Poppe H. Fibrous dysplasia in the light of new diagnostic methods. Arch Orthop Trauma Surg 1979;94:255.

100. Levine MA. Clinical implications of genetic defects in G proteins: oncogenic mutations in G alpha s as the molecular basis for the McCune-Albright syndrome. Arch Med Res 1999;30(6):522–31.

101. Waldron CA. Fibro-osseous lesions of the jaws. J Oral Surg 1970;28:58.

102. Hamner JE III, Scofield HH, Cornyn J. Benign fibro-osseous jaw lesions of periodontal membrane origin. Cancer 1968;22:861.

103. Waldron CA, Giansanti JS. Benign fibro-osseous lesions of the jaws: a clinico-radiologic-histologic review of sixty-five cases: I. Fibrous dysplasia of the jaws. II. Benign fibro-osseous lesions of periodontal ligament origin. Oral Surg Oral Med Oral Pathol 1973;35:190, 340.

104. Eversole LR, Sabes WR, Rovin S. Fibrous dysplasia: a nosologic problem in the diagnosis of fibro-osseous lesions of the jaws. J Oral Pathol 1972;1:189.

105. Zachariades N, Vairakteris E, Mezitis M, et al. Aneurysmal bone cyst of the jaws. Review of the literature and report of 2 cases. Int J Oral Maxillofac Surg 1986;15:534.

106. Toljanic JA, Lechewski E, Hervos AG, et al. Aneurysmal bone cysts of the jaw: a case study and review of the literature. Oral Surg Oral Med Oral Pathol 1987;64:72.

107. Kaugars GE, Cale AE. Traumatic bone cyst. Oral Surg Oral Med Oral Pathol 1987;63:318.

108. Correll RW, Jensen JC, Rhyne RR. Lingual cortical mandibular defects: a radiographic incidence study. Oral Surg Oral Med Oral Pathol 1980;50:287.

109. Barker GR. A radiolucency of the ascending ramus of the mandible associated with invested parotid salivary gland material and analogous with a Stafne bone cavity. Br J Oral Maxillofac Surg 1988;26:81.

110. Friedman E, Eisenbud L. Surgical and pathological complications in cherubism. Int J Oral Surg 1981;10(Suppl 1):52–7.

111. Zacharides N, Papanicolaou S, Xypolyta A, et al. Cherubism. Int J Oral Surg 1985;14:138.

112. Hamner JE III, Ketcham AS. Cherubism: an analysis of treatment. Cancer 1969;23:1133.

113. DeThomasi DC, Hann JR, Stewart HM. Cherubism: report of a nonfamilial case. J Am Dent Assoc 1985;111:455.

114. Dunlap C, Neville B, Vickers RA, et al. The Noonan syndrome/cherubism association. Oral Surg Oral Med Oral Pathol 1989;67:698.

115. Ramon Y, Berman W, Bubis JJ. Gingival fibromatosis combined with cherubism. Oral Surg Oral Med Oral Pathol 1967;24:436.

116. Roediger WE, Spitz L, Schmaman A. Histogenesis of benign cervical teratomas. Teratology 1974;10:111.

117. Arcand P, Granger J, Brochu P. Congenital dermoid cyst of the oral cavity with gastric choristoma. J Otolaryngol 1988;17:219.

118. Black EE, Leathers RD, Youngblood D. Dermoid cyst of the floor of the mouth. Oral Surg Oral Med Oral Pathol 1993;75:556.

119. Zeltser R, Milhem I, Azaz B, Hasson O. Dermoid cysts of floor of the mouth: report of four cases. Am J Otolaryngol 2000;21:55–60.

120. Shear M. Cysts of the oral region. 3rd ed. Oxford: Wright/Butterworth-Heinemann Ltd.; 1992.

121. Pindborg JJ, Kramer IRH, Torloni H. Histologic typing of odontogenic tumors, jaw cysts and allied lesions. WHO International Classification of Tumours series No. 5. Geneva: World Health Organization; 1971.

122. Kramer IRH, Pindborg JJ, Shear M. Histological typing of odontogenic tumors. 2nd ed. WHO International Histological Classification of Tumours series. Berlin: Springer Verlag; 1992.

123. Main DMG. Epithelial jaw cysts: 10 years of the WHO classification. J Oral Pathol 1985;14:1.

124. Shear M. Cysts of the jaw: recent advances. J Oral Pathol 1985;14:43.

125. Browne RM. Investigative pathology of the odontogenic cysts. Boca Raton: CRC Press, Inc.; 1991.

126. Marmary Y, Kutiner G. A radiographic survey of periapical jaw bone lesions. Oral Surg Oral Med Oral Pathol 1986;61:405.

127. Thawley SE, Panje WR, Batsakis JG, Lindberg RD. Comprehensive management of head and neck tumors. Philadelphia: W.B. Saunders; 1987.

128. Miles DA, van Dis M, Kaugars GF, Lovas JGL. Oral and maxillofacial radiology: radiologic/pathologic correlations. Philadelphia: W.B. Saunders; 1991.

129. Gardner DG, Sapp JP, Wysocki GP. Odontogenic and "fissural" cysts of jaws. Pathol Annu 1978;13(Pt I):177.

130. Browne RM. The pathogenesis of odontogenic cysts: a review. J Oral Pathol 1975;4:31.

131. Maxymiw WG, Wood RE. Carcinoma arising in a dentigerous cyst: a case report and review of the literature. J Oral Maxillofac Surg 1991;49:639.

132. Al-Talabani NG, Smith CJ. Experimental dentigerous cysts and enamel hypoplasia: their possible significance in explaining the pathogenesis of human dentigerous cysts. J Oral Pathol 1980;9:82.

133. Struthers PJ, Shear M. Root resorption produced by the enlargement of ameloblastomas and cysts of the jaws. Int J Oral Surg 1976;5:128.

134. Gardner DG. Plexiform unicystic ameloblastoma: a diagnostic problem in dentigerous cysts. Cancer 1981;47:1358.

135. Berenholz L, Gottlieb RD, Cho SY, Lowry LD. Squamous cell carcinoma arising in a dentigerous cyst. Ear Nose Throat J 1988;67:764.

136. Vedtofte P, Practorius F. Recurrence of the odontogenic keratocyst in relation to clinical and histological features. A 20 year follow-up study of 72 patients. Int J Oral Surg 1979;8:412.

137. Blanas N, Freund B, Schwartz M, Furst IM. Systematic review of the treatment and prognosis of the odontogenic keratocyst. Oral Surg Oral Med Oral Pathol Oral Radiol Endod 2000;90(5):553–8.

138. Swanson AE. The recalcitrant keratocyst. Int J Oral Maxillofac Surg 1986;15:451.

139. Koppang HS, Johannessen S, Haugen LK, et al. Glandular odontogenic cyst (sialo-odontogenic cyst): report of two cases and literature review of 45 previously reported cases. J Oral Pathol Med 1998;27:455–62.

140. Ohba T, Ogawa Y, Hiromatsu T, Shinohara Y. Experimental comparison of radiographic techniques in the detection of maxillary sinus disease. Dentomaxillofac Radiol 1990;19:13.

141. Scaccia FJ, Strauss M, Arnold J, Maniglia AJ. Maxillary ameloblastoma: case report. Am J Otolaryngol 1991;12:20.

142. Stewart JCB. Odontogenic tumors. In: Regezi JA, Sciubba JJ, editors. Oral pathology: clinical-pathologic correlations. 2nd ed. Philadelphia: W.B. Saunders; 1993.

143. Inoue N, Shimojyo M, Iwai H, et al. Malignant ameloblastoma with pulmonary metastasis and hypercalcemia. Report of an autopsy case and review of the literature. Am J Clin Pathol 1988;90:474.

144. Walsh KM. Classification of epithelial odontogenic tumors (domestic animals). J Comp Pathol 1987;97:503.

145. Hong SP, Ellis GL, Hartman KS. Calcifying odontogenic cyst. A review of ninety-two cases with reevaluation of their nature as cysts or neoplasms, the nature of ghost cells, and sub-classification. Oral Surg Oral Med Oral Pathol 1991;72:56.

146. Buchner A, Merrell PW, Hangen LS, Leider AS. Peripheral (extraosseous) calcifying odontogenic cyst. Oral Surg Oral Med Oral Pathol 1991;72:65.

147. Gardner DG. A pathologist's approach to the treatment of ameloblastoma. J Oral Maxillofac Surg 1984;42:161.

148. Muller H, Stootweg P. The ameloblastoma, the controversial approach to therapy. J Maxillofac Surg 1985;13:79.

149. Li TJ, Wu YT, Yu SF, Yu GY. Unicystic ameloblastoma: a clinicopathologic study of 33 Chinese patients. Am J Surg Pathol 2000;24(10):1385–92.

150. Waldron C, El-Mofty S. A histopathologic study of 116 ameloblastomas with reference to the desmoplastic variety. Oral Surg Oral Med Oral Pathol 1987;63:441.

151. Corio R, Goldblatt L, Edwards S, et al. Ameloblastic carcinoma: a clinicopathologic study and assessment of eight cases. Oral Surg Oral Med Oral Pathol 1987;64:570.

152. Slootweg P, Muller H. Malignant ameloblastoma or ameloblastic carcinoma. Oral Surg Oral Med Oral Pathol 1984;57:168.

153. Baden E, Doyle JL, Petriella V. Malignant transformation of peripheral ameloblastoma. Oral Surg Oral Med Oral Pathol 1993;75:214.

154. Gardner DG, O'Neill PA. Inability to distinguish ameloblastomas from odontogenic cysts based on expression of blood cell carbohydrates. Oral Surg Oral Med Oral Pathol 1988;66:480.

155. Philipsen HP, Reichart PA. Adenomatoid odontogenic tumour: facts and figures. Oral Oncol 1999;35(2):125–31.

156. Giansanti JS, Someren A, Waldron CA. Odontogenic adenomatoid tumor (adenoameloblastoma). Survey of 3 cases. Oral Surg Oral Med Oral Pathol 1970;30:69.

157. Krolls SO, Pindborg JJ. Calcifying epithelial odontogenic tumor. A survey of 23 cases and discussion of histomorphologic variations. Arch Pathol 1974;98:206.

158. Philipsen HP, Reichart PA. Calcifying epithelial odontogenic tumour: biological profile based on 181 cases from the literature. Oral Oncol 2000;36(1):17–26.

159. Buchner A, Sciubba JJ. Peripheral epithelial odontogenic tumors: a review. Oral Surg Oral Med Oral Pathol 1987;63:688.

160. Reichart PA, Philipsen HP. Squamous odontogenic tumor. J Oral Pathol Med 1990;19:226.

161. Eversole L, Belton C, Hansen L. Clear cell odontogenic tumor: histochemical and ultrastructural features. J Oral Pathol 1985;14:603.

162. Happonen RP, Peltola J, Yipaavaluiemi P, Lamberg M. Myxoma of the jaws. An analysis of 13 cases. Proc Finn Dent Soc 1988;84:45–52.

163. Dunlap C, Barker B. Central odontogenic fibroma of the WHO type. Oral Surg Oral Med Oral Pathol 1984;57:390.

164. Allen CM, Hammond HL, Stimson PG. Central odontogenic fibroma WHO type. A report of three cases with an unusual associated giant cell reaction. Oral Surg Oral Med Oral Pathol 1992;73:62.

165. Melrose R, Abrams A, Mills B. Florid osseous dysplasia. Oral Surg Oral Med Oral Pathol 1976;41:62.

166. El-Mofty SK. Cemento-ossifying fibroma and benign cementoblastoma. Semin Diagn Pathol 1999;16(4):302–7.

167. Wilcox LR, Walton RE. Case of mistaken identity: periapical cemental dysplasia in an endodontically treated tooth. Endodod Dent Traumatol 1989;5:298–301.

168. Tanaka H, Yoshimoto A, Toyama Y. Periapical cemental dysplasia with multiple lesions. Int J Oral Maxillofac Surg 1987;16:757.

169. Eliasson S, Halvarsson C, Ljungheimer G. Periapical condensing osteitis and endodontic treatment. Oral Surg Oral Med Oral Pathol 1984;57:195.

170. Neville BW, Albenesius RJ. The prevalence of benign fibro-osseous lesions of periodontal ligament origin in black women: a radiographic survey. Oral Surg Oral Med Oral Pathol 1986;62:340.

171. Chaudhry AP, Spink JH, Gorlin RJ. Periapical fibrous dysplasia (cementoma). J Oral Surg 1958;16:483.

172. Puterman M, Fliss DM, Sidi J, Zirkin H. Giant cementoblastoma simulating a peridental infection. J Laryngol Otol 1988;102:264.

173. Schneider LC, Mesa ML. Differences between florid osseous dysplasia and chronic diffuse sclerosing osteomyelitis. Oral Surg Oral Med Oral Pathol 1990;70:308.

174. Groot RH, van Merkesteyn JP, Bras J. Diffuse sclerosing osteomyelitis and florid osseous dysplasia. Oral Surg Oral Med Oral Pathol Oral Radiol Endod 1996;81:333–42.

175. Regezi J, Kerr D, Courtney R. Odontogenic tumors: an analysis of 706 cases. J Oral Surg 1978;36:771.

176. Slootweg PJ. An analysis of the interrelationship of the mixed odontogenic tumors—ameloblastic fibroma, ameloblastic fibro-odontoma, and the odontomas. Oral Surg Oral Med Oral Pathol 1981;51:266.

177. Katz RW. An analysis of compound and complex odontomas. ASCD J Dent Child 1989;56:445.

178. Swan RH. Odontomas. A review, case presentation and periodontal considerations in treatment. J Periodontol 1987;58:856.

179. Wong GB. Surgical management of a large complex mandibular odontoma by unilateral sagittal split osteotomy. J Oral Maxillofac Surg 1989;47:179.

180. Smith KT, Campo MS. The biology of papillomaviruses and their role in oncogenesis. Anticancer Res 1985;5:31.

181. Pindborg JJ, Praetorius F. Oral human papillomavirus infections. Tandlaegebladet 1987;91:404–9.

182. Scully C, Fox MF, Prime SS, Maitland NJ. Papillomaviruses: the current status in relation to oral disease. Oral Surg Oral Med Oral Pathol 1988;65:526.

183. Scully C, Epstein J, Porter S, Cox M. Viruses and chronic disorders involving the human oral mucosa. Oral Surg Oral Med Oral Pathol 1991;72:537.

184. Williamson AL, Dennis SJ. The use of the polymerase chain reaction for the detection of human papillomavirus type 13. J Virol Methods 1991;31:57.

185. Maitland NJ, Cox MF, Lynas C, et al. Detection of human papillomavirus DNA in biopsies of human oral tissue. Br J Cancer 1987;56:245.

186. Steele C, Shillitoe EJ. Viruses and oral cancer. Crit Rev Oral Biol Med 1991;2:153.

187. Luomanen M. Oral focal epithelial hyperplasia removed with CO2 laser. Int J Oral Maxillofac Surg 1990;19:205.

188. Jenson AB, Lancaster WD, Hartmann D-P, Shaffer EL. Frequency and distribution of papillomavirus structural antigen in verrucae, multiple papillomas and condylomata of the oral cavity. Am J Pathol 1982;107:212.

189. Archard HO, Heck JW. Stanley HR. Focal epithelial hyperplasia: an unusual oral mucosal lesion in Indian children. Oral Surg Oral Med Oral Pathol 1965;20:201.

190. Praetorius-Clausen F, Willis JM. Papova virus-like particles in focal epithelial hyperplasia. Scand J Dent Res 1971;79:362.

191. Greenspan D, deVilliers EM, Greenspan JS, et al. Unusual HPV types in oral warts in association with HIV infection. J Oral Pathol 1988;17:482.

192. Matis WL, Triana A, Shapiro R, et al. Dermatologic findings associated with human immunodeficiency virus infection. J Am Acad Dermatol 1987;17:746.

193. Whitaker SB, Wiegand SE, Budnick SD. Intraoral molluscum contagiosum. Oral Surg Oral Med Oral Pathol 1991;72:334.

194. Buller RM, Palumbo GT. Poxvirus pathogenesis. Microbiol Rev 1991;55:80.

195. Smoller BR, Kwan TH, Said TW, et al. Keratoacanthoma and squamous cell carcinoma of the skin: immunohistochemical localization of involucrin and keratin proteins. J Am Acad Dermatol 1986;14:226.

196. Kohn MW, Eversole LR. Keratoacanthoma of the lower lip: report of cases. J Oral Surg 1972;30:522.

197. Svirsky JA, Freedman PD, Lumerman H. Solitary intraoral keratoacanthoma. Oral Surg Oral Med Oral Pathol 1977;43:116.

198. Iverson RE, Vistnes LM. Keratoacanthoma is frequently a dangerous diagnosis. Am J Surg 1974;37:202.

199. Fitzpatrick TB, Eisen AZ, Wolff K, editors. Dermatology in general medicine. 4th ed. New York: McGraw-Hill; 1993.

200. Bologna J, Braverman IM. Skin manifestations of internal disease. In: Wilson JD, Braunwald E, Isselbacher KJ, et al, editors. Harrison's principles of internal medicine. 12th ed. New York: McGraw-Hill; 1991. p. 332.

201. McLean DI, Haynes HA. Cutaneous manifestations of internal malignant disease. In: Fitzpatrick TB, Eisen AZ, Wolff K, editors. Dermatology in general medicine. 4th ed. New York: McGraw-Hill; 1993.

202. Habif TP. Clinical dermatology. A color guide to diagnosis and therapy. In: Cutaneous manifestations of internal diseases. 2nd ed. St Louis: CV Mosby; 1990.

203. Roach ES. Diagnosis and management of neurocutaneous syndromes. Semin Neurol 1988;8:83.

204. Rubenstein A. Neurofibromatosis, a review of the problem. Ann N Y Acad Sci 1986;486:1.

205. Rasmussen SA, Friedman JM. NF1 gene and neurofibromatosis 1. Am J Epidemiol 2000;151(1):33–40.

206. Pomerance B. The elephant man. New York: Grove Press Inc.; 1979.

207. Shapiro S, Abramovitch K, van Dis M, et al. Neurofibromatosis: oral and radiographic manifestations. Oral Surg Oral Med Oral Pathol 1984;58:493.

208. Scriver CR, Beaudet AL, Sly WS, editors. Metabolic basis of inherited disease. 6th ed. New York: McGraw-Hill; 1989.

209. Jones K, Korzcak P. The diagnostic significance and management of Gardner's syndrome. Br J Oral Maxillofac Surg 1990;28:80.

210. Antoniades K, Eleftheriades I, Karakasis D. The Gardner syndrome. Int J Oral Maxillofac Surg 1987;16:480.

211. Little JB, Nove J, Weichselbaum RR. Abnormal sensitivity of diploid skin fibroblasts from a family with Gardner's syndrome to the lethal effects of X-radiation, ultraviolet light and mitomycin-C. Mutat Res 1980;70:241.

212. Fine G, Ma CK. Alimentary tract. In: Kissano JM, editor. Anderson's pathology. 8th ed. St Louis: CV Mosby; 1985.

213. Lowe NJ. Peutz-Jeghers syndrome with pigmented oral papillomas. Arch Dermatol 1975;111:503.

214. Fenoglio-Preiser CM, Lantz PE, Davis M, et al. Polyposis. In: Gastrointestinal pathology. An atlas and text. New York: Raven Press; 1989.

215. Bussey H, Morson B. Familial polyposis coli. In: Lipman M, Good R, editors. Gastrointestinal Tract Cancer. New York: Plenum Press; 1978.

216. Aaltonen LA. Hereditary intestinal cancer. Semin Cancer Biol 2000;10:289–98.

217. Johnson RL, Rothman AL, Xie J, et al. Human homolog of patched, a candidate gene for the basal cell nevus syndrome. Science 1996;272(5268):1668–71.

218. Gorlin RJ. Nevoid basal-cell carcinoma syndrome. Medicine 1987;66:98.

219. Brondum N, Jensen VJ. Recurrence of keratocysts and decompression treatment. A longterm follow-up of forty-four cases. Oral Surg Oral Med Oral Pathol 1991;72:265.

220. Bale SJ, Falk RT, Rogers GR. Patching together the genetics of Gorlin syndrome. J Cutan Med Surg 1998;3(1):31–4.

221. Regezi JA, Sciubba JJ, editors. Cysts of the oral region. In: Oral pathology. Clinico-pathologic correlations. 2nd ed. Philadelphia: W.B. Saunders; 1993.

222. McGuigan JE. Peptic ulcer and gastritis. In: Wilson JD, Braunwald E, Isselbacher KJ, et al, editors. Harrison's principles of internal medicine. 12th ed. New York: McGraw-Hill; 1991. p. 1241.

223. Steiner AL, Goodman AD, Powers SR. Study of a kindred with pheochromocytoma, medullary thyroid carcinoma, hyperparathyroidism and Cushing's disease: multiple endocrine meoplasia, type 2. Medicine 1968;47:371.

224. Khairi MR, Dexter RN, Burzynski NJ, et al. Mucosal neuroma, pheochromocytoma and medullary thyroid carcinoma: multiple endocrine neoplasia type 3. Medicine 1975;54:89.

225. Edwards M, Reid JS. Multiple endocrine neoplasia syndrome type IIb: a case report. Int J Paediatr Dent 1998;8:55–60.

226. Rubin MM, Delgado EB, Cozzi GM, Palladino VS. Tuberous sclerosis complex and a calcifying epithelial odontogenic tumor. Oral Surg Oral Med Oral Pathol 1987;64:207.

227. Ragan MR, Baughman RA. Tuberous sclerosis with orocutaneous manifestations. Ear Nose Throat J 1988;67:276.

228. Papanayotou P, Vezirtzi E. Tuberous sclerosis with gingival lesions. Report of a case. Oral Surg Oral Med Oral Pathol 1975;39:578.

229. Morisaki I, Kato K, Sobue S, Ishida T. Epulis in a child with tuberous sclerosis. J Pedod 1987;11:385–90.

230. Ramirez-Amador V, Esquivel-Pedraza L, Caballero-Mendoza E, et al. Oral manifestations as a hallmark of malignant acanthosis nigricans. J Oral Pathol Med 1999;28:278-81.

231. Merkow RL, Lane JM. Paget's disease of bone. In: Lane JM, editor. Pathologic fractures in metabolic bone disease. Orthop Clin North Am 1990;21:171.

232. Vuillemin-Bodaghi V, Parlier-Cuau C, Cywiner-Golenzer C, et al. Multifocal osteogenic sarcoma in Paget's disease. Skeletal Radiol 2000;29:349–53.

233. Carter LC. Paget's disease: important features for the general practitioner. Compendium 1990;11:662.

234. Mills BG, Holst PA, Stabile EK, et al. A viral antigen bearing cell line derived from culture of Paget's bone cells. Bone 1986;6:257.

235. Mirra JM, Bauer FC, Grant TT. Giant cell tumor with viral-like intranuclear inclusions associated with Paget's disease. Clin Orthop 1981;158:243.

236. Basle MF, Fournier JG, Rosenblatt S, et al. Measles virus RNA detected in Paget's disease bone tissue by in situ hybridization. J Gen Virol 1986;67:907.

237. Hosking DJ. Advances in the management of Paget's disease of bone. Drugs 1990;40:829.

238. Upchurch KS, Simon LS, Schiller AL, et al. Giant cell reparative granuloma of Paget's disease of bone. A unique clinical entity. Ann Intern Med 1983;98:35.

239. Carnisa C, Bikowski JB, McDonald SG. Cowden's disease. Association with squamous cell carcinoma of the tongue and perianal basal cell carcinoma. Arch Dermatol 1984;120:677.

240. Eng C. Will the real Cowden syndrome please stand up: revised diagnostic criteria. J Med Genet 2000;37:828–30.

241. Scriver, Beaudet AL, Sly WS, editors. Metabolic basis of inherited disease. Part 7, Lipoprotein and lipid metabolism disorders. 6th ed. New York: McGraw-Hill 1989. p. 1129.

242. Raffle EJ, Hale DC. Xanthomatosis presenting with oral lesions. Br Dent J 1968;125:62.

243. Travis WD, Davis GE, Tsokos M, et al. Multifocal verruciform xanthoma of the upper aerodigestive tract in a child with a systemic lipid storage disease. Am J Surg Pathol 1989;13:309.

244. Neville B. The verruciform xanthoma. A review and report of eight new cases. Am J Dermatopathol 1986;8:247.

245. Fredrickson DS, Altrocchi PH, Avioli LV, et al. Tangier disease: combined staff conference at the National Institute of Health. Ann Intern Med 1961;55(6):1016.

246. Wilson DE, Floweres CM, Hershgold EJ, et al. Multiple myeloma, cryoglobulinemia and xanthomatosis. Distinct clinical syndromes in two patients. Am J Med 1975;59:721.

247. Thomas JA, Janossy G, Chilosi M, et al. Combined immunological and histochemical analysis of skin and lymph node lesions in histocytosis X. J Clin Pathol 1982;35:327.

248. Haynes BF. Enlargement of lymph nodes and spleen. In: Wilson JD, Braunwald E, Isselbacher KJ, et al, editors. Harrison's principles of internal medicine. 12th ed. New York: McGraw-Hill; 1991.

249. Wood GS, Turner RR, Shiurba RA, et al. Human dendritic cells and macrophages. In situ immunophenotype definition of subsets that exhibit specific morphologic and microenvironmental characteristics. Am J Pathol 1985;119:73.

250. Headington JT. The histocyte. In memoriam. Arch Dermatol 1986;122:532–3.

251. Dagenais M, Pharoah MJ, Sikorski PA. The radiographic characteristics of histiocytosis X. A study of 29 cases that involve the jaws. Oral Surg Oral Med Oral Pathol 1992;74:230.

252. Pringle GA, Daley TD, Veinot LA, Wysocki GP. Langerhans' cell histiocytosis in association with periapical granulomas and cysts. Oral Surg Oral Med Oral Pathol 1991;74:186.

253. Harsanyi BB, Larsson A. Xanthomatous lesions of the mandible: osseous expression of non-X histiocytosis and benign fibrous histiocytoma. Oral Surg Oral Med Oral Pathol 1988;65:551.

254. Crainin AM, Gross ER. Severe oral and perioral amyloidosis as a primary complication of multiple myeloma. Oral Surg Oral Med Oral Pathol 1967;23:153.

255. Flick WG, Lawrence FR. Oral amyloidosis as initial symptom of multiple myeloma. Oral Surg Oral Med Oral Pathol 1980;49:18.

256. Kornblut AD, editor. Symposium on granulomatous disorders of the head and neck. Otolaryngol Clin North Am 1982;15:1.

257. Adams DO, Hamilton TA. Phagocytic cells. Cytotoxic activities of macrophages. In: Gallin JI, Goldstein IM, Snyderman R, editors. Inflammation: basic principles and clinical correlates. New York: Raven Press; 1988. p. 471.

258. Happonen RP. Immunocytochemical diagnosis of cervicofacial actinomycosis: with special emphasis on periapical inflammatory lesions [dissertation]. Medical Faculty, University of Turku, Finland; 1986.

259. Howell A, Stephan RM, Paul F. Prevalence of *Actinomyces israelii, A. naeslundii, Bacterionema matruchotii,* and *Candida albicans* in selected areas of the oral cavity and saliva. J Dent Res 1962;41:1050.

260. Mitchell RH. Actinomycosis and the dental abscess. Br Dent J 1966;120:423.

261. Glahn M. Cervico-facial actinomycosis—typical and non-typical. Acta Chir Scand 1950;99:537.

262. Borssen E, Sundquist G. *Actinomyces* of infected dental root canals. Oral Surg Oral Med Oral Pathol 1981;51:643.

263. O'Grady JF, Reade PC. Periapical actinomycosis involving *Actinomyces israelii.* J Endod 1988;14:147.

264. Gonor S, Allard M, Boileau GR. Appendicovesical fistula caused by ileocecal actinomycosis. Can J Surg 1982;25:23.

265. Valicenti JF Jr, Pappas AA, Graber CD, et al. Detection and prevalence of IUD-associated *Actinomyces* colonization and related morbidity. A prospective study of 69,925 cervical smears. JAMA 1982;247:1149.

266. Brignall ID, Gilhooly N. Actinomycosis of the tongue. A diagnostic dilemma. Br J Oral Maxillofac Surg 1989;27:249.

267. Laforgia P, Mangini F. Nodular isolated actinomycosis of the tongue—a case report. Dent Surv 1979;55(4):48.

268. Happonen RP, Viander M, Pelliniemi L, Aitasalo K. *Actinomyces israelii* in osteoradionecrosis of the jaws. Histopathologic and immunocytochemical study of five cases. Oral Surg Oral Med Oral Pathol 1983;55:580.

269. Bazhanov NN, Kasparova BV, Kapnik VI, et al. Application of hyperbaric oxygenation in the treatment of actinomycosis of the maxillofacial region. Stomatologiia (Mosk) 1980;59(2):28–9.

270. Wein JC, Buck WH. Periapical actinomycosis. Oral Surg Oral Med Oral Pathol 1982;54:336.

271. Martin IC, Harrison JD. Periapical actinomycosis. Br Dent J 1984;54:169.

272. Freeman LR, Zimmerman E, Ferrillo PJ. Conservative treatment of periapical actinomycosis. Oral Surg Oral Med Oral Pathol 1981;51:205.

273. Norman J. Cervicofacial actinomycosis. Oral Surg Oral Med Oral Pathol 1970;29:735.

274. Edmunds DH. *Actinomyces* organisms associated with a tooth intentionally reimplanted two years previously. A case report. Oral Surg Oral Med Oral Pathol 1991;71:100.

275. Wear DJ, Margileth AM, Hadfield TL, et al. Cat-scratch disease: a bacterial infection. Science 1983;221:1403.

276. Zangwill KM, Hamilton DH, Perkins BA, et al. Cat scratch disease in Connecticut. Epidemiology, risk factors, and evaluation of a new diagnostic test. N Engl J Med 1993;329:8.

277. Mintz SM, Anavi Y. Cat-scratch fever presenting as a substantial swelling. J Oral Maxillofac Surg 1988;46:1015.

278. Premachandra DJ, Milton CM. Cat-scratch disease in the parotid gland presenting with facial paralysis. Br J Oral Maxillofac Surg 1990;28:413.

279. Jawad AS, Amen AA. Cat-scratch disease presenting as the oculoglandular syndrome of Parinaud: a report of two cases. Postgrad Med J 1990;66:467.

280. Margileth AM, Wear DJ, English CK. Systemic cat-scratch disease. Report of 23 patients with prolonged or recurrent, systemic bacterial infection. J Infect Dis 1987;155:390.

281. MacGregor RR. Infections caused by animal bites and scratches. In: Wilson JD, Braunwald E, Isselbacher KJ, et al, editors. Harrison's principles of internal medicine. 12th ed. New York: McGraw-Hill; 1991. p. 551.

282. Schlossberg D, Morad Y, Krouse TB, et al. Culture-proved disseminated catscratch disease in acquired immunodeficiency syndrome. Arch Intern Med 1989;149:1437.

283. Reich CV. Leprosy: cause, transmission, and a new theory of pathogenesis. Rev Infect Dis 1987;9:589.

284. Epker BN, Via WF. Oral and perioral manifestations of leprosy. Oral Surg Oral Med Oral Pathol 1969;28:342.

285. Lighterman I, Watanabe Y, Hidaka T. Leprosy of the oral cavity and adnexa. Oral Surg Oral Med Oral Pathol 1962;15:1178.

286. Alfieri N, Fleury RN, Opromolla DVA, et al. Oral lesions in borderline or reactional tuberculoid leprosy. Oral Surg Oral Med Oral Pathol 1983;55:52.

287. Oliver ID, Pickett AB. Cheilitis glandularis. Oral Surg Oral Med Oral Pathol 1990;49:526.

288. Rogers RS. Granulomatous cheilitis, Melkersson-Rosenthal syndrome, and orofacial granulomatosis. Arch Dermatol 2000;136(12):1557–8.

289. Brook IM, King DJ, Miller ID. Chronic granulomatous cheilitis and its relationship to Crohn's disease. Oral Surg Oral Med Oral Pathol 1983;56:405.

290. Worsaac N, Pindborg JJ. Granulomatous gingival manifestations of Melkersson-Rosenthal syndrome. Oral Surg Oral Med Oral Pathol 1980;49:131.

291. Williams PM, Greenberg MS. Management of cheilitis granulomatosa. Oral Surg Oral Med Oral Pathol 1991;72:436.

292. Lindhe J. Textbook of clinical periodontology. 2nd ed. Copenhagen: Munksgaard; 1989.

293. Philstrom B, McHugh R, Oliphant T, et al. Comparison of surgical and non-surgical treatment of periodontal disease. A review of current studies and additional results after six and one half years. J Clin Periodontol 1984;10:524.

294. Emslie RD, Massler M, Zwemer JD. Mouth breathing: I. Etiology and effects (a review). J Am Dent Assoc 1952;44:506.

295. Bolger WE, West CB Jr, Parsons DS, Gates GA. Upper airway obstruction due to massive gingival hyperplasia. A case report and description of a new surgical treatment. Int J Pediatr Otorhinolaryngol 1990;19:63.

296. Hassell TM. Epilepsy and the oral manifestations of epilepsy. Monogr Oral Sci 1981;9:116.

297. Anonymous. Panel discussion: the oral manifestations of gingival hyperplasia. Compendium 1990;Suppl 14:S515–8.

298. Hassell TM, Hefti AF. Drug-induced gingival overgrowth: old problem, new problem. Crit Rev Oral Biol Med 1991;2:103.

299. Hall WB. Dilantin hyperplasia: a preventable lesion? Compendium 1990;Suppl 14:S502–5.

300. Pihlstrom BL. Prevention and treatment of Dilantin-associated gingival enlargement. Compendium 1990;Suppl 14:S506.

301. Schraeder PL. The risks of having epilepsy. Compendium 1990;Suppl 14:S497.

302. Nally FF. Gingival hyperplasia due to Primidone ("Mysoline"). J Ir Dent Assoc 1967;13:113–4.

303. Russell BG, Bay LM. Oral use of chlorhexidine toothpaste in epileptic children. Scand J Dent Res 1978;86:52.

304. Klipstein FA. Subnormal serum folate and macrocytosis associated with anticonvulsant drug therapy. Blood 1964;23:68.

305. Drew HJ, Vogel RI, Molofsky W, et al. Effect of folate on phenytoin hyperplasia. J Clin Periodontol 1987;14:330.

306. Jensen ON, Olesen OV. Subnormal serum folate due to anticonvulsive therapy. A double-blind study of the effect of folic acid treatment to patients with drug-induced subnormal serum folate. Arch Neurol 1970;22:181.

307. Butler RT, Kalkwarf KL, Kaldahl WB. Drug-induced gingival hyperplasia: phenytoin, cyclosporin and nifedipine. J Am Dent Assoc 1987;144:56.

308. Wysocki GP, Gretzinger HA, Lanpacis A, et al. Fibrous hyperplasia of the gingiva: a side effect of cyclosporine A therapy. Oral Surg Oral Med Oral Pathol 1983;55:274.

309. Pernu HE, Oikarinen K, Hietanen J, Knuutila M. Verapamil-induced gingival overgrowth; a clinical, histologic, and biochemic approach. J Oral Pathol Med 1989;18:422.

310. Bowman J, Levy BA, Grubb RV. Gingival overgrowth induced by diltiazem. Oral Surg Oral Med Oral Pathol 1988;65:183.

311. Lucas RM, Howell LP, Wall BA. Nifedipine-induced gingival hyperplasia: a histochemical and ultra-structural study. J Periodontol 1985;56:211.

312. Barak S, Engelberg IS, Hiss J. Gingival hyperplasia caused by nifedipine. Histopathologic findings. J Periodontol 1987;58:639.

313. Brown RS, Sein P, Corio R, Bottomley WK. Nitrendepine-induced gingival hyperplasia. First case report. Oral Surg Oral Med Oral Pathol 1990;70:593.

314. Nyska A, Waner T, Pirak M, et al. Gingival hyperplasia in rats induced by oxodipine—a calcium channel blocker. J Periodontal Res 1990;25:65.

315. Galiano A. Oxodipine. Drugs of the Future 1987;12:633.

316. Hassell T, Sobhani S. Effects of dihydropyridines on connective tissue cells in vitro. J Dent Res 1987;66:282.

317. Yamasaki A, Rose GG, Pinero GJ, Mahan CJ. Ultra-structure of fibroblasts in cyclosporin A-induced hyperplasia. J Oral Pathol 1987;16:129.

318. Clark D. Gingival fibromatosis and its related syndromes, a review. J Can Dent Assoc 1987;53:137.

319. Witkop CJ Jr. Heterogeneity in gingival fibromatosis. Birth Defects 1971;7:212.

320. Holmes LB, Moser HW, Halldorsson S, et al. Mental retardation. An atlas of diseases associated with physical abnormalities. New York: Macmillan; 1972.

321. Cuestos-Carnero R, Bornancini CA. Hereditary generalized gingival fibromatosis associated with hypertrichosis. Report of five cases in one family. J Oral Maxillofac Surg 1988;46:415.

322. Anavi Y, Lerman P, Mintz S, Kiviti S. Idiopathic familial gingival fibromatosis associated with mental retardation, epilepsy and hypertrichosis. Dev Med Child Neurol 1989;31:538.

323. Houston I, Shoots N. Rutherford's syndrome: a familial oculodental disorder. Acta Pediatr Scand 1966;55:233.

324. Henefer EP, Kay LA. Congenital idiopathic gingival fibromatosis in the deciduous dentition. Oral Surg Oral Med Oral Pathol 1967;24:65.

325. Chodirker BN, Chudley AE, Toffler MA, Reed MH. Zimmerman-Laband syndrome and profound mental retardation. Am J Med Genet 1986;25:543.

326. Bazopoulou-Kyrkanidou E, Papagianoulis L, Papanicolaou S, Mavrou A. Laband syndrome: a case report. J Oral Pathol Med 1990;19:385.

327. Hartsfield JK Jr, Bixler D, Hazen RH. Gingival fibromatosis with sensorineural hearing loss. An autosomal dominant trait. Am J Med Genet 1985;22:623.

328. Hall EH, Terezhalmy GT. Focal dermal hypoplasia syndrome. J Am Acad Dermatol 1983;9:443.

329. Wechsler MA, Papa CM, Haberman F, Marion RW. Variable expression in focal dermal hypoplasia. An example of differential X-chromosome inactivation. Am J Dis Child 1988;142:297.

330. Aldred MJ, Crawford PJM. Juvenile hyaline fibromatosis. Oral Surg Oral Med Oral Pathol 1987;63:71.

331. Quintal D, Jackson R. Juvenile hyaline fibromatosis. A 15-year follow-up. Arch Dermatol 1985;121:1062.

332. Remberger K, Krieg T, Kunze D, et al. Fibromatosis hyalinica multiplex (juvenile hyaline fibromatosis). Light microscopic, electron microscopic, immunohistochemical and biochemical findings. Cancer 1985;56:614.

333. Cross HE, McKusick VA, Breen W. A new oculocerebral syndrome with hypopigmentation. J Pediatr 1967;70:398.

334. Salinas CF. Orodental findings and genetic disorders. Birth Defects 1982;18:79.

335. Galili D, Yatziv S, Russell A. Massive gingival hyperplasia preceding dental eruption in I-cell disease. Oral Surg Oral Med Oral Pathol 1974;37:533.

336. Terashima Y, Tsuda K, Isomura S, et al. I-cell disease. Report of three cases. Am J Dis Child 1975;129:1083.

337. Whelan DT, Chang PL, Cockshott PW. Mucolipidosis II. The clinical, radiological and histochemical features in three cases. Clin Genet 1983;24:90.

338. Brown HM, Gorlin RJ. Oral mucosal involvement in nevus unius lateralis (ichthyosis hystrix). Arch Dermatol 1960;81:509.

339. Reichart PA, Lubach D, Becker J. Gingival manifestations in linear nevus sebaceous syndrome. Int J Oral Surg 1983;12:437.

8

ORAL CANCER

JOEL B. EPSTEIN, DMD, MSD, FRCD(C)

▼ EPIDEMIOLOGY

Worldwide, oral carcinoma is one of the most prevalent cancers and is one of the 10 most common causes of death. Of the more than one million new cancers diagnosed annually in the United States, cancers of the oral cavity and oropharynx account for approximately 3%.[1] If oral cancers and cancers of the nasopharynx, pharynx, larynx, sinus, and salivary glands are combined, these sites represent more than 5% of total body cancers. In males, oral cancer represents 4% of total body cancers; in females, 2% of all cancers are oral. Oral cancer accounts for 2% of cancer deaths in males and 1% of cancer deaths in females.[1] The statistics are similar throughout North America but vary throughout the world; in French men, the incidence is up to 17.9 cases per 100,000 population, and high rates are reported in India and other Asian countries. Higher rates in these countries also are reported in females, with the highest rate in Singapore (5.8 cases per 100,000 population).[1] The majority of oral cancers are squamous cell cancers. Other malignant diseases that can occur in the head and neck include tumors of the salivary glands, thyroid gland, lymph nodes, bone, and soft tissue. However, these cancers are much less common, and this chapter thus focuses on squamous cell cancer.

Oral cancer is a disease of increasing age: approximately 95% of cases occur in people older than 40 years, with an average age at diagnosis of approximately 60 years.[2,3] The age-related incidence suggests that time-dependent factors result in the initiation and promotion of genetic events that result in malignant change. The majority of oral cancers involve the tongue, oropharynx, and floor of the mouth.[1–3] The lips, gingiva, dorsal tongue, and palate are less common sites. Primary squamous cell carcinoma of bone is rare; however, a tumor may develop from epithelial rests and from the epithelium of odontogenic lesions, including cysts and ameloblastoma. Individuals who have had a previous cancer are at high risk of developing a second oropharyngeal cancer.[4–8] African Americans in the United States have a higher risk of developing oropharyngeal cancer than do Caucasians.[2,9,10] The increased risk appears to be due to environmental factors; possible genetic factors have not been determined.

▼ ETIOLOGY AND RISK FACTORS

Evidence of the etiologic factors of squamous cell carcinoma is based on studies of at-risk groups, differences in incidence of disease, laboratory studies of malignant tissues, and animal studies. The incidence of oral cancer is clearly age related, which may reflect declining immune surveillance with age, time for the accumulation of genetic changes, and duration of exposure to initiators and promoters (these include chemical and physical irritants, viruses, hormonal effects, cellular aging, and decreased immunologic surveillance). Evidence from long-term follow-up of immunosuppressed patients after organ and bone marrow transplantation shows that immunosuppression increases the risk of the development of squamous cell carcinoma.

Tobacco and alcohol are acknowledged risk factors for oral and oropharyngeal cancer.[2,3,11–13] Tobacco contains potent carcinogens, including nitrosamines (nicotine), polycyclic aromatic hydrocarbons, nitrosodicthanolamine, nitrosoproline, and polonium. Nicotine is a powerful and addicting drug. Tobacco smoke contains carbon monoxide, thiocyanate, hydrogen cyanide, nicotine, and metabolites of these constituents. Epidemiologic studies have shown that of people with oral cancer, more than half smoke.[12,14] One study demonstrated that 80% of patients with cancer were smokers.[4] In addition to the risk of primary cancers, the risk of subsequent primary oral cancers has been related to the continuing of smoking after treatment.[4–8,15–17] Of patients who were observed for 1 year, 18% developed a second primary oral cancer, and those who continued to smoke had a 30% risk of second cancers.[4] The effect of smoking on cancer risk diminishes 5 to 10 years after quitting. Smoking has declined in North America, particularly in adults; approximately 30% of adults smoke. Unfortunately, this trend is not seen worldwide and is not shown in teenagers and young adults. The incidence of oral squamous cell cancer varies worldwide and may be explained partly by differences in the use of tobacco products. In parts of Asia where the use of tobacco, betal nuts, or lime to form a quid is widespread (e.g., India), the incidence of oral cancer is high.[2]

Most studies have focused on cigarette use; however, other forms of tobacco use have been associated with oral cancers. The use of smokeless tobacco products (chewing tobacco and snuff) is of increasing concern due to the increase in their use and to their use at a young age.[18–23] Benign hyperkeratosis and epithelial dysplasia have been documented after short-term use, and it is likely that chronic use will be associated with an increasing incidence of malignant lesions.[2,12,24]

All forms of alcohol, including "hard" liquor, wine, and beer, have been implicated in the etiology of oral cancer. In some studies, beer and wine may be associated with greater risk than is hard liquor.[12,13] The combined effects of tobacco and alcohol result in a synergistic effect on the development of oral cancer.[11–14,16,25–28] The mechanism(s) by which alcohol and tobacco act synergistically may include dehydrating effects of alcohol on the mucosa, increasing mucosal permeability, and the effects of carcinogens contained in alcohol or tobacco. Secondary liver dysfunction and nutritional status also may play a role.

Factors for which no evidence of a role in oral cancer has been documented include denture use, denture irritation, irregular teeth or restorations, and chronic cheek-biting habits.[2,3,29,30] However, it is possible that chronic trauma, in addition to other carcinogens, may promote the transformation of epithelial cells, as demonstrated in animal studies in which chronic trauma in addition to carcinogen application promotes tumor development.[31] In lip cancer, sun exposure, fair skin and a tendency to burn, pipe smoking, and alcohol are identified risk factors.[13] The decreasing incidence of lip cancer may reflect greater public awareness of the potential damaging effects of the sun.[2] High alcohol content in mouthwashes has been implicated in oral cancer. However, it has been suggested that smokers may use mouthwash more frequently; thus, the correlation between regular use of high-alcohol mouthwash and oral cancer may be confounded by alcohol and tobacco use.[13] In contrast with the well-documented risk associated with the use of alcohol and tobacco products, the role of other environmental agents (such as pollution)requires future study.

Pathogenesis

Oral squamous cell cancer (SCC) is the result of a multistage process from normal to dysplastic lesions and ultimately to SCC. A premalignant or precancerous lesion is defined by the World Health Organization as a morphologically altered tissue in which cancer is more likely to occur and includes oral leukoplakia, oral erythroplakia, and possibly oral lichen planus. Leukoplakia is a white patch of oral mucosa that cannot be characterized clinically or pathologically as any other diagnosed disease. Lesions should be defined by their probable cause, such as traumatic or tobacco-associated leukoplakia.

Dysplastic lesions have been categorized as mild, moderate, or severe, based on histomorphologic criteria. Mild dysplasia has dysplastic cells that are limited to the basal layer of the epithelium; moderate dysplasia and severe dysplasia involve increasing changes in cellular morphology and increasing thickness of the epithelium. Carcinoma in situ is a lesion in which abnormal cells involve the entire epithelium without invasion through the basement membrane, and carcinoma is diagnosed when there is disruption of the basement membrane and invasion into connective tissue.

The presence and severity of dysplasia is thought to have an impact on the malignant risk of premalignant lesions. Silverman and colleagues[32] found a mean of 7.2 years from diagnosis of leukoplakia to SCC although more than one-third of dysplastic lesions will progress to SCC whereas progression was seen in 15% of nondysplastic lesions. The current "gold standard" for predicting the malignant potential of premalignant lesions is the presence and degree of dysplasia. The risk of progression of leukoplakia varies from 0.13 to 24%, depending on the patients and the follow-up period.[32–34] The majority of leukoplakias (epithelial hyperplasia, mild dysplasia) do not progress to malignancy. *Candida* colonization has been associated with an increased risk of progression.[35]

Molecular Changes in Oral Cancer and Premalignancy

Carcinogenesis is a genetic process that leads to a change in morphology and in cellular behavior. The assessment of changes at the molecular level may become the primary means of diagnosis and may guide management since these changes mediate morphologic changes that occur after genetic changes, and knowledge of current morphologic changes is based on the subjective assessment of clinical and histopathologic changes. Major genes involved in head and neck squamous cell carcinoma (HNSCC) include proto-oncogenes and tumor suppressor genes (TSGs). Other factors that play a role in the progression of disease may include allelic loss at other chro-

mosome regions, mutations to proto-oncogenes and TSGs, or epigenetic changes such as deoxyribonucleic acid (DNA) methylation or histone deacetylation. Cytokine growth factors, angiogenesis, cell adhesion molecules, immune function, and homeostatic regulation of surrounding normal cells could also play a role.

While proto-oncogenes increase cell growth and differentiation and are likely involved in carcinogenesis, few have been reported in HNSCC. Proto-oncogenes may function in coding for growth factors, growth factor receptors, protein kinases, signal transducers, nuclear phosphoproteins, and transcription factors. Proto-oncogenes associated with HNSCC include ras (rat sarcoma), cyclin-D1, myc, erb-b (erythroblastosis), bcl-1, bcl-2 (B-cell lymphoma), int-2, CK8, and CK19.[36]

TSGs negatively regulate cell growth and differentiation. Functional loss of TSGs is common in carcinogenesis.[37] Both copies of a TSG must be inactivated or lost (loss of heterozygosity [LOH]) for loss of function (the "two-hit" hypothesis). TSGs involved in HNSCC are *p53*, *Rb* (retinoblastoma), and *p16INK4A*. Other candidates include *FHIT* (fragile histidine triad), *APC* (adenomatous polyposis coli), *DOC1 VHL* (gene for von Hippel-Lindau syndrome), and *TGF-βR-II* (gene for transforming growth factor type II receptor).[38–41] Chromosomes are numbered (1 to 23), and the arms of each chromosome are divided by the centromere into a short arm (designated P) and a long arm (designated Q). These TSGs have been associated with sites of chromosome abnormalities where LOH has been reported to commonly involve chromosome arms 3p, 4q, 8p, 9p, 11q, 13q, and 17p.

Loss on 3p and 9p are early and common events in oral carcinogenesis. Chromosome arm 3p may code for *FHIT* and is involved in epithelial cancers. Diadenosine tetraphosphate may accumulate in the absence of *FHIT*, which may lead to DNA synthesis and cell replication. TSGs at another site of 3p may include the *VHL* gene, which encodes membrane proteins that function in signal transduction and cell adhesion. LOH on 9p is seen in 72% of lesions and may represent the site for *p16*, which encodes a cell cycle protein that inhibits cyclin-dependent kinases and that arrests the cell cycle at the G_1–S phase, and loss may lead to cell proliferation.

Later changes are seen on chromosomes 13 and 17 and are highly associated with progression to malignancy. LOH on 13q is identified in more than 50% of HNSCC.[36,42] The putative TSGs are near the interferon locus and are close to the *Rb* locus. LOH on 13q has been associated with lymph node metastasis in HNSCC. LOH on 17p (the region of the *p53* gene) is found in 50% of cases of HNSCC. The p53 protein functions in transcription activation, DNA repair, apoptosis, senescence, and G_1 and G_2 cell cycle inhibition.

Other genetic changes have been identified on chromosomes 4, 8, and 11.[43–47] Loss on chromosome 4 occurs in up to 80% of HNSCC cases; the putative TSG may be the epidermal growth factor (*EGF*) gene. Loss on 8p occurs in up to 67% of HNSCCs and is associated with a higher stage and a poor prognosis; the related TSG is unknown. Loss on chromosome 11 is present in up to 61% of HNSCCs; the common site lost may code the *cyclin D1* gene. There is increasing evidence of the prognostic value of LOH in HNSCC.[42,48] LOH on 13q correlates with lymph node metastases and recurrence in HNSCC.

Molecular staging may provide more precise predictions of the malignant potential than conventional clinicopathologic features do as it represents the fundamental biologic characteristics of each tumor. The current model of carcinogenesis is a multistage process, with loss occurring on chromosome arms 3p and 9p early in the lesion's progress from benign to dysplastic, with additional losses later in the disease, often involving 8p, 13q, and 17p. Putative TSGs at these sites of loss are *p16* loss at 9p and *p53* gene loss at 17p (Figure 8-1). Molecular markers are likely to become important clinical markers in diagnosis and staging and in treatment planning.

Earlier studies focused on LOH in SCC; currently, there is increasing study of LOH in premalignant lesions.[36,39,44,45,49,50] LOH may predict the malignant risk of low-grade dysplastic oral epithelial lesions.[51,52] This is of importance as the majority of oral premalignant lesions (hyperplasia, mild and moderate dysplasia) do not progress to cancer. Lesions that progress to SCC appear to differ genetically from nonprogressing lesions although they may not differ on the basis of histomorphologic findings. Progressing early lesions (low-grade dysplastic lesions and hyperplasia without dysplasia) are genetically different from morphologically similar nonprogressing lesions and molecular

analysis may therefore become necessary in diagnosis. LOH at 3p and/or 9p occurs early in the majority of hyperplasias and mild dysplasias, and LOH on 17p occurs later. LOH on 8p occurs in 27% of dysplastic lesions and in 67% of invasive oral and laryngeal SCCs. LOH on 3p and/or 9p is seen in virtually all progressing cases and also in some nonprogressing cases. LOH on 3p and/or 9p (but no other chromosome arms) has a 3.8 times relative risk for developing SCC, and if additional sites of LOH are present (4q, 8p, 11q, 13q, or 17p), a 33-fold increase in risk of progression to cancer is seen. Accumulation of allelic loss is seen in progressing lesions, and the majority of progressing dysplasias have LOH on more than one arm (91%, vs 31% of nonprogressing dysplasias); 57% have loss on more than two arms (vs 20% of dysplasias without progression). LOH at 3p and/or 9p may be a prerequisite for the progression of oral premalignant lesions. LOH on 4q, 8p, 11q, 13q, and 17p is common in severe dysplasia/carcinoma-in-situ (CIS) or SCC.

The importance of the study of TSG loss (LOH) is that both the tumor and the precancer have an increasing aggressive nature with increasing molecular changes. Molecular changes predate the current morphologic criteria for diagnosis and for determining margins. It may be possible to assess risk based on TSG loss, to predict risk for metastases and recurrences of lesions, and to guide current therapy by indicating treatment volumes (margins). In the future, treatment may be directed at

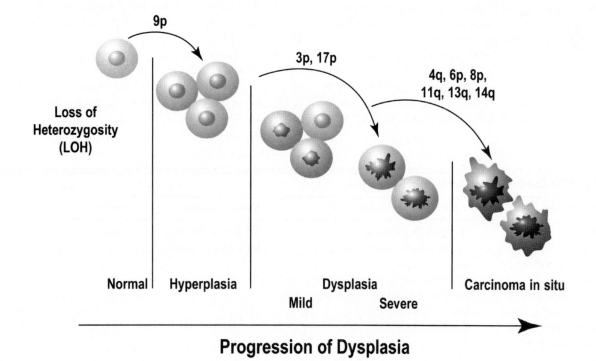

Molecular Model of Dysplasia and Carcinogenesis

FIGURE 8-1   Molecular model with early and late changes that accumulate over time leading to cancer.

the function of proto-oncogenes or TSGs rather than to current therapies with their associated toxicities. TSG changes may provide tools for prognosis and may serve as intermediate markers in assessing treatment and prevention outcomes.

▼ PROGNOSIS

The American Joint Committee on Cancer (AJCC) has developed the tumor, node, metastasis (TNM) system of cancer classification.[53] The AJCC classification is principally a clinical description of the disease but also includes imaging in the classification. The TNM staging of tumors of the oral cavity is shown in Table 8-1. In the oral cavity, T is determined by the size of the primary tumor, N indicates the presence of tumor in lymph nodes, and M indicates distant metastasis. The staging system has combined the T, N, and M to classify lesions as stages 1 to 4. However, when these factors are combined for staging, tumors with different behaviors may be staged similarly; therefore, classification by TNM description is now more common than combining these factors into the four staging groups. For example, there may be differences in biology and response to treatment between a stage 3 tumor that is classified as T1 N1 M0 and a stage 3 tumor that is classed as T3 N0 M0.

Local or regional spread of oral SSC is common and affects the choice of therapy and prognosis. Metastases to cervical lymph nodes are common, but distant metastases below the clavicle are rare. Oral cancer occurring in the posterior aspect of the oral cavity and oropharynx and inferior in the mouth tends to be associated with a poorer prognosis, which may be explained by diagnosis occurring with advanced disease and by a higher incidence of spread to lymph nodes at the time of diagnosis. Ipsilateral lymph node metastases are frequent; however, spread to contralateral nodes also occurs and is more common with midline and posterior lesions.

The most important factor in survival is the stage of disease at diagnosis. Unfortunately, the majority of oral cancers are diagnosed after becoming symptomatic.[3] Since 1960, some progress has been seen with an increase in 5-year survival rates from 45 to 53%.[1] African Americans have had a poorer 5-year survival rate and continue to have a survival rate of less than one-third as compared to caucasians, who have a 5-year survival rate of 53%.[1,2,9,10] These survival rates may be conditioned by physical and social environment; lack of knowledge; risk-promoting lifestyle, attitude, and behavior; and limited access to health care. At least half of the difference in survival in the poor has been attributed to late diagnosis.[9,10]

The incidence of spread is influenced by tumor size. Lesions classed as T1 may show regional spread in 10 to 20% of cases, T2 lesions in 25 to 30% of cases, and T3 to T4 tumors in 50 to 75%.[54–56] A 3-year follow-up with no evidence of disease occurs with approximately 75 to 85% of T1 lesions, 50 to 60% of T2 lesions, and 20 to 30% of T3 to T4 lesions.[57] For patients without lymph node involvement, the overall 3-year no-evidence-of-disease rate is approximately 50 to 60%; however, with lymph node involvement, the rate of cure is approximately 33 to 50%.[58]

Review of the report of the National Cancer Data Base[59] indicated that patients with localized tumors of the oral cavity and pharynx have an overall survival rate of 70%. The database showed an 81% survival rate for those who were treated with surgery alone, a 70% survival rate for those treated with surgery and radiation combined, and a 55% survival rate for those treated with radiation alone. For patients with regional disease, overall survival was 46%; survival rates were 60% for those treated with surgery alone, 58% for those treated with combined surgery and radiation, and 39% for those treated with radiation alone. For patients with distant metastases, overall survival was 33%.

The National Cancer Institute's Surveillance, Epidemiology and End Results program shows relative survival rates of 51% over a 5-year period and a 10-year survival rate of 41%.[60] Progress in the control of oral and pharyngeal cancer has been seen in years of life lost due to cancer: 23.1 years in 1970 and 19.9 years in 1985.[61]

There is rarely a second chance for a cure; therefore, the initial approach to therapy is critical. Death from head and neck cancer may be due to erosion of major vessels, erosion of the cranial base, cachexia, and secondary infection of the respiratory tract.

TABLE 8-1 TNM Classification of Tumors of the Oral Cavity

T (Size of Primary Tumor)	N (Cervical Lymph Node Metastases)	M (Distant Metastases)	Staging
T1s: carcinoma in situ	N0: no node involvement detected	M0: no known metastases	Stage 1: T1 N0 M0
T1: tumor < 2 cm	N1: single ipsilateral node < 3 cm	M1: metastases present	Stage 2: T2 N0 M0
T2: tumor > 2 cm and < 4 cm	N2a: single ipsilateral node < 6 cm		Stage 3: T3 N0 M0;
T3: tumor > 4 cm	N2b: multiple ipsilateral nodes > 3 cm and < 6 cm		T1,T2, or T3 N1 M0
T4: tumor > 4 cm with invasion of	N2c: bilateral or contralateral lymph nodes < 6 cm		Stage 4: T4 any N M0; any T N2
adjacent structures (ie, through	N3a: ipsilateral node > 6 cm		or N3 M0; any T or N, with M1
cortical bone; deep into extrinsic	N3b: bilateral nodes > 6 cm		
muscles of tongue, maxillary sinus,			
and skin)			

A thorough understanding of each treatment modality, its efficacy, and its side effects is needed, which has led to the need for a team approach that may include surgeons, radiation oncologists, medical oncologists, dentists, and adjunctive health care workers.

▼ PRECANCEROUS LESIONS

Leukoplakia and Erythroplakia

CLASSIFICATION AND DIAGNOSIS

Histomorphologic classifications of oral leukoplakia have been proposed, to assist in predicting which oral lesions are at increased risk of progression to cancer. The more recent proposals are similar to each other (Table 8-2).[62,63] The classifications include histologic findings and the clinical description, site, and size of the lesion. The site of the lesion has been associated with increased risk and is included in the more complex classification, as shown.

Early detection of dysplastic and malignant lesions is a continuing goal. Thorough head and neck and intraoral examination is a prerequisite. Aids to oral examination include vital tissue staining using toluidine blue and (more recently) computer-assisted cytology of oral brush biopsy specimens.[64]

TABLE 8-2 Classification and Staging for Oral Leukoplakia

Provisional (clinical) diagnosis

    L: extent of leukoplakia
        L0, no evidence of lesion
        L1, ≤ 2 cm
        L2, 2–4 cm
        L3, ≥ 4 cm
        Lx, not specified

    S: site of leukoplakia
        S1, all sites excluding FOM, tongue
        S2, FOM and/or tongue
        Sx, not specified

    C: clinical aspect
        C1, homogenous
        C2, nonhomogenous
        Cx, not specified

Definitive (histopatholgic) diagnosis

    P: histopathologic features
        P1, no dysplasia
        P2, mild dysplasia
        P3, moderate dysplasia
        P4, severe dysplasia
        Px, not specified

Staging
    1: any L, S1, C1, P1 or P2
    2: any L, S1 or S2, C2, P1 or P2
    3: any L, S2, C2, P1 or P2
    4: any L, any S, any C, P3 or P4

Adapted from Pindborg JJ et al;[62] Schepman KP et al.[63]
FOM = floor of the mouth.

Toluidine blue can be applied directly to suspicious lesions or used as an oral rinse. A study of the application of toluidine blue to a consecutive series of patients who had prior head and neck cancer and in whom all lesions were examined by biopsy revealed 100% of the carcinomas in situ and SCCs (no false-negatives; sensitivity was 100%) whereas clinical findings would not have led to biopsy being performed on 28% of these malignant lesions ($p = .02$).[65] Toluidine blue has documented clinical use in choosing biopsy sites, may guide surgical treatment of malignant lesions, and facilitates the decision to perform a biopsy. The assessment of dye uptake depends on clinical judgment and experience (Figures 8-2 and 8-3). Positive retention of toluidine blue (particularly in areas of leukoplakia, erythroplakia, and uptake in a peripheral pattern of an ulcer) may indicate the need for biopsy. False-positive dye retention may occur in inflammatory and ulcerative lesions, but false-negative retention is uncommon.[65] A return appointment in 14 days, providing time for inflammatory lesions to improve, may lead to a decrease in false-positive results. However, the definitive test is biopsy, and any suspicious lesion should not remain undiagnosed. Toluidine blue provides guidance for the selection for the biopsy site and indicates sites that are at risk for malignancy in wide areas of leukoplakia. Toluidine blue can provide additional aid in determining the margins of a lesion for treatment purposes. In postradiotherapy follow-up, the retention of toluidine blue may act as a guide indicating the distinction between chronic nonhealing ulcers and persistent or recurrent disease.

Computer-assisted analysis of oral brush cytology is completed on Pap-stained exfoliated cells, scanned by computer for abnormal cell morphology and keratinization, and a final diagnosis is made by an examining pathologist on the basis of standard histomorphologic criteria. This approach was evaluated in 945 patients, of whom only approximately one-third underwent biopsy, and true positives were reported in 100% of the lesions that were positive by brush cytology (sensitivity, 100%; no false-negatives); unfortunately, not all patients underwent biopsy, and false-negative results are not evaluable

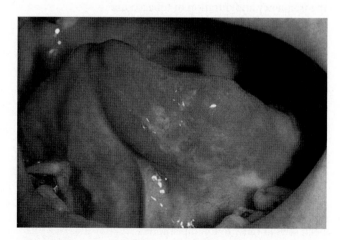

FIGURE 8-2 Undiagnosed lesion presenting with irregular erythema and erosion involving the ventral surface of the tongue.

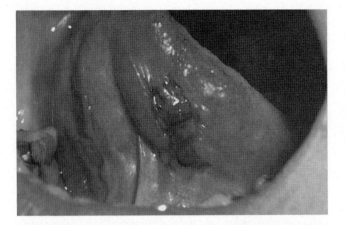

FIGURE 8-3 The same case shown in Figure 8-2 following application of toluidine blue. Dye retention was consistent with dysplasia or carcinoma and indicated the best site for biopsy. The biopsy specimen was reported as squamous cell carcinoma.

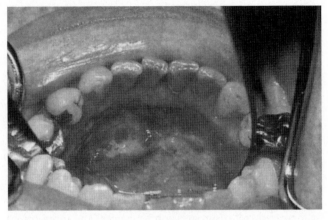

FIGURE 8-4 Irregular leukoplakia involves the floor of the mouth and extends to the attached gingiva of the lingual aspect of the mandible. Histopathologic interpretation was of severe dysplasia with areas of carcinoma in situ; no invasion of connective tissue was seen.

for the whole group. Of importance, 4.5% of clinically benign lesions that were positive on brush cytology were subsequently evaluated by biopsy and diagnosed as dysplasia or SCC. Brush cytology may be useful, and it can be used in conjunction with vital staining.[64] Future developments may include studies of exfoliated cells by using molecular markers of dysplasia or carcinoma to improve the diagnostic and prognostic value. A recent study showed that exfoliative epithelial cells have the same genetic changes associated with dysplasia and cancer as did paired biopsy specimens.[66]

CLINICAL FEATURES

Leukoplakia is a white lesion that involves the oral mucosa, cannot be removed by rubbing, and cannot be classified as any other lesion following histopathologic examination (Figures 8-4 and 8-5). Leukoplakia can affect any area of the oral mucosa and most commonly represents benign keratosis. Leukoplakia has been associated with trauma and tobacco use. A dose-response relationship exists between leukoplakia and the frequency and duration of tobacco use.

At the time of identification of leukoplakia, biopsy reveals dysplasia in 12 to 25% of patients and reveals carcinoma in 3 to 10%.[32,67–72] Dysplasia is present more frequently in leukoplakia that involves the tongue, lips, and floor of the mouth and less frequently in leukoplakia that involves the palate and retromolar regions. The presence of dysplasia within a leukoplakia lesion implies an increased risk of malignant transformation. In studies with a mean follow-up of more than 7 years, the incidence of malignant transformation of leukoplakia has varied from less than 1% to 17.5%, with the most common range being 2 to 6%.[32,73,74] Leukoplakia associated with tobacco use is frequently reversible with the discontinuance of tobacco use. Spontaneous regression of leukoplakia also has been seen in these follow-up studies.

Proliferative verrucous leukoplakia (PVL) is a unique verrucous form of oral leukoplakia that is associated with a high

risk of progression to squamous cell carcinoma. The lesion is more common in males. In one study, the mean age was more than 62 years, and over 70% of the lesions progressed to carcinoma.[75] PVL has been associated with human papillomavirus (HPV) type 16.[76] Aggressive management and close follow-up is needed.

Leukoplakia has been regarded as the most common oral presentation of cancer; however, it has been shown that erythroplakia and irregular erythroleukoplakia are at a greater risk of being dysplastic or malignant than are white lesions.[2,3,72] Erythroplakic lesions may be malignant or dysplastic in up to 80% of tissue biopsy specimens[3,72] (Figure 8-6). In a study of asymptomatic oral cancers, 60% were mixed leukoerythroplakic, one third were erythroplastic, and 4.9% were white lesions.[77] The risk of malignant transformation of erythroplakia has been shown to have four to seven times the risk of change in leukoplakia.[32,70,72,73,78,79]

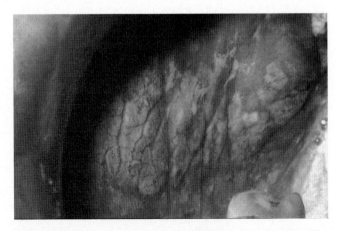

FIGURE 8-5 Extensive leukoplakia involving the buccal mucosa. The multiple plaquelike pattern and the fine delicate pattern of leukoplakia have been associated with tobacco use.

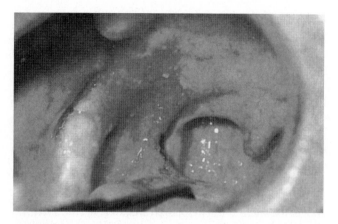

FIGURE 8-6 Erythroplakia with a minimal white component. Histopathologic interpretation was invasive squamous cell carcinoma.

The use of smokeless tobacco has increased and has been associated with oral leukoplakia[24,72,80,81] (Figure 8-7). The presence of leukoplakia in adolescent users of smokeless tobacco is related to years of use, frequency of use, and the amount used.[80] Malignant transformation of leukoplakia may occur in 0.5 to 6.2% of individuals[80,81] and is expected to increase with years of use (Figure 8-8). A 50-fold increased risk of oral carcinoma has been estimated for female snuff dippers.[24] A cocarcinogenic effect of smokeless tobacco and HPV[56] and extracts from smokeless tobacco and herpes simplex virus infection has been shown in vitro.[82,83] Leukoplakia is less common in people who do not use tobacco products. Paradoxically, leukoplakia in individuals who do not use tobacco has a greater risk of malignant transformation, which suggests other etiologic factors in these cases.

Candida is often associated with leukoplakia, and a higher prevalence has been seen in erythroplakia.[2,72] The presence of *Candida* may represent secondary colonization. While there is little evidence to implicate *Candida* in the causing of squamous cell carcinoma, further study is required because some biotypes may transform carcinogenic nitrosamines from precursors.[72]

Lichen Planus

Lichen planus is an immunologically mediated mucocutaneous disease primarily seen in adults, more commonly in women. Chronic lichen planus has been shown to present a low but measurable risk of cancer,[2,72] and oral cancer has been identified as arising from areas of erythematous atrophic lichen planus.[72,84–87] Malignant transformation of lichen planus has been reported in 0.4 to 2.5% of cases in long-term studies, which represents a 50-fold or greater increase in risk. Other reports have questioned the prevalence of malignant transformation of lichen planus because of the lack of detail and uniformity of diagnosis presented in the literature and because the epidemiology suggests that the majority of cases of SCC would be related to the transformation of lichen planus, if above estimates are correct.[88]

Syphilis and Submucous Fibrosis

A relationship between syphilis and oral cancer has been discussed, but the evidence is equivocal.[2] The oral lesions of syphilis may need to be differentiated from oral malignant lesions.

Submucous fibrosis is a disease of the oral mucosa, characterized by epithelial atrophy and fibrosis of the submucosa. Submucous fibrosis is most common among East Indians. While the etiology is unknown, consumption of spices and irritants has been suspected to be the cause. Squamous cell carcinoma has been described in up to one-third of patients with submucous fibrosis.

Oral Hairy Leukoplakia

Oral hairy leukoplakia presents as a vertical folded white patch most frequently seen on the lateral borders of the tongue (Figure 8-9). It may occur in patients with chronic immunosuppression and is associated with the presence of Epstein-Barr virus. While most common in people with human immunodeficiency virus (HIV) infection, it has been reported in

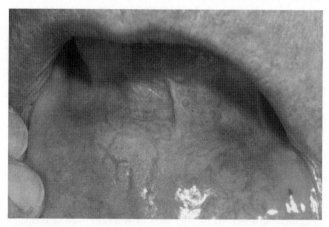

FIGURE 8-7 Leukoplakia involving the labial mucosa and vestibule in a young adult who was a user of smokeless tobacco. Pathologic review reported hyperkeratosis without dysplasia.

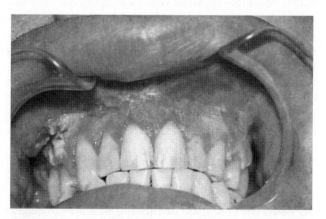

FIGURE 8-8 Extensive leukoplakia in an adult who used snuff for many years. The leukoplakia demonstrated dysplasia, and in the right maxillary gingiva, invasive squamous cell carcinoma was diagnosed. In the area of carcinoma, increased thickening, ulceration, and palpable thickness were noted.

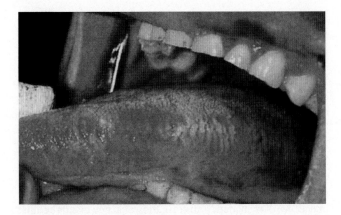

FIGURE 8-9   Hairy leukoplakia of the lateral border of the tongue in an HIV-positive adult man. The vertical folding and corrugated appearance of the lesion are characteristic.

patients after organ and bone marrow transplantation. When *Candida* is associated with the lesion, it colonizes secondarily. Evidence of premalignant potential, abnormal keratin, and dysplasia has not been seen in hairy leukoplakia.

Management of Leukoplakia

In managing leukoplakia, risk factors must be eliminated if at all possible. If leukoplakia is not reversed, treatment may be indicated. Therapy is needed when dysplasia is seen on biopsy specimens. Treatment may include excision and topical therapies. Laser excision/ablation using carbon dioxide laser and neodymium:yttrium-aluminum-garnet (Nd:YAG) laser has been reported as effective although recurrence of lesions is not uncommon.[89] The potential advantage of laser therapy is improved healing of the treated area; however, a potential disadvantage is the inability to carefully assess histologic margins. Topical application of vitamin A acid may achieve remission in cases of mild dysplasia;[2,90–92] however, lesions often recur when therapy is discontinued. Systemic retinoids (analogues of vitamin A) have antiproliferative and differentiating effects on human squamous epithelial cells. In addition, retinoids may play a role in reducing the risk of recurrence or second primary lesions although recurrence of the lesion is common if the retinoid is discontinued.[93,94] Bleomycin has been applied in a topical solution of dimethyl sulfoxide and has shown reduction and elimination of oral lesions in short- and long-term follow-ups.[95,96] Close follow-up is needed for persistent leukoplakia as some of these lesions will progress to SCC. If changes in behavior or appearance occur, a repeat biopsy is indicated.

▼ VIRUSES IN ORAL CANCER

The potential role of viruses in oral cancer is under continuing study. The interaction of viruses with other carcinogens and oncogenes may be an important mechanism of disease.

Herpes simplex virus (HSV) has been shown to produce a number of mutations in cells.[97] A cocarcinogenic effect between HSV and chewing tobacco has been demonstrated

in animal studies.[82,83,98] Smokers demonstrate higher antibody titers to HSV, suggesting reactivation.[99,100] Neutralizing antibodies to HSV are present in the serum of patients with oral cancer at higher titers in those who have advanced cancer, and antibody response to HSV antigen is greater in patients than in controls.[99,100] However, HSV has not been detected in human squamous cell carcinoma.[97,101] If HSV is etiologic, it is likely that the virus has an effect which leaves no evidence of its presence after its oncogenic effect (a "hit-and-run" effect).[97,102]

HPVs are being studied in oral cancer. In laboratory studies, HPVs can transform cells. The association of HPV with anogenital and cervical dysplasia, carcinoma in situ, and invasive carcinoma has been well established.[72,97,103,104] The sensitivity of methods and the sequences of DNA selected for study may explain the variability of findings in the study of HPV in oral squamous cell carcinoma. In some studies, approximately one-half of oral squamous cell carcinomas contain HPV types 16 or 18 (HPV-16 or -18).[72,105–108] When studied by using polymerase chain reaction, 90% of oral carcinomas were found to contain HPV-16 or HPV-18.[108] However, additional study is needed due to inconsistent findings in some studies with respect to the presence of HPV or the presence of fragments of the HPV genome.[72,104,108–112]

▼ TUMOR BIOLOGY

Studies of the repair mechanisms of cellular damage may play a role in the understanding of malignant disease and in its therapy in the future.[72,113] Oncogene amplification has been seen in oral carcinoma. Genetic risk and cocarcinogenesis are continuing to be investigated (see above). The role of cytokines, including epidermal and transforming growth factors, may be relevant in oral squamous cell carcinoma.[72,113,114] Changes in cell surface receptors and major histocompatibility class I and class II antigens have been seen and may indicate that immune surveillance and immune function may be affected in patients with oral cancer.[114] The changes noted in human leukocyte antigen expression may be useful in the prognosis of tumor behavior. Other cell surface changes include a loss of cytoplasmic membrane binding of lectins, which has been shown to correlate to the degree of cellular atypia. Cell surface markers are altered in neoplastic dedifferentiation; examples are the loss of ABO blood group antigens, beta$_2$-microglobulin, and involucrin and a loss of reaction to pemphigus antisera. Alterations in cell-bound immunoglobulins and circulating immunocomplexes are detectable, but the importance of these changes in pathogenesis is unclear. Carcinoembryonic antigens are elevated in patients with oral cancer. Intracellular enzymes also are altered or lost, commensurate with the degree of cellular dysplasia.

The development of malignant disease in immunosuppressed patients indicates the importance of an intact immune response. Mononuclear cell infiltration correlates with prognosis, and more aggressive disease is associated with limited inflammatory response. Total numbers of T cells are decreased in patients with head and neck cancer. The mixed lymphocyte reaction is reduced in some patients, and a diminished migration of macrophages has been demonstrated. Cluster designation 8 (CD8) lymphocytes (T suppressor cells) predominate in the infiltrate, suggesting an evolving immunosuppression with progression to invasive carcinoma. Langerhans' cells (intraepithelial macrophages) are slightly increased in neoplastic epithelium; however, in animal models of chemical-induced carcinogenesis, Langerhans' cells are decreased. Further understanding of immune function and the response to SCC may lead to the development of new therapies that modulate the immune response.[113]

Squamous cell carcinoma primarily spreads by direct local extension and by regional extension through the lymphatics. Regional spread in the oral mucosa may occur by direct extension and sometimes by submucosal spread, which may result in wide areas of involvement. Bone involvement occurs when the periosteal barrier is violated. Production of type I collagenase and other proteinases, prostaglandin E_2, and interleukin-1 may affect the extracellular matrix, and motility of epithelial cells may allow invasion.[72,91,114] Changes in the basement membrane, such as the breakdown of laminin and collagen, occur with invasion. Understanding the biology of invasion by malignant cells may lead to additional approaches to diagnosis and management.

▼ NUTRITION: RISK AND PROPHYLAXIS

Vitamin A may play a role in oral cancer.[2,115–118] This hypothesis is based on population studies in which deficiency was associated with risk of squamous cell carcinoma, on population studies of vitamin A and carotenoid supplementation, and on studies of reduction in carcinogenesis in animal models. Vitamin A may cause regression of premalignant leukoplakia, and the prophylactic use of supplementation in patients at high risk of recurrent or new secondary squamous cell carcinoma is being studied.

A review (based on a study conducted by the National Toxicology Program) of the benefits and risks of fluoride use demonstrated equivocal evidence of carcinogenicity of fluoride in male rats.[119] The evidence was based on the finding of a few cases of osteosarcoma in male rats, but in female rats and in male and female mice, no malignant disease was seen.[119] Other animal studies have not confirmed these results. There is no epidemiologic evidence of an association between fluoride and osteosarcoma or other malignant disease in humans.[72,119,120]

▼ PRESENTING SIGNS AND SYMPTOMS

Oral cancer is initially asymptomatic, and unfortunately, patients are most often identified only after the development of symptoms and after progression of disease. Discomfort is the most common symptom that leads a patient to seek care

and is present at the time of diagnosis in up to 85% of patients.[2,121] Patients also may present with an awareness of a mass in the mouth or neck. Dysphagia, odynophagia, otalgia, limited movement, and oral bleeding occur less frequently.

The oral cavity should be examined following a careful assessment of the cervical and submandibular lymph nodes. Examination of the oral cavity should not neglect any area, but the high-risk sites for oral carcinoma must be most carefully examined. The patient should be assessed for tissue changes that may include a red, white, or mixed red-and-white lesion; a change in the surface texture of the lesion, producing a smooth, granular, rough, or crusted lesion; or the presence of a mass or ulceration (Figures 8-10 to 8-14). The lesion may be flat or elevated and ulcerated or nonulcerated, and it may be minimally palpable or indurated. Loss of function involving the tongue can affect speech, swallowing, and diet.

Lymphatic spread of oral carcinoma usually involves the submandibular and digastric nodes, the upper cervical nodes, and finally the remaining nodes along the cervical chain. The nodes most commonly involved are those that are on the same side as the primary tumor although the closer the tumor is to the midline and the more posterior it is in the oral cavity or oropharynx, the more common is the involvement of the bilateral and contralateral nodes. Lymph node involvement may not occur in an orderly fashion, and thorough examination is mandatory. Lymph nodes associated with cancer become enlarged and firm to hard in texture. The nodes are not tender unless they are associated with secondary infection or unless an inflammatory response is present, such as may occur after a biopsy. The fixation of nodes to adjacent tissue due to invasion of cells through the capsule is a late occurrence. The fixation of the primary tumor to adjacent tissue overlying bone suggests the involvement of periosteum and possible spread to bone. Spread of tumor is critical for prognosis and for selection of treatment. It is critical that the status of the lymph nodes be carefully assessed before a biopsy is performed. The understaging of nodes by cursory assessment or the overstaging of nodes following a biopsy, when an inflammatory component may be present, has dramatic effects on the selection of treatment. Therefore, accurate node examination is needed before biopsy, and the individual who is performing the procedure must be experienced in lymph node palpation.

▼ IMAGING

Imaging, including routine radiology, computed tomography (CT), nuclear scintiscanning, magnetic resonance imaging (MRI), and ultrasonography, can provide evidence of bone involvement and can indicate the extent of some soft-tissue lesions.

Bone involvement is important in staging, selecting therapy, and determining the prognosis. Determination of bone involvement is based on imaging and on clinical and histologic findings. Imaging to determine bone involvement may be done by routine radiology, CT, and bone scanning (Figures 8-15 to 8-21). Nuclear scintiscanning may provide evidence

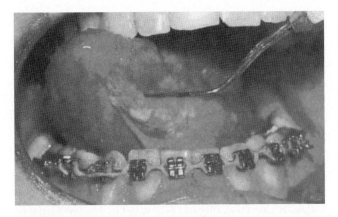

FIGURE 8-10 Irregular leukoerythroplakia involving the ventral surface of the tongue in a 15-year-old. Biopsy revealed invasive squamous cell carcinoma.

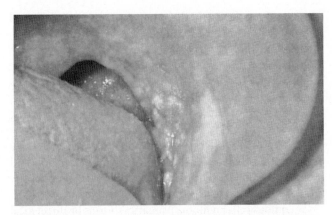

FIGURE 8-11 Irregular leukoerythroplakia involving the anterior pillar of the fauces. Biopsy revealed invasive squamous cell carcinoma.

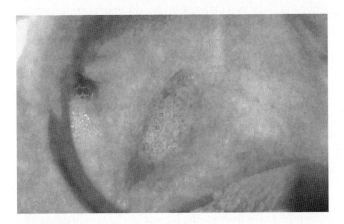

FIGURE 8-12 Shallow ulcer involving the soft palate. The margins were rolled and palpably thickened. The differential diagnosis may include traumatic ulcer, tumor of salivary gland, necrotizing sialometaplasia, and squamous cell carcinoma. Squamous cell carcinoma was demonstrated on biopsy.

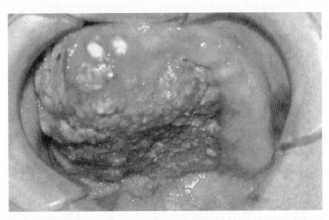

FIGURE 8-13 Extensive firm mass filling the hard palate was diagnosed on biopsy as squamous cell carcinoma. The tumor mass had caused destruction of the alveolar bone and invaded the antrum.

of bone involvement by tumor and bony necrosis following radiation therapy. MRI is of limited value in determining bone involvement but may show distortion of bony trabeculae. Future developments may include monoclonal antibodies linked to a radiolabel to enhance the sensitivity and specificity of the imaging.

Soft-tissue involvement of the antrum and nasopharynx can be assessed with CT and MRI. Panoramic radiography of patients with antral carcinoma may document the lesion in a large number of such cases. MRI is rapidly replacing CT as the imaging technique of choice for the head and neck.[122] Each MRI image should include T1-weighted images, which demonstrate normal anatomy with detail and soft-tissue definition, and T2-weighted images, which demonstrate the tumor in comparison to adjacent muscle and other soft tissues. MRI will allow more accurate distinctions between tumor and benign inflammatory disease than CT allows and may be useful in assessing the sinus. Motion distortion can

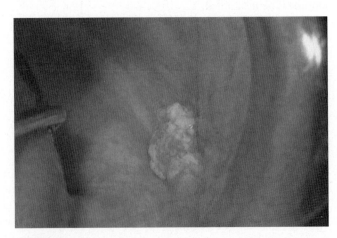

FIGURE 8-14 Exophytic firm mass with an irregular erythroleukoplakic surface. Pathology revealed squamous cell carcinoma. The mass was not mobile, which suggested bone involvement.

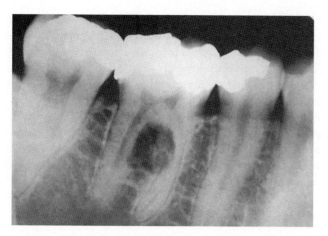

FIGURE 8-15 Periapical radiograph demonstrating bone destruction in the furcation of the first molar tooth and associated resorption of the root. A subsequent biopsy specimen demonstrated squamous cell carcinoma, which was diagnosed as a primary intra-alveolar lesion.

limit its imaging, particularly in moving tissues, but the continuing development of MRI is resulting in less time being needed for imaging.

CT and MRI aid in determining the status of the cervical lymph nodes. There is evidence that imaging will enhance the findings of expert clinical examination when positive lymph nodes are being sought.[123] Small-part ultrasonography may be

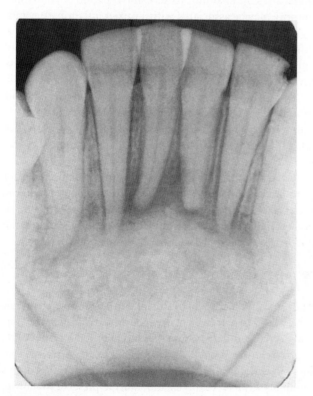

FIGURE 8-16 Periapical radiograph demonstrating an irregular radiolucency involving the bone of the apical region of the mandibular anterior teeth, without change in root anatomy. The teeth tested vital. The radiographic finding was the first indication of involvement of the boney adenocarcinoma.

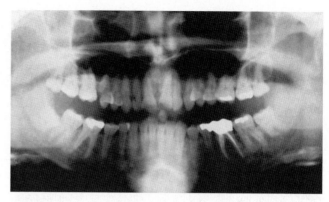

FIGURE 8-17 Panoramic radiograph taken at the time of diagnosis of adenocarcinoma.

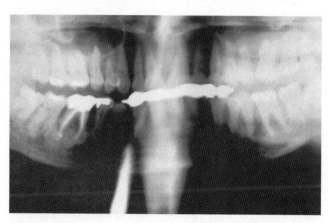

FIGURE 8-18 Massive bone destruction of the mandible, shown after 5 years of follow-up in a case of adenocarcinoma (see Figures 8-16 and 8-17) extending to the molar regions bilaterally. The anterior teeth had been lost due to progressive destruction of the anterior mandible and floor of the mouth.

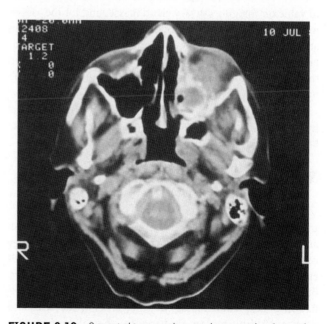

FIGURE 8-19 Computed tomography scan demonstrating destruction of the medial wall of the antrum and opacification of the antrum. Additional views suggested that the opacification represented a tissue mass that was consistent with tumor.

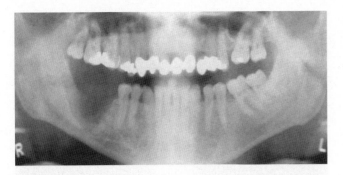

FIGURE 8-20 Panoramic radiograph showing bony destruction of the molar region of the right mandible due to invasion of contiguous tumor. Paresthesia of the right lip was present at the time of diagnosis.

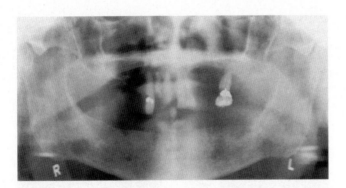

FIGURE 8-21 Panoramic radiograph demonstrating a destructive lesion of the right mandible overlying the mandibular canal. Anesthesia of the mandibular nerve and jaw pain were present. The bone biopsy specimen was consistent with metastatic colon carcinoma, which was subsequently diagnosed.

of value for imaging salivary gland masses and for the assessment of lymph nodes; however, differentiation between benign and malignant nodes may not be possible. The ultrasonographically guided needle biopsy technique may be useful in the assessment of head and neck masses, including lymph nodes.

In the assessment of metastases to the lung, conventional radiography will detect advanced involvement (> 1 cm); detection of smaller masses or lymph nodes is possible with CT.

▼ ACQUISITION OF A TISSUE SPECIMEN

In addition to the standard biopsy techniques of incision and excision, tissue also can be acquired for histopathology by using fine-needle aspiration (FNA). Open biopsy of enlarged lymph nodes is not recommended; in such cases, FNA biopsy should be considered. FNA also may aid the evaluation of suspicious masses in other areas of the head and neck, including masses that involve the salivary glands, tongue, and palate.

Exfoliative cytology is of limited value in the assessment of cancer because squamous mucosa is difficult to sample to the

basal epithelium (which is needed to assess dysplasia) and because only keratin may be acquired in keratinized mucosa. Thus, false-negative results may provide a false sense of comfort and may delay diagnosis. However, if the entire thickness of the epithelium (including basal cells) can be sampled (as has been suggested as possible by using a brush cytology technique), improved diagnostic value may be achieved. An additional means of improving diagnostic value may be the application of molecular markers to exfoliated cells since LOH at sites of putative TSGs in exfoliated cells has been shown to reflect those found on biopsy.[66]

▼ HISTOPATHOLOGY

Microscopic examination is required for diagnosis. Dysplasia or atypia describes a range of cellular abnormalities that includes changes in cell size and morphology, increased mitotic figures, hyperchromatism, and alteration in normal cellular orientation and maturation. The descriptions of mild, moderate, and severe dysplasia refer to epithelial abnormality of varying severity. When the abnormality does not involve the full thickness of the epithelium, the diagnosis is carcinoma in situ. When the basement membrane is violated and connective-tissue invasion occurs, carcinoma is diagnosed. Well-differentiated carcinoma may retain some anatomic features of epithelial cells and may retain the ability to produce keratin whereas poorly differentiated carcinoma loses the anatomic pattern and function of epithelium. Tumors may be associated with a mixed inflammatory infiltrate. Inflammatory and reactive lesions can be difficult to differentiate from dysplasia, and the experience of the pathologist becomes important with the need for clinical reassessment and repeat investigation.

Recognition of tumor invasion may be assisted by a study of type IV collagen (basement membrane collagen) by immunocytochemistry.[114] Invasion of lymphatics, blood vessels, and perineural spaces is of critical importance but is difficult to determine.[114]

Currently, diagnosis is based on the interpretation of histomorphologic changes. However, these changes appear following molecular change, and it is possible that when molecular markers become automated, they will provide additional information and may ultimately become the gold standard in diagnosis.

▼ TREATMENT OF ORAL CANCER

The principle objective of treatment is to cure the patient of cancer. The choice of treatment depends on such factors as cell type and degree of differentiation; the site, size, and location of the primary lesion; lymph node status; the presence of bone involvement; the ability to achieve adequate surgical margins; the ability to preserve speech; the ability to preserve swallowing function; the physical and mental status of the patient; a thorough assessment of the potential complications of each therapy; the experience of the surgeon and radiotherapist; and the personal preferences and cooperation of the patient. If the lesion is not cured by the initial therapy, the options for treatment may be limited, and the likelihood of cure may be reduced.

Surgery or radiation are used with curative intent in the treatment of oral cancer. Chemotherapy is an adjunct to the principal therapeutic modalities of radiation and surgery. Either surgery or radiation may be used for many T1 and T2 lesions; however, combined surgery and radiation is usually needed for more advanced disease. For advanced disease, chemotherapy is used in combination with either or both of the primary treatment modalities.

Surgery

Surgery may be the primary treatment or may be part of combined treatment with radiation therapy. Surgery is indicated (1) for tumors involving bone, (2) when the side effects of surgery are expected to be less significant than those associated with radiation, (3) for tumors that lack sensitivity to radiation, and (4) for recurrent tumor in areas that have previously received a maximum dose of radiotherapy. Surgery also may be used in palliative cases to reduce the bulk of the tumor and to promote drainage from a blocked cavity (eg, antrum). Surgery may fail due to incomplete excision, inadequate margins of resection, tumor seeding in the wound, unrecognized lymphatic or hematogenous spread, neural invasion, or perineural spread. Adequate surgical margins are required but may not be attainable due to the size and location of the tumor. Surgery results in a necessary sacrifice of structure, which may have important esthetic and functional considerations. Future advances in treatment may include surgery combined with systemic chemotherapy and immunotherapy, and there also may be advances in reconstruction.

Surgical management of clinically positive cervical nodes is the treatment of choice. Surgery is needed when bone is involved, and radiotherapy alone cannot be considered adequate to produce a cure. In some cases with minimal bone involvement of the alveolar crest, a partial mandibulectomy may allow the continuity of the mandible to be maintained. However, in many cases, mandibulectomy and resection in continuity with the involved nodes are required.

Radical neck dissection may be conducted as part of an en bloc resection of tumor with lymph node metastases and can be combined with radiation therapy when the primary tumor is treated by radiotherapy. Neck dissection can be used in salvage treatment of cancer that has recurred in the neck. Tumors with node involvement should be treated aggressively due to the poorer prognosis that is seen with positive nodes.

Surgical excision of dysplastic and malignant lesions can be accomplished with laser therapy. Laser therapy for these lesions is well tolerated and usually decreases the period of hospitalization but has the disadvantage of limiting the assessment of the margins for histopathologic confirmation.

Advances in surgical management have taken the form of new surgical approaches and new approaches to reconstruction, such as vascularized flaps and free microvascular reconstruction.[123] Reconstruction with the use of osseointegrated implants offers the ability to provide stable prostheses and enhanced functional results. The ability to place implants in irradiated bone has increased options for rehabilitation.

Radiation Therapy

Radiation therapy may be administered with intent to cure, as part of a combined radiation-surgery and/or chemotherapy management, or for palliation. Radical radiotherapy is intended to cure. The total dose is high, the course of radiation is prolonged, and early and late radiation effects are common. In palliative care, radiation may provide symptomatic relief from pain, bleeding, ulceration, and oropharyngeal obstruction. Hyperfractionation of radiation (usually twice-daily dosing) is being used more extensively as chronic complications appear to be reduced although acute complications are more severe.

Radiation kills cells by interaction with water molecules in the cells, producing charged molecules that interact with biochemical processes in the cells. DNA is disrupted, and chromosomal damage occurs. The affected cells may die or remain incapable of division. Due to a greater potential for cell repair in normal tissue than in malignant cells and a greater susceptibility to radiation due to the higher growth fraction of cancer cells, a differential effect is achieved. To result in an enhanced therapeutic effect, radiation therapy is delivered in daily fractions for a planned number of days. The relatively hypoxic central tumor cells are less susceptible to radiotherapy, but they may become better oxygenated as peripheral cells are affected by radiation and are thus more susceptible to subsequent fractions of radiation.[124]

The biologic effect of radiation depends on the dose per fraction, the number of fractions per day, the total treatment time, and the total dose of radiation. Methods for representing the factors of dose, fraction size, and time of radiation with a single calculation using the time-dose fraction (TDF) and the nominal standard dose (NSD) calculations have been described.[124–126] When comparing studies of radiation effect and when describing the results of studies of cancer patients treated with radiotherapy, reporting the total dose is inadequate because of the importance of fraction size and the time of therapy (which are not available for comparison). The use of the TDF or the NSD will facilitate the understanding of the biologic effect. The tolerance of the vascular and connective tissues to radiation influences both the success of tumor control and the development of treatment complications. The late complications of radiotherapy are due to effects on vascular, connective, and slowly proliferating parenchymal tissues. Late effects are related to the number of fractions, the fraction size, the total dose, the tissue type, and the volume of tissue irradiated. An increase in fraction size or a reduction in the number of fractions with the same total dose results in increased late complications, including tissue fibrosis and soft-tissue and bone necrosis.[127]

It is well known that a relationship exists between the dose of radiation and the survival of a cell population. Cell survival is influenced by the repair of sublethal damage, oxygenation of the cells, total dose, fraction size, and the type of radiation used. Standard single-fraction irradiation protocols deliver 1.8 to 2 Gy to tissue, without significant complications.

SSCs are usually radiosensitive, and early lesions are highly curable. In general, the more differentiated the tumor, the less rapid will be the response to radiotherapy. Exophytic and well-oxygenated tumors are more radiosensitive whereas large invasive tumors with small growth fractions are less responsive. SSC that is limited to the mucosa is highly curable with radiotherapy; however, tumor spread to bone reduces the probability of cure with radiation alone. Small cervical metastases may be controlled with radiation therapy alone although advanced cervical node involvement is better managed with combined therapy.

Radiation therapy has the advantage of treating the disease in situ and avoiding the need for the removal of tissue, and it may be the treatment of choice for many T1 and T2 tumors. Radiation may be administered to a localized lesion by using implant techniques (brachytherapy) or to a region of the head and neck by using external-beam radiation. External-beam therapy can be provided in such a way as to protect adjacent uninvolved tissues, with enhanced effects by using smaller boost fields or by combining external-beam and interstitial techniques. Three-dimensional conformal radiation therapy also enhances the sparing of nonmalignant tissue. Primary tumors of the posterior third of the tongue, oropharynx, and tonsillar pillar are best treated by external-beam radiotherapy, and surgery is reserved for the treatment of tumors with node involvement. Larger radiation fields result in increased patient complications. Smaller fields may be used to boost the dose to the central portion of the tumor since control of peripheral well-oxygenated cells may be possible at a lower dose than that used for the central-less-well-oxygenated tumor mass.

RADIATION SOURCES

For treatment of superficial tumors, radiation with a low penetration may be used. Low-kilovolt radiation (50 to 300 kV) can be used in the treatment of skin and lip lesions. Electron beam therapy provides superficial radiation and has largely replaced low-kilovolt x-ray machines because electrons produce a rapid dose buildup and a sharp falloff of dose; thus, the depth of penetration can be relatively controlled. Electrons may be useful in providing radiation to skin lesions, parotid tumors, and cervical nodes. Deep-seated tumors may be treated with heavy-particle irradiation, such as neutron beam radiation.

Megavoltage radiation using cobalt 60 or the use of a linear accelerator of ≥ 4 MeV is reported to be skin and bone sparing. The linear accelerator provides variable penetration due to its ability to vary the energy of the photons.

TREATMENT PLANNING

The radiation treatment plan is determined by tumor site, tumor size, the total volume to be radiated, the number of treatment fractions, the total number of days of treatment, and the tolerance of the patient. Treatment planning in radiation therapy includes planning for the sparing of uninvolved tissues or organs. The dose to the eye or spinal cord, salivary glands, alveolar bone, and soft tissue can be limited through the selection of the radiation source, field set-up, and shielding and by moving the uninvolved tissue out of the field.

For repeated doses of radiation to be applied to the site of treatment, the patient and the area of treatment must be immobilized. The head can be immobilized by using various techniques and materials, including head holders; bandages; laser positioning, using head and neck "landmarks" or tattoos; and custom acrylic shells (mould room technique). These techniques may be combined with an oral device to position the mandible, allowing the maxilla or mandible to be moved into or out of the radiation field (Figures 8-22 to 8-24). The oral device can incorporate a tongue depressor to position the tongue in or out of the treatment field. This device can be made by using an acrylic tube around which wax is placed. Impressions in warmed baseplate wax can be readily accomplished with bite pressure. The tube serves as a handle and can

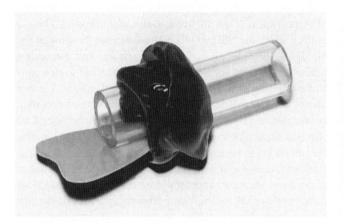

FIGURE 8-22 Tongue and mandibular positioning device. The tube is clear acrylic; the tongue deflector is acrylic but cut to shape and attached by baseplate wax that has been softened and formed to the dentition or residual alveolar ridge.

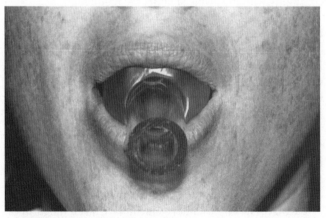

FIGURE 8-23 Tongue and mandibular positioning device placed intra-orally. The wax impression and tube displace the soft tissue minimally to reduce the local irritation that can occur during irradiation.

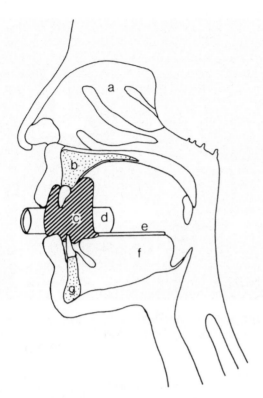

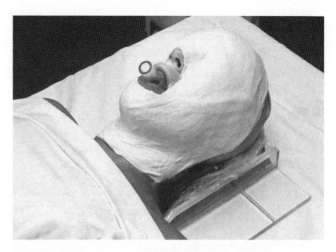

FIGURE 8-25 A patient positioned on a head support. An oral positioning device is in place, and plaster bandages have been placed to form an impression.

FIGURE 8-24 Schematic diagram of the positioning device placed intraorally. (a = nasal cavity; b = upper alveolus; c = wax impression; d = acrylic tube; e = acrylic tongue depressor; f = tongue; g = lower alveolus.)

facilitate respiration. The device can be left as wax or can be processed in acrylic.

Treatment planning requires localization of the tumor and radiation planning. The margins of the tumor can be marked with radiopaque gold seeds or lead wire. If a shell is used, markings can be placed on the shell, or entrance and exit sites can be marked by a tattoo on the skin (Figures 8-25 to 8-27). The contours of the radiation field can be estimated by computer modeling, and alterations can be made as needed.

For most epithelial malignancies, radiation is commonly delivered in 1.8 to 2 Gy per fraction for 5 weeks to a total dose of 6,000 to 6,500 cGy. Hyperfractionation protocols vary, but 100 to 150 cGy often are delivered twice daily. Therapy can be accelerated to produce a total dose of 5,000 cGy in 3 weeks. Lymphomas in the head and neck usually are treated to a total dose of 3,500 to 5,000 cGy delivered at 180 to 200 cGy per day.

In external-beam therapy, the two principal field arrangements are parallel opposed fields (bilateral) and wedged-pair fields. The wedged-pair field allows a therapeutic dose to unilateral disease while sparing a high dose to the opposite side (Figure 8-28). When a large tumor or midline lesion is present, a parallel opposed-field set-up or three-field set-up may be needed, which produces relatively uniform exposure for midline disease. Fields are often modified by placing wedges in the beam to accommodate the variation in tissue contour in the head and neck. A more complex set-up may be needed in some situations and may include three-field techniques, boost fields,

and sequential-field set-ups to maximize therapeutic effects and reduce complications (Figure 8-29). Specific portions of fields such as the orbit, spinal cord, and portions of the alveolus may be blocked with lead (Figure 8-30).

BRACHYTHERAPY

Interstitial and intracavitary implants are used to treat primary cancers in the head and neck. Brachytherapy may the primary treatment modality for localized tumors in the anterior two-thirds of the oral cavity, for boosted doses of radiation to a specific site, or for treatment following recurrence. The isotopes used include cesium, iridium, and gold. Directly implanted sources may be used to deliver radiation, or an afterloading technique may be used in which the radiation source is placed by using previously inserted guide tubes.

The frequency of tissue necrosis is related to the treated volume and to the proximity of the implant to bone. Tissue deflectors can be made to deflect the tongue so that an implant designed to treat a cancer of the tongue does not expose adjacent alveolar bone. These devices can be fabricated by using a double layer of flexible mouth guard material or by using heat-cured acrylic (Figure 8-31). Lead foil can be added to the surface of the deflector if needed. Similarly, devices can be made to keep radiation from superficial treatment of the lip from affecting the alveolar bone (Figure 8-32). Lead cutouts can be made and placed on the skin to isolate the lesion; these may be used in combination with an intraoral device that can shield the intraoral tissues (Figure 8-33).

Future developments in radiotherapy include investigations of radiation sources, radiation fractionation, radiosensitizers, radioprotectors, and combined therapy.[91,128] Advances in radiotherapy that are currently being studied include the use of heavy charged particles (ie, neutrons), which may provide a more focused distribution of cellular damage and which are less sensitive to hypoxia than are conventional radiation sources. Methods of protecting tissues from late radiation

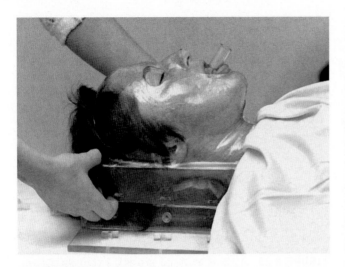

FIGURE 8-26   The acrylic shell or mold is made following removal of the plaster impression. A plaster facial model is poured, and the shell is formed to the model by means of a vacuform technique. The shell and the oral positioning device are used to place the patient in a reproducible position on the machine.

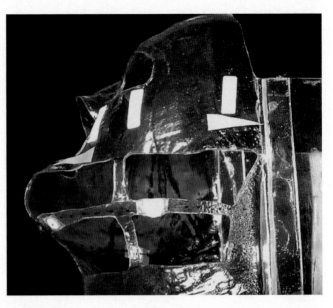

FIGURE 8-27   The final shell with cutouts, field markings, and identification wedges prior to radiation treatment.

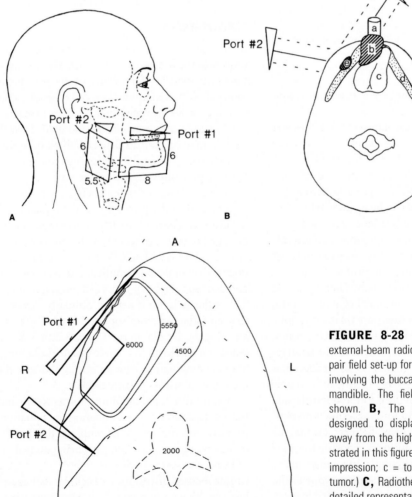

FIGURE 8-28 A, Treatment plan for external-beam radiotherapy using a wedged-pair field set-up for squamous cell carcinoma involving the buccal mucosa adjacent to the mandible. The field size and wedges are shown. **B,** The positioning device was designed to displace the tongue laterally away from the high-dose volume, as demonstrated in this figure. (a = acrylic tube; b = wax impression; c = tongue; d = mandible; e = tumor.) **C,** Radiotherapy treatment plan with detailed representation of the field set-up and isodose calculations.

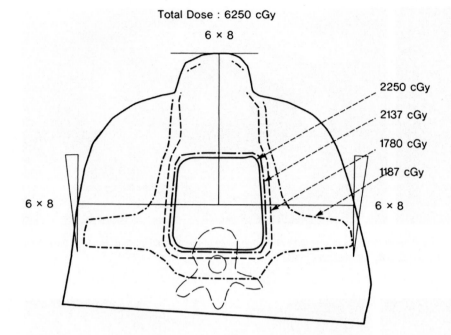

Total Dose : 6250 cGy

6 × 8

2250 cGy

2137 cGy

1780 cGy

1187 cGy

6 × 8   6 × 8

FIGURE 8-29 Treatment plan for radiation treatment of nasopharyngeal carcinoma to a total dose of 6,250 cGy, using a three-field technique. The plan shows the isodose pattern generated, and wedges in the lateral fields are shown.

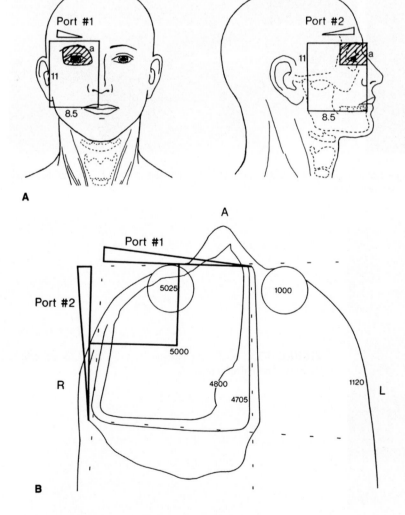

FIGURE 8-30 A, Wedged-pair treatment plan for radiotherapy for squamous cell carcinoma of the antrum in the case demonstrated on CT scan in Figure 8-19. The two-field set-up is shown with a lead blockout for the eye. **B,** Isodose calculations; they indicate the need for the placement of lead shielding.

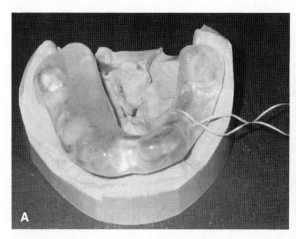
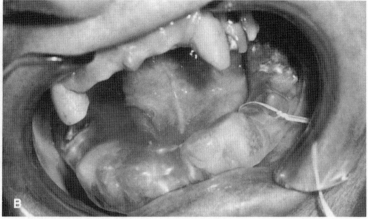

FIGURE 8-31   A, Tongue deflector, fabricated by using three thicknesses of vacuform vinyl on the side of the planned implant. The vinyl provides a smooth soft surface to displace the tongue away from the alveolus. **B,** The appliance in situ.

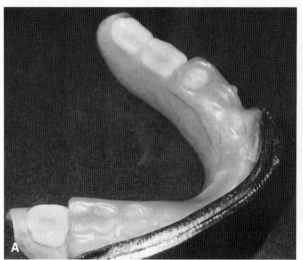
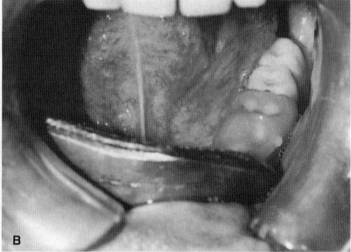

FIGURE 8-32   A, A denture that has been modified with a double thickness of lead shielding attached with baseplate wax. **B,** The modified appliance, shown in situ, prevents exposure of the alveolus to the radiation source.

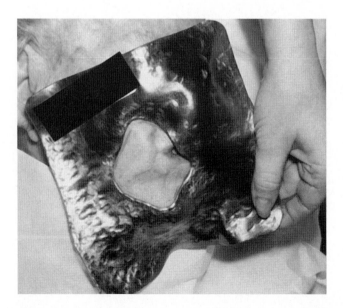

FIGURE 8-33   Lead cutout designed to shield the tissue adjacent to the tumor from radiation exposure.

effects (such as those that compromise the vasculature) are under study. Hyperfractionation (ie, the use of more than one fraction of radiation each day of therapy) may result in improved tumor control with a reduction in late complications; however, increased severity of oral mucositis is reported.[124,129] Thus, efforts to prevent or palliate mucositis will reduce one of the treatment-limiting complications associated with hyperfractionation of radiation therapy. The development of in vitro clonagenic assays to determine tumor cell kinetics and susceptibility to therapy may lead to improvements in the selection of treatment.

Chemotherapy

Chemotherapy has been considered for treatment of individuals with advanced tumors or recurrent disease in whom surgery or radiation is unlikely to result in cure. Chemotherapy is used as induction therapy prior to local therapies, as simultaneous chemoradiotherapy, and as adjuvant chemotherapy after local treatment.[91,130,131] Combined chemotherapy and radiotherapy protocols are being investigated; regression of tumor has been seen, but no improvement in 5-year survival has been seen consistently.[128] The objective of adding chemotherapy is to promote initial tumor reduction and to provide early treatment of micrometastases. The potential toxic effects of chemotherapy include mucositis, nausea, vomiting, and bone marrow suppression. The principal agents that have been studied alone or in combination are methotrexate, bleomycin, taxol and its derivatives, cisplatin and platinum derivatives, and 5-fluorouracil. Chemotherapy for head and neck cancer may result in a temporary reduction in tumor size, but this has not translated into increased survival, control of the primary tumor, or a decreased incidence of metastasis.[2,91,128,132,133] The initial tumor response to chemotherapy prior to radiotherapy may predict tumor responsiveness to radiation. Research will continue and may include investigations into increasing the number of drugs used in combination; increasing the number of courses of chemotherapy provided; using modulators of chemotherapeutics, such as 5-fluorouracil and leucovorin; and modifying administration, such as by intermittent and continuous infusion.

Combined Radiation and Surgery

Advantages of radiotherapy is its ability to eradicate well-oxygenated tumor cells at the periphery of a tumor and to manage subclinical regional disease. Surgery more readily manages tumor masses with relatively radiation-resistant hypoxic cells and tumor that involves bone. Thus, combined therapy can result in improved survival in cases of advanced tumors and tumors that show aggressive biologic behavior.[123] Radiation can be used preoperatively, postoperatively, or with a planned split-course approach. There is no consensus on the best approach to combined therapy with preoperative or postoperative radiation. The advantages of preoperative radiation are the destruction of peripheral tumor cells, the potential control of subclinical disease, and the possibility of converting inoperable lesions into operable lesions. The disadvantages

include difficulty in defining the exact tumor extent, delayed surgery, and delayed postsurgical healing. Surgery prior to radiotherapy can be used to remove the bulk of the tumor containing hypoxic cells. Postoperative radiotherapy can be used to treat cells that remain at the margin of resection and to control subclinical disease. Postoperative radiotherapy is chosen in specific cases, such as extensive carcinoma (in which a delay in healing due to preoperative radiotherapy could be critical), tumor that extends to the margin of the specimen, and extracapsular extension of tumor. Local control of the primary disease appears to be similar with preoperative or postoperative radiotherapy, but in some series, the incidence of metastases was lower in the postoperative group.[134,135] Well-controlled clinical trials are needed to guide the choice of preoperative versus postoperative radiotherapy.

▼ OTHER HEAD AND NECK CANCERS

Malignant Tumors of the Salivary Glands

Tumors of the salivary glands, the majority of which involve the parotid glands, represent less than 5% of all head and neck tumors. Approximately two-thirds of these tumors are benign mixed tumors (pleomorphic adenomas). When tumors involve the submandibular or sublingual glands, there is a high probability that they will be malignant. In order of decreasing frequency, the malignant salivary gland tumors are mucoepidermoid carcinoma, adenoid cystic carcinoma, adenocarcinoma, squamous cell carcinoma, malignant pleomorphic adenoma, undifferentiated carcinoma, lymphoma, melanoma, and a mixed group of sarcomas. Most salivary gland tumors spread by local infiltration, by perineural or hematogenous spread, and (less commonly) through lymphatics. Rarely, metastases from other malignancies may involve the parotid glands. The cause of salivary gland tumors remains obscure, but ionizing radiation has been identified as a risk factor.

Malignant salivary gland tumors most commonly present as a mass that may be ulcerated. Neurologic involvement may lead to discomfort; with parotid gland tumors, involvement of the facial nerve may cause facial paralysis. Most small malignant lesions are indistinguishable from benign lesions. The majority of minor salivary gland tumors are malignant. The most common site is the posterior hard palate, but other sites in the oral cavity or upper respiratory tract may be involved. The presentation is usually a painless mass. The staging of salivary gland tumors is shown in Table 8-3.

Necrotizing sialometaplasia is a self-limiting non-neoplastic inflammatory condition of unknown etiology that affects the palatal salivary glands. The painful lesion occurs in sites of mucus-secreting glands and produces an ulceration with rolled borders. Clinical and histologic differentiation may be difficult, but accurate diagnosis is critical because necrotizing sialometaplasia will resolve spontaneously, usually within 1 to 2 months.

Biopsy of masses in the major glands may be accomplished by FNA, and diagnosis may be made without open biopsy. However, surgical biopsy may be necessary if FNA is not diagnostic. In masses involving minor glands, biopsy can be performed with routine techniques.

TREATMENT OF SALIVARY GLAND TUMORS

Surgery is the principle treatment of the primary tumor. Radiotherapy at a high dose is effective in malignant salivary gland tumors.[128] Postoperative radiation can contribute to cure and to improved local control and is indicated for patients with residual disease following surgery, extensive perineural involvement, lymph node involvement, high-grade malignant disease, tumors with more than one local recurrence after surgery, inoperable tumors, or malignant lymphoma and for those who refuse surgery. Doses and fractionation similar to those used in the treatment of squamous cell carcinoma are usually employed.

PROGNOSIS

The prognosis of salivary gland tumors is related to tumor type, tumor size, lymph node involvement, and extension of disease.[136] Small tumors, acinic cell tumor, low-grade mucoepidermoid carcinoma, and mixed tumors have a high probability of cure. Tumors with a poor prognosis include large tumors, adenocarcinoma, adenoid cystic carcinoma, high-grade mucoepidermoid carcinoma, poorly differentiated carcinoma, and squamous cell carcinoma. Histologic findings that correlate with lymph node involvement include deep (> 8 mm) and diffuse invasion of stromal tissue and invasion of lymphatics.[123] Adenoid cystic carcinoma has a high incidence of progression, and 10- and 15-year survivals must be examined due to late progression (recurrence may be seen after 10-15 years, therefore 10-15 year survivals should be assessed).

Malignant Lesions of the Jaw

Osteogenic sarcoma is the most common malignancy of bone.[2,137] Its treatment requires surgery, possibly in combination with radiotherapy. Primary squamous cell carcinoma of the jaw is rare and may arise from epithelial rests or from the epithelium of odontogenic lesions.

Tumor metastatic to the jaw most often involves the posterior mandible. Metastases are rare, representing approximately 1% of all oral malignant tumors.[138] Common tumors that metastasize to the jaw are adenocarcinomas (of the breast, prostate, and gastrointestinal tract) and renal carcinoma. Other reported sites of primary tumors that metastasize include the thyroid, testes, bladder, ovary, and uterine cervix. Symptoms associated with metastases to the jaw may include pain, paresthesia, anesthesia, mobility of teeth, and swelling. Destruction of bone may be visualized with imaging (see Figure 8-21). Lesions in periapical regions can be mistaken for dental disease. Gingival masses can occur as signs of metastatic tumor; however, metastases to soft tissue are extremely rare, representing less than 0.1% of oral tumors.[138] Diagnosis requires biopsy. Multiple myeloma may cause radiolucent lesions in multiple bones, including the jaw. Multiple myeloma may cause periapical lesions and (because pain may be associated with the disease) must be distinguished from dental disease.

These conditions require definitive diagnosis before it is assumed that the lesions represent other than a dental pathosis. The practitioner must arrive at a definitive diagnosis before embarking on routine dental treatment.

Nasopharyngeal Carcinoma

Nasopharyngeal cancer has implications in dental practice because patients may present with complaints that may mimic temporomandibular disorders and because radiation therapy includes all major saliva glands, leading to hyposalivation and oral complications post treatment. Symptoms associated with nasopharyngeal carcinoma include pain, limited jaw opening, earache, and other ear complaints. The most common symptoms are nasal stuffiness, nosebleed, and neck mass.

Risk factors for nasopharyngeal carcinoma include Epstein-Barr virus infection, smoking, childhood consumption of salted fish and other preserved foods that are common in a Cantonese diet, and origin from southern China.[13,113,139-141] Long-term survival is approximately 50% because most patients are identified after the tumor has spread regionally and after lymph nodes are involved.[141,142] FNA can provide tissue diagnosis, and the sensitivity can be enhanced by DNA amplification (polymerase chain reaction) of the Epstein-Barr virus genome, which is commonly associated with nasopharyngeal carcinoma but which is rare in other head and neck cancers.[143]

Treatment requires radiation therapy and is increasingly combined with chemotherapy. A three-field set-up for radiotherapy is shown in Figure 8-29. Surgery may play a role in involved neck nodes but not in the treatment of the primary tumor. Chemotherapy and immunotherapy in combination with radiation therapy have been reported.[141] Radiation therapy will result in radiation exposure of all of the salivary glands and in severe xerostomia.

Basal Cell Carcinoma

Basal cell carcinoma is a locally destructive cancer that may occur in the head and neck. Sun exposure is considered the principal etiologic factor. Basal cell carcinoma presents as persistent keratotic lesions (indurated papules) that may develop rolled borders and ulcerate. If advanced, they may lead to locoregional tissue necrosis and ulceration. Treatment may involve local excision or topical chemotherapy. While basal cell carcinoma rarely metastasizes, recurrence or second primary lesions are common. Dental workers have the opportunity to identify basal cell lesions on the head and neck if routine extraoral examination is conducted with care.[144]

Malignant Melanoma

Melanoma may present as an area of altered pigmentation involving the skin. Oral malignant melanoma is extremely rare[145] (2% of all melanomas). Among 65 patients with head and neck melanoma, two-thirds of the patients were in their sixth decade, and only 10% of cases involved the oral mucosa.[145] However, among Japanese people, oral lesions account for 14% of all cases of melanoma.[72] The oral lesions may present as tissue masses or ulceration that may be pigmented, but nonpigmented lesions are often reported. Most intraoral cases occur in the maxillary mucosa, presenting as a mass or flat lesions that may ulcerate and that may be associated with bleeding. Melanoma is an aggressive malignant disease; metastasis through lymphatic and hematogenous routes is common, and the prognosis is poor. Aggressive therapy of the primary tumor and careful investigation for metastases are required.

Intraoral and Head and Neck Sarcoma

Intraoral sarcoma is a very rare disease with a poor prognosis. It may constitute approximately 1% of all head and neck cancers and only 0.14% of intraoral malignancies.[146] The lesions are most often identified as a mass, and the most common malignancy is rhabdomyosarcoma. Chondrosarcoma and osteosarcoma may involve the jaw, the commonest presentation being as a mass.[147] Treatment is wide surgical excision although combined chemoradiotherapy to improve the prognosis is being examined.

Head and Neck Malignant Disease in AIDS

HIV infection that leads to immunosuppression increases the risk of the development of neoplastic disease.[148] Advances in the management of HIV infection have lead to a reduction in the prevalence of manifestations of immunosuppression, but it is usually anticipated that HIV disease will ultimately progress and that oral findings will be identified. Kaposi's sarcoma (KS) is the most common neoplastic disease of acquired immunodeficiency syndrome (AIDS). Lymphoma is the most rapidly increasing malignant disease of AIDS. Non-Hodgkin's lymphoma, most commonly of B-cell origin, may present with central nervous system involvement but also may present with head, neck, or oral lesions. The lymphomas are aggressive and carry a poor prognosis. Oropharyngeal squamous cell carcinoma has been reported in patients with HIV disease; however, prevalence rates have not been determined.

KS is a multicentric neoplastic proliferation of endothelial cells. KS may occur in up to 55% of homosexual males with AIDS and may be the first sign of progression to AIDS or may occur during the course of the disease. KS is less common in AIDS patients whose risk factor is not sexual transmission, suggesting that KS is associated with a sexually transmitted agent, which has now been identified as human herpesvirus type 8 (HHV-8). As increasing numbers of intravenous drug abusers are affected, the frequency of KS has decreased. KS can involve any oral site but most frequently involves the attached mucosa of the palate, gingiva, and dorsum of the tongue. Lesions begin as blue purple or red purple flat discolorations that can progress to tissue masses that may ulcerate (Figures 8-34 to 8-36). The lesions do not blanch with pressure. Nondiscolored KS also has been reported in the oral cavity. Initial lesions are asymptomatic but can cause discomfort and interfere with speech, denture use, and eating when lesions progress. The differential diagnosis includes ecchymosis, vascular lesions, and salivary gland tumors. Definitive diagnosis requires biopsy. Because KS is a multicentric neoplastic disease,

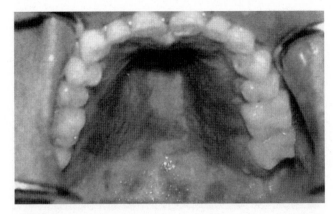

FIGURE 8-34 Bilateral involvement of the hard palate with purple discolorations consistent with Kaposi's sarcoma. The lesion possesses some thickness on the left but appears to be nonthickened on the right. Blue-red discoloration in isolated Kaposi's lesions is present on the soft palate.

multiple sites of involvement can occur, including skin, lymph nodes, gastrointestinal tract, and other organ systems.

Intralesional chemotherapy for treatment of oral KS has shown effective palliation.[145,148–150] Intralesional treatment with vinblastine and interferon has been reported. The lesions can be treated with the injection of vinblastine (0.2 mg/mL) under local anesthesia. The effect of treatment may continue for several weeks and may result in palliation for approximately 4 months (see Figure 8-36). Repeat injection can be completed with similar efficacy. KS is radiosensitive, and radiation can be palliative for regional disease. Fractionated radiotherapy (for a total dose of 25 to 30 Gy over 1 to 2 weeks) may be provided for oral KS. Severe mucositis can follow radiotherapy for oral KS although this may be less severe with fractionated treatment. If KS progresses at multiple sites, systemic chemotherapy may be needed. New approaches to management that are being investigated include the use of cytokines that reduce angiogenesis and the use of antiviral agents for HHV-8 infection.

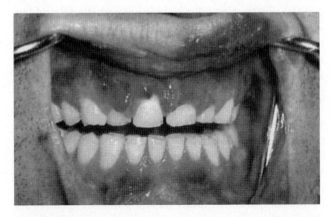

FIGURE 8-35 Multiple blue-red masses of Kaposi's sarcoma involving the attached gingiva and lip.

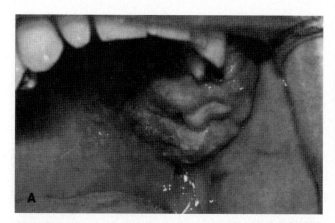
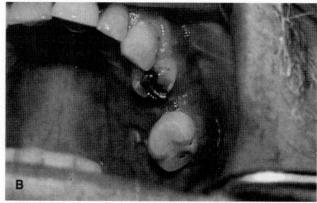

FIGURE 8-36 A and **B,** Kaposi's sarcoma treated with intralesional vinblastine injection, resulting in successful palliation with elimination of discomfort and mobility of the involved teeth, reduction in tissue mass, and persistence of discoloration.

▼ PRETREATMENT ORAL AND DENTAL ASSESSMENT

Detailed oral and dental assessment is necessary prior to cancer treatment. The oral assessment is needed to identify conditions that should be treated prior to cancer therapy, to (1) reduce the risk or severity of complications, (2) reduce the risk of infection involving the dentition and mucosa, and (3) minimize and manage the complications of hyposalivation. The assessment also will aid the institution of a program for preventing caries. The acquisition of baseline data will allow assessment of the progress of the patient's oral condition during and following cancer therapy.

The essential aspects of a pretreatment oral examination have been reviewed.[151] Pretreatment interventions are directed at the maintenance of mucosal and bony integrity, dental and periodontal health, salivary gland function and the prevention of potential complications of therapy.[152] The patient's history should review past dental care, current oral or dental symptoms, and the presence and condition of prostheses. The assessment must be comprehensive and must include head and neck examination (with attention to the presence of lymphadenopathy), intraoral mucosal examination, and periodontal and dental examination. The periodontal examination must include full periodontal probing. Periodontal attachment loss is greater in radiated fields, and this future attachment loss should be considered in preradiotherapy treatment planning.[153] Definitive dental diagnosis and management must be provided prior to radiation therapy because periodontal disease may require periodontal surgery or extractions, which are fraught with risk if the teeth involved were within the high-dose fraction. Radiographic examination should allow detailed evaluation of the teeth and periapical regions and should include imaging of any bone pathosis. Saliva production should be measured prior to therapy, to document any change in flow rate, which may predict a risk of oral complications. Study models should be acquired for the provision of gel carriers, for construction of surgical prostheses if indicated, and for permanent records. Cultures for

patients with suspected infections of the mucosa (eg, *Candida*) are indicated throughout the course of treatment. Culture of cariogenic bacteria in xerostomic patients is important for the diagnosis of cariogenic risk and indicates the need for therapy (see "Caries," later in this chapter). A shift to cariogenic flora occurs due to hyposalivation and is not seen during radiation therapy in patients who are provided with fluoride and in those maintaining plaque control.[154] Plaque control and gingivitis at first examination provide evidence of past oral care habits, and unless it is believed that a true change in habits can be achieved, past practices should be expected to predict future care.

Prior to radiation therapy, teeth to be maintained should be scaled and root planed. Sites of potential mechanical irritation should be eliminated. The prevention of osteoradionecrosis requires the extraction of nonrestorable or questionable teeth, root tips, and periodontally involved teeth in the planned radiation field (see "Tissue Necrosis," later in this chapter). If time permits, asymptomatic periapical radiolucent lesions can be managed; however, endodontics can be performed following radiation if expert management is accomplished. Detailed review of oral hygiene, oral care during radiation therapy, and oral care following radiotherapy is an important part of long-term care.

▼ COMPLICATIONS OF CANCER TREATMENT

Acute reactions occur during the course of radiotherapy because of direct tissue toxicity and possibly secondary bacterial irritation resulting in ulcerative mucositis; these reactions resolve over several weeks following the completion of therapy. Chronic complications or late radiation reactions occur due to change in the vascular supply, fibrosis in connective tissue and muscle, and change in the cellularity of tissues. These complications develop slowly over months to years following treatment. The effect on the mucosa is one of epithelial atrophy, altered vascular supply, and fibrosis in connective tissue, resulting in an atrophic and friable mucosa. The connective tissue and musculature may demonstrate increased fibrosis. Fibrosis in muscle and joint tissue may result in limited function. In salivary glands, loss of acinar cells, alteration in duct epithelium, fibrosis, and fatty degeneration occur. In bone, hypovascularity and hypocellularity lead to the risk of osteoradionecrosis. Surgical treatment of the malignant disease results in acute pain and may result in chronic complications due to structural change, fibrosis, and neurologic changes. Hyperfractionation of radiation therapy may reduce the late complications but may increase the severity of the acute reactions. The antiprostaglandin effects and the effects of acetylsalicyclic acid (ASA) and nonsteroidal analgesics on platelet adhesion may reduce the vascular complications following radiation therapy.[155,156] Low-dose ASA has been shown to increase stromal tolerance by 20%[156] and has the potential to reduce the severity of late radiation complications.

Mucositis

Ulcerative oral mucositis is a painful and debilitating condition that is a dose- and rate-limiting toxicity of cancer therapy. The potential sequelae of mucositis consist of severe pain, increased risk for local and systemic infection, compromised oral and pharyngeal function, and oral bleeding that affect quality of life, may lead to hospitalization or increase the duration of hospitalization, and may increase the cost of care.

Mucositis is the most common cause of pain during the treatment of cancer. Pain due to oropharyngeal mucositis frequently requires the use of opioid analgesics, which is associated with increased costs and side effects. The increasing use of more aggressive therapy to improve cancer cure rates has increased the frequency and severity of oral complications. In neutropenic patients, the risk of systemic infection due to oral opportunistic and acquired flora is increased with mucosal ulceration. Increased risk of mucositis has been associated with poor oral hygeine, tobacco use, hyposalivation at baseline, and older age.[157–162] Hyperfractionation, combined chemoradiotherapy, and the use of radiosensitizers cause increased severity of oral mucositis. The plasma level of glutamyl-cysteinyl-glycine (GSH) has been shown to predict the severity of acute radiation mucositis,[163] suggesting that GSH has a radioprotective role due to protection against either membrane lipid oxidation or DNA damage.

The literature does not provide definitive evidence for direct management of mucositis, but research is continuing. Most studies of oral mucositis involve small numbers of patients, many studies are preliminary rather than randomized placebo-controlled trials, and many suffer from the use of outcome measures that lack sensitivity and that are not validated. The wide variation in the quality of studies of mucositis makes the assessment of outcomes difficult and requires that reviewers carefully assess the methods employed in the study.

ASSESSMENT

Radiation-associated mucositis is virtually a universal complication in patients with head and neck cancer. The reported incidence and severity of mucositis depends on the methods used for oral assessment, as demonstrated in a study in which a chart review and an interview were conducted and in which mucositis was respectively identified in 30% and 69% of the same patients.[164] Clinical examination of tissue change and assessments of symptoms are the principal means of assessing mucositis. A recent study assessed and validated the use of the Oral Mucositis Assessment Scale (OMAS) and showed that the OMAS was easily used and demonstrated intrarater and interobserver reproducibility and temporal changes with treatment.[165] Other markers of mucositis may become available. Current investigations include cell morphology and viability of exfoliated buccal cells; the viability of cells was determined by the trypan blue dye exclusion test, and a shift from mature to immature cells was seen as mucositis developed.[166] Oral symptoms, function scales and validated measures of tissue damage currently represent the best means of assessing the outcome of treatment interventions.

PATHOGENESIS

Cytotoxic chemotherapy and radiation therapy have direct effects on mucosal epithelial cells, resulting in thinning of the epithelium and ultimately to loss of the barrier (see Table 8-1). Connective tissue and vascular elements are also affected. Mucositis may include an initial inflammatory/vascular and epithelial phase that is followed by an ulcerative/bacteriologic phase and ultimately a healing phase.[167] In the initial phase, changes in cell surface molecules,[168] and epidermal growth factor (EGF) may increase the risk of mucositis, and cytokines that reduce epithelial cell proliferation may decrease the severity of tissue damage.[169] Interaction with cytokines produced in the connective tissue may affect tissue damage. The oral microflora appear to play a role in the development of ulceration and pseudomembrane, as suggested in studies of gram-negative bacterial flora in patients with radiation-induced mucositis.[167,170] Shifts in the oral microflora include the development of a flora that is high in Streptococcus mutans, lactobacilli, Candida, and gram-negative bacilli, which may result in oral infections and may aggravate mucositis (Figure 8-37). Resolution of mucositis is dependent on epithelial cell regeneration and angiogenesis and may also be dependent on white blood cell function and the production of growth factors. Pain associated with mucositis is dependent on the degree of tissue damage, the sensitization of pain receptors, and the elaboration of inflammatory and pain mediators. Oral defenses compromised due to irradiation include decreased mucosal cell turnover, increased permeability and loss of the mucosal barrier, changes in saliva secretion, reduced levels of antimicrobial factors in saliva, loss of protective mucins, and diluting effects. Impairment of the mobility of oral structures may lead to reduced clearing of local irritants and food products.

The first signs of mucositis may be a white appearance to the mucosa, caused by hyperkeratinization and intraepithelial edema, or a red appearance due to hyperemia and epithelial thinning (Figure 8-38). Pseudomembrane formation represents ulceration with a fibrinous exudate with oral debris and

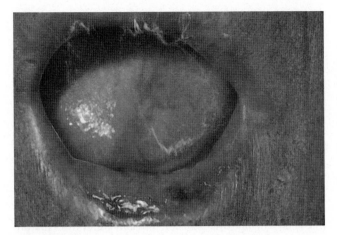

FIGURE 8-37   Radiation mucositis complicated by candidiasis, resulting in increased severity of mucositis and angular cheilitis.

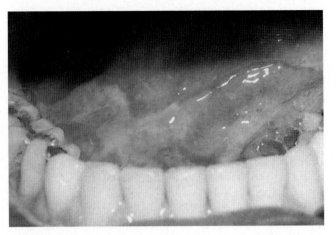

FIGURE 8-39   Increasing ulceration of radiation mucositis, seen after 3 weeks of treatment in a planned 6-week course.

microbial components (Figures 8-39 and 8-40). Radiation has more marked effects on rapidly proliferating epithelium, and mucositis therefore involves the nonkeratinized mucosa first. Late changes in the mucosa reflect endarteritis and vascular changes associated with hypovascularity and with hyalinization of collagen[171] (Figure 8-41). With common fractions of 180 to 220 cGy per day, mucositis with erythema is noted in 1 to 2 weeks and increases throughout the course of therapy (often to a maximum in 4 weeks) with persistence until healing occurs 2 or more weeks after the completion of therapy.[172] Metallic dental restorations and appliances may produce secondary radiation when in the path of the radiation beam; this may increase the effect of irradiation on adjacent tissue, resulting in increased mucositis and risk of late effects. Thus, removable dental appliances should be removed during radiation; however, metal restorations are not removed, and their significance in complications is not well documented. The increasing use of dental implants will require consideration in future treatment planning for patients with head and neck cancer.

HYPOSALIVATION

Bilateral exposure of the major salivary glands to radiation therapy will predictably result in xerostomia. In patients who receive radiotherapy for treatment of Hodgkin's disease (ie, mantle fields), saliva production is affected when the upper limit of the field is at the chin to the mastoid; below this level, minimal long-term effects are seen.[173] Individuals who receive radiation doses greater than a total dose of 3,000 cGy are at risk if all major glands are in the field. Irreversible effects occur at a total dose of 6,000 Gy for 5 weeks. Radiation results in acinar cell atrophy and necrosis, changes in the vascular connective tissue, and altered neurologic function. During radiation, the serous acini are affected earlier than the mucinous acini, resulting in a thick viscous secretion that can be upsetting to the patient. Saliva production rapidly decreases and can be reduced by 50% after 1 week of standard fractionated radiation. Depending on the amount of salivary tissue included in the field, xerostomia may resolve within 6 months, but in many cases, the loss of function is permanent. A review of patients at 3 years post radiation therapy that

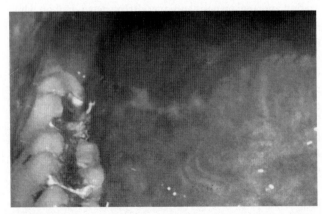

FIGURE 8-38   Early mucositis of the floor of the mouth seen after 2 weeks of radiation therapy, with increasing erythema of nonkeratinized mucosa in the treatment field and developing ulceration.

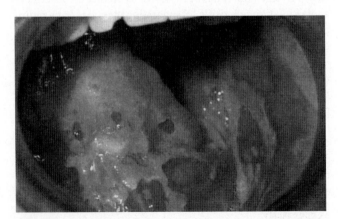

FIGURE 8-40   Extensive ulceration and pseudomembrane formation involving the buccal mucosa, floor of the mouth, and ventral surface of the tongue due to severe mucositis.

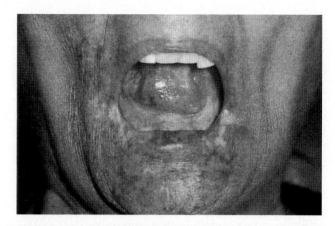

FIGURE 8-41 Late complications of radiation therapy are demonstrated. Atrophy of mucosa, altered vascular pattern with telangiectasia, fibrosis leading to limited jaw opening and limited oral aperture, and irregular pigmentation of the skin are present in this case.

included the major glands in the field showed a 95% reduction in saliva volume.[174] Xerostomia in such patients may be lifelong, and prevention of oral complications may therefore need to be continued indefinitely.

Changes in the composition of saliva also occur. Decreases in secretory immunoglobulin A, buffering capacity, and acidity are seen.[175–177] These changes affect the microbial flora and the remineralizing potential of teeth. The goals in the management of xerostomia are to stimulate the remaining salivary gland function and (if such stimulation is not achieved) to palliate xerostomia, prevent tooth demineralization and caries, and manage microbial shifts.

RADIATION THERAPY–RELATED MUCOSITIS AND FUNGAL AND VIRAL COLONIZATION

Radiotherapy-related mucositis is the most frequent complication in patients receiving irradiation for head and neck cancers. Chronic oral sensitivity frequently continues after treatment, due to mucosal atrophy (33%) and neurologic syndromes attributed to de-afferentation (16%).[178,179]

Oral colonization by *Candida* spp and candidiasis is common during and following radiotherapy and is related to hyposalivation and to denture and tobacco use.[154,180] The role of fungal colonization and infection in radiation mucositis is not clearly understood. In a group of patients receiving head and neck irradiation, patients who were on fluconazole developed 1 mycotic infection and had 14 nonscheduled breaks in radiation therapy, compared to 19 infections and 30 breaks in radiation therapy for those who were not provided with fungal prophylaxis.[181] However, an association between candidiasis or oral colonization and mucositis during irradiation has not been confirmed by other studies.[182] The potential role of the reactivation of HSV during head and neck radiation therapy is unclear, and reactivation of HSV infection does not appear to commonly complicate radiation mucositis.[183]

SYSTEMIC APPROACHES TO MANAGEMENT

Pain Management. Management of severe oropharyngeal mucositis often requires the use of systemic opioids (Table 8-4). Systemic analgesics should be prescribed by following the World Health Organization (WHO) analgesic "ladder," which suggests the use of non-opioid analgesics, alone or in combination with opioids and adjunctive medications, for increasing pain.[184] Analgesics should be provided on a time-contingent basis, with provision for breakthrough pain. While there may be patient and professional concerns regarding the use of opioids for cancer pain, difficulty in stopping the analgesic does not occur if pain resolves, and addiction is not a concern in oncology patients. Rather, the concern is with the underuse of analgesics and with underdosing that leads to poor pain control.[184]

There has been limited study of the use of adjunctive approaches to pain management in patients with oral mucositis. Relaxation, imagery, biofeedback, hypnosis, and transcutaneous electrical nerve stimulation have the potential to provide adjunctive approaches for the management of cancer pain.[184] The use of hypnosis has been shown to be a valuable adjunct,[185,186] and relaxation and imagery reduce the pain experience.[187]

Systemic prednisone provided to patients with head and neck cancer in a double-blind protocol resulted in a trend to reduced severity and duration of mucositis, and fewer treatment interruptions occurred.[188] However, the use of steroids may result in increased risk of infection. Systemic β-carotene administered during a combined course of chemotherapy and radiotherapy for patients with advanced head and neck squamous carcinoma has been reported to reduce the severity of mucositis.[189]

Radioprotectors. Amifostine (Ethyol) is a sulfhydryl compound that acts by scavenging free radicals generated in tissues exposed to radiation and that promotes repair of damaged DNA. Amifostine has been shown to protect a variety of tissues, including mucosa, cardiac tissue, renal tissue, bone marrow, and neuro- and ototoxicity when administered prior to irradiation and chemotherapy. There is reduced uptake of amifostine into tumor, and tumor protection is not seen. Trials are under way to assess the use of amifostine in patients with cancer (including head and neck cancer) who are being treated with chemoradiotherapy. Side effects include nausea, vomiting, and reversible hypotension. Administration requires prehydration, and intravenous administration is necessary prior to each fraction of irradiation. In initial studies of patients receiving chemoradiotherapy for head and neck cancer, those who received amifostine (compared to those who received no intervention) had reduced mucositis[190–192] and xerostomia.[190–193] Amifostine has been approved in the United States for reduction of renal toxicity secondary to cisplatin administration and for reduction of xerostomia in patients who are treated with radiotherapy. This agent has potential for reducing the effects of the acute and chronic toxicity of cancer therapy, including mucositis. However, further study including cost-benefit analysis is needed.

Biologic Response Modifiers. Extensive studies have been conducted on biologic response modifiers. These are molecules that affect cellular function, including growth and tissue repair. Early findings on the effect of granulocyte colony-stimulating factor (G-CSF) upon reducing oral mucositis have been described although this has not been confirmed in other studies.[194] Granulocyte-macrophage colony-stimulating factor (GM-CSF) has shown benefits in a number of initial clinical trials in patients treated with chemoradiotherapy.[195–198] Keratinocyte growth factor (KGF), a member of the fibroblast growth factor family, binds to KGF receptor, accelerating the healing of wounds.[199] Systemic KGF modifies the proliferation and differentiation of epithelial cells and may protect the cells from damage. Animal studies have shown the potential of KGF to reduce mucositis caused by radiation and chemotherapy.[199–201] Double-blind controlled trials are in progress.

TOPICAL APPROACHES TO MANAGEMENT

The effect of oral hygiene and the elimination of local irritants may have an impact on the development of mucositis. Maintaining good oral hygiene has been shown to reduce the severity of oral mucositis and does not increase the risk of septicemia in neutropenic patients.[93] Mucositis is not reduced with the use of chlorhexidine rinses during radiation therapy.[170,202,203] This may be due to the inactivation of chlorhexidine by saliva, the lack of an etiologic role for gram-positive bacteria (which are suppressed by chlorhexidine) in mucositis, and a limited effect of chlorhexidine on gram-negative organisms that may be important in the development of ulcerative mucositis. Other studies, using an oral lozenge containing polymyxin, tobramycin, and amphotericin B, have shown an effect on *Candida* colonization and gram-negative bacilli, and a reduction in mucositis was reported.[170,204]

Palliation of mucositis may be achieved by the use of bland oral rinses and topical anesthetic and coating agents; however, controlled studies are lacking (see Table 8-4). Saline, bicarbonate, dilute hydrogen peroxide, and water also have been suggested for hydrating and diluting by rinsing. Lip applica-

tions with water-based lubricants (eg, lubricating jelly, such as K-Y Jelly [Johnson & Johnson]) or preparations that contain lanolin have been suggested rather than the use of oil-based products because the chronic use of oil-based products (eg, Vaseline) results in the atrophy of epithelium and the risk of infection under occlusion of the application. A study comparing saline and hydrogen peroxide rinses in radiation therapy found no significant differences among patients with mucositis although oral sensitivity was greater in those using peroxide.[205] Coating agents used as oral rinses, such as milk of magnesia, liquid Amphogel, and Kaopectate (Pharmacia Corp., Peapack, N.J.) are often recommended but have not been subjected to double-blind studies.[184] Viscous lidocaine is frequently recommended although there are no studies that assess its benefit or its potential for toxicity in cancer patients. Lidocaine may cause local symptoms that include burning and that eliminate taste and affect the gag reflex. Potent topical anesthetic agents should be used with caution due to their potential for decreasing the gag reflex, causing central nervous system depression or excitation and causing cardiovascular effects that may follow excessive absorption. Local applications of topical anesthetic creams or gels may be useful for local painful mucosal ulcerations. A combination of agents that may include a coating agent and an analgesic or anesthetic agent also have been suggested, but no randomized controlled studies of mixtures of agents have been reported.

Benzydamine hydrochloride (Tantum, Riker-3M, Canada; Diflam, UK) is a nonsteroidal agent that possesses analgesic anti-inflammatory properties and is mildly anesthetic. Benzydamine may stabilize cell membranes, inhibit the degranulation of leukocytes, affect cytokine production, and alter the synthesis of prostaglandins. Signs and symptoms of oral mucositis are reduced when benzydamine is used prophylactically throughout the course of radiation therapy.[170,172,203,206–209] However, another study, comparing the use of chlorhexidine and benzydamine, did not show less severe mucositis in patients using benzydamine rinse.[210] Benzydamine is currently available in Europe and Canada and is under review by the US Food and Drug Administration (FDA).

Sucralfate is a cytoprotective agent that is available for the management of gastrointestinal ulceration. The agent may form a barrier on the surface of ulcerated mucosa in acidic

TABLE 8-3   Staging for Salivary Gland Cancer

T (Size of Primary Tumor)	N (Lymph Node Involvement)	M (Distant Metastases)
T1: tumor < 2 cm	N0: no nodal involvement	M0: no metastases
T2: tumor > 2 and < 4 cm	N1: ipsilateral lymph node involvement < 3 cm	MI: distant metastases
T3: tumor > 4 and < 6 cm	N2: ipsilateral lymph node involvement > 3 cm or multiple ipsilateral nodes	
T4: tumor > 6 cm	N2a: single ipsilateral node > 3 and < 6 cm	
T1–T4a: no local extension	N2b: multiple ipsilateral nodes < 6 cm	
T1–T4b: local extension (clinical or	N2c: bilateral or contralateral nodes < 6 cm	
macroscopic extension to skin, bone, nerve)	N3: lymph > 6 cm	

Reproduced with permission from American Joint Committee on Cancer. Manual for staging of cancer. 3rd ed. Philadelphia: J.B. Lippincott; 1988.

conditions and may stimulate the release of prostaglandins. Sucralfate suspension has been studied in patients with mucositis, and less severe mucositis has been reported in some studies[211] but not in the majority of studies.[212–214] However, reduced oral pain was reported for sucralfate users compared to placebo users.[212,213] Another potential benefit is a reduction in potentially pathogenic oral organisms in patients with mucositis.[212,215,216] Because of its coating and protective effects, sucralfate may be useful in the palliation of established mucositis. A comparison of sucralfate and a diphenhydramine-plus-kaolin-pectin suspension did not show a greater efficacy for either suspension, but reduced mucositis was seen in both groups when compared to historic controls.[216]

Misoprostol is a synthetic prostaglandin E analogue that is used for the prevention of gastric ulcers for patients on nonsteroidal anti-inflammatory medication, due to its antisecretory and mucosal protective effects. Topical application of misoprostol in head and neck cancer patients treated with irradiation has been reported to be beneficial in one of two centers studied.[217] Further study is continuing.

Hydroxypropyl cellulose has been applied to isolated ulcers and may form a barrier on the surface, reducing symptoms.[218] Hydroxypropyl cellulose also has been combined with topical anesthetic agents (eg, benzocaine), with clinical reports of efficacy. Further research is needed to provide evidence of efficacy of its topical application in the management of oral complications of cancer patients.

Chlorhexidine has been assessed in radiotherapy patients,[203,219] and the majority of studies do not demonstrate a prophylactic impact on mucositis.[220,221] The effects of chlorhexidine on plaque levels, gingival inflammation, caries, and oral streptococcal colonization have not been the primary end points in these studies, but they may be valuable during cancer therapy. A prospective study of patients treated with chemoradiotherapy for head and neck cancer showed that mucositis was reduced in those who received oral applications of povidone iodine, compared to those who received sterile water rinses.[221] However, the impact of oral hygiene may be a confounding factor in these studies.

Studies of the use of a nonabsorbable antimicrobial lozenge that combines polymixin, tobramycin, and amphotericin B in conjunction with radiation therapy for head and neck cancer have shown the medication to reduce gram-negative bacterial colonization and to prevent oral ulcers.[195,222] A double-blind placebo-controlled trial of 112 patients found that patients' self-reports of severe mucositis were lessened but that mucositis scores were not different.[222] Studies of topical antimicrobials for prevention of mucositis are continuing.

Oral capsaicin in a taffylike candy vehicle produced temporary partial pain reduction in 11 patients with oral mucositis pain.[223] The findings suggest that some of the pain of mucositis is mediated by substance P.

Radiation shields to protect normal tissue from radiation exposure are often suggested during radiation therapy. They were shown to be effective, with patients experiencing less weight loss, fewer hospitalizations for nutritional support, and

a trend toward fewer treatment interruptions when compared with control patients.[242]

Interest in the use of cytokines in the prevention and treatment of mucositis is increasing. An animal model of mucositis has been used to assess the potential of growth factors to affect oral mucositis.[225–230] In this model, epidermal growth factor (EGF) increased the severity of mucosal damage when given concurrently with chemotherapy.[230] Transforming growth factor beta-3 (TGF-β3), which reduces the proliferation of epithelial cells, reduced the incidence, severity, and duration of mucositis; however, this finding has not been confirmed in human trials to date.[227,228] The use of interleukin-11 (IL-11) resulted in a statistically significant reduction in mucositis.[225,226,229] A rat model of inflammatory bowel disease also showed a reduction in gross and microscopic damage to the colon in animals treated with IL-11.[229]

Due to hyposalivation, the quantity of EGF in saliva decreased in people receiving head and neck irradiation, and its concentration in saliva decreased as mucositis increased.[168] EGF may represent a marker for mucosal damage and has the potential to promote the resolution of radiation-induced mucositis. A double-blind trial of EGF mouthwash used in patients treated with chemotherapy showed no differences in the healing of established ulcers, but a delay in onset and reduced severity were seen in recurrent ulceration, suggesting that topical EGF may protect the mucosa from toxicity.[231] Several preliminary studies have assessed the effect of GM-CSF on oral mucositis,[195,232,233] and a less severe or reduced duration of mucositis was seen in several trials.

Low-energy helium-neon laser has been reported to reduce the severity of oral mucositis in patients receiving head and neck radiation therapy.[234] The mechanism of action is unknown but has been suggested to be due to cytokine release following laser exposure.

CURRENT MANAGEMENT

Current management of mucositis in radiotherapy patients (see Table 8-4) includes an emphasis on good oral hygiene, the use of frequent oral rinses for wetting the surfaces and diluting oral contents, avoidance of irritating foods and oral care products, avoidance of tobacco products, and the use of benzydamine (in countries where it is available). The management of oropharyngeal pain in cancer patients frequently requires systemic analgesics, adjunctive medications, physical therapy, and psychological therapy, in addition to local measures, oral care, and topical treatments.

Biologic response modifiers offer the potential to prevent oral mucositis and to speed the healing of damaged mucosa. Antimicrobial approaches have met with conflicting results; chlorhexidine and systemic antimicrobials have little effect in preventing mucositis in radiation patients, but there is increasing evidence of the effectiveness of topical antimicrobials that affect gram-negative oral flora. Thiol derivatives, including amifostine, have been associated with radioprotection and have potential for clinical application. Other approaches that require further study include low-energy lasers and (possibly) anti-inflammatory medications.

Xerostomia

STIMULATION OF SALIVARY FUNCTION

The use of sialagogues offers the advantage of stimulating saliva secretion, which may include all normal components which provide the protective functions of saliva. Measurement of saliva flow rates to determine the amount of residual function should be conducted before prescribing a sialagogue. If no saliva is collected under resting or stimulated conditions, it is unlikely that a systemic agent will be effective. The use of sugarless gum or candies also may assist the stimulation of residual gland function.

Pilocarpine is the best studied sialagogue.[2,235–239] Pilocarpine is a parasympathomimetic agent and has its major effects at the muscarinic cholinergic receptor of salivary gland acinar cells. In doses of up to 15 mg/d, increased secretion of saliva occurs, and few cardiovascular side effects have been noted. Anetholetrithione (Paladin Laboratories Inc, Montreal, Canada) has been reported to be beneficial in the management of dry mouth.[237] The mechanism of action may be to increase the number of cell surface receptors on salivary acinar cells. Because pilocarpine stimulates the receptors and because anetholetrithione may act by stimulating the formation of receptor sites, synergistic effects may result with the combined use of these drugs.[237]

Bethanechol and bromhexine have received limited study.[2,236] Bethanechol (75 to 200 mg/d in divided doses), which stimulates the parasympathetic nervous system, has been reported to have potential benefits without causing gastrointestinal upset. Bromhexine has been studied in patients with dry mouth due to Sjögren's syndrome, without evidence of an increase in saliva volume; however, no studies of bromhexine have been conducted in cancer patients.

Stimulation of the salivary glands during radiation therapy has been suggested as a possible means of reducing damage to the glands. Patients who begin radiation therapy with higher initial flow rates retain more residual flow.[173] Preliminary study of the prophylactic use of pilocarpine (5 mg qid) in patients receiving radiation therapy suggests that parotid gland function may be better preserved; however, this effect was not demonstrated in submandibular and sublingual gland saliva following treatment.[175] Amifostine, which is administered intravenously prior to radiation exposure, has been licensed by the FDA for prevention of salivary gland dysfunction and may reduce the severity of oral mucositis; however, additional study is needed to determine its impact on mucositis and its cost versus benefit.

PALLIATION

Mouth-wetting agents or saliva substitutes may be used when it is not possible to stimulate salivary function.[236] Frequent sipping of water and a moist diet are mandatory. The desired characteristics of saliva substitutes are excellent lubrication, surface wetting, inhibition of overgrowth of pathogenic microorganisms, maintenance of the hardness of dental structure, pleasant taste, long duration of effect, extended shelf life, and low cost. The majority of products currently available are based on carboxymethylcellulose. Animal mucins have been incorporated into some European products. Most commercial products are more viscous than saliva and do not simulate the non-newtonian viscoelastic properties of saliva. They also do not contain the complex enzyme systems and antibodies of natural saliva. Many of the commercial products being marketed have not been subjected to controlled clinical study.

Candidiasis

In radiated patients, the most common clinical infection of the oropharynx is candidiasis. During radiation therapy, the number of patients colonized by *Candida*, quantitative counts, and clinical infection all increase[151,154,159,202,238–240] (see Figure 8-37). These changes persist in patients, with continuing hyposalivation. The role of *Candida* spp in oral mucositis associated with radiation therapy is not known. Candidiasis may enhance the discomfort of mucositis and may be associated with discomfort and changes in taste after treatment.

Patients who receive radiation therapy should be managed with topical antifungals because oral candidiasis produces oral discomfort but does not lead to systemic infection unless the patient is immunocompromised.[241] When prescribing topical antifungal drugs, the presence of sucrose in the product must be known because frequent use of sucrose-sweetened products may promote caries, particularly in patients with dry mouth.

Caries

Caries associated with hyposalivation typically affect the gingival third and the incisal cusp tips of the teeth (Figure 8-42). The etiology is related to a lack of production of saliva, resulting in loss of remineralizing potential, loss of buffering capacity, increased acidity, and a change in the bacterial flora. Treatment of each component of the caries process must be addressed.

Oral hygiene must be scrupulously maintained. Hyposalivation should be managed, and thorough trials of sialagogues should be conducted. The tooth structure may be hardened by the use of fluorides, and remineralization may be enhanced by the use of fluorides and remineralizing products.[170,242–246] The effects of topical products may be enhanced by increased contact time on the teeth which can be achieved by applying them with occlusive vacuform splints or gel carriers, which should extend over the gingival margins of the teeth. Custom vinyl trays are most useful for the application of fluoride to prevent and control caries in high-risk patients.[151,170,174,244,245] A comparison of neutral sodium fluoride gel in carriers with a twice-daily fluoride rinse protocol suggested a similar efficacy of the rinse protocol, but this was not a controlled comparative study.[246] Further studies are needed to define the simplest effective protocol. However, until controlled studies are available, treatment should remain fluoride application in gel carriers; for those who do not comply with carrier application, high-potency brush-on fluoride dentrifice may be suggested as it is simpler and

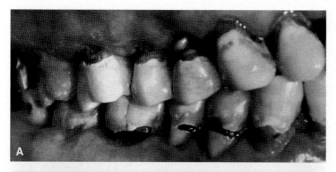

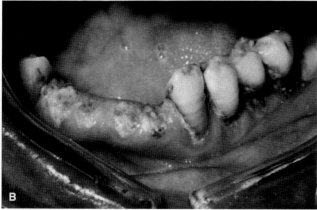

FIGURE 8-42 A, Ravages of xerostomia-associated caries, seen with decalcification of enamel and loss of structure in the gingival third. **B,** Dental caries with decalcification of the teeth, structural loss undermining the crowns of the teeth, and amputation of the crowns of the mandibular teeth.

as it may reduce demineralization and caries. Continuing reinforcement of topical fluoride use is needed and will enhance patient compliance.

A shift to a cariogenic flora has been well documented in patients following head and neck radiation therapy. A high risk of caries that is associated with *Streptococcus mutans* and *Lactobacillus* spp has been demonstrated in cancer patients.[247,248] Assessment of quantities of cariogenic organisms should be carried out before considering whether antimicrobials are needed. A high risk of caries is reported if more than 10^5 *Streptococcus mutans* and more than 10^4 *Lactobacillus* colony-forming units per milliliter of saliva are present. Topical fluorides and chlorhexidine rinses may reduce levels of *Streptococcus mutans*.[247,248] A 2% chlorhexidine gel applied in mouth guards demonstrated an enhanced ability to control cariogenic flora in cancer patients with xerostomia.[249]

Tissue Necrosis

Soft-tissue necrosis may involve any oral site, including the cheeks and tongue. Involvement of tissue overlying bone that has received high-dose radiation may predispose to necrosis of soft tissue and bone (Figure 8-43). Postradiation osteonecrosis (PRON) may be chronic or progressive. A classification of PRON for identifying stages of the condition for research and clinical purposes and for guiding therapy has been described[250,251] (Table 8-4). Radiation therapy causes endar-

teritis that affects vascularity, resulting in hypovascular, hypocellular, and hypoxic tissue that is unable to repair or remodel itself effectively when a challenge occurs (Figure 8-44). The challenge may take the form of trauma (such as from surgical procedures), active periodontal disease or denture trauma, and idiopathic or spontaneous necrosis for which no known cause is identified. While PRON may be secondarily infected, the infection is not etiologic. Symptoms and signs may include discomfort or tenderness at the site, bad taste, paresthesia and anesthesia, extraoral and oroantral fistulae, secondary infection, and pathologic fracture. The primary risk factor for the development of PRON is radiation therapy, in which dose, fraction, and numbers of fractions result in the biologic effect (eg, a high risk when TDF > 109). The volume of bone included in the field of irradiation increases the risk. The presence of teeth in a high-dose radiation field represents a risk factor for PRON, probably in relation to dental or periodontal disease or irritation. The risk of necrosis is lifelong and may occur many years after irradiation. The risk of developing PRON has been estimated in the last 20 years as between 2.6 and 15%.[250,215] The mandible is most commonly involved although cases can occur in the maxilla.

The prevention of PRON begins with the preradiation dental examination and with radiotherapy treatment planning. Teeth in the high-dose fraction with questionable prognosis (particularly when due to periodontal disease and when excellent compliance with regular oral care is unlikely) should be extracted prior to radiotherapy. If extractions are planned, it is desirable to allow as much healing time as possible; 7 to 14 days and up to 21 days have been suggested as healing times prior to radiotherapy.[251,252] The time required may depend on the nature of the extraction, and expert atraumatic extraction will require less healing time.

When PRON develops, management should include having the patient avoid mucosal irritants, discontinue the use of dental appliances if they contact the area of the lesion, maintain nutritional status, and stop smoking, and eliminate alcohol consumption. Topical antibiotic (ie, tetracycline) or antiseptic (chlorhexidine) rinses may reduce the potential local irritation from the microbial flora. For chronic persisting PRON (stage II), this therapy and regular follow-up may be the best approach to treatment. Hyperbaric oxygen (HBO) therapy increases the oxygenation of tissue, increases angiogenesis, and promotes osteoblast and fibroblast function. In cases associated with symptoms of pain and progression (stage III), HBO is an important part of therapy. Appropriate analgesia should be provided. HBO therapy and surgical guidelines have been established.[252,253] HBO therapy is usually prescribed as 20 to 30 dives at 100% oxygen and 2 to 2.5 atmospheres of pressure. Sequestra may be managed with limited resection or may require mandibulectomy. If surgery is required, postsurgical HBO therapy of 10 dives is recommended. The mandible can be reconstructed to provide continuity for esthetics and function. Prophylactic HBO therapy may be considered (1) when surgery is required after radiation therapy, (2) when the patient is felt to be at extreme risk due to high-dose radiation to the bone with a high biologic effect (TDF > 109), and (3) when

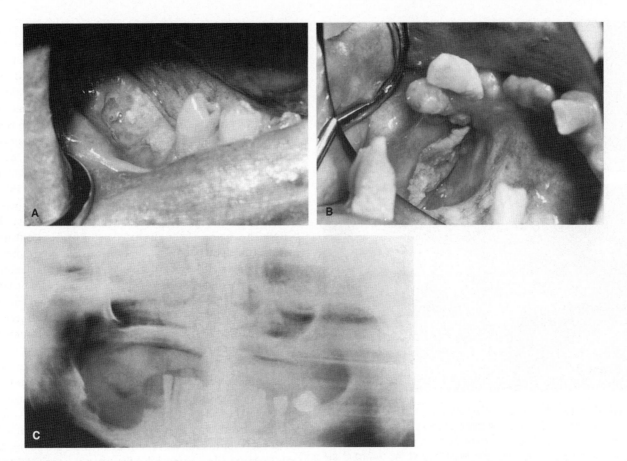

FIGURE 8-43 A, Chronic exposure of bone in the mandibular region, following radiation therapy. There was local discomfort, and the area was tender to palpation. **B,** Another case of exposure of mandibular bone due to postradiation osteonecrosis. Involvement extends to the periodontal support of the bicuspid and to the molar region of the lingual plate. The adjacent tissue of the floor of the mouth shows the telangiectatic appearance of late radiation changes. **C,** Panoramic radiograph of a case of postradiation osteonecrosis, demonstrating bone destruction approaching the inferior border of the mandible, leading to an increased risk of pathologic fracture.

extensive surgery is required. However, if expert atraumatic extraction is performed, HBO therapy may be considered only if delayed healing occurs. In a select population of patients referred for HBO therapy and surgery, prophylactic HBO therapy was suggested.[252] In a general cancer clinic, however, extractions were managed with expert surgery, and approximately 5% of extractions were associated with delayed healing; it was recommended that in most cases, HBO therapy should be reserved for those in whom osteonecrosis developed.[251]

A number of studies have reported the effect of HBO on necrosis, and several have concluded that HBO therapy is an important part of the comprehensive management of necrosis following radiation therapy.[254–256] A long-term follow-up of patients after their first episode of necrosis showed that in 20 of the 26 patients who were available for follow-up, 10% experienced a recurrence of necrosis following HBO therapy.[255] In 60% of these patients, the condition remained stable, and no recurrence of signs and symptoms of necrosis occurred; in 10%, a further improvement occurred over time while 20% of the patients continued to demonstrate persisting (stage 2) necrosis. This study supports the potential value of HBO therapy in managing initial episodes of necrosis and

TABLE 8-4 Management of Mucositis

Diluting agents
  Saline, bicarbonate rinses, frequent water rinses, dilute hydrogen peroxide rinses
Coating agents
  Kaolin-pectin, aluminum chloride, aluminum hydroxide, magnesium hydroxide, hydroxypropyl cellulose, sucralfate
Lip Lubricants
  Water-based lubricants, lanolin
Topical anesthetics
  Dyclonine HCl, xylocaine HCl, benzocaine HCl, diphenhydramine HCl
Analgesic agents
  Benzydamine HCl

HCl = hydrochloride.

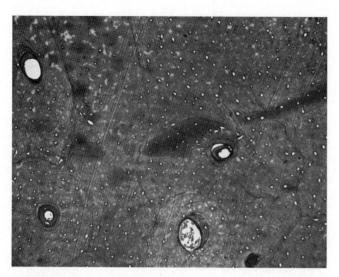

FIGURE 8-44 Histopathologic appearance of bone with empty lacunae and haversian canals of nonvital bone, representative of the lack of viability of bone in postradiation osteonecrosis.

in potentially preventing the recurrence of second episodes. In addition, the findings indicate that stage 2 chronic necrosis may remain stable and without progression over extended periods following initial treatment with HBO therapy. A number of studies have reported the effect of HBO therapy on necrosis, and several have concluded that HBO therapy is an important part of the comprehensive management of necrosis following radiation therapy.[150,254–256]

Speech and Mastication

Abnormal speech may follow surgery or radiation because of hyposalivation and fibrosis that affects tongue mobility, mandibular movement, and soft-palate function (Figure 8-45). Maxillectomy that produces a palatal defect must be managed with prostheses to allow function in speech, mastication, and deglutition. Speech therapy and prostheses are the principal means of managing these complications.

Nutrition

Radiation therapy produces changes in the patient's perceptions of taste and smell.[257] Taste may be affected directly due to an effect on the taste buds, or indirectly, due to hyposalivation and secondary infections. A total fractionated dose of > 3,000 Gy reduces the acuity of all tastes (ie, sweet, sour, bitter, and salty).[258] Taste often will recover slowly over several months, but permanent alteration may result.[2] Zinc supplementation (zinc sulfate, 220 mg twice daily) may be useful for some patients who experience taste disturbances.[2,259]

Nutritional counseling in which the focus is on the maintenance of caloric and nutrient intake may be required during therapy. Following treatment and when mucositis has resolved, nutritional counseling must consider the long-term complications that may occur. These include hyposalivation, an altered ability to chew, difficulty in forming the food bolus, and

dysphagia. Consideration must be given to taste, texture, moisture, and caloric and nutrient content.

Mandibular Dysfunction

Musculoskeletal syndromes may arise due to fibrosis of muscles, which may follow radiation and surgery. Limited opening has been related to radiation exposure of the upper head of the lateral pterygoid muscle. Mandibular discontinuity following surgery and the emotional stress associated with malignant disease and its treatment may influence musculoskeletal syndromes and pain. Mandibular stretching exercises and prosthetic aids may reduce the severity of fibrosis and limited mandibular movement when conducted before severe limitation has developed, but few benefits are seen after such limitation has developed. The management of temporomandibular disorders in this population may present additional difficulties due to major discontinuity of the mandible, with severe limitation of function and emotional reaction. There is no research that documents the best choices of therapy for these patients. Therapy may include occlusal stabilization appliances, physiotherapy, exercises, trigger point injections and analgesics, muscle relaxants, tricyclic medications, and other chronic pain management strategies.[260] Management of pain is discussed later in this chapter.

Dentofacial Abnormalities

When children receive radiotherapy to the facial skeleton, future growth and development may be affected.[261] Agenesis of teeth, agenesis of roots, abnormal root forms, or abnormal calcification may occur (Figure 8-46). Despite these dental abnormalities, teeth will erupt even without root formation and may be retained for years. Growth of the facial skeleton in the radiated field may be affected, which can result in micrognathia, retrognathia, altered growth of the maxilla, and asymmetric growth (Figure 8-47). Altered growth and development may occur if treatment affects the pituitary gland. Trismus occur in patients secondary to fibrosis of muscles.

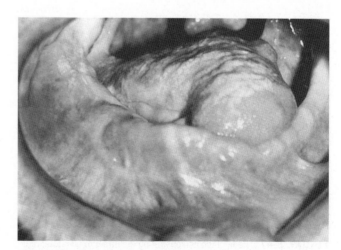

FIGURE 8-45 Results of a partial glossectomy that has led to functional impairment of speech and manipulation of food and to difficulty in retaining the mandibular denture.

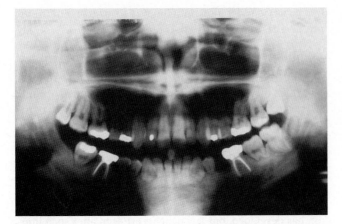

FIGURE 8-46 Radiograph showing the effects of radiation on the development of the dentition. Agenesis, shortened root forms, lack of root development, and premature closure of apical foramina are seen in teeth that were in the primary radiation field and that were in the process of development during radiation therapy.

The dental abnormalities pose significant management challenges due to these effects on dental development and skeletal growth.

Pain

Head, neck, and oral pain may be caused by the tumor or by cancer therapy or may be unrelated to cancer[260] (Table 8-6). Pain, whether related to the tumor, recurrence or progression of tumor, treatment of tumor, or unrelated to the cancer, often is interpreted as being due to the disease and is influenced by an emotional response caused by fear of cancer. The important emotional components of the reaction to pain must be considered in the patient's complaint and in management. Pain at diagnosis of head and neck cancer is common, is reported in up to 85% of those seeking treatment, and is usually described

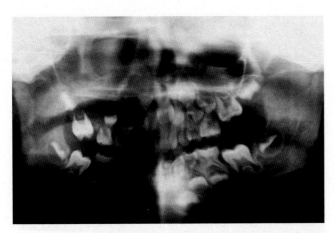

FIGURE 8-47 Radiograph demonstrating the effect of unilateral radiation that was required during dentofacial development. Asymmetric development of height and width of the ramus and body of the mandible and dentition resulted.

TABLE 8-5 Classification of Postradiation Osteonecrosis

Stage	Description	Treatment
I	Resolved, healed	Prevention of recurrence
Ia	No pathologic fracture	
Ib	Past pathologic fracture	
II	Chronic, nonprogressive	Local wound care; HBO if indicated
IIa	No pathologic fracture	
IIb	Pathologic fracture	
III	Active, progressive	Local wound care
IIIa	No pathologic fracture	HBO and surgery if indicated*
IIIb	Pathologic fracture	

Reproduced with permission from Epstein et al.[250]

HBO = hyperbaric oxygen therapy.

*Combined surgery and HBO described by Marx RE.[253]

as low-grade discomfort.[260] Acute pain following radiotherapy and surgery is universal.

Health care providers have been criticized for the needless suffering of patients caused by the providers' lack of understanding of the use of analgesics and adjuvant medications, lack of attention to the emotional and social aspects of pain, and failure to use adjunctive physical and psychological treatment. The management of cancer pain requires attention to the potential multiple causes of pain (see Table 8-6).

Dental and periodontal disease that causes pain may be controlled with analgesics and antibiotics; however, definitive dental management is needed. Management of mucositis is discussed earlier in this chapter. Bacterial, fungal, and viral infections are managed with specific antimicrobial agents. In mucosal infection, topical antifungals and antiseptics may be effective, but if resolution does not occur, systemic medications may be needed.

Neurologic pain states, including neuropathic pain and neuralgia-like pain, may require the use of antidepressants and anticonvulsants, respectively. Management of osteonecrosis is discussed in this chapter. In all cases of persisting pain, chronic pain management approaches including counseling, relaxation therapy, imagery, biofeedback, hypnosis, and transcutaneous nerve stimulation may be needed. Pain associated with musculoskeletal syndromes is described in the section entitled "Mandibular Dysfunction."

Analgesics should be provided according to the level of pain, the drug's pharmacologic action, and the duration of action of the drug. They should be combined with adjuvant medications according to the multiple causes of pain and the secondary effects of pain (Table 8-7). Analgesics, when required, should be provided on a regularly scheduled or time-contingent basis, not on an as-needed basis. Improved pain control requiring lower total doses of analgesics can be achieved with medication provided on a time-contingent basis. In general, non-narcotic analgesics should be provided to all patients even if potent opioids are required because this

TABLE 8-6 Head, Neck, and Oral Pain in Cancer Patients

Pain due to tumor
  Loss of epithelial barrier; ulceration; exposure of nerves
  Tumor necrosis; secondary infection
  Chemosensitization of nerves; pressure on nerves
  Tumor infiltration of bone, muscle, nerve, blood vessels
  Exacerbation of dental or periodontal disease

Pain due to cancer therapy
  Pain following surgery
  Acute surgical injury
  Secondary infection
  Myofascial or musculoskeletal syndromes
  Neuroma; deafferentation pain

Pain due to radiotherapy
  Mucositis
  Necrosis of soft tissue or bone
  Myofascial or musculoskeletal syndromes
  Exacerbation of dental or periodontal disease

Pain due to chemotherapy
  Mucositis
  Peripheral neuropathy
  Infection
  Exacerbation of dental or periodontal disease

Pain unrelated to cancer or cancer therapy

may allow a lower dose of narcotic medication. Adjuvant medications such as tricyclics anti-depressants may enhance the analgesic effects of other agents, possesses analgesic potential themselves, and promotes sleep, which is often disrupted by pain. Adjuvant medications directed at the etiology of the pain should be used whenever possible. For example, for neuralgia-like pain, anticonvulsant medications should be included. Possible side-effects, such as constipation due to opioids, should be anticipated and treated. Reassessments of the efficacy of pain control, with an awareness of toxicity and side effects, should be conducted on a regular basis. Medications should not be used alone but should be part of a pain control strategy that also includes physical therapy, counseling, relaxation therapy, biofeedback, hypnosis, and transcutaneous nerve stimulation.

TABLE 8-7 Pain Management in Head and Neck Cancer

Category of Medication	Action
Topical anesthetic	Topical anesthesia
Analgesic	Elevate pain threshold
Anti-inflammatory	Reduce inflammation; mild to moderate analgesic
Antimicrobial	Modify pathologic process
Anticonvulsant	Modify pathologic process
Anxiolytic	Antianxiety
Antidepressant	Reduce depression; analgesic effect; promote sound sleep
Muscle relaxant	Reduce muscle tension or spasm

▼ CONCLUSION

Oral and dental care is important in all phases of the diagnosis and treatment of the patient with head and neck cancer. Early recognition and diagnosis are important for improving survival and for limiting the complications of therapy. Prevention of the oral complications that arise during or after therapy and management of the complications when they occur require the involvement of a knowledgeable practitioner. Dental providers are a part of the health care team and must be involved in the care of the head and neck cancer patient. Continuing research is needed in the epidemiology, pathogenesis, etiology, prevention, diagnosis, and management of head and neck cancer.

▼ REFERENCES

1. Landis SH, Murray MT, Bolden S, Wingo PA. Cancer statistics. CA Cancer J Clin 1999;49:8–31.
2. Silverman S Jr. Oral Cancer. American Cancer Society. Hamilton (ON): B.C. Decker; 1998.
3. Mashburg A, Samit AM. Early detection, diagnosis and management of oral and oropharyngeal cancer. CA Cancer J Clin 1989;39:67–88.
4. Silverman S Jr, Gorsky M, Greenspan D. Tobacco usage in patients with head and neck carcinomas: a follow-up study on habit changes and second primary oral/oropharyngeal cancers. J Am Dent Assoc 1983;106:33–7.
5. Cahan WG, Castro EB, Rosen PP, Strong EW. Separate primary carcinomas of the esophagus and head and neck region in the same patient. Cancer 1976;37:85–9.
6. Tepperman BS, Fitzpatrick PJ. Second respiratory and upper digestive tract cancers after oral cancer. Lancet 1981;2:547–9.
7. Newell GR, Krementz ET. Multiple malignant neoplasms in the Charity Hospital of Louisiana Tumor Registry. Cancer 1977;40:1812–20.
8. Wynder EL, Mushinski MH, Spivak JC. Tobacco and alcohol consumption in relation to the development of multiple primary cancers. Cancer 1977;40:1872–8.
9. Mahboubi E. The epidemiology of oral cavity, pharyngeal and esophageal cancer outside of North America and Western Europe. Cancer 1977;40:1879–86.
10. Freeman HP. Cancer in the socioeconomically disadvantaged. CA Cancer J Clin 1989;39:266–88.
11. Feldman JG, Hazan M, Nagarajan M, Kissen B. A case-control investigation of alcohol, tobacco, and diet in head and neck cancer. Prev Med 1975;4:444–63.
12. Mashburg A, Garfinkel L, Harris S. Alcohol as a primary risk factor in oral squamous carcinoma. CA Cancer J Clin 1981;31:146–55.
13. Boyle P, Zheng T, Macfarlane GJ, et al. Recent advances in the etiology and epidemilogy of head and neck cancer. Curr Opin Oncol 1990;2:539–45.
14. Graham S, Dayal H, Rohrer T, et al. Dentition, diet, tobacco and alcohol in the epidemiology of oral cancer. J Natl Cancer Inst 1977;59:1611–8.
15. Moore C. Cigarette smoking and cancer of the mouth, pharynx and larynx. A continuing study. JAMA 1971;218:553–8.
16. Johnston WD, Ballantyne AJ. Prognostic effect of tobacco and alcohol use in patients with oral tongue cancer. Am J Surg 1977;134:444–7.

17. Wynder EL, Hoffman D. Tobacco and health: a societal change. N Engl J Med 1979;300:894–903.

18. Spitz MR, Fueger JJ, Goepfert H, et al. Squamous cell carcinoma of the upper aerodigestive tract. A case comparison analysis. Cancer 1988;61:203–8.

19. Greer RO Jr, Poulson TC. Oral tissue alterations associated with the use of smokeless tobacco by teenagers. Part 1. Clinical findings. Oral Surg Oral Med Oral Pathol 1983;56:275–84.

20. Squier CA. The nature of smokeless tobacco and patterns of use. CA Cancer J Clin 1988;38:226–9.

21. Connolly GN, Winn DM, Hecht SS, et al. The reemergence of smokeless tobacco. N Engl J Med 1984;314:1020–7.

22. Holmstrup P, Pindborg JJ. Oral mucosal lesions in smokeless tobacco users. CA Cancer J Clin 1988;38:230–5.

23. Winn DM. Smokeless tobacco and cancer: the epidemiologic evidence. CA Cancer J Clin 1988;38:236–43.

24. Winn DM, Blot WJ, Shy CM, et al. Snuff dipping and oral cancer among women in the southern United States. N Engl J Med 1981;304:745–9.

25. Schmidt W, Popham RE. The role of drinking and smoking in mortality from cancer and other causes in male alcoholics. Cancer 1981;47:1031–41.

26. Rothman K, Keller A. The effect of joint exposure to alcohol and tobacco on risk of cancer of the mouth and pharynx. J Chronic Dis 1972;25:711–6.

27. Kissin B, Kaley M, Su WH, Lerner R. Head and neck cancer in alcoholics: the relationship to drinking, smoking and dietary patterns. JAMA 1973;224:1174–5.

28. Keller AZ. Alcohol, tobacco and age factors in the relative frequency of cancer among males with and without liver cirrhosis. Am J Epidemiol 1977;106:194–202.

29. Gorsky M, Silverman S Jr. Denture wearing and oral cancer. J Prosthet Dent 1984;52:164–6.

30. Browne RM, Camsey MC, Waterhouse JAH, Manning GL. Etiological factors in oral squamous cell carcinoma. Community Dent Oral Epidemiol 1977;5:301–6.

31. Fujita K, Kaku T, Sasaki M, Onoe T. Experimental production of lingual carcinomas in hamsters by local application of 9,10-dimethyl-1, 2 benzanthracene. J Dent Res 1973;52:327–32.

32. Silverman S, Jr, Gorsky M, Lozada F. Oral leukoplakia and malignant transformation. A follow-up study of 257 patients. Cancer 1984;53:563–8.

33. Papadimitrakoulou V, Izzo J, Lippman SM, et al. Frequent inactivation of p16/INK4a in oral premalignant lesions. Br J Cancer 1997b;14:1799–803.

34. Lummerman H, Freedman P, Kerpel S. Oral epithelial dysplasia and the development of invasive squamous cell carcinoma. Oral Surg Oral Med Oral Pathol 1995;79:321–9.

35. Van der Waal I, Schepman KP, van der Meij HE, Smeele LE. Oral leukoplakia: a clinicopathological review. Oral Oncol 1997;33(5):291–301.

36. Scully C, Field J. Genetic aberrations in squamous cell carcinoma of the head and neck (SCCHN), with reference to oral carcinoma (review). Int J Oncol 1996;10:5–21.

37. Leis JF, Livingston DM. The tumor suppressor genes and their mechanisms of action. In: Bishop JM, Weinberg RA, editors. Molecular oncology. Scientific American Inc.; 1996. p. 111–41.

38. Croce CM, Sozzi G, Huebner K. Role of FHIT in human cancer. J Clin Oncol 1999;17:1618–24.

39. Mao L, El-Naggar AK, Papadimitrakopoulou V, et al. Phenotype and genotype of advanced premalignant head and neck lesions after chemopreventive therapy. J Natl Cancer Inst 1998;90(20):1545–51.

40. Uzawa K., Suzuki H, Komiya A, et al. Evidence for two distinct tumor-suppressor gene loci on the long arm of chromosome 11 in human oral cancer. Int J Cancer 1996;67:510–4.

41. Uzawa N, Yoshida MA, Hosoe S, et al. Functional evidence for involvement of multiple putative tumor suppressor gene on the short arm of chromosome 3 in human oral squamous cell carcinogenesis. Cancer Genet Cytogenet 1998;107:125–31.

42. Nawroz H, van der Riet P, Hruban RH, et al. Allelotype of head and neck squamous cell carcinoma. Cancer Res 1994;54(5):1152–5.

43. Bockmuhl U, Schwendel A, Dietel M, Petersen I. Distinct patterns of chromosomal alterations in high- and low-grade head and neck squamous cell carcinomas. Cancer Res 1996; 56:5325–9.

44. Califano J, Westra WH, Koch W, et al. Unknown primary head and neck SCC: molecular identification of the site of origin. J Natl Cancer Inst 1999;91(7):599–604.

45. El-Naggar AK, Hurr K, Batsakis JG, et al. Sequential loss of heterozygosity at microsatellite motifs in preinvasive and invasive head and neck squamous carcinoma. Cancer Res 1995;55(12):2656–9.

46. Field J, Kiaris H, Risk J, et al. Allelotype of squamous cell carcinoma of the head and neck: fractional allele loss correlates with survival. Br J Cancer 1995;72:1180–8.

47. Perhouse MA, El-Naggar AK, Hurr K, et al. Deletion mapping of chromosome 4 in head and neck squamous cell carcinoma. Oncogene 1997;14:369–73.

48. Lydiatt WM, Davidson BJ, Shah J, et al. The relationship of loss of heterozygosity to tobacco exposure and early recurrence in head and neck squamous cell carcinoma. Am J Surg 1994;168:437–40.

49. Califano J, van der Riet P, Westra W, et al. Genetic progression model for head and neck cancer: implications for field cancerization. Cancer Res 1996;56:2488–92.

50. Emilion G, Langdon JD, Speight P, Partridge M. Frequent gene deletions in potentially malignant oral lesions. Br J Cancer 1996;73(6):809–13.

51. Mao E, Oda D, Haigh W, Beckman A. Loss of the adenomatous polyposis coli gene and human papillomavirus infection in oral carcinogenesis. Eur J Cancer Oral Oncol 1996;32B:260–3.

52. Zhang L, Michelsen C, Cheng X, et al. Molecular analysis of oral lichen planus: a premalignant lesion? Am J Pathol 1997;8:323–7.

53. American Joint Committee on Cancer. Manual for staging of cancer. 4th ed. Philadelphia: J.B. Lippincott; 1992. p. 27–52.

54. Ballard BR, Suess GR, Pickren JW, et al. Squamous cell carcinoma of the floor of the mouth. Oral Surg Oral Med Oral Pathol 1978;45:568–79.

55. Kolson H, Spiro RH, Roswit B, Lawson W. Epidermoid carcinoma of the floor of the mouth. Analysis of 108 cases. Arch Otolaryngol 1971;93:280–3.

56. Lindberg R. Distribution of cervical lymph node metastases from squamous cell carcinoma of the upper respiratory and digestive tracts. Cancer 1982;29:1446–9.

57. Weller SA, Goffinet DR, Goode RL, et al. Carcinoma of the oropharynx: results of megavoltage radiation therapy in 305 patients. AJR Am J Roentgenol 1976;126:236–47.

58. Wang CC. Oral cancer. In: Wang CC, editor. Radiation therapy for head and neck neoplasms. Chicago: Year Book Medical Publishers; 1990. p. 110–206.

59. Menck HR, Garfinkel L, Dodd GD. Preliminary report of the National Cancer Data Base. CA Cancer J Clin 1991;41:7–18.

60. Meyers MH, Gloeckler-Ries LA. Cancer patient survival rates: SEER program for 10 years of follow-up. CA Cancer J Clin 1989;39:21–32.

61. Mettlin C. Trends in years of life lost to cancer: 1970 to 1985. CA Cancer J Clin 1989;39:33–9.

62. Axell T, Pindborg JJ, Smith CJ, van der Waal I. Oral white lesions with special reference to precancerous and tobacco-related lesions: conclusions of an international symposium held in Upsala, Sweden. May 18–21, 1994. International Collaborative Group of White Oral Lesions. J Oral Pathol Med 1996;25:49–54.

63. Schepman KP, van der Meij EH, Smeele LE, van der Waal I. Prevalence study of oral white lesions with special reference to a new definition of oral leukoplakia. Eur J Cancer B Oral Oncol 1996;32(B):410–9.

64. Scuibba JJ. Improving detection of precancerous and cancerous oral lesions: computer-assisted analysis of the oral brush biopsy. J Am Dent Assoc 1999;130:1445–57.

65. Epstein JB, Oakley C, Millner A, et al. The utility of toluidine blue application as a diagnostic aid in patients previously treated for upper oropharyngeal carcinoma. Oral Surg Oral Med Oral Pathol Oral Radiol Endod 1997;83:537–47.

66. Rosin MP, Epstein JB, Berean K, et al. The use of exfoliative cell samples to map clonal genetic alterations in the oral epithelium of high-risk patients. Cancer Res 1997;57:5258–60.

67. Pindborg JJ, Renstrup G, Poulsen HE, et al. Studies in oral leukoplakias. V. Clinical and histologic signs of malignancy. Acta Odontol Scand 1963;20:407–11.

68. Silverman S Jr, Rozen RD. Observations on the clinical characteristics and natural history of oral leukoplakia. J Am Dent Assoc 1968;76:772–6.

69. Banoczy J, Csiba A. Occurrence of epithelial dysplasia in oral leukoplakia. Analysis and follow-up of 12 cases. Oral Surg Oral Med Oral Pathol 1976;42:766–74.

70. Waldron CA, Shafer WG. Leukoplakia revisited. A clinicopathologic study of 3,256 oral leukoplakias. Cancer 1975;36:1386–92.

71. Pindborg JJ, Daftary DK, Mehta FS. A follow-up study of sixty-one oral dysplastic precancerous lesions in Indian villagers. Oral Surg Oral Med Oral Pathol 1977;43:383–90.

72. Eversole LR. Lichen planus. Erythroplakia. Leukoplakia. Squamous cell carcinoma. In: Millard HD, Mason DK, editors. 1988 World workshop on oral medicine. Chicago: Year Book Medical Publishers; 1989. p. 60–65, 99–122.

73. Banoczy J. Follow-up studies in oral leukoplakia. J Maxillofac Surg 1977;5:69–75.

74. Gupta PC, Mehta FS, Daftary DK, et al. Incidence rates of oral cancer and natural history of oral precancerous lesions in a 10-year follow-up study of Indian villagers. Community Dent Oral Epidemiol 1980;8:283–333.

75. Silverman S Jr, Gorsky M. Proliferative verrucous leukoplakia: a follow-up study of 54 cases. Oral Surg Oral Med Oral Pathol Oral Radiol Endod 1997;84:154–7.

76. Palefsky JM, Silverman S Jr, Abdel-Salaam M, et al. Association between proliferative verrucous leukoplakia and infection with human papillomavirus type 16. J Oral Pathol Med 1995; 24:193–7.

77. Mashberg A, Feldman LJ. Clinical criteria for identifying early oral and oropharyngeal carcinoma: erythroplasia revisited. Am J Surg 1988;156:273–5.

78. Mashberg A. Erythroplasia: the earliest sign of asymptomatic oral cancer. J Am Dent Assoc 1978;96:615–20.

79. Mashberg A, Morissey JB, Garfinkle L. A study of the appearance of early asymptomatic oral squamous carcinomas. Cancer 1973;32:1436–45.

80. Creath CJ, Cutter G, Bradley DH, Wright JT. Oral leukoplakia and adolescent smokeless tobacco use. Oral Surg Oral Med Oral Pathol 1991;72:35–41.

81. US Department of Health and Human Services. The health consequences of using smokeless tobacco: a report to the Advisory Committee to the Surgeon General. Public Health Service. Washington (DC): US Government Printing Office; 1986. NIH publication No. 86–2874.

82. Dokko H, Min PS, Cherrick HM, Park NH. Effect of smokeless tobacco and tobacco-related chemical carcinogens on survival of ultraviolet light-inactivated herpes simplex virus. Oral Surg Oral Med Oral Pathol 1991;71:464–8.

83. Park N-H, Herbosa EG, Sapp JP. Effect of tar condensate from smoking tobacco and water-extract of snuff on the oral mucosa of mice with latent herpes simplex virus. Arch Oral Biol 1987;32:47–53.

84. Silverman S Jr, Griffith M. Studies on oral lichen planus. II. Follow-up on 200 patients, clinical characteristics and associated malignancy. Oral Surg Oral Med Oral Pathol 1974;37:705–10.

85. Silverman S Jr, Gorsky M, Lozada-Nur F. A prospective follow-up study of 570 patients with oral lichen planus: persistence, remission and malignant association. Oral Surg Oral Med Oral Pathol 1985;60:30–4.

86. Holmstrup P, Pindborg JJ. Erythroplakic lesions in relation to oral lichen planus. Acta Derm Venereol 1979;59 Suppl 85:77–84.

87. Fulling HJ. Cancer development in oral lichen planus: a follow-up study of 327 patients. Arch Dermatol 1973;108:667–9.

88. van der Meij EH, Schepman KP, Smeele LE, et al. A review of the recent literature regarding malignant transformation of oral lichen planus. Oral Surg Oral Med Oral Pathol Oral Radiol Endod 1999;88:307–10.

89. Schoelch ML, Sekandari N, Regezi JA, Silverman S Jr. Laser management of oral leukoplakias: a follow-up study of 70 patients. Laryngoscope 1999;109:949–53.

90. Hong WK, Endicott J, Itri LM, et al. 13-Cisretinoic acid in the treatment of oral leukoplakia. N Engl J Med 1986;315:1501–5.

91. Vermorken JB. Chemotherapy and new treatments in squamous cell carcinoma of the head and neck. Curr Opin Oncol 1990;2:578–84.

92. Epstein JB, Gorsky M. Topical application of vitamin A to oral leukoplakia: a clinical case series. Cancer 1999;86:921–7.

93. Kaugers GE, Silverman S Jr, Lovas JG, et al. Use of antioxidant supplements in the treatment of human oral leukoplakia. Oral Surg Oral Med Oral Pathol Oral Radiol Endod 1996;81:5–14.

94. Kaugers GE, Silverman S Jr, Lovas JG, et al. A clinical trial of antioxidant supplements in the treatment of oral leukoplakia. Oral Surg Oral Med Oral Pathol 1994;78:462–8.

95. Wong F, Epstein J, Millner A. Treatment of oral leukoplakia with topical bleomycin. Cancer 1989;64:361–5.

96. Epstein JB, Gorsky M, Wong FLW, Milner A. Topical bleomycin for the treatment of dysplastic oral leukoplakia. Cancer 1998;83:629–34.

97. Shillitoe EJ. Relationship of viral infection to malignancies. Curr Opin Dent 1991;1:398–403.

98. Hirsch JM, Johansson SL, Vahlne A. Effect of snuff and herpes simplex virus I on rat oral mucosa. Possible association with development of squamous cell carcinoma. J Oral Pathol 1984;13:52–62.

99. Shillitoe EJ, Greenspan D, Greenspan JS, et al. Neutralizing antibody to herpes simplex virus type I in patients with oral cancer. Cancer 1982;49:2315–20.

100. Shillitoe EJ, Greenspan D, Greenspan JS, Silverman S Jr. Antibody to early and late antigens of herpes simplex virus type I in patients with oral cancer. Cancer 1984;54:266–73.

101. Shillitoe EJ, Hwang CBC, Silverman S Jr, Greenspan JS. Examination of oral cancer tissue for the presence of the proteins ICP4, ICP5, ICP6, ICP8 and gB of herpes simplex virus type I. J Natl Cancer Inst 1986;76:371–4.

102. Galloway DA, McDougall JK. The oncogenic potential of herpes simplex viruses: evidence for a "hit-and-run" mechanism. Nature 1983;302:21–4.

103. Lorinez AT, Temple GF, Kurman RJ, et al. Oncogenic association of specific human papillomavirus types with cervical neoplasia. J Natl Cancer Inst 1987;79:671–7.

104. Eversole R. The human papillomaviruses and oral mucosal disease. Oral Surg Oral Med Oral Pathol 1991;71:700.

105. Greer RO, Douglas JM, Breese P, Crosby LK. An evaluation of oral and laryngeal specimens for human papillomavirus (HPV) DNA by dot blot hybridization. J Oral Pathol Med 1990;19:35–8.

106. Milde K, Loning T. Detection of papillomavirus DNA in oral papillomas and carcinomas: application of in situ hybridization with biotinylated HPV 16 probes. J Oral Pathol 1986;15:292–6.

107. Maitland NJ, Cox MF, Lynas C, et al. Detection of human papillomavirus DNA in biopsies of human oral tissue. Br J Cancer 1987;56:245–50.

108. Watts SL, Brewer EE, Fry TL. Human papillomavirus DNA types in squamous cell carcinomas of the head and neck. Oral Surg Oral Med Oral Pathol 1991;71:701–7.

109. Shroyer KR, Greer RO. Detection of human papillomavirus DNA by in situ-DNA hybridization and polymerase chain reaction in premalignant and malignant oral lesions. Oral Surg Oral Med Oral Pathol 1991;71:708–13.

110. Zeus SM, Miller CS, White DK. In situ hybridization analysis of human papillomavirus DNA in oral mucosal lesions. Oral Surg Oral Med Oral Pathol 1991;71:714–20.

111. Tsuchiya H, Tomita Y, Shirasawa H, et al. Detection of human papillomavirus in head and neck tumors with DNA hybridization and immunohistochemical analysis. Oral Surg Oral Med Oral Pathol 1991;71:721–5.

112. Young SK, Min KW. In situ DNA hybridization analysis of oral papillomas, leukoplakias and carcinomas for human papillomavirus. Oral Surg Oral Med Oral Pathol 1991;71:726–9.

113. Schantz SP. Experimental head and neck oncology. Curr Opin Oncol 1990;2:546–51.

114. Carter RL. Pathology of squamous cell carcinomas of the head and neck. Curr Opin Oncol 1990;2:552–6.

115. Hennekens CH, Mayrent SL, Willett W. Vitamin A, carotenoids and retinoids. Cancer 1986;58:1837–41.

116. Stich HF, Mathew B, Sankaranarayanan R, Nair MK. Remission of precancerous lesions in the oral cavity of tobacco chewers and maintenance of the protective effect of B-carotene or vitamin A. Am J Clin Nutr 1991;53:298(s)–304(s).

117. Tsiklalkis K, Papadakou A, Angelopoulos AP. The therapeutic effect of an aromatic retinoid (RO-109359) on hamster buccal pouch carcinomas. Oral Surg Oral Med Oral Pathol 1987;64:327–32.

118. Kandarkar SV, Sirsat SM. Periodic histopathological and ultrastructural changes of excess vitamin A on oral carcinogenesis. Indian J Exp Biol 1990;28:10–7.

119. Ad Hoc Subcommittee on Fluoride, Public Health Service. Review of fluoride benefits and risks. Dept. of Health and Human Services; 1991 February.

120. McGuire SM, Vanable ED, McGuire M, et al. Is there a link between fluoridated water and osteosarcoma. J Am Dent Assoc 1991;122:39–45.

121. Epstein JB, Schubert MM, Scully C. Evaluation and treatment of pain in patients with orofacial cancer: a review. Pain Clinic 1991;4:3–20.

122. Castelijns JA. Diagnostic radiology in head and neck oncology. Curr Opin Oncol 1990;2:557–61.

123. Strong EW. Surgical treatment in head and neck cancer. Curr Opin Oncol 1990;2:562–72.

124. Wang CC. Biologic concepts of radiation therapy. In: Wang CC, editor. Radiation therapy for head and neck neoplasms. Chicago: Year Book Medical Publishers; 1990. p. 17–27.

125. Ellis F. Nominal standard dose and the RET. Br J Radiol 1971;44:101–8.

126. Orton CG, Ellis F. A simplification of the use of NSD concept in practical radiotherapy. Br J Radiol 1973;46:529–37.

127. Thomas F, Ozanne F, Mamelle G, et al. Radiotherapy alone for oropharyngeal carcinomas: the role of fraction size (2 Gy vs 2.5 Gy) on local control and early and late complications. Int J Radiat Oncol Biol Phys 1988;15:1097–102.

128. Eschwege F, Lartigau E. Radiotherapy and combined chemoradiotherapy in head and neck carcinoma. Curr Opin Oncol 1990;2:573–7.

129. Withers HR. Biologic basis for altered fractionation scheme. Cancer 1985;55:2086–95.

130. Al-Sarraf M. New approaches to the management of head and neck cancer: the role of chemotherapy. Adv Oncol 1990;6:11–4.

131. Volkes EE. Concomitant chemoradiotherapy for head and neck cancer. Adv Oncol 1990;6:24–9.

132. Hong WK, Bromer HR, Amato DA, et al. Patterns of relapse in locally advanced head and neck cancer patients who achieved complete remission after combined modality therapy. Cancer 1985;56:1242–5.

133. Jacobs C, Goffinet DR, Kohler M, et al. Chemotherapy as a substitute for surgery and in the treatment of advanced resectable head and neck cancer: a report from the Northern California Oncology Group. Cancer 1987;60:1178–83.

134. Vandenbrouck C, Sancho H, LeFur R, et al. Results of a randomized clinical trial of preoperative irradiation versus postoperative irradiation in treatment of tumors of the hypopharynx. Cancer 1977;39:1445–9.

135. Snow JB, Gelber RD, Kramer S, et al. Randomized preoperative and postoperative radiation therapy for patients with carcinoma of the head and neck. Laryngoscope 1980;90:930–45.

136. Spiro RH, Dubner S. Salivary gland tumors. Curr Opin Oncol 1990;2:589–95.

137. Clark JL, Unni KK, Dahlin DC, Devine KD. Osteosarcoma of the jaw. Cancer 1983;51:2311–6.

138. Epstein JB, Knowling MA, LeRiche JC. Multiple gingival metastases from angiosarcoma of the breast. Oral Surg Oral Med Oral Pathol 1987;64:554–7.

139. Pearson GR, Weiland LH, Neel HB, et al. Application of Epstein-Barr virus (EBV) serology to the diagnosis of North American nasopharyngeal carcinoma. Cancer 1983;51:260–8.

140. Mabuchi K, Bross DS, Kessler II. Cigarette smoking and nasopharyngeal carcinoma. Cancer 1985;55:2874–6.

141. Fee WE. Nasopharyngeal carcinoma. Curr Opin Oncol 1990;2:585–8.

142. Wang DC, Cai WM, Hu YH, Gu XZ. Longterm survival of 1035 cases of nasopharyngeal carcinoma. Cancer 1988;61:2338–41.

143. Feinmesser R, Miyazaki I, Cheung R, et al. Diagnosis of nasopharyngeal carcinoma by DNA amplification of tissue obtained by fine-needle aspiration. N Engl J Med 1992;326:17–21.

144. Rishiraj B, Epstein JB. Basal cell carcinoma: what dentists need to know. J Am Dent Assoc 1999;130:375–80.

145. Epstein JB. Treatment of oral Kaposi sarcoma with intralesional vinblastine. Cancer 1993;71:1722–5.

146. Gorsky M, Epstein JB. Head and neck and intra-oral soft tissue sarcomas. Oral Oncol 1998;34:292–6.

147. Gorsky M, Epstein JB. Craniofacial osseous and chondromatous sarcomas in British Columbia—a review of 34 cases. Oral Oncol 1999;36:27–31.

148. Epstein JB, Silverman S Jr. Head and neck malignancies associated with HIV infection. Oral Surg Oral Med Oral Pathol 1992;73:193–200.

149. Epstein JB, Lozada-Nur F, Mcleod WA, Spinelli J. Oral Kaposi's sarcoma in acquired immunodeficiency syndrome. Review of management and report of the efficacy of intralesional vinblastine. Cancer 1989;64:2424–30.

150. Epstein JB, Scully C. Intralesional vinblastine for oral Kaposi's sarcoma in HIV infection. Lancet 1989;ii:1100–1.

151. Stevenson-Moore P. Essential aspects of a pretreatment oral examination. Natl Cancer Inst Monogr 1990;9:33–6.

152. Wright WE. Pretreatment oral health care interventions for radiation patients. Natl Cancer Inst Monogr 1990;9:57–9.

153. Epstein JB, Lunn R, Le N, Stevenson-Moore P. Periodontal attachment loss in patients after head and neck radiation therapy. Oral Surg Oral Med Oral Pathol Oral Radiol Endod 1998;86:715–9.

154. Epstein JB, Chin EA, Jacobson JJ, et al. The relationships among fluoride, cariogenic oral flora and salivary flow rate during radiation therapy. Oral Surg Oral Med Oral Pathol Oral Radiol Endod 1998;86:286–92.

155. Goldberg RI. Protection of irradiated parotid by prostaglandin synthesis inhibitors. J Am Dent Assoc 1986;112:179–81.

156. Ludgate CM. Preliminary report: acetylsalicylic acid therapy in the treatment of complications following abdominal radiation. J Can Assoc Radiol 1985;36:138–40.

157. Schubert MM, Izutsu KT. Iatrogenic salivary gland dysfunction. J Dent Res 1987;66:680–8.

158. Borowski B, Benhamou E, Pico JL, et al. Prevention of oral mucositis in patients treated with high-dose chemotherapy and bone marrow transplantation: a randomised controlled trial comparing two protocols of dental care. Eur J Cancer B Oral Oncol 1994;30B(2):93–7.

159. McCarthy GM, Awde JD, Ghandi H, et al. Risk factors associated with mucositis in cancer patients receiving 5-fluorouracil. Oral Oncol 1998;34:484–90.

160. Berger AM, Eilers J. Factors influencing oral cavity status during high-dose antineoplastic therapy: a secondary data analysis. Oncol Nurs Forum 1998;25:1623–6.

161. Larson PJ, Miaskowski C, MacPhail L, et al. The PRO-SELF Mouth Aware program: an effective approach for reducing chemotherapy-induced mucositis. Cancer Nurs 1998; 21:263–8.

162. Dodd MJ, Miaskowski C, Shiba GH, et al. Risk factors for chemotherapy-induced oral mucositis: dental appliances, oral hygiene, previous oral lesions and history of smoking. Cancer Invest 1999;17:278–84.

163. Bhattathiri VN, Sreelekha TT, Sebastian P, et al. Influence of plasma GSH level on acute radiation mucositis of the oral cavity. Int J Radiat Oncol Biol Phys 1994;29:383–6.

164. Dodd MJ, Facione NC, Dibble SL, MacPhail L. Comparison of methods to determine the prevalence and nature of oral mucositis. Cancer Pract 1996;4:312–8.

165. Sonis ST, Eilers JP, Epstein JB, et al. Validation of a new scoring system for the assessment of clinical trial research of oral mucositis induced by radiation or chemotherapy. Cancer 1999;85:2103–13.

166. Wymenga AN, van der Graaf WE, Spijkervet FL, et al. A new in vitro assay for quantitation of chemotherapy-induced mucositis. Br J Cancer 1997;76:1062–6.

167. Sonis ST. Mucositis as a biologic process: a new hypothesis for the development of chemotherapy-induced stomatotoxicity. Oral Oncol 1998;34:39–43.

168. Handschel J, Prott FJ, Meyer U, et al. Prospective study of the pathology of radiation-induced mucositis. Mund Kiefer Gesichtschir 1998;2:131–5.

169. Epstein JB, Emerton S, Guglietta A, Le N. Assessment of epidermal growth factor in oral secretions of patients receiving radiation therapy for cancer. Oral Oncol 1997;33:359–63.

170. Spijkervet FKL, van Saene HK, van Saene JJ, et al. Effect of selective elimination of oral flora in irradiated head and neck cancer patients. J Surg Oncol 1991;46:167–73.

171. Squier CA. Mucosal alterations. Natl Cancer Inst Monogr 1990;9:169–72.

172. Epstein JB, Stevenson-Moore P, Jackson S, et al. Prevention of oral mucositis in radiation therapy: a controlled study with benzydamine hydrochloride rinse. Int J Radiat Oncol Biol Phys 1989;16:1571–5.

173. Mira JG, Westcott WB, Starke EN, et al. Some factors influencing salivary function when treated with radiotherapy. Int J Radiat Oncol Biol Phys 1981;7:535–41.

174. Dreizen S, Daley TE, Drane JB, et al. Oral complications of cancer radiotherapy. Postgrad Med 1984;61:85–92.

175. Wolff A, Atkinson JC, Macynski AA, Fox PC. Pretherapy interventions to modify salivary dysfunction. Natl Cancer Inst Monogr 1990;9:87–90.

176. Anderson MW, Izutsu KT, Rice JC. Parotid gland pathophysiology after mixed gamma and neutron irradiation of cancer patients. Oral Surg Oral Med Oral Pathol 1981;52:495–500.

177. Marks JE, Davis CC, Gottsman VL, et al. The effects of radiation on parotid salivary function. Int J Radiat Oncol Biol Phys 1981;7:1013–9.

178. Epstein JB, Stewart KH. Radiation therapy and pain in patients with head and neck cancer. Eur J Cancer B Oral Oncol 1993;29B(3):191–9.

179. Withers HR, Peters LJ, Taylor JMG, et al. Late normal tissue sequelae from radiation therapy for carcinoma of the tonsil: patterns of fractionation study of radiobiology. Int J Radiat Oncol Biol Phys 1995;33:563–8.

180. Ramirez-Amador V, Silverman S Jr, Mayer P, et al. Candidal colonization and oral candidiasis in patients undergoing oral and pharyngeal radiation therapy. Oral Surg Oral Med Oral Pathol Oral Radiol Endod 1997;84:149–53.

181. Gava A, Ferrarese F, Tonetto V, et al. Can the prophylactic treatment of mycotic mucositis improve the time of performing radiotherapy in head and neck tumors? Radiol Med (Torino) 1996;91(4):452–5.

182. Epstein JB, Freilich MM, Le ND. Risk factors for oropharyngeal candidiasis in patients who receive radiation therapy for

malignant conditions of the head and neck. Oral Surg Oral Med Oral Pathol 1993;76:169–74.

183. Oakely C, Epstein JB, Sherlock CH. Reactivation of oral herpes simplex virus: implications for clinical management of herpes simplex virus recurrence during radiotherapy. Oral Surg Oral Med Oral Pathol Oral Radiol Endod 1997;84:272–8.

184. Epstein JB, Schubert MM. Management of orofacial pain in cancer patients. Eur J Cancer B Oral Oncol 1993;29B:243–50.

185. Koerner ME. Using hypnosis to relieve pain of terminal cancer. Hypnosis 1977;20:39–46.

186. Barber J, Gritelson J. Cancer pain: pyschological management using hypnosis. Cancer 1980;30:130–5.

187. Syrjala KL, Donaldson GW, Davis MW, et al. Relaxation and imagery and cognitive-behavioral training reduce pain during cancer treatment: a controlled clinical trial. Pain 1995;63(2):189–98.

188. Leborgne JH, Leborgne F, Zubizarreta E, et al. Corticosteroids and radiation mucositis in head and neck cancer. A double-blind placebo-controlled randomized trial. Radiother Oncol 1998;47:145–8.

189. Mills EED. The modifying effect of beta-carotene on radiation and chemotherapy-induced oral mucositis. Br J Cancer 1988;57:416–7.

190. Buntzel J, Kuttner K, Frohlich D, Glatzel M. Selective cytoprotection with amifostine in concurrent radiochemotherapy for head and neck cancer. Ann Oncol 1998;9:505–9.

191. Hospers GA, Eisenhauer EA, de Vries EG. The sulfhydryl containing compounds WR-2721 and glutathione as radio- and chemoprotective agents. A review, indications for use and prospects. Br J Cancer 1999;80:629–38.

192. Taylor SE, Miller EG. Preemptive pharmacologic intervention in radiation-induced salivary dysfunction. Proc Soc Exp Biol Med 1999;221:14–26.

193. McDonald S, Meyerowitz C, Smudzin T, Rubin P. Preliminary results of a pilot study WR-2721 before fractionated irradiation of the head and neck to reduce salivary gland dysfunction. Int J Radiat Oncol Biol Phys 1994;29:747–54.

194. Mascarin M, Franchin G, Minatel E, et al. The effect of granulocyte colony-stimulating factor on oral mucositis in head and neck cancer patients treated with hyperfractionated radiotherapy. Oral Oncol 1999;35:203–8.

195. Chi K-H, Chen C-H, Chan W-K, et al. Effect of granulocyte-macrophage colony-stimulating factor on oral mucositis in head and neck cancer patients after cisplatin, fluorouracil and leucovorin chemotherapy. J Clin Oncol 1995;13:2620–8.

196. Kannan V, Bapsy PP, Anantha H, et al. Efficacy and safety of granulocyte macrophage-colony stimulating factor (GM-CSF) on the frequency and severity of radiation mucositis in patients with head and neck carcinoma. Int J Radiat Oncol Biol Phys 1997;37:1005–10.

197. Rosso M, Blasi G, Ghrelone E, Rosso R. Effect of granulocyte-macrophage colony-stimulating factor on prevention of mucositis in head and neck cancer patients treated with chemo-radiotherapy. J Chemother 1997;9:382–5.

198. Wagner W, Alfrink M, Haus U, Matt J. Treatment of irradiation-induced mucositis with growth factors (rhGM-CSF) in patients with head and neck cancer. Anticancer Res 1999;19:799–803.

199. Danilenko DM. Preclinical and early clinical development of keratinocyte growth factor, an epithelial-specific tissue growth factor. Toxicol Pathol 1999;27:64–71.

200. Farrell CL, Rex KL, Kaufman SA, et al. Effects of keratinocyte growth factor in the squamous epithelium of the upper aerodigestive tract of normal and irradiated mice. Int J Radiat Biol 1999;75:609–20.

201. Farrell CL, Bready JV, Rex KL, et al. Keratinocyte growth factor protects mice from chemotherapy and radiation-induced gastrointestinal injury and mortality. Cancer Res 1998;58:933–9.

202. Spijkervet RKL, Van Saene HKF, Panders AK, et al. Effect of chlorhexidine rinsing on the oropharyngeal ecology in patients with head and neck cancer who have irradiation mucositis. Oral Surg Oral Med Oral Pathol 1989;67:154–61.

203. Samaranayake LP, Robertson AG, MacFarlane TE, et al. The effect of chlorhexidine and benzydamine mouthwashes on mucositis induced by therapeutic irradiation. Clin Radiol 1988;39:291–4.

204. Symonds RP, McIlroy P, Khorrami J, et al. The reduction of radiation oral mucositis by selective decontamination antibiotic pastilles: a placebo-controlled double-blind trial. Br J Cancer 1996;74:312–7.

205. Garfunkel AA, Tager N, Chausu S, et al. Oral complications in bone marrow transplantation patients: recent advances. Isr J Med Sci 1994;30(1):120–4.

206. Prada A, Chiesa F. Effects of benzydamine on the oral mucositis during antineoplastic radiotherapy and/or intra-arterial chemotherapy. Int J Tissue React 1987;9:115–9.

207. Kim JH, Chu FCH, Lakshmi V, et al. Benzydamine HCL, a new agent for the treatment of radiation mucositis of the oropharynx. Am J Clin Oncol 1986;9:132–4.

208. Epstein JB, Stevenson-Moore P, Jackson S, et al. Prevention of oral mucositis in radiation therapy: a controlled study with benzydamine hydrochloride rinse. Int J Radiat Oncol Biol Phys 1989;16:1571–5.

209. Epstein JB, Stevenson-Moore P. Benzydamine hydrochloride in prevention and management of pain in oral mucositis associated with radiation therapy. Oral Surg Oral Med Oral Pathol 1986;62:145–8.

210. Samaranayake LP, Robertson AG, MacFarlane TW, et al. The effect of chlorhexidine and benzydamine mouthwashes on mucositis induced by therapeutic irradiation. Clin Radiol 1988;39:291–4.

211. Adams S, Toth B, Dudley BS. Evaluation of sucralfate as a compounded oral suspension for the treatment of stomatitis. Clin Pharmacol Ther 1985;2:178.

212. Epstein JB, Wong FL. The efficacy of sucralfate suspension in the prevention of oral mucositis due to radiation therapy. Int J Radiat Oncol Biol Phys 1994;28(3):693–8.

213. Makkonen TA, Bostrom P, Vilja P, Joensuu H. Sucralfate mouth washing in the prevention of radiation-induced mucositis: a placebo-controlled double-blind randomized study. Int J Radiat Oncol Biol Phys 1994;30:177–82.

214. Meridith R, Salter M, Kim R, et al. Sucralfate for radiation mucositis: results of a double-blind randomized trial. Int J Radiat Oncol Biol Phys 1997;37:275–9.

215. Shenep JL, Kalwinsky DK, Huston PR, et al. Efficacy of oral sucralfate suspension in prevention and treatment of chemotherapy-induced mucositis. J Pediatr 1988;113:758–63.

216. Barker G, Loftus L, Cuddy P, Barker B. The effects of sucralfate suspension and diphenhydramine syrup plus kaolin-pectin on radiotherapy-induced mucositis. Oral Surg Oral Med Oral Pathol 1991;71:288–93.

217. Hanson WR, Marks JE, Reddy SP, et al. Protection from radiation-induced oral mucositis by misoprostol prostaglandin E1 analog: a placebo controlled double blind clinical trial. Am J Ther 1995;2:850–7.

218. Oguchi M, Shikama N, Saskai S, et al. Mucosa-adhesive water-soluble polymer film for treatment of acute radiation-induced oral mucositis. Int J Radiat Oncol Biol Phys 1998;40:1033–7.

219. Foote RL, Loprinzi CL, Frank AR, et al. Randomized trial of a chlorhexidine mouthwash for alleviation of radiation-induced mucositis. J Clin Oncol 1994;12:2630–3.

220. Dodd MJ, Larson PJ, Dibble SL, et al. Randomized clinical trial of chlorhexidine versus placebo for prevention of oral mucositis in patients receiving chemotherapy. Oncol Nurs Forum 1996;23:921–7.

221. Adamietz IA, Rahn R, Bottcher HD, et al. Prophylaxis with povidone-iodine against induction of oral mucositis in radiochemotherapy. Support Care Cancer 1998;6:373–7.

222. Okuno SH, Foote RL, Loprinzi CL, et al. A randomized trial of a nonabsorbable antibiotic lozenge given to alleviate radiation-induced mucositis. Cancer 1997;79:2193–9.

223. Berger A, Henderson M, Nadoolman W, et al. Oral capsaicin provides temporary relief for oral mucositis pain secondary to chemotherapy/radiation therapy. J Pain Symptom Manage 1995;10(3):243–8.

224. Perch SJ, Machtay M, Markiewicz DA, Kligerman MM. Decreased acute toxicity by using midline mucosa-sparing blocks during radiation therapy for carcinoma of the oral cavity, oropharynx, and nasopharynx. Radiology 1995;197(3):863–6.

225. Sonis S, Muska A, O'Brien J, et al. Alteration in the frequency, severity and duration of chemotherapy-induced mucositis in hamsters by interluekin-11. Eur J Cancer Oral Oncol 1995;31B:261–6.

226. Sonis ST, Van Vugt AG, McDonald J, et al. Mitigating effects of interleukin 11 on consecutive courses of 5-fluorouracil-induced ulcerative mucositis in hamsters. Cytokine 1997;9:605–12.

227. Sonis ST, Van Vugt AG, Brien JP, et al. Transforming growth factor-beta 3 mediated modulation of cell cycling and attenuation of 5-fluorouracil induced oral mucositis. Oral Oncol 1997;33:47–54.

228. Sonis ST, Lindquist L, Van Vugt A, et al. Prevention of chemotherapy-induced ulcerative mucositis by transforming growth factor beta 3. Cancer Res 1994;54:1135–8.

229. Keith JC Jr, Albert L, Sonis ST, et al. IL-11, a pleiotropic cytokine: exciting new effects of IL-11 on gastrointestinal mucosal biology. Stem Cells 1994;12 Suppl 1:89–90.

230. Sonis ST, Costa JW Jr, Evitts SM, et al. Effect of epidermal growth factor on ulcerative mucositis in hamsters that receive cancer chemotherapy. Oral Surg Oral Med Oral Pathol 1992;74:749–55.

231. Girdler NM, McGurk M, Aqual S, Prince M. The effect of epidermal growth factor mouthwash on cytotoxic-induced oral ulceration. A phase I clinical trial. Am J Clin Oncol 1995;18:403–6.

232. Bez C, Demarosi F, Sardella A, et al. GM-CSF mouthrinses in the treatment of severe oral mucositis: a pilot study. Oral Surg Oral Med Oral Pathol Oral Radiol Endod 1999;88:311–5.

233. Nicolatou O, Sotiropoulou-Lontou A, Skarlatos J, et al. A pilot study of the effect of granulocyte-macrophage colony-stimulating factor on oral mucositis in head and neck cancer patients during X-radiation therapy: a preliminary report. Int J Radiat Oncol Biol Phys 1998;42:551–6.

234. Bensadoun RJ, Franquin JC, Ciais G, et al. Low-energy He/Ne laser in the prevention of radiation-induced mucositis. Support Care Cancer 1999;7:244–52.

235. Fox PC, Atkinson JC, Macynski AA, et al. Pilocarpine treatment of salivary gland hypofunction and dry mouth (xerostomia). Arch Intern Med 1991;151:1149–52.

236. Greenspan D. Management of salivary dysfunction. Natl Cancer Inst Monogr 1990;9:159–61.

237. Epstein JB, Schubert MM. Synergistic effect of sialogogues in management of xerostomia after radiation therapy. Oral Surg Oral Med Oral Pathol 1987;64:179–82.

238. Silverman S Jr, Luangjarmekorn L, Greenspan D. Occurrence of oral Candida in irradiated head and neck cancer patients. J Oral Med 1984;39:194–6.

239. Rossie KM, Taylor J, Beck FM, et al. Influence of radiation therapy on oral Candida albicans colonization: a quantitative assessment. Oral Surg Oral Med Oral Pathol 1987;64:698–701.

240. Epstein JB. Infection prevention in bone marrow transplantation and radiation patients. Natl Cancer Inst Monogr 1990;9:73–85.

241. Epstein JB. Antifungal therapy in oropharyngeal mycotic infections. Oral Surg Oral Med Oral Pathol 1990;69:32–41.

242. Dreizen S, Brown LR, Daly TE, Drane JB. Prevention of xerostomia-related dental caries in irradiated cancer patients. J Dent Res 1977;56:99–104.

243. Wei SHY. Clinical uses of fluorides: a state-of-the-art conference on the use of fluorides in clinical dentistry. J Am Dent Assoc 1984;109:472–4.

244. Anonymous. Oral complications of cancer therapies: diagnosis, prevention and treatment. NIH Consens Statement 1989;7:1–11.

245. Jansma J, Vissink A, Gravenmade EJ. In vivo study on the prevention of postirradiation caries. Caries Res 1989;23:172–8.

246. Meyerowitz C, Featherstone JDB, Billings RJ, et al. Use of an intra-oral model to evaluate 0.05% sodium fluoride mouthrinse in radiation-induced hyposalivation. J Dent Res 1991;70:894–8.

247. Epstein JB, Loh R, Stevenson-Moore P, et al. Chlorhexidine rinse in prevention of dental caries in patients following radiation therapy. Oral Surg Oral Med Oral Pathol 1989;68:401–5.

248. Keene HJ, Fleming TJ. Prevalence of caries-associated microflora after radiotherapy in patients with cancer of the head and neck. Oral Surg Oral Med Oral Pathol 1987;64:421–6.

249. Epstein JB, McBride BC, Stevenson-Moore P, et al. The efficacy of chlorhexidine gel in reduction of Streptococcus mutans and Lactobacillus species in patients treated with radiation therapy. Oral Surg Oral Med Oral Pathol 1991;71:172–8.

250. Epstein JB, Wong FLW, Stevenson-Moore P. Osteoradionecrosis: clinical experience and a proposal for classification. J Oral Maxillofac Surg 1987;45:104–10.

251. Epstein JB, Rea G, Wong FLW, Stevenson-Moore P. Osteonecrosis: study of the relationship of dental extractions in patients receiving radiotherapy. Head Neck Surg 1987;10:48–54.

252. Myers RA, Marx RE. Hyperbaric oxygen in postradiation head and neck surgery. Natl Cancer Inst Monogr 1990;9:151–7.

253. Marx RE. A new concept in the treatment of osteoradionecrosis. J Oral Maxillofac Surg 1983;41:283–8.

254. McKenzie MR, Wong FLW, Epstein JB, Lepawsky M. Hyperbaric oxygen and postradiation osteonecrosis of the mandible. Eur J Cancer Oral Oncol 1993;29B(3):201–7.

255. Epstein JB, van der Meij E, McKenzie M, et al. Postradiation osteonecrosis of the mandible: a long-term follow-up study. Oral Surg Oral Med Oral Pathol Oral Radiol Endod 1997;83:657–62.

256. van Merkesteyn JP, Bakker DJ, Borgmeijer-Hoelen AM. Hyperbaric oxygen treatment of osteoradionecrosis of the mandible: experience in 29 patients. Oral Surg Oral Med Oral Pathol 1995;80:12–6.

257. Bartoshuk LM. Chemosensory alterations and cancer therapies. Natl Cancer Inst Monogr 1990;9:179–84.

258. Conger AD. Loss and recovery of taste acuity in patients irradiated to the oral cavity. Radiat Res 1973;53:338–47.

259. Silverman S Jr, Thompsom JS. Serum zinc and copper in oral/oropharyngeal carcinoma. A study of seventy-five patients. Oral Surg Oral Med Oral Pathol 1984;57:34–6.

260. Epstein JB, Schubert MM, Scully C. Evaluation and treatment of pain in patients with orofacial cancer: a review. Pain Clinic 1991;4:3–20.

261. Rosenberg SW. Chronic dental complications. Natl Cancer Inst Monogr 1990;9:173–8.

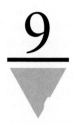

9

SALIVARY GLAND DISEASES

MARGARET M. GRISIUS, DDS
PHILIP C. FOX, DDS

Patients with salivary gland disease most frequently present with complaints of oral dryness, swelling, or a mass in a gland. This chapter first reviews briefly the anatomy and physiology of the salivary glands and then outlines a diagnostic approach to the patient who has signs and symptoms that are suggestive of salivary gland dysfunction. The examination of a patient with dry mouth is described, and the approach to the patient with a salivary mass is reviewed. Each of the major salivary gland disorders are described. At the end of the chapter, treatment options for the patient with salivary gland dysfunction are discussed.

▼ SALIVARY GLAND ANATOMY AND PHYSIOLOGY

There are three major salivary glands: parotid, submandibular, and sublingual. These are paired glands that secrete a highly modified saliva through a branching duct system. Parotid saliva is released through Stenson's duct, the orifice of which is visible on the buccal mucosa adjacent to the maxillary first molars. Sublingual saliva may enter the floor of the mouth via a series of short independent ducts, but will empty into the submandibular (Wharton's) duct about half of the time. The orifice of Wharton's duct is located sublingually on either side of the lingual frenum. There are also thousands of minor salivary glands throughout the mouth, most of which are named for their anatomic location (labial, palatal, buccal, etc). These minor glands are located just below the mucosal surface and communicate with the oral cavity with short ducts.

Saliva is the product of the major and minor salivary glands dispersed throughout the oral cavity. It is a highly complex mixture of water and organic and non-organic components. Most of the constituents are produced locally within the glands; others are transported from the circulation. The three major salivary glands share a basic anatomic structure. They are composed of acinar and ductal cells arranged much like a cluster of grapes on stems. The acinar cells (the "grapes" in this analogy) make up the secretory endpiece and are the sole sites of fluid transport into the glands. The acinar cells of the parotid gland are serous, those of the sublingual gland are mucous, and those of the submandibular gland are of a mixed mucous and serous type. The duct cells (the "stems") form a branching system that carries the saliva from the acini into the oral cavity. The duct cell morphology changes as it progresses from the acinar junction toward the mouth, and different distinct regions can be identified.

While fluid secretion occurs only through the acini, proteins are produced and transported into the saliva through both acinar and ductal cells. The primary saliva within the acinar endpiece is isotonic with serum but undergoes extensive modification within the duct system, with resorption of sodium and chloride and secretion of potassium. The saliva, as it enters the oral cavity, is a protein-rich hypotonic fluid.

The secretion of saliva is controlled by sympathetic and parasympathetic neural input. The stimulus for fluid secretion is primarily via muscarinic cholinergic receptors, and the stimulus for protein release occurs through β-adrenergic receptors. Ligation of these receptors induces a complex signaling and signal transduction pathway within the cells, involving numerous transport systems.[1] An important point to consider is that loss of acini, as occurs in a number of clinical conditions, will limit the ability of the gland to transport fluid and to produce saliva. Also, muscarinic agonists will have the greatest effect in increasing saliva output as they are primarily responsible for the stimulus of fluid secretion. These points have implications for the treatment of salivary gland dysfunction.

▼ DIAGNOSTIC APPROACHES TO THE PATIENT WITH SALIVARY GLAND DISEASE

Evaluation of Dry Mouth

The subjective feeling of oral dryness is termed xerostomia. Xerostomia is a symptom, not a diagnosis or disease. The term is used to encompass the spectrum of oral complaints voiced by patients with dry mouth. It is important to recognize that a patient complaining of dry mouth cannot automatically be assumed to have a salivary dysfunction. While oral dryness is most commonly the result of salivary gland dysfunction, it may have other causes. Patients need careful objective examination to identify the basis of their problem. Since individuals with salivary gland dysfunction are at risk for a variety of oral and systemic complications due to alterations in normal salivary performance, they should be identified, and appropriate treatment should be implemented.

There are a number of nonsalivary causes of oral dryness complaints that should be considered, such as dehydration. Although dehydration may secondarily affect salivary gland output, changes in body water can affect mucosal hydration, which may lead to changes in the perception of wetness in the mouth. Central cognitive alterations and oral sensory disturbances can lead to a sense of mucosal dryness. There are also psychological conditions that can lead to the complaint of dry mouth.

Dysfunction of the salivary glands, however, is the most common cause of complaints of dry mouth. It is important to recognize that changes in salivary composition may be as important as a reduction in salivary output in some cases. Therefore, the demonstration of seemingly adequate salivary flow alone is not a guarantee of normal salivary gland function.

The differential diagnosis of xerostomia and salivary gland dysfunction is lengthy. The optimal approach to diagnosis is a sequential plan that first establishes the cause of the complaint, then determines the extent of salivary gland hypofunction that is present, and finally assesses the potential for treatment. An initial evaluation should include a past and present medical history, an oral examination, and an assessment of salivary function. Further techniques that may be indicated are salivary imaging, biopsy, and clinical laboratory assessment of hematologic variables. These are described below in more detail.

SYMPTOMS OF SALIVARY GLAND DYSFUNCTION

Symptoms in the patient with salivary gland hypofunction are related to decreased fluid in the oral cavity. Patients complain of dryness of all the oral mucosal surfaces, including the throat, and also of difficulty chewing, swallowing, and speaking. Many patients report a need to drink fluids while eating to help swallowing or report an inability to swallow dry foods. Most will carry fluids at all times for oral comfort and to aid speaking and swallowing. Pain is a common complaint. The mucosa may be sensitive to spicy or coarse foods, which limits the patient's enjoyment of meals.[2]

PAST AND PRESENT MEDICAL HISTORY

A critical first step is a thorough history. If the past and present medical history reveals medical conditions or medications that are known to be associated with salivary gland dysfunction, a diagnosis may be obvious. Examples would be a patient who has received radiotherapy for a head and neck malignancy or an individual who has recently started taking a tricyclic antidepressant. A recent survey found 1,500 drugs that are reported to have some incidence of dry mouth as a side effect. A complete history of all medications being taken (including over-the-counter medications, supplements, and herbal preparations) is critical. Often the temporal association of symptom onset with the treatment is a valuable clue. When the history does not suggest an obvious diagnosis, further detailed exploration of the symptomatic complaint should be undertaken. Unfortunately, the general complaint of oral dryness is not well correlated with decreased salivary function, but specific symptoms may be.[2] For example, while complaints of oral dryness at night or on awakening have not been found to be associated reliably with reduced salivary function, the complaints of oral dryness while eating, the need to sip liquids to swallow dry food, or difficulties in swallowing dry food have all been highly correlated with measured decreases in secretory capacity. These complaints focus on oral activities (eg, swallowing and eating) that rely on stimulated salivary function. Patients should also be questioned concerning dryness at other body sites. A patient's report of eye, throat, nasal, skin, or vaginal dryness, in addition to xerostomia, may be a significant indication of a systemic condition, such as Sjögren's syndrome.[3,4]

CLINICAL EXAMINATION

Most patients with advanced salivary gland hypofunction have obvious signs of mucosal dryness. The lips are often cracked, peeling, and atrophic. The buccal mucosa may be pale and corrugated in appearance, and the tongue may be smooth and reddened, with loss of papillation. Patients may report that their lips stick to the teeth, and the oral mucosa may adhere to the dry enamel. There is often a marked increase in erosion and caries, particularly decay on root surfaces and even cusp tip involvement. The decay may be progressive, even in the presence of vigilant oral hygiene. One should look for active caries and determine whether the caries' history and current condition are consistent with the patient's oral hygiene. While caries are unquestionably increased, it has not been determined definitively whether increased prevalence or severity of periodontal pathology is associated with salivary gland hypofunction. Candidiasis, most commonly of the erythematous form, is frequent. Two additional indications of oral dryness that have been gleaned from clinical experience are the "lipstick" and "tongue blade" signs. In the former, the presence of lipstick or shed epithelial cells on the labial surfaces of the anterior maxillary teeth is indicative of reduced saliva (saliva would normally wet the mucosa and aid in cleansing the teeth). To test for the latter sign, the examiner can hold a tongue blade against the buccal mucosa; in a dry mouth, the tissue will adhere to the tongue blade as the blade is lifted away. Both signs suggest that the mucosa is not sufficiently moisturized by the saliva.

Enlargement of the salivary glands is seen frequently. In these cases, one must distinguish between inflammatory, infectious, or neoplastic etiologies. The major salivary glands should be palpated to detect masses and also to determine if saliva can be expressed via the main excretory ducts. Normally, saliva can be expressed from each major gland orifice by compressing the glands with bimanual palpation and by pushing towards the orifice. The consistency of the secretions should be examined. The expressed saliva should be clear, watery, and copious. Viscous or scant secretions suggest chronically reduced function. A cloudy exudate may be a sign of bacterial infection although some patients with very low salivary function will have hazy flocculated secretions that are sterile. In these cases, there may be mucoid accretions and clumped epithelial cells, which lend the saliva a cloudy appearance. The exudate should be cultured if it does not appear clear, particularly in the case of an enlarged gland. Palpation should be painless. Enlarged painful glands are indicative of infection or acute inflammation. The consistency of the gland should be slightly rubbery but not hard, and distinct masses within the body of the gland should not be present.[3–5]

SALIVA COLLECTION

Salivary flow rates provide essential information for diagnostic and research purposes. Salivary gland function should be determined by objective measurement techniques. Salivary flow rates can be calculated from the individual major salivary glands or from a mixed sample of the oral fluids, termed "whole saliva."

Whole saliva is the mixed fluid contents of the mouth. The main methods of whole saliva collection include the draining, spitting, suction, and absorbent (swab) methods. The draining method is passive and requires the patient to allow saliva to flow from the mouth into a preweighed test tube or graduated cylinder for a timed period. In the spitting method, the patient allows saliva to accumulate in the mouth and then expectorates into a preweighed graduated cylinder, usually every 60 seconds for 2 to 5 minutes. The suction method uses an aspirator or saliva ejector to draw saliva from the mouth into a test tube for a defined time period. The absorbent method uses a preweighed gauze sponge that is placed in the patient's mouth for a set amount of time. After collection, the sponge is weighed again, and the volume of saliva is determined gravimetrically.

The suction and absorbent (swab) methods give a variable degree of stimulation of secretion and are therefore less reproducible. The draining and the spitting methods are more reliable and reproducible for unstimulated whole saliva collection. If a stimulated whole saliva collection is desired, a standardized method of stimulation should be used. Chewing unflavored gum base or an inert material such as paraffin wax or a rubber band at a controlled rate is a reliable and reproducible means of inducing saliva secretion. One can also apply 2% citric acid to the tongue at regular intervals.[6,7]

It is difficult to determine a "normal" value for salivary output as there is a large amount of interindividual variability and consequently a large range of normal values. However, with the collection methods described above, most experts do agree on the minimal values necessary to consider salivary output normal. Unstimulated whole saliva flow rates of < 0.1 mL/min and stimulated whole saliva flow rate's of < 1.0 mL/min are considered abnormally low and indicative of marked salivary hypofunction. It is important to recognize that greater levels of output do not guarantee that function is normal. Indeed, they may represent marked hypofunction for some individuals. These values represent a lower limit of normal and a guide for the clinician.

Individual parotid gland saliva collection is performed by using Carlson-Crittenden collectors. The collectors are placed over the Stensen duct orifices and are held in place with gentle suction. Saliva from individual submandibular and sublingual glands is collected with an aspirating device or an alginate-held collector called a segregator. When using the suction device, gauze is placed sublingually to dry and isolate the sublingual region. The gauze and tongue are gently retracted away from the duct orifice. Gentle suction is used to collect the saliva as it is produced. The segregator is positioned over Wharton's ducts and is then held in place by alginate. As saliva is produced, it flows through tubing and is collected in a preweighed vessel.[6,8]

Stimulated saliva from individual glands is obtained by applying a sialagogue such as citric acid to the dorsal surface of the tongue. Preweighed tubes are used for individual salivary gland collections and for some of the whole saliva collection techniques, and flow rates are determined gravimetrically in milliliters per minute per gland, assuming that the specific gravity of saliva is 1 (ie, 1 g equals 1 mL of saliva). Samples to be retained for compositional analysis should be collected on ice and frozen until tested.[9–12]

Flow rates are affected by many factors. Patient position, hydration, diurnal variation, and time since stimulation can all affect salivary flow. Whichever technique is chosen for saliva collection, it is critical to use a well-defined, standardized, and clearly documented procedure. This allows meaningful comparisons to be made with other studies and with repeat measures in an individual over time. It is best to collect saliva in the morning. To insure an unstimulated sample, patients should refrain from eating, drinking, or smoking for 90 minutes prior to the collection.[9,12]

For a general assessment of salivary function, unstimulated whole saliva collection is the most valuable method of collection. It is easy to accomplish and is accurate and reproducible if carried out with a consistent and careful technique. Ideally, dentists would determine baseline values for unstimulated whole saliva output at an initial examination. This would allow later comparisons if patients begin to complain of oral dryness or present with other signs and symptoms of salivary dysfunction. For research purposes, or if more specific functional information is required for one particular gland, individual gland collection techniques should be used. These are not difficult but require specialized equipment and more time to accomplish.

SALIVARY GLAND IMAGING

A number of imaging techniques are useful in the evaluation of the salivary glands. For a full description of imaging techniques, see chapter 3, "Maxillofacial Imaging." The following describes specific techniques as they relate to the diagnosis of salivary gland disorders. Depending on the technique used, imaging can provide information on salivary function, anatomic alterations, and space-occupying lesions within the glands. This section discusses plain-film radiography, sialography, ultrasonography, radionuclide imaging, magnetic resonance imaging, and computed tomography (Table 9–1).

Plain-Film Radiography. Since the salivary glands are located relatively superficially, radiographic images may be obtained with standard dental radiographic techniques. Symptoms suggestive of salivary gland obstruction (swelling of the gland and pain) warrant plain-film radiography of the major salivary glands in order to visualize possible radiopaque sialoliths (stones) (Figure 9–1). Panoramic or lateral oblique and anteroposterior (AP) projections are used to visualize the parotid glands. Panoramic views overlap anatomic structures that can mask the presence of a salivary stone. A standard occlusal film can be placed intraorally adjacent to the parotid duct to visualize a stone close to the gland orifice. However, this technique will not capture the entire parotid gland. Sialoliths obstructing the submandibular gland can be visualized by panoramic, occlusal, or lateral oblique views.

Smaller stones or poorly calcified sialoliths may not be visible radiographically. If a stone is not evident with plain-film radiography but clinical evaluation and history are suggestive of salivary gland obstruction, then additional images are necessary.

Sialography. Sialography is the radiographic visualization of the salivary gland following retrograde instillation of soluble contrast material into the ducts (Figure 9–2). Sialography is one of the oldest imaging procedures and was first mentioned by Carpy in 1902. In 1925, Barsony and Uslenghi separately described sialography as a diagnostic tool. Sialography is the recommended method for evaluating intrinsic and acquired abnormalities of the ductal system because it provides the clearest visualization of the branching ducts and acinar end-

TABLE 9–1   Salivary Gland Imaging Modalities: Indications, Advantages, and Disadvantages

Imaging Modality	Indications	Advantages	Disadvantages
Ultrasonography	Biopsy guidance; mass detection	Noninvasive; cost-effective	No quantification of function; observer variability; limited visibility of deeper portions of gland; no morphologic information
Sialography	Stone, stricture; R/O autoimmune or radiation-induced sialadenitis	Visualizes ductal anatomy/ blockage	Invasive; requires iodine dye; no quantification
Radionuclide imaging	R/O autoimmune sialadenitis; sialosis, tumor	Quantification of function	Radiation exposure; no morphologic information
Computed tomography	R/O calcified structure; tumor	Differentiates osseous structures from soft tissue	No quantification; contrast dye injection; radiation exposure
Magnetic resonance imaging	R/O soft-tissue lesion	Soft-tissue resolution excellent, with ability to differentiate osseous structures from soft tissue; no radiation burden	Dental scatter; contraindicated with pacemaker or metal implant; no quantification

R/O = rule out

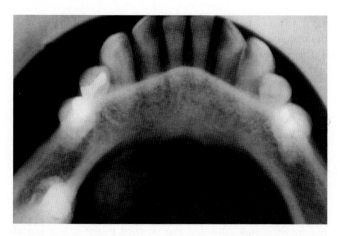

Figure 9–1 This roentgenogram occlusal view demonstrates a calcified deposit in Wharton's duct.

pieces. Salivary ductal obstruction, whether by a sialolith or stricture, can be easily recognized by sialography. When patients present with a history of rapid-onset, acute, painful swelling of a single gland (typically brought on by eating), sialography is the indicated imaging technique. Potential neoplasms are better visualized by cross-sectional imaging techniques such as computerized tomography or magnetic resonance imaging.

The two contraindications to sialography are active infection and allergy to contrast media. Sialography performed during active infection may further irritate and potentially rupture the already inflamed gland. Additionally, the injection of contrast material might force bacteria throughout the ductal structure and worsen the infection. The iodine in the contrast media may induce an allergic reaction and also can

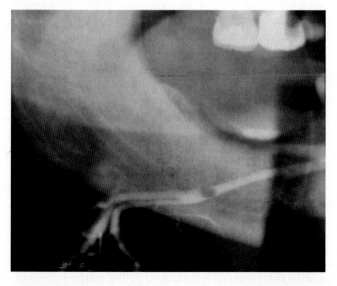

Figure 9–2 This is a sialogram of the submandibular gland demonstrating an uncalcified sialolithiasis in Wharton's duct, which can be visualized where the submandibular duct overlies the inferior alveolar canal. Courtesy of Dr. Eisa Mozaffari, University of Pennsylvania.

interfere with thyroid function tests and with thyroid cancer evaluation by nuclear medicine.

Sialography can be performed on both the submandibular and parotid glands. Initial plain-film radiography is recommended for visualizing radiopaque stones and potential bony destruction from malignant lesions, as well as for providing a background for interpreting the sialogram. Oil- and water-based contrast media are available. Both contain iodine and are therefore contraindicated in patients with iodine sensitivity.[13,14]

Oil-based contrast material is not diluted in saliva or absorbed across the mucosa, which allows for maximum opacificaton of the ductal and acinar structures. However, if extravasation into the glandular tissue occurs, the residual contrast material will remain at the site and may interfere with subsequent computed tomography (CT) images. Inflammatory responses and even the formation of granulomas have been reported following sialography using oil-based contrast. Injection of oil-based contrast medium requires more pressure because of its viscosity.

Water-based dyes are soluble in saliva and can diffuse into the glandular tissue, which can result in decreased radiographic density and poor visualization of peripheral ducts, compared to oil-based contrast. Higher-viscosity water-soluble contrast agents that allow better visualization of the ductal structures are available and are recommended.

Routine radiography includes panoramic, lateral oblique, AP, and "puffed-cheek" AP views. The normal ductal architecture has a "leafless tree" appearance. As the ductal structure branches through the major glands, the submandibular gland demonstrates a more abrupt transition in ductal diameter whereas the parotid gland demonstrates a gradual decrease in ductal diameter. Ductal stricture, obstruction, dilatation, ductal ruptures, and stones can be visualized by sialography. Nonopaque sialoliths appear as voids. Sialectasis is the appearance of focal collections of contrast medium within the gland, seen in cases of sialadenitis and Sjögren's syndrome. The progression of severity is classified as punctate, globular, and cavitary. Sialography is the imaging technique of choice for delineating ductal anatomy and for identifying and localizing sialoliths. It also may be a valuable tool in presurgical planning prior to the removal of salivary masses.[13,14]

Following the procedure, the patient should be encouraged to massage the gland and/or to suck on lemon drops to promote the flow of saliva and contrast material out of the gland. Postprocedure radiography is done approximately 1 hour later. If a substantial amount of contrast material remains in the salivary gland at that time, follow-up visits should be scheduled until the contrast material empties or is fully resorbed. Incomplete clearing can be due to obstruction of salivary outflow, extraductal or extravasated contrast, collection of contrast material in abscess cavities, or impaired secretory function.

Ultrasonography. Due to their superficial locations, the parotid and submandibular glands are easily visualized by ultrasonography although the deep portion of the parotid

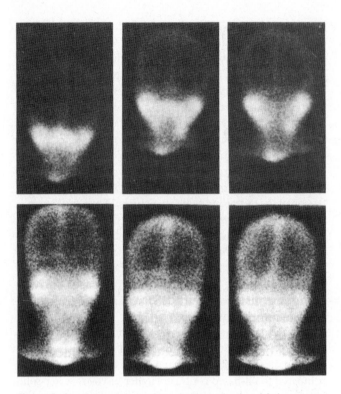

Figure 9–3   Anteroposterior view scintigrams developed during sequential salivary scintigraphy of the parotid gland for a normal patient (top row) and a patient with acute sialadenitis following administration of phenylbutazone (bottom row). Both illustrations on the left are at 10 minutes postintravenous injection of ^{99m}Tc pertechnetate, those in the middle at 30 minutes, and those on the right at 60 minutes. At 10 minutes, the isotope is already concentrated in the parotid and submandibular areas in contrast to that in the bloodstream, as reflected in the fainter outline of the cranium and sagittal venous sinuses. The thyroid gland, which also concentrated the isotope, also is intensely marked at the base of each scintigram. Normal and abnormal scintigrams show little difference at the time. In the normal scintigram at 30 minutes, an additional spot has appeared between the two parotid spots, corresponding to the secretion and accumulation of secreted isotope in the mouth and pharynx. By contrast, in the patient with acute sialadenitis who had markedly diminished salivary secretion, the parotid spots have intensified without development of a central spot. At 60 minutes, the xerostomia patient still retains a high level of radioactivity in the glands without a central secretory spot, whereas in the normal patient, the parotid spots are fading in contrast to the central spot. Because of the short half-life of this isotope of 6 hours, all radioactivity will have essentially disappeared from the scintigram by the next day, allowing the technique to be repeated if necessary. (Garfunkel AA, et al. Phenylbutazone-induced sialadenitis. Oral Surg. 1974; 38:223.)

gland is difficult to visualize because the mandibular ramus lies over the deep lobe. Ultrasonography is best at differentiating between intra- and extraglandular masses as well as between cystic and solid lesions. In general, solid benign lesions present as well-circumscribed hypoechoic intraglandular masses. Ultrasonography can demonstrate the presence of an abscess in an acutely inflamed gland, as well as the presence of sialoliths, which appear as echogenic densities that exhibit acoustic shadowing. Makula and colleagues studied a group of patients with Sjögren's syndrome and reported the appearance of parenchymal inhomogeneity. They also noted good agreement between ultrasonographic, sialographic, and scintigraphic results in this patient group. Ultrasonography is a noninvasive and cost-effective imaging modality that can be used in the evaluation of masses occurring in the submandibular gland and the superficial lobe of the parotid gland.[15–17]

Radionuclide Salivary Imaging.   Scintigraphy with technetium (Tc) 99m pertechnetate is a dynamic and minimally invasive diagnostic test to assess salivary gland function and to determine abnormalities in gland uptake and excretion. Scintigraphy is the only salivary imaging technique that provides information on the functional capabilities of the glands (Figure 9–3). Technetium is a pure gamma ray–emitting radionuclide that is taken up by the salivary glands (following intravenous injection), transported through the glands, and then secreted into the oral cavity. Uptake and secretion phases can be recognized on the scans. Uptake of Tc 99m by a salivary gland indicates that there is functional epithelial tissue present. The Tc-99m scan can be used as a measure of secretory function as it has been shown to correlate well with salivary output. Tc 99m is capable of substituting for chloride (Cl^-) in the sodium-potassium (Na^+/K^+)/$2Cl^-$ salivary transport pump and serves as a measurement of fluid movement in the salivary acinar glands. Duct cells can also accumulate Tc 99m. Scintigraphy is indicated for the evaluation of patients when sialography is contraindicated or cannot be performed (such as in cases of acute gland infection or iodine allergy) or when the major duct cannot be cannulated successfully. It has also been used to aid in the diagnosis of ductal obstruction, sialolithiasis, gland aplasia, Bell's palsy and Sjögren's syndrome.[18–23]

Salivary imaging is performed following the injection of 10 to 20 mCi of Tc 99m pertechnetate. The uptake, concentration, and excretion of the pertechnetate anion by the major salivary glands and other organs is imaged with a gamma detector that records both the number and the location of gamma particles released in a given field during a period of time. This information can be stored in a computer for later analysis or recorded directly on film from the gamma detector, to give static images.

Several rating scales exist for the evaluation of salivary scintiscans; however, no standard rating method presently exists. Current approaches to functional assessment include visual interpretation, time-activity curve analysis, and numeric indices. Most radiologists read Tc 99m scans by using visual interpretation and clinical judgment. A semiquantitative method exists in which Tc 99m uptake and secretion is calculated by computer analysis of a user-defined region of interest (ROI). Time-activity ROI studies are time-consuming and are more commonly used for research.

Radionuclide imaging can provide information regarding salivary gland function by generating a time-activity curve. A normal time-activity curve has three phases: flow, concentration, and washout. The flow phase is about 15 to 20 seconds in duration and represents the phase immediately following injection when the iostope is equilibrating in the blood and accumulating in the salivary gland at a submaximal rate. The concentration phase represents the accumulation of Tc 99m pertechnetate in the gland through active transport. This phase starts about 1 minute after administration of the tracer and increases over the next 10 minutes. With normal salivary function, tracer activity should be apparent in the oral cavity without stimulation after 10 to 15 minutes. Approximately 15 minutes after administration, tracer begins to increase in the oral cavity and decrease in the salivary glands. A normal image should demonstrate uptake of Tc 99m by both the parotid and submandibular glands, and the uptake should be symmetrical.

The last phase is the excretory or washout phase. During this phase, the patient is given a lemon drop, or citric acid is applied to the tongue to stimulate secretion. Normal clearing of Tc 99m should be prompt, uniform, and symmetrical. Activity remaining in the salivary glands after stimulation is suggestive of obstruction, certain tumors, and inflammation.

With few exceptions, neoplasms arising within the salivary glands do not concentrate Tc 99m. However, Warthin's tumor and oncocytomas, which arise from ductal tissue, are capable of concentrating the tracer. They retain Tc 99m because they do not communicate with the ductal system, and they appear as areas of increased activity on static images. The difference is accentuated during the washout phase, when normal tissue activity decreases with stimulation and activity is retained in the tumors. Other salivary tumors may appear as areas of decreased activity on scintiscans.[18–26]

Computed Tomography and Magnetic Resonance Imaging.
Computed tomography (CT) images are produced by radiographic beams that penetrate the tissues (Figure 9–4). Computerized analysis of the variance of absorption produces a reconstructed image of the area. Coronal and axial images are usually obtained. The varying water content of tissues allows for magnetic resonance imaging (MRI) to distinguish tissue types. Tissues absorb and then re-emit electromagnetic energy when exposed to a strong electromagnetic field. Analysis of the net magnetization by radiofrequency is reconstructed to provide an image. Images are described as T1- or T2-weighted images, according to the rate constant with which magnetic polarization or relaxation occurs.

CT and MRI are useful for evaluating salivary gland pathology, adjacent structures, and the proximity of salivary lesions to the facial nerve. The retromandibular vein, carotid artery, and deep lymph nodes also can be noted on CT.

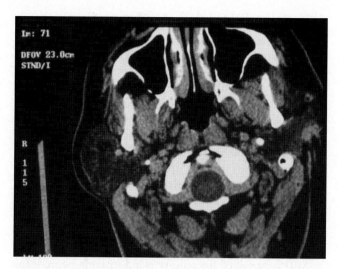

Figure 9–4 This is an axial view of a CT image soft tissue window demonstrating a tumor of the right parotid. Courtesy of Dr. Mel Mupparapu, University of Pennsylvania.

Osseous erosions and sclerosis are better visualized by CT than by MRI. Since calcified structures are better visualized by CT, this modality is especially useful for the evaluation of inflammatory conditions that are associated with sialoliths. Abscesses have a characteristic hypervascular wall that is evident with CT imaging. CT also provides definition of cystic walls, making it possible to distinguish fluid-filled masses (ie, cyst) from abscess.

CT images of salivary glands should be obtained by using continuous fine cuts through the involved gland. Axial-plane cuts should include the superior aspect of the salivary glands, continuing to the hyoid bone and visualizing potentially enlarged lymph nodes in the suprahyoid neck region. Dental restorations may interfere with CT imaging and may require repositioning the patient to a semiaxial position.

Non-enhanced and enhanced CT images are routinely obtained. The initial non-enhanced scans are reviewed for the presence of sialoliths, masses, glandular enlargement and/or asymmetry, nodal involvement, and loss of tissue planes. Glandular damage from chronic disease often alters the density of the salivary glands and makes the identification of masses more difficult. Contrast-enhanced images are more defined and accentuate pathology. Tumors, abscesses, and inflamed lymph nodes have abnormal enhancement compared to that of normal structures.

Ultrafast CT and three-dimensional–image CT sialography have been reported by Szolar and colleagues to be an effective method of visualizing masses that are poorly defined on MRI; they also advocate ultrafast CT for patients who are unable to lie still long enough for adequate MRI (pediatric, geriatric, claustrophobic, and mentally or physically challenged patients) and for patients for whom MRI is contraindicated. The disadvantages of CT include radiation exposure, administration of intravenous iodine-containing contrast media for enhancement, and potential scatter from dental restorations.

MRI has become the imaging modality of choice for pre-operative evaluation of salivary gland tumors because of its excellent ability to differentiate soft tissues and its ability to provide multiplanar imaging. It provides images for evaluating salivary gland pathology, adjacent structures, and proximity to the facial nerve. In T1-weighted images, the normal parotid gland has greater intensity than muscle and lower intensity than fat or subcutaneous tissue. In T2-weighted images, the parotid has greater intensity than adjacent muscle and lower intensity than fat. Structures and conditions that are dark on both T1- and T2-weighted images include calcifications, rapid blood flow, and fibrous tissue. The use of intravenous MRI contrast can improve imaging and aid in defining neoplastic processes, but its uses are specific, and indications should be discussed with the radiologist.

MRI is preferred for salivary gland imaging because (a) patients are not exposed to radiation, (b) no intravenous contrast media are required routinely, and (c) there is minimal artifact from dental restorations. MRI is contraindicated for patients with pacemakers or metallic implants such as aneurysmal bone clips. Patients who have difficulty maintaining a still position or patients with claustrophobia may have difficulty tolerating the MRI procedure, which may result in poor image quality.[27–33]

The advantages and disadvantages of each method of imaging, as well as their indications for imaging the salivary glands, are listed in Table 9–1.

SALIVARY GLAND BIOPSY

Definitive diagnosis of salivary pathology may require tissue examination. When Sjögren's syndrome is suspected, the labial minor salivary gland is the most frequently sampled site. This procedure is considered to be the most accurate sole criterion for diagnosis of the salivary component of this disorder. Standardized histopathologic grading systems are used to assess the extent of changes (this is described in greater detail in the section of this chapter detailing Sjögren's syndrome). Biopsy of minor glands can also be used to diagnose amyloidosis. Biopsy of a minor gland of the lower lip is a minimal operative procedure that can be done with limited morbidity, using appropriate techniques. The incision is made on the inner aspect of the lower lip so that it is not externally visible. Six to ten minor gland lobules from just below the mucosal surface are removed and submitted for examination. The incision should be made through normal-appearing tissue, avoiding areas of trauma or inflammation of the lip that could influence the appearance of the underlying minor glands.

Biopsy of the major salivary glands requires an extraoral approach. There is increased morbidity, and major gland biopsy has not been shown to offer diagnostic superiority to the minor gland procedure in patients with Sjögren's syndrome. When major gland biopsy is indicated, such as for the evaluation of a distinct salivary mass, fine-needle aspiration can be attempted. If this does not yield an adequate sample for diagnosis, an open biopsy procedure should be done. In cases of suspected lymphoma, immunophenotyping of the tissue is essential for diagnosis.[34–36]

SEROLOGIC EVALUATION

Laboratory blood studies are helpful in the evaluation of dry mouth, particularly in suspected cases of Sjögren's syndrome. The presence of nonspecific markers of autoimmunity, such as antinuclear antibodies, rheumatoid factors, elevated immunoglobulins (particularly immunoglobulin G [IgG]), and erythrocyte sedimentation rate, or the presence of antibodies directed against the more specific extractable nuclear antigens SS-A/Ro or SS-B/La are important contributors to the definitive diagnosis of Sjögren's syndrome. Approximately 80% of patients with Sjögren's syndrome will display antinuclear antibodies, and about 60% will have antibodies against anti-SS-A/Ro. This latter autoantibody is considered the most specific marker for Sjögren's syndrome although it may be found in a small percentage of patients with systemic lupus erythematosus or other autoimmune connective-tissue disorders.[37,38] Another serologic marker that may prove useful for the diagnosis of salivary gland disorders is serum amylase. This is frequently elevated in cases of salivary gland inflammation. Determination of amylase isoenzymes (pancreatic and salivary) will allow the recognition of salivary contributions to the total serum amylase concentration.

Evaluation of a Salivary Mass or Enlarged Salivary Gland

PRESENTATION

Salivary gland tumors most commonly present as an asymptomatic mass. Pain is not a reliable indicator of malignancy. Cystic enlargement, hemorrhage, or infection can cause pain in benign tumors. Malignant tumors often enlarge without symptoms, but when pain occurs, it is often the result of neural involvement and carries a worse prognosis. If nasal obstruction is also present, the clinician should suspect a tumor in the nasal or paranasal sinuses, possibly arising from a minor salivary gland.

PHYSICAL EXAMINATION OF THE SALIVARY GLANDS

The major salivary glands are palpated, and the orifices of the ducts are observed for saliva output. Normally, clear saliva should be expressed when the gland is pressed and "milked." The facial nerve is assessed for any decrease in motor function, and regional lymph nodes are palpated. Intraorally, any masses noted on the soft or hard palate are evaluated for ulceration of mucosa and invasion of associated structures.

Tumors of the parotid gland will typically present as solitary painless mobile masses, most often located at the tail of the gland. It is important to document function of the facial nerve when evaluating parotid tumors, because the nerve runs through the gland, and evidence of decreased motor function of the nerve thus has diagnostic significance. Facial nerve paralysis is usually indicative of malignancy. Rarely, benign tumors may cause paralysis by either sudden rapid growth or the presence of an infection. Other findings suggesting malignancy include multiple masses, a fixed mass with invasion of surrounding tissue, and the presence of cervical lymphadenopathy.

Tumors in the submandibular or sublingual glands usually present as painless solitary slow-growing mobile masses. Bimanual palpation, with one hand intraorally on the floor of the mouth and the other extraorally below the mandible, is necessary to evaluate the glands adequately. Tumors of the minor salivary glands are usually smooth masses located on the hard or soft palate. Ulceration of the overlying mucosa should raise suspicion of malignancy.

Other lesions may mimic the presentation of salivary gland tumors. Inflammatory diseases, infections, and nutritional deficiencies may present as diffuse glandular enlargement (usually of the parotid gland). Patients who are seropositive for human immunodeficiency virus (HIV) may develop cystic lymphoepithelial lesions that may be confused with tumors. Both melanoma and squamous cell carcinoma can metastasize to the parotid gland and appear similar to a primary salivary tumor. Chronic sialadenitis in the submandibular glands can commonly be confused with a tumor. In the minor salivary glands, necrotizing sialometaplasia can be confused with squamous cell carcinoma. This can have significant adverse consequences since the treatments for these two lesions are so different.

IMAGING

Plain-film radiography of the mandible or maxilla may be performed as a rapid and inexpensive way to determine if salivary tumors involve adjacent bony structures. The bone is assessed for compression by slow expansion or erosion by aggressive invasion.

CT and MRI both image the salivary glands well, but they do not differentiate reliably between benign and malignant tumors. These modalities are not cost-effective for the initial evaluation of salivary gland lesions and are not recommended for the routine evaluation of salivary gland masses. Frequently, these imaging techniques are reserved for presurgical treatment planning, and initial evaluation is plain-film radiography followed by biopsy. If malignancy is known or suspected, scans can provide useful information about nodal involvement. Central necrosis of a lymph node is indicative of metastatic involvement.

Technetium scanning is useful for diagnosing salivary gland tumors containing oncocytes, such as Warthin's tumor and oncocytoma. These lesions appear as bright masses on the scan, indicating active uptake and retention of the radionuclide. Technetium scanning also provides information on the functional capabilities of the major salivary glands.

FINE-NEEDLE ASPIRATION BIOPSY

Fine-needle aspiration (FNA) biopsy is a simple and effective technique that aids the diagnosis of solid lesions. It may be particularly useful for elderly patients who can not tolerate an excisional biopsy because of medical considerations. A syringe is used to aspirate cells from the lesion for cytologic examination. To establish a diagnosis accurately, it is important to have a well-trained cytopathologist who is familiar with salivary cytology read the specimen. FNA biopsies do not provide a specimen with anatomic structure. The cytologist will examine the individual cells aspirated from the lesion and will offer a diagnosis based on the cellular characteristics of different lesions. Even if an exact diagnosis is not made, it may be possible to determine if a lesion is benign or malignant. Knowing the biologic aggressiveness of the tumor prior to definitive surgery is helpful in planning optimal treatment.[39]

OPEN SURGICAL BIOPSY

A preoperative surgical biopsy is rarely indicated for salivary masses. In almost all salivary gland tumors, the treatment of choice is an excisional biopsy. In the parotid gland, this most often consists of a superficial parotidectomy, with careful preservation of the facial nerve. In small well-localized tumors of the parotid gland, local excision may be performed. Enucleation of tumors or local excision, however, is associated with a high recurrence rate in the parotid gland and is infrequently recommended. Tumors in the submandibular gland require the total removal of the gland. For tumors in the minor salivary glands, total excision with a margin of normal tissue is required. This approach is both diagnostic and curative in the majority of salivary gland tumors.

Analysis of frozen sections should be performed at the time of surgery, to establish a diagnosis and guide the surgical approach. More than 80% of the time, the diagnosis based on the frozen section agrees with the final pathologic diagnosis from fixed and stained tissue. Most errors involve a failure to recognize malignant lesions. Malignant tumors are incorrectly called benign 5 to 24% of the time, but benign tumors are incorrectly diagnosed as malignant only 0 to 2% of the time. If frozen sections reveal a malignant tumor, the surgical margins may require extension.[40,41]

STAGING OF SALIVARY GLAND TUMORS

A single tumor-node-metastasis (TNM) staging system (Table 9–2) is used for tumors of the parotid and submandibular glands. The letter "T" denotes tumor size as well as extension into adjacent tissue; the letter "N" indicates nodal involvement. Local lymph nodes that are commonly involved by tumors of the parotid gland include the intraparotid, intra-auricular, and preauricular nodes. The submandibular gland drains locally to the submandibular, upper cervical, and internal jugular lymph nodes. The letter "M" signifies metastases. Any nodal involvement other those mentioned above is considered a distant metastasis.

▼ SPECIFIC DISEASES AND DISORDERS OF THE SALIVARY GLANDS

Developmental Abnormalities

The absence of salivary glands is rare although it may occur together with other developmental defects, especially malformations of the first brachial arch, which manifest with various craniofacial anomalies. Patients with salivary gland aplasia

Table 9–2 Staging for Major Salivary Gland Cancer

T_x	Primary tumor can not be assessed
T_0	No evidence of primary tumor
T_1	Tumor < 2 cm in greatest dimension
T_2	Tumor 2–4 cm in greatest dimension
T_3	Tumor 4–6 cm in greatest dimension
T_4	Tumor >6 cm in greatest dimension

All categories are subdivided: (a) no local extension, (b) local extension.
Local extension is clinical/macroscopic invasion of skin, soft tissue, bone or nerve.
Microscopic evidence alone is not considered local extension for classification
    purposes.

N_x	Regional nodes cannot be assessed
N_0	No regional lymph node metastases
N_1	Single ipsilateral node < 3 cm in diameter
N_{2a}	Single ipsilateral node 3–6 cm in diameter
N_{2b}	Multiple ipsilateral node, none > 6 cm
N_{2C}	Bilateral or contralateral nodes, none > 6 cm
N_3	Metastasis in a lymph node > 6 cm
M_x	Presence of distant metastases cannot be assessed
M_0	No distant metastases
M_1	Distant metastases

Stage	T	N	M
Stage I	T_{1a}	N_0	M_0
	T_{2a}	N_0	M_0
Stage II	T_{1b}	N_0	M_0
	T_{2b}	N_0	M_0
	T_{3a}	N_0	M_0
Stage III	T_{3b}	N_0	M_0
	T_{4a}	N_0	M_0
	Any T (except T_{4b})	NI	M_0
Stage IV	T_{4b}	Any N	M_0
	Any T	$N_2 N_3$	M_0
	Any T	Any N	M_1

Adapted from the American Joint Committee for Cancer Staging and End Results
Reporting: manual staging of cancer. Chicago 1988

experience xerostomia and increased dental caries. Indeed, rampant dental caries in children who have no other symptoms has led to the diagnosis of congenitally missing salivary glands. Enamel hypoplasia, congenital absence of teeth, and extensive occlusal wear are other oral manifestations of salivary agenesis.[42,43]

Parotid gland agenesis has been reported in conjunction with several congenital conditions, including hemifacial microstomia, mandibulofacial dysostosis, cleft palate, lacrimoauriculodentodigital syndrome, Treacher Collins syndrome, and anophthalmia. Hypoplasia of the parotid gland has been associated with Melkersson-Rosenthal syndrome. Congenital fistula formation within the ductal system has been associated with brachial cleft abnormalities, accessory parotid ducts, and diverticuli.[43–51]

"Aberrant" salivary glands are salivary tissues that develop at unusual anatomic sites. Aberrant salivary glands have been reported in a variety of locations, including the middle-ear cleft, external auditory canal, neck, posterior mandible, anterior mandible, pituitary, and cerebellopontine angle. These are usually incidental findings and do not require intervention.[52-56]

When the submandibular salivary gland sits within a depression on the lingual posterior surface of the mandible, it is referred to as Staphne's cyst. Staphne's cyst is usually located between the angle of the mandible and the first molar below the level of the inferior alveolar nerve. The gland is usually asymptomatic and appears on radiographs as a round unilocular well-circumscribed radiolucency. The characteristic location and radiographic appearance make Staphne's cyst easily recognized. Palpation of the salivary gland is possible sometimes, and sialography has been used to aid in diagnosis. Surgical intervention is recommended only in atypical situations in which the diagnosis is unclear and a tumor is suspected. Less commonly, anterior lingual submandibular salivary glands have been reported.[56–60]

Aberrant salivary glands occur rarely in the anterior mandible and are difficult to diagnose. They may give rise to radiolucent lesions at the apex of teeth, at extraction sites, and below and between the roots of teeth. The differential diagnosis includes the numerous unilocular radiolucent lesions of the mandible, and definitive diagnosis usually requires surgical intervention. FNA biopsy may be attempted and can yield sufficient tissue for diagnosis.[60–61]

Accessory Salivary Ducts

Accessory ducts are common and do not require treatment. In a study of 450 parotid glands by Rauch and Gorlin, half of the patients had accessory parotid ducts. The most frequent location was superior and anterior to the normal location of Stenson's duct.[42]

Diverticuli

By definition, a diverticulum is a pouch or sac protruding from the wall of a duct. Diverticuli in the ducts of the major salivary glands often lead to pooling of saliva and recurrent sialadenitis. Diagnosis is made by sialography. Patients are encouraged to regularly milk the involved salivary gland and to promote salivary flow through the duct.[63–64]

Darier's Disease

Salivary duct abnormalities have been reported in Darier's disease. Sialography of parotid glands in this condition revealed duct dilation, with periodic stricture affecting the main ducts. Symptoms of occasional obstructive sialadenitis have been reported. Progressive involvement of the salivary ducts in Darier's disease may be more common than previously reported.[63,64]

Sialolithiasis (Salivary Stones)

The true prevalence of sialolithiasis is difficult to determine since many cases are asymptomatic. Sialoliths are calcified and organic matter that form within the secretory system of the major salivary glands. The etiology of sialolith formation is still unknown; however, there are several factors that contribute to stone formation. Inflammation, irregularities in the duct system, local irritants, and anticholinergic medications may cause pooling of saliva within the duct, which is thought to pro-

TABLE 9–3 Causes of Salivary Gland Hypofunction

Pharmaceuticals

Radiation therapy
    External-beam radiation
    Internal radionuclide therapy

Oncologic chemotherapy

Systemic diseases
    Sjögren's syndrome (primary and secondary)
    Granulomatous diseases (sarcoidosis, tuberculosis)
    Graft-versus-host disease
    Cystic fibrosis
    Bell's palsy
    Diabetes
    Amyloidosis
    Human immunodeficiency virus infection
    Thyroid disease (hyper- and hypofunction)
    Late-stage liver disease

Psychological factors (affective disorder)

Malnutrition (anorexia, bulimia, dehydration)

Idiopathic disorders

mote stone formation. It is believed that a nidus of salivary organic material becomes calcified and gradually forms a sialolith. Researchers have investigated the possibility of altered salivary hydrogen ion concentration (pH), abnormal serum calcium and phosphorous levels, and diet as causes of sialolith formation, but consistent alterations have not been detected. Frequently, there is no clear explanation for stone formation. Since the underlying cause is unknown and uncorrected in most patients, the recurrence rate is ≈20%.[65–67]

It is known that the structure of sialoliths is crystalline and that sialoliths are primarily composed of hydroxyapatite. The chemical composition is calcium phosphate and carbon, with trace amounts of magnesium, potassium chloride, and ammonium. Fifty percent of parotid gland sialoliths and 20% of submandibular gland sialoliths are poorly calcified. This is clinically significant because such sialoliths are not radiographically detectable.[66–69]

The submandibular gland is the most common site of involvement, and 80 to 90% of sialoliths occur in this gland. The parotid gland is involved in 5 to 15% of cases, and 2 to 5% of cases occur in the sublingual or minor salivary glands. It is believed that the higher rate of sialolith formation in the submandibular gland is due to (1) the torturous course of Wharton's duct, (2) higher calcium and phosphate levels, and (3) the dependent position of the submandibular glands, which leave them prone to stasis.[65–67]

Gout can cause salivary calculi composed of uric acid. However, patients with a history of renal stone formation do not have an increased incidence of salivary gland stone formation. There is one report of obstructive sialadenitis by intraparotid deposits of gold salts in a patient receiving sodium aurothiomalate (gold salt compound) treatment for rheumatoid arthritis.[70]

CLINICAL PRESENTATION AND EVALUATION

Patients with sialoliths most commonly present with a history of acute, painful, and intermittent swelling of the affected major salivary gland. The degree of symptoms is dependent on the extent of salivary duct obstruction and the presence of secondary infection. Typically, eating will initiate the salivary gland swelling. The stone totally or partially blocks the flow of saliva, causing salivary pooling within the ducts and gland body. Since the glands are encapsulated, there is little space for expansion, and enlargement causes pain. If the calculus partially blocks the duct, then the swelling subsides as salivary stimulation is removed and output decreases, and saliva seeps past the partial obstruction.[71,72]

The involved gland is usually enlarged and tender. Stasis of the saliva may lead to infection, fibrosis, and gland atrophy. Fistulae, a sinus tract, or ulceration may occur over the stone in chronic cases. An examination of the soft tissue surrounding the duct may show a severe inflammatory reaction. Palpation along the pathway of the duct may confirm the presence of a stone. Bacterial infections may or may not be superimposed and are more common with chronic obstructions. Other complications from sialoliths include acute sialadenitis, ductal stricture, and ductal dilatation.[72]

Radiographic examination is often necessary since the stone may not be accessible to bimanual palpation. However, as stated earlier, poorly calcified sialoliths will not be visible radiographically (see Figure 9–1). An occlusal view is the recommended view for radiography of submandibular glands. Stones in the parotid gland can be more difficult to visualize due to the superimposition of other anatomic structures; therefore, requesting proper radiographic views is important. An anteroposterior view of the face is useful for visualization of a parotid stone. One can also place an occlusal film intraorally adjacent to the duct. CT may be used for the detection of sialoliths and has 10 times the sensitivity of plain-film radiography for detecting calcifications.

Calcified phleboliths are stones that lie within a blood vessel; they can be easily mistaken radiographically for sialoliths. Phleboliths occur outside the ductal structure, and sialography can therefore aid in differentiating these lesions.

Stanley and colleagues reported using FNA of the submandibular gland as a diagnostic tool in 5 patients who did not present with classic symptoms of sialolithiasis. In 3 of the 5 cases, stone fragments were identified, and the patients were diagnosed with sialolithiasis. In the other 2 patients, FNA samples did not reveal stone fragments but showed foam cells and metaplastic squamous cells in a mucoid background that resembled low-grade mucoepidermoid carcinoma. Surgical excision of the glands was performed, and stones were found, which emphasizes that FNA cytology should be interpreted cautiously in this situation.[72]

TREATMENT

During the acute phase, therapy is primarily supportive. Standard care includes analgesics, hydration, antibiotics, and antipyretics, as necessary. In pronounced exacerbations, surgical intervention for drainage is sometimes required. Stones at or near the orifice of the duct can often be removed transorally by milking the gland, but deeper stones require surgery. Once the acute phase subsides, surgical treatment can be performed. Location within the duct determines the type of surgery required for removal of the stone. If the stone lies in the intraglandular portion of the duct, it is recommended that the entire gland be removed. As much as 75% of normal function can return if the stone can be removed from within the duct, without entering the body of the gland.

Lithotripsy is gaining popularity because it offers a noninvasive treatment for sialoliths. Current protocols use ultrasonography to detect the stone and extracorporeal lithotripsy to fragment the stone. Several treatments may be needed, and a stone with a diameter of > 2 mm is required for detection with ultrasonography. Reported complications associated with this procedure include transient hearing changes, hematoma at the site, and pain. There have been initial reports of intraductal lithotripsy, but this technique requires specialized equipment and has been performed at only a few centers.[73–76]

Mucoceles

"Mucocele" is a clinical term that describes swelling caused by the accumulation of saliva at the site of a traumatized or obstructed minor salivary gland duct. Mucoceles are classified as extravasation types and retention types. A large form of mucocele located in the floor of the mouth is known as a ranula[77] (Figure 9–5).

EXTRAVASATION AND RETENTION MUCOCELES

Etiology. The formation of an extravasation mucocele is believed to be the result of trauma to a minor salivary gland excretory duct. Laceration of the duct results in the pooling of saliva in the adjacent submucosal tissue and consequent swelling. The extravasation type of mucocele is more common than the retention form. Although often termed a cyst, the extravasation mucocele does not have an epithelial cyst wall or a distinct border. In contrast, the retention mucocele is caused by obstruction of a minor salivary gland duct by calculus or possibly by the contraction of scar tissue around an

injured minor salivary gland duct. The blockage of salivary flow causes the accumulation of saliva and dilation of the duct. Eventually, an aneurysm-like lesion forms, which can be lined by the epithelium of the dilated duct.

Clinical Presentation. Extravasation mucoceles most frequently occur on the lower lip, where trauma is common. The buccal mucosa, tongue, floor of the mouth, and retromolar region are other commonly traumatized areas where mucous extravasation may be found. Mucous retention cysts are more commonly located on the palate or the floor of the mouth.

A common clinical sequence is a history of a traumatic event, followed by the development of the lesion. Mucoceles often present as discrete painless smooth-surfaced swellings that can range from a few millimeters to a few centimeters in diameter. Superficial lesions frequently have a characteristic blue hue. Deeper lesions can be more diffuse and can be covered by normal-appearing mucosa without the distinctive blue color. The lesions may vary in size over time. Patients will frequently traumatize a superficial mucocele, allowing it to drain and deflate. In these circumstances, the mucocele will recur (see Figure 9–5; Figure 9–6).

Although the development of a bluish lesion after trauma is highly suggestive of a mucocele, other lesions (including salivary gland neoplasms, soft-tissue neoplasms, vascular malformation, and vesiculobullous diseases) should be considered.

Treatment. The treatment of choice for mucoceles is surgical excision. Removal of the associated salivary glands is essential to prevent recurrence. Aspiration of the fluid only does not provide long-term benefit. Managing of mucoceles can be difficult because surgical removal may cause trauma to other adjacent minor salivary glands and lead to the development of a new mucocele. Intralesional injections of corticosteroids have been used successfully to treat mucoceles.

RANULAS

A ranula is a large mucocele located on the floor of the mouth. Ranulas may be either mucous extravasation phenomena or

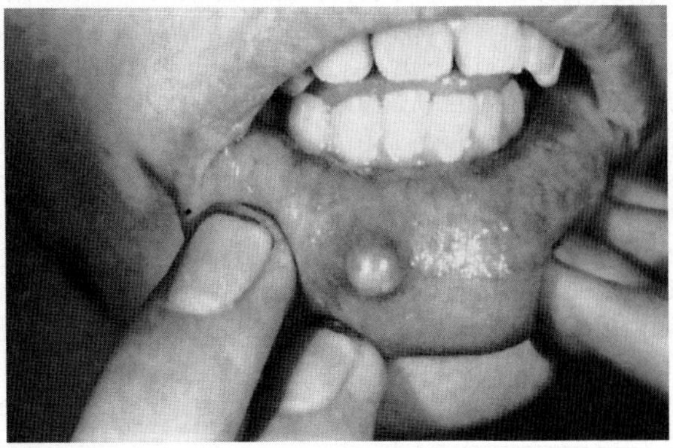

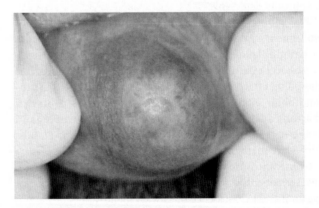

Figure 9–5 Mucocele. Mucous extravasation phenomenon involving the lower lip.

Figure 9–6 With time, fibrosis occurs, replacing the acinar functional cells with connective tissues. The inflammatory components disappear, and a sessile, firm mass is observed on the lower lip with normal mucous membrane.

mucous retention cysts and are most commonly associated with the sublingual salivary gland duct (Figure 9–7).

Etiology. The most common cause of ranula formation is trauma. Other causes include an obstructed salivary gland or a ductal aneurysm. A sarcoid-associated ranula also has been reported.

Clinical Presentation. The term "ranula" is used because this lesion often resembles the swollen abdomen of a frog. The lesion most commonly presents as a painless, slow growing, soft, and movable mass located in the floor of the mouth. Usually, the lesion forms to one side of the lingual frenum; however, if the lesion extends deep into the soft tissue, it can cross the midline. Like mucoceles, superficial ranulas can have a typical bluish hue, but when the lesion is deeply seated, the mucosa may have a normal appearance. The size of the lesions can vary, and larger lesions can cause deviation of the tongue. A deep lesion that herniates through the mylohyoid muscle and extends along the fascial planes is referred to as a plunging ranula and may become large, extending into the neck. Radiography should be performed to rule out a sialolith as a cause of duct obstruction. Radiopaque material instilled into the ranula cavity may be helpful in delineating the borders and full extent of the lesion.

Treatment. Ranulas are usually treated sugically. A marsupialization procedure that unroofs the lesion is the initial treatment of choice, especially for smaller lesions. Recurrences have been noted with the marsupialization technique alone, and in these cases, excision of the lesion (including the gland) is recommended. Intralesional injections of corticosteroids have been used succsessfully in the treatment of ranulas.

Inflammatory and Reactive Lesions

NECROTIZING SIALOMETAPLASIA

Etiology. Necrotizing sialometaplasia is a benign self-limiting reactive inflammatory disorder of the salivary tissue. Clinically, this lesion mimics a malignancy, and failure to recognize this lesion has resulted in unnecessary radical surgery. It is widely accepted that necrotizing sialometaplasia is initiated by a local ischemic event.

Clinical Presentation. Necrotizing sialometaplasia has a rapid onset. Lesions occur predominately on the palate; however, lesions can occur anywhere salivary gland tissue exists, including the lips and the retromolar pad region. Lesions initially present as a tender erythematous nodule. Once the mucosa breaks down, a deep ulceration with a yellowish base forms. Even though lesions can be large and deep, patients often describe only a moderate degree of dull pain.

Lesions often occur shortly after oral surgical procedures, restorative dentistry, or administration of local anesthesia although lesions also may develop weeks after a dental procedure or trauma. It is not uncommon for lesions to develop in

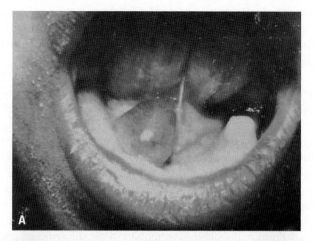

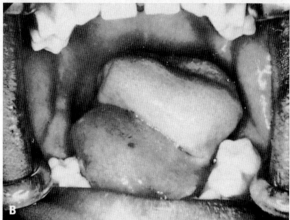

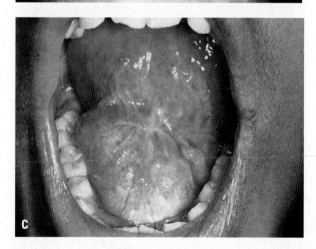

Figure 9–7 **A,** Blockage of Wharton's duct at the salivary orifice on the lingual frenum induces acute cystic dilation of the proximal portion of the duct as the secretory pressure from a functional gland is directed at the point of blockage. The ranula may be caused by blockage of this duct and is manifested by acute swelling in the floor of the mouth. **B,** When blockage is extensive and complete, the swollen mass extends posteriorly throughout the course of the submandibular salivary duct. The tongue may be elevated by this fluctuant mass, with associated pain and discomfort. Note the prominent vasculature, indicating the stretching of the sublingual tissues. **C,** Frequently some form of drainage is spontaneously achieved, but the cystic enlargement of the distal section of duct proximal to the blockage persists, with changes in the tissue architecture of the entire sublingual space.

an individual with no obvious history of trauma or oral habit. Necrotizing sialometaplasia has been reported along with induced vomiting practiced by patients suffering from bulimia.[78–83]

Treatment. It is important for the clinician to understand the etiology and biologic behavior of this lesion and for the pathologist to have expertise on oral lesions. In addition to the specimen, a complete clinical history should be provided to the pathologist to aid in distinguishing this lesion from squamous cell carcinoma.

An adequate biopsy specimen is essential since the histologic features of this lesion are unique. Necrosis of the salivary gland, pseudoepitheliomatous hyperplasia of the mucosal epithelium, and squamous metaplasia of the salivary ducts are seen. Histopathologic examination will reveal that there are no malignant cells and that the lobular architecture is preserved even though necrosis is present.[74–77]

Necrotizing sialometaplasia is self-limiting, lasts approximately 6 weeks, and heals by secondary intention. No specific treatment is required, but débridement and saline rinses may help the healing process. Recurrence and impairment are not usually encountered.

RADIATION-INDUCED PATHOLOGY

Effects of External-Beam Radiation. External-beam radiation is standard treatment for head and neck tumors, and the salivary glands are often within the field of radiation. Doses of ≥ 50 Gy will result in permanent salivary gland damage and symptoms of oral dryness. The exact mechanism of the destruction of salivary gland tissue by radiation is not fully understood.

Clinical Presentation. Radiotherapy is usually delivered in fractionated doses 5 days per week for 6 to 8 weeks. Acute effects on salivary function can be recognized within a week of beginning treatments at doses of approximately 2 Gy daily and patients will often voice complaints of oral dryness by the end of the second week. Mucositis is a very common consequence of treatment and can become severe enough to alter the radiation therapy regimen. If permanent salivary dysfunction develops, patients are at risk of the full range of associated oral complications. Typically, at doses > 50 Gy, salivary dysfunction is severe and permanent. Difficulty in speaking, dysphagia, and increased dental caries are common complaints that dramatically affect the quality of life for patients with radiation-induced salivary gland dysfunction. Saliva is minimal, and the saliva that is present tends to be thick and ropy.[84–86]

"Radiation caries" is the term commonly used to describe these patients' rapidly advancing caries, which characteristically occur at the incisal or cervical aspect of the teeth and wrap around the teeth in an "apple core" fashion. In spite of meticulous oral hygiene, the caries rate is often difficult to control and poses a challenge to even the experienced restorative dentist.

This patient population is susceptible to other oral complications, including candidiasis and sialadenitis. Clinicians should always be aware of the risk of osteonecrosis and the increased incidence of salivary gland neoplasms in postradiation patients. Osteonecrosis is a lifelong risk due to the decreased vascularity following the exposure of bone to radiation. There is also an increased incidence of second primary tumors involving the radiated tissues.

Treatment. Radiation planning is key to the effective preservation of salivary gland tissue. Eisbrush and colleagues reported that when three-dimensional comformal radiation therapy was used in patients receiving bilateral head and neck radiation with the goal of limiting salivary exposure, 50% of salivary gland function was preserved. Tumor control and complications are still being assessed, but this technique appears to offer real benefit.[86,87]

In addition to improvements in the planning and delivery of radiation therapy, radioprotective agents may help limit radiation therapy–induced salivary gland damage. Starting in the 1970s, studies have investigated the radioprotective properties of amifostine; however, not until 1999 was amifostine approved as a radioprotective agent by the Food and Drug Administration. This agent is useful for the preservation of salivary function and for the reduction of dry mouth in patients undergoing radiation treatment for head and neck cancer when the radiation port includes a substantial portion of the parotid glands. The proposed mechanism of action involves the scavenging of free oxygen radicals. Following administration, amifostine is dephosphorylated in the circulation by alkaline phosphatase to a pharmacologically active free thiol metabolite. The thiol metabolite scavenges free oxygen species generated by radiation. Normal tissue is more vascular than the tumor and has higher capillary levels of alkaline phosphatase. Therefore, the concentration of the active thiol metabolite is higher in normal tissue and thus will protect the normal tissue but not the cancer. Amifostine is administered intravenously 15 to 30 minutes prior to each fractionated radiation treatment. Major side effects include hypotension, hypocalemia, nausea, and vomiting. Reversible episodes of loss of consciousness and rare incidences of seizures have been reported. This drug should be used with close supervision in patients taking hypertension medications. Its safety for patients with cardiovascular disease or cerebrovascular conditions has not been studied.[88–92]

Since patients undergoing radiation therapy have reduced salivary flow, they are susceptible to oral fungal and bacterial infections. Candidal infections can be difficult to treat and resistant to therapy. Due to the increased risk of caries, antifungal agents should be free of sugar. Vaginal clotrimazole troches and dissolved nystatin powder may be used orally as sugar-free antifungal agents. Since xerostomic patients may have too little saliva to dissolve troches, antifungal oral rinses are preferred. Daily prescription-strength topical fluoride (which can be brushed on or administered in trays) is recommended to help control caries.

Symptomatic treatment for postradiation patients is discussed in detail later in this chapter, in the section on the treatment of xerostomia. Alternative medicine is gaining popularity in Western culture and medical curricula. Studies investigating acupuncture treatment for radiation-induced xerostomia have reported varying results. Chi gong and herbal medications are alternative therapies that are reported to increase salivary flow. More controlled trials of these therapeutic modalities are needed.[93]

Effects of Internal Radiation Therapy. *Etiology.* Disseminated thyroid cancer (DTC) is treated by the removal of the thyroid gland. To insure that all remnants of thyroid tissue are destroyed, patients are given radioactive iodine 131 (^{131}I) after surgery. Radioactive iodine is taken up not only by thyroid tissue but also by the oncocytes in salivary gland tissue. Radioactive iodine can cause permanent salivary gland damage and fibrosis resulting in salivary gland hypofunction. Mandel and colleagues recently reported changes in saliva composition following ^{131}I therapy. It is believed that salivary gland damage is related to the dose of ^{131}I administered.[94,95]

Clinical Presentation. Patients with DTC treated with ^{131}I may experience xerostomia and decreased salivary gland function. However, ^{131}I treatment is less caustic than external-beam radiation therapy and generally causes less destruction to the salivary glands.

Treatment. Following administration of ^{131}I, patients should suck on lemon drops or chew gum to stimulate salivary flow. This will aid in clearing the radioactive iodine from the salivary glands and will potentially decrease salivary gland damage. Patients with ^{131}I-induced salivary gland hypofunction should be treated with the same measures as patients who have salivary gland damage from other causes.

ALLERGIC SIALADENITIS

Enlargement of the salivary glands has been associated with exposure to various pharmaceutical agents and allergens. Cases that are without rash or other signs of allergy have been reported. The characteristic feature of such an allergic reaction is acute salivary gland enlargement, often accompanied by itching over the gland. It is unclear whether all of the reported cases are true allergic reactions or some represent secondary infections resulting from medications that reduced salivary flow. Compounds have salivary gland enlargement as a potential side effect include phenobarbital, phenothiazine, ethambutol, sulfisoxazole, iodine compounds, isoproterenol, and heavy metals. The diagnosis of allergic reaction should be made judiciously, especially when salivary gland enlargement is not accompanied by other signs of an allergic reaction. The possibility of infection or autoimmune disease should be considered. Allergic sialadenitis is self-limiting. Avoiding the allergen, maintaining hydration, and monitoring for secondary infection are recommended.[96]

Viral Diseases

Viruses have been associated with acute nonsuppurative salivary gland enlargement. This section focuses on the viruses responsible for the majority of cases of virally induced salivary gland enlargement: *Paramyxovirus, Cytomegalovirus* (CMV), HIV, and hepatitis C virus (HCV). Echoviruses, Epstein-Barr virus, parainfluenza virus, and choriomeningitis virus infections have been linked to occasional reports of nonsuppurative salivary gland enlargement.

MUMPS (EPIDEMIC PAROTITIS)

Etiology. Mumps is caused by a ribonucleic acid (RNA) *Paramyxovirus* and is transmitted by direct contact with salivary droplets. The United States and Canada have recommended the mumps vaccine since the 1970s and monitor vaccinations at school admission. An attenuated live vaccine is available and is indicated for immunization against mumps in children aged 12 months or older. The incidence of mumps in developed countries has significantly decreased; in the United States, 906 cases were reported in 1995.[97] The Centers for Disease Control and Prevention (CDC) published modifications to the Recommended Childhood Immunization Schedule in 1998. The CDC currently recommends an initial vaccination at 12 to 18 months of age and a second dose at 4 to 6 years of age. Mumps virus vaccine is not recommended for severely immunocompromised children because the protective immune response often does not develop, and risk of complications exists.[97,98] There has been speculation that the measles-mumps-rubella (MMR) vaccine might be linked to autism and inflammatory bowel disease, which raised parental concern. Although epidemiologic studies demonstrate no evidence for a causal association between MMR administration and these conditions, many parents have refused vaccination for their children.[99–102] This raises public health concerns as it results in a susceptible population and the possibility of the re-emergence of mumps in the United States. International travelers who have not had mumps or been vaccinated can import the virus. In 1997, an outbreak of mumps among adults (ages 17 to 40 years) attending "rave" parties was reported in Vancouver, British Columbia.[100–102] Therefore, this infection must be considered in cases of acute nonsuppurative salivary gland inflammation in unvaccinated patients who have not had mumps.

Clinical Presentation. Ordinarily, mumps occurs in children between the ages of 4 and 6 years. The diagnosis of mumps in adults can be more difficult. The incubation period is 2 to 3 weeks; this is followed by salivary gland inflammation and enlargement, preauricular pain, fever, malaise, headache, and myalgia. The majority of cases involve the parotid glands, but 10% of the cases involve the submandibular glands alone. The skin over the involved glands is edematous. The salivary gland enlargement is sudden and painful to palpation. The salivary gland ducts are inflamed but without purulent discharge. If partial duct obstruction occurs, the patient may experience pain when eating. One gland can become symptomatic 24 to 48 hours before another gland does so. Swelling is usually bilateral and lasts approximately 7 days[99–102] (Figure 9–8).

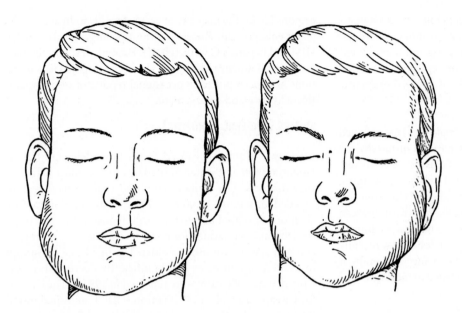

Figure 9–8 *Left,* Typical location and configuration of swelling associated with mumps. *Right,* Usual location and configuration of swelling associated with abscessed mandibular molars.

The diagnosis is made by the demonstration of antibodies to the mumps S and V antigens and to the hemagglutination antigen. Serum amylase levels may be elevated.

Complications of mumps include mild meningitis and encephalitis. Deafness, myocarditis, thyroiditis, pancreatitis, and oophoritis occur less frequently. Males can experience epididymitis and orchitis, resulting in testicular atrophy and infertility if the disease occurs in adolescence or later.

Treatment. The treatment of mumps is symptomatic, and vaccination is important for prevention. Rare fatalities have occurred from viral encephalitis, myocarditis, and neuritis.

CYTOMEGALOVIRUS INFECTION

Etiology. Human CMV is a beta herpesvirus that infects only humans. CMV may remain latent after initial exposure and infection. Although its reactivation can occur in healthy individuals without clinical illness, reactivation in immunocompromised individuals can be life threatening.[103–104]

CMV can be cultured from blood, saliva, feces, respiratory secretions, urine, and other body fluids. A large percentage of healthy adults have serum antibodies to the virus. CMV is the major cause of non-Epstein-Barr virus infectious mononucleosis in the general population. Horizontal transmission can occur through blood transfusion, allograft transplants, and sexual contact. Particularly high rates of seropositivity are found in homosexual males, intravenous drug users, prostitutes, and individuals who have undergone multiple transfusions.[108–111]

Transmission from children to adults or between children is more common through fomites, urine, and respiratory secretions. Transplacental spread of CMV may result in congenital infection and malformations. Perinatal infection occurs in 3% of all live births and is thought to be due to transmission from breast milk, saliva, fomites, or urine. Infection in newborns and young children can be fatal.[110,111]

Clinical Presentation. CMV mononucleosis often occurs in the young adult population and presents as an acute febrile illness that includes salivary gland enlargement. Diagnosis is based on an elevated titer of antibody to CMV, and the prognosis for healthy adults is excellent. There is one report (by Guntinas-Lichius and colleagues) of acute severe CMV sialadenititis in a 57-year-old immunocompetent male who required hospitalization for 30 days.[106]

It is important to detect CMV infections in pregnant women. Transplacental transmission of CMV can result in prematurity, low birth weight, and various congenital malformations. Infected newborns and young children suffer from hepatitis, myocarditis, hematologic abnormalities, pneumonitis, and nervous system damage. The infection is often fatal; those children who do survive frequently experience permanent nerve damage resulting in mental retardation and seizure disorders.[108–112]

Infection in adults can occur by reactivation of the latent virus or by primary infection. An impaired immune system allows the virus to replicate and allows disseminated infection to occur. Patients taking immunosuppressive medications and patients with hematologic abnormalities or HIV infection are susceptible to severe CMV infections. In fact, CMV is considered a clinical marker for acquired immunodeficiency syndrome (AIDS). The CDC's surveillance case definition for AIDS includes CMV infection of the salivary glands that lasts longer than 1 month in adult patients. CMV infection also is strongly associated with an increased incidence of fungal and bacterial infections, particularly from gram-negative organisms.

The advent of highly active antiretroviral therapy (HAART) for treating HIV infection has resulted in a decline of CMV end-organ damage. Deayton and colleagues reported that HAART (including a protease inhibitor) suppresses CMV viremia in HIV-infected patients who are not receiving specific anti-CMV therapy. There are no published reports addressing the incidence of CMV-related salivary gland pathology in HIV-infected patients since the widespread adoption of HAART.[102]

The diagnosis of CMV infection may be difficult because of the issues of viral latency in many individuals, past virus infection versus acute clinical disease, and reactivation. The classic method for detection is histologic examination of infected tissue. CMV-infected tissue contains large atypical cells with inclusion bodies. These cells can be two times the normal size and have eccentrically placed nuclei, resulting in an "owl-like" appearance. Tissue necrosis and nonspecific inflammation may also be seen histologically.

Current methods for diagnosis include culture, antigen detection, and CMV deoxyribonucleic acid (DNA) detection. Diagnosis of primary infection in an immunocompetent patient uses a combination of immunoglobulin M (IgM) anti-CMV antibody seropositivity, IgG seroconversion, and viral culture. Antibodies to CMV are less useful diagnostically in immunocompromised individuals. Anti-CMV antibodies can be falsely negative in transplantation patients and falsely positive in patients with autoimmune disease. The virus can be detected directly in body fluids or tissue by culture, antigen assay, or CMV DNA assay. The presence of IgG antibodies against CMV is used to detect past CMV infection in immunocompetent patients who are being screened for blood or organ donation.[108–110]

Treatment. Immunocompetent patients are treated symptomatically. Immunocompromised patients require aggressive management and may be treated with intravenous gancyclovir, foscarnet, or cidofovir. A live attenuated vaccine is in clinical trials and has demonstrated partial protection in seronegative women exposed to seropositive infants and in seronegative kidney transplant recipients who received organs from seropositive donors. It is speculated that vaccine-induced immunity will be less effective against sexually transmitted CMV infection, in which re-infection with wild virus strains occurs.[108–112]

HIV INFECTION

Etiology. Neoplastic and non-neoplastic salivary gland lesions occur with increased frequency in HIV-infected patients. Clinicians should consider AIDS-related tumors such as Kaposi's sarcoma and lymphoma. A Sjögren's syndrome–like phenomenon is also seen in HIV-infected patients. A variety of terms have been used to describe this condition; "HIV salivary gland disease" (HIV-SGD) is the preferred term. HIV-SGD describes xerostomia and benign (unilateral or bilateral) salivary gland enlargement in HIV-positive patients. The prevalence of HIV-SGD is ≈1.0% in adult HIV-infected patients but has been reported to be as high as 19% in pediatric patients. Adult African Americans experience lesions more frequently than Caucasians based on data in the US. Homosexual persons and intravenous drug users experience gland enlargement more frequently than patients infected by other routes of transmission. The etiol-

ogy of HIV-SGD is not understood, but the reactivation of a latent virus has been hypothesized. Changes in the incidence of parotid hypertrophy since the advent of HAART have not been reported.[115–119]

HIV-SGD is associated with a cluster designation 8 (CD8) cell lymphocytosis of the salivary glands and with the diffuse infiltrative lymphocytosis syndrome (DILS). In this condition, lymphocytic infiltration is found in the salivary glands, lungs, gastrointestinal tract, and liver.

Modest changes in salivary function without enlargement have also been reported. Greenberg and colleagues studied two groups of HIV-infected patients: one group with xerostomia and one group without xerostomia. Both groups were evaluated for the presence of CMV in saliva, blood, labial minor salivary glands, and peripheral blood mononuclear cells.[115] Xerostomia and reduced salivary flow were associated with the presence of CMV. These results suggest a potential link between CMV in saliva and salivary gland dysfunction in HIV-infected patients.[120]

Clinical Manifestations. The most notable symptom of HIV-SGD is salivary gland swelling, which may or may not be accompanied by xerostomia. The parotid glands are involved in 98% of reported cases, and 60% of patients have bilateral enlargement[115–117] (Figure 9–9).

HIV-SGD frequently resembles Sjögren's syndrome and must be distinguished from this disorder by appropriate evaluation including salivary flow rates, ophthalmologic evaluation (with assessments of lacrimal function and the tear film), and autoimmune serologies. Ten percent of HIV-infected patients have a reduced lacrimal flow. Salivary flow rates may be reduced, and salivary immunoglobulin A (IgA) may be elevated both in patients with Sjögren's syndrome and in patients with HIV-SGD. Peripheral blood changes can resemble the changes seen in cases of Sjögren's syndrome and include hypergammaglobulinemia, circulating immune complexes, and rheumatoid factors. However, anti-SS-A and anti-SS-B autoantibodies are usually negative in the HIV-SGD population. A minor salivary gland biopsy may be indicated, and histologic findings resemble changes seen in cases of Sjögren's syndrome (including focal mononuclear cell infiltration) with routine tissue examination. Using immunohistochemical stains to differentiate the infiltrating cells, one finds a preponderance of CD8-positive (+) cells in HIV-SGD, as compared to the CD4+ infiltrates that predominate in Sjögren's syndrome. If there is involvement of the major salivary glands, they can be imaged with ultrasonography, CT, or MRI. Multiple cystic masses are characteristic of HIV-associated benign lymphoepithelial hypertrophy. With persistent enlargement of a major gland, a biopsy of the affected tissue may be necessary to exclude neoplasia. Of particular concern are lymphoma and Kaposi's sarcoma, both of which have been reported in the salivary glands of HIV-infected individuals. A biopsy specimen from an HIV-SGD–involved major gland demonstrates hyperplastic lymph nodes, lymphocytic infiltates, and cystic cavities.[115–118]

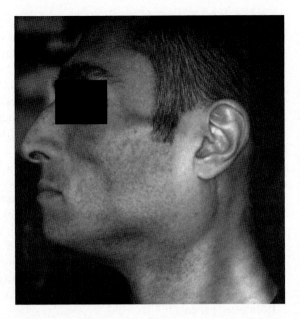
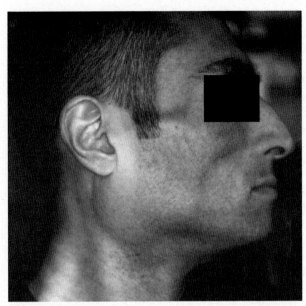

Figure 9–9   The patient demonstrates the bilateral salivary gland enlargement often associated with HIV. Courtesy of Dr. Michael Glick, University Medicine and Dentistry, New Jersey.

When assessing the HIV infected patient who has salivary complaints, it is important to consider that this patient group also frequently experiences medication-induced xerostomia. When salivary gland enlargement is present, bacterial infection should also be considered.

Treatment.   Treatment of neoplastic lesions is addressed below, under "Salivary Gland Tumors." Treatment for HIV-SGD is primarily symptomatic. Xerostomia may be relieved by sipping water, using saliva substitutes, chewing sugar-free gum, or sucking sugar-free candy. Topical fluoride is suggested for control of caries. (For a fuller discussion, see the section "Treatment of Xerostomia," below.)

Benign parotid enlargement is an esthetic concern for some patients, and surgery has been performed for cosmetic reasons. Treatment of the enlargement with external radiation therapy has also been attempted, but only 1 of 12 HIV-infected patients with parotid hypertrophy who were treated with 8 to 10 Gy of radiotherapy to the affected gland had a reduction in gland size. In 68% of patients, 24 Gy delivered in 1.5 Gy doses was effective, and 70% of those cases had a clinical benefit lasting 2 years. The potential for radiation-induced malignancy does exist, and clinicians must schedule regular follow-up visits to monitor for malignant changes. Radiation therapy also may increase the degree of xerostomia. It is speculated that systemic anti-HIV treatment may augment radiation therapy. However, antiretroviral treatments alone have shown minimal effects on enlarged parotid glands.[121,122]

Two other methods of treatment include the aspiration of cysts and tetracycline sclerosis. The injection of a tetracycline solution into cystic areas will sometimes induce an inflammatory reaction and eventual sclerosis. Formal studies with long-term follow-up have not been reported for these methods.[123]

HEPATITIS C VIRUS INFECTION

Etiology.   Viruses have been considered potential triggers of autoimmune diseases for many years. Retroviruses are known to infect cells of the immune system and to disrupt immunoregulation. Sicca symptoms mimicking Sjögren's syndrome have been described in diseases caused by retroviruses (see discussion of HIV-SGD, above). Hepatitis C virus (HCV) DNA has been detected in the saliva of patients with chronic hepatitis C infection, and it has been demonstrated that the saliva of HCV carriers is infective. A number of reports from European centers have suggested an association between HCV and Sjögren's syndrome.[124–128] Subsequent investigations reported conflicting results. King and colleagues examined 48 Sjögren's syndrome patients and reported them negative for HCV.[122] Marrone and colleagues found that none of their 100 well-characterized Sjögren's syndrome patients had evidence of acute or chronic HCV infection.[127] In contrast, Pawlotsky and colleagues looked at a series of HCV-infected patients and found that 14% had a salivary gland pathology that resembled Sjögren's syndrome.[129]

These differences in results may be due to population variability and differing case definitions. The prevalence of asymptomatic HCV infection is higher in Europe than in the United States. Also, different authors have used less stringent diagnostic criteria for Sjögren's syndrome. When stringent diagnostic criteria have been applied and studies have been done in populations with relatively low endemic HCV infection, an increase of HCV infection in Sjögren's syndrome has not been found. However, the potential relationship between HCV and autoimmune disease remains an area of continuing debate.

Although a causal relationship between autoimmune disease and HCV is unlikely, salivary gland pathology can be noted in HCV-infected patients. Haddad and colleagues reported that 16 of 28 HCV-infected patients in their study had sialadenitis resembling Sjögren's syndrome.[130] Scott and colleagues performed biopsies of labial minor salivary glands in HCV-infected patients and found lymphoid aggregates, duct ectasia, lymphocytic infiltrates, and acinar depletion.[131] Pirisi and colleagues reported that specimens from lip biopsies from 17 of 22 HCV-positive patients demonstrated inflammatory changes similar to those seen in patients with Sjögren's syndrome. The inflammation seen in the HCV-infected population was described as mild compared to that seen in Sjögren's syndrome patients.[132]

Clinical Manifestations. HCV infection has many extrahepatic manifestations, including salivary gland enlargement. Patients may report xerostomia along with chronic major salivary gland enlargement.[133–141] Both Scott and colleagues and Haddad and colleagues reported that females with chronic HCV infection had a greater tendency for sialadenitis.[130,131] Clinical manifestations and salivary histologic lesions generally are significantly milder in patients with chronic HCV infection than in patients with Sjögren's syndrome.[135,136] It is worth noting that HCV-infected patients do not commonly experience dry eyes along with xerostomia. The diagnosis of HCV infection is made by the detection of anti-HCV antibodies and HCV DNA.[133,134]

Treatment. Hepatitis-associated sialadenitis is treated symptomatically.

BACTERIAL SIALADENITIS

Etiology. Bacterial infections of the salivary glands are most commonly seen in patients with reduced salivary gland function(Figure 9–10 and 9–11). This condition was formerly referred to as "surgical parotitis" because postsurgery patients often experienced gland enlargement from ascending bacterial infections. This was thought to relate to the markedly decreased salivary flow during anesthesia, often as the result of administered anticholinergic drugs and relative dehydration due to restricted fluids. With the administration of prophylactic antibiotics and routine perioperative hydration, this condition now occurs much less frequently.[142] Raad and colleagues reported only three instances in 300,000 cases occurring postoperatively.[143]

Today, the majority of bacterial infections occur in patients with disease- or medication-induced salivary gland hypofunction. The reduction of salivary flow results in diminished mechanical flushing, which allows bacteria to colonize the oral cavity and then to invade the salivary duct and cause acute bacterial infection. Studies have shown that poor oral hygiene contributes to salivary gland bacterial infections. The geriatric population is particularly suseptible to bacterial sialadenitis due to the frequent combination of medication-induced xerostomia and poor oral hygiene (Figure 9–12). The habit of fecal ingestion also has been associated with sialadenitis.[142–144]

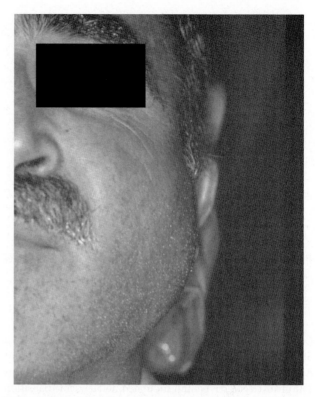

Figure 9–10 This patient demonstrates parotid swelling due to a bacterial infection.

Although sialoliths occur more frequently in the submandibular glands, bacterial sialadenitis occurs more frequently in the parotid glands. It is theorized that the submandibular glands may be protected by the high level of mucin in the saliva, which has potent antimicrobial activity. Anatomy may also play a protective role; tongue movements tend to clear the floor of the mouth and protect Wharton's duct. In contrast, the orifice of Stenson's duct is located adjacent to the molars, where heavy bacterial colonization occurs.[142–144]

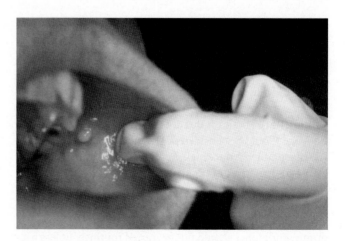

Figure 9–11 The expression of purulence from Stenson's duct seen in this patient is one of the signs of acute parotitis. Culture and sensitivity testing will produce guidance to appropriate antibiotics.

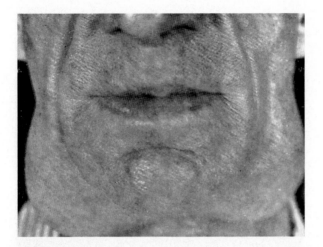

Figure 9-12 Bilateral chronic submaxillary sialadenitis in a dehydrated patient. (King HA, Koerner TA. JAMMA. 167:1813.)

Clinical Presentation. Patients usually present with a sudden onset of unilateral or bilateral salivary gland enlargement. Approximately 20% of the cases present as bilateral infections. The involved gland is painful, indurated, and tender to palpation. The overlying skin may be erythematous. A purulent discharge may be expressed from the duct orifice, and samples of this exudate should be cultured for aerobes and anaerobes (Figure 9–11). A second specimen should be sent for testing with Gram's stain.

The most commonly cultured organisms include coagulase-positive *Staphylococcus aureus, Streptococcus viridans, Streptococcus pneumoniae, Escherichia coli,* and *Haemophilus influenzae.* Institutionalized individuals are particularly susceptible to infections caused by methicillin-resistant *Staphylococcus aureus.*

Due to the dense capsule surrounding the salivary glands, it is difficult to determine, based on physical examination alone, whether an abscess has formed. Ultrasonography or CT is recommended for visualizing possible cystic areas.[142–144]

Treatment. If a purulent discharge is present, empiric intravenous administration of a penicillinase- resistant antistaphylococcal antibiotic is indicated. Patients should be instructed to "milk" the involved gland several times throughout the day. Increased hydration and improved oral hygiene are required. With these measures, significant improvement should be noted within 24 to 48 hours. If this does not occur, then incision and drainage should be considered. The mortality rate for bacterial sialadenitis was once high, but the availability of a selection of broad-spectrum antibiotics has eliminated mortality in noncritically ill patients.

As salivary gland enlargement may be nonbacterial in origin, such as in virally induced swelling or in Sjögren's syndrome, antibiotics should not be started routinely unless bacterial infection is clinically obvious. In any case, purulent discharge from the salivary gland should be cultured to confirm the diagnosis and determine antibiotic sensitivity.[142–144]

Systemic Conditions with Salivary Gland Involvement

Many systemic diseases are manifested by salivary gland dysfunction. Systemic conditions with associated salivary gland involvement are listed in Table 9–4. The most prominent example is Sjögren's syndrome. Xerostomia, the symptom of oral dryness, has been reported in association with many additional systemic conditions. In some instances, it is unclear whether these symptoms and the salivary gland changes are part of the disease process or whether they result from treatment of the disease.

Metabolic Conditions

Sialadenitis most often involves the parotid gland. The underlying systemic metabolic disorders that are commonly associated with salivary gland disease include diabetes, anorexia nervosa, bulimia, and alcoholism.[145–147] The parotid gland is not often involved.

DIABETES

Diabetes mellitus is a common endocrine disease, especially in the geriatric population. Multiple metabolic abnormalities take place, and long-term complications such as renal hypertension, neuropathies, and ophthalmic disease can occur.

TABLE 9–4 Systemic Conditions with Salivary Gland Involvement

Infectious disorders
    Actinomycosis
    Grandulomatous disease (sarcoidosis, tuberculosis)
    Tuberculosis

Viral infection
    HIV-SGD
    Hepatitis
    CMV infection

Metabolic disorders
    Sjögren's syndrome
    Thyroid disease
    Granulomatous disease (sarcoidosis, tuberculosis)
    Alcoholism
    Malnutrition
    Eating disorders (anorexia, bulimia)
    Diabetes (uncontrolled)

Neoplasms
    Benign
        Pleomorphic adenoma
        Monomorphic adenoma
        Ductal papilloma
    Malignant
        Lymphoma
        Mucoepidermoid carcinoma
        Adenoid cystic carcinoma
        Acinic cell carcinoma
        Squamous cell carcinoma
        Adenocarcinoma

CMV = *Cytomegalovirus*; HIV-SGD = human immunodeficiency syndrome salivary gland disease.

Patients with uncontrolled diabetes often report dry mouth, which is believed to be due to polyuria and poor hydration. Research results regarding salivary flow and compositional changes in diabetic patients are contradictory. One study reported that salivary flow rates in children with poorly controlled diabetes mellitus were decreased when compared to flow rates in well-controlled pediatric diabetic patients and normal controls.[148] However, other investigators found that salivary flow rates were normal but that salivary compositional changes occurred in pediatric diabetic patients.[149] Ship and colleagues[150] conducted a clinical trial comparing adult diabetes type 2 patients with normal controls. They found that patients with poorly controlled diabetes had lower salivary flow rates when compared to patients with well-controlled diabetes and to normal controls. Of interest, these investigators also found that there was no difference between these populations in the frequency of xerostomic complaints, and further, that salivary dysfunction may be present in older diabetic patients who do not complaint of xerostomia.[150–152]

The etiology of diabetic salivary gland dysfunction is unclear.[153–155] (Figure 9–13). Sreebny and colleagues suggested that poor glycemic control directly effects salivary gland metabolism.[146] It has also been suggested that autonomic nervous system dysfunction may play a role. Meurman and colleagues reported no change in flow rates between non-insulin-dependent diabetic patients and normal controls.[154] However, they found the effects of xerostomic medications on salivary flow rates to be stronger in the diabetic patients. They postulated that this was due to documented autonomic nervous system dysfunction in the diabetic population.

ANOREXIA NERVOSA/BULIMIA

Salivary gland enlargement and dysfunction can occur in patients with anorexia nervosa and bulimia.[156] The enlargement appears to be related to nutritional deficiencies and to the habit of induced vomiting. One case study reported that histologic examination of the involved salivary gland revealed acinar enlargement and reduced interstitial fat. Salivary gland

enlargement usually resolves when patients return to normal weight and discontinue unhealthy eating habits. However, benign hypertrophy may persist and be a cosmetic concern. While superficial parotidectomy will reduce salivary hypertrophy, some surgeons believe that surgical management is contraindicated for a patient with an eating disorder, because of the increased risk associated with the patient's metabolic imbalance and psychological profile.

Total and salivary specific amylase levels are increased with bulimia. Salivary amylase tends to increase with the frequency of binge eating, but the correlation is not strong enough to include salivary amylase levels as an index of disease severity.[157,158]

Eating disorders are difficult to diagnose because of the secretive nature of the condition. To facilitate early diagnosis and treatment, dentists should be aware of the common oral findings (enamel erosion, xerostomia, salivary gland enlargement, mucosal erythema, and cheilitis). Patients should be questioned directly if an eating disorder is suspected. Eating disorders must be considered in the differential diagnosis of salivary gland dysfunction and hypertrophy.

CHRONIC ALCOHOLISM

Chronic alcoholism is associated with salivary gland dysfunction and bilateral salivary (usually parotid) gland enlargement. The exact etiology is unclear, but the decreased salivary flow is believed to be due to dehydration and poor nutrition. Enlarged salivary glands in alcoholic patients demonstrate fatty-tissue changes on histologic examination.[159,160] (Figure 9–14).

Medication-Induced Salivary Dysfunction

There are over 400 medications that are listed as having dry mouth as an adverse event. However, there are relatively few drugs that have been shown objectively to reduce salivary function. The reason for this disparity is unclear. It may be due to unrecognized alterations in saliva composition that lead to the perception of oral dryness in spite of an apparently unchanged volume of saliva. Drugs that have been shown to result in sali-

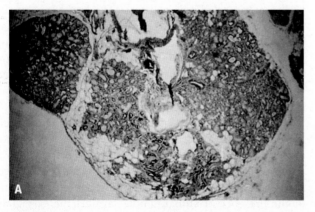 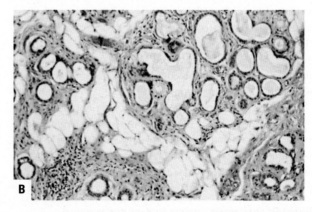

Figure 9-13 Histologic section of biopsy of minor salivary gland from lip of patient with complaints of dry, sore mouth; persistent salty taste; and evidence of chronic pansialadenitis, diabetes mellitus, and type II hyperlipoproteinemia, H & E stain. **A,** Low-power view showing chronic sialadenitis affecting entire gland with fatty replacement of some area fibrosis and atrophy of the gland parenchyma and cystic dilation of ducts. **B,** High-power view to illustrate the same features.

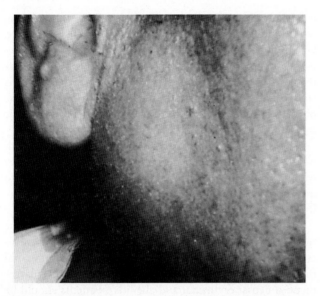

Figure 9-14   Sialadenosis. Asymptomatic parotid swelling in an alcoholic. Salivary secretion is normal.

vary dysfunction include anticholinergics, antidepressants (particularly tricyclics), antihypertensives, and antihistaminics. Medication-induced salivary hypofunction usually affects the unstimulated output, leaving stimulated function intact. When the causative drug is withdrawn, function often returns to normal.[12,65,85]

Immune Conditions

BENIGN LYMPHOEPITHELIAL LESION (MIKULICZ'S DISEASE)

The etiology of benign lymphoepithelial lesion is unknown. It has been speculated that autoimmune, viral, or genetic factors are the trigger. This condition predominantly affects middle-aged women.

Patients present with unilateral or bilateral salivary gland swelling due to a benign lymphoid infiltration. Reduced salivary flow makes these patients susceptible to salivary gland infections. The differential diagnosis includes Sjögren's syndrome, lymphoma, sarcoidosis, and other diseases associated with salivary gland enlargement. Diagnosis is based on findings of salivary gland biopsy and the absence of the abnormalities in peripheral blood counts and autoimmune serologies seen in Sjögren's syndrome.[161, 162]

Treatment is palliative. The possibility of neoplastic transformation is a concern. The detection of a monoclonal lymphocytic infiltrate is thought to be suggestive of a low-grade lymphoma. Treatment is controversial; some clinicians advocate irradiation therapy whereas others recommend monitoring when the disease is limited to the salivary glands.

SJÖGREN'S SYNDROME (PRIMARY AND SECONDARY)

Sjögren's syndrome (SS) is a chronic autoimmune disease characterized by symptoms of oral and ocular dryness and lymphocytic infiltration and destruction of the exocrine

glands. The etiology of SS is unknown, and there is no cure. The salivary and lacrimal glands are primarily affected, but other exocrine tissues, including the thyroid, lungs, and kidney, may also be involved. SS patients also frequently experience arthralgias, myalgias, peripheral neuropathies, and rashes. Autoimmune-associated anemia, hypergammaglobulinemia, and other serologic abnormalities are frequent in this patient population.[163,164]

SS primarily affects postmenopausal women (the female-to-male ratio is 9:1) and is classified as primary or secondary. Patients with secondary SS have salivary and/or lacrimal gland dysfunction in the setting of another connective-tissue disease. Primary SS is a systemic disorder that includes both lacrimal and salivary gland dysfunctions without another autoimmune condition.

Clinical Manifestations.   Patients with SS experience the full spectrum of oral complications that result from decreased salivary function. Virtually all patients complain of dry mouth and the need to sip liquids throughout the day. Oral dryness causes difficulty with chewing, swallowing, and speaking without additional fluids. Patients often have dry cracked lips and angular cheilitis. Intraorally, the mucosa is pale and dry, minimal salivary pooling is noted, and the saliva that is present tends to be thick and ropy. Mucocutaneous candidal infections are common in this patient population. As noted previously, decreased salivary flow results in increased dental caries and erosion of the enamel structure.[165]

Patients with SS can experience chronic salivary gland enlargement. (Figure 9–15). They are also susceptible to salivary gland infections and/or gland obstructions that present as acute exacerbations of chronically enlarged glands.[164,165] (Figure 9–16).

Diagnosis.   There are no universally accepted diagnostic criteria for SS, and multiple criteria sets have been published.[164–169] The strictest criteria include objective measurement of decreased salivary and lacrimal gland function, positive autoimmune serologies, and a minor salivary gland biopsy specimen that demonstrates focal mononuclear cell infiltration in a periductal pattern (focus score > 1 [see below]). Less stringent criteria, which rely partly on symptomatic reports, exist and are commonly used by clinicians.[166] At present, a criteria set created by a European Community SS multicenter study group and validated by large-scale clinical testing is gaining wider acceptance.[167] Efforts are being made to establish an internationally accepted diagnostic criteria set for SS. Most investigators accept the premise that a definitive diagnosis of primary SS requires either the presence of a salivary gland biopsy specimen demonstrating characteristic histopathologic findings or the presence of autoantibodies against the extractable nuclear antigens SS-A/Ro or SS-B/La, in addition to objective evidence of lacrimal dysfunction.

The minor salivary gland biopsy specimen finding is considered to be the best sole diagnostic criterion for the salivary

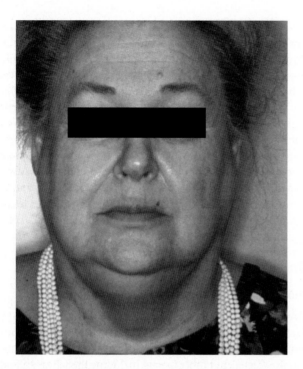

Figure 9-15 This patient demonstrates bilateral parotid enlargement secondary to Sjögren's syndrome.

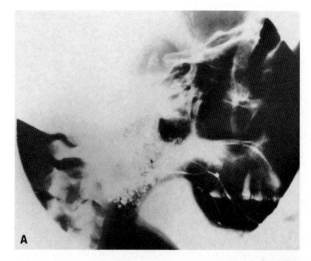

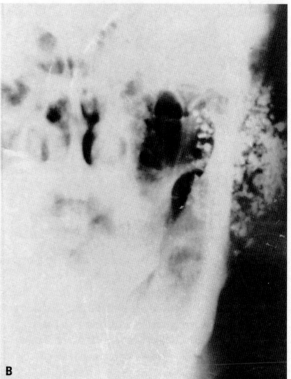

Figure 9–16 Retrograde sialogram of patient with Sjögren's syndrome. **A,** Lateral view; **B,** Anteroposterior view. Note the absence of fine arborization and the presence of many larger dye-filled spaces (sialectasis) on the posterior view. Also note dilatation of major intraglandular duct in lateral view. (Nichols CN, Brightman VJ. Parotid calcifications and cementomas in a patient with Sjögren's syndrome and idiopathic thrombocytopenic purpura. J Oral Pathol 1977; 6:51.)

component of SS. A grading system exists for quantifying the salivary histologic changes seen in the minor glands in SS, as follows: (1) the numbers of infiltrating mononuclear cells are determined, with an aggregate of 50 or more cells being termed a focus; (2) the total number of foci and the surface area of the specimen are measured; and (3) the number of foci per 4 mm^2 is calculated. This constitutes the focus score. The range is from 0 to 12, with 12 denoting confluent infiltrates. A focus score of 1 is considered positive for SS in some criteria although others require the score to be > 1. Acinar degeneration, with the relative preservation of ductal structures, is also noted[157] (Figure 9–17).

Imaging of the salivary glands is discussed earlier in this chapter. Sialography shows characteristic changes and may be useful in the evaluation of SS. MRI or CT can be helpful also, particularly in the assessment of enlarged glands and potential lymphadenopathies. MRI is preferable to CT, unless a stone or other calcified structure requires visualization as MRI provides better resolution of soft tissue. Some clinicians use Tc-99m radionuclide studies to determine salivary gland function.

Treatment. Treatment for SS is limited. As the causes of SS and the mechanisms of salivary damage are not fully understood, available treatment modalities are primarily symptomatic. Management of the oral consequences of salivary dysfunction in SS is not different than in other causes of secretory damage. Symptomatic therapies include artificial saliva, oral rinses and gels, and water sipping (see "Treatment of Xerostomia," below). Patients with remaining salivary

function can also stimulate salivary flow by chewing sugarfree gum or by sucking on sugarfree candies. Corticosteroids and nonsteroidal anti-inflammatory drugs (NSAIDs) have not been shown to improve salivary flow in SS patients.[170–172] Systemic cholinergic medications that stimulate salivary flow in functioning salivary glands include pilocarpine and cevimeline.[173,174] Multicenter clinical trials of interferon-α

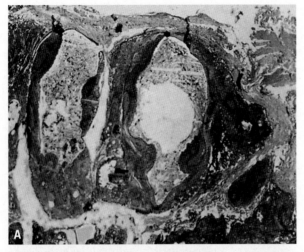

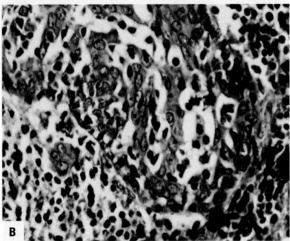

Figure 9–17   Histologic section of excised parotid gland from patient with Sjögren's syndrome, H & E stain. **A,** Low-power view of two cystlike spaces with development of lymphoid follicles in their walls. Elsewhere parotid gland parenchyema is obliterated and replaced by lymphoid tissue. **B,** High-power view of lymphoepithelial proliferation within an area of lymphoid infiltration. (Nichols CN, Brightman VJ. Parotid calcifications and cementomas in a patient with Sjögren's syndrome and idiopathic thrombocytopenia purpura. J Oral Pathol 1977; 6:51.)

lozenges as a treatment for the salivary component of SS are taking place.[175] Other biologics are also being investigated as possible therapeutic agents. The role of sex hormones in SS is an area of active research, and there is an ongoing clinical trial investigating the use of dehydroepiandrosterone (DHEA), a systemically administered nonvirilizing androgen, as a therapy for SS.

There is a recognized increased incidence of malignant lymphomas in SS.[176,177] These tumors often involve the salivary glands. It has been hypothesized that salivary gland enlargement in SS may progress from a benign sialadenitis with polyclonal lymphocytic infiltration to an oligoclonal infiltration and that monoclonal lymphoid malignancy may later

develop. Chronic salivary gland enlargement or any lymphadenopathy in SS patients should be viewed with caution. Routine monitoring is required and should include regular physical evaluation and assessment of immunoglobulin levels. Laboratory studies should determine if a monoclonal gammopathy is present. Suspicious lesions can be assessed by cytologic examination of FNA biopsy specimens for clonality of lymphoid cells. Histologic findings dictate the degree of intervention. An oncologist should be consulted when lymphoma or a monoclonal gammopathy is detected. Often, salivary lymphomas in SS are indolent and progress very slowly, and the recommended treatment is close monitoring. However, lesions can be aggressive, and this must be considered when exploring treatment options.

Granulomatous Conditions

TUBERCULOSIS

Tuberculosis (TB) is a chronic bacterial infection, caused by *Mycobacterium tuberculosis*, that leads to the formation of granulomas in the infected tissues. The lungs are most commonly affected, but other tissues, including the salivary glands, may be involved. Patients with TB may experience xerostomia and/or salivary gland swelling, with granuloma or cyst formation within the affected glands. Salivary gland enlargement usually presents as part of a characteristic symptom complex; however, salivary gland changes have been reported in the absence of systemic symptoms.

The worldwide increase in mycobacterial diseases and their association with immunocompromised patients must be considered when developing a differential diagnosis. Diagnosis depends on the identification of *Mycobacterium*. Treatment of the salivary involvement is encompassed in standard multidrug anti-TB chemotherapy. Patients who have not responded to appropriate chemotherapy regimens have required surgical intervention to address persistent salivary gland pathology.[178,179]

SARCOIDOSIS

Sarcoidosis is a chronic condition in which T lymphocytes, mononuclear phagocytes, and granulomas cause destruction of involved tissue. The etiology of the disease is unknown. Onset primarily occurs in the third or fourth decades of life. Women are affected more often than men, and African Americans are affected more often than Caucasians. Heerfordt's syndrome (uveoparotid fever) is a form of sarcoid that can occur in the presence or absence of systemic sarcoidosis. The syndrome is defined by the triad of inflammation of the uveal tract of the eye, parotid swelling, and facial palsy.[180]

Sarcoidosis affects the salivary glands in 1 of 20 cases. Patients usually present with bilateral, painless, and firm salivary gland enlargement. Unilateral salivary gland enlargement has been reported. Decreased salivary function is usually noted in the involved glands. Examination of a minor salivary gland biopsy specimen can confirm the diagnosis of sarcoidosis. Serum laboratory chemistries including calcium level, autoimmune serologies, and angiotensin I–converting enzyme concentration aid in the diagnosis.[180–182]

The treatment of the salivary component of sarcoidosis is primarily palliative. Depending on the extent of disease affecting other tissues or during exacerbations, corticosteroids may be administered. Chloroquine has also been used, alone or in combination with corticosteroids. Immunosuppressive and immunomodulatory medications have been administered to patients who failed to respond to corticosteroids.[180,181]

▼TREATMENT OF XEROSTOMIA

Treatment that is available for the dry mouth patient can be divided into four main categories: (1) preventive therapy, (2) symptomatic treatment, (3) local or topical salivary stimulation, and (4) systemic salivary stimulation. Effective treatment of an underlying systemic disorder associated with salivary gland dysfunction may correct the salivary complaint as well.

Preventive Therapy

The use of topical fluorides in a patient with salivary gland hypofunction is absolutely critical to control dental caries. There are many different fluoride therapies available (eg, over-the-counter fluoride rinses, brush-on forms, and highly concentrated prescription fluorides that can be applied by brush or in a custom carrier). The frequency of application (from daily to once per week) should be modified, depending on the severity of the salivary dysfunction and the rate of caries development.

It is essential that patients maintain meticulous oral hygiene. Patients will require more frequent dental visits (usually every 4 months) and must work closely with the dentist to maintain good dental health. When salivary function is compromised, there may be an increase in demineralization, speeding the loss of tooth structure. Remineralizing solutions may be used to alleviate some of the effects of the loss of normal salivation.

Patients with dry mouth also experience an increase in oral infections, particularly mucosal candidiasis. This may take an erythematous form (without the easily recognized pseudomembranous plaques), and the patient may present with redness of the mucosa and complaints of a burning sensation of the tongue or other intraoral soft tissues. A high index of suspicion should be maintained, and appropriate antifungal therapies should be instituted as necessary. Patients with salivary gland dysfunction may require prolonged treatment periods and re-treatment to eradicate oral fungal infections.[171]

Symptomatic Treatment

Several symptomatic treatments are available. Water is by far the most important. Patients should be encouraged to sip water throughout the day; this will help to moisten the oral cavity, hydrate the mucosa, and clear debris from the mouth. The use of water with meals can make chewing and forming the food bolus easier, will ease swallowing, and will improve taste perception. An increase in environmental humidity is exceedingly important. The use of room humidifiers, particularly at night, may lessen discomfort markedly. As part of the normal diurnal variation, salivary flow drops almost to zero during rest. In individuals who have any degree of secretory hypofunction, the dessication of the mucosa is particularly troublesome at night and may interfere with restorative sleep.

There are a number of oral rinses and gels available. Patients should be cautioned to avoid products containing alcohol, sugar, or strong flavorings that may irritate sensitive dry mucosa. Moisturizing creams are important. The frequent use of products containing aloe vera or vitamin E should be encouraged. Persistent cracking and erythema at the corners of the mouth should be investigated for a fungal cause.

There are many commercially available salivary substitutes. However, saliva replacements (artificial salivas) are not well accepted by most patients. While there is clearly a role for the use of saliva replacements, particularly in individuals who have no residual salivary gland function, it must be recognized that this is not a highly effective symptomatic therapy.[170,171]

Salivary Stimulation

LOCAL OR TOPICAL STIMULATION

Several approaches are available for stimulating salivary flow. Chewing will stimulate salivary flow effectively, as will sour and sweet tastes. The combination of chewing and taste, as provided by gums or mints, can be very effective in relieving symptoms for patients who have remaining salivary function. Patients with dry mouth must be told not to use products that contain sugar as a sweetener, due to the increased risk for dental caries in this group. Electrical stimulation has also been used as a therapy for salivary hypofunction but has been inadequately investigated clinically. A device that delivers a very-low-voltage electrical charge to the tongue and palate has been described although its effect was modest in patients with dry mouth.

SYSTEMIC STIMULATION

The use of systemic secretogogues for salivary stimulation has also been examined, with mixed results. More than 24 agents have been proposed as means of stimulating salivary output systemically. Four have been examined extensively in controlled clinical trials; these are bromhexine, anetholetrithione, pilocarpine hydrochloride (HCl), and cevimeline HCl.

Bromhexine is a mucolytic agent used in Europe and the Middle East. The proposed mechanism of action for salivary stimulation is unknown. No proven benefit to salivary function has been shown by objective and controlled clinical trials. Bromhexine may stimulate lacrimal function in patients with Sjögren's syndrome although this is controversial.[183,184]

Anetholetrithione is a mucolytic agent that has been shown to increase salivary output in clinical trials. The mechanism of action is not definitively known, but it has been suggested that anetholetrithione may up-regulate muscarinic receptors. In patients with mild salivary gland hypofunction, anetholetrithione significantly increased saliva flow. However, it was ineffective in patients with marked salivary gland hypofunction. The adverse effects are mild. One study suggested a possible synergistic effect of anetholetrithione in combination with pilocarpine.[185,186]

Pilocarpine HCL is approved specifically for the relief of xerostomia. Current indications are for patients with dryness following radiotherapy for head and neck cancers and for those with Sjögren's syndrome. Pilocarpine HCL is a parasympathomimetic drug, functioning as a muscarinic cholinergic agonist. Pilocarpine increases salivary output, stimulating any remaining gland function. The adverse effects of pilocarpine in human studies are very common and are usually mild. They are consistent with the known mechanism of action of the drug. Sweating is the most common side effect. Other frequently reported side effects are hot flashes, urinary frequency, diarrhea, and blurred vision.[172,173,187,188]

After the administration of pilocarpine, salivary output increases fairly rapidly, usually reaching a maximum within 1 hour. The best-tolerated doses are those of 5.0 to 7.5 mg, given three or four times daily. The duration of action is approximately 2 to 3 hours. Pilocarpine is contraindicated for patients with pulmonary disease, asthma, cardiovascular disease, glaucoma, or urethral reflux. Patients do not appear to develop tolerance to pilocarpine following prolonged use. Pilocarpine has been shown to be a safe and effective therapy for patients with diminished salivation but who have some remaining secretory function that can be stimulated.[172,173,187,188]

Cevimeline HCl is another parasympathomimetic agonist that has been recently approved for the treatment of symptoms of oral dryness in Sjögren's syndrome. This medication reportedly specifically targets the muscarinic receptors of the salivary and lacrimal glands. It still must be used with caution in patients with a history of glaucoma or cardiovascular, respiratory, or gall bladder disease and in patients who use various medications. Its side effects are similar to those of pilocarpine. To date, there have been few published reports of clinical trials with cevimeline.[174,189]

Pilocarpine HCl and cevimeline HCl are the only systemic sialagogues that are available in the United States. Medical consultation prior to prescribing these drugs for patients with significant medical conditions may be indicated. Increased understanding of the causes of xerostomia and salivary gland hypofunction undoubtedly will lead to improvement in the available treatments through the design and testing of more rational and specific therapies.

▼ SIALORRHEA

"Sialorrhea" refers to excess saliva production. Medications (eg, pilocarpine and cevimeline) can cause increased salivation. Often, the report of increased salivation is due to changes in oral perception or decreased swallowing efficiency rather than to an increase in salivation. Patients with neurologic changes may note an onset of sialorrhea. This commonly occurs after a cerebral vascular accident or in various neuromuscular diseases (eg, Parkinson's disease). Patients who have undergone extensive oral surgical procedures (eg, for oral cancer) may also report changes in salivary flow. A patient with a severe neurologic deficit may experience drooling due to the inability to swallow effectively. Drooling can be socially akward and can affect the patient's quality of life.

A complete past medical history and a history of present illness are important for determining the etiology of sialorrhea. Saliva collection is helpful in diagnosing hypersalivation and gives an objective measurement of salivary flow. The complaint of increased salivation can be due to decreased swallowing efficiency. Swallowing studies aid in diagnosis and evaluate the risk of aspiration.

The treatment of sialorrhea varies. If the patient is experiencing difficulty in swallowing, speech pathology study and therapy are recommended. Informing the patient about oral perception changes and therapy often provide sufficient relief. Depending on the patient's medical condition and the severity of the problem, a mild xerostomia-inducing medication (such as an antihistamine) may be helpful. A temporary reduction in salivary flow has been reported after the injection of botulinum toxin into the parotid glands of patients with neurologic disease. Injection of botulinum toxin should be done by experienced clinicians who are familiar with the side effects of botulinum toxin.[190]

▼ SALIVARY GLAND TUMORS

The majority of salivary gland tumors (about 80%) arise in the parotid glands. The submandibular glands account for 10 to 15% of tumors, and the remaining tumors develop in the sublingual or minor salivary glands. Approximately 80% of parotid gland tumors and 50% of submandibular gland tumors are benign. In contrast, more than 60% of tumors in the sublingual and minor salivary glands are malignant. The risk of malignancy increases as the size of the tumor decreases. Over 85% of salivary gland tumors occur in adults. Salivary tumors in children are most often located in the parotid glands, and about 65% of all salivary tumors found in children are benign.[191–198]

Benign Tumors

PLEOMORPHIC ADENOMA

Etiology. The pleomorphic adenoma is the most common tumor of the salivary glands; overall, it accounts for about 60% of all salivary gland tumors. It is often called a mixed tumor because it consists of both epithelial and mesenchymal elements. About 85% of these tumors are found in the parotid glands, 8% are found in the submandibular glands, and the remaining tumors are found in the sublingual and minor salivary glands. This tumor represents the most common neoplasm in each of the salivary glands and accounts for about 50% of salivary tumors in the minor salivary glands.[192,193]

Pleomorphic adenomas may occur at any age, but the highest incidence is in the fourth to sixth decades of life. It also represents the most common salivary neoplasm in children. There is a slight predilection for female gender.[194]

Clinical Presentation. On clinical examination, these tumors will appear as painless, firm, and mobile masses that rarely ulcerate the overlying skin or mucosa. In the parotid gland, these neoplasms are slow growing and usually occur in the posterior inferior aspect of the superficial lobe. Mixed tumors in the submandibular glands present as well-defined palpable masses. It is difficult to distinguish these tumors from malignant neoplasms and indurated lymph nodes. Intraorally, the mixed tumor most often occurs on the palate, followed by the upper lip and buccal mucosa.

Pleomorphic adenomas can vary in size, depending on the gland in which they are located. In the parotid gland, the tumors are usually several centimeters in diameter but can reach much larger sizes if left untreated. When observed in situ, the tumors are encased in a pseudocapsule and exhibit a lobulated appearance.[194–196]

Pathology. The gross appearance of pleomorphic adenoma is that of a firm smooth mass within a pseudocapsule. Histologically, the lesion demonstrates both epithelial and mesenchymal elements. The epithelial cells make up a trabecular pattern that is contained within a stroma. The stroma may be chondroid, myxoid, osteoid, or fibroid. The presence of these different elements accounts for the name pleomorphic tumor or mixed tumor. Myoepithelial cells are also present in this tumor and add to its histopathologic complexity. One characteristic of a pleomorphic adenoma is the presence of microscopic projections of tumor outside of the capsule. If these projections are not removed with the tumor, the lesion will recur.

Treatment. The treatment of this lesion consists of surgical removal with adequate margins. Because of its microscopic projections, this tumor requires a wide resection to avoid recurrence. In spite of the capsule, close excision should not be attempted. A superficial parotidectomy is sufficient for the majority of these lesions. A small tumor in the tail of the parotid gland may be removed with a wide margin of normal tissue, sparing the remainder of the superficial lobe. Lesions that occur in the submandibular gland are treated by the removal of the entire gland.[194–196]

MONOMORPHIC ADENOMA

A monomorphic adenoma is a tumor that is composed predominantly of one cell type, as opposed to a mixed tumor (pleomorphic adenoma), in which different elements are present.[196] Management is the same as pleomorphic adenoma.

PAPILLARY CYSTADENOMA LYMPHOMATOSUM

Papillary cystadenoma lymphomatosum, also known as Warthin's tumor, is the second most common benign tumor of the parotid gland. It represents about 6 to 10% of all parotid tumors and is almost always located in the parotid gland, most commonly in the inferior pole of the gland, posterior to the angle of the mandible. The tumor demonstrates a slight predilection toward males, and it usually occurs between the fifth and eighth decades. These tumors occur bilaterally in about 6 to 12% of patients.[192–194,197]

Clinical Presentation. This tumor presents as a well-defined slow growing mass in the tail of the parotid gland. It is usually painless unless it becomes superinfected. Because this tumor contains oncocytes, it will take up technetium and will be visible on technetium scintiscans.

Pathology. The gross appearance of this tumor is smooth, with a well-defined capsule. Cutting a specimen reveals cystic spaces filled with thick mucinous material. Histologically, the tumor consists of papillary projections lined with eosinophilic cells that project into cystic spaces. The projections are characterized by a lymphocytic infiltrate. Oncocytes are present within this tumor, and because they can concentrate technetium, these tumors are visible with Tc-99m nuclear imaging.

Treatment. Papillary cytadenoma lymphomatosum is most often located in the tail of the parotid gland and is easily removed with a margin of normal tissue. Larger tumors that involve a significant amount of the superficial lobe of the parotid gland are best treated by a superficial parotidectomy. Recurrences and malignant degeneration of this tumor are rare.[192,193,197]

ONCOCYTOMA

Oncocytomas are less common benign tumors that make up less than 1% of all salivary gland neoplasms. The name of the tumor is derived from the fact that it contains oncocytes, which are large granular acidophilic cells. This tumor occurs almost exclusively in the parotid glands and is equally distributed in both men and women. The sixth decade is the most common time of presentation.[199–202]

Clinical Presentation. Oncocytomas are usually solid round tumors that can be seen in any of the major salivary glands but that are extremely rare intraorally. These lesions can be found commonly in the superficial lobe of the parotid gland. Bilateral presentation of this tumor can occur, and it is the second most common salivary gland tumor that occurs bilaterally (after Warthin's tumor).

Pathology. On gross examination, these tumors appear noncystic and firm. Histologically, they consist of brown granular eosinophilic cells. The oncocytes within this tumor concentrate technetium, and this tumor can be visualized by Tc-99m scintigraphy. Malignant oncocytomas can occur, and these are aggressive lesions.

Treatment. Oncocytomas demonstrate a very slow growth rate and a benign course. Superficial parotidectomy with preservation of the facial nerve is the treatment of choice for parotid gland tumors. Removal of the gland is the treatment of choice for tumors in the submandibular gland, and gland removal with a normal cuff of tissue is the treatment of choice for oncocytomas of the minor salivary glands. Recurrence is rare.[195,196,199–202]

BASAL CELL ADENOMAS

Basal cell adenomas are slow growing and painless masses and account for approximately 1 to 2% of salivary gland adenomas. This lesion has a male predilection (the male-to-female ratio is 5:1). Seventy percent of basal cell adenomas occur in the parotid gland, and the upper lip is the most common site for basal cell adenomas of the minor salivary glands.

Pathology. Histologically, three varieties of basal cell adenomas exist: solid, trabecular-tubular, and membranous. The solid form consists of islands or sheets of basaloid cells. Nuclei have a normal size and are basophilic, with minimal cytoplasmic material. The trabecular-tubular form consists of trabecular cords of epithelium. The membranous form is multilocular, and 50% of the lesions are encapsulated. The membranous form tends to grow in clusters interspersed between normal salivary tissue.

Treatment. Lesions are removed, with conservative surgical excision extending to normal tissue. In general, lesions do not recur; however, the membranous form has a higher recurrence rate.[200]

CANALICULAR ADENOMA

Canalicular adenomas predominantly occur in persons older than 50 years of age and occur mostly in women. Eighty percent of cases occur in the upper lip. The lesions are slow growing, movable, and asymptomatic.

Pathology. This lesion is composed of long strands of basaloid tissue, usually arranged in a double row. The supporting stroma is loose, fibrillar, and highly vascular.

Treatment. Treatment is surgical excision with a margin of normal tissue. Recurrence is rare but has been reported; thus, patients should be monitored periodically.[195,196,200,201]

MYOEPITHELIOMA

Most myoepitheliomas occur in the parotid gland; the palate is the most common intraoral site. No gender predilection exists, and lesions tend to occur in adults, with the average age being 53 years. Lesions present as a well-circumscribed asymptomatic slow-growing mass.

Pathology. Myoepitheliomas consist of spindle-shaped cells, plasmacytoid cells, or a combination of the two. Diagnosis is based on the identification of myoepithelial cells. Growth patterns vary from a solid to a loose stroma formation with myoepithelial cells. This tumor is epithelial in origin; however, it functionally resembles smooth muscle and is demonstrated by immunohistochemical staining for actin, cytokeratin, and S-100 protein.

Treatment. Standard surgical excision, including a border of normal tissue, is recommended. Recurrence is uncommon.[195,196,198,200,201]

SEBACEOUS ADENOMA

Sebaceous adenomas are rare. These lesions are derived from sebaceous glands located within salivary gland tissue. The parotid gland is the most commonly involved gland.

Pathology. Cells derived from sebaceous glands are present. Benign forms contain well-differentiated sebaceous cells whereas malignant forms consist of more poorly differentiated cells.

Treatment. Removal of the involved gland is the treatment of choice. Intraoral lesions are surgically removed with a border of normal tissue.[195,196,200,201]

DUCTAL PAPILLOMA

Ductal papillomas form a subset of benign salivary gland tumors that arise from the excretory ducts, predominantly of the minor salivary glands. The three forms of ductal papillomas are simple ductal papilloma (intraductal papilloma), inverted ductal papilloma, and sialadenoma papilliferum.

Simple Ductal Papilloma. The simple ductal papilloma presents as an exophytic lesion with a pedunculated base. The lesion often has a reddish color. Microscopic examination reveals epithelium-lined papillary fronds projecting into a cystic cavity without proliferating into the wall of the cyst. Local surgical excision is the recommended treatment. A minimal recurrence rate is reported.[188,186,190–191]

Inverted Ductal Papilloma. The inverted ductal papilloma occurs in the minor salivary glands. It presents clinically as a submucosal nodule that is similar to a fibroma or lipoma. The inverted ductal papilloma histologically resembles the sialadenoma. This form of ductal papilloma also consists of projections of ductal epithelium that proliferate into surrounding stromal tissue, forming clefts. The lesion is treated by surgical excision. A low recurrence rate is reported.[195,196,200–204]

Sialadenoma Papilliferum. The sialadenoma papilliferum form of ductal papilloma is analogous to the syringocystadenoma papilliferum of the skin. An adult male predilection exists, and most lesions occur between the fifth and eighth decades of life. This lesion occurs primarily on the palate and buccal mucosa and presents as a painless exophytic mass. Clinically, the lesion resembles a papilloma. Microscopic examination shows epithelium-lined papillary projections supported by fibrovascular connective tissue, forming a series of clefts within the lesion. Local surgical excision is the recommended treatment. Recurrence is rare.[195,196,200–202]

Malignant Tumors

MUCOEPIDERMOID CARCINOMA

Mucoepidermoid carcinoma is the most common malignant tumor of the salivary glands. It is the most common malignant tumor of the parotid gland and the second most common malignant tumor of the submandibular gland, after adenoid cystic carcinoma. Approximately 60 to 90% of these lesions occur in the parotid gland; the palate is the second most common site. Men and women are affected equally by this tumor, and the highest incidence occurs in the third to fifth decades of life.

As its name suggests, mucoepidermoid carcinoma consists of both epidermal and mucous cells. The tumor is classified as of either a high grade or a low grade, depending on the ratio of epidermal cells to mucous cells. The low-grade tumor has a higher ratio and is a less aggressive lesion. Although low-grade tumors have the ability for metastasis and local invasion, they behave more like benign tumors. The high-grade form is considered to be a more malignant tumor and has a poorer prognosis.[195,196,202–204]

Clinical Presentation. The clinical course of this lesion depends on its grade. It is not uncommon for low-grade tumors to undergo a long period of painless enlargement. In contrast, high-grade mucoepidermoid carcinomas often demonstrate rapid growth and a higher likelihood for metastasis. Pain and ulceration of overlying tissue are occasionally associated with this tumor. If the facial nerve is involved, the patient may exhibit a facial palsy.

Pathology. Macroscopically, low-grade mucoepidermoid carcinomas are usually small and partially encapsulated. The high-grade tumors are less likely to demonstrate a capsule because of the more rapid growth and local tissue invasion. After sectioning, the low-grade tumors usually demonstrate a mucinous fluid, but the high-grade lesions are usually solid in appearance.

Microscopically, the low-grade lesions consist of regions of mucoid cells with interspersed epithelial strands. The high-grade tumors consist primarily of epithelial cells, with very few mucinous cells. In fact, special stains are necessary to differentiate between high-grade mucoepidermoid carcinoma and squamous cell carcinoma.

Treatment. A low-grade mucoepidermoid carcinoma can be treated with a superficial parotidectomy if it involves only the superficial lobe. Usually, the facial nerve can be spared. High-grade lesions should be treated aggressively to avoid recurrence. A total parotidectomy is performed, with facial nerve preservation if possible. If there is any possibility that the tumor involves the facial nerve, the nerve is resected with the tumor. Immediate nerve reconstruction can be performed at the time of tumor extirpation. Neck dissections may be performed for lymph node removal and staging in high-grade lesions. Postoperative radiation therapy has been shown to be a useful adjunct in treating the high-grade tumor. With high-grade lesions, recurrence with metastases can occur in up to 60% of patients. The survival rate for patients with low-grade lesions is about 95% at 5 years; for patients with high-grade lesions, this rate drops to approximately 40%.[195,196,198–204]

ADENOID CYSTIC CARCINOMA

Adenoid cystic carcinomas make up about 6% of all salivary gland tumors and are the most common malignant tumors of the submandibular and minor salivary glands. They make up 15 to 30% of submandibular gland tumors, 30% of minor salivary gland tumors, and 2 to 15% of parotid gland tumors. Approximately 50% of adenoid cystic carcinomas occur in the minor salivary glands. The tumor affects men and women equally and usually occurs in the fifth decade of life.[195,196,198,204–207]

Clinical Presentation. Adenoid cystic carcinoma usually presents as a firm unilobular mass in the gland. Occasionally, the tumor is painful, and parotid tumors may cause facial nerve paralysis in a small number of patients. This tumor has a propensity for perineural invasion; thus, tumor tissue often can extend far beyond the obvious tumor margin. Unfortunately, the tumor's slow growth may delay diagnosis for several years, allowing perineural invasion to be advanced at the time of surgical extirpation. An intraoral adenoid cystic carcinoma may exhibit mucosal ulceration, a feature that helps distinguish it from a benign mixed tumor. Radiographically, the tumor reveals extension into adjacent bone. Metastases into the lung are more common than regional lymph node metastasis.

Pathology. On gross examination, the tumor is unilobular and either partially encapsulated or non-encapsulated. There is often evidence of invasion into adjacent normal tissue. Microscopically, the individual cells are small and cuboidal. Nuclear atypia and mitotic figures are not seen, but chromatin aggregation is dense. Pseudocystic spaces filled with acellular material are a characteristic feature of this tumor. Also, microscopic evidence of perineural or intraneural invasion is a distinguishing feature of adenoid cystic carcinoma.

Treatment. Because of the ability of this lesion to spread along the nerve sheaths, radical surgical excision of the lesion is the appropriate treatment. Even with aggressive surgical margins, tumor cells can remain, leading to long-term recurrence. Frozen pathologic sections of the nerve sheath can help the surgeon achieve a clear margin. Some clinicians feel that a more conservative surgical resection and radiation therapy can provide adequate treatment. Neutron beam radiation has been shown to be more effective than photon beam therapy for the treatment of this tumor. Because of this tumor's capability for long-term recurrence, patients need to be observed indefinitely. Factors affecting the long-term prognosis are the size of the primary lesion, its anatomic location, the presence of metastases at the time of surgery, and facial nerve involvement.[195,196,198,204–211]

ACINIC CELL CARCINOMA

Acinic cell carcinoma represents about 1% of all salivary gland tumors. About 90 to 95% of these tumors are found in the parotid gland; almost all of the remaining tumors are located in the submandibular gland. The distribution of acinic cell carcinoma reflects the location of acinar cells within the different glands. This tumor occurs with a higher frequency in women and is usually found in the fifth decade of life. It is the second most common malignant salivary gland tumor in children, second only to mucoepidermoid carcinoma.

Clinical Presentation.   These lesions often present as slow-growing masses. Pain may be associated with the lesion but is not indicative of the prognosis. The superficial lobe and the inferior pole of the parotid gland are common sites of occurrence. Bilateral involvement of the parotid gland has been reported in approximately 3% of cases.

Pathology.   The gross specimen is a well-defined mass that is often encapsulated. Microscopically, two types of cells are present; cells similar to acinar cells in the serous glands are seen adjacent to cells with a clear cytoplasm. These cells are positive on periodic acid–Schiff (PAS) staining. Lymphocytic infiltration is often found.

Treatment.   Acinic cell carcinomas initially undergo a relatively benign course. Unfortunately, long-term survival is not as favorable, and the 20-year survival rate is about 50%. Treatment consists of superficial parotidectomy, with facial nerve preservation if possible. When these tumors are found in the submandibular gland, total gland removal is the treatment of choice.[205-208]

CARCINOMA EX PLEOMORPHIC ADENOMA

Carcinoma ex pleomorphic adenoma is a malignant tumor that arises within a pre-existing pleomorphic adenoma. The malignant cells in this tumor are epithelial in origin. This tumor represents 2 to 5% of all salivary gland tumors.

Clinical Presentation.   These tumors are slow growing and have usually been present for 15 to 20 years before they suddenly increase in size and become clinically apparent. Carcinoma ex pleomorphic adenoma occurs more often in pleomorphic adenomas that have been left untreated for long periods of time (It is for this reason that early removal of pleomorphic adenomas is recommended).

Pathology.   Macroscopically, these tumors are nodular or cystic, without encapsulation. The sectioned tumor appears similar to pleomorphic adenoma except for the presence of necrosis and hemorrhage associated with the malignant tumor.

Histologically, the tumor appears as a squamous cell carcinoma, adenocarcinoma, or undifferentiated carcinoma located within a benign mixed tumor. It may appear as a small focus of malignancy within the pleomorphic adenoma, or the malignant cells can almost completely replace the mixed tumor, making its appearance similar to that of a primary malignant tumor. Destructive infiltrative growth is usually seen around the malignancy.

Treatment.   This is a malignant salivary gland tumor that has an aggressive course and that carries a very poor prognosis. Local and distant metastases are common. Surgical

removal with postoperative radiation therapy is the recommended treatment. Early removal of benign parotid gland tumors is recommended to avoid the development of this lesion.[195,196,202,204,208]

ADENOCARCINOMA

Any tumors arising from salivary duct epithelium are, by definition, adenocarcinomas. This group of neoplasms has been divided into discrete entities based on structure and behavior. The term "adenocarcinoma" is often used as a catchphrase to refer to lesions that do not meet the specific criteria for other lesions (such as polymorphous low-grade adenocarcinoma, epimyoepithelial carcinoma, or salivary duct carcinoma). Clarification of the type of adenocarcinoma with a histologic description should be obtained in order to determine an appropriate treatment approach.[195,196,204,208]

LYMPHOMA

By definition, "primary lymphoma" describes a situation in which a salivary gland is the first clinical manifestation of the disease. Primary lymphoma of the salivary glands probably arises from lymph tissue within the glands. However, primary lymphoma of the salivary glands is rare.

The major forms of lymphoma are non-Hodgkin's lymphoma (NHL) and Hodgkin's disease. NHL is less curable and is often disseminated at diagnosis. There is an increased incidence of NHL in patients with autoimmune disease, as was described earlier in this chapter (see section on Sjögren's syndrome). The parotid gland is the most commonly involved gland, followed by the submandibular gland.

Clinical Presentation.   This lesion commonly presents as painless gland enlargement or adenopathy.

Treatment.   Superficial parotidectomy is recommended for isolated asymptomatic parotid gland masses. A staging workup is required to determine treatment. An initial phase of observation is not uncommon for patients with asymptomatic low-grade disease. Appropriate treatment includes radiation therapy, chemotherapy, or a combination of the two, depending on the staging of the lymphoma.[208,212]

Surgical Treatment

PAROTIDECTOMY

Since most tumors of the parotid gland occur in the tail region, superficial to the facial nerve, surgical treatment most commonly consists of superficial parotidectomy. The facial nerve is identified at surgery in order to avoid damage. If a tumor is very small, it may be excised with an adequate margin of tissue, leaving the remainder of the superficial lobe. Superficial parotidectomy is also the treatment of choice in cases of low-grade malignant salivary tumors.

For high-grade malignant salivary tumors, a total parotidectomy is performed. Unless there is intimate involvement of the tumor with the facial nerve, the nerve may be spared. If the tumor does invade the nerve, resection of the nerve is performed, with immediate reconstruction. Biopsies of any suspicious regional lymph nodes are performed; if the results are positive for malignancy, a modified neck dissection is performed immediately. There is no evidence to support prophylactic neck dissection for malignant tumors of the salivary glands.[198,202,204,208,213]

Complications can occur after parotidectomy. Permanent partial or total facial nerve paralysis occurs in less than 3% of patients, and temporary nerve palsies can occur in 10 to 30% of patients. A salivary fistula or sialocele is a relatively common complication after parotid gland surgery. A sialocele occurs when an edge of the parotid gland capsule is cut and the gland continues to leak fluid, leading to a palpable collection. Pressure dressings can be applied, and an anti-sialagogue such as glycopyrolate can be given if there are no contraindications. In cases of chronic sialoceles, serial aspirations or drain placement may be carried out in an attempt to expedite resolution.[213]

Frey's syndrome is a relatively common complication of parotidectomy. This syndrome presents as gustatory sweating. When regenerating postganglionic secretory parasympathetic fibers from the parotid gland become mixed with the post-ganglionic sympathetic fibers to the sweat glands, a condition in which a patient will flush or sweat with salivary stimulation results. Minor's starch-iodine test can be used to demonstrate the area of gustatory sweating. Iodine is applied to the patient's face and is allowed to dry. Starch is then lightly applied to the regions of interest. After a sialagogue is administered, the patient will begin to sweat in the areas of involvement. Wetting the starch and iodine, the sweat will turn the involved areas black. This test aids in delineating the distribution of affected area. Frey's syndrome can occur in as many as 30 to 60% of patients who have undergone parotidectomy. The treatment of this disorder consists of the topical application of antiperspirants or anticholinergics. Botulinum toxin injections have been used to treat Frey's syndrome. However, it is recommended that only experienced clinicians attempt this treatment.[214]

SUBMANDIBULAR, SUBLINGUAL, AND MINOR SALIVARY GLAND SURGERY

Tumors of the submandibular and sublingual glands are treated by total removal of the gland. The loss of salivary flow from a single submandibular gland is negligible, and patients tolerate this procedure well. The risks associated with the removal of the submandibular gland include hemorrhage, infection, and injury to the hypoglossal, lingual, or marginal mandibular nerves.

The treatment of tumors of the minor salivary glands depends on the location and extent of disease. Complete excision is usually sufficient for benign tumors. Complications from the treatment of benign lesions are few.[200,202,208,209,211] In contrast, the treatment of malignant tumors may involve maxillectomy or composite resection.

▼ REFERENCES

1. Baum BJ. Principles of saliva secretion. Ann N Y Acad Sci 1993;694:17–23.
2. Fox PC, Busch KA, Baum BJ. Subjective reports of xerostomia and objective measures of salivary gland performance. J Am Dent Assoc 1987;115:581–4.
3. Valdez IH, Fox PC. Diagnosis and management of salivary dysfunction. Crit Rev Oral Biol Med 1993;4:271–7.
4. Mandel ID. Sialochemistry in diseases and clinical situations affecting salivary glands. Crit Rev Clin Lab Sci 1980;12:321–66.
5. Fox PC, Brennan MJ, Pillemer S, et al. Sjögren's syndrome: a model for dental care in the 21st century. J Am Dent Assoc 1988;129:719–28.
6. Navazesh M. Methods for collecting saliva. Ann N Y Acad Sci 1993;694:72–4.
7. Kohler PF, Winter ME. A quantitative test for xerostomia: the Saxon test, an oral equivalent of the Schirmers. Arthritis Rheum 1985;28(10);1128–32.
8. Carlson AV, Crittenden AL. The relation of ptyalin concentration to the diet and to the rate of secretion of saliva. Am J Physiol 1910;26:169–77.
9. Ship JA, Fox PC, Baum BJ. How much saliva is enough? Normal function defined. J Am Dent Assoc 1991;122:63–9.
10. Sreebny LM, Schwartz SS. A reference guide to drugs and dry mouth. Gerodontology 1986;5:75–102.
11. Tylenda CA, Ship JA, Fox PC, Baum BJ. Evaluation of submandibular salivary flow rate in different age groups. J Dent Res 1988;67(9);1225–8.
12. Mason DK, Chisolm DM. Salivary glands in health and disease. London: W.B. Saunders; 1975. p. 37–69.
13. Becker TS. Salivary gland imaging. In: Bailey B, editor. Head and neck surgery-otolaryngology. Philadelphia: J.B. Lippincott, 1993. p. 455–74.
14. Del Balso A. Salivary imaging. Oral Maxillofac Surg Clin North Am 1995;7(3);387–422.
15. Murray ME, Buckenham TM, Joseph AEA. The role of ultrasound in screening patients referred for sialography: a possible protocol. Clin Otolaryngol 1996;21:21–3.
16. Shimizu M, Ussmuller J, Hartwein J. Statistical study for sonographic differential diagnosis of tumorous lesions in the parotid gland. Oral Surg Oral Med Oral Pathol Oral Radiol Endod 1999;88:226–33.
17. Makula E, Pokorny G, Rajtar M, Kiss I. Parotid gland ultrasonography as a diagnostic tool in primary Sjogren's syndrome. Br J Rheumatol 1996;35:972–7.
18. Weber AL. Imaging of the salivary glands. Curr Opin Radiol 1992;4:117–22.
19. Sigal R. Oral cavity, oropharynx and salivary glands. Neuroimaging Clin N Am 1996;6(2):379–400.
20. Klutmann S, Bohuslavizki KH, Kroger S, etal. Quantitative salivary gland scintigraphy. J Nucl Med Technol 1999;27:20–6.
21. Mermann GA, Vivino FB, Shnier D. Diagnostic accuracy of salivary scintigraphic indices in xerostomic populations. Clin Nucl Med 1999;24(3):167–72.
22. Umehara I, Yamada I, Murata Y. Quantitative evaluation of salivary gland scintigraphy in Sjogren's syndrome. J Nucl Med 1999;40(1):64–9.
23. Bohuslavizki KH, Brenner W, Lassmann S. Quantitative salivary gland scintigraphy in the diagnosis of parenchymal damage after treatment with radioactive iodine. Nucl Med Commun 1996;17:681–6.

24. Helman J, Turner RJ, Fox PC, Baum BJ. Tc-pertechnetate uptake in parotid acinar cells by the Na+/K+/Cl- co-transport system. J Clin Invest 1987;79:1310–3.

25. Kohn WG, Ship JA, Atkinson JC, et al. Salivary gland Tc-scintigraphy: a grading scale correlation with major salivary gland flow rates. J Oral Pathol Med 1992;21:70–4.

26. Baum BJ, Fox PC, Neuman RD. The salivary glands. In: Harbert JC, Eckelman WC, Neuman RD, editors. Nuclear medicine. New York: Theime Medical Publishers, 1996. p. 439–44.

27. Casselman JW, Mancuso AA. Major salivary gland masses: comparison of MR imaging and CT. Radiology 1987;165(1):183–9.

28. Del Balso AM, Williams E, Tane TT. Parotid masses: current modes of diagnostic imaging. J Oral Surg 1982;54(3):360–4.

29. Yousem DM, Chalian AA. Oral cavity and pharynx. Radiol Clin North Am 1998; 36(5):967–1014.

30. Kaneda T, Minami M, Ozawa K. MR of the submandibular gland: normal and pathologic states. Am J Neuroradiol 1996; 17:1575–81.

31. Keyes JW, Harkness BA, Greven KM. Salivary gland tumors: pretherapy evaluation with PET. Radiology 1994;192:99–102.

32. Noyek AM, Fliss DM, Kassel EE. Diagnostic imaging. In: Bailey B, editor. Head and neck surgery-otolaryngology. Philadelphia: J.B. Lippincott, 1993. p. 83–91.

33. Silvers AR, Som PM. Salivary glands. Radiol Clin North Am 1998;36(5):942–66.

34. Fox RI, Saito I. Criteria for diagnosis of Sjogren's syndrome. Rheum Dis Clin North Am 1994;20(2):391–407.

35. Daniels TE. Labial salivary gland biopsy in Sjogren's syndrome: assessment as a diagnostic criterion in 362 suspected cases. Arthritis Rheum 1984;27:147–56.

36. Fox PC. Simplified biopsy technique for labial minor salivary glands. Plast Reconstr Surg 1985;75(4):592–3.

37. Williams RC Jr. Immunologic markers for differentiation of autoimmune responses. Adv Dent Res 1996;10:41–3.

38. Fox RI, Kang HI. Pathogenesis of Sjogren's syndrome. Rheum Dis Clin North Am 1992;18:517–38.

39. Jayaram N, Ashim D, Rajwanshi A, et al. The value of fine needle aspiration biopsy in the cytodiagnosis of salivary gland lesions. Diagn Cytopathol 1989;5:349.

40. Truelson JM. Controversies in salivary gland disease. In: Bailey BJ, editor. Head and neck surgery-otolaryngology. Vol. 2. J.B. Lippincott Co.: Philadelphia; 1993. p. 882–8.

41. Wheelis RF, Yarington CT. Tumors of the salivary glands. Arch Otolaryngol 1984;110:76.

42. Rauch S, Gorlin RJ. Diseases of the salivary glands. In: Gorlin RJ, Goldman HM, editors. Thomas's oral pathology. 6th ed. St. Louis: C.V. Mosby; 1970. p. 968.

43. Matsuda C, Matsui Y, Ohno K, Michi K. Salivary gland aplasia with cleft lip and palate: a case report and review of the literature. Oral Surg Oral Med Oral Pathol 1999;87(5):594–9.

44. Bhide VN, Warshawsky RJ. Agenesis of the parotid gland: association with ipsilateral accessory parotid tissue. AJR Am J Roentgenol 1998; 170(6):1670–1.

45. Powenell PH, Brown OE, Pransky SM, Manning SC. Congenital abnormalities of the submandibular duct. Int J Pediatr Otorhinolaryngol 1992;24(2):161–9.

46. Kubo S, Abe K, Ureshino T, Oka M. Aplasia of the submandibular gland. A case report. J Craniomaxillofac Surg 1990; 18(3):119–21.

47. Gomez RS, Aguiar MJ, Ferreira AP, Castro WH. Congenital absence of parotid glands and lacrimal puncta. J Clin Pediatr Dent 1998;22(3):247–8.

48. Nordgarden H, Johannessen S, Storhaug K, Jensen JL. Salivary gland involvement in hypohidrotic ectodermal dysplasia. Oral Dis 1998;4(2):152–4.

49. O'Mallet AM, Macleod RI, Welbury RR. Congenital aplasia of the major salivary glands in a 4 year old child. Int J Paediatr Dent 1993;3(3):141–4.

50. Milunsky JM, Lee VW, Siegal BS, Milunsky A. Agenesis or hypoplasia of major salivary and lacrimal glands. Am J Med Genet 1991;41(2):269–70.

51. Gelbier MJ, Winter GB. Absence of salivary glands in children with rampant dental caries: a report of seven cases. Int J Paediatr Dent 1995;5:253–7.

52. Rice DH. Salivary gland disorders: neoplastic and nonneoplastic. Otolaryngology for the internist. Med Clin North Am 1999;83(1):197–221.

53. Banerjee AR, Soames JV, Birchall JP, et al. Ectopic salivary gland tissue in the palantine and lingual tonsil. Int J Pediatr Otorhinolaryngol 1993;27(2):159–62.

54. Bottrill ID, Chawla OP, Ramsay AD. Salivary gland choristoma of the middle ear. J Laryngol Otol 1992;106(7):630–2.

55. Hinni ML, Beatty CW. Salivary gland choristoma of the middle ear: report of a case and review of the literature. Ear Nose Throat J 1996;75:422-4.

56. Stene T, Pederson KN. Aberrant salivary gland tissue in the anterior mandible. J Oral Surg 1977;44:75.

57. Shira RB. Anterior lingual mandibular salivary gland defect: evaluation of 24 cases. Oral Surg Oral Med Oral Pathol 1991;71:131–6.

58. Steelman R, Weisse M, Ramadan H. Congenital ranula. Clin Pediatr 1998;37(3):205–6.

59. Salman L, Chaudhry AP. Malposed sublingual gland in the anterior mandible: a variant of Staphne's idiopathic bone cavity. Compendium 1991;12(1):40,42–3.

60. Myers MA, Youngberg RA, Bauman JM. Congenital absence of the major salivary glands and impaired lacrimal secretion in a child: case report. J Am Dent Assoc 1994;125(2):210–2.

61. Carney AS, Sharp JF, Cozens NJA. Atypically located submandibular gland diagnosed by Doppler ultrasound. J Laryngol Otol 1996;110(12):1171–2.

62. Rauch S, Gorlin RJ. Diseases of the salivary glands. In: Gorlin RJ, Goldman HM, editors. Thoma's oral pathology. 6th ed. St. Louis: C.V. Mosby; 1970. p.968.

63. Blitzer A. Inflammatory and obstructive disorders of salivary glands. J Dent Res 1987;66:675–81.

64. Adams AM, Macleod RI, Munro CS. Symptomatic and asymptomatic salivary duct abnormalities in Darier's disease: a sialographic study. Dentomaxillofac Radiol 1994;23:25–8.

65. Mandel ID, Wotmans. The salivary secretions in health and disease. Oral Sci Rev 1976;8:25–47.

66. Haring JI. Diagnosing salivary stones. J Am Dent Assoc 1991;122(6):75–6.

67. Levy DM, Remine WH, Devine KD. Salivary gland calculi. JAMA 1962;181:1115–9.

68. Burstein LS, et al. The crystal chemistry of submandibular and parotid salivary gland stones. J Oral Pathol 1979;8:284.

69. Strubel G, Rzepka-Glinder V. Structure and composition of sialoliths. J Clin Chem Clin Biochem 1989;27:244.

70. Zuazua JS, Garcia de la Fuente AM, Rodriguez JCM, et al.

Obstructive sialadenitis caused by intraparotid deposits of gold salts. Oral Surg Oral Med Oral Pathol Oral Radiol Endod 1996;81:649–51.

71. Lustman J, Regeve E, Melamed Y. Sialolithiasis: a survey of 245 patients and review of the literature. Int J Oral Maxillofac Surg 1990;19:135.

72. Stanley MW, Bardales RH, Beneke J, et al. Sialolithiasis differential diagnostic problems in fine-needle aspiration cytology. Am J Clin Pathol 1996;106(2):229–33.

73. Iro H, Zenk J, Benzel W. Laser lithotripsy of salivary duct stones. Adv Otorhinolaryngol 1995;49:148–52.

74. Kater W, Meyer WW, Wehrmann T, et al. Efficacy, risks and limits of extracorporeal shock wave lithotripsy for salivary gland stones. J Endourol 1994;8(1):21–4.

75. Aidan P, de Kerviler E, Le Duc A, Monteil JP. Treatment of salivary stones by extracorporeal lithotripsy. Am J. Otolaryngol 1996;17:246-50.

76. Escudier MP, Drage NA. The management of sialolithiasis in 2 children through use of extracorporeal shock wave lithotripsy. Oral Surg Oral Med Oral Pathol Oral Radiol Endo 1999;88:44-9.

77. Wilcox JW, Hickory R. Nonsurgical resolution of mucoceles. J Oral Surg 1978;36:478.

78. Brannon RB, Fowler CB, Hartman KS. Necrotizing sialometaplasia. A clinicopathologic study of sixty nine cases and review of the literature. Oral Surg Oral Med Oral Pathol 1991;72:317–25.

79. Imbery TA, Edwards PA. Necrolizing sialometaplasia: literature review and case. J Am Dent Assoc 1996;127(7):1087–92.

80. Schroeder WA. Necrolizing sialometaplasia. Otolaryngol Head Neck Surg 1994; 111(3 pt 1): 328–9.

81. Sneige N, Batsakis JG. Necrotizing sialometaplasia. Ann Otol Rhinol Laryngol 1992;101(3):282–4.

82. Schoning H, Emshoff R, Kreczy A. Necrotizing sialometaplasia in two patients with bulimia and chronic vomiting. Int J Oral Maxillofac Surg 1998;27:463–5.

83. Mandel L, Kaynar A, DeChiara S. Necrotizing sialometaplasia in a patient with sickle-cell anemia. J Oral Maxillofac Surg 1991;49(7):757–9.

84. Shannon IL, Trodahl JN, Starcke EN. Radiosensitivity of the human parotid gland. Proc Soc Exp Biol Med 1978;157:50–3.

85. Schubert MM, Izutsu KT. Iatrogenic causes of salivary gland dysfunction. J Dent Res 1987;66:680–7.

86. Toljanic JA, Saunders VW. Radiation therapy and management of the irradiated patient. J Prosthet Dent 1984;52:852–8.

87. Dreizen S, Brown LR, Daly TE, Drane JB. Prevention of xerostomia-related dental caries in irradiated cancer patients. J Dent Res 1977;56:99–104.

88. Mehta M. Amifostine and combined-modality therapeutic approaches. Semin Oncol 1999;26(2 Suppl 7):95–101.

89. Wasserman T. Radioprotective effects of amifostine. Semin Oncol 1999;26(2 Suppl 7):89–94.

90. Shaw LM, Bonner HS, Schuchter L, et al. Pharmacokinetics of amifostine: effects of dose and method of administration. Semin Oncol 1999;26(2 Suppl 7):34–6.

91. Taylor SE, Miller EG. Preemptive pharmacologic intervention in radiation-induced salivary dysfunction. Proc Soc Exp Biol Med 1999;221(1):14–26.

92. Johnson JT, Ferretti GA, Nethery WJ, et al. Oral pilocarpine for postirradiation induced xerostomia in patients with head and neck cancer. N Engl J Med 1993;329:390–5.

93. Andersen SW, Machin D. Acupuncture treatment of patients with radiation-induced xerostomia. Oral Oncol 1997;33(2):146–7.

94. Maier H, Bihl H. Effects of radioactive iodine therapy on parotid gland function. Acta Otolaryngol 1987;103:318–24.

95. Mandel SJ, Mandel L. Persistent sialadenitis after radioactive iodine therapy: report of two cases. J Oral Maxillofac Surg 1999;57:738.

96. Harkness P. Submandibular salivary disease: a proposed allergic aetiology. J Laryngol Otol 1995;109:66–7.

97. Caplan CE. Mumps in the era of vaccines. Can Med Assoc J 1999;160(6);856–66.

98. Measles immunization in HIV-infected children. American Academy of Pediatrics. Committee on Infectious Diseases and Committee on Pediatric AIDS. Pediatrics 1999;103 (5 Pt1);1057–60.

99. Buxton J, Craig C, Daly P, et al. An outbreak of mumps among young adults in Vancouver, British Columbia, associated with "rave"parties. Can J Public Health 1999:90(3):160–3.

100. Bhatt R. Autism, inflammatory bowel disease, and MMR vaccine. Lancet 1998;35:1357.

101. Mumps and mumps vaccine: a global view. Bull World Health Organ 1999;77(1):3–14.

102. Chochi SI. Perspective on the relative resurgence of mumps in the United States. Am J Dis Child 1988;142;499–502.

103. Schubert MM, Sullivan KM, Morton TH, et al. Oral manifestations of chronic graft-vs-host disease. Arch Intern Med 1984;144:1591–5.

104. Woo SB, Lee SJ, Schubert MM. Graft versus host disease. Crit Rev Oral Biol Med 1997;8(2):201–16.

105. Mariette X, Cazals-Hatem D, Agbalika F, et al. Absence of *Cytomegalovirus* and Epstein-Barr virus expression in labial salivary glands of patients with chronic graft-versus-host disease. Bone Marrow Transplant 1996 17(4):607–10.

106. Guntinas-Lichius O, Wagner M, Kruegar GF, Stennert E. Severe CMV sialadenitis in adults is not always an opportunistic infection of AIDS. Int J STD AIDS. 1997;8(3):206–7.

107. O'Sullivan CE, Drew WL, McMullen DJ, et al. Decrease of *Cytomegalovirus* replication in human immunodeficiency virus infected patients after treatment with highly active antiretroviral therapy. J Infect Dis 1999;18(93):847–9.

108. Drew WL, Lalezari JP. *Cytomegalovirus*: disease syndromes and treatment. Curr Clin Top Infect Dis 1999;19:16–29.

109. Zaia JA. Diagnosis of CMV. Pediatr Infect Dis J 1999; 18(2):153–4.

110. Rawlinson WD. Broadsheet number 50: diagnosis of human *Cytomegalovirus* infection and disease. Pathology 1999;31(2):109–15.

111. Zanghellini F, Boppana SB, Emery VC, et al. Asymptomatic primary *Cytomegalovirus* infection; virologic and immunologic features. J Infect Dis 1999;180(3):702–3.

112. Bowen EF. *Cytomegalovirus* reactivation in patients infected with HIV; the use of polymerase chain reaction in prediction and management. Drugs 1999;57(5):735–41.

113. Hayashi T, Lee S, Ogasawara H, et al. Exacerbation of systemic lupus erythematosus related to *Cytomegalovirus* infection. Lupus 1998;7(8):561–4.

114. Maitland N, Flint S, Scully C. Detection of *Cytomegalovirus* and Epstein-Barr virus in labial salivary glands in Sjögren's syndrome and non-specific sialadenitis. J Oral Pathol Med 1995;24:293–8.

115. DiGiuseppe JA, Corio RL, Westra WH. Lymphoid infiltrates of the salivary glands: pathology, biology, and clinical signifi-

cance. Curr Opin Oncol 1996;8:232–7.

116. Fox PC. Saliva and salivary gland alterations in HIV infection. J Am Dent Assoc 1991;122(12):46–8.

117. Schiodt M, Greenspan D, Levy JA, et al. Does HIV cause salivary gland disease? AIDS 1989;3(12):819–22.

118. Schiodt M, Greenspan D, Daniels TE, et al. Parotid gland enlargement and xerostomia associated with labial sialadenitis in HIV-infected patients. J Autoimmun 1989;2(4);415–25.

119. Craven DE, Duncan RA, Stram JR, O'Hara CJ. Response of lymphoepithelial parotid cysts to antiretroviral treatment in HIV-infected adults. Ann Intern Med 1998;128:455–9.

120. Greenberg MS, Glick M, Nghiem L, et al. Relationship of *Cytomegalovirus* to salivary gland dysfunction in HIV infected patients. Oral Surg Oral Med Oral Pathol Oral Radiol Endod 1997;83(3):334–9.

121. Beitler JJ, Smith RV, Brook A, et al. Benign parotid hypertrophy in +HIV patients: limited late failures after external beam radiation. Int J Radiat Oncol Biol Phys 1999;45(2):451–5.

122. Goldstein J, Rubin J, Silver C, et al. Radiation therapy as a treatment for benign lymphoepithelial parotid cysts in patients infected with human immunodeficiency virus-1. Int J Radiat Oncol Biol Phys 1992;23:1045–50.

123. Lustig LR, Lee KC, Murr A, et al. Doxycycline sclerosis of benign lymphoepithelial cysts in patients infected with HIV. Laryngoscope 1998:108:1199–205.

124. Taliani G, Domenico C, Conetta M, et al. Hepatitis C virus infection of salivary gland epithelial cell: lack of evidence. J Hepatol 1997;26;1200–6.

125. Wanchu A, Bambery P, Sud A, et al. Autoimmune hepatitis in a patient with primary Sjögren's syndrome and selective IgA deficiency. Trop Gastroenterol 1998;19(2):62–3.

126. Font J, Tassies D, Garcia-Carrasco M, et al. Hepatitis G virus infection in primary Sjögren's syndrome: analysis in a series of 100 patients. Ann Rheum Dis 1998;57(1):42–4.

127. King PD, McMurray RW, Becherer PR. Sjogren's syndrome with mixed cryoglobulinemia is not associated with hepatitis C virus infection. Am J Gastroenterol 1994;89:1047–50.

128. Marrone A, DiBisceglie AM, Fox P. Absence of hepatitis C viral infection among patients with primary Sjogren's syndrome. J Hepatol 1995;22(5):599.

129. Pawlotsky JM, Roudot-Thoraval F, Simmonds P, et al. Extrahepatic manifestations in chronic hepatitis C and hepatitis C virus serotypes. Ann Intern Med 1995;122:169–73.

130. Haddad J, Deny P, Munz-Gotheil C, et al. Lymphocytic sialadenitis associated with chronic hepatitis C virus liver diseases. Lancet 1992;339:321–3.

131. Scott CA, Avellini C, Desinan L, et al. Chronic lymphocytic sialadenitis in HCV-related chronic liver disease: comparison with Sjogren's syndrome. Histopathology 1997;30:41–8.

132. Pirisi M, Scott C, Ferracciolo G, et al. Mild sialadenitis: a common finding in patients with hepatitis C virus infection. Scand J Gastroenterol 1994;29:940–2.

133. Glick M. Know thy hepatitis: A through TT. J Calif Dent Assoc 1999;27(5):376–85.

134. Lodi G, Porter SR, Scully C. Hepatitis C virus infection: review and implications for the dentist. Oral Surg Oral Med Oral Pathol Oral Radiol Endod 1998;86(1):8–22.

135. Coll J, Gambus G, Corominas J, et al. Immunohistochemistry of minor salivary gland biopsy specimens from patients with Sjögren's syndrome with and without hepatitis C virus. Ann Rheum Dis 1997;56(6):390–2.

136. Lichen planus and Sjögren's-type sicca syndrome in patients with chronic hepatitis C. J Dermatol 1997;24(1):20–7.

137. Gordon SC. Extrahepatic manifestations of hepatitis. Dig Dis 1996;14(3):157–68.

138. Biasi D, Colombari R, Achille A, et al. HCV RNA detection in parotid gland biopsy in a patient with liver disease. Acta Gastroenterol Belg 1995;58(5–6):465–9.

139. Lindgren S, Manthorpe R, Eriksson S. Autoimmune liver disease in patients with Sjögren's syndrome. J Hepatol 1994;20(3):354–8.

140. Durand JM, Lefevre P, Kaplanski G, et al. Sjögren's syndrome and hepatitis C virus infection. Clin Rheumatol 1995;14(5):570–1.

141. Sorrentino D, Ferraccioli GF, DeVita S, et al. Hepatitis C virus infection and gastric lymphoproliferatation in patients with Sjögren's syndrome. Blood 1997;90(5):2116–7.

142. Fox PC. Bacterial infections of salivary glands. Curr Opin Dent 1991;1:411–4.

143. Raad II, Sabbagh MF, Caranasos GJ. Acute bacterial sialadenitis: a study of 29 cases and review. Rev Infect Dis 1990;12(4);591–601.

144. Goldberg MH, Bevilacqua RG. Infections of salivary glands. Oral Maxillofac Surg Clin North Am 1995;7(3):423–30.

145. Mandel ID. Sialochemistry in diseases and clinical situations affecting salivary glands. Crit Rev Clin Lab Sci 1980;12:321–66.

146. Fox PC. Salivary monitoring in oral diseases. Ann N Y Acad Sci 1993;694:234-7.

147. Mandel ID, Wotman S. The salivary secretions in health and disease. Oral Sci Rev 1976;8:25-47. Colevas AD. Sialedenosis: a presenting sign in bulimia. Head Neck 1999;21:582.

148. Harrison R, Bowen WH. Flow rate and organic constituents of whole saliva in insulin-dependent diabetic children and adolescents. Pediatric Dent 1987;9(4):287–91.

149. Twentman S, Nederfors T, Stahl B, Aronson S. Two-year longitudinal observations of salivary status and dental caries in children with insulin-dependent diabetes mellitus. Pediatr Dent 1992;14:184–8.

150. Ship et al

151. Chavez EM, Taylor GW, Borrell LN, Ship JA. Salivary function and glycemic control in older persons with diabetes. Oral Surg Oral Med Oral Pathol Oral Radiol Endod 2000;89(3);305–11.

152. Cherry-Peppers G, Sorkin J, Andres R, et al. Salivary gland function and glucose metabolic status. J Gerontol 1992; 47(4):M130–4.

153. Sreebny LM, Yu A, Green A, Valdini A. Xerostomia in diabetes mellitus. Diabetes Care 1992;15(7):900–4.

154. Meurman JH, Collin HL, Niskanen L, et al. Saliva in non-insulin dependent diabetic patients and control subjects: a role of the autonomic nervous system. Oral Surg Oral Med Oral Pathol Oral Radiol Endod 1998;86(1):69–76.

155. Dodds M, Dodds A. Effects of glycemic control on salivary flow rates and protein composition in non-insulin dependent diabetes mellitus. Oral Surg Oral Med Oral Pathol Oral Radiol Endod 1997;83:465-70.

156. Coleman H, Altini M, Nayler S, Richards A. Sialadenosis: a presenting sign in bulimia. Head Neck 1998;20(8):758–62.

157. Metzger ED, Levine JM, McArdle CR, Wolfe BE. Salivary gland enlargement and elevated serum amylase in bulimia nervosa. Biol Psychiatry 1999 45(11):1520–2.

158. Kinzl J, Biebl W, Herold M. Significance of vomiting for hyperamylasemia and sialadenosis in patients with eating disorders. Int J Eat Disord 1993;13(1):117–24.

159. Dutta SK, Orestes M, Vengulekur S, Kwo P. Ethanol and human saliva: effects of chronic alcoholism on flow rate, composition, epidermal growth factor. Am J Gastroenterol 1992;87(3):350–4.

160. Dutta SK, Dukehart M, Narang A, Latham PS. Functional and structural changes in parotid glands of alcoholic cirrhotic patients. Gastroenterology 1988;16(4):215–8.

161. Anavi Y, Mintz S. Benign lymphoepithelial lesion of the sublingual gland. J Oral Maxillofac Surg 1992;50(10):1111–3.

162. Lee ST, Raman R, Tay A. Benign lymphoepithelial lesion of the submandibular glands. Otolaryngol Head Neck Surg 1987;97(6):580–2.

163. Fox RI, Kang HI. Pathogenesis of Sjögren's syndrome. Rheum Dis Clin North Am 1992;18:517-38.

164. Greenspan J, Daniels T, Talal N, Sylvester R. The histopathology of Sjögren's syndrome in labial salivary gland biopsies. Oral Surg Oral Med Oral Pathol 1974;37:217–29.

165. Atkinson JC, Travis WD, Pillemer SR, et al. Major salivary gland function in primary Sjögren's syndrome and it's relationship to clinical features. J Rheumatol 1990;17:318–22.

166. Fox RI, Saito I. Criteria for diagnosis of Sjogren's syndrome. Rheum Dis Clin North Am 1994;20(2):391–407.

167. Vitali C, Moutsopoulos HM, Bombardieri S. The European Community Study Group on diagnostic criteria for Sjogren's syndrome. Sensitivity and specificity of tests for ocular and oral involvement in Sjogren's syndrome. Ann Rheum Dis 1994;53:637–47.

168. Fox R. Classification criteria for Sjogren's syndrome. Rheum Dis Clin North Am 1994;20:391–407.

169. Fox RI, Howell FV, Bone RC, Michelson P. Primary Sjögren's syndrome and immunologic features. Semin Arthritis Rheum 1984;14:77-105.

170. Fox PC, Brennan M, Pillemer S, et al. Sjogren's syndrome: a model for dental care in the 21st century. J Am Dent Assoc 1988;129:719–28.

171. Atkinson JC. Sjogren's syndrome: oral and dental considerations. J Am Dent Assoc 1993;124:74–86.

172. Fox PC. Systemic therapy of salivary gland hypofunction. J Dent Res 1987;66:689–92.

173. Johnson JT, Ferretti GA, Nethery WJ. Oral pilocarpine for postradiation induced xerostomia in patients with head and neck cancer. N Engl J Med 1993;11:149–56.

174. Fox RI, Petrone D, Condemi J, Fife R. Randomized placebo controlled trial of SNI-2011, a novel M3 muscarinic receptor agonist for the treatment of Sjogren's syndrome. Arthritis Rheum 1998;41(9):580.

175. Ship JA, Fox PC, Michalek JE, et al. Treatment of primary Sjogren's syndrome with low dose natural interferon-alpha administered by the oral mucosal route: a phase II clinical trial. J Interferon Cytokine Res 1999;19:943–51.

176. Daniels TE. Labial salivary gland biopsy in Sjogren's syndrome: assessmant as a diagnostic criterion in 362 suspected cases. Arthritis Rheum 1984;27:147–56.

177. Kassan SS, Thomas TL, Moutosopoulos HM, et al. Increased risk of lymphoma in sicca syndrome. Ann Intern Med 1978;89:888–92.

178. Rowe-Jones JM, Vowles R, Leighton SE, Freedman AR. Diffuse tuberculous parotitis. J Laryngol Otol 1992;106(12):1094–5.

179. Weiner GM, Pahor AL. Tuberculous parotitis: limiting the role of surgery. J Laryngol Otol 1996;110(1):96–7.

180. James DG, Sharma OP. Parotid gland sarcoidosis. Sarcoidosis Vasc Diffuse Lung Dis 2000;17(1):27–32.

181. Beely JA, Chisholm DM. Sarcoidosis with salivary gland involvement: biochemical studies on parotid saliva. J Lab Clin Med 1976;88:276–81.

182. Harvey J, Catoggio L, Gallagher PJ, Maddison PJ. Salivary gland biopsy in sarcoidosis. Sarcoidosis 1989;6(1):47–50.

183. Frost-Larsen K, Isager H, Manthorpe R. Bromhexine treatment of Sjogren's syndrome: effect on lacrimal and salivary secretion and on proteins in tear fluid and saliva. Scand J Rheumatol 1981;10:177–80.

184. Prause JV, Frost-Larsen K, Hoj L. Lacrimal and salivary secretion in Sjogren's syndrome: the effect of systemic treatment with bromhexine. Acta Opthalmol 1984;62:189–97.

185. Lelard G, Mercat C, Fuseiller C. Action favourable du trithioparamethoxyphenylpropene sur le complications salivaries des traitments psychotrope. Rev Med Tours 1969;3:343–4.

186. De Buck R, Titeca R, Pelc I. Etude controlee de l'action de l'Anetholtrithione sur les aisialies et les hyposialies provoquees par les medicaments psychotropices. 1973;73:510–9.

187. Valdez IH, Wolff A, Atkinson JC. Use of pilocarpine during head and neck radiation therapy to reduce xerostomia and salivary gland dysfuction. Cancer 1993;71(50):1848–52.

188. Fox PC, Vander ven PF, Baum BJ. Pilocarpine for the treatment of xerostomia associated with salivary gland dysfuction. J Oral Surg 1986;61:243–8.

189. Iwabuchi Y, Masuhara T. Sialogogic activities of SNI–2011 compared with those of pilocarpine and Mcn=A-343 in rat salivary glands. Identification of a potential therapeutic agent for treatment of Sjogren's syndrome. Gen Pharmacol 1994; 25(1):123–9.

190. Marks L, Turner K, O'Sullivan J, et al. Drooling in Parkinson's disease: a novel speech and language therapy intervention. Int J Lang Commun Disord 2001;36 Suppl:282–7.

191. Spiro RH. Diagnosis and pitfalls in the treatment of parotid tumors. Semin Surg Oncol 1991;7:20–4.

192. Carlson ER. Salivary gland tumors: classification, histogenesis, and general considerations. Oral Maxillofac Surg Clin North Am 1995;7(3):519–27.

193. Everson JW, Cawson RA. Salivary gland tumors. A review of 2,410 cases with particular reference to histologic type, site, age, and sex distribution. J Pathol 1985;146:51–8.

194. Main JHP, Orr JA, McGurk FM, et al. Salivary gland tumors: review of 643 cases. J Oral Pathol 1976;5:88–102.

195. Eisele DW, Johns ME. Salivary gland neoplasms. In: Bailey BJ, editor. Head and neck surgery-otolaryngology. Vol. 2. Philadelphia: J.B. Lippincott Co.; 1993. p. 1125–47.

196. Salivary gland disease. In: Regazi J, Sciubba J, editors. Oral pathology. Philadelphia: W.B. Saunders Co.; 1993. p. 239–302.

197. Batsakis JG, Brannon RB, Sciubba JJ. Monomorphic adenomas of salivary glands: a histologic study of 96 tumors. Clin Otolaryngol 1981;6:129–43.

198. Spiro RH. Salivary neoplasms: overview of a 35 year experience with 2,807 patients. Head Neck Surg 1986;8:177–84.

199. Johns ME, Regazi JA, Batsakis JG. Oncocytic neoplasms of the salivary glands. Laryngoscope 1977;87:862.

200. Spiro RH, Dubner S. Salivary gland tumors. Curr Opin Oncol 1990;2:589–95.

201. Rice DH. Salivary gland disorders: neoplastic and nonneoplastic. Med Clin North Am 1999;83(1):197–218.

202. Spiro RH. Changing trends in the management of salivary tumors. Semin Surg Oncol 1995;11;240–5.

203. Calearo C, Storchi OF, Pastore A, Polli G. Parotid gland carci-

noma: analysis of prognostic factors. Ann Otol Rhinol Laryngol 1998;107:969–73.

204. Stafford ND, Wilde A. Parotid cancer. Surg Oncol 1997; 6(4):209–13.

205. Szanto P, Luna M, Tortoledo ME, White RA. Histopathologic grading of adenoid cystic carcinoma of the salivary glands. Cancer 1984;54:1062.

206. Virkam B, Strong EW, Shah JP, Spiro RH. Radiation therapy in adenoid cystic carcinoma. Int J Radiat Oncol Biol Phys 1984;10:221.

207. Van der Waal JE, Snow GB, Karim AB, Van der Waal I. Intraoral adenoid cystic carcinoma. The role of postoperative radiotherapy in local control. Head Neck 1989;11(6):497–9.

208. Mehle M, Kraus D, Wood BG, et al. Lymphoma of the parotid gland. Laryngoscope 1993;103;17–21.

209. Parsons JT, Mendenhall WM, Stringer SP, et al. Management of minor salivary gland carcinomas. Int J Radiat Oncol Biol Phys 1996;35(3):443-54.

210. Eschwege F. Management of minor salivary gland carcinomas. Int J Radiat Oncol Biol Phys 1996;35(3):631-2.

211. Lopes MA, Kowalski LP, da Cunha Santos G, Paes de Almeida O. A clinicopathologic study of 196 intraoral minor salivary gland tumours. J Oral Pathol Medicine 1999;28(6):264-7.

212. Spiro RH. Management of malignant tumors of the salivary glands. Oncology 1998;12:671–80.

213. Moody AB, Avery CME, Taylor J, Langdon JD. A comparison of one hundred and fifty consecutive parotidectomies for tumors and inflammatory disease. J Oral Maxillofac Surg 1999;28:211–5.

214. Tugnoli V, Anna AS, Marchese Ragona R, et al. Treatment of Frey syndrome with botulinum toxin type F. Arch Otolaryngol Head Neck Surg 2001;127(3):339–40.

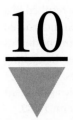

10

TEMPOROMANDIBULAR DISORDERS

BRUCE BLASBERG, DMD, FRCD(C)
MARTIN S. GREENBERG, DDS

This chapter focuses on the assessment and management of disorders of the masticatory system. The masticatory apparatus is a specialized unit that performs multiple functions, including those of suckling, speaking, cutting and grinding food, and swallowing. The loss of these functions in association with pain is characteristic of masticatory system disorders and causes significant distress that can be severely disabling.

In the past, disorders of the masticatory system were generally treated as one condition or syndrome, with no attempt to differentiate subtypes of muscle and joint disorders. With increased understanding, the ability to identify different muscle or joint disorders has become possible; this should lead to a better understanding of the natural course, more accurate predictions on prognosis, and more effective treatments of temporomandibular disorders (TMD). The term "temporomandibular disorders" (TMD), used in this chapter, is a collective term embracing a number of clinical problems that involve the masticatory musculature, the temporomandibular joint (TMJ) and associated structures, or both.[1] These disorders are characterized by (1) facial pain in the region of the TMJ and/or the muscles of mastication, (2) limitation or deviation in the mandibular range of motion, and (3) TMJ sounds during jaw movement and function.[2]

The cause of most TMD remains unknown although numerous hypotheses have been proposed. The relationship of occlusal disharmony and TMD became a focus after Costen reported that a group of patients with multiple complaints around the jaws and ears improved after their occlusal-vertical dimension was altered.[3] The occlusal hypothesis was then expanded to include other occlusal discrepancies in addition to loss of vertical dimension.[4] During the 1950s and 1960s, a muscular cause not directly related to occlusion was proposed.[5–7] In the late 1970s, advances in diagnostic imaging resulted in a better understanding of the intracapsular problems associated with TMD.[8,9] The lack of a clear understanding with regard to cause, the existence of multiple hypotheses,

and strongly held beliefs by some clinicians have resulted in a wide spectrum of treatments being offered. Standardized methods for assessment, classification, and treatment do not exist, and this has impeded the ability to interpret the existing research and make comparisons between studies. This chapter presents a general approach to the diagnostic assessment and nonsurgical management of the most common TMD.

▼ FUNCTIONAL ANATOMY

Temporomandibular Joint

The TMJ articulation is classified as a ginglymodiarthrodial joint, namely, a joint that is capable of hinge-type movements (ginglymos) and gliding movements, with the bony components enclosed and connected by a fibrous capsule. The mandibular condyle forms the lower part of the bony joint and is generally elliptical although variations in shape are common.[10] The articulation is formed by the mandibular condyle occupying a hollow in the temporal bone (the mandibular or glenoid fossa) (Figures 10-1 and 10-2). The S-shaped form of the fossa and eminence develops at about 6 years of age and continues into the second decade.[11] During wide mouth opening, the condyle rotates around a hinge axis and glides, causing it to move beyond the anterior border of the fossa, the articular eminence.[12] The TMJ has a rigid end point when the teeth contact.

The capsule is lined with synovium and the joint cavity is filled with synovial fluid. Synovial tissue is a vascular connective tissue lining the fibrous joint capsule and extending to the boundaries of the articulating surfaces. Both upper and lower joint cavities are lined with synovium. Synovial fluid is a filtrate of plasma with added mucins and proteins. Its main constituent is hyaluronic acid. Fluid forms on the articulating surfaces, decreasing friction during joint compression and motion.[13] Joint lubrication is achieved by mechanisms described as weeping lubrication and boundary lubrication. Weeping lubrica-

FIGURE 10-1 The S-shaped form of the fossa and eminence develops at about 6 years and continues into the second decade. The mandibular condyle occupies the space of the fossa, with enough room to both rotate and translate during mandibular movements.

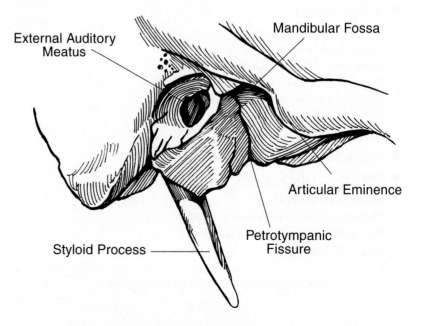

External Auditory Meatus

Mandibular Fossa

Articular Eminence

Styloid Process

Petrotympanic Fissure

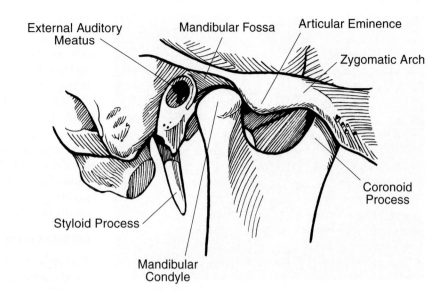

FIGURE 10-2 The articulation is formed by the mandibular condyle occupying a hollow in the temporal bone (the mandibular or glenoid fossa) during wide mouth opening, the condyle rotates around an axis and glides, causing it to move beyond the anterior border of the fossa, the articular eminence.

tion occurs as fluid is forced laterally during compression and expressed through the unloaded fibrocartilage. As the adjacent areas become loaded, this weeping lubrication aids in reducing friction. Boundary lubrication is a function of water physically bound to the cartilaginous surface by a glycoprotein.

The distinguishing features of this joint include a covering of fibrocartilage over the articulating surfaces, rather than hyaline cartilage and its bilaterality. Fibrocartilage is less distensible than hyaline cartilage due to a greater number of collagen fibers. The matrix and chondrocytes are decreased because of the larger irregular bundles of collagen fibers. Fibrocartilage derives its nutrition from the diffusion of nutrients into the synovial fluid; these then diffuse through the dense matrix to the chondrocytes.

ARTICULAR DISK

The space between the condyle and mandibular fossa is occupied by collagenous fibrous tissue of variable thickness, called the articular disk (Figures 10-3 and 10-4). The disk consists of collagen fibers, cartilage-like proteoglycans[14] and elastic fibers.[15] The disk contains variable numbers of cartilage cells and is referred to as a fibrocartilage. The collagen fibers in the center of the disk are oriented perpendicular to its transverse axis. The collagen fibers become interlaced as they approach the anterior and posterior bands, and many fibers are oriented parallel to the mediolateral aspect of the disk. The cartilage-like proteoglycans contribute to the compressive stiffness of articular cartilage.[16] The disk is attached to the lateral and medial poles of the condyle by ligaments consisting of collagen and elastic fibers.[17] These ligaments permit rotational movement of the disk on the condyle during the opening and closing of the jaw. The disk is thinnest in its center and thickens to form anterior and posterior bands. This arrangement is considered to help stabilize the condyle in the glenoid fossa. The disk is primarily avascular and has little sensory nerve penetration.

The disk provides an interface for the condyle as it glides across the temporal bone. The disk and its attachments divide

the joint into upper and a lower compartments that normally do not communicate. The passive volume of the upper compartment is estimated to be 1.2 mL, and that of the lower compartment is estimated to be 0.9 mL.[17] The roof of the superior compartment is the mandibular fossa whereas the floor is the superior surface of the disk. The roof of the inferior compartment is the inferior surface of the disk, and the floor is the artic-

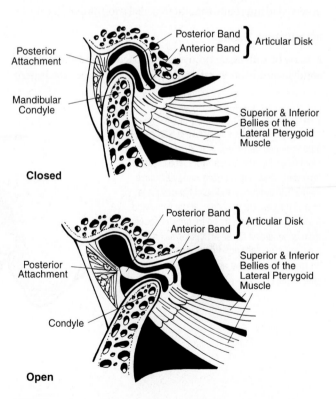

FIGURE 10-3 The temporomandibular joint is a ginglymoarthrodial joint that is capable of hinge-type movements and gliding movements. The articular disk has ligamentous attachments to the mandibular fossa and condyle. The disk's attachments create separate superior and inferior joint compartments.

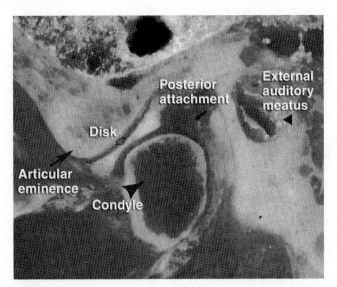

FIGURE 10-4 A cadaver section through the temporomandibular joint shows the relationship of the condyle, fossa, and articular disk.

ulating surface of the mandibular condyle.[17] At its margins, the disk blends with the fibrous capsule. Muscle attachments inserting into the anterior aspect of the disk have been observed.[18] Fibers of the posterior one-third of the temporalis muscle and deep masseter muscle may attach on the anterolateral aspect.[18] Fibers of the superior head of the lateral pterygoid have been observed to insert into the anteromedial two-thirds of the disk.[18]

RETRODISCAL TISSUE

A mass of soft tissue occupies the space behind the disk and condyle and is often referred to as the posterior attachment.

The posterior attachment is a loosely organized system of collagen fibers, branching elastic fibers, fat, blood and lymph vessels, and nerves. Synovium covers the superior and inferior surfaces. The attachment has been described as being arranged in two laminae of dense connective tissue,[19] but this has been challenged.[20] Between the laminae, a loose areolar, highly vascular, and well-innervated tissue has been described. The superior lamina arises from the posterior band of the disk and attaches to the squamotympanic fissure and consists primarily of elastin.[19] The inferior lamina arises from the posterior band of the disk and inserts into the inferior margin of the posterior articular slope of the condyle and is composed mostly of collagen fibers.[19]

CAPSULAR LIGAMENT

The capsular ligament is a thin inelastic fibrous connective-tissue envelope that attaches to the margins of the articular surfaces (Figure 10-5). The fibers are mainly oriented vertically and do not restrain joint movements.

TEMPOROMANDIBULAR LIGAMENT

The temporomandibular ligament is the main ligament of the joint, lateral to the capsule but not easily separated from it by dissection. Its fibers pass obliquely from bone lateral to the articular tubercle in a posterior and inferior direction and insert in a narrower area below and behind the lateral pole of the condyle (see Figure 10-5). In earlier literature, this ligament was identified as an oblique band from the condylar neck to the anterosuperior region on the eminence and as a horizontal band from the lateral condylar pole to an anterior attachment of the eminence.[17] A recent study was unable to confirm two distinct structures separate from the capsule.[21]

FIGURE 10-5 The capsular ligament is a thin inelastic fibrous connective-tissue envelope, oriented vertically, that attaches to the margins of the articular surfaces. The capsular ligament does not restrain condylar movements. The temporomandibular ligament is lateral to the capsule but is not easily separated from it by dissection. Its fibers pass obliquely from bone lateral to the articuular tubercle in a posterior and inferior direction to insert in a narrower area below and behind the lateral pole of the condyle.

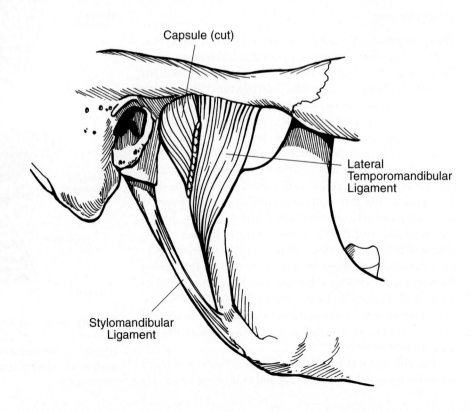

Muscles Associated with Mandibular Movement and Function

MUSCLES OF MASTICATION

The muscles of mastication are the paired masseter, medial and lateral pterygoid, and temporalis muscles (Figures 10-6, 10–7, and 10-8). Mandibular movements toward the tooth contact position are performed by contraction of the masseter, temporalis, and medial pterygoid muscles. Masseter contraction also contributes to moving the condylar head toward the anterior slope of the mandibular fossa. The posterior part of the temporalis contributes to mandibular retrusion, and unilateral contraction of the medial pterygoid contributes to a contralateral movement of the mandible. The masseter and medial pterygoid muscles have their insertions at the inferior border of the mandibular angle. They join together to form a sling that cradles the mandible and produces the powerful forces required for chewing. The masseter is divided into a deep portion and a superficial portion.

The temporalis muscle is broadly attached to the lateral skull and has been divided into anterior, middle, and posterior parts. The muscle fibers converge into a tendon that inserts on the coronoid process and anterior aspect of the mandibular ramus. The anterior and middle fibers are generally oriented in a straight line from their origin on the skull to their insertion on the mandible. The posterior part traverses anteriorly then curves around the anterior root of the zygomatic process before insertion.

The lateral pterygoid is the main protrusive and opening muscle of the mandible. It is arranged in parallel-fibered units whereas the other muscles are multipennated. This arrangement allows greater displacement and velocity in the lateral pterygoid and greater force generation in the jaw-closing muscles.[22] The lateral pterygoid muscle is divided into two parts. The inferior part arises from the outer surface of the lateral pterygoid plate of the sphenoid and the pyramidal process of the palatine bone. The superior part originates from the greater wing of the sphenoid and the pterygoid ridge. The fibers of the upper and lower heads course posteriorly and laterally, fusing in front of the condyle.[23] They insert into the anteromedial aspect of the condylar neck. Some of the fibers insert into the most anterior medial portion of the disk, but most of the lateral pterygoid fibers insert into the condyle.[23] Debate continues about the functional anatomy of the lateral pterygoid. The superior head is thought to be active during closing movements, and the inferior head is thought to be active during opening and protrusive movements.[24–26] Translation of the condylar head onto the articular eminence is produced by contraction of the lateral pterygoid.

ACCESSORY TO MASTICATORY MUSCLES

The digastric muscle is a paired muscle with two bellies. The anterior belly attaches to the lingual aspect of the mandible at the parasymphysis and courses backward to insert into a

FIGURE 10-6 The masseter and medial pterygoid muscles have their insertions at the inferior border of the mandibular angle. They join together to form a sling that cradles the ramus of the mandible and produces the powerful forces required for chewing. The masseter muscle has been divided into a deep portion and a superficial portion.

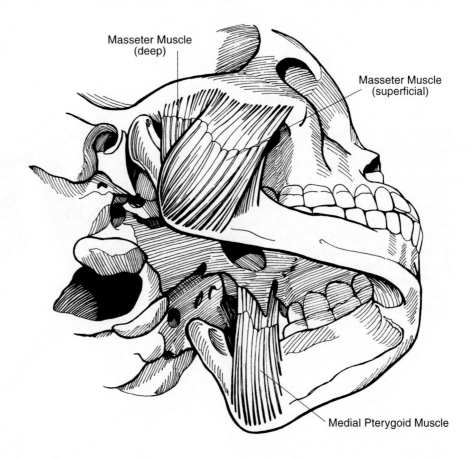

Masseter Muscle (deep)

Masseter Muscle (superficial)

Medial Pterygoid Muscle

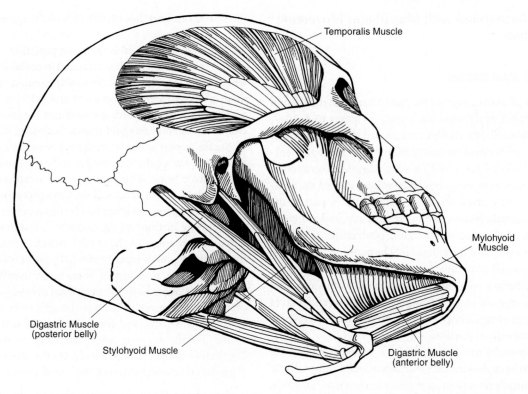

FIGURE 10-7   The digastric muscle is a paired muscle with two bellies. The anterior belly attaches to the lingual aspect of the mandible at the parasymphysis and courses backward to insert into a round tendon attached to the hyoid bone. Contraction produces a depression and retropositioning of the mandible. The mylohyoid and geniohyoid muscles contribute to depressing the mandible when the infrahyoid muscles stabilize the hyoid bone during mandibular movement. These muscles may also contribute to retrusion of the mandible. The temporalis muscle is broadly attached to the lateral skull. The muscle fibers converge to insert on the coronoid process and anterior aspect of the mandibular ramus. The posterior part traverses anteriorly then curves around the anterior root of the zygomatic process before insertion. The posterior part of the temporalis contributes to mandibular retrusion.

FIGURE 10-8   The lateral pterygoid muscle is the main protrusive and opening muscle of the mandible. It is arranged in parallel-fibered units that allow for greater displacement and velocity than that of the multipennated closing muscles. The lateral pterygoid muscle is divided into two parts. The inferior part arises from the outer surface of the lateral pterygoid plate of the sphenoid and the pyramidal process of the palatine bone. The superior part originates from the greater wing of the sphenoid and the pterygoid ridge. The fibers of the upper and lower heads course posteriorly and laterally, fusing in front of the temporomandibular joint. They insert into the anteromedial aspect of the condylar neck. Some of the fibers insert into the most anterior medial portion of the disk, but most of the lateral pterygoid fibers insert into the condyle. Translation of the condylar head onto the articular eminence is produced by contraction of the lateral pterygoid.

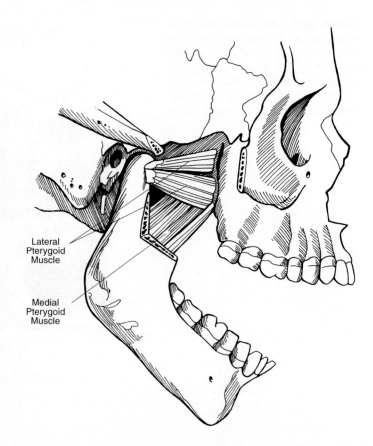

round tendon attached to the hyoid bone. Contraction produces a depression and retropositioning of the mandible. The mylohyoid and geniohyoid muscles contribute to depressing the mandible when the infrahyoid muscles stabilize the hyoid bone during mandibular movement. These muscles may also contribute to retrusion of the mandible. The buccinator attaches inferiorly along the facial surface of the mandible, just behind the mental foramen and superiorly high on the alveolar surface behind the zygomatic process. The fibers are arranged horizontally. Anteriorly, fibers insert into mucosa, skin, and lip. The buccinator helps position the cheek during chewing movements of the mandible.

Vascular Supply of Temporomandibular Structures

The external carotid artery is the main blood supply for the temporomandibular structures. The artery leaves the neck and courses superiorly and posteriorly, embedded in the substance of the parotid gland. The artery sends two important branches, the lingual and facial arteries, to supply the region. At the level of the condylar neck, the external carotid bifurcates into the superficial temporal artery and the internal maxillary artery. These two arteries supply the muscles of mastication and the TMJ. Arteries within the temporal bone or mandible may also send branches to the capsule.

Nerve Supply of Temporomandibular Structures

The masticatory structures are innervated primarily by the trigeminal nerve, but cranial nerves VII, IX, X, and XI and cervical nerves 2 and 3 also contribute. The peripheral nerves synapse with nuclei in the brainstem that are associated with touch, proprioception, and motor function. The large spinal trigeminal nucleus occupies a major part of the brainstem and extends to the spinal cord. The spinal trigeminal nucleus is thought to be the main site for the reception of impulses from the periphery involved in pain sensation. The mandibular division of the trigeminal supplies motor innervation to the muscles of mastication and the anterior belly of the digastric muscle. Branches of the auriculotemporal nerve supply the sensory innervation of the TMJ; this nerve arises from the mandibular division in the infratemporal fossa and sends branches to the capsule of the joint (Figure 10-9). The deep temporal and masseteric nerves supply the anterior portion of the joint. These nerves are primarily motor nerves, but they contain sensory fibers distributed to the anterior part of the TMJ capsule. The autonomic nerve supply is carried to the joint by the auriculotemporal nerve and by nerves traveling along the superficial temporal artery.

JAW JERK REFLEX

The jaw jerk reflex is analogous to the knee jerk reflex. It is a stretch reflex whereby stretching the jaw-closing muscles (by applying a downward tap on the chin) produces a reflex contraction of these muscles. It demonstrates the existence of a feedback loop from the jaw-closing muscles to their own motor neurons in the central nervous system. This reflex is thought to relate to the fine control of jaw movements to take into account different consistencies of food.[27]

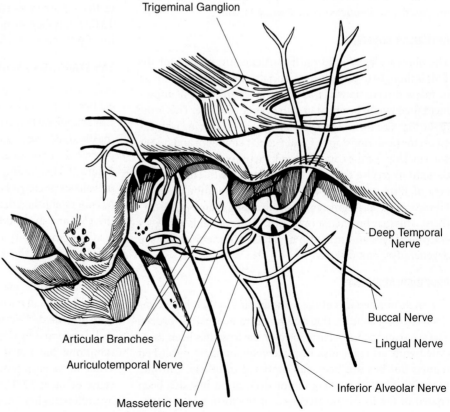

FIGURE 10-9 Branches of the auriculotemporal nerve supply sensory innervation of the TMJ. This nerve arises from the mandibular division in the infratemporal fossa and sends branches to the capsule of the joint.

Trigeminal Ganglion

Deep Temporal Nerve

Buccal Nerve

Lingual Nerve

Inferior Alveolar Nerve

Articular Branches

Auriculotemporal Nerve

Masseteric Nerve

JAW-OPENING REFLEX

Stimulating mechanoreceptors within the mouth or nociceptors from the mouth or face triggers the jaw-opening reflex. The pathway is polysynaptic; the first synapse is in either the trigeminal sensory nuclei or the adjacent reticular formation, and the final synapse is in the trigeminal motor nucleus. The reflex results in an inhibition of the activity of the jaw-closing muscles. This reflex is thought to help prevent injury when biting or chewing objects that may cause damage.[27]

Anatomy of Clinical Interest

REST POSITION

When the mandible is not functionally active, it adopts a rest position in which the condyle occupies a relatively central position in the glenoid fossa and in which the teeth are separated. This position varies for a number of reasons (including head posture and levels of muscle activity) and is not an exact position.

RANGE OF MANDIBULAR MOVEMENT

The position of widest mouth opening is associated with the condyle moving to the crest of the articular eminence or beyond. A wide variation in mandibular movement exists. Incisor displacement remains the most common diagnostic indicator.[28] The temporomandibular, sphenomandibular, and stylomandibular ligaments, together with the articular eminence, have been suggested as the main constraints of jaw opening.[29] Muscular constraint of jaw opening has also been proposed as a significant contributing factor.[30]

ARTICULAR COVERING

The fibrocartilage found on the articulating surfaces of the TMJ is thought to provide more surface strength against forces in many directions while allowing more freedom of movement than would be possible with hyaline cartilage. This is the tissue that also forms the articular disk. This covering is thickest on the posterior slope of the articular eminence and on the anterior slope of the condylar head; these are the areas that are thought to receive the greatest functional load. The thinnest area of fibrocartilage is the roof of the mandibular fossa. Fibrocartilage has a greater repairing ability than hyaline cartilage. This may be a factor in how the TMJ responds to degenerative changes and may also be a factor in the treatment of degenerative joint disease.[31]

DISK DISPLACEMENTS

The angle or steepness of the mandibular fossa has been considered to be a contributing factor in intra-articular disorders. The steep and more vertical form of the fossa has been associated with articular disk displacements in some published reports but has not been substantiated in others. Chronic recurring condyle subluxation or dislocation has also been related to the form and steepness of the fossa and articular eminence. Surgical treatments that increase the steepness or flatten the eminence have been proposed.

Demonstration of the lateral pterygoid's attachment to the anterior articular disk has led to the theory that at least some anterior disk displacements may be related to lateral pterygoid-muscle dysfunction. The theory suggests that hyperactivity of the superior head of the lateral pterygoid may be capable of pulling the disk forward, displacing it from its normal position over the mandibular condyle.[32] Research on cadaver specimens has indicated that muscle fibers inserting into the disk or the condyle are not differentiated into inferior and superior heads.[23,33] The fibers that do insert into the disk are located primarily at the medial portion. Carpentier postulated that the two heads did not have distinct independent actions and that the lateral pterygoid was not a significant cause of disk displacement.[23] While "clicking" has been described as the most common irregularity detected during clinical examination, disk displacement may occur in the absence of clinical findings.[34]

OCCLUSION

The intercuspal position is a position of the mandible in which maximum intercuspation of opposing teeth occurs.[35] Occlusal stability has been defined as "the equalization of contacts that prevents tooth movement after closure."[36] A physiologic occlusion has been defined as "an occlusion in which a functional equilibrium or state of homeostasis exists between all tissues of the masticatory system."[37] There is general agreement that occlusal forces at the intercuspal position are best directed toward the long axes of teeth.[38,39] A reduced number of contacting teeth in the intercuspal position and loss of posterior teeth have been reported as risk factors for the development of TMD,[40] but they are not likely to be major causes in the majority of patients with TMD.

EAR SYMPTOMS ASSOCIATED WITH TMD

A ligament between the disk and the malleolus of the middle ear has been observed in some anatomic specimens. The superior retrodiscal lamina has been considered to be a remnant of the discomalleolar ligament of the fetus, connecting the lateral pterygoid tendon to the malleus through the squamotympanic fissure.[41] This finding has been used to speculate about the prevalence of ear or hearing symptoms in TMD, but research has not established that this is a functioning ligament between the TMJ and the middle ear.[42]

Close proximity of the auriculotemporal nerve to the medial aspect of the condyle has been described. Extension of the medial wall of the fossa, exposing the auriculotemporal nerve to possible mechanical irritation in circumstances in which the articular disk becomes displaced medially, has also been described.[43] Nerve entrapment or compression was originally proposed by Costen as the explanation for pain and ear symptoms but was discounted by subsequent investigators. While nerve entrapment or compression is probably not the cause of most TMD, it reflects the need to review existing hypotheses in light of new information.

INJECTION SITES

TMJ injections may be part of diagnostic assessment or therapy. The site of injection should be anterior to the tragus to minimize the risk of intravascular injection of the external carotid artery or the accompanying vein. Because the auriculotemporal nerve enters the capsule from the medial aspect, injections (normally given from the lateral aspect) may not completely anesthetize the joint.[44]

PALPATION EXAMINATION

Examination of the lateral pterygoid muscle by intraoral palpation has been challenged because of the inaccessibility of the muscle (Figure 10-10).[45] The technique is likely to cause discomfort in individuals without a TMD, diminishing its value as a diagnostic test.[46]

The fibers of the deep masseter muscle are intimately related to the lateral wall of the joint capsule. This makes differentiating pain to palpation of this area difficult.[47,48]

JAW JERK REFLEX AND THE SILENT PERIOD

A prolonged period of electrical inactivity on electromyography recordings has been observed in TMD patients.[49] This "silent period" never evolved into a clinically useful test.

▼ ETIOLOGY, EPIDEMIOLOGY, AND CLASSIFICATION

Etiology

The etiology of the most common TMD is unknown. Two hypotheses, occlusal disharmony and psychological distress, have dominated the literature, but neither has been supported by the literature.[50] Research studying discrepancies between centric relation and centric occlusion, nonworking side interferences, and Angle's classification has not shown a strong association in myofascial-pain patients when compared to controls.[51–53] Studies of patients with myofascial pain and control subjects have failed to demonstrate significant differences in occlusion although there may be some cases in which occlusal problems are an initiating factor.[54] A relationship between tooth loss and osteoarthrosis has been found in patient studies[55] but has not been observed in nonpatient studies.[56] No difference between a symptomatic and control population was found when attempting to correlate incisal relationships, condylar position, and joint sounds.[57] An observed relationship between severe overbite and TMD symptoms has been reported but has not been consistently observed.[58,59] Alternatively, there is some experimental evidence to suggest that some observed occlusal changes could be produced by masticatory-muscle pain.[60] Anterior open-bite malocclusion may result from severe TMJ involvement in patients with rheumatoid arthritis.[61]

Masticatory-muscle hyperactivity progressing to a "vicious cycle" has been proposed as the cause of myofascial pain. The diagnostic terms of "myospasm," "muscle spasm," and "reflex splinting" have been used to describe these conditions. A link between muscle hyperactivity and the pain disorder has not been demonstrated.[62–66] Differences between resting electromyographic activity in painful jaw-closing muscles and nonpainful muscles have not been found.[67] Tooth attrition signaling dental wear due to bruxing has not been associated with TMJ clicking or tenderness or with masticatory-muscle tenderness.[68]

The results of a number of experimental studies of myofascial pain are consistent with the hypothesis of pain caused by altered central nervous system processing,[69–73] but these findings could also be interpreted as a consequence of the pain rather than the cause of the pain.

The psychological hypothesis proposes that the disorder evolves as a consequence of psychological distress that is usually due to the individual's stressful environment; the psychological distress leads to parafunctional habits (tooth clenching and grinding) that result in muscle pain.[74–76] A challenge that is continually faced in chronic pain disorders is determining how much of the psychological distress is a cause or is a consequence of the chronic pain.[77] The weight of the evidence suggests that in most cases, the emotional distress is more a consequence than a cause of pain.[78]

The lack of a clear single cause has resulted in the proposal of a multifactorial etiology.[75] These factors may contribute to the initiation, aggravation, and/or perpetuation of the disorder. Some of the factors proposed are the following:

1. Parafunctional habits (eg, nocturnal bruxing, tooth clenching, lip or cheek biting)[79,80]
2. Emotional distress[81,82]
3. Acute trauma from blows or impacts[83]
4. Trauma from hyperextension (eg, dental procedures, oral intubation for general anesthesia, yawning, hyperextension associated with cervical trauma)[84]
5. Instability of maxillomandibular relationships[85]
6. Laxity of the joint[86]
7. Comorbidity of other rheumatic or musculoskeletal disorders[87]
8. Poor general health and an unhealthy lifestyle[88]

The frequency and the importance of these factors as causes are unknown.

Epidemiology

Between 65 and 85% of people in the United States experience some symptoms of TMD during their lives, and approximately 12% experience prolonged pain or disability that results in chronic symptoms.[89] Although the prevalence of one or more signs of mandibular pain and dysfunction is high in the population, only about 5 to 7% have symptoms severe enough to need treatment.[89,51,90] TMD patients are similar to headache and back pain patients with respect to disability, psychosocial profile, and pain intensity, chronicity, and frequency.[91,92] The lower prevalence of TMD signs and symptoms in older age groups supports the probability that most TMD are self-limiting.

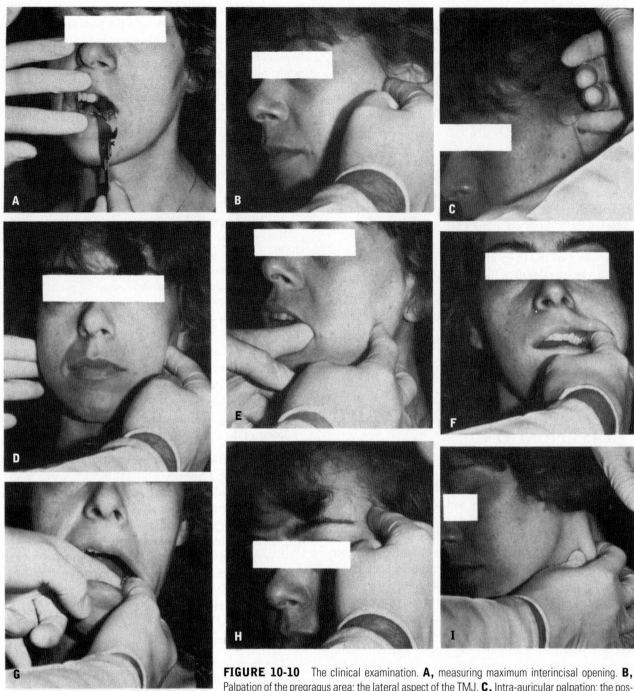

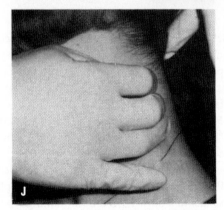

FIGURE 10-10   The clinical examination. **A,** measuring maximum interincisal opening. **B,** Palpation of the pregragus area; the lateral aspect of the TMJ. **C,** Intra-auricular palpation; the posterior aspect of the TMJ. **D,** Palpation of the masseter muscles. **E,** Bi-manual palpation of the masseter muscle. **F,** Palpation of the lateral pterygoid muscle. **G,** Palpation of the medial pterygoid muscle. **H,** Palpation of the temporalis muscle. **I,** Palpation of the sternocleidomatoid muscle. **J,** Palpation of the trapezius muscle. Note that the lateral and medial pterygoid muscle palpations are from an intra-oral approach. Access to these muscles is limited and the procedure may produce an unacceptable rate of false positives (pain on palpation). The results of lateral and medial pterygoid palpation should be interpreted with caution.

Available evidence indicates that TMD are most prevalent between the ages of 20 and 40 years and predominantly affect women. The reason why women make up the majority of patients presenting for treatment is still unclear. In a community-based study, a greater likelihood of developing TMD was found if oral contraceptives were used and, in women over 40 years of age, if estrogen replacement was used.[93]

While the prevalence of TMD is highest in the 20- to 40-year age range, signs and symptoms of masticatory-muscle and joint dysfunction are commonly observed in children.[94-96] Belfer reported on a group of 40 children, aged 10 to 16 years, presenting with signs and symptoms of TMD; 14 (35%) of the 40 were diagnosed as having acute reactive depression.[97] In another study, arthrography and computed tomography were performed on 31 pediatric patients complaining of TMJ pain and dysfunction.[98] Twelve were diagnosed with disk displacement with reduction, and 17 were found to have disk displacement without reduction. In 12 of the 29 patients with internal derangement, the problem was thought to be due to a previous injury. In a survey of 1,000 12-year-old children, 1% had a maximum mouth opening of less than 40 mm, and few children presented with clinical findings severe enough to warrant treatment.[99]

A number of studies have been performed to investigate a possible relationship between orthodontic treatment and the development of TMD, but the results do not support a causal relationship between orthodontic treatment and the subsequent development of TMD.[100,101]

Classification

Due to the uncertainty about etiology, current diagnostic classifications of TMD are based on signs and symptoms. Earlier classifications characterized disorders as intracapsular (TMJ) or extracapsular (muscle) disorders and were often not versatile enough to allow for multiple diagnoses of masticatory muscle and TMJ abnormalities. More recent classifications do allow for more than one diagnosis, and this better reflects the clinical reality.[102,103] Arthrographic techniques have provided evidence resulting in more-accurate descriptions of intracapsular disorders in relation to presenting clinical features.[63,104] Disk disorders are now differentiated on the basis of arthrographic or magnetic resonance imaging findings.

In 1989, Clark and colleagues published a classification system that was useful to the practicing clinician (Table 10-1).[105]

TABLE 10-2 Diagnostic Classification of Temporomandibular Disorders

Diagnostic Category	Diagnoses
Cranial bones (including the mandible)	Congenital and developmental disorders: aplasia, hypoplasia, hyperplasia, dysplasia (eg, 1st and 2nd branchial arch anomalies, hemifacial microsomia, Pierre Robin syndrome, Treacher Collins syndrome, condylar hyperplasia, prognathism, fibrous dysplasia)
	Acquired disorders (neoplasia, fracture)
Temporomandibular joint disorders	Deviation in form
	Disk displacement (with reduction; without reduction)
	Dislocation
	Inflammatory conditions (synovitis, capsulitis)
	Arthritides (osteoarthritis, osteoarthrosis polyarthritides)
	Ankylosis (fibrous, bony)
	Neoplasia
Masticatory-muscle disorders	Myofascial pain
	Myositis
	Spasm
	Protective splinting
	Contracture

Adapted from McNeill C.[87]

The American Academy of Orofacial Pain (AAOP) has published a general classification of disorders that affect the cranial bones, temporomandibular joints, and masticatory muscles[87] (Table 10-2). This classification system is useful because it attempts to define the diagnostic terms and provide diagnostic criteria. This classification has not been subjected to testing for validity. It represents an attempt by experts to apply available knowledge to the development of a more acceptable and useful system for clinical practice. Table 10-3 provides a partial list of the diagnostic terms and their diagnostic criteria. This classification does provide the clinician with an aid in clinical decision making. A number of other clinical findings, described as possibly accompanying the diagnosis, are listed in the latest AAOP publication on orofacial pain guidelines.[1] The supporting signs in disk disorders may have additional clinical value and are listed in Table 10-3 as "clinical findings that may support the diagnosis."

TABLE 10-1 Classification for Diagnosing Temporomandibular Disorders

Diagnostic Category	Diagnoses
Muscle and facial disorders	Myalgia; muscle contracture; splinting; hypertrophy; spasm; dyskinesia; forceful jaw closure habit; myositis (bruxism)
TMJ disorders	Disk condyle incoordination; osteoarthritis; disk condyle restriction; inflammatory polyarthritis; open dislocation; traumatic articular disease; arthralgia
Disorder of mandibular mobility	Ankylosis; adhesions (intracapsular); fibrosis of muscular tissue; coronoid elongation-hypermobility of TMJ
Disorders of maxillomandibular growth	Masticatory-muscle hypertrophy/atrophy; neoplasia (muscle, maxillomandibular or condylar); maxillomandibular or condylar hypoplasia/hyperplasia

Adapted from Clark GT et al.[105]

TMJ = temporomandibular joint.

TABLE 10-3 Diagnostic Terms and Clinical Criteria for Temporomandibular Disorders

Diagnostic Terms	Clinical Criteria
Deviation in form (painless mechanical dysfunction or altered function due to irregularities or aberrations in form of the intracapsular soft and hard articular tissues)	Complaint of faulty or compromised joint mechanics Reproducible joint noise, usually at the same position during opening and closing Radiographic evidence of structural bony abnormality or loss of normal shape
Disk displacement with reduction (abrupt alteration or interference of the disk-condyle structural relation during mandibular translation with mouth opening and closing; from a closed-mouth position, the "temporarily" misaligned disk reduces or improves its structural relation with the condyle when mandibular translation occurs with mouth opening, which produces joint noise described as clicking or popping)	Pain (when present) is precipitated by joint movement. Reproducible joint noise, usually at variable positions during opening and closing mandibular movements Soft-tissue imaging reveals displaced disk that improves its position during jaw opening. Clinical findings that may support the diagnosis: pain (when present) precipitated by joint movement; deviation during movement coinciding with a click; no restriction in mandibular movement (episodic and momentary catching of smooth jaw movements during mouth opening [< 35 mm] that self-reduces with voluntary mandibular repositioning).
Disk displacement without reduction (altered or misaligned disk-condyle structural relation that is maintained during mandibular translation)	Pain precipitated by function Marked limited mandibular opening Straight-line deviation to the affected side on opening Marked limited laterotrusion to the contralateral side Soft-tissue imaging reveals displaced disk without reduction. Clinical findings that may support the diagnosis: pain precipitated by forced mouth opening; history of clicking that ceases with the locking; pain with palpation of the affected joint; ipsilateral hyperocclusion
Synovitis or capsulitis (inflammation of the synovial lining or capsular lining)	Localized pain at rest exacerbated by function, especially with superior and posterior joint loading Limited range of motion secondary to pain T2-weighted MRI may show joint fluid
Osteoarthrosis (degenerative noninflammatory condition of the joint, characterized by structural changes of joint surfaces secondary to excessive straining of the remodeling mechanism)	Crepitus Limited range of motion causes deviation to the affected side on opening. Radiographic evidence of structural bony change (subchondral sclerosis, osteophyte formation) and joint-space narrowing
Osteoarthritis (degenerative condition accompanied by secondary inflammation [synovitis] of the TMJ)	Same as for osteoarthritis, plus crepitus or multiple joint noises, pain with function due to inflammation, and point tenderness on palpation
Myofascial pain (regional dull aching pain and presence of localized tender spots [trigger points] in muscle, tendon, or fascia that reproduce pain when palpated and may produce a characteristic pattern of regional referred pain and/or autonomic symptoms on provocation)	Regional pain, usually dull Localized tenderness in firm bands of muscle and/or fascia Reduction in pain with local muscle anesthetic injection or vapocoolant spray and stretch of muscle trigger points
Myositis, delayed onset (painful condition due to intermittent overuse that results in interstitial inflammation)	Increased pain with mandibular movement Onset following prolonged or unaccustomed use (up to 48 hours afterward)
Myositis, generalized (constant, acutely painful, and generalized inflammation and swelling, usually of the entire muscle)	Pain usually acute in localized area Localized tenderness over entire region of the muscle Increased pain with mandibular movement Moderately to severely limited range of motion, due to pain and swelling Onset following injury or infection
Protective muscle splinting (restricted or guarded mandibular movement due to cocontraction of muscles as a means of avoiding pain caused by movement of the parts)	Severe pain with function but not at rest Marked limited range of motion without significant increase on passive stretch
Contracture (chronic resistance of a muscle to passive stretch, as a result of fibrosis of the supporting tendon, ligaments, or muscle fibers themselves)	Limited range of motion Unyielding firmness on passive stretch History of trauma or infection

Adapted from McNeill C.[87]

MRI = magnetic resonance imaging; TMJ = temporomandibular joint.

The interpretation of the TMD literature and advances in knowledge have been impeded by the lack of widely accepted methods or standards for selecting or describing patients who are part of clinical research projects. Dworkin and colleagues developed a classification for the most common TMD, to provide a system that could be used in clinical research. The Research Diagnostic Criteria for TMD (RDC/TMD) were published as a system "offered to allow standardization and replication of research into the most common forms of muscle- and joint-related TMD."[28] The classification scheme is intended to provide a means for standardizing data collection and for comparing findings among clinical investigators. Because of the chronicity of TMD, a classification system that reflects psychological, behavioral, and social issues is as important as an accurate description of the physical pathology. The RDC/TMD classification has a separate axis that assesses psychosocial status to create profiles of disability, depression, anxiety, and preoccupation with other physical symptoms. The RDC/TMD classification has not yet been subjected to the research required for validation.

The classifications published by Clark and the AAOP were designed for clinical practice and are more comprehensive. The RDC/TMD classification was developed for research purposes but is useful in clinical practice for the types of TMD most likely to present to a dentist. The classification does not include the conditions that are less common but still likely to present to clinicians. The RDC/TMD system allows for multiple diagnoses for each individual but only one muscle diagnosis and allows for each joint only one disk disorder diagnosis and one articular bone diagnosis. The terms used are clearly defined, and the criteria required to meet the diagnosis are detailed although the validation of these criteria and the classification system will have to await further research. To allow greater use in the research environment, the criteria do not include diagnostic imaging. While the clinician will likely not adhere to all the guidelines or diagnoses, the assessment and classification system serves as a useful method of organizing clinical information for the most commonly presenting TMD[28] (Tables 10-4 and 10-5). The reliance on clinical findings for diagnosis is consistent with the research purpose, but diagnostic imaging would likely be required to establish a disk disorder diagnosis such as "disk displacement without reduction, without limited opening." The clinician should add diagnostic imaging as part of the assessment whenever the diagnosis, treatment choice, or outcome may benefit. If the RDC/TMD classification system is used more frequently in research, clinicians who are familiar with it will be in a better position to evaluate the published research. (The reader is referred to the publication by Dworkin and colleagues.)[28] Muscle conditions (such as myositis, contracture, and myospasm) and joint conditions associated with systemic arthritis, acute trauma, hyperplasia, and neoplasia are not part of the defined conditions.

Schiffman and colleagues compared clinical findings and tomographic findings to define criteria for intra-articular disorders and presented criteria for the classification of articular disorders.[106] No single sign or symptom was consistently accurate for establishing a diagnosis, but the patterns listed in Table 10-6 show 75% agreement when compared to findings by arthrotomography.[106] The diagnosis of articular disk displacement without reduction, chronic (similar to RDC/TMD articular disk displacement without reduction and without limited opening), may be the most problematic diagnosis without imaging. Other clinical findings may support the diagnosis and include pain, markedly reduced from the acute stage and usually presenting as a

TABLE 10-4   Research Diagnostic Criteria for Clinical Temporomandibular Disorder Conditions, Axis 1[28]

Clinical Location	RDC/TMD Diagnoses
Muscle	Myofascial pain Myofascial pain with limited opening
Disk displacement	Disk displacement with reduction Disk displacement without reduction, with limited opening Disk displacement without reduction, without limited opening
Articular bone	Arthralgia Osteoarthritis of the TMJ Osteoarthrosis of the TMJ

RDC/TMD = Research Diagnostic Criteria for temporomandibular disorders; TMJ = temporomandibular joint.

feeling of stiffness; a history of clicking that resolves with the sudden onset of the locking; and gradual resolution of limited mouth opening.

▼ ASSESSMENT

Present examination methods have not yet demonstrated the ability to differentiate accurately persons with a TMD from those without a TMD.[107] The most valuable aspects of the diagnostic assessment are a thorough history and physical examination.[108] Most of the tests used to assess TMD patients have not been validated and are not standardized, and an ideal method for classification has not been established.[109] Diagnostic tests such as ultrasonographic analysis of joint sounds, thermography, jaw-tracking devices, and electromyography do not offer the assurance of a more accurate diagnosis.[110] These tests require sophisticated instrumentation that increases health care costs to the patient. In most cases, the correct diagnostic classification can be reached by using the self-reporting of the patient and the findings on clinical examination.[106,111] Diagnostic imaging is of value in selected conditions but not as part of a standard assessment. Diagnostic imaging can increase accuracy in the detection of internal derangements and abnormalities of articular bone.

While pain is a characteristic feature of TMD, it may also be associated with serious undetected disease. Muscle or joint pain may be a secondary feature of other disease or may mimic a TMD, and a diagnosis may be missed or delayed.[112,113] Severe throbbing temporal pain associated with a palpable nodular temporal artery, increasingly severe headache associated with nausea and vomiting, and documented altered sensation or hearing loss are all indications of serious disease requiring timely diagnosis and management.

Assessment should result in a diagnosis of a TMD and an estimation of psychological distress and pain-related disability. The lack of a direct relationship between (a) physical pathology and intensity of pain and (b) subsequent disability emphasizes the need to assess the psychological and behavioral effects of the disorder. Fricton recommends developing

TABLE 10-5 Definitions and Clinial Criteria for Temporomandibular Disorders

Definitions*	Clinical Criteria*
Myofascial pain (pain of muscle origin, including complaint of pain associated with localized areas of tenderness to palpation in muscle)	Report of pain or ache in jaw, temples, face, preauricular area, or inside ear at rest or during function, and pain on palpation in three or more muscle sites
Myofascial pain with limited opening	Myofascial pain, pain-free unassisted mandibular opening of < 40 mm, and a maximum assisted opening of ≥ 5 mm greater than the pain-free unassisted opening
Disk displacement with reduction (disk is displaced from its position between the condyle and eminence to an anterior and medial or lateral position but is reduced in full opening, usually resulting in a noise)	Click on both vertical opening and closing that occurs at a point at least 5 mm (interincisal opening) greater than on closing, is eliminated on protrusive opening, and is reproducible in two of three consecutive trials or click on opening or closing and click on lateral excursion or protrusion, reproducible in two of three consecutive trials
Disk displacement without reduction, with limited opening (disk is displaced from normal position between condyle and fossa to an anterior and medial or lateral position, associated with limited opening)	History of significant limitation of opening Maximum unassisted opening ≤ 35 mm, passive stretch increases opening by ≤ 4 mm, and contralateral excursion < 7 mm and/or uncorrected deviation to the ipsilateral side on opening Absence of joint sounds or sounds that do not meet criteria for disk displacement with reduction
Disk displacement without reduction without limited opening (disk is displaced from its position between condyle and eminence to an anterior and medial or lateral position, not associated with limited opening)	History of significant limitation of mandibular opening Maximum unassisted opening > 35 mm, passive stretch increases opening by ≥ 5 mm over maximum unassisted opening, contralateral excursion ≥ 7 mm, and presence of joint sounds not meeting criteria for disk displacement with reduction
Arthralgia (pain and tenderness in joint capsule and/or synovial lining of the TMJ)	Pain in one or both joint sites and self-report of pain in region of joint Pain in joint during maximum opening (assisted or unassisted) Pain in joint during lateral excursion
Osteoarthritis of the TMJ (inflammatory condition within the joint, resulting from a degenerative condition of joint structures)	Arthralgia and coarse crepitus or imaging showing one or more of the following: erosion of normal cortical outlines, sclerosis of parts or all of condyle and articular eminence, flattening of joint surfaces, osteophyte formation
Osteoarthrosis of the TMJ (degenerative joint disorder in which joint form and structure are abnormal)	Absence of arthralgia Coarse crepitus or imaging showing one or more of the following: erosion of normal cortical outlines, sclerosis of parts or all of condyle and articular eminence, flattening of joint surfaces, osteophyte formation

TMJ = temporomandibular joint.
* For the complete description, refer to Dworkin S, LeResche L.[28]

a problem list of the contributing factors associated with TMD.[114] Contributing factors may affect the symptom control and the long-term success of any treatment program. No one individual can be expected to manage or address the var-

ious lifestyle emotional, cognitive, and social issues that may have an impact on the chronic pain. The importance of these factors to TMD pain and to the patient's general health needs to be assessed; an appropriate plan to address them can then

TABLE 10-6 Clinical Findings of Disk Disorders, Correlating with Arthrotomography

Assessment Procedure	Clinical Findings			
	Normal	ADD with Reduction	Acute ADD without Reduction	Chronic ADD without Reduction
History	None	None	Positive for mandibular limitation	Positive for TMJ noise
Physical examination	Reciprocal click No coarse crepitus Passive stretch ≥ 40 mm Lateral movements ≥ 7 mm If S-curve present, joint is silent	Reciprocal click or popping No coarse crepitus Passive stretch ≥ 35 mm	No reciprocal click No coarse crepitus Maximum opening ≤ 35 mm Passive stretch < 40 mm Contralateral movement < 7 mm No S-curve deviation	No reciprocal click Coarse crepitus or joint sounds other than reciprocal clicking
Tomography	No decreased translation in ipsilateral condyle No osseous change	None	Decreased translation of ipsilateral condyle	Decreased translation of ipsilateral condyle or positive osseous changes

Adapted from Schiffman et al.[106]

ADD = articular disk displacement; TMJ = temporomandibular joint.

TABLE 10-7   Problem List of Contributing Factors Associated with Temporomandibular Disorders

Lifestyle	Emotional Factors	Cognitive Factors	Biologic Factors	Social Factors
Diet	Prolonged anger	Negative self-image	Other illnesses	Work stresses
Sleep	Anxiety	Unrealistic expectations	Past trauma	Unemployment
Alcohol	Excessive worry	Inadequate coping	Past jaw surgery	Family stresses
Smoking	Depression			Litigation
Overwork				Financial difficulty

Adapted from Fricton.[114]

be developed. Table 10-7 lists some of the contributing factors discussed by Fricton.[114]

A validated and empirically derived classification of TMD patients, based on psychosocial and behavioral parameters, has identified three unique subgroups: dysfunctional patients, interpersonally distressed patients, and adaptive copers.[115] TMD is not unique in the psychosocial and behavioral parameters; TMD patients and back pain patients have demonstrated similar profiles.[91,116] Interventions targeting pain and psychological distress are of equal importance to the pathophysiology of temporomandibular structures in managing a chronic TMD. Psychosocial assessment should provide the clinician with an appreciation of the extent to which pain and dysfunction interfere with or diminish the patient's quality of life. The assessment should identify patients with psychological distress that warrants further investigation and possible treatment by a psychologist or psychiatrist. In addition to assessments of pain intensity and emotional state, an assessment of limitation in activity will provide a reflection of the magnitude of the condition.[117,118] In one report, approximately 16% of TMD patients experienced significant activity limitation, compared to approximately 3% of controls.[119] A systematic method of screening is necessary because dentists have been found to be inaccurate in identifying psychological problems in TMD patients.[120] The RDC/TMD uses a questionnaire partly developed for this classification system and from previously used scales to assess pain intensity and disability, depression, and nonspecific physical symptoms. (The reader is referred to the publication by Dworkin and colleagues.)[28]

History

The most common symptom related to TMD is pain. This pain usually shows some relation to mandibular function, or an alternative diagnosis should be suspected. A "pain diary" can be a useful tool for identifying events or times of increased and decreased pain; it may also serve to identify behaviors or situations that are contributing to the persistence of symptoms. A pain diagram of the head and neck is helpful in defining the extent of pain and may also be used to assess treatment progress. A diagram that includes the whole body may help identify patients who have multiple sites of pain, which suggests a more systemic disorder. Table 10-8 lists questions that are useful (as part of the history) for assessing mandibular function.

Physical Examination

No one physical finding can be relied on to establish a diagnosis, but a pattern of abnormalities may suggest the source of the problem and a possible diagnosis. Masticatory-muscle tenderness on palpation (see Figure 10-10) is the most consistent examination feature present in cases of TMD.[102] The clinical features that distinguish patients from controls are

1. passive mouth opening,[121]
2. masticatory-muscle tenderness on palpation and maximal mouth opening,[122] and
3. an uncorrected deviation on maximum mouth opening and tenderness on palpation.[89]

Components of the physical examination that are discussed in this section are summarized in Table 10-9.

TABLE 10-8   History: Questions to Ask when Evaluating a Patient for Mandibular Dysfunction*

Do you have pain in the face, in front of the ear and temple areas?

Do you get headaches, earaches, neckache, or cheek pain?

When is pain at its worst (morning [on awakening] or as day progresses [toward evening])?

Do you experience pain when using the jaw (opening wide, yawning, chewing, speaking, or swallowing)?

Do you experience pain in the teeth?

Do you experience joint noises when moving your jaw or when chewing (clicking, popping, or crepitus)?

Does your jaw ever lock or get stuck (locking in the open position or locking in the closed position)?

Does your jaw motion feel restricted?

Have you had an abrupt change in the way your teeth meet together?

Does your bite feel "off" or uncomfortable?

Have you had any jaw injuries?

Have you had treatment for the jaw symptoms? If so, what was the effect?

Do you have any other muscle, bone, or joint problem such as arthritis or fibromyalgia?

Do you have pain in any other body sites?

*Miscellaneous symptoms are sometimes reported in association with temporomandibular dysfunction and may include dizziness; nausea; fullness or ringing in the ears; diminished hearing; facial swelling; redness of the eyes; nasal congestion; altered sensation such as numbness, tingling, or burning; altered vision; and muscle twitching.

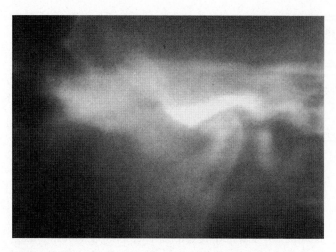

FIGURE 10-11 Temporomandibular joint tomogram displaying flattening of the condylar head in degenerative joint disease.

RANGE OF MANDIBULAR MOVEMENT

Interincisor separation plus or minus the incisor overlap in centric occlusion provides the measure of mandibular movement. Maximum opening should be measured without pain, as wide as possible even with pain, and after opening with clinician assistance. Assisting the jaw during mouth opening is accomplished by applying mild to moderate pressure against the upper and lower incisors with the thumb and index finger. Assisted opening should be measured. Passive stretching is a technique for assessing and differentiating restrictions due to muscle or joint. It results in a measure to be compared with active opening and an experience of the quality of resistance at the end of the movement. Muscle restrictions are associated with a soft-end feel, and a mouth opening increase of > 5 mm can often be achieved. Joint disorders such as acute nonreducing disk displacements are described as having a hard-end feel and characteristically restrict assisted opening to < 5 mm. The normal maximum mouth opening is ≥ 40 mm. In a study of 1,160 adults, the mean maximum mouth opening was 52.8 mm (with a range of 38.7 to 67.2 mm) for men and 48.3 mm (with a range of 36.7 to 60.4 mm) for women.[123] Measures of lateral movement are made with the teeth slightly separated, measuring the displacement of the lower midline from the maxillary midline and adding or subtracting the lower-midline displacement at the start of movement. Protrusive movement is measured by adding the horizontal distance between the upper and lower central incisors and adding the distance the lower incisors travel beyond the upper incisors. Normal lateral and protrusive movements are ≥ 7 mm.[62,124–126] Measures of the mandibular range of movement are similarly performed in children. The mean maximum mouth opening recorded in 75 boys and 75 girls aged 6 years was 44.8 mm.[127] A study of 189 individuals with a mean age of 10 years reported similar values (a mean maximum opening of 43.9 mm, with a range of 32 to 64 mm).[128] The means of left,

right, and protrusive maximal movements were each approximately 8 mm.

PALPATION OF MASTICATORY MUSCLES

The primary finding related to masticatory-muscle palpation is pain. The methods for palpation are not standardized in clinical practice. The amount of pressure to apply and the exact sites that are most likely associated with TMD are unknown. Some clinicians have recommended attempting to establish a baseline (to serve as a general guide or reference) by squeezing the muscle between the index finger and thumb or by applying pressure in the center of the forehead or thumbnail to gauge what pressure becomes uncomfortable. The RDC/TMD guidelines recommend 1 lb of pressure for the joint and 2 lb of pressure for the muscles.[28] The RDC/TMD pressures have been established for research purposes. In the clinical setting, a greater range of pressures is probably required. All of the examination procedures should be accompanied by questioning the patient about the production of pain and the site of pain during the particular examination procedure. Reproducing the site and the character of the pain during the examination procedure helps identify the possible anatomic site of the pain. This may also provide insight into the possibility of referred pain as a factor. Palpation of the joint and the muscles for pain should be done with the muscles in a resting state. There are no standardized methods of assessing the severity of palpable pain, and the patient should be asked to rate the severity by using a scale (eg, a numerical scale from 1 to 10, a visual analogue

TABLE 10-9 Physical Examination Directed Toward Mandibular Dysfunction

Examination Component	Observations
Inspection	Facial asymmetry, swelling, and masseter- and temporal-muscle hypertrophy Opening pattern (corrected and uncorrected deviations, uncoordinated movements, limitations)
Assessment of range of mandibular movement	Maximum opening with comfort, with pain, and with clinician assistance Maximum lateral and protrusive movements
Palpation examination	Masticatory muscles Temporomandibular joints Neck muscles and accessory muscles of the jaw Parotid and submandibular areas Lymph nodes
Provocation tests	Static pain test (mandibular resistance against pressure) Pain in the joints or muscles with tooth clenching Reproduction of symptoms with chewing (wax, sugarless gum)
Intraoral examination	Signs of parafunction (cheek or lip biting, accentuated linea alba, scalloped tongue borders, occlusal wear, tooth mobility, generalized sensitivity to percussion, thermal testing, multiple fractures of enamel and restorations)

scale, or a ranking such as none, mild, moderate, or severe). The RDC/TMD recommend using the categories of pressure only, mild pain, moderate pain, and severe pain. These ratings may be useful as part of the process of assessing treatment progress. Palpation may reproduce the patient's pain symptoms or may produce pain referred to a distant site such as the molar teeth, which may help in differential diagnosis. Abnormalities such as trigger points and taut bands in muscle have not been sufficiently characterized in the masticatory muscles to always enable the clinician to distinguish these sites anatomically from normal muscle.

PALPATION OF CERVICAL MUSCLES

Patients with TMD/MPD often have musculoskeletal problems in other regions that are particularly associated with the neck.[129,130] The sternocleidomastoid and trapezius muscles are often part of a neck muscle disorder and may refer pain to the face and head. Other muscle groups to palpate include the paravertebral (scalene) and suboccipital muscles.

PALPATION OF THE TMJ

Palpation of the TMJ will reveal pain and irregularities during condylar movement, described as clicking or crepitus. The lateral pole of the condyle is most accessible for palpation during mandibular movements. Palpating just anterior and posterior to the lateral pole should detect pain associated with the TMJ capsular ligaments. In addition to joint noises and pain, there may be palpable differences in the form of the condyle when comparing right and left. The condyle that does not translate may not be palpable during mouth opening and closing. The click that occurs on opening and closing and that is eliminated by bringing the mandible into a protrusive position before opening is most often associated with articular disk displacement with reduction.

PROVOCATION TESTS

Provocation tests are designed to elicit the described pain. Since pain is often aggravated by jaw use, a positive response adds support for a diagnosis of TMD. The static pain test involves having the mandible slightly open and remaining in one position while the patient resists the slowly increasing manual force applied by the examiner in a lateral, upward, and downward direction. If the mandible remains in a static position during the test, it is the muscles that will be subjected to activation. However, the ability of this test to discriminate between muscle and joint pain is not known. Clenching the teeth or chewing wax or gum is expected to load the joints and muscles. According to one report, approximately 50% of TMD patients who chewed one-half of a leaf of gauge-28 green casting wax for 3 minutes reported an increase in pain, but 30% reported decreased pain, and 20% reported no change.[131]

Assessment of Parafunctional Habits

It is difficult to determine the presence of active severe oral habits, and only indirect means are generally available. The patient is often unaware of tooth clenching or other behaviors contributing to jaw hyperactivity while awake. Self-reports, instructions for checking jaw activity during the day, and reports by sleeping partners of tooth-grinding noises are helpful. Examination for tooth wear, soft-tissue changes (lip or cheek chewing, a hyperplastic occlusal line, and scalloped tongue borders), and hypertrophic jaw-closing muscles may suggest hyperactivity.

Diagnostic Imaging

When the clinical presentation suggests a progressive pathologic condition of the TMJ, imaging should be part of the assessment. Recent injury, sensory or motor abnormality, severe restriction in mandibular motion, and acute alterations of the occlusion are clinical findings for which imaging is indicated. The most frequent abnormalities that are imaged in TMD patients are degenerative changes of bone and disk displacement. TMJs can be examined by using plain-film radiography, tomography, arthrography, computerized tomography (CT), magnetic resonance imaging (MRI), single-photon emission computed tomography, and radioisotope scanning. MRI has become the imaging method of choice to assess disk position. For the majority of TMDs, diagnostic imaging has not proven to be a valuable test for directing treatment or for predicting outcome and long-term course. No differences were found in joint-space narrowing in the centric occlusion position in symptomatic and asymptomatic patients by transcranial plain-film radiography and tomography.[132,133] A large variation exists in condylar position in plain-film radiographic and tomographic studies, making the condyle-fossa relationship of little value in the diagnosis or treatment of TMD.[134] Using plain films (such as in transcranial radiography) to determine condylar position or using the condylar position on these films to assess disk position is not recommended.[132,133,135] Imaging such as tomography and CT is relied on to document osteodegenerative joint disease. CT provides detail for bony abnormalities and is an appropriate study when considering ankylosis, fractures, tumors of bone, and osteodegenerative joint disease. MRI is the method of choice for establishing alterations in articular disk position in the open- and closed-mouth positions. MRI studies in asymptomatic volunteers have shown disk abnormalities in approximately one-third of subjects.[34,136] With the use of T2-weighted MRI, a correlation between joint pain and joint effusion has been suggested, but the results are conflicting.[137,138] Radioisotope scanning for detecting increases in metabolic activity has been used to detect condylar hyperplasia. Bone scanning is a sensitive indicator of metabolic bone activity and may therefore show a positive result in a joint that is undergoing physiologic remodeling as well. Radioisotope scanning in combination with other imaging and clinical findings (including findings on periodic examinations) is usually effective in diagnosing continued condylar change due to hyperplasia.

Diagnostic Local Anesthetic Nerve Blocks

Injections of anesthetics into the TMJ or selected masticatory muscles may help to confirm a diagnosis. A positive test may result in the elimination of pain and improved jaw motion.

Diagnostic injections may also be helpful in differentiating pain arising from joints or muscle. In situations in which a joint procedure is being considered, local anesthetic injection of the joint may confirm the joint as the source of pain. Lidocaine (2%) without a vasoconstrictor can be used. Injecting trigger points or tender areas in the muscle should eliminate pain from that site and should also eliminate referred pain associated with the injected tender or trigger point.[139] These tests, like all others, require interpretation in the context of all the diagnostic information since a positive result does not insure a specific diagnosis.

Prediction of Chronicity

While most TMD patients respond to nonsurgical management that can be provided or coordinated by a dentist, some individuals develop chronic pain and disability. This group experiences great psychological distress and disruption of their normal daily activities, as well as the need to access ongoing health care resources. Predicting the cases that are likely to become chronic is important to provide alternative or additional interventions.

Psychological factors seem to be more important than peripheral injury or physical disease of the masticatory system in predicting chronicity.[140–144] Epker and colleagues found that the combination of high pain intensity (as measured by RDC/TMD scales) and a myofascial pain diagnosis (reported pain on palpation of muscles) was predictive of persisting TMD symptoms in their population.[145]

Comorbidity with widespread musculoskeletal pain is likely to contribute to the persistence of TMD symptoms. The prevalence of fibromyalgia in masticatory myofascial pain patients is higher than in the general population.[146,147] The presence of pain in other body sites in myofascial pain dysfunction (MPD) patients is high[129] and may indicate that the musculoskeletal problem affecting the jaws is part of a more generalized problem. In a follow-up study on MPD patients, the group that self-reported the coexistence of fibromyalgia had a higher frequency of chronic TMD symptoms.[148]

Trauma associated with the onset of TMD has always been considered to be a factor likely to increase severity and extend the course of the disorder. In a comparison of treatment between groups with TMD associated with trauma and without trauma, there was no difference to the treatment outcome, suggesting that trauma may not be an important factor; but more research is needed to draw conclusions.[149]

Referral to a Pain Specialist

While the majority of patients with TMD are responsive to treatment and are appropriately managed by dental professionals in association with psychologists, physiotherapists, and other health care professionals, a small group of patients may be more appropriately managed by a pain specialist. This may be indicated when (1) the disability greatly exceeds what is expected on the basis of physical findings, (2) the patient makes excessive demands for tests and treatments that are not indicated, (3) the patient displays significant psychological distress (eg, depression), or (4) the patient displays aberrant behavior, such as continual nonadherence to treatment.[150]

▼ GENERAL CLINICAL CHARACTERISTICS

The most important feature of TMD is pain. Pain may be present at rest, may be continuous or intermittent, and characteristically increases with jaw functions such as chewing or opening wide. Other common findings include pain reported during palpation of the TMJ and/or muscles of mastication; a restricted range of mandibular movement or uncoordinated movements; and irregularities in the joints during movement, characterized by clicking or grating sounds. Myofascial pain is the most common TMD[102] and may present with or without restricted mouth opening. Pain causes the jaw-closing muscles to co-contract, so that the pain itself may influence the degree of mandibular restriction in cases of MPD.[151,152] Chronic TMD pain (like all chronic pain) results in psychological, behavioral, and social disturbances. The assessment and the treatment of these problems are equally important to the physical pathology.

Treatment goals for TMD are to control pain and to return mandibular motion and function to normal or as close to normal as possible. Clinical case studies suggest that the majority of individuals with TMD respond to conservative noninvasive therapy, making the use of invasive procedures unwarranted as initial therapy. No one treatment has emerged as superior although many of the treatments studied have shown some beneficial effect.[153] The symptoms of TMD tend to be intermittent, fluctuate over time, and are often self-limiting.[154–156] The process of deciding whether to treat and how aggressively to treat should include an assessment of the course of symptoms. Patients who are improving at the time of assessment may require a minimum of care and monitoring, compared to the individual whose symptoms are becoming progressively more severe and disabling.

The variations in treatment recommended by dentists have been explained by the gap between published information in the medical and dental literature and the individual beliefs and attitudes of practicing dentists.[157,158] These observations suggest that the treatment effect may be nonspecific and related more to the therapeutic relationship established between therapist and patient than to the specific treatment.[159]

Patients with irreversible anatomic abnormalities such as disk disorders are still able to regain painless jaw function.[160,161] Decreasing pain and improved physical findings are not directly related.[162] The presence of joint noises and deviations from the ideal in occlusion, in maxillomandibular relationships, and in the morphology of bony structures such as the condyle are relatively common in the general population. Evidence indicating prophylactic treatment of these anatomic abnormalities when no pain, impairment of function, or disability exists is lacking. Rather, treatment should be based on the severity of pain and disability and should be directed toward those factors that are considered to be important in initiating, aggravating, or perpetuating the disorder.

Episodes of pain and dysfunction may recur even after successful symptom control. Re-injury or factors that contributed to earlier episodes of symptoms may be responsible. Recurrence should not be considered a treatment failure, and initiating previous treatment that was successful should be considered first. In one study, myogenous disorders required recurrent treatment more frequently than did articular disorders.[163]

For the smaller group of patients in whom TMD progresses to a chronic pain disorder, treatment becomes more complex. These patients may still benefit from local therapies but will also require more comprehensive management to address the emotional and behavioral disabilities that result from chronic pain. The drug therapy may also be complex, requiring knowledge and experience that are not common in general dental practice. These patients are often at risk for unnecessary investigations or treatments that may be harmful and that may further complicate their problems.[164,165]

At a recent National Institutes of Health conference on TMD therapy, the following conclusions were published:[166]

1. Significant problems exist with present diagnostic classifications because these classifications appear to be based on signs and symptoms rather than on etiology.
2. No consensus has been developed regarding which TMD problems should be treated and when and how they should be treated.
3. The preponderance of the data does not support the superiority of any method for initial management, and the superiority of such methods to placebo controls or to no treatment controls remains undetermined.
4. Because most individuals will experience the improvement or relief of symptoms with conservative treatment, the vast majority of TMD patients should be initially managed with noninvasive and reversible therapies.
5. The efficacy of most treatment approaches for TMD is unknown because most have not been adequately evaluated in long-term studies and because virtually none have been studied in randomized controlled group trials.
6. Therapies that permanently alter the patient's occlusion cannot be recommended on the basis of current data.
7. Surgical intervention should be considered for the small percentage of patients with persistent and significant pain and dysfunction who show evidence of pathology or evidence that an internal derangement of the TMJ is the source of their pain and dysfunction and for whom more conservative treatment has failed.
8. Relaxation and cognitive-behavioral therapies are effective approaches to managing chronic pain.

▼ SPECIFIC DISORDERS AND THEIR MANAGEMENT

Myofascial Pain of the Masticatory Muscles

The term most commonly used for muscle pain that occurs with palpation is "myofascial pain." The ability to diagnose and explain the pathology associated with muscle pain is still a challenge for further research. Since treatment cannot be designed to address a particular cause, multiple therapies for controlling symptoms and restoring range of movement and jaw function are usually combined in a management plan. These therapies are more effective when used together than when used alone.[103,167–171]

Most of the research on the natural course of this disorder suggests that for most individuals, symptoms are intermittent and usually do not progress to chronic pain and disability. The dentist is the appropriate clinician to manage these patients, using conservative methods. The principles of treating this disorder are based on a generally favorable prognosis and an appreciation of the lack of clinically controlled trials indicating the superiority, predictability, and safety of the treatments that are presently being recommended. The literature suggests that most treatments can be expected to have some beneficial effect although this effect may be nonspecific and not directly related to the particular treatment. Treatments that are relatively accessible, not prohibitive due to expense, safe, and reversible should be given priority. Treatments with these characteristics include education, self-care, physical therapy, intraoral appliance therapy, short-term pharmacotherapy, behavioral therapy, and relaxation techniques (Table 10-10). There is evidence to suggest that combining treatments produces a better outcome.[172] Occlusal therapy continues to be recommended by some clinicians as an initial treatment or as a requirement to prevent recurrent symptoms. Research does not support occlusal abnormalities as a significant etiologic factor. The evaluation of occlusion and the correction of occlusal abnormalities are an important part of dental practice but should not be a standard treatment of TMD.

EDUCATION AND INFORMATION

A source of great anxiety for the patient is the possibility that the problem is a progressive and degenerative one that will lead to much greater pain and loss of function in the future. Patients may have sought prior consultations from other physicians and dentists who were not able to establish a diagnosis or explain the nature of the problem. This often leads to fears of a more catastrophic problem such as a brain tumor or other life-threatening disease. Explaining where the pain comes from and the varied nature of the symptoms that may occur is effective in reducing the patient's anxiety. Education is the basis for the self-care activities that patients can perform to aid in symptom control. This requires enough time in an unhurried environment for health care workers to provide information and to allow the patient to express his or her concerns and also to ask questions. This interaction is the basis for the therapeutic relationship and provides the patient with the understanding and ability to perform daily activities and to make choices about using the jaw. The patient has to participate in developing strategies to avoid stresses that aggravate symptoms or interfere with the ability to manage therapy.

SELF-CARE AND HABIT REVERSAL

Attention to jaw activities that are unrelated to function (such as tooth clenching, jaw posturing habits, jaw-muscle tensing,

TABLE 10-10 Initial Treatment of Myofascial Pain

Treatment Component	Description
Education	Explanation of the diagnosis and treatment Reassurance about the generally good prognosis for recovery and natural course Explanation of patient's and doctor's roles in therapy Information to enable patient to perform self-care
Self-care	Eliminate oral habits (eg, tooth clenching, chewing gum) Provide information on jaw care associated with daily activities
Physical therapy	Education regarding biomechanics of jaw, neck, and head posture Passive modalities (heat and cold therapy, ultrasound, laser, and TENS). Range-of-motion exercises (active and passive) Posture therapy Passive stretching, general exercise, and conditioning program
Intraoral appliance therapy	Cover all the teeth on the arch the appliance is seated on Adjust to achieve simultaneous contact against opposing teeth Adjust to a stable comfortable mandibular posture Avoid changing mandibular position Avoid long-term continuous use
Pharmacotherapy	NSAIDs, acetaminophen, muscle relaxants, antianxiety agents, tricyclic antidepressants, clonazepam
Behavioral/relaxation techniques	Relaxation therapy Hypnosis Biofeedback Cognitive-behavioral therapy

NSAIDs = nonsteroidal anti-inflammatory drugs; TENS = transcutaneous electrical nerve stimulation.

and leaning on the jaw) is a critical beginning. Those behaviors associated with hyperactivity need to be replaced with restful jaw postures, and this should be part of any initial therapy. Habit control was found to be helpful in reducing pain in myofascial pain patients.[173] Dispensing a set of instructions to patients can help focus their attention on habits that are contributing to the aggravation or persistence of symptoms (Table 10-11). Instructions for habit reversal and for resting the jaw should also be accompanied by physical therapy that can be performed at home without specialized equipment (eg, the application of moist heat to the affected areas for 15 to 20 minutes twice daily, range-of-motion exercises that stay within the comfort zone, and the occasional use of ice for pain control or for relief of an acute injury superimposed over a chronic TMD [ice or a cold compress 10 minutes every 2 hours during an acute episode may be helpful]).

PHYSIOTHERAPY

While clinical trials necessary to confirm the effectiveness of physiotherapy are lacking, the clinical literature suggests that physiotherapy is a reasonable part of initial therapy.[174] Physiotherapy has been shown to be better than placebo, but no differences between various physical therapies have been shown.[175] Both passive and active treatments are commonly included as part of therapy. Posture therapy has been recommended to avoid forward head positions that are thought to adversely affect mandibular posture and masticatory-muscle activity.

Passive modalities such as ultrasound, laser, and transcutaneous electrical nerve stimulation (TENS) are often used to start physical therapy, reduce pain, and allow the patient to perform jaw exercises that promote recovery. TENS uses a low-voltage biphasic current of varied frequency and is designed for sensory counterstimulation for the control of pain. It is thought to increase the action of the modulation that occurs in pain processing at the dorsal horn of the spinal cord and (in the case of the face) the trigeminal nucleus of the brainstem. Ultrasound therapy relies on high-frequency oscillations that are produced and converted to heat as they are transmitted through tissue; it is a method of producing deep heat more effectively than the patient could achieve by using surface warming.

TABLE 10-11 Instructions to Patients for Self-Care As Part of Initial Therapy

Be aware of habits or patterns of jaw use.
  Avoid tooth contact except during chewing and swallowing.
  Notice any contact the teeth make.
  Notice any clenching, grinding, gritting, or tapping of teeth or any tensing or rigid holding of the jaw muscles.
  Check for tooth clenching while driving, studying, doing computer work, reading, or engaging in athletic activities and also when at work or in social situations and when experiencing overwork, fatigue, or stress.

Position the jaw to avoid tooth contacts.
  Place the tip of the tongue behind the top teeth, and keep the teeth slightly apart; maintain this position when the jaw is not being used for functions such as speaking and chewing.

Modify your diet.
  Choose softer foods and only those foods that can be chewed without pain.
  Cut foods into smaller pieces; avoid foods that require wide mouth opening and biting off with the front teeth or foods that are chewy and sticky and that require excessive mouth movements.
  Do not chew gum.

Do not test the jaw.
  Do not open wide or move the jaw around excessively to assess pain or motion.
  Avoid habitually maneuvering the jaw into positions to assess its comfort or range.
  Avoid habitually clicking the jaw if a click is present.

Avoid certain postures.
  Do not lean on or cup the chin when performing desk work or at the dining table.
  Do not sleep on the stomach or in postures that place stress on the jaw.
  Avoid elective dental treatment while symptoms of pain and limited opening are present.

Adopt other helping practices.
  During yawning, support the jaw by providing mild pressure underneath the chin with the thumb and index finger or with the back of the hand.
  Apply moist hot compresses to the sides of the face and to the temple areas for 10 to 20 min twice daily.

Exercises include exercises for increasing the range of motion in the comfort zone, passive stretching to increase mandibular motion, and isotonic and isometric exercises. Mouth-opening and mouth-closing exercises in a straight line in front of a mirror and/or with the tongue in contact with the palate are common controlled mouth-opening exercises.

Some physiotherapists apply mobilization techniques to increase mandibular motion. These are done passively under the control of the physiotherapist and will usually include distraction and some combination of lateral and protrusive gliding movements. The choice of treatment and timing is an individual consideration since the literature is not developed enough to provide specific guidelines.

INTRAORAL APPLIANCES

Intraoral appliances (splints, orthotics, orthopedic appliances, bite guards, nightguards, or bruxing guards) are used in TMD treatment, and their use is considered to be a reversible part of initial therapy. A number of studies on splint therapy have demonstrated a treatment effect although researchers disagree as to the reason for the effect.[156,172,176,177] In a review of the literature on splint therapy, Clark found a reported improvement of 70 to 90%.[178] A decrease in masticatory-muscle activity has been associated with splint therapy.[179,180] Other studies suggest that the treatment effect cannot be specifically attributed to appliance therapy.[181] Theories that explain the effects include occlusal disengagement, altered vertical dimension, re-aligned maxillomandibular relationship, mandibular condyle repositioning, and cognitive awareness of mandibular posturing and habits.[182] This question will require further research; for the present, however, intraoral appliance therapy is considered to be a reversible treatment and is often included in initial treatment. The choice of material for the construction of an appliance remains one of individual preference. A study comparing a hard and soft material during a 3-month trial found no difference in outcome when either the hard or the soft appliance was used.[183] Long-term continuous wearing of an occlusal appliance is a risk for a permanent change in the occlusion.[184] This is a greater concern with appliances that provide only partial coverage or that occlude only on selected opposing teeth.

General dentists and dental specialists commonly use appliance therapy. Many designs and materials are used, but in a survey, a flat-plane splint made of hard acrylic was used more frequently than any other design or material.[185] The most common purposes advocated for appliance therapy are to provide joint stabilization, protect the teeth, redistribute forces, relax elevator muscles, and decrease bruxism.[182] The appliance most commonly used is described as a stabilization appliance or muscle relaxation splint. Such appliances are designed to cover a full arch and are adjusted to avoid altering jaw position or placing orthodontic forces on the teeth. The appliance should be adjusted to provide bilateral even contact with the opposing posterior teeth on closure and in a comfortable mandibular posture. Anterior guidance in the canine or incisor area is preferred and can usually be achieved with an appro-

priate acrylic contour. During the period of treatment as symptoms improve, the appliance should be re-examined periodically and re-adjusted as necessary to accommodate changes in mandibular posture or muscle function that may affect the opposing tooth contacts on the appliance. At the beginning of appliance therapy, a combination of appliance use during sleep and for periods during the waking hours is appropriate. This should be monitored to determine the most effective schedule for appliance use. Factors such as tooth-clenching when driving or exercising or pain symptoms that tend to increase as the day progresses may be better managed by increasing splint use during these times. To avoid the possibility of occlusal change, the appliance should not be worn continuously (ie, 24 hours per day) over prolonged periods. Many patients continue to wear stabilization splints during sleep with periodic monitoring. Full-coverage appliance therapy during sleep is a common practice to reduce the effects of bruxing and is not usually associated with occlusal change.

Splints that reposition the mandible anteriorly have been used effectively in treating disk displacements,[186] but they increase the risk of permanently altering the occlusion and should be used with caution. These splints have been made for the upper or lower arch although the maxillary appliance is better able to maintain a forward mandibular posture by using a ramp extending from the anterior segment that guides the mandible forward during closure. These appliances were used with greater frequency in the past to correct disk position as a step toward more permanently altering mandibular position through permanent changes in the occlusion. This approach was associated with great technical difficulties, and the treatment failed to correct disk displacement in a significant percentage of patients. Repositioning appliances used for short periods intermittently can be useful in controlling symptoms arising from the mechanical instability of the disk-condyle relationship. Short-term intermittent repositioning therapy may be helpful when transient episodes of jaw locking occur due to disk displacement and are accompanied by pain and dysfunction.

PHARMACOTHERAPY

Mild analgesics, nonsteroidal anti-inflammatory drugs (NSAIDs), antianxiety agents, tricyclic antidepressants, and muscle relaxants are medications used as part of initial treatment. The long-acting benzodiazepine clonazepam was effective in a pilot study of TMD treatment.[187] Opioids are generally reserved for complex chronic pain disorders or (briefly) for acute injuries to the TMJ or muscles. Drug therapy as part of TMD management should follow the general principles of analgesic therapy and be used on a fixed dose schedule rather than as needed for pain. Drug therapy requires a thoughtful assessment of the potential risks relative to the benefits, including the clinician's own professional ability and confidence in using the particular drug or drugs.

NSAIDs are commonly prescribed for pain control in TMD therapy. There are a number of classes of NSAIDs, and the selective cyclo-oxygenase (cox-2) inhibitors celecoxib and rofecoxib offer the same analgesic effect, with a reduced risk of gastrointestinal injury. These drugs should be used for a period of 2 weeks on a fixed dose schedule to assess their effectiveness. Other NSAIDs in common use include ibuprofen (400 mg four times daily, obtainable without a prescription), naproxen, diclofenac, and nabumetone. Diclofenac has been incorporated into a gel (pluronic lecithin organogel) and is applied externally on the skin over the painful muscle or joint. Capsaicin cream (0.025% or 0.075%) has also been used as an analgesic and can be applied to the skin in the painful area four times daily. Capsaicin has a burning quality on application that sometimes limits its usefulness.

Antianxiety agents are useful, especially during acute exacerbations of muscle pain. They are best used at night to avoid daytime sedation, and their potential for dependence is another limiting factor in their usefulness.

Muscle relaxants are a class of drugs that act in the central nervous system, inhibiting interneurons and depressing motor activity. They also have sedative effects that may contribute to their affect on symptoms. These drugs include carisoprodol, methocarbamol, chlorzoxazone, orphenadrine, and the tricyclic derivative cyclobenzaprine. Because their sedative effects will interfere with daily activities, these medications are best taken at night, before sleep.

Tricyclic antidepressants, particularly amitriptyline, have proven to be effective in managing chronic orofacial pain. Amitriptyline is analgesic at low doses, has sedative effects, and promotes restful sleep; all of these effects can be helpful in treatment. It is the anticholinergic effects of the drug (dry mouth, weight gain, sedation, and dysphoria) that often make it intolerable. An effective dose can be as low as 10 mg at night but can be increased gradually to 75 to 100 mg, depending on the patient's tolerance of the side effects.

Drug therapy with an NSAID and a benzodiazepine or cyclobenzaprine, along with the other components of initial therapy, may contribute to symptom control.[188] NSAIDs and benzodiazepines have adverse effects that require caution and monitoring of the drug therapy. A 2-week course with re-evaluation as initial therapy is a reasonable trial. TMD symptoms that are more chronic may require long-term medication use. The choice of drugs and their management as a part of a complex chronic pain disorder is different and is not covered in this chapter.

BEHAVIORAL THERAPY AND RELAXATION TECHNIQUES

Integrating behavioral therapy and relaxation techniques in chronic pain management is effective.[189] In some cases, self-care and awareness of habits may not be sufficient to change behaviors that are contributing to symptoms. A more structured program supervised by a clinician who is competent in behavioral therapy offers a greater chance of addressing issues that are contributing factors. There is general agreement in the literature that behavioral and educational therapies are effective in the management of chronic pain disorders although the existing research is not sufficient to conclude that any one technique is superior. Relaxation techniques, biofeedback, hypnosis, and cognitive-behavioral therapy have all been used

to reduce symptoms in patients with TMD.[190] The mechanism of action with these techniques is unclear.

Relaxation techniques generally decrease sympathetic activity and (possibly) arousal. Deep methods include autogenic training, meditation, and progressive muscle relaxation.[189] These techniques are aimed at producing comforting body sensations, calming the mind, and reducing muscle tone. Brief methods for relaxation use self-controlled relaxation, paced breathing, and deep breathing. Hypnosis produces a state of selective or diffuse focus in order to induce relaxation. The technique includes pre- and postsuggestion and is used to introduce specific goals. Individuals vary greatly in their susceptibility to hypnosis and suggestion. Hypnosis does not effect endorphin production, and its effect on catecholamine production is not known.

Cognitive-behavioral therapy, which often includes relaxation techniques, changes patterns of negative thoughts. Hypnosis and cognitive-behavioral therapy have been hypothesized to block pain from entering consciousness, by activating the frontal limbic attention system to inhibit pain impulse transmission from the thalamic to the cortical structures.[189] Biofeedback is a treatment method that provides continuous feedback, usually by monitoring the electrical activity of muscle with surface electrodes or by monitoring peripheral temperature. The monitoring instruments provide patients with physiologic information that allows them to reliably change physiologic functions to produce a response similar to that produced by relaxation therapies. The patient performs relaxation exercises that are aimed at either lowering the electrical activity of the muscle or raising peripheral temperature. Repetitive practice using the biofeedback instrumentation provides the training for the patient to achieve a more relaxed state and also a greater sensitivity to the activities that have adverse effects.

Barriers to integrating behavioral and relaxation therapy exist in standard medical and dental care. The biomedical model of disease is emphasized in medical and dental education. The biomedical model explains disease in anatomic and pathophysiologic terms and does not stress psychosocial issues or the importance of the patient's experience of disease. Behavioral therapies can be time-intensive and may also not be supported by insurance companies.

For the patient who does not respond to initial treatment and who continues to have significant pain and disability, additional therapies beyond those described above are usually required. These patients are characterized more as having a chronic pain disorder than as having an anatomic abnormality that is unique to the masticatory system. Treatments used in the management of chronic pain are indicated for this group. Multidisciplinary pain clinic management may be required. The use of chronic pain medications, including opioids and the drugs described as adjuvant analgesics (tricyclic antidepressants, anticonvulsants, membrane stabilizers, and sympatholytics), may be part of a long-term management plan. Chronic pain disorders cause psychosocial changes that require management to reduce the associated disability.

A greater focus on behavioral therapies and coping strategies may provide additional benefits. Sleep disorders may require the use of hypnotics or other drug combinations to increase restorative sleep. Depression commonly accompanies chronic pain. Surgery for a chronic muscle pain disorder has no value.

TRIGGER POINT THERAPY

Trigger point therapy has used two modalities: the cooling of skin over the involved muscle and stretching and the direct injection of local anesthetic into the muscle.

Spray and stretch therapy is performed by cooling the skin with fluoromethane (a refrigerant spray) and then gently stretching the involved muscle. The cooling is done to allow the stretching to take place without the pain leading to a reactive contraction or strain. This technique is described in detail by Travell,[139] who introduced the method as a treatment of MPD. Patients who respond to this therapy can use a variation at home by first warming the muscle, then briefly icing it, and then gently stretching the jaw passively.

Intramuscular trigger point injections have been performed by injecting local anesthetic, saline, or sterile water or by dry needling without depositing a drug or solution. The choice of solution for injection exists because of the lack of established benefits of any one method.[191] Injection of sterile water was associated with greater injection pain than was injection of saline[192] and should thus probably be avoided. In a study in which MPD patients were treated with injection of lidocaine or with dry needling, both groups reported decreased pain immediately after injection, but the group that received dry needling experienced greater soreness 48 hours after the procedure.[193] Procaine diluted to 0.5% with saline has been recommended because of its low toxicity to the muscle,[194] but lidocaine (2% without vasoconstrictor) is also used, with a standard dental syringe. There are no tested protocols for trigger point injection therapy, but the injections are often given to a muscle group in a series of weekly treatments for 3 to 5 weeks; this may be continued with modification of the intervals between injections, depending on the response.[195] If there is no response to the initial series of injections, this treatment should be abandoned. Hopwood and Abram analyzed treatment outcomes for 197 patients who received trigger point injection therapy for myofascial pain.[196] They found that (1) unemployment due to pain increased the odds of treatment failure threefold, (2) a longer duration of pain and greater change in social activity increased the risk of failure twofold, and (3) constant pain (versus intermittent pain) increased the likelihood of treatment failure by 80%. These results emphasize that chronic pain is a multidimensional and complex problem and that a variety of factors not directly related to the specific treatment effect will influence the outcome. Botulinum toxin has also been injected in trigger points for myofascial pain, but clinical trials to assess its effectiveness have not been performed.

Oral Health Care Delivery in TMD Patients

Patients who require elective dental treatment should defer such procedures until the MPD symptoms have resolved or are under reasonable control. Patients who develop active dental disease requiring treatment while they are suffering from myofascial pain are likely to have increased myofascial pain after dental procedures. The dentist should attempt to minimize the effect of a procedure on myofascial pain by using a variety of measures, as outlined in Table 10-12.

Other TMD Treatments

This section has highlighted only the most common treatment methods and has not addressed many treatments that have been applied in the management of TMD. Acupuncture has received attention in chronic pain management. There are few clinical trials using acupuncture to treat TMD. Acupressure, different forms of injection therapy using natural substances, massage therapy, naturopathic and homeopathic remedies, and herbal remedies are just a few of the treatments that patients may pursue. There are also treatment systems for which there are several Web sites that provide patients with information for determining whether the system or product may be of value to them. There is a present need (which will increase in the future) for dentists to help patients interpret the treatments and products that are promoted, to avoid harm to patients and unnecessary expense in pursuing treatment to control a distressing disorder. Most of these treatments lack a significant literature that is even descriptive in relation to TMD treatment. This fact, coupled with the present lack of clarity in the scientific research about causes and about the effect of treatment, makes the need to establish a trusting doctor-patient relationship critical.

Bruxism

Nocturnal bruxing is thought to aggravate or contribute to the persistence of pain symptoms associated with TMD. The etiology is not understood, but the evidence suggests that occlusal

---

TABLE 10-12 Managing Temporomandibular Disorder Patients Requiring Dental Procedures

Prior to the procedure
  Use hot compresses to masseter and temporalis areas 10 to 20 minutes two to three times daily for 2 days
  Use a minor tranquilizer or skeletal-muscle relaxant (eg, lorazepam, 1 mg; cyclobenzaprine, 10 mg) on the night and day of the procedure.
  Start a nonsteroidal anti-inflammatory analgesic the day of the procedure, before the procedure.

During the procedure
  Use a child-sized surgical rubber mouth prop to support the patient's comfortable opening; remove periodically to reduce joint stiffness.
  Consider intravenous sedation and/or inhalation analgesia.
  Provide frequent rest periods to avoid prolonged opening.
  Apply moist heat to masticatory muscles during rest breaks.
  Gently massage masticatory muscles during rest breaks.
  Perform the procedure in the morning, when reserve is likely to be greatest.

After the procedure
  Extend the use of muscle relaxant and NSAID medication as necessary.
  Apply cold compresses to the TMJ and muscle areas during the 24 hours after the procedure.

NSAID = nonsteroidal anti-inflammatory drug; TMJ = temporomandibular joint.

abnormalities are not the cause.[197,198] Occlusal appliances may protect the teeth from the effects of bruxism but cannot be expected to prevent or decrease the bruxing activity.[199] When bruxing is considered to be the cause or a factor of TMD symptoms, oral appliance therapy is effective, but symptoms are likely to return when appliance therapy is withdrawn.[200] In one report, nocturnal aversive biofeedback and splint therapy caused a decrease in the frequency and duration of bruxing, but bruxing activity returned after treatment was withdrawn.[201] Occlusal splints worn during sleep have not been found to stop bruxing but do reduce the signs of bruxing.[202]

Recently, case reports of bruxism and symptoms of facial pain, earache, and headache associated with the onset of therapy with selective serotonin reuptake inhibitors (SSRIs) for depression have been published.[203] Symptoms of bruxing resolved when the dosage was decreased or when buspirone was added.[204] Buspirone has a postsynaptic dopaminergic effect and may act to partially restore suppressed dopamine levels associated with the use of SSRIs.

Tan injected severe bruxers in the masseter muscles with botulinum toxin in an open-label prospective trial and reported significant improvement in symptoms and minimal adverse effects.[205] The treatment effect lasted approximately 5 months and had to be repeated. Botulinum toxin exerts a paralytic effect on the muscle by inhibiting the release of acetylcholine at the neuromuscular junction.

Intracapsular Disorders of the TMJ: Articular Disk Disorders

Intracapsular disorders affecting the TMJ are divided into two broad categories: arthritis and articular disk disorders. Either of these disorders may be present with or without symptoms. It is important for the clinician treating patients with TMD to distinguish between clinically significant intracapsular disorders that require therapy from those that are an incidental finding in a patient with facial pain from other causes.

Articular disk displacement (ADD) is an abnormal relationship between the disk, the mandibular condyle, and the articular eminence, resulting from the stretching or tearing of the attachment of the disk to the condyle and glenoid fossa. ADD may result in abnormal joint sounds, limitation in mandibular range of motion, and pain during mandibular movement, but the majority of cases of ADD occur without significant pain or joint dysfunction. MRI studies have demonstrated that ADD is present in 25 to 35% of the normal asymptomatic adult population.[206,207] This is similar to the finding of asymptomatic clinically insignificant disk displacement that is well documented in the knee and spine.[208,209] ADD of the TMJ does not appear to effect children below the age of 5 years.[210]

Loosened disks become displaced anterior to the mandibular condyle in a vast majority of cases. It is theorized that ADD occurs more frequently when the superior head of the lateral pterygoid muscle attaches to the disk. This attachment would pull a loosened disk anterior and medial to the condyle. Posterior disk displacement (when a portion of the disk is found posterior to the top of the condyle) does occur occasionally.[211]

The specific etiology of the majority of cases of disk displacement is poorly understood. Some cases result from direct trauma to the joint from a blow to the mandible. It is also generally believed that chronic low-grade microtrauma resulting from long-term bruxism or clenching of the teeth is a major cause of ADD, and studies using arthroscopic examination of the TMJ have demonstrated a relationship between intracapsular disorders and bruxism.[212] There is also evidence that ADD may be associated with a generalized laxity of joints, and studies have demonstrated a significantly higher incidence of generalized joint laxity in ADD patients than in normal controls.[213] Craniofacial morphology may also play a role in ADD.[214]

Clinicians have also theorized that indirect trauma from cervical flexion extension injuries or certain types of malocclusion may also predispose an individual to disk displacement. These theories are not proven, and the specific series of events that commonly result in ADD is unknown. It is likely that a combination of mechanisms related to the anatomy of the joint and the facial skeleton, connective-tissue chemistry, and chronic loading of the joint increases the susceptibility of certain individuals to a disturbance of the restraining ligaments and displacement of the disk. ADD results in significant pain or dysfunction when accompanied by capsulitis, synovitis, and joint effusions.

CLINICAL MANIFESTATIONS

Disk displacement is divided into stages based on signs and symptoms combined with the results of imaging studies. A simple classification system divides ADD into (1) anterior disk displacement with reduction (clicking joint), (2) anterior disk displacement with intermittent locking, and (3) anterior disk displacement without reduction (closed lock).

Anterior Disk Displacement with Reduction. This condition is caused by an articular disk that has been loosened because of elongation or tearing of restraining ligaments and has moved from its normal position on the top of the condyle. Alteration in the form of the disk may also cause movement from the normal position. A reducing disk displacement is common in the general population, and a clicking or popping joint is of little clinical significance unless the clicking is accompanied by pain or unless the patient experiences dysfunction due to intermittent locking. There are occasional patients who seek professional advice regarding treatment of an audible click that is not accompanied by pain but that may be socially embarrassing.

The clinician who is treating disk displacement in patients with jaw pain must distinguish the patient with myofascial pain and a co-incidental clicking joint from the patient whose pain is related directly to disk displacement. Clinicians should also be aware that symptoms of pain and dysfunction associated with anterior disk displacement with reduction resolve over time with minimal noninvasive therapy in the majority of cases.[215]

Patients with clinically significant anterior disk displacement with reduction will complain of pain during mandibular movement; the pain is most noticeable at the time of the click. Palpation and auscultation of the TMJ will reveal a clicking or popping sound during both opening and closing mandibular movements (the so-called reciprocal click). The clicking or popping sound due to anterior disk displacement with reduction is characterized by a click that occurs at a different point during opening and closing. For example, the opening click may be present at 25 mm of opening, and the closing click may be present at 10 mm. This is due to movement of the disk as the condyle moves it forward during mandibular opening. Clinicians examining patients with ADD may observe a deflection of the mandible early in the opening cycle, with correction towards the midline after the click. Tenderness will be present when ADD is accompanied by capsulitis or synovitis. TMJ effusion may be noted on a T2-weighted MRI scan.[216]

Anterior Disk Displacement without Reduction (Closed Lock). Closed lock may be the first sign of TMD occurring after trauma or severe long-term nocturnal bruxism. It is detected more frequently in patients with clicking joints that progress to intermittent brief locking and then permanent locking. A patient with an acute closed lock will often have a history of a long-standing TMJ click that suddenly disappears with a sudden restriction in mandibular opening. This limited mandibular opening occurs when the disk interferes with the normal translation of the condyle along the glenoid fossa. Other findings include pain directly over the joint during mandibular opening (especially at maximum opening) and limited lateral movement to the side away from the ADD since disks are most frequently displaced medially as well as anteriorly. During maximum mandibular opening, the mandible will deviate towards the side of the displacement. Palpation of the joints will reveal decreased translation of the condyle on the side of the disk displacement.

Posterior Disk Displacement. Posterior disk displacement has been described as the condyle slipping over the anterior rim of the disk during opening, with the disk being caught and brought backward in an abnormal relationship to the condyle when the mouth is closed. The disk is folded in the dorsal part of the joint space, preventing full mouth closure.[217] The clinical features are (1) a sudden inability to bring the upper and lower teeth together in maximal occlusion, (2) pain in the affected joint when trying to bring the teeth firmly together, (3) displacement forward of the mandible on the affected side, (4) restricted lateral movement to the affected side, and (5) no restriction of mouth opening.[217]

MANAGEMENT

Longitudinal studies demonstrate that most symptoms associated with ADD resolve over time either with no treatment or with minimal conservative therapy.[218] For example, one study of patients with symptomatic anterior disk displacement without reduction showed that symptoms had resolved without treatment in 75% of cases after 2.5 years.[219] A long-term study

reported 87% of patients to be without pain or restricted movement 30 years after ADD was initially documented. Since symptoms associated with anterior disk displacement with and without reduction tend to decrease with time, the clinician should not treat patients on the assumption that asymptomatic clicking will inevitably progress to painful clicking or locking. Painful clicking or locking should initially be treated with conservative therapy

Recommended treatments for symptomatic ADD include splint therapy, manual manipulation and other forms of physical therapy, anti-inflammatory drugs, arthrocentesis, arthroscopic lysis and lavage, arthroplasty, and vertical ramus osteotomy. Many of these nonsurgical and surgical techniques are effective in decreasing pain and in increasing the range of mandibular motion although the abnormal position of the disk is not corrected.[220]

Anterior Disk Displacement with Reduction. Patients with TMJ clicking or popping that is not accompanied by pain do not require therapy. Flat-plane stabilization splints that do not change mandibular position and anterior repositioning splints have both been used to treat painful clicking. Anterior repositioning splints maintain the mandible in an anterior position, preventing the condyle from closing posterior to the disk. One meta-analysis that summarized results of previous studies concluded that repositioning splints were more effective than stabilization splints in eliminating both clicking and pain in patients with ADD.[221] Clinicians must weigh the potential benefits of using repositioning splints against the potential side effects of these appliances, which include tooth movement and open bite. Clinicians have advocated techniques that are designed to "recapture" the disk to its normal position, but studies have indicated that splint therapy, arthrocentesis, or arthroscopy rarely replaces the disk in a normal position. The painful symptoms resolve although the disk remains displaced.

Anterior Disk Displacement without Reduction. Some patients with closed lock may present with little or no pain whereas others have severe pain during mandibular movement. Treatment options should depend on the degree of pain associated with the ADD. Management of a locked TMJ may be nonsurgical or surgical. The goals of successful therapy are to eliminate pain and to restore function by increasing the range of mandibular motion. Replacing the disk in a normal position is not necessary to achieve these goals.

Patients who present with restricted movement but minimal pain frequently benefit from manual manipulation of the mandible and from an exercise program that is designed to increase mandibular range of motion by using manual methods or commercially available mandibular range-of-motion devices. Many practitioners will also use a flat-plane occlusal stabilization appliance to decrease the adverse effects of bruxism. Sato and colleagues reported that a combination of a flat-plane stabilization splint and anti-inflammatory drugs was successful in reducing pain and increasing the range of motion in over 75% of patients.[222] The success of this therapy was attributed to decreased inflammation and to the gradual elongation of the posterior attachment, permitting increased movement of the condyle in the fossa. This therapy was also helpful in reducing secondary muscle pain. Patients with severe pain on mandibular movement may benefit from either arthrocentesis or arthroscopy. Flushing the joint with intra-articular corticosteroids to decrease inflammation or with sodium hyaluronate to increase joint lubrication and decrease adhesions has also been reported to help in decreasing the pain associated with nonreducing disk displacement.[216]

▼ ARTHRITIS OF THE TEMPOROMANDIBULAR JOINT

Degenerative Joint Disease (Osteoarthritis)

Degenerative joint disease (DJD), also referred to as osteoarthrosis, osteoarthritis, and degenerative arthritis, is primarily a disorder of articular cartilage and subchondral bone, with secondary inflammation of the synovial membrane. It is a localized joint disease without systemic manifestations. The process begins in loaded articular cartilage, which thins and clefts (fibrillation) and then breaks away during joint activity. This leads to sclerosis of underlying bone, subcondylar cysts, and osteophyte formation.[223] It is essentially a response of the joint to chronic microtrauma or pressure. The microtrauma may be in the form of continuous abrasion of the articular surfaces as in natural wear associated with age or as increased loading forces possibly related to chronic parafunctional activity. The fibrous tissue covering in patients with degenerative disease is preserved.[224] This may be a factor in remodeling and the recovery that is usually expected in osteoarthrosis and osteoarthritis. The relationship between internal derangements and DJD is unclear, but a higher frequency of radiographic signs of DJD was observed in subjects with disk displacement without reduction.[225]

Degenerative joint disease may be categorized as primary or secondary although both are similar on histopathologic examination. Primary degenerative joint disease is of unknown origin, but genetic factors play an important role. It is often asymptomatic and is most commonly seen in patients above the age of 50 years, although early arthritic changes can be observed in younger individuals. Secondary degenerative joint disease results from a known underlying cause, such as trauma, congenital dysplasia, or metabolic disease.

CLINICAL MANIFESTATIONS

DJD of the TMJ begins early and has been observed in over 20% of joints in individuals over the age of 20 years.[226] A study of patients below the age of 30 years presenting to a TMD clinic demonstrated that two-thirds of the patients had degenerative changes detected on tomograms.[227] The incidence of degenerative changes increases with age, and such changes are found in over 40% of patients over 40 years of age. Richards and Brown observed a direct relationship, irrespective of age, between the rate and extent of dental attrition and degenerative disease of the TMJs in cadavers of aboriginal humans.[228] They also noted that the temporal bone exhibited more changes than did the condyle. Many patients with mild to moderate DJD of the TMJ have no symptoms although arthritic changes are observed on radiographs. The presence of pain in patients with DJD is associated with inflammation and joint effusions.

Degenerative changes of the TMJ detected on radiographic examination may be incidental and may not be responsible for facial pain symptoms or TMJ dysfunction; however, some degenerative changes may be underdiagnosed by conventional radiography because the defects are confined to the articular soft tissue. These soft-tissues changes are better visualized with MRI.[229]

Patients with symptomatic DJD of the TMJ experience unilateral pain directly over the condyle, limitation of mandibular opening, crepitus, and a feeling of stiffness after a period of inactivity. Examination reveals tenderness and crepitus on intra-auricular and pretragus palpation with deviation of the mandible to the painful side. Radiographic findings in degenerative joint disease may include narrowing of the joint space, irregular joint space, flattening of the articular surfaces, osteophytic formation, anterior lipping of the condyle, and the presence of Ely's cysts. These changes may be seen best on tomograms or CT scans (Figure 10-11). The presence of joint effusion is most accurately detected in T2-weighted MRI images.

Treatment. Degenerative joint disease of the TMJ can usually be managed by conservative treatment. Significant improvement is noted in many patients after 9 months, and a "burning out" of many cases occurs after 1 year.[230] It seems prudent to manage a patient with conservative treatment for 6 months to 1 year before considering surgery unless severe pain or dysfunction persists after an adequate trial of nonsurgical therapy.

Conservative therapy includes nonsteroidal anti-inflammatory medications; heat; soft diet; rest; and occlusal splints that allow free movement of the mandible. It also may be necessary to concomitantly treat myofascial pain or meniscal defects. Intra-articular steroids can be used during acute episodes, but there is concern that repeated injections may cause degenerative bony changes.[231] Preliminary reports suggest that the anti-inflammatory effects of doxycycline therapy may be helpful in reducing pain associated with TMJ DJD.[232] When TMJ pain or significant loss of function persists and when distinct radiographic evidence of degenerative joint changes exists, surgery is indicated.[233] An arthroplasty, which limits surgery to the removal of osteophytes and erosive areas, is commonly performed. Artificial TMJs have been developed to treat patients with advanced degenerative changes of the TMJ.

Synovial Chondromatosis

CHONDROMETAPLASIA

Synovial chondromatosis (SC) is an uncommon benign disorder characterized by the presence of multiple cartilagenous nodules of the synovial membrane that break, off resulting in clusters of free-floating loose calcified bodies in the joint. It is theorized that SC originates from embryonic mesenchymal remnants of the subintimal layer of the synovium that become metaplastic, calcify, and break off into the joint space.[234,235] SC most commonly involves one joint, but cases of multiarticular SC have been reported.[236] Some cases appear to be triggered by trauma whereas others are of unknown etiology. The knee and elbow are most commonly involved, and less than 100 cases of SC of the TMJ have been reported in the world medical literature.

More sophisticated imaging techniques, such as CT, and arthroscopy have revealed cases of SC that previously would have received other diagnoses, causing authors of recent publications to suspect that SC is more common than previously believed.[237–240] Extension of SC from the TMJ joint to surrounding tissues (including the parotid gland, middle ear, or middle cranial fossa) may occur.[241]

CLINICAL MANIFESTATIONS

Slow progressive swelling in the pretragus region, pain, and limitation of mandibular movement is the most common presenting clinical picture. TMJ clicking, locking, crepitus, and occlusal changes may also may be present.[235] The extension of the lesion from the joint capsule and involvement of surrounding tissues may make diagnosis difficult, causing SC to be confused with parotid, middle-ear, or intracranial tumors. Cases of SC which were mistaken for a chondrosarcoma have been reported. Intracranial extension may lead to neurologic deficits such as facial nerve paralysis. Conventional radiography may not lead to the diagnosis, due to superimposition of cranial bones that may obscure the calcified loose bodies.[242] A CT scan should be obtained if SC is suspected after clinical evaluation. The lesion may appear as a single mass or as many small loose bodies.[237] Arthroscopy may be necessary for accurate diagnosis, particularly when the loose bodies are not calcified and cannot be visualized by conventional radiology or CT.[241]

TREATMENT

Treatment should be conservative and consist of removal of the mass of loose bodies. This may be done arthroscopically when only a small lesion is present, but arthrotomy is required for larger lesions. The synovium and articular disk should be removed when they are involved. Lesions that extend beyond the joint space may require extensive resection.

Rheumatoid Arthritis

The percentage of rheumatoid arthritis (RA) patients with TMJ involvement ranges from 40 to 80%, depending on the group studied and the imaging technique used.[229, 243–245]

Studies using conventional radiography and tomography find fewer abnormalities than CT finds.[229] For example, Goupille, using CT, found TMJ changes in 88% of RA patients, but changes were also detected in more than 50% of controls.[245] CT changes did not correlate with clinical complaints. Avrahami detected condylar changes in approximately 80% of RA patients, using high-resolution CT.[229] Ackerman and colleagues, using tomography, detected erosive condylar changes in two-thirds of RA patients and stated that symptoms were related to the severity of radiographic changes.[246] The disease process starts as a vasculitis of the synovial membrane. It progresses to chronic inflammation marked by an intense round cell infiltrate and subsequent formation of granulation tissue. The cellular infiltrate spreads from the articular surfaces eventually to cause an erosion of the underlying bone.

CLINICAL MANIFESTATIONS

The TMJs are usually bilaterally involved in RA. The most common symptoms include limitation of mandibular opening and joint pain. Pain is usually associated with the early acute phases of the disease but is not a common complaint in later stages. Other symptoms often noted include morning stiffness, joint sounds, and tenderness and swelling over the joint area.[247] The symptoms are usually transient in nature, and only a small percentage of patients with RA of the TMJs will experience permanent clinically significant disability.

The most consistent clinical findings include pain on palpation of the joints and limitation of opening. Crepitus also may be evident. Micrognathia and an anterior open bite are commonly seen in patients with juvenile RA. Larheim attributes the micrognathia to a combination of direct injury to the condylar head and altered orofacial muscular activity.[248] Ankylosis of the TMJ related to RA is rare. Radiographic changes in the TMJ associated with RA may include a narrow joint space, destructive lesions of the condyle, and limited condylar movement. There is little evidence of marginal proliferation or other reparative activity in RA in contrast to the radiographic changes often observed in degenerative joint disease. High-resolution CT of RA patients' TMJs will show erosions of the condyle and glenoid fossae that cannot be seen by conventional radiography.[229]

TREATMENT

Involvement of the TMJ by RA is usually treated by anti-inflammatory drugs in conjunction with the therapy for other affected joints.[249] The patient should be placed on a soft diet during acute exacerbation of the disease process, but intermaxillary fixation is to be avoided because of the risk of fibrous ankylosis. Use of a flat plane occlusal appliance may be helpful, particularly if parafunctional habits are exacerbating the symptoms. An exercise program to increase mandibular movement should be instituted as soon as possible after the acute symptoms subside. When patients have severe symptoms, the use of intra-articular steroids should be considered. Prostheses appear to decrease symptoms in fully or partially edentulous patients.[250]

Surgical treatment of the joints including placement of prosthetic joints, is indicated in patients who have severe functional impairment or intractable pain not successfully managed by other means.

Psoriatic Arthritis

Psoriatic arthritis (PA) is an erosive polyarthritis occurring in patients with a negative rheumatoid factor who have psoriatic skin lesions.[251] The skin lesions precede the joint involvement by several years. PA affects 5 to 7% of patients with psoriasis. Investigators suspect that the cutaneous and joint manifestations of the disease may be traced to the same immunologic abnormality.[252] PA commonly involves the fingers and spine. Pitting of the nails is observed in 85% of patients.

TMJ involvement was once considered rare in PA, with only 28 cases having been reported in the world literature, but recent studies by Könönen and Kilpinen suggest that TMJ involvement is more common than previously believed.[253]

CLINICAL MANIFESTATIONS

The symptoms of PA of the TMJ are similar to those noted in RA, except that the signs and symptoms are likely to be unilateral.[254] Limitation of mandibular movement, deviation to the side of the pain, and tenderness directly over the joint may be observed on examination. Radiographic findings show erosion of the condyle and glenoid fossae rather than proliferation. Coronal CT is particularly useful in showing TMJ changes of PA.[256]

TREATMENT

The management of PA is similar to the treatment of RA, with an emphasis on physical therapy and NSAIDS that control both pain and inflammation in many cases. Antimalarial drugs should not be used because they may cause severe skin reactions in patients with psoriasis. Immunosuppressive drugs, particularly methotrexate, are used for patients with severe disease that does not respond to conservative treatment. Only when there is intractable TMJ pain or disabling limitation of mandibular movement is surgery indicated. Arthroplasty or condylectomy with placement of costochondral grafts has been performed successfully.[251] Surgery may be complicated by psoriasis forming in the surgical scar (Koebner effect).[255]

Septic Arthritis

Septic arthritis of the TMJ most commonly occurs in patients with previously existing joint disease such as rheumatoid arthritis, or underlying medical disorders (particularly diabetes). Patients receiving immunosuppressive drugs or long-term corticosteroids also have an increased incidence of septic arthritis. The infection of the TMJ may result from bloodborne bacterial infection or by extension of infection from adjacent sites such as the middle ear, maxillary molars, and parotid gland.[256] Gonococci are the primary bloodborne agents causing septic arthritis in a previously normal TMJ

while *Staphylococcus aureus* is the most common organism involved in previously arthritic joints.[257]

CLINICAL SYMPTOMS

Symptoms of septic arthritis of the TMJ include trismus, deviation of the mandible to the affected side, severe pain on movement, and an inability to occlude the teeth, owing to the presence of inflammation in the joint space. Examination reveals redness and swelling in the region of the involved joint. In some cases, the swelling may be fluctuant and extend beyond the region of the joint.[258] Large tender cervical lymph nodes are frequently observed on the side of the infection; this helps to distinguish septic arthritis from more common types of TMJ disorders. Diagnosis is made by detection of bacteria on Grams stain and culture of aspirated joint fluid.

Serious sequelae include osteomyelitis of the temporal bone, brain abscess, and ankylosis. Facial asymmetry may accompany septic arthritis of the TMJ, especially in children. Of the 44 cases of ankylosis of the TMJ reviewed by Topazian, 17 resulted from infection.[259] The primary sources of these infections were the middle ear, teeth, and the hematologic spread of gonorrhea.

Evaluation of patients with suspected septic arthritis must include a review of signs and symptoms of gonorrhea, such as purulent urethral discharge or dysuria. The affected TMJ should be aspirated and the fluid obtained tested by Grams stain and specially cultured for *Neisseria gonorrhoeae*.

TREATMENT

Treatment of septic arthritis of the TMJ consists of surgical drainage, joint irrigation, and 4 to 6 weeks of antibiotics.

Gout and Pseudogout

Gouty arthritis is caused by long-term elevation of serum urate levels, which results in the deposition of crystals in a joint, triggering an acute inflammatory response. Acute pain in a single joint (monoarticular arthritis) is the characteristic clinical manifestation of gouty arthritis. Gouty arthritis of the TMJ appears to be very rare although crystal deposition may be apparent in tissues adjacent to the joint. An attack of gouty arthritis is most accurately diagnosed by examination of aspirated synovial fluid from the involved joint by polarized light microscopy. The detection of monosodium urate crystals confirms the diagnosis of gout.

An acute attack of gout may be successfully treated with colchicine, NSAIDS, or the intra-articular injection of corticosteroids.

The deposition of other crystals, such as calcium pyrophosphate dihydrate (CPPD) or calcium hydroxyapatite, may cause a syndrome that resembles gout and that has been referred to as pseudogout.[260] This disorder most frequently effects elderly individuals, and involvement of the TMJ has been reported in cases documented by the demonstration of characteristic CPPD crystals in synovial fluid.[261] Pseudogout of the TMJ has been successfully treated with colchicine or arthrocentesis.

▼ DEVELOPMENTAL DEFECTS AND TRAUMA

Developmental Defects

Developmental disturbances involving the TMJ may result in anomalies in the size and shape of the condyle. Hyperplasia, hypoplasia, agenesis, and the formation of a bifid condyle may be evident on radiographic examination of the joint. Local factors, such as trauma or infection, can initiate condylar growth disturbances.

True condylar hyperplasia usually occurs after puberty and is completed by 18 to 25 years of age. Limitation of opening, deviation of the mandible to the side of the enlarged condyle, and facial asymmetry may be observed. Pain is occasionally associated with the hyperplastic condyle on opening.

Facial asymmetry often results from disturbances in condylar growth because the condyle is considered to be a site for compensatory growth and adaptive remodeling. The facial deformities associated with condylar hyperplasia involve the formation of a convex ramus on the affected side and a concave shape on the normal side. If the condylar hyperplasia is detected and surgically corrected at an early stage, the facial deformities may be prevented.

Deviation of the mandible to the affected side and facial deformities also are associated with unilateral agenesis and hypoplasia of the condyle. Rib grafts have been used to replace the missing condyle to minimize the facial asymmetry in agenesis. In cases of hypoplasia, there is a short wide ramus, shortening of the body of the mandible, and antegonial notching on the affected side, with elongation of the mandibular body and flatness of the face on the opposite side. Early surgical intervention is again emphasized to limit facial deformity.

Trauma

FRACTURES

Fractures of the condylar head and neck often result from a blow to the chin (Figure 10-12). The patient with a condylar fracture usually presents with pain and edema over the joint area and limitation and deviation of the mandible to the injured side on opening. Bilateral condylar fractures may result in an anterior open bite. The diagnosis of a condylar fracture is confirmed by radiographic examination. Intracapsular nondisplaced fractures of the condylar head are usually not treated surgically. Early mobilization of the mandible is emphasized to prevent bony or fibrous ankylosis.

DISLOCATION

In dislocation of the mandible, the condyle is positioned anterior to the articular eminence and cannot return to its normal position without assistance. This disorder contrasts with subluxation, in which the condyle moves anterior to the eminence during wide opening but is able to return to the resting position without manipulation. It has been demonstrated that subluxation is a variation of normal function and

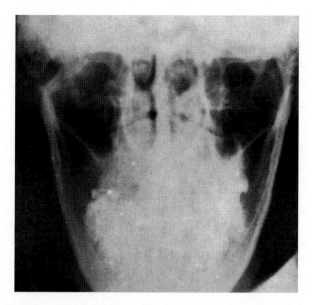

FIGURE 10-12 Fractured and medially displaced condyle.

that the normal range of motion of the condyle is not limited to the fossa.

Dislocations of the mandible usually result from muscular incoordination in wide opening during eating or yawning and less commonly from trauma; they may be unilateral or bilateral. The typical complaints of the patient with dislocation are an inability to close the jaws and pain related to muscle spasm. On clinical examination, a deep depression may be observed in the pretragus region corresponding to the condyle being positioned anterior to the eminence.

The condyle can usually be repositioned without the use of muscle relaxants or general anesthetics. If muscle spasms are severe and reduction is difficult, the use of intravenous diazepam (approximately 10 mg) can be beneficial. The practitioner who is repositioning the mandible should stand in front of the seated patient and place his or her thumbs lateral to the mandibular molars on the buccal shelf of bone; the remaining fingers of each hand should be placed under the chin. The condyle is repositioned by a downward and backward movement. This is achieved by simultaneously pressing down on the posterior part of the mandible while raising the chin. As the condyle reaches the height of the eminence, it can usually be guided posteriorly to its normal position.

Postreduction recommendations consist of a decrease in mandibular movement and the use of aspirin or nonsteroidal anti-inflammatory medications to lessen inflammation. The patient should be cautioned not to open wide when eating or yawning because recurrence is common, especially during the period initially after repositioning. Long periods of immobilization are not advised due to the risk of fibrous ankylosis.

Chronic recurring dislocations have been treated with surgical and nonsurgical approaches. Injections of sclerosing solutions are not used as often now because of difficulty in controlling the extent of fibrosis and condylar limitation. Various surgical procedures have been advocated for treating recurrent dislocations of the mandible; these include bone grafting to the eminence, lateral pterygoid myotomy, eminence reduction, eminence augmentation with implants, shortening the temporalis tendon by intraoral scarification, plication of the joint capsule, and repositioning of the zygomatic arch.

Ankylosis

True bony anklyosis of the TMJ involves fusion of the head of the condyle to the temporal bone. Trauma to the chin is the most common cause of TMJ ankylosis although infections also may be involved.[258] Children are more prone to ankylosis because of greater osteogenic potential and an incompletely formed disk. Ankylosis frequently results from prolonged immobilization following condylar fracture. Limited mandibular movement, deviation of the mandible to the affected side on opening, and facial asymmetry may be observed in TMJ ankylosis. Osseous deposition may be seen on radiographs. Ankylosis has been treated by several surgical procedures. Gap arthroplasty using interpositional materials between the cut segments is the technique most commonly performed.

▼ REFERENCES

1. Okeson J, editor. Orofacial pain: guidelines for assessment, diagnosis, and management. Chicago: Quintessence Publishing Co., Inc.; 1996.
2. American Dental Association. The president's conference on the examination, diagnosis and management of temporomandibular disorders. Chicago: American Dental Association; 1983.
3. Costen J. A syndrome of ear and sinus symptoms dependent upon disturbed function of the temporomandibular joint. Ann Otol 1934;43:1–15.
4. Schuyler C. Fundamental principles in the correction of occlusal disharmony, natural and artificial. J Am Dent Assoc 1935;22:1193–202.
5. Travell J, Rinzler S. The myofascial genesis of pain. Postgrad Med 1952;11:425–34.
6. Schwartz L. Pain associated with the temporomandibular joint. J Am Dent Assoc 1955;51:394–7.
7. Laskin D. Etiology of the pain-dysfunction syndrome. J Am Dent Assoc 1969;79:147–53.
8. Dolwick M, Katzberg RW, Helms CA, Bales DJ. Arthrotomographic evaluation of the temporomandibular joint. J Oral Surg 1979;37:793–9.
9. Katzberg R, Dolwick MF, Helms CA, et al. Arthrotomography of the temporomandibular joint. AJR Am J Roentgenol 1980;134:995–1003.
10. Yale S, Allison B, Hauptfuehrer J. An epidemiological assessment of mandibular condyle morphology. Oral Surg Oral Med Oral Pathol Oral Radiol Endod 1966;21:169–77.
11. Wright D, Moffett BC Jr. The postnatal development of the human temporomandibular joint. Am J Anat 1974;141:235–49.
12. Muto T, Kohara M, Kanazawa M, Kawakami J. The position of the mandibular condyle at maximal opening in normal subjects. J Oral Maxillofac Surg 1994;52:1269–72.
13. Isreal H. Current concepts in surgical management of temporomandibular joint disorders. J Oral Maxillofac Surg 1994;52:289–94.
14. Granstrom G, Linde A. Glycosaminoglycans of temporomandibular articular discs. Scand J Dent Res 1973;81:462–6.
15. Griffin C, Sharpe C. Distribution of elastic tissue in the human temporomandibular meniscus especially in respect to "compression" areas. Aust Dent J 1962;7:72–8.
16. Mills D, Fiandaca D, Scapino R. Morphologic, microscopic and immunohistochemical investigations into the function of the primate TMJ disc. J Orofac Pain 1994;8:136–54.
17. Griffen C, Hawthorn R, Harris R. Anatomy and histology of the human temporomandibular joint. Monogr Oral Sci 1975;4:1–26.
18. Velasco JM, Vazquez JR, Collado JJ. The relationships between the temporomandibular disc and related masticatory muscles in humans. J Oral Maxillofac Surg 1993;51:390–5.
19. Rees A. The structure and function of the mandibular joint. Br Dent J 1954;96:125–33.
20. Kino K, Ohmura Y, Amagasa T. Reconsideration of the bilaminar zone in the retrodiskal area of the temporomandibular joint. Oral Surg Oral Med Oral Pathol 75:410–21.
21. Schmolke C. The relationship between the temporomandibular joint capsule, articular disc and jaw muscles. J Anat 1994;184:335–45.
22. Van Eijden TM, Korfage J, Brugman P. Architecture of the human jaw-closing and jaw-opening muscles. Anat Rec 1997;248:464–74.
23. Carpentier P, Yung JP, Marguelles-Bonnet R, Meunissier M. Insertion of the lateral pterygoid muscle. J Oral Maxillofac Surg 1988;46:477–82.
24. Wilkenson T. The relationship between the disck and lateral pterygoid muscle in the human temporomandibular joint. J Prosthet Dent 1988;60:715–24.
25. Mahan P, Wilkinson TM, Gibbs CH, et al. Superior and inferior bellies of the lateral pterygoid muscle EMG activity at basic jaw positions. J Prosthet Dent 1983;50:710–8.
26. Lipke D, Gay T, Gross B. An electromyographic study of the human lateral pterygoid muscle. J Dent Res 1977;56:230.
27. Mckay G, Yemm R, Cadden S. The structure and function of the temporomandibular joint. Br Dent J 1992;173:127–32.
28. Dworkin S, LeResche L. Research Diagnostic Criteria for Tempormandibular Disorders: review, criteria, examinations, and specifications, critique. J Craniomandib Disord 1992; 6:301–35.
29. Osborn J. A model to describe how ligaments may control symmetrical jaw opening movements in man. J Oral Rehabil 1993;20:585–604.
30. Peck C. Dynamic musculoskeletal biomechanics in the human jaw. Department of Oral Biology. Vancouver: University of British Columbia; 1999. p. 266.
31. Meikle M. Remodeling. In: Sarnat B, Laskin D, editors. The temporomandibular joint: a biological basis for clinical practice. Philadelphia: W.B. Saunders Co.; 1992. p. 93–107.
32. McNamara JA Jr. The independent functions of the two heads of the lateral pterygoid muscle. Am J Anat 1973;1387:197–206.
33. Carpentier P. Microscopic study of the superior lateral pterygoid muscle attachment. J Dent Res 1986;65:1033.
34. Westesson P, Eriksson L, Kurita K. Reliability of a negative clinical temporomandibular joint examination: prevalence of disk displacement in asymptomatic temporomandibular joints. Oral Surg Oral Med Oral Pathol 1989;68:551–4.
35. The glossary of prosthodontic terms. The Academy of Prosthodontics. J Prosthet Dent 1994;71:88.

36. Principles, concepts and practices committee. The Academy of Prosthodontics. J Prosthet Dent 1995;73:73–94.

37. McNeill C. Fundamental treatment goals. In: McNeill C, editor. Science and practice of occlusion. Chicago: Quintessence Publishing Co., Inc.; p. 306–22.

38. Okeson J. Management of temporomandibular disorders and occlusion. 1998. St. Louis: Mosby-Year Book, Inc.; 1998. p. 253–6.

39. Jordan R, Abrams L. Kraus' dental anatomy and occlusion. St. Louis: Mosby; 1992.

40. McNamara D. Variance of occlusal support in temporomandibular pain and dysfunction patients. J Dent Res 1982; 61:350.

41. Pinto O. A new structure related to the temporomandibular joint and middle ear. J Prosthet Dent 1962;12:95–103.

42. Eckerdal O. The petrotympanic fissure: a link connecting the tympanic cavity and the temporomandibular joint. Cranio 1991;9:15–22.

43. Johansson A-S, Isberg A, Isacsson G. A radiographic and histologic study of the topographic relations in the temporomandibular joint region: implications for a nerve entrapment mechanism. J Oral Maxillofac Surg 1990;49:953–61.

44. Friedman MH. Anatomic relations of the medial aspect of the temporomandibular joint. J Prosthet Dent 1988;59:495–8.

45. Johnstone D. The feasibility of palpating the lateral pterygoid muscle. J Prosthet Dent 1980;44:318.

46. Naidoo L. Lateral pterygoid muscle and its relationship to the meniscus of the temporomandibular joint. Oral Surg Oral Med Oral Pathol Oral Radiol Endod 1996;82:4–9.

47. Meyenberg K, Kubik S, Palla S. Relationship of the muscles of mastication to the articular disc of the temporomandibular joint. Helv Odontol Acta 1986;30:1–20.

48. Axelsson S, Fitins D, Hellsing G, Holmlund A. Arthrotic changes and deviation in form of the temporomanbibular joint — an autopsy study. Swed Dent J 1987;11:195–200.

49. Bessette R, Bishol B, Mohl N. Duration of masseteric silent period in patients with TMJ syndrome. J Appl Physiol 1971;30:864–59.

50. Seligman D, Pullinger A. The role of intercuspal relationships in temporomandibular disorders. J Craniomandib Disord 1991;5:96–106.

51. Greene C, Marbach J. Epidemiologic studies of mandibular dysfunction: a critical review. J Prosthet Dent 1982;48:184–90.

52. Solberg W, Flint R, Brentner J. Temporomandibular joint pain and dysfunction: a clinical study of emotional and occlusal components. J Prosthet Dent 1972;28:412–22.

53. Mohl N, Ohrbach R. The dilemma of scientific knowledge versus clinical management of temporomandibular disorders. J Prosthet Dent 1992;67:113–20.

54. Clark N. Occlusion and myofascial pain dysfunction: is there a relationship. J Am Dent Assoc 1982;104:443.

55. Kopp S. Clinical findings in temporomandibular joint osteoarthrosis. Scand J Dent Res 1977;85:434–43.

56. Kerveskari P, Alanen P. Association between tooth loss and TMJ dysfunction. J Oral Rehabil 1985;12:189–94.

57. Tallents R, Catania J, Sommers E. Temporomandibular joint findings in pediatric populations and young adults: a critical review. Angle Orthod 1991;61:7–16.

58. Runge M, Sadowsky C, Sakols E. The relationship between temporomandibular joint sounds and malocclusion. Am J Orthod 1989;96:36–42.

59. Seligman D, Pullinger A, Solberg W. Temporomandibular disorders. Part III: Occlusal and articular factors associated with muscle tenderness. J Prosthet Dent 1988;59:483–9.

60. Obrez A, Stohler C. Jaw muscle pain and its effect on gothic arch tracings. J Prosthet Dent 1996;75:393–8.

61. Akerman S, Kopp S, Nilner M. Relationship between clinical and radiologic findings of the temporomandibular joint in rheumatoid arthritis. Oral Surg Oral Med Oral Pathol 1988;66:639-43.

62. Farrar W. Characteristics of the condylar path in internal derangements of the TMJ. J Prosthet Dent 1978;39:319–23.

63. Farrar W, McCarty WL Jr. Inferior joint space arthrography and characteristics of condylar paths in internal derangements of the TMJ. J Prosthet Dent 1979;41:548–55.

64. Rasmussen O. Description of populations and progress of symptoms in a longitudinal study of temporomandibular arthropathy. Scand J Dent Res 1981;89:196–203.

65. Magnusson T, Egermark-Eriksson I, Carlsson G. Five-year longitudinal study of signs and symptoms of mandibular dysfunction in adolescents. Cranio 1986;4:338–44.

66. Roberts C, Tallents RH, Katzberg RW, et al. Clinical and arthrographic evaluation of temporomandibular joint sounds. Oral Surg Oral Med Oral Pathol 1986;62:373–6.

67. Lund J, Widmer C. An evaluation of the use of surface electromyography in the diagnosis, documentation and treatment of dental patients. J Craniomandib Disord 1989;3:125–37.

68. Seligman D, Pullinger A, Solberg W. The prevalence of dental attrition and its association with factors of age, gender, occlusion, and TMJ symptomatology. J Dent Res 1988; 67:1323–33.

69. McNulty W, Gevirtz RN, Hubbard DR, Berkoff GM. Needle electromyographic evaluation of trigger point response to a psychological stressor. Psychophysiology 1994;31:313–6.

70. Jensen R, Olesen J. Initiating mechanisms of experimentally induced tension-type headache. Cephalagia 1996;16:175–82.

71. Svensson P, et al. Human mastication modulated by experimental trigeminal and extra-trigeminal painful stimuli. J Oral Rehabil 1996;23:838–48.

72. Fillingim R, et al. Pain sensitivity in patients with temporomandibular disorders: relationship to clinical and psychological factors. Clin J Pain 1996;12:260–9.

73. Granges G, Littlejohn G. Pressure pain threshold in pain-free subjects, in patients with chronic regional pain syndromes, and in patients with fibromyalgia syndrome. Arthritis Rheum 1993;36:642–6.

74. Greene C, Olson R, Laskin D. Psychological factors in the etiology, progression and treatment of MPD syndrome. J Am Dent Assoc 1982;105:443–8.

75. Rugh J, Solberg W. Psychological implications in temporomandibular pain and dysfunction. Oral Sci Rev 1976;7:3–30.

76. Scott D, Gregg J. Myofascial pain of the temporomandibular joint: a review of the behavioral-relaxation therapies. Pain 1980;9:231–41.

77. Lipowski Z. Somatization: the concept and its clinical application. Am J Psychiatry 1988;145:1358–68.

78. Gamsa A. Is emotional disturbance a precipitator or a consequence of chronic pain? Pain 1990;42:183–95.

79. Moss R, et al. Oral habits and TMJ dysfunction in facial pain and non-pain subjects. J Oral Rehabil 1995;22:79–81.

80. Rugh J, Harlan J. Nocturnal bruxism and temporomandibular disorders. Adv Neurol 1988;49:329–41.

81. Southwell J, Deary I, Geissler P. Personality and anxiety in temporomandibular joint syndrome patients. J Oral Rehabil 1990;17:239–43.

82. Flor H, et al. Stress-related electromyographic responses in patients with chronic temporomandibular pain. Pain 1991;46:145–52.

83. Isacsson G, Linde C, Isberg A. Subjective symptoms in patients with temporomandibular joint disk displacement versus patients with myogenic craniomandibular disorders. J Prosthet Dent 1989;61:70–7.

84. Braun B, et al., A cross-sectional study of temporomandibular joint dysfunction in post-cervical trauma patients. J Craniomandib Disord 1992;6:24–31.

85. Riolo M, Brandt D, Have TT. Associations between occlusal characteristics and signs and symptoms of TMJ dysfunction in children and young adults. Am J Orthod Dentofacial Orthop 1987;92:467–77.

86. Buckingham R, Braun T, Harinstein DA, et al. Temporomandibular joint dysfunction syndrome: a close association with systemic joint laxity (the hypermobility syndrome). Oral Surg Oral Med Oral Pathol 1991;72:514–9.

87. McNeill C, editor. Temporomandibular disorders: guidelines for classification, assessment, and management. Chicago: Quintessence Books; 1993.

88. Parker M. A dynamic model of etiology in temporomandibular disorders. J Am Dent Assoc 1990;120:283–90.

89. Dworkin Huggins KJ, LeResche L, et al. Epidemiology of signs and symptoms in temporomandibular disorders: clinical signs in cases and controls. J Am Dent Assoc 1990;120:273–81.

90. Schiffman E, Fricton JR, Haley DP, Shapiro BL. The prevalence and treatment needs of subjects with temporomandibular disorders. J Am Dent Assoc 1990;120:295–303.

91. Turk D, Rudy T. Toward an empirically derived taxonomy of chronic pain patients: integration of psychological assessment data. J Consult Clin Psychol 1988;56:233–8.

92. Rudy TE, Turk DC, Berna SF, et al. Quantification of biomedical findings of chronic pain patients: development of an index of pathology. Pain 1990;42:167–82.

93. LeResche L, Saunders K, Von Korff MR, et al. Use of exogenous hormones and risk of temporomandibular disorder pain. Pain 1997;69:153–60.

94. Egermark-Eriksson I, Carlsson G, Ingervall B. Prevalence of mandibular dysfunction and orofacial parafunction in 7, 11 and 15 year-old Swedish children. Eur J Orthod 1981;3:163–72.

95. Williamson E. Temporomandibular dysfunction in pretreatment adolescent patients. Am J Orthod 1977;72:429–33.

96. Grosfeld O, Jackowska M, Czarnecka B. Results of epidemiological examinations of temporomandibular joint in adolescents and young adults. J Oral Rehab 1985;12:95–105.

97. Belfer M, Kaban L. Temporomandibular joint dysfunction with facial pain in children. Pediatrics 1982;69:564–7.

98. Katzberg R, Tallents RH, Hayakawa K, et al. Internal derangements of the temporomandibular joint: findings in the pediatric age group. Radiology 1985;154:125–7.

99. Mohlin B, Pilley J, Shaw W. A survey of craniomandibular disorders in 1000 12-year-olds. Study design and baseline data in a follow-up study. Eur J Orthod 1991;13:111–23.

100. Sadowsky C, Polson A. Temporomandibular disorders and functional occlusion after orthodontic treatment: results of two long-term studies. Am J Orthod 1984;86:386–90.

101. Larsson E, Ronnerman A. Mandibular dysfunction symptoms in orthodontically treated patients ten years after completion of treatment. Eur J Orthod 1981;3:89–94.

102. Truelove E, Sommers EE, LeResche L, et al. Clinical diagnostic criteria for TMD, new classification permits multiple diagnoses. J Am Dent Assoc 1992;123:47–54.

103. Fricton J, Kroening R, Hathaway K. TMJ and craniofacial pain: diagnosis and management. St. Louis: Ishiyaku EuroAmerica; 1988.

104. Wilkes C. Arthrography of the temporomandibular joint in patients with TMJ pain-dysfunction syndrome. Minn Med 1978;61:645–52.

105. Clark GT, Seligman DA, Solberg WK, Pullinger AG. Guidelines for the examination and diagnosis of temporomandibular disorders. J Craniomandib Disord 1989;3:7–14.

106. Schiffman E, Anderson G, Fricton J, et al. Diagnostic criteria for intra-articular TM disorders. Community Dent Oral Epidemiol 1989;17:252–7.

107. Widmer C. Physical characteristics associated with temporomandibular disorders. In: Sessle B, Bryant P, Dionne R, editors. Temporomandibular disorders and related pain conditions. Seattle: IASP Press: 1995. p. 161–74.

108. Lund J, Widmer C, Feine J. Validity of diagnostic and monitoring tests used for temporomandibular disorders. J Dent Res 1995;74:1133–43.

109. Clark G, Delcanho R, Goulet J-P. The utility and validity of current diagnostic procedures for defining temporomandibular disorder patients. Adv Dent Res 1993;7:97–112.

110. Widmer C, McCall W, Lund J. Adjunctive diagnostic tests. In: Zarb G, et al, editors. Temporomandibular joint and masticatory muscle disorders. Copenhagen: Munksgaard; 1994

111. Lundeen T, Levitt S, McKinney M. Clinical application of the TMJ Scale. Cranio 1988;6:339–45.

112. Gobetti J, Turp J. Fibrosarcoma misdiagnosed as a temporomandibular disorder: a cautionary tale. Oral Surg Oral Med Oral Pathol Oral Radiol Endod 1998;85:404–9.

113. Roistacher S, Tanenbaum D. Myofascial pain associated with oropharyngeal cancer. Oral Surg Oral Med Oral Pathol 1986;61:459–62.

114. Fricton J. Establishing the problem list: an inclusive conceptual model for chronic illness. In: Fricton J, Kroening R, Hathaway K, editors. TM disorders and craniofacial pain: diagnosis and management. St. Louis: Ishiyaku EuroAmerica: 1988.7 p. 21–6.

115. Rudy TE, Turk DC, Zaki HS, Curtin HD. An empirical taxometric alternative to traditional classification of temporomandibular disorders. Pain 1989;36:311–20.

116. Turk D. Strategies for classifying chronic orofacial pain patients. Anesth Prog 1990;37:155–60.

117. Fordyce W. Learning process in pain. In: Sternbach R, editor. The psychology of pain. New York: Raven Press; 1986. p. 49–65.

118. Keefe F, Gil K. Behavioral concepts in the analysis of chronic pain syndromes. J Consult Clin Psychol 1986;54:776–83.

119. Korff MV, Dworkin S, LeResche L. Graded chronic pain status: an epidemiologic evaluation. Pain 1990;40:279–91.

120. Oakley ME, McCreary CP, Flack VF, et al. Dentists' ability to detect psychological problems in patients with temporomandibular disorders and chronic pain. J Am Dent Assoc 1989;118:727–30.

121. Lobbezoo-Scholte A, Steenks MH, Faber JA, Bosman F. Diagnostic value of orthopedic tests in patients with temporomandibular disorders. J Dent Res 1993;72:1443–53.

122. Cacchiotti D, Plesh O, Blanchi P, McNeill C. Signs and symptoms in samples with and without temporomandibular disorders. J Craniomandib Disord 1991;5:167–72.

123. Mexitis M, Rallis G, Zachariades N. The normal range of mouth opening. J Oral Maxillofac Surg 1989;47:1028–9.

124. Helkimo M. Studies on function and dysfunction of the masticatory system. Proc Finn Dent Soc 1974;70:37–49.

125. Eriksson L, Westesson P. Clinical and radiographic study of patients with anterior disc displacement of the temporomandibular joint. Swed Dent J 1983;7:55–64.

126. Westesson P, Bronstein S, Liedburg J. Internal derangement of the temporomandibular joint. Morphologic description with correlation to joint function. Oral Surg Oral Med Oral Pathol 1985;43:194–200.

127. Agerberg G. Maximal mandibular movements in children. Acta Odontol Scand 1974;32:147–59.

128. Rothenberg L. An analysis of maximum mandibular movements, craniofacial relationships and temporomandibular joint awareness in children. Angle Orthod 1991;61:103–12.

129. Blasberg B, Chalmers A. Temporomandibular pain and dysfunction syndrome associated with generalized musculoskeletal pain: a retrospective study. J Rheumatol Suppl 1989;19:87–90.

130. Clark G, Green EM, Dornan MR, Flack VF. Craniocervical dysfunction level in a patient sample from a temporomandibular joint clinic. J Am Dent Assoc 1987;115:251–6.

131. Dao T, Lund J, Lavigne G. Pain responses to experimental chewing in myofascial pain patients. J Dent Res 1994;73:1163–7.

132. Bean L, Thomas C. Significance of condylar positions in patients with temporomandibular disorders. J Am Dent Assoc 1987;114:76–7.

133. Katzberg R, DA Keith, Ten Lick WR. Internal derangements of the temporomandibular joint: an assessment of condylar position in centric occlusion. J Prosthet Dent 1983;49:250–4.

134. Westesson P-L. Reliability and validity of imaging diagnosis of temporomandibular joint disorder. Adv Dent Res 1993; 7:137–51.

135. Eckerdal O, Lundberg M. Temporomandibular joint relations as revealed by conventional radiographic techniques. Dentomaxillofac Radiol 1979;8:65–70.

136. Kircos LT, Ortendahl DA, Mark AS, Arakawa M. Magnetic resonance imaging of the TMJ disc in asymptomatic volunteers. J Oral Maxillofac Surg 1987;45:852–4.

137. Schellhas K, Wilkes C. Temporomandibular joint inflammation: comparison of MR fast scanning with T1- and T2-weighted imaging techniques. AJR Am J Roentgenol 1989; 153:93–8.

138. Marakami K, Nishida M, Bessho K, et al. MRI evidence of high signal intensity and temporomandibular arthralgia and relating pain. Does the high signal correlate to the pain? Br J Oral Maxillofac Surg 1996;34:220–4.

139. Travell J, Simons D. Myofascial pain and dysfunction, the trigger point manual. Baltimore: Williams and Wilkens; 1983.

140. Ohrbach R, Dworkin S. Five-year outcomes in TMD: relationship of changes in pain to changes in physical and psychological variables. Pain 1998;74:315–26.

141. Garofalo JP, Gatchel RJ, Wesley AL, Ellis E 3rd. Predicting chronicity in acute temporomandibular joint disorders using the research diagnostic criteria. J Am Dent Assoc 1998;129:438–47.

142. Faucett J. Depression in painful chronic disorders: the role of pain and conflict about pain. J Pain Symptom Manage 1994;9:520–6.

143. Gallagher RM, Marbach JJ, Raphael KG, et al. Myofascial face pain: seasonal variability in pain intensity and demoralization. Pain 1995;61:113–20.

144. Zautra AJ, Marbach JJ, Raphael KG, et al. The examination of myofascial face pain and its relationship to psychological distress among women. Health Psychol 1995;14:223–31.

145. Epker J, Gatchel R, Ellis E. A model for predicting chronic TMD: practical application in clinical settings. J Am Dent Assoc 1999;130:1470–5.

146. Plesh O, Wolfe F, Lane N. The relationship between fibromyalgia and temporomandibular disorders: prevalence and symptom severity. J Rheumatol 1996;23:1948–52.

147. Wolfe F, Ross K, Anderson J, et al. The prevalence and characteristics of fibromyalgia in the general population. Arthritis Rheum 1995;38:19–28.

148. Raphael K, Marbach J, Klausner J. Myofascial pain — clinical characteristics of those with regional vs. widespread pain. J Am Dent Assoc 2000;131:161–71.

149. Greco CM, Rudy TE, Turk DC, et al. Traumatic onset of temporomandibular disorders: positive effects of a standardized conservative treatment program. Clin J Pain 1997;13:337–47.

150. Turk D. Assess the person, not just the pain. Pain Clin Updates 1993;1(3):1–4.

151. Lund JP, Donga R, Widmer CG, Stohler CS. The pain-adaptation model: a discussion of the relationship between chronic musculoskeletal pain and motor activity. Can J Physiol Pharmacol 1991;69:683–94.

152. Stohler C, Ashton-Miller J, Carlson D. The effects of pain from the mandibular joint and muscles on masticatory motor behavior in man. Arch Oral Biol 1988;33:175–82.

153. Korff MV, Howard J, Truelove E. Temporomandibular disorders. Variations in clinical practice. Med Care 1988;26:307–14.

154. Pullinger A, Seligman D. TMJ osteoarthrosis: a differentiation of diagnostic subgroups by symptom history and demographics. J Craniomandib Disord 1987;1:251–6.

155. Randolph C, Greene CS, Moretti R, et al. Conservative management of temporomandibular diosrders: a post treatment comparison between patients from a university clinic and from private practice. Am J Orthod Dentofacial Orthop 1990;98:77–82.

156. Carlsson G. Long-term effects of treatment of craniomandibular disorders. Cranio 1985;3:337–42.

157. LeResche L, Truelove E, Dworkin S. Temporomandibular disorders: a survey of dentists' knowledge and beliefs. J Am Dent Assoc 1993;124:90–106.

158. Glaros A, Glass E, McLaughlin L. Knowledge and beliefs of dentists regarding temporomandibular disorders and chronic pain. J Orofac Pain 1994;8:216–21.

159. Goodman P, Greene C, Laskin D. Response to patients with myofascial pain-dysfunction syndrome to mock equilibration. J Am Dent Assoc 1976;92:755.

160. Helkimo E, Westling I. History, clinical findings and outcome of treatment of patients with anterior disc displacement. Cranio 1987;5:270–6.

161. Vichaichalermvong S, Nilner M. Clinical followup of patients with different disc positions. J Orofac Pain 1993;7:61–7.

162. Dworkin S, LeResche L, Korff MV. Studying the natural hisotry of TMD: epidemiologic perspectives on physical and psychological findings. In: Vig K, Vig P, editors. Clinical research as the basis of clinical practice. Ann Arbor: University of Michigan; 1991.

163. Scholte A, Steenks M, Bosman F. Characteristics and treatment outcome of diagnostic subgroups of CMD patients: retrospective study. Community Dent Oral Epidemiol 1993; 21:215–20.

164. Remick R, Blasberg B, Barton JS, et al. Ineffective dental and surgical treatment associated with atypical facial pain. Oral Surg Oral Med Oral Pathol 1983;55:355–8.

165. Loeser J. Mitigating the dangers of pursuing cure. In: Cohen M, Campbell J, editors. Pain treatment centers at a crossroads. Seattle: IASP Press; 1996. p. 101–8.

166. National Institutes of Health. Management of temporomandibular disorders: NIH technology assessment statement. 1996.

167. Farrar W. Differentiation of temporomandibular joint dysfunction to simplify treatment. J Prosthet Dent 1972; 28:555–629.

168. Block S. Differential diagnosis of craniofacial-cervical pain. In: Sarnat B, Laskin D, editors. The temporomandibular joint. Springfield: Charles C. Thomas; 1980. p. 348–421.

169. Eversole L, Machado L. Temporomandibular joint internal derangements and associated neuromuscular disorders. J Am Dent Assoc 1985;110:69–79.

170. Bell W. Temporomandibular disorders: classification, diagnosis and management. 2nd ed. Chicago: Year Book Medical Publishers; 1986.

171. McNeill C. Temporomandibular disorders: guidelines for evaluation, diagnosis, and management. 2nd ed. Chicago: Quintessence Publishing Co.; 1993.

172. Turk D, Zaki H, Rudy T. Effects of intraoral appliances and biofeedback/stress management alone and in combination in treating pain and depression in patients with temporomandibular disorders. J Prosthet Dent 1993;70:158–64.

173. Gramling S, Neblette J, Grayson R, Townsend D. Temporomandibular disorder: efficacy of an oral habit reversal treatment program. J Behav Ther Exp Psychiatry 1996; 27:245–55.

174. Clark G, Adachi N, Dornan M. Physical medicine procedures affect temporomandibular disorders: a review. J Am Dent Assoc 1990;121:151–61.

175. Gray R, Quayle AA, Hall CA, Schofield MA. Physiotherapy in the treatment of temporomandibular joint disorders: a comparative study of four treatment methods. Br Dent J 1994;176:257–61.

176. Linde C, Isacsson G, Jonsson B. Outcome of 6-week treatment with transcutaneous electric nerve stimulation compared with splint on symptomatic temporomandibular joint disc displacement without reduction. Acta Odontol Scand 1995; 53:92–8.

177. Davies S, Gray R. The pattern of splint usage in the management of two common temporomandibular disorders. Part II: the stabilization splint in the treatment of pain dysfunction syndrome. Br Dent J 1997;183:247–51.

178. Clark G. A critical evaluation of orthopedic interocclusal appliance therapy: design, theory and overall effectiveness. J Am Dent Assoc 1984;108:359–64.

179. Clark G, et al. Nocturnal electromyographic evaluation of myofascial pain dysfunction in patients undergoing splint therapy. J Am Dent Assoc 1979;99:607.

180. Clark G. Management of muscular hyperactivity. Int Dent J 1982;31:216.

181. Dao T, et al. The efficacy of oral splints in the treatment of myofascial pain of the jaw muscles: a controlled clinical trial. Pain 1994;56:85–94.

182. Clark G. A critical evaluation of orthopedic interocclusal appliance therapy: effectiveness for specific symptoms. J Am Dent Assoc 1984;108:364–8.

183. Pettengill C, Growney MR Jr, Schoff R, Kenworthy CR. A pilot study comparing the efficacy of hard and soft stabilizing appliances in treating patients with temporomandibular disorders. J Prosthet Dent 1998;79:165–8.

184. Abbot D, Bush F. Occlusions altered by removable appliances. J Am Dent Assoc 1991;122:79–81.

185. Pierce CJ, Weyant RJ, Block HM, Nemir DC. Dental splint prescription patterns: a survey. J Am Dent Assoc 1995;126:248–54.

186. Tallents RH, Katzberg RW, Macher DJ, Roberts CA. Use of protrusive splint therapy in anterior disk displacement of the temporomandibular joint: a 1- to 3-year follow-up. J Prosthet Dent 1990;63:336.

187. Harkins S, Linford J, Cohen J. Administration of clonazepam in the treatment of TMD and associated myofascial pain: a double blind pilot study. J Craniomandib Disord 1991; 5:179–86.

188. Denucci D, Dionne R, Dubner R. Identifying a neurobiologic basis for drug therapy in TMDs. J Am Dent Assoc 1996; 127:581–93.

189. Natonal Institutes of Health. Integration of behavioral and relaxation approaches into the treatment of chronic pain and insomnia. In: National Institutes of Health technology assessment conference statement. 1995.

190. Millard H, Mason D, editors. 3rd world workshop on oral medicine. Ann Arbor: University of Michigan Continuing Dental Education School of Dentistry; 2000. p. 258–64.

191. Tschopp K, Gysin C. Local injection therapy in 107 patients with myofascial pain syndrome of the head and neck. ORL J Otorhinolaryngol Relat Spec 1996;58:306–10.

192. Wreje U, Brorsson B. A multicenter randomized controlled trial of injections of sterile water and saline for chronic myofascial pain syndromes. Pain 1995;61:441–4.

193. Hong C. Lidocaine injection versus dry needling to myofascial trigger points. The importance of the local twitch response. Am J Phys Med Rehabil 1994;73:256–63.

194. Ritchie J, Greene N. Local anesthetics. In: Goodman A, Goodman L, Rall T, editors. Goodman and Gilman's the pharmacologic basis of therapeutics. New York: McMillan; 1985. p. 302–22.

195. Phero J, Raj P, McDonald J. Transcutaneous electrical nerve stimulation and myoneural injection therapy for management of chronic myofascial pain. Dent Clin North Am 1987; 31:703–23.

196. Hopwood M, Abram S. Factors associated with failure of trigger point injections. Clin J Pain 1994;10:227–34.

197. Rugh J, Barghi N, Drago C. Experimental occlusal discrepancies and nocturnal bruxism. J Prosthet Dent 1984;51:548–53.

198. Kardachi B, Bailey J, Ash M. A comparison of biofeedback and occlusal adjustment on bruxism. J Periodontol 1978; 49:367–72.

199. Holmgren K, Sheikholeslam A, Riise C. Effect of a full-arch maxillary occlusal splint on parafunctional activity during sleep in patients with nocturnal bruxism and signs and symptoms of craniomandibular disorders. J Prosthet Dent 1993;69:293–7.

200. Sheikholeslam A, Holmgren K, Riise C. Therapeutic effects of the plane occlusal splint on signs and symptoms of craniomandibular disorders in patients with nocturnal bruxism. J Oral Rehabil 1993;20:473–82.

201. Pierce C, Gale EN. A comparison of different treatments for nocturnal bruxism. J Dent Res 1988;67:597–607.

202. Yap A. Effects of stabilization appliances on nocturnal parafunctional activities in patients with and without signs of temporomandibular disorders. J Oral Rehabil 1998;25:64–8.

203. Ellison J, Stanziani P. SSRI-associated nocturnal bruxism in four patients. J Clin Psychiatry 1993;54:432–4.

204. Bostwick J, Jaffee M. Buspirone as an antidote to SSRI-induced bruxism in 4 cases. J Clin Psychiatry 1999;60:857–60.

205. Tang E-K, Jankovic J. Treating severe bruxing with botulinum toxin. J Am Dent Assoc 2000;131:211–6.

206. Katzberg RW, Westesson PL, Tallents RH, Drake CM. Anatomic disorders of the temporomandibular joint disc in asymptomatic subjects. J Oral Maxillfac Surg 1996;54:147.

207. Kirkos LT, Ortendahl DA, Mark AS, Arakawa M. Magnetic resonance imaging of the TMHJ disc in asymptomatic volunteers. J Oral Maxillofac Surg 1987;45:852.

208. Boden SD, Davis DO, Dina TS, et al. A prospective and blinded investigation of magnetic resonance imaging of the knee. Abnormal findings in asymptomatic subjects. Clin Orthop 1992;282:177.

209. Boden SD, McCowin PR, Davis DO, et al. Abnormal magnetic resonance scans of the cervical spine in asymptomatic subjects. J Bone Joint Surg 1990;72:1178.

210. Paesani D, Salas E, Martinez A, Isberg A. Prevalence of temporomandibular joint disk displacement in infants and young children. Oral Surg Oral Med Oral Path Oral Radiol Endod 1999;87:15–9.

211. Westesson PL, Larheim TA, Tanaka H. Posterior disc displacement in the temporomandibular joint. J Oral Maxillofac Surg 1998;56:1266.

212. Israel HA, Diamond B, Saed-Nejad F, Ratcliffe A. The relationship between parafunctional masticatory activity and arthroscopically diagnosed temporomandibular joint pathology. J Oral Maxillofac Surg 1999;57:1034.

213. Perrini F, Tallents RH, Katzberg RW, et al. Generalized joint laxity and temporomandibular disorders. J Orofac Pain 1997;11:215–21.

214. Nebbe B, Major PW, Prasad Ng. Female adolescent facial pattern associated with TMJ disk displacement and reduction in disk length: part 1. Am J Orthod Dentofacial Ortho 1999;116:168.

215. Kurita K, Westesson P-L, Yuasa M, et al. Natural course of untreated symptomatic temporomandibular joint disc displacement without reduction. J Dent Res 1998;77:361.

216. Takahashi T, Nagai H, Seki H, Fukuda M. Relationship between joint effusion, joint pain, and protein levels in joint lavage fluid of patients with internal derangements of the temporomandibular joint. J Oral Maxillofac Surg 1999;57:1187.

217. Blankestun J, Boering G. Posterior dislocation of the temporomandibular disc. Int J Oral Surg 1985;14:437–43.

218. Emshoff R, Rudisch A, Bosch R, Ganer R. Effect of arthrocentesis and hydraulic distension on the temporomandibular joint disk position. Oral Surg Oral Med Oral Pathol Oral Radiol Endod 2000;89:271.

219. Sato S, Takahashi K, Kawamura H, Motegi K. The natural course of nonreducing disk displacement of the temporomandibular joint. Int J Oral Maxillofac Surg 1998;27:173.

220. Kai S, Kai H, Tabata O, et al. Long term outcomes of nonsurgical treatment in nonreducing anteriorly displaced disk of the temporomandibular joint. Oral Surg Oral Med Oral Pathol Oral Radiol Endod 1998;85:258.

221. Santacatterina A, Paoli R, Peretta A, et al. A comparison between horizontal splint and repositioning splint in the treatment of disc dislocation with reduction: literature meta-analysis. J Oral Rehabil 1998;25:81.

222. Sato S, Sakamoto M, Kawamura H, Motegi K. Disc position and morphology in patients with nonreducing disc displacement treated by injection of sodium hyaluronate. Int J Oral Maxillofac Surg 1999;28:253

223. Boering G, Stegenga B, deBont LG. Temporomandibular joint osteoarthrosis and internal derangement. Part I: Clinical course and initial treatment. Int Dent J 1990;40:339

224. Pullinger A, Basdioceda F, Bibb C, Relationship of TMJ articular soft tissue to underlying bone in young adult condyles. J Dent Res 1990;69:1512–18.

225. Katzberg RW, Keith DA, Guralnick WC, et al. Internal derangement and arthritis of the temporomandibular joint. Radiology 1982;146:107–12.

226. Oberg T, Carlsson GE, Fajers CM. The temporomandibular joint. A morphologic study on a human autopsy material. Acta Odontol Scand 1971;29:349.

227. Wiberg B, Wanman A. Signs of osteoarthritis of the temporomandibular joint in young patients: a clinical and radiographic study. Oral Surg Oral Med Oral Pathol Oral Radiol Endod, 1998;86:158.

228. Richards LC, Brown T. Dental attrition and degenerative arthritis of the temporomandibular joint. J Oral Rehabil 1981;8:293.

229. Avrahami E, Segal R, Solomon A. Direct coronal high resolution computed tomography of the temporomandibular joints in patients with rheumatoid arthritis. J Rheumatol 1989;16:298.

230. Toller PA. Osteoarthrosis of the mandibular condyle. Br Dent J 1973;134:223.

231. Toller PA. Use and misuse of intra-articular corticosteroids in treatment of temporomandibular joint pain. Proc R Soc Med 1977;70:461.

232. Isreal HA, Ramamurthy NS, Greenwald R, Golub L. The potential role of doxycycline in the treatment of osteoarthritis of the temporomandibular joint. Adv Dent Res 1998;12: 51–5

233. Stegenga B, Dijkstra PV, deBont LG, Boering G. Temporomandibular joint osteoarthrosis and internal derangement. Part II. Additional treatment options. Int Dent J 1990;40:347.

234. Musgrove B, Moody G. Synovial chondromatosis of the temporomandibular joint. Int J Oral Maxillofac Surg 1991;20:93.

235. Gusenbauer A, White G. Synovial chondromatosis of the TMJ: case report and review of literature. Can Dent Assoc J 1989;55:897.

236. Reinish E, Feinberg SE, Devaney K. Primary synovial chondromatosis of the temporomandibular joint with suspected traumatic etiology. Report of a case. Int J Oral Maxillofac Surg 1997;26:419.

237. Herzog S, Mafee M. Synovial chondromatosis of the TMJ: MR and CT findings. AJNR Am J Neuroradiol 1990;11:742.

238. Nitzan DW, Marmary Y, Field SI, Shteyer A. The diagnostic value of computed tomography in temporomandibular joint synovial chondromatosis. Comput Med Imaging Graphics 1991;15:53.

239. Chossegros C, Gola R, Waller PY, et al. Synovial chondromatosis of the temporomandibular joint. Apropos of 3 cases. Rev Stomatol Chir Maxillofac 1990;91:417.

240. Sun S, Helmy E, Bays R. Synovial chondromatosis with intracranial extension: a case report. Oral Surg 1990;70:5.

241. Ikebe T, Nakayama E, Shinohara M, et al. Synovial chondromatosis of the temporomandibular joint: the effect of interleukin-1 on loose body derived cells. Oral Surg Oral Med Oral, Pathol, Oral Radiol Endod, 1998;85:526.

242. Nussenbaum B, Roland PS, Gilcrease MZ, Odell DS. Extraarticular synovial chondromatosis of the temporomandibular joint: pitfalls in diagnosis. Arch Otolaryngol 1999;125:1394.

243. Olson L, Eckerdal O, Hallonsten AL, et al. Craniomandibular function of juvenile chronic arthritis. A clinical and radiographic study. Swed Dent J 1991;15:71.

244. Kreiborg S, Holm K, Nodal M, Pedersen FK. Juvenile chronic arthritis. A clinical and radiographic study of the chewing apparatus. Tandlaegernes Tidsskr 1991;6:168.

245. Goupille P, Pouquet B, Cotty P, et al. The temporomandibular joint in rheumatoid arthritis. Correlations between clinical and computer tomography features. J Rheumatol 1990;17:1285.

246. Ackerman S, Kopps, Nilner M, et al. Relationship between clinical and radiographic findings of the temporomandibular joint in rheumatoid arthritis. Oral Surg 1988;66:639.

247. Stabrun AE, Larheim TA, Hyeraal HM. Temporomandibular joint involvement in juvenile rheumatoid arthritis. Clinical diagnostic criteria. Scand J Rheum 1989;18:197.

248. Larheim TA. Comparison between three radiographic techniques for examination of the temporomandibular joints in juvenile rheumatoid arthritis. Acta Radiol (Diagn) 1981;22:195.

249. Tabeling HG, Dolwick MF. Rheumatoid arthritis: diagnosis and treatment. Fla Dent J 1985;56:1.

250. Sato H, Fujii H, Takada H, Yamada N. The temporomandibular joint in rheumatoid arthritis—a comparative clinical and tomographic study pre and postprosthesis. J Oral Rehab 1990;17:165.

251. Wilson AW, Brown JS, Ord RA. Psoriatic arthropathy of the temporomandibular joint. Oral Surg 1990;70:555.

252. Koorbusch GF, Zeitler DL, Fotos PG, Doss JB. Psoriatic arthritis of the temporomandibular joints with ankylosis. Oral Surg 1991;71:267.

253. Könönen M, Kilpinen E. Comparison of three radiographic methods in screening of temporomandibular joint involvement in patients with psoriatic arthritis. Acta Odontol Scand 1990;48:271.

254. Miles DA, Kaugars GA. Psoriatic involvement of the temporomandibular joint. Oral Surg 1991;71:770.

255. Laurent R. Psoriatic arthritis. Clin Rheumatol 1985;11:65.

256. Bounds GA, Hopkins R, Sugar A. Septic arthritis of the temporomandibular joint—a problematic diagnosis. Br J Oral Maxillofac Surg 1987;25:61

257. Hekkenberg RJ, Piedade L, Mock D, et al. Septic arthritis of the temporomandibular joint. Otolaryngol. Head neck Surg,1999, 120:780.

258. Hincapie JW, Tobon D, Diaz-Reyes GA. Septic arthritis of the temporomandibular joint. Otolaryngol Head Neck Surg 1999;121:836.

259. Topazian RG. Etiology of ankylosis of the temporomandibular joint: analysis of 44 cases. J Oral Surg 1964;22:227.

260. Nakagawa Y, Ishii H, Shimoda S, Ishibashi K. Pseudogout of the temporomandibular joint: a case report. Int J Oral Maxillofac Surg 1999;28:26.

261. Strobl H, Emshoff R, Kreczy A. Calcium pyrophosphate dihydrate crystal deposition disease of the temporomandibular joint. Oral Surg Oral Med Oral Pathol Oral Radiol Endod 1998,85:349.

11

OROFACIAL PAIN

BRUCE BLASBERG, DMD, FRCD(C)
MARTIN S. GREENBERG, DDS

Orofacial pain (OFP) is the presenting symptom of a broad spectrum of diseases. As a symptom, it may be due to disease of the orofacial structures, generalized musculoskeletal or rheumatic disease, peripheral or central nervous system disease, or psychological abnormality; or the pain may be referred from other sources (eg, cervical muscles or intracranial pathology). OFP may also occur in the absence of detectable physical, imaging, or laboratory abnormalities. Some of these disorders are easily recognized and treated whereas others defy classification and are unresponsive to present treatment methods. The possible causes of orofacial pain are considerable and cross the boundaries of many medical and dental disciplines. An interdisciplinary approach is often required to establish a diagnosis and for treatment.

This chapter discusses new developments that have led to a better understanding of chronic pain and reviews the diagnosis and treatment of OFP disorders. Disorders of the musculoskeletal system that cause OFP are discussed in Chapter 10, "Temporomandibular Disorders".

▼ DEFINING PAIN

In this century, the concept of pain has evolved from that of a one-dimensional sensation to that of a multidimensional experience encompassing sensory-discriminative, cognitive, motivational, and affective qualities. The most recent definition of pain, produced by the Task Force on Taxonomy of the International Association for the Study of Pain (IASP) is, *"An unpleasant sensory and emotional experience associated with actual or potential tissue damage, or described in terms of such damage."*[1]

An accompanying explanatory note emphasizes the subjective and emotional nature of pain as well as the lack of correlation between pain and tissue damage.

"Note: Pain is always subjective. Each individual learns the application of the word through experiences related to injury in early life. Biologists recognize that those stimuli which cause pain are liable to damage tissue. Accordingly, pain is that experience we associate with actual or potential tissue damage. It is unquestionably a sensation in a part or parts of the body, but it is also always unpleasant and therefore also an emotional experience. Experiences which resemble pain but are not unpleasant, eg, pricking, should not be called pain. Unpleasant abnormal experiences (dysesthesias) may also be pain but are not necessarily so because, subjectively, they may not have the usual sensory qualities of pain.

Many people report pain in the absence of tissue damage or any likely pathophysiological cause; usually this happens for psychological reasons. There is usually no way to distinguish their experience from that due to tissue damage if we take the subjective report. If they regard their experience as pain and if they report it in the same ways as pain caused by tissue damage, it should be accepted as pain. This definition avoids tying pain to the stimulus. Activity induced in the nociceptor and nociceptive pathways by a noxious stimulus is not pain, which is always a psychological state, even though we may well appreciate that pain most often has a proximate physical cause."[1]

Pain, in the medical model, is considered a symptom of disease, to be diagnosed and treated. Unfortunately, a cause and a diagnosis cannot always be established. Repeated attempts to identify a physical cause may result in unnecessary and sometimes harmful investigations and treatments. Establishing a precise diagnosis and providing effective treatment have become major challenges in medicine and dentistry. This has led to the development of a biobehavioral or biopsychosocial model to explain the phenomena observed in patients experiencing chronic pain. In this model, pain is not divided into physical versus psychological components. Instead, physical, psychological, and social factors are viewed as mutually influential forces with the potential to create an infinite number of unique pain experiences.[2] The biologic system deals with the anatomic, structural, and molecular substrates of disease. The psychological system deals with the effects of motivation and personality on the experience of illness and on reactions to illness. The social system deals with cultural, environmental, and familial influences on the expression and experience of illness. Each system affects and is affected by all of the others.[3]

The words "pain" and "suffering" have often been used synonymously, but the experience of suffering has been differentiated from pain. Suffering has been defined as including the experience of pain but as also including vulnerability, dehumanization, a lost sense of self, blocked coping efforts, lack of control over time and space, and an inability to find meaning or purpose in the painful experience.[2] The term "suffering" attempts to convey the experience of pain beyond sensory attributes.

Anatomic Considerations

Cranial nerve V (CN V), the trigeminal nerve, is the dominant nerve that relays sensory impulses from the orofacial area to the central nervous system. The facial (CN VII), glossopharyngeal (CN IX), and vagus (CN X) nerves and the upper cervical nerves (C2 and C3) also relay sensory information from the face and surrounding area (Table 11-1). (For a more detailed study of this topic, the reader is referred to the sources listed in the "Suggested Readings" section at the end of this chapter.)

Primary sensory neurons associated with pain (nociceptors) are characterized by small-diameter axons with slow conduction velocities (ie, finely myelinated A delta fibers and unmyelinated C fibers) (Figure 11-1). Nociceptors are activated by intense or noxious stimuli. Some are unimodal and respond only to thermal or mechanical stimuli; others are polymodal and respond to mechanical, thermal, and chemical stimuli. Nociceptors encode the intensity, duration, and quality of a noxious stimulus.

Information associated with pain is carried in the three divisions of the trigeminal nerve to the trigeminal sensory ganglion. The central processes of these neurons enter the pons, where they descend in the brainstem as the spinal trigeminal tract. Fibers from the spinal trigeminal tract synapse in the adjacent trigeminal nucleus that extends parallel to the tract in the brainstem. The spinal nucleus of CN V extends

TABLE 11-1 Cranial and Cervical Nerves That Provide Somatic and Visceral Sensation to the Orofacial Area

Nerve	General Area Served
V: Trigeminal	Skin of face, forehead and scalp as far as the top of the head; conjunctiva and bulb of the eye; oral and nasal mucosa; part of the external aspect of the tympanic membrane; teeth; anterior two-thirds of tongue; masticatory muscles; TMJ; meninges of anterior and middle cranial fossae
VII: Facial	Skin of the hollow of the auricle of the external ear; small area of skin behind the ear
IX: Glossopharyngeal	Mucosa of the pharynx; fauces; palatine tonsils; posterior one-third of the tongue; internal surface of the tympanic membrane; skin of the external ear
X: Vagus	Skin at the back of the ear; posterior wall and floor of external auditory meatus; tympanic membrane; meninges of posterior cranial fossa; pharynx; larynx
Cervical nerve 2	Back of the head extending to the vertex; behind and above the ear; submandibular, anterior neck
Cervical nerve 3	Lateral and posterior neck

TMJ = temporomandibular joint.

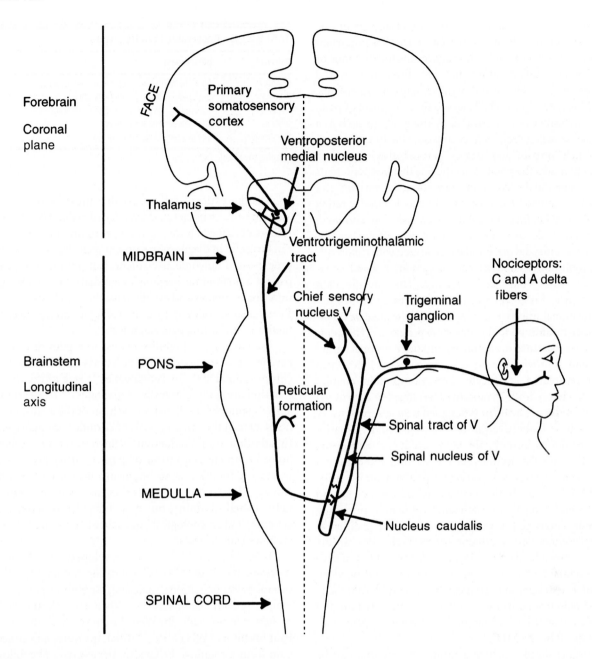

FIGURE 11-1 Nociceptive transmission associated with the trigeminal nerve.

from the chief sensory nucleus of CN V to the spinal cord, where it merges with the dorsal gray matter. The spinal nucleus is divided into three nuclei; the most caudal, the nucleus caudalis, is continuous with and resembles the dorsal horn of the cervical spinal cord.[4] Morphologic, clinical, and electrophysiologic observations indicate that the nucleus caudalis is the principal site in the brainstem for nociceptive information.[5–7] Axons from the spinal nucleus of CN V cross to the opposite side and ascend to the ventral posteromedial nucleus of the thalamus and also project to the reticular formation and the medial and intralaminar thalamic nuclei. From the thalamus, neurons course and end at the somatosensory cortex.

Measurement of Pain and Disability

There is no simple method of measuring pain. The intensity of an individual's pain is based on what is verbally or nonverbally communicated about the experience. Patients often express difficulty describing pain, and two people may have very different descriptions for pain that accompanies a similar injury. Within a specific diagnosis, great variability exists regarding the disabling effects of pain on an individual's life. Adding to this complexity is the lack of a direct correlation between the severity of a chronic pain disorder and the magnitude of the anatomic or pathologic change described by the clinical diagnosis.[8] In assessing OFP patients, pain intensity, emotional distress, and associated disability are important and cannot be captured with one scale or questionnaire. This has important implications for treatment because addressing the anatomic or pathologic abnormality alone may not eliminate pain and restore health. Individuals with cognitive impairment, infants, and children pose special challenges to the assessment of pain.

Pain intensity can be measured by using ratings such as a visual analog scale (VAS). A VAS consists of a 10 cm line on which 0 cm is "no pain" and 10 cm is "pain as bad as it could be." The patient marks the point along the line that best represents his or her pain, and the score is measured from the "no pain" end of the scale. Numeric scales (eg, 1 to 10) and descriptive rating scales (eg, no pain, mild, moderate, severe pain) are also used. Visual analog scales are sensitive to treatment effects,[9] can be incorporated into pain diaries, and can be used with children.[10]

The multidimensional aspects of pain are not well measured by scales that rate intensity. The McGill Pain Questionnaire (MPQ) (Figure 11-2) was created to measure the motivational-affective and the cognitive-evaluative qualities of pain, in addition to the sensory experience.[11] The questionnaire was designed to capture the multidimensional nature of pain and to provide quantitative measures of clinical pain that can be treated statistically. The questionnaire enables patients to choose from 78 adjectives (arranged in 20 groups) that describe pain. The form is designed to assess the sensory (groups 1 to 10), affective (groups 11 to 15), and evaluative (group 16) dimensions of pain and to produce a pain-rating index. There are also sections for the location and temporal characteristics of pain and a rating for present pain intensity.

The MPQ is used both by clinicians and researchers and has been helpful in pain research and treatment by providing a common language for assessing and comparing different pain experiences and treatment effects. Verbal descriptors have been shown to discriminate between reversible and irreversible damage of nerve fibers in a tooth[12] and between trigeminal neuralgia and atypical facial pain.[13] Toothache pain and pain from burning mouth syndrome were found to be equal in magnitude but significantly different in pain quality as assessed by the MPQ.[12]

Clinicians should include a rating or scale that can be used initially and during treatment to provide a reference for the course of the disorder and the treatment progress. Visual analog scales and numeric scales require no specific forms and are easily administered. The MPQ is available from the International Association for the Study of Pain (IASP) and is used in pain clinics and by clinicians focusing on pain management.

Patients experiencing pain may display a broad range of observable behaviors that communicate to others that they are experiencing pain (Table 11-2). These may be observable during the diagnostic interview or in response to physical examination procedures. An awareness of pain behaviors is valuable, but their presence or absence in any given situation is not necessarily diagnostic. These behaviors are often diminished or absent in patients with chronic pain and cannot be correlated with the presence or absence of pain or pain intensity.

TABLE 11-2 Observable Pain Behaviors

Behavior	Observations
Guarding	Abnormally slow, stiff, or interrupted movement
Bracing	Stiff, pain-avoidant posturing while in a static position
Rubbing	Touching, rubbing, or holding of the painful area
Sighing	Pronounced exhalation of air
Grimacing	Obvious facial expression of pain

Adapted from Keefe F et al.[14]

It is the patient's self-report that must be relied on for assessing the character and severity of pain. The scales and ratings described above are attempts to provide a rating that can be useful in diagnosis, treatment planning, and treatment progress and outcome assessment. Pain ratings also give the patient a method for keeping a pain diary to provide insight into what activities and events make the pain better or worse. Visual analog scales and numerical scales are relatively easy methods of charting pain intensity.

Assessments of disability related to a pain disorder and psychological status are important parts of any evaluation of chronic pain. Disability is defined as "a lack of the ability to function normally, physically or mentally."[15] The level of disability cannot be predicted on the basis of the anatomic diagnosis. One of the primary goals of chronic pain management (in addition to pain reduction) is the restoration of function. Since complete resolution of pain is often not possible, increasing function is an important measure of treatment success. There is no universally accepted method of assessing pain-related disability, but pain-related interference with activities and psychological impairments associated with pain are important aspects.

Turk and Rudy[8,16] have developed the Multiaxial Assessment of Pain (MAP) classification and have tested it on several pain populations, including a group of patients with temporomandibular disorders.[17] Their assessment included a 61-item questionnaire, the West Haven-Yale Multidimensional Pain Inventory (WHYMPI),[18] which measures adjustment to pain from a cognitive-behavioral perspective. The following three distinct profiles emerged: (1) "dysfunctional, characterized by patients who perceived the severity of their pain to be high, reported that pain interfered with much of their lives, reported a higher degree of affective distress, and maintained low levels of activity; (2) interpersonally distressed, characterized by a common perception that 'significant others' were not very understanding or supportive of the patient's problems; and (3) adaptive copers, patients with high levels of social support, relatively low levels of pain, perceived interference, affective distress, and higher levels of activity and perceived control".[19] Turk and Rudy found that when they used the MAP profiles, psychosocial and behavioral response patterns to pain were similar despite different medical and dental diagnoses. An assessment in this domain can be combined with any classification scheme related to OFP disorders, to provide a more comprehensive profile of the presenting problem. Establishing

MEASUREMENT OF PAIN

McGill Pain Questionnaire

Patient's Name _____ Date _____ Time_____am/pm

PRI: S_____ A_____ E_____ M_____ PRI(T)_____ PPI_____
    (1-10)   (11-15)   (16)   (17-20)   (1-20)

1 FLICKERING ___
  QUIVERING ___
  PULSING ___
  THROBBING ___
  BEATING ___
  POUNDING ___

2 JUMPING ___
  FLASHING ___
  SHOOTING ___

3 PRICKING ___
  BORING ___
  DRILLING ___
  STABBING ___
  LANCINATING ___

4 SHARP ___
  CUTTING ___
  LACERATING ___

5 PINCHING ___
  PRESSING ___
  GNAWING ___
  CRAMPING ___
  CRUSHING ___

6 TUGGING ___
  PULLING ___
  WRENCHING ___

7 HOT ___
  BURNING ___
  SCALDING ___
  SEARING ___

8 TINGLING ___
  ITCHY ___
  SMARTING ___
  STINGING ___

9 DULL ___
  SORE ___
  HURTING ___
  ACHING ___
  HEAVY ___

10 TENDER ___
   TAUT ___
   RASPING ___
   SPLITTING ___

11 TIRING ___
   EXHAUSTING ___

12 SICKENING ___
   SUFFOCATING ___

13 FEARFUL ___
   FRIGHTFUL ___
   TERRIFYING ___

14 PUNISHING ___
   GRUELLING ___
   CRUEL ___
   VICIOUS ___
   KILLING ___

15 WRETCHED ___
   BLINDING ___

16 ANNOYING ___
   TROUBLESOME ___
   MISERABLE ___
   INTENSE ___
   UNBEARABLE ___

17 SPREADING ___
   RADIATING ___
   PENETRATING ___
   PIERCING ___

18 TIGHT ___
   NUMB ___
   DRAWING ___
   SQUEEZING ___
   TEARING ___

19 COOL ___
   COLD ___
   FREEZING ___

20 NAGGING ___
   NAUSEATING ___
   AGONIZING ___
   DREADFUL ___
   TORTURING ___

PPI
0 NO PAIN ___
1 MILD ___
2 DISCOMFORTING ___
3 DISTRESSING ___
4 HORRIBLE ___
5 EXCRUCIATING ___

BRIEF ___	RHYTHMIC ___	CONTINUOUS ___
MOMENTARY ___	PERIODIC ___	STEADY ___
TRANSIENT ___	INTERMITTENT ___	CONSTANT ___

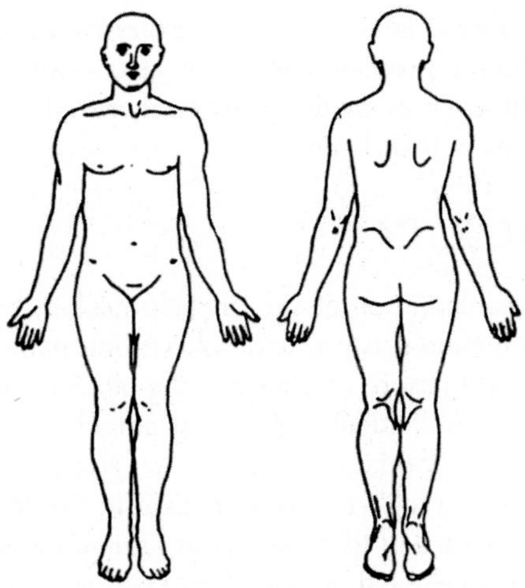

E = EXTERNAL
I = INTERNAL

COMMENTS:

FIGURE 11-2 The McGill Pain Questionnaire.

a specific OFP diagnosis and assessing the psychosocial and behavioral issues is critical in the treatment and prognosis of chronic pain.

Dworkin, LeResche, and colleagues have developed a method for assessing dysfunctional chronic pain as part of a classification system, the Research Diagnostic Criteria.[20] They used the Graded Chronic Pain Severity scale,[21] the depression and vegetative-symptom scales from the symptom checklist-90-revised (SCL-90-R),[22] and a "jaw disability checklist." All three of these scales are based on questionnaires that are completed by the patient. The criteria were developed to advance the research in temporomandibular disorders. The criteria require validation, but the design of the classification makes it applicable to clinical practice. The Graded Chronic Pain Severity scale has four grades of disability and pain intensity based on seven questions, of which three are related to pain intensity and four are related to disability. The SCL-90-R depression scales are used to identify patients who may be experiencing significant depression, a problem commonly associated with chronic pain. These issues are discussed further in the section on assessment in this chapter.

▼ CHRONIC PAIN

Although a precise definition of chronic pain has not been established, a distinction between acute and chronic pain has emerged. The somatosensory system serves the valuable function of warning the individual of actual or potential tissue damage. Nociceptors, specialized recptors that signal tissue damage, terminate in a highly ordered manner in the dorsal horn of the spinal cord and its homologous subnucleus caudalis in the spinal trigeminal nucleus. Information is transferred directly or through relay to the ventrobasal thalamus and then to the cortex. In the spinal cord, other pathways from the dorsal horn pass to the ventral horn and activate flexor motor neurons, generating the withdrawal flexion reflex.

This model draws attention to the protective aspect of the sensation of pain and is consistent with the qualities of acute pain. In other circumstances following peripheral tissue or nerve injury, a pathologic state may develop, resulting in persistent pain long after the injured tissue has healed. In this state, pain no longer represents a warning signal of potential or actual tissue damage; pain itself becomes the disorder.

Chronic pain is now recognized as a complex disorder that is influenced by biologic factors and by a range of psychosocial factors, including emotion, psychological distress, family and work environment, cultural background, the meaning of the pain, and appraisals of the controllability of the pain. Chronic pain has been defined as pain that persists past the normal time of healing,[23] but this may not be an easy determination. Alternatively, chronic pain has been related to duration (ie, pain that lasts longer than 6 months). Recently, pain lasting longer than 3 months has been used to define chronic pain. In the IASP publication on classification, Merskey describes chronic pain as "a persistent pain that is not amenable, as a rule,

to treatments based on specific remedies, or to the routine methods of pain control such as non-narcotic analgesics."[1]

As pain persists, psychosocial issues (including depression, maladaptive beliefs about pain, medication abuse, strained interpersonal relationships, and ineffective coping strategies) become prominent aspects of the disorder.[24,25] The term "chronic pain syndrome" has been used to describe a condition that may have started because of an organic cause but is now compounded by psychological and social problems. The term has been criticized since it may obscure more-accurate physical and psychiatric diagnoses. It has sometimes been used pejoratively and has been interpreted by some to suggest a pain disorder that is psychological.[1] Originally, this label was used in an attempt to characterize a disorder that (regardless of its original cause) had evolved into a condition in which psychological and social problems were contributing to the persistence or exacerbation of the illness and in which significant disability was present.

In situations in which no ongoing peripheral injury was present to explain the pain, it was assumed that the pain was psychological. Patients need to be educated about the psychological distress and depression that can be a consequence of chronic pain. This is an important issue for clinicians and patients because of the demoralization and doubt patients develop about the condition and about their mental health.

Pathophysiology

The gate-control theory, introduced by Melzak and Wall in 1965,[26] articulated a model that explained the pain experience as a multidimensional process with many modulating influences. The proposed explanation for the persistence of pain after healing relates to changes (neuroplasticity) in the central nervous system.[27] Neurons are thought to be capable of altering their structure and function in response to stimuli, resulting in new stimulus-response relationships. This sensitization does not require ongoing peripheral input but is a consequence of changes in the sensitivity of neurons in the spinal cord.[28] These changes include the following:

1. A reduction of the stimulation threshold, with the result that the neurons no longer require a noxious stimulus in order to be activated
2. An alteration in the temporal pattern of the response, so that a transient stimulus evokes a sustained burst of activity
3. An increase in the general responsiveness of the motor neurons, so that a noxious stimulus produces a greater effect
4. The expansion of receptive fields, with the result that responses are evoked over a much wider area.

The clinical manifestations of these changes include hyperalgesia (an increased response to a stimulus that is normally painful); allodynia (pain due to a stimulus that does not normally provoke pain); and spontaneous, radiating, and referred pain.

The interaction between the sympathetic and somatosensory nervous systems has been associated with chronic pain and thought to be the cause of many but not all cases of complex regional pain syndrome (CRPS). The relationship may be a coupling mediated by the neurotransmitter noradrenaline, which is released from sympathetic nerve endings acting on α-adrenoreceptors in the membrane of afferent neurons, causing depolarization. The mechanism is thought to be more likely a sensitivity of the somatosensory system than a hyperactivity of the sympathetic efferent system.[29]

Behavioral Issues

The observation that some individuals with high levels of pain continue to work while others are completely disabled led to the exploration of behavioral assessment and theories as a possible explanation.[30] Behavioral theories suggest that pain behaviors influence and are influenced by the patient's social environment.[30,31] The behavioral model views the pain behavior and associated disability as being as important as the underlying pathophysiology. A major goal in therapy is to modify pain behavior, thus improving function even when pain itself cannot be treated directly. Behavior therapy focuses on eliminating or reducing maladaptive behavior without theorizing about inner conflicts. It is based on principles of learning theory, particularly operant and classic conditioning.[3]

Pain itself can be viewed as a stress. The consequences of chronic pain (eg, loss of income, marital difficulties) are also significant stressors. Emotional distress is a component of pain, but it is also a consequence of pain, a cause of pain, or a concurrent problem with independent sources. These distinctions have not always been made clear, and there has been debate and confusion concerning whether emotional processes should be conceptualized as causes or consequences of pain.[32] The belief that chronic pain is a psychological disorder arose from two unproven assumptions: (1) chronic pain patients are a homogeneous group whose pain can be explained in terms of a more or less consistent constellation of personality characteristics, and (2) psychosocial disturbances (such as anxiety, depression, and social isolation) in pain patients reflect life events before the pain and are thus significant in explaining its onset.

The prevalence of depression is substantially higher in chronic pain patients compared to individuals without pain, but the majority of chronic pain patients are not depressed.[33] An association between chronic pain and depression exists, but no one hypothesis has emerged or has been proven to explain the relationship. Theories proposed include the following:

1. Depression causes hypersensitivity to pain.
2. Pain is a "masked" form of depression.
3. Depression is caused by the stress of chronic pain.

Depression, anxiety, and anger frequently coexist with chronic illness, but these reactions are not necessarily "psychopathological."[34] The literature suggests that in general, pain is more likely to cause emotional disturbances than to be precipitated by them.[35] The fourth edition of the *Diagnostic and Statistical Manual of Mental Disorders* (DSM-IV) uses the classification "mood disorder due to a general medical condition" to describe this. This classification is not considered to be a mental disorder.

A substantial group of chronic pain patients can be characterized as "dysfunctional" because of a consistent pattern of high levels of pain severity, affective distress, life interference, and lower-than-average levels of life control and activity.[36] The loss of customary roles at work, in the family, and in social settings, accompanied by the realization that neither one's own best efforts nor the interventions of highly respected health care professionals have been effective, is a major stressor. Challenges to the legitimacy of the complaints also represent a major source of stress. Excess use of medical services, hospitalizations for surgery, and abuse of medications are part of the profile of patients with dysfunctional chronic pain.

Treatment

Treatment that is specific to a particular pain disorder is discussed in a later section. The following is a discussion of general principles of treatment.

Even though it may occur in different locations, chronic pain tends to have certain characteristics regardless of the anatomic diagnosis or site. This tendency has led to the development of treatments to address the effects of chronic pain and to restore activity. These therapies are applied in multidisciplinary pain clinics (MPCs) regardless of whether pain is arising from the jaw, neck, back, or other anatomic site. MPCs have been organized in response to the recognition that pain is a complex physiologic, psychological, and sociologic experience beyond the expertise of any individual or discipline. Interdisciplinary therapy includes education, counseling, medication, pain management techniques (eg, electrical nerve stimulation techniques, nerve-blocking procedures, and acupuncture), psychological therapy (eg, cognitive, behavioral), relaxation training (eg, biofeedback, mental imagery, yoga, and meditation), hypnosis, occupational therapy, physical therapy modalities (eg, thermal and ultrasonic therapies, postural training), and stretching, strengthening, and conditioning programs. Treatment goals usually focus on managing medication misuse or abuse, increasing function, reducing the use of medical resources, decreasing pain intensity, and managing associated depression and anxiety. Behavioral therapy has been shown to be effective at reducing pain and improving function at work and at home.[37]

Pain reduction is a primary goal, but it is not always achieved. Published studies of pain reduction after treatment in pain clinics report pain reduction ranges of from 14[38] to 60%,[39] with an average pain reduction of between 20 and 30%.[40] Other treatment outcome criteria include reductions in addictive medication, reductions in the use of health care services, increased activity (including return to work), and closures of disability claims.[41] Providing effective treatment of chronic pain is challenging, and many of the treatments that are effective for acute pain fail to relieve chronic pain. Individuals suffering from chronic pain often seek care from many different practitioners and may be willing to submit to treatments that may complicate the problem or be harmful. This can result in more suffering and disability.

Chronic pain management is often seen as a low priority among health care providers; it is perceived as complicated, time-intensive, and often ineffective.[2] Ineffective medications are often overprescribed, repetitive examinations are conducted in an attempt to find a simple anatomic problem that is causing the pain, and comorbidities are ignored.[36] The failure to understand that chronic pain is a relevant clinical entity with physiologic and psychological consequences has been a barrier to improved care. This is complicated by a reluctance of patients to learn pain management or coping techniques, because their energy and attention is usually focused on finding a cure.

COGNITIVE THERAPY

Cognitive therapy is based on the theory that an individual's affect and behavior are largely determined by the manner in which she or he structures the world. A person's structuring of the world is based on ideas and assumptions (developed from previous experiences). For example, "I am stronger if I don't need medicine" is a cognition that contributes to poor adherence to prescribed medication.[3]

In chronic OFP practice, it is not unusual to encounter patients who express ideas that are based on faulty assumptions. Examples include the following:

1. A firm belief that an allergy or an undiscovered or low-grade infection is the cause of pain. Diagnostic testing that fails to find evidence of infection or allergy is not always sufficient to re-direct a patient's energy and attention to the pursuit of other factors or treatment. Infection and allergies are possible causes of pain, but when clinical findings are not supportive, the patient's persistent beliefs or attitudes may become a barrier to effective treatment.

2. Acceptance of the possibility that the pain is not a signal of ongoing or increasing tissue damage or life-threatening disease. This often prompts the patient to seek several consultations and to submit to invasive tests or procedures in an attempt to find a cause and (ultimately) a cure.

3. Anxiety about the possibility of further injury when pain increases with activity, resulting in deconditioning, inactivity, and increased emotional distress and limiting the potential for restored function and activity.

4. A focus on an orofacial structure or on a deviation from the ideal in respect to teeth and jaws, even though it is not responsible for the pain. This may complicate the situation and make it more difficult for the patient to accept a more multidisciplinary approach that includes behavioral management.

These are examples of maladaptive thoughts that lead to behaviors that contribute to the disability. Cognitive therapy is an effective method of exploring these thoughts and addressing them as part of the management. Cognitive-behavioral therapy attempts to alter patterns of negative thoughts and dysfunctional attitudes in order to foster more healthy and adaptive thoughts, emotions, and actions.[44] The cognitive-behavioral model suggests that patients develop negative and distorted convictions regarding their functional capacities, diagnoses, prognoses, and futures. These convictions about illness affect behavior and are reinforced when activity or reconditioning proves to be painful. Cognitive therapy interventions share four basic components: education, skill acquisition, cognitive and behavioral rehearsal, and generalization and maintenance.[42] Treatment is intended to identify and reframe negative cognitions while increasing the patient's range of activity.[34]

RELAXATION THERAPY

Relaxation techniques are used for nondirected calming rather than for achieving a specific therapeutic goal. They do not always reduce pain intensity and are recommended as an adjunctive treatment. The results of relaxation therapy may be more significant in reducing the distress associated with pain. Other benefits may include improved sleep, reduced skeletal-muscle tension, and decreased fatigue. Guided imagery, sometimes considered a relaxation technique, involves the recall of a pleasant or peaceful experience. Patients should be reassured that they are receiving this therapy not because "the pain is imaginary and they just need to relax," but because the therapy addresses an important area of distress that arises from having chronic pain.

Relaxation techniques share two basic components:[42] (1) a repetitive focus on a word, sound, prayer, phrase, body sensation, or muscular activity, and (2) the adoption of a passive attitude toward intruding thoughts and a return to focus.

Relaxation training produces physiologic affects that are opposite to those of anxiety (ie, slower heart rate, increased peripheral blood flow, and decreased muscle tension or activity). Relaxing muscle groups in a fixed order (progressive relaxation), imagining oneself in a place associated with pleasant relaxed memories (guided imagery), and doing yoga are examples. The reader is referred to the references listed in "Suggested Readings" at the end of this chapter for a more detailed discussion and for specific exercises that can be applied in management.

DRUG THERAPY

Drug therapy continues to be a significant part of chronic pain management. Analgesics are generally divided into three groups: non-opioids, opioids, and adjuvants. (Adjuvants are drugs that have been approved for use for conditions other than pain; anticonvulsants are an example.) The drugs in these groups have different pharmacologic actions although their analgesic actions are often not well understood. With the exception of clonazepam, benzodiazepines are not thought to be analgesic and are not recommended for long-term chronic pain management although they may be helpful for relief of muscle pain due to tension or spasm. Drug therapy for chronic pain often involves the simultaneous use of more than one drug. This takes advantage of the different mechanisms of action of different drugs. It may also allow the use of smaller doses and may reduce adverse effects or risks. The most common example of this in dentistry is the combination of an opioid (such as codeine) with aspirin or acetaminophen, in which each drug acts at different sites.

Choosing the analgesic group (or groups) and the specific drugs is the first step in management. Drug therapy requires the individualizing of regimens for the greatest effect. In chronic pain management, a drug should also be selected to deal with "breakthrough" pain, an episode of increased pain that the regular regimen is not able to control. This drug is usually a μ-receptor agonist (e.g. oxycodone) with a relatively rapid rate of onset for a brief period. The oral route is preferred for compliance and convenience, and the drug dose requires titration to establish the appropriate regimen. An analgesic is most likely to be effective when given before pain increases and is usually best prescribed with a fixed dose schedule that does not require an increase in pain to signal the need for analgesia.

Non-opioid Analgesics. This group consists primarily of acetaminophen and the large group of nonsteroidal anti-inflammatory drugs (NSAIDs). Acetaminophen is dispensed over the counter and is also available in controlled formulations in combination with codeine and other opioids. Acetaminophen generally has fewer adverse effects when compared to NSAIDs. It does not affect platelet function, rarely causes gastrointestinal (GI) disturbances, and can be given to patients who are allergic to aspirin or other NSAIDs. Caffeine has been shown to enhance the effectiveness of non-opioid drugs and is often added to the analgesic.[43] The mechanism of action of acetaminophen is different from that of the NSAIDs but remains unknown; there is some evidence that suggests a central action.[44] Acetaminophen is generally used for mild pain of all types and is also combined with opioids for an additive analgesic effect or to reduce the amount of opioid required. Due to its potential to cause liver damage, it may pose a danger to patients with liver disease, patients who regularly consume moderate to large amounts of alcohol, and patients who are fasting.[45] Acetaminophen has an analgesic "ceiling," and the recommended maximum dose in a 24-hour period is 4 grams.[46]

NSAIDs are thought to work primarily at the site of injury by inhibiting the enzyme cyclo-oxygenase (COX), which is required for the synthesis of prostaglandins, substances that sensitize peripheral sensory nerves and contribute to the experience of pain. Users of NSAIDs do not exhibit tolerance or physical dependence, but these drugs do have an analgesic ceiling. Patients may vary in their response to NSAIDs, and if appropriate dosage adjustment does not produce an analgesic effect after several days to 1 week, it is appropriate to switch to a different NSAID. It is inadvisable to prescribe two different NSAIDs at the same time; rather, one NSAID should be used and its dose and timing adjusted for maximum analgesic effect. Combinations of NSAIDs increase the risk of side effects. Several NSAIDs (aspirin, ibuprofen, ketoprofen, and naproxen) are available in nonprescription formulations. The usual starting dose for these drugs is the dose recommended by the manufacturer. Titrating doses by starting at a lower dose and assessing incremental effects every 5 to 7 days has been recommended to achieve the greatest effect with the lowest dose.[47]

Prostaglandins (PGs) perform other functions in the body, and this is responsible for many of the side effects. PGs maintain the protective layer of gastric mucosa, and the loss of this layer makes the mucosa more vulnerable to erosion. The longer NSAIDs are administered, the greater the risk of GI bleeding. This effect is a systemic one and is not avoided by administering the drug by other routes (eg, rectal suppository). NSAIDs should be taken with food or at least with a full glass of water. Coadministration of misoprostol (a PG analogue) has resulted in a reduced risk of GI bleeding.[48] Risk factors that are indications for using misoprostol include age of more than 60 years, concurrent steroid therapy, high doses of the NSAID, and a history of ulcer disease. While all NSAIDs pose a risk of GI bleeding, ibuprofen and diclofenac are considered to pose a lower risk, and ketoprofen and piroxicam are considered to pose a higher risk.[49] Nabumatone is also considered to be less likely to cause GI effects.[50] With any NSAID, the risk increases when high doses are prescribed.

NSAIDs are available that selectively inhibit only one of the isoforms of COX, namely, COX-2. The inhibition of COX-2 seems to be related to the anti-inflammatory and analgesic effects whereas the inhibition of COX-1 is thought to be responsible for many of the side effects. The COX-2 inhibitors celecoxib and rofecoxib pose less risk of GI bleeding and do not inhibit platelet aggregation.

Opioids. The largest group of opioids that are commonly used for analgesia consists of the morphine-like agonists. Their most important effects are on the central nervous system and GI system. These drugs bind to μ opioid receptors, resulting in actions that lead to the analgesic effects. Opioids exert a number of effects after binding to receptor sites. Effects at the membrane level include opening potassium channels and inhibiting voltage-gated calcium channels, leading to a decrease in neuronal excitability. Opioids increase activity in some neuronal pathways (such as the descending inhibitory pathways) but may do so by suppressing the firing of inhibitory interneurons. At the spinal level, morphine inhibits the transmission of nociceptive impulses through the dorsal horn.[51] All μ agonists relieve pain by the same mechanism, but patients may vary in their responsiveness to the analgesic and to the adverse effects of specific agents. The use of opioid therapy in moderate to severe acute pain and cancer pain is well established. There has been an increased interest in the use of opioid analgesics for chronic nonmalignant pain. The practice remains controversial, and concern about addiction and behavior is the argument presented against opioid use. The concern relates to the risk of additional disability and antisocial behavior with long-term opioid use. The anecdotal literature suggests that in certain circumstances, opioids are an effective part of management and do not cause the predicted problems of addiction and antisocial behavior.[52] An agreement between the patient and doctor along with close monitoring minimizes potential misuse.

Agonist-antagonist drugs such as buprenorphine, butorphanol, and pentazocine are used to treat moderate to severe acute pain. As a group, they have a more limited role than the μ agonists. Agonist-antagonist drugs may cause withdrawal symptoms in patients who are taking μ agonists, and they are more likely to cause psychotomimetic effects such as agitation, dysphoria, and confusion. Butorphanol nasal spray (Stadol [Bristol-Myers Squibb, New York, N.Y.]) is used for the treatment of migraine headache.

Adjuvant Drugs. This group of drugs has been approved for use in conditions other than pain. Alone or in combination with other analgesics and adjuvants, they have been found to be of value in pain management. Sequential trials are often necessary due to the variability of side effects and treatment responses; this may mean trying different drugs in the same group and in different groups. In controlled clinical trials, carbamazepine (an anticonvulsant) has proven to be effective for the treatment of trigeminal neuralgia.[53]

Amitriptyline (a tricyclic antidepressant), the antidepressant that has been most frequently studied in clinical trials, has been proven to be effective in chronic OFP treatment.[54,55] A patient with chronic pain who is receiving an antidepressant is considered to be better off than 74% of chronic pain patients who are receiving a placebo.[56] The magnitude of the analgesic effect was not different (1) for pain having an organic or psychogenic basis, (2) in the presence or absence of depression (masked or manifest), (3) in the presence or absence of an antidepressant effect, (4) in normal doses and in doses smaller than those that are usually effective in depression, and (5) for sedating and nonsedating drugs.

Information relating to pain from the periphery crosses a common synaptic pathway in the dorsal horn of the spinal cord and its homologue, the spinal trigeminal nucleus in the brainstem. The neurotransmitters serotonin and norepinephrine are thought to play a role in the descending inhibitory transmissions from the brain to the dorsal horn, modulating nociceptive impulses. Tricyclic antidepressants (TCAs) block the reuptake of serotonin and norepinephrine (NE), and this is thought to enhance the central inhibitory system in pain processing. These effects occur at doses that are lower than those required for an antidepressant effect, but further evidence is still required to explain the mechanism. TCAs are usually introduced at low doses and are gradually increased in an attempt to reduce the adverse effects, which can be intolerable even at low doses. Side effects such as dry mouth, increased appetite and weight gain, cardiac effects, sedation, and dysphoria may prevent the use of these drugs.

Anticonvulsant drugs are effective in the treatment of trigeminal neuralgia and diabetic neuropathy and for migraine prophylaxis.[57] There have been no clinical trials for the treatment of other OFP disorders with anticonvulsants. These drugs frequently produce side effects (including sedation, dizziness, ataxia, and mood changes) that can limit their usefulness. Newer anticonvulsants (specifically felbamate,[58] lamotrigine,[59] and gabapentin[60,61]) are receiving attention as possible therapies for pain. Gabapentin has become commonly used in pain management partly because of its relatively few side effects.[62] Movement disorders have been reported with gabapentin. The disorders resolve after administration of the drug is stopped.[63]

A variety of other drugs are used in the treatment of chronic pain although there is little research involving chronic OFP. These drugs include mexiletine,[64] clonidine,[65] clonazepam,[66] and alprazolam.[67]

Topical Medications. Topical analgesic therapy on the skin or oral mucosa has the advantage of reduced systemic absorption and thus a reduced risk of side effects. Capsaicin used as a topical cream has been the most researched drug in this field. It is effective in treating postherpetic neuralgia. Capsaicin is a natural product (extracted from the pungent red chili pepper) that has been used topically to treat a variety of pain conditions.[68] In a single application, neurogenic inflammation occurs and causes a burning sensation, followed by hyperalgesia. After multiple applications, the burning and hyperalgesia resolve. Topical application blocks C-fiber conduction, inactivates the release of neuropeptides from peripheral nerve endings,[69] and subsequently depletes the stores of substance P from sensory neurons.[70] The therapeutic effect is thought to be due to the depletion of substance P in C fibers,[68] decreasing their input to the central nervous system (CNS) neurons. Topical NSAIDs have been demonstrated to be effective for musculoskeletal pain.[71] Doxepin, clonidine, ketamine, cyclobenzaprine, and carbamazepine have been used topically in a variety of vehicles but have not been subjected to controlled trials.

Drug therapy for chronic pain is complex and often involves multiple drugs with different routes of administration. Patients often express anxiety about dependence on medication and may sometimes feel that drug therapy is used or recommended in place of "getting to the real cause" of the pain. When using drug therapy to treat the pain as the disorder, patients need information and education about the potential value of drug therapy as part of the comprehensive management of chronic pain.

▼ CLASSIFICATION OF OROFACIAL PAIN

Classification is more than an academic exercise as it provides researchers and practitioners with a way of communicating and understanding groups of individuals who share a set of relevant characteristics. An understanding of the mechanisms of a disorder, the prescription of treatment, and the prognosis are important clinical issues that can be addressed in an effective classification system. Most of the present classifications are based on a consensus of existing knowledge and on unstructured examination findings or assumptions about the consistency of signs and symptoms. This weakness was illustrated in a study of 35 patients who were diagnosed with atypical facial pain and whose findings were compared to the criteria established by the International Headache Society (IHS). Bilateral pain, pain-free periods, and paroxysms of pain were common in the patient group but were inconsistent with the criteria.[72]

Current Classification Schemes

Chronic pain classifications that address the physical, psychological, and social aspects of chronic pain provide a more comprehensive view of the disorder. Turk and Rudy proposed the Multiaxial Assessment of Pain (MAP), which integrates physical, psychosocial, and behavioral data.[8] They also developed a classification of chronic pain patients that is based on psychosocial and behavioral data alone.[16] They hypothesized that certain patterns exist in chronic pain patients regardless of the medical diagnosis. Three different response patterns emerged: dysfunctional patients, interpersonally distressed patients, and adaptive copers. The study indicated that despite differences in medical/dental diagnoses, patients had similar psychosocial and behavioral responses. A classification such as the MAP may be useful when combined with a classification that focuses on biomedical or physical conditions. The TMJ Scale,[73] the computer-based assessment system for psychosocial and behavioral issues (IMPATH),[74] and the Research Diagnostic Criteria (RDC)[75] are assessment systems for OFP that include psychosocial parameters.

The IHS, the American Academy of Orofacial Pain (AAOP), and the IASP have all produced classification schemes that include OFP. The IASP classification, originally published in 1986 and revised in 1994, is composed of five axes[1] (Table 11-3). The IASP has categorized OFP within the section termed "Relatively Localized Syndromes of the Head and Neck" (Table 11-4); listed within this section are 67 different disorders. The IASP publication includes a comparison between the IASP and IHS diagnostic categories that shows that there are significant differences between these two systems.

Two of thirteen categories in the IHS classification[76] specifically relate to OFP disorders: category 11, "headache or facial pain associated with disorders of cranium, neck, eyes, ears, nose, sinuses, teeth, mouth or other facial or cranial structures," and category 12, "cranial neuralgias, nerve trunk pain, and de-afferentation pain." Category 11 includes temporomandibular joint disease and disorders of teeth, jaws, and related structures. Disorders in category 12 are listed in Table 11-5. The AAOP has used the IHS classification as the basis for a classification on OFP disorders.[77] A separate axis (not included in the publication) is recommended for defining psychosocial factors and diagnosing mental disorders. OFP disorders in this classification are listed in Table 11-6.

Classification of Idiopathic Facial Pain

ATYPICAL FACIAL PAIN

The use of the term "atypical facial pain" as a diagnostic classification has been recently discouraged.[1,77] Originally, the term was used to describe patients whose response to neurosurgical procedures was not "typical."[78] The term has been

applied to various facial pain problems and has been considered to represent a psychological disorder although no specific diagnostic criteria have ever been established.

Atypical facial pain (AFP) is defined more by what it is not than by what it is. Feinmann characterized AFP as a nonmuscular or joint pain that has no a detectable neurologic cause.[54] Truelove and colleagues described AFP as a condition characterized by the absence of other diagnoses and causing continuous, variable-intensity, migrating, nagging, deep, and diffuse pain.[79] In the TMD classification of the AAOP, AFP is listed in the glossary of terms and is defined as "a continuous unilateral deep aching pain sometimes with a burning component." AFP was not included as a diagnostic category.[80] The IHS classification (IHS 12.8) uses the term, "facial pain not fulfilling other criteria" for AFP[81] (Table 11-7). Recent advances in the understanding of chronic pain suggest that at least a portion of patients who have been diagnosed with AFP may be experiencing neuropathic pain.

ATYPICAL ODONTALGIA

Atypical odontalgia (AO), described as a chronic pain disorder characterized by pain localized to teeth or gingiva,[1] has been considered to be a variant of AFP. The condition has also been called "phantom tooth pain" and defined as persistent pain in endodontically treated teeth or edentate areas for which there is no explanation to be found by physical or radiographic

---

TABLE 11-3 Scheme for Coding Chronic Pain Diagnoses*

Axis	Definition
1	Regions (eg, head, face, and mouth)
2	Systems (eg, nervous system)
3	Temporal characteristics of pain (eg, continuous, recurring irregularly, paroxysmal)
4	Patient's statement of intensity: time since onset of pain (eg, mild, medium, severe; 1 month or less; more than 6 months)
5	Etiology (eg, genetic, infective, psychological)

Adapted from Merskey H, Bogduk N.[1]
*International Association for the Study of Pain (IASP) classification.

TABLE 11-4 Classification of Localized Syndromes of the Head and Neck*

Neuralgias of the head and face

Craniofacial pain of musculoskeletal origin

Lesions of the ear, nose, and oral cavity

Primary headache syndromes, vascular disorders, and cerebrospinal fluid syndromes

Pain of psychological origin in the head, face, and neck

Suboccipital and cervical musculoskeletal disorders

Visceral pain in the neck

Adapted from Merskey H, Bogduk N.[1]
*International Association for the Study of Pain (IASP) classficiation.

TABLE 11-5   Classification of Cranial Neuralgias, Nerve Trunk Pain, and De-afferentation Pain*

IHS Category	Specific Disorders or Definition
12.1 Persistent (in contrast to ticlike) pain of cranial origin	Compression or distortion of cranial nerves and 2nd or 3rd cervical roots Demyelination of cranial nerves (optic neuritis) Infarction of cranial nerves (diabetic neuritis) Inflammation of cranial nerves (herpes zoster and postherpetic neuralgia) Tolosa-Hunt syndrome Neck-tongue syndrome
12.2 Trigeminal neuralgia (TN)	Idiopathic TN Symptomatic TN (caused by demonstrable structural lesion)
12.3 Glossopharyngeal neuralgia (GN)	Idiopathic GN Symptomatic GN (caused by demonstrable structural lesion)
12.4 Nervus intermedius neuralgia	Rare disorder characterized by brief paroxysms of pain felt deeply in the auditory canal
12.5 Superior laryngeal neuralgia	Rare disorder characterized by severe pain in the lateral aspect of the throat, submandibular region, and underneath the ear, precipitated by swallowing, shouting, or turning the head
12.6 Occipital neuralgia	Paroxysmal jabbing pain in the distribution of the greater or lesser occipital nerves, accompanied by diminished sensation or dysesthesia in the affected area; commonly associated with tenderness over the nerve concerned
12.7 Central causes of head and facial pain other than tic douloureux	Anesthesia dolorosa: painful anesthesia or dysesthesia, often related to surgical trauma of the trigeminal ganglion, evoked most frequently after rhizotomy or thermocoagulation for treatment of idiopathic TN Thalamic pain: unilateral facial pain and dysesthesia, attributed to a lesion of the quintothalamic pathway or thalamus
12.8 Facial pain not fulfilling criteria in groups 11 and 12 (previously used terms: atypical facial pain, atypical odontalgia)	Persistent facial pain that does not have the characteristics of the cranial neuralgias classified above and is not associated with physical signs or a demonstrable organic cause

Reproduced with permission from Olesen J.[76]

*International Headache Society (IHS) classification.

examination.[82] In the AAOP classification, AO is listed within the category "facial pain not fulfilling other criteria" and is considered to be a de-afferentation pain.[77] AO appears in the IASP classification under "lesions of the ear, nose, and oral cavity" and is defined as a severe throbbing pain in the teeth in the absence of a major pathology.

In an attempt to identify chronic OFP due to neuropathic injury, Lynch and Elgeneidy suggested additional categories to the IASP taxonomy.[83] They also recom-

mended replacing AFP with the term "not otherwise specified." This is the terminology used in the DSM-IV for a condition that does not conform to criteria in another category.[84] While the term "atypical facial pain" has a long history and has been associated with a number of different etiologies, it still is used by clinicians to identify an OFP disorder that does not meet other diagnostic criteria and that is characterized by its chronicity and lack of response to most treatments. The term may fade away as new knowl-

TABLE 11-6   Differential Diagnosis of Orofacial Pain*

Intracranial pain disorders	Neoplasm, aneurysm, abscess, hemorrhage, hematoma, edema
Primary headache disorders (neurovascular disorders)	Migraine, migraine variants, cluster headache, paroxysmal hemicrania, cranial arteritis, carotodynia, tension-type headache
Neurogenic pain disorders	Paroxysmal neuralgias (trigeminal, glossopharyngeal, nervus intermedius, superior laryngeal) Continuous pain disorders (de-afferentation, neuritis, postherpetic neuralgia, post-traumatic and postsurgical neuralgia) Sympathetically maintained pain
Intraoral pain disorders	Dental pulp, periodontium, mucogingival tissues, tongue
Temporomandibular disorders	Masticatory muscle, temporomandibular joint, associated structures
Associated structures	Ears, eyes, nose, paranasal sinuses, throat, lymph nodes, salivary glands, neck

Reproduced with permission from Okeson J.[77]

*American Academy of Orofacial Pain classification.

TABLE 11-7 Classification of Idiopathic Orofacial Pain*

Daily pain that is deep and poorly localized, persisting for most or all of the day

Pain at onset confined to a limited area on one side of the face and that may spread to the upper and lower jaws or a wider area of the face or neck

Pain not associated with sensory loss or other physical signs, and laboratory investigations (including radiography of face and jaws) do not demonstrate relevant abnormality.

Reproduced with permission from Committee on Headache Classification, International Headache Society.[81]

*International Headache Society (IHS) classification 12.8: Facial Pain Not Fulfilling Other Criteria.

edge identifies causes for these disorders and allows for better classifications and treatment.

NEURALGIA-INDUCING CAVITATIONAL OSTEONECROSIS

Ischemic osteonecrosis of the jaws has been presented as a cause of idiopathic facial pain. The term given to describe this disorder is "neuralgia-inducing cavitational osteonecrosis" (NICO). The pain is described as slowly progressive over time and spreading. It may be intermittent and may vary in extent, location, and character. This disorder has been described as occurring at a wide range of ages but is more frequent in the fourth and fifth decades of life. It is thought to occur most frequently in the mandibular molar area. Most NICO sites are thought to involve edentulous areas or areas associated with radiographically successful endodontic procedures. No specific imaging criteria are diagnostic.[85] There continues to be significant debate about NICO as a cause of facial pain.[86] Treatment by surgically entering and curretting these cavities raises a concern about the possibility of exacerbating the disorder rather than controlling it. Procedures that risk nerve injury are generally not recommended for patients with persistent neuropathic pain. The lack of clearly defined criteria for the diagnosis of these conditions raises the risk of additional injury and aggravation of the symptoms.

▼ EXAMINATION AND ASSESSMENT OF THE PATIENT WITH CHRONIC OROFACIAL PAIN

The examination and assessment of patients with chronic OFP is challenging for all clinicians. In most disorders, no specific biologic marker, validated diagnostic criteria, or "gold standard" exists. Biologic markers, including tyramine,[87] oxygen free radicals,[88] and metabolites of neurotransmitters in lumbar cerebrospinal fluid,[89] have been studied in a limited manner in regard to OFP and are not applicable in diagnosis. Even test procedures that are considered objective, such as local anesthetic nerve blocking[90] and the testing of sensation after nerve damage,[91] have yielded inconsistent results. A systematic approach for collecting diagnostic information is needed to minimize the risk of missing critical information. A formal and

systematic approach increases the probability of identifying disease that occurs from time to time and is life threatening.[92]

History, physical examination, and behavioral assessment usually serve as the basis for diagnosis. Frequent re-evaluation, including assessment of the effects of treatment, is an important part of this process. In circumstances in which treatment is ineffective or only partially successful, patients are at risk of seeking additional and alternative treatments that may be inappropriate and potentially dangerous.[93] Even when a diagnosis is uncertain or when previous treatment has failed, the clinician can make a valuable contribution by coordinating the further use of medical and dental services and by being available to advise the patient about possible treatments. Validating patients' feelings and symptoms in these times is critically important and serves to reduce suffering.

History

Evaluation of OFP symptoms must include all of the standard components of a medical interview: chief complaint, history of present illness, past medical history, medications, review of systems, and family and social history. A diagnosis can sometimes be made on the basis of the history, or the possibilities can be significantly narrowed. Since there are a number of OFP disorders that do not produce physical abnormalities, the history and description of pain may serve as the basis for the diagnosis.

HISTORY OF THE PRESENT ILLNESS

A history of the present illness should include a detailed description of the pain and its location (Table 11-8). The VAS or numeric scale described above can be used to assess intensity, and a questionnaire such as the MPQ can capture the multidimensional experience of the pain. Details of previous injuries, surgeries, and radiation therapy should be obtained. Questions about habits such as gum chewing and tooth clenching or grinding may reveal important contributing factors of which the patient is unaware. The effects of eating, opening the mouth wide, rest, exercise, and heat and cold on pain should be explored. Referred pain to the orofacial region is an important clinical consideration. The location of pain,

TABLE 11-8 Pain Characteristics

Intensity

Quality

Location

Onset

Associated events at onset

Duration and timing of pain

Course of symptoms since onset

Activities or experiences that increase pain

Activities or experiences that decrease pain

Associated symptoms (eg, altered sensation, swelling)

Previous treatments and their effects

therefore, will not always correspond to its source. A mechanism that has been proposed to explain referred pain is convergence,[94–96] in which primary afferent fibers from different sites converge on the same second-order neuron in the brainstem nucleus. Patients should mark the location and extent of pain on a diagram.

PAST MEDICAL HISTORY AND REVIEW OF SYSTEMS

The past medical history and review of systems should help provide an insight into the general health of the patient and may provide clues regarding the present pain complaint. Pain may be a presenting feature or an ongoing complaint in systemic disease (eg, connective-tissue disease, demyelinating disease of the CNS, metastatic disease).

The patient's use of medication (including over-the-counter preparations, naturopathic and homeopathic remedies, and prescription drugs) should be recorded. Prescription medication is often used incorrectly; therefore, the directions as well as the actual usage should be determined. The medication list may uncover a medical condition that the patient failed to mention in other questioning. Drug effects such as fatigue, dizziness, anxiety, insomnia, or depression may affect the patient's pain complaints. The use of tobacco, alcohol, caffeine, or illicit drugs should be explored.

FAMILY, SOCIAL, AND OCCUPATIONAL HISTORY

Chronic pain can have disastrous effects on one's ability to maintain daily activities and fulfill responsibilities. Pain has profound and often negative effects on family and social relationships, and it is important to assess the level of dysfunction that may have occurred. Traumatic events or emotional distress prior to the onset of pain, a history of other close family members with chronic illness or pain, and changes in work and or marital status should be explored because these can be significant stressors.

Physical Examination

The physical examination may identify an abnormality that explains the cause of pain. It can also help eliminate from diagnosis the presence of serious disease related to the pain. The examination should include the following:

1. Inspection of the head and neck, skin, topographic anatomy, and swelling or other orofacial asymmetry
2. Palpation of masticatory muscles, tests for strength and provocation
3. Assessment and measurement of the range of mandibular movement
4. Palpation of soft tissue (including lymph nodes)
5. Palpation of the temporomandibular joint
6. Palpation of cervical muscles and assessment of cervical range of motion
7. Cranial nerve examination (Table 11-9)
8. General inspection of the ears, nose, and oropharyngeal areas
9. Examination and palpation of intraoral soft tissue
10. Examination of the teeth and periodontium (including occlusion)

MUSCLE EXAMINATION

Pain that is reproduced or increases as a result of muscle palpation may point to the source of the pain and to a diagnosis. The degree of finger pressure will influence the result of the palpation examination, and patients' responses to palpation may vary with time. Pressure algometers have been used in research to help standardize examination procedures[97] but are not commonly used in clinical practice. Muscle palpation has been shown to yield reliable scores among examiners, but the diagnostic validity and reliability of muscle palpation has not been established. The masseter and temporalis muscles can be palpated bilaterally to identify differences in size or firmness. The suprahyoid muscles, mylohyoid, and anterior belly of the digastric should be included in the palpation examination. Intraoral techniques have been described for palpating the medial and lateral pterygoids. The ability to perform a meaningful palpation examination of the lateral pterygoid has been questioned.[98] Palpation techniques have been described, but it may be difficult to distinguish tenderness associated with the procedure from an actual muscle abnormality.[99] The temporalis tendon, where it inserts onto the coronoid process, can also be reached intraorally for palpation. Testing muscles against resistance in a static position and having the patient clench on separators to prevent the teeth from coming together may help identify the source of pain.[100]

Palpation of cervical muscles and a general assessment of the cervical range of motion may indicate an abnormality contributing to the pain complaint. Pain localized to the orofacial region can be referred from neck muscles.[94] The cervical muscles to be palpated include the trapezii and the sternocleidomastoid and the muscles that lie deeper between them, including the capitus and scalene muscles and the levator scapulae.

RANGE OF MOTION ASSESSMENT

Mandibular and cervical ranges of motion should be assessed. Movements with and without pain should be noted. Mandibular movements with comfort, with pain, and with examiner assistance should be measured and recorded. Cervical motion can be examined during active, passive, and resisted motions. When restrictions in movement are thought to be caused by muscle guarding, the application of a vapocoolant spray such as Fluori-Methane Spray (Gebauer Co., Cleveland, Ohio) followed by stretching may significantly increase range, confirming a muscle cause. Alternatively, injection of a local anesthetic into muscle may block pain and thus identify the source of the pain and the restricted movement.

INTRAORAL EXAMINATION

A systematic intraoral inspection looking for changes in form, symmetry, color, and surface texture should be carried out. The examination should include manipulation of the tongue and mandible to clearly visualize all areas. Pooling of saliva on the floor of the mouth should be observed. The palate and tongue should be examined at rest and during function to detect underlying masses that might displace or alter the normal structures. The examiner's finger should palpate the alveolar processes, lateral and posterior parts of the tongue, floor

TABLE 11-9 Summary of Cranial Nerve Examination

Cranial Nerve	Function	Usual Complaint	Test of Function	Physical Findings
I (Olfactory)	Smell	None or loss of "taste" if bilateral	Sense of smell with each nostril	No response to olfactory stimuli
II (Optic)	Vision	Loss of vision	Visual acuity Visual fields of each eye	Decreased visual acuity or loss of visual field
III (Oculomotor)	Eye movement Pupillary constriction	Double vision	Pupil and eye movement	Failure to move eye in field of motion of muscle Pupillary abnormalities
IV (Trochlear)	Eye movement	Double vision, especially on down and medial gaze	Ability to move eye down and in	May be difficult to detect anything if 3rd nerve intact
V (Trigeminal)	Facial, nasal, and oral sensation Jaw movement	Numbness Paresthesia	Light touch and pinprick sensation on face Corneal reflex Masseter contraction	Decreased pin and absent corneal reflex Weakness of masticatory muscles
VI (Abducens)	Eye movement	Double vision on lateral gaze	Move eyes laterally	Failure of eye to abduct
VII (Facial)	Facial movement	Lack of facial movement, eye closure Dysarthria	Facial contraction Smiling	Asymmetry of facial contraction
VII (Auditory and vestibular)	Hearing Balance	Hearing loss Tinnitus Vertigo	Hearing test Nystagmus Balance	Decreased hearing Nystagmus Ataxia
IX (Glossopharyngeal)	Palatal movement	Trouble with swallowing	Elevation of palate	Asymmetric palate
X (Vagus)	Vocal cords	Trouble swallowing	Vocal cords	Brassy voice
XI (Spinal accessory)	Turns neck	None	Contraction of sternocleidomastoid and trapezius	Paralysis of sternocleidomastoid muscle
XII (Hypoglossal)	Moves tongue	Dysarthria	Protrusion of tongue	Wasting and fasciculation or deviation of tongue

of the mouth, buccal mucosa, and hard and soft palate to identify abnormalities that may not be readily observed. The finger should not meet significant resistance as it moves across a normally lubricated mucosa. The openings of the submandibular and parotid salivary gland ducts should be isolated and dried with cotton; the glands should then be "milked" to verify a clear flow of saliva.

The dentition should be examined for wear, damaged teeth, and evidence of caries. This inspection should be followed by probing, palpation for tooth mobility, and percussion of teeth. If a pulpal problem is suspected, thermal and vitality tests should be included. Applying differential pressure on the teeth by having the patient bite down on cotton rolls, wooden bite sticks, or one of the commercially available instruments designed to apply concentrated pressure on cusps may identify pain associated with a vertical crown or root fracture. Periodontal structures should be examined for color changes suggestive of inflammation, altered gingival architecture that occurs with chronic disease, swelling, or other surface changes. Periodontal probing should be performed to identify bleeding points and pocket depths. Tooth contacts in the maximum intercuspal position, in centric relation, and during excursive movements should be identified. Heavy contacts or interferences in association with tooth mobility or tooth sensitivity may indicate conditions contributing to occlusal trauma.

Pain-Related Disability and Behavioral Assessment

An interview most often serves as the basis for a behavioral assessment. Self-report questionnaires and instruments that include methods of scoring are also in use to assess disability and psychological factors. The assessment should explore the following:[101]

1. Events that precede and follow exacerbation of pain
2. The patient's daily activities
   — How time is spent during the day and in the evening
   — Activities that have been performed more often or less often since the onset of pain
   — Activities that have been modified or eliminated since the onset of pain
3. Relatives or friends that suffer chronic pain or disabilities of a similar nature
4. The degree of affective disturbance
   — Change in mood or outlook on life
   — Satisfaction level with friends and family relationships

— Vegetative signs of depression (sleep disturbance, change in food intake, decreased sexual desire)

While psychosocial factors are of great importance in pain disorders, studies indicate that physicians and dentists do not always adequately recognize psychological problems.[102–104] One of the problems dentists face is the lack of formal training in psychological assessment. A great deal of study has been focused on the use of questionnaires to assess psychosocial status. Inventories that are completed by the patient, such as the Minnesota Multiphasic Personality Inventory (MMPI), the Beck Depression Inventory,[105] the Zung Self-Rating Depression Scale, the Personality Diagnostic Questionnaire,[106] and the General Health Questionnaire,[107] are examples of self-report questionnaires used for psychological assessment. The TMJ Scale,[73] IMPATH,[74] and (more recently) the RDC[20] are instruments designed for evaluating OFP, and they include behavioral assessments. No one method has gained widespread acceptance for evaluating OFP patients. One strategy for addressing the lack of psychological assessment skills among physicians and dentists is to provide a method of screening that identifies OFP patients who might benefit from a more thorough behavioral assessment. Gale and Dixon[108] found that the following two questions correlated with lengthier questionnaires:

1. How depressed are you?
2. Do you consider yourself more tense than calm or more calm than tense?

Oakley et al used a five-item questionnaire that allows patients to rate levels of depression, anxiety, and recent life stresses showed moderate to strong association with results from extensive psychological testing.[109] Two of the questions were similar to those used by Gale and Dixon.

Being asked open-ended questions about common areas of life experience provides the patient with an opportunity to express concerns or problems that may not otherwise be communicated, such as what the patient feels may be the cause of pain; activities or problems in the common areas of life (work, love, and play); and complaints of current or previously diagnosed or undiagnosed pain elsewhere in the body. Responses to these questions may be helpful in identifying abnormal thought patterns, external stressors, or other symptoms that are suggestive of a more generalized pain disorder. Recent research indicates that the prevalence of a history of physical and sexual abuse in patients with chronic pain is higher than expected, but how to identify patients who should be referred to experienced therapists remains a challenge.[101]

Self-report instruments are used for clinical and research purposes to assess psychological variables associated with pain. They provide standardized assessments and are sensitive to treatment-related changes. Instruments such as the Minnesota Multiphasic Personality Inventory (MMPI) and the revised MMPI (MMPI-2) have been used to evaluate psychological distress in chronic pain patients. The use of the MMPI or MMPI-2[110] with chronic pain patients has been questioned because the subjects who were used to standardize the inventories were not chronic pain patients.[111–113] In chronic pain patients, elevations on the hypochondriasis, depression, and hysteria scales have been associated with severe pain, affective disturbance, and disability.[114,115] MMPI profiles have been unable to predict treatment outcomes.[101] Other shorter and simpler instruments such as the Beck Depression Inventory are used in place of the MMPI.[116] The shorter inventories are likely to get better patient compliance as well. Questionnaires such as the SCL-90-R,[22] the Millon Behavioral Health Inventory,[118] and the Illness Behavior Questionnaire[117] are examples of shorter inventories that take less time to complete. A universally accepted assessment instrument for chronic pain patients does not exist.

Dworkin and colleagues[20] have published (as part of the RDC) a classification for assessing pain-related disability, identifying depression, and characterizing limitations related to mandibular functioning. The RDC were produced to increase the standardization of assessment and classification applied to clinical research on TMD. While this assessment/classification requires further validation, it may be of value to clinicians. The pain-related disability assessment is based on the "Graded Chronic Pain Status," a seven-item questionnaire, and specific scoring.[21] An explanation of the scoring and the scale can be found in Von Korff's article.[21] The assessment method, scoring, and discussion of the pain-related disability status have been published by Dworkin, LeResche, and colleagues.[20]

From the discussion above, it should be apparent that there is no universal standard that can be relied on to provide a screening assessment of behavioral and pain-related disability. Table 11-10 lists questions discussed in this section that may be valuable as part of this assessment. These questions may be posed during the interview to explore possible behavioral, psychological, or other systemic problems that may have an impact on the diagnosis and management of an OFP disorder. This is not a scale or instrument with scoring but questions that may provide an opportunity for the patient to communicate issues

---

TABLE 11-10 Questions to Consider for Screening Assessment

What events precede and follow increased episodes of pain?

How is time spent during the day and the evening?

What activities are performed more often or less often since the onset of pain?

What activities have been modified or eliminated since the onset of pain?

Do relatives or friends suffer chronic pain or disabilities of a similar nature?

Do you characterize yourself as depressed?

Do you have changes in sleep pattern, food habits, sexual desire (vegetative signs of depression)?

Have there been changes in your relationships with friends, family, co-workers?

Do you characterize yourself as being anxious or tense?

Do you think you have experienced a lot of stressful situations over the past year?

What do you think is causing the pain?

Do you presently have any diagnosed or undiagnosed pain complaints elsewhere in the body?

that may be important to the complaint. The threshold for deciding when the information obtained indicates a more thorough investigation is a clinical judgment. There are no well-defined rules to govern this decision.

When psychosocial issues are thought to be significant and to require assessment and possible management by a psychologist or psychiatrist, the patient should be so advised. This should be done in a conversation that allows the patient to respond and that asks for feedback since the patient may have some insight into the issue. The interviewer's opinion may help to validate the patient's own assessment, and the possibility of successfully addressing these issues may be increased. Communicating with the patient's general physician or referring the patient to his or her general physician to explore this further may be an effective method of managing the situation.

When a psychiatric disorder is suspected, a direct referral to a psychiatrist or psychologist may be indicated.[119] The patient may resist this referral for the following reasons:

1. Perception of the referral as a judgment that the problem is only psychological or as a personal rejection
2. Beliefs about the legitimacy of psychiatric therapy and about the kind of people who consult psychologists or psychiatrists
3. Beliefs about the condition that do not include the possibility of a psychological or emotional component

A patient is most likely to accept a recommendation if a trusting relationship is present. The following are suggestions that may facilitate the referral:

1. Make the referral a part of the evaluation. Inform the patient that the consultation is part of your complete evaluation and that it will be part of the other clinical findings for determining the diagnosis and management.
2. Arrange the appointment at the same time that the patient is in the office if the patient agrees. This will facilitate the process.
3. Provide the patient with information about what the consultation will involve.
4. Schedule a follow-up appointment to review the findings and discuss treatment.

Diagnostic Imaging

Imaging can be used to confirm a suspected abnormality, to screen or rule out possible abnormalities that are not detectable by other methods, or to establish the extent of an identified disorder. It is the best method for evaluating a suspected tumor, infection, or ongoing inflammation in sites that are not easily accessible. Many OFP disorders do not produce abnormalities demonstrable with imaging, and its greatest value may be to rule out serious life-threatening disease.

Diagnostic Nerve Blocks

Nerve blocks interrupt the transmission of nociceptive impulses through specific pathways. If pain relief occurs, it is presumed to be due to the interruption of the nerves via the pathways suspected of being involved. Conversely, the absence of pain after a successful block suggests the possibility of a central process.[120] False-positive results may occur due to systemic effects of local anesthetics, blockade of afferent pathways other than those intended, and placebo effects. Conversely, lack of pain relief may be due to technical or anatomic factors.[121] Diagnostic nerve blocks are a valuable part of an assessment, but the results can be equivocal and do not always contribute to an accurate diagnosis. There is a high frequency of placebo response to local anesthetic blocking, even among patients diagnosed with neuropathic pain.[90]

Nerve blocks to diagnose sympathetically maintained pain include local anesthetic block of the sympathetic chain (eg, stellate ganglion), regional guanethedine block (intravenous injection into an arm or leg), and intravenous phentolamine to block the α-adrenoreceptor, preventing the excitation of afferent nociceptors by noradrenaline. The interpretation of these tests has been challenged because of the lack of placebo-controlled procedures and because of a high placebo response,[122,123] but the weight of evidence supports the hypothesis that the sympathetic nervous system contributes to chronic pain in some circumstances.

Local anesthetic blocking should be considered in the context of all of the clinical findings. Topical, intraligament, infiltration, and regional block anesthesia may identify a peripheral site that is responsible for pain. A complete resolution of pain after local anesthetic application or injection should prompt an investigation for a local cause. The injection of local anesthesia may produce ambivalent results when patients report a change in symptoms but not necessarily resolution of pain. In these circumstances, one should consider a more central cause of pain.

Laboratory Tests

Laboratory tests have limited value except in special circumstances. Most OFP disorders do not cause abnormalities that can be identified in laboratory specimens. Exceptions include temporal arteritis, in which the erythrocyte sedimentation rate is elevated and temporal artery biopsy is abnormal and collagen vascular diseases that cause detectable immunologic abnormalities.

Consultation and Referral

Referral and consultation are recommended for a number of reasons, and there are few rigid rules. For a complex pain problem, it may be necessary to include examinations by other dental specialists, otolaryngologists, neurologists, psychologists or psychiatrists, and internists. Referrals may be of value when (1) the referral is for confirming or establishing a suspected or unknown diagnosis, (2) the referral is for the purpose of treatment after a diagnosis has been made, and (3) the referral is for obtaining a second opinion to review an established diagnosis or treatment recommendation.

Suggesting referral to a patient may be met with ambivalence and anxiety. Concerns about the seriousness of the problem, financial issues, time commitments, and having to establish a new relationship with another health care provider may be sources of resistance. The practitioner may feel pressure to do something before a diagnosis is established, and this may lead to ineffective and inappropriate treatment.

Special Circumstances in Assessment of Orofacial Pain Patients

OFP DISORDERS POSSIBLY CONFUSED WITH TOOTHACHE

Patients who choose to consult a dentist regarding a pain complaint do so because they believe it may be a tooth-related problem. Several OFP disorders have characteristics that may be confused with those of a toothache (Table 11-11). This confusion may occur because of (1) the location of the pain, (2) the quality of pain that suggests an inflammatory process, or (3) increased pain associated with stimulation of the teeth or surrounding tissues.

OFP SYMPTOMS INDICATING SERIOUS DISEASE

Presenting signs or symptoms may suggest the possibility of a serious or life-threatening disorder and indicate an urgent need to establish a diagnosis. These conditions may warrant referral as part of a thorough and timely evaluation (Table 11-12).[124]

HEADACHE AND OFP SYMPTOMS ASSOCIATED WITH SYSTEMIC DISEASE

For most of the systemic diseases that manifest in the oral cavity, there is little information on the frequency with which signs and symptoms identified in the oral cavity lead to the recognition and diagnosis of systemic disease. Table 11-13 lists systemic diseases that have been associated with headache and OFP.[125–133] The literature in this area is primarily case reporting and is a poor guide to the likelihood of finding evidence that implicates a previously undiagnosed systemic disease process as the cause of a patient's unexplained facial OFP. Hyperparathyroidism and metastatic disease will eventually produce radiologic findings that lead to a diagnosis. In other situations, physical signs or laboratory evidence will direct the diagnostic process, but in the early

TABLE 11-11 Orofacial Disorders That May Be Confused with Toothache

Trigeminal neuralgia
Trigeminal neuropathy (due to trauma or tumor invasion of nerves)
Atypical facial pain and atypical odontalgia
Cluster headache
Acute and chronic maxillary sinusitis
Myofascial pain of masticatory muscles

stage of disease, pain (with or without altered sensation) may be the first indication of the disorder.

Diseases such as diabetes mellitus (which occurs with some frequency in the population) will often be found, but evidence associating the systemic disease and the oral symptoms may be harder to find. Clinical investigation of the majority of patients referred after initial evaluation by dentists and physicians for an unsolved oral complaint only rarely detects undiagnosed systemic disease. More often, abnormal blood values such as glucose or iron levels have been noted at earlier examinations. Treating the abnormality, does not always eliminate the oral symptoms. Alternatively, both patient and physician are aware of the presence of the systemic disease, but the methods used to control it have been inadequate. Referral consultations for unexplained oral complaints may thus result in recommendations for additional treatment of systemic disease noted at the time of consultation. In many cases, however, these conditions are not specifically related to the oral complaint.

Despite the time and money invested in extensive searches for systemic disease that only rarely find a possible cause of unexplained oral symptoms, such searches are sometimes justified. Unexplained chronic oral symptoms generate considerable anxiety in addition to the discomfort experienced by the patient, and a "leave no stone unturned" approach often seems necessary to allay these anxieties. Patients with problems sometimes demand a continued bat-

TABLE 11-12 Orofacial Pain Symptoms That Indicate Serious Disease

Orofacial Pain Symptom	Disease Indicated
Pain at the angle of the mandible, brought on by exertion, relieved by rest	Cardiac ischemia
New onset; localized progressive headache; superficial temporal artery swelling, tenderness, and lack of pulse; severe throbbing temporal pain; transient visual abnormalities; systemic symptoms of fever, weight loss, anorexia, malaise, myalgia, chills, sweating	Temporal arteritis
New onset of headache in adult life; increasing severe headache, nausea, and vomiting not explained by systemic illness or migraine; nocturnal occurrence; precipitated or increased by changes in posture; confusion, seizures, or weakness; any abnormal neurologic sign	Intracranial tumor
Earache, trismus, altered sensation in the mandibular branch distribution	Carcinoma of the infratemporal fossa
Trigeminal neuralgia in a person less than 50 years of age	Multiple sclerosis
Pain associated with altered sensation confirmed by physical examination	Neurogenic disorder; tumor invasion of nerve

TABLE 11-13 Systemic Diseases Associated with Headache and Orofacial Pain

Paget's disease

Metastatic disease

Hyperthyroidism

Multiple myeloma

Hyperparathyroidism

Vitamin B deficiencies

Systemic lupus erythematosus

Vincristine therapy for cancer

Folic acid and iron deficiency anemias

tery of sophisticated studies. In these circumstances, the clinician's judgment is needed to prevent the unnecessary repetition of tests and to advise the patient on the likelihood of a particular procedure providing additional useful diagnostic information.

ABSENCE OF A CONVINCING PHYSICAL EXPLANATION FOR SYMPTOMS

Patients who have no convincing physical explanation for their symptoms are the most difficult patients for the practitioner. The resultant problems are not restricted to oral medicine, and all who practice medicine and dentistry usually become aware of them early in their careers. Such patients are seen with greater frequency in specialty practices, simply because unresolved problems commonly lead to a referral for further diagnostic testing. For residents in specialty training, it is often a discovery that a considerable number of patients will not be concerned with clearly defined pathologic states that are amenable to treatment. Patients with unexplained oral sensory abnormalities still require management and some form of treatment even when a thorough diagnostic search fails to find an explanation.

RESPONSES TO UNEXPLAINED SYMPTOMS

The assumption underlying all diagnostic procedures is that an explanation will be found for the patient's complaint of pain. When extensive and reasonably adequate diagnostic investigations fail to find such an explanation, the initial response by the patient and doctor is that further testing to probe for more unusual conditions is needed. When this approach fails, the doctor may begin to assume that the symptoms are not real and that they represent exaggeration for some secondary gain or represent a psychiatric abnormality. Alternatively, the doctor may judge that a borderline abnormality found by palpation or by diagnostic imaging might be more serious than was first considered and might represent evidence of a lesion. Both of these responses on the doctor's part may be exaggerated, and they represent two pitfalls that may complicate the diagnostic and treatment process. First, concluding that symptoms are evidence of a psychiatric abnormality may deny the patient the opportunity for further

diagnostic testing that may provide an explanation and solution to the unusual symptoms. Second, performing surgical treatment (even when there are only minimal physical findings) risks complications from the surgical procedure. While all clinicians are vulnerable to these errors, awareness of these pitfalls does help prevent such extremes of response on the doctor's part.

Patients may respond to the lack of an adequate explanation and treatment by requesting further tests or consultation or by independently seeking further consultation. Considering the wide variety of training and traditions that exist in the health professions, it is not difficult to appreciate that a patient will find a practitioner who will provide some treatment that the patient feels might alleviate the symptoms. Multiple consultation and heavy use of surgical services are characteristic features of patients with chronic disorders, especially among those whose symptoms remain unexplained.[134–138] In three separate studies, OFP patients averaged 5, 6, and 7.5 physician/dentist consultations.[72,139,140]

ORAL SYMPTOMS OUT OF PROPORTION TO RECOGNIZED ORAL LESIONS

Patients with unexplained oral symptoms do not always present completely free of dental, periodontal, and mucosal lesions that might be considered possible causes for the unusual symptoms. The evaluation of these patients commonly involves decisions as to whether a degenerating pulp, a coarsely fissured tongue, or muscle tension, for example, may explain complaints of chronic pain or a burning and painful tongue. When possible, treatment of the abnormality by root canal therapy, increased oral and tongue hygiene, or administration of muscle relaxants (in the situations just described) may resolve the question. However, when symptoms persist in the face of apparently adequate treatment, the clinician must decide whether the patient's symptoms possibly arise from another cause or whether they represent an exaggerated response to the particular oral abnormality that has been found and presumably adequately treated.

Among patients with unexplained oral symptoms, there is a group of patients whose salient features are the atypical or exaggerated response to the pain focus and (perhaps) the length of time their symptoms have persisted. It is important to identify the patient whose problem appears to be an inability to cope with minor oral sensory abnormality and who reacts to chronic low-grade pain in the same manner as he or she reacts to pain of greater intensity. Although this identification must be made cautiously and must be reviewed from time to time as treatment progresses, it does help focus treatment on the behavioral component of the patient's pain problem and help reduce continued and unnecessary diagnostic searches.

PSYCHOLOGICAL AND EMOTIONAL FACTORS

Clues that a patient may be reacting in an unusual fashion to abnormal sensory stimuli of low intensity can come from a variety of inquiries during the diagnostic interview. Patients may reveal evidence of a thought disorder during the interview. Patients may reveal the inability to provide clear and consistent statements about symptoms or events that can be checked with reasonable certainty. Confusion between symptoms and an emotionally charged event or personal relationship; the use of bizarre, mechanical, or animalistic explanations for oral symptoms; and the patient's inability to separate him- or herself from real or imaginary objects or people indicate a need for further psychological evaluation. The dentist also will recognize those who express marked paranoia (eg, the pain that is due to an object purposely left behind by the surgeon, who is acting as the agent of God or any enemy of the patient).

None of these phenomena alone substantiates a diagnosis of mental disease. Specific diagnoses (such as schizophrenia, paranoia, and depression) made by the dentist on this basis are unjustified, but the dentist who becomes aware of compromised mental ability in his or her patient should consider the likelihood that abnormal psychological factors may be complicating the diagnostic situation. Such mental confusion may involve organic or functional mental disease that will require further consultation and assessment.

Mental disease, mental retardation, and the inability to conform to society do not produce oral symptoms, but they may affect the individual's ability to handle sensory abnormality. Conversely, pain and other abnormal oral sensations also are experienced by mentally ill persons in response to physical causes, and the clinician must always be on guard against discounting oral symptoms in mentally ill individuals in favor of a psychological explanation without thorough examination of the patient. Table 11-14 lists the IASP classification categories of "pain of psychological origin in the head, face, and neck."[1]

The DSM-IV[84] includes the classification entitled "pain disorder" within a larger category of "somatoform disorders." Somatoform disorders are characterized by the presence of physical symptoms that suggest a general medical condition but that are not fully explained by the medical condition, the direct effects of a substance, or another mental disorder. A pain disorder is characterized by "pain as the predominant focus of clinical attention where psychological factors are judged to have an important role in its onset, severity, exacerbation, or maintenance".

The majority of patients for whom emotional factors obviously complicate their oral symptoms do not have diagnosable mental disease although they may often be referred to as "crazy." Periods of increased emotional stress, whether brought about by interpersonal conflicts, external pressure from work or family, or an individual's own physical and personal drives, are normal for everyone, but such episodes also frequently reduce pain tolerance and the ability to handle chronic low-grade sensory abnormality. To the observer, the influence of the patient's emotions on the oral symptoms may at times be quite evident; for the patient, the interaction of emotional distress and physical disease may be impossible to manage, and he or she may be unable to control either aspect without assistance from the clinician. The following factors are clues that may provide insight into complicating emotional factors:

1. *The setting of the story.* The time of onset of the symptoms may have occurred in a period of increased personal, family, or work stress.

2. *A history of extensive medical/dental treatment.* Unusually extensive and (perhaps) multiple surgical procedures and the use of many medications despite minimal signs of "disease" that others tolerate as part of life indicate "increased help-seeking behavior" that may be maladaptive.[141]

3. *The "naive" or medically inexperienced patient.* Patients who have been free of oral disease until adulthood and who then need dental procedures may respond with excessive anxiety.[142] Paradoxically, those who have suffered painful traumatic and surgical episodes in childhood and have learned excessively apprehensive or other maladaptive responses within their families[143] may also become intolerant of the discomfort associated with dental procedures.

4. *The presence of a psychiatric illness or personality disorder.* An association exists between chronic pain and psychiatric illness.[144,145] However, this does not confirm an etiologic relationship; rather, it is important to

---

TABLE 11-14 Classification of Pain of Psychological Origin*

Pain of Psychological Origin Classification	Definition
Muscle Tension	Virtually continuous pain in any part of the body due to sustained muscle contraction and provoked by persistent overuse of particular muscles
Delusional or hallucinatory	Pain of psychological origin and attributed by the patient to a specific delusional cause
Hysterical, conversion, or hypochondriacal	Pain specifically attributable to the thought process, emotional state, or personality of the patient in the absence of an organic or delusional cause or tension mechanism
Associated with depression	Pain occurring in the course of a depressive illness usually not preceding the depression and not attributable to any other cause. (Note: not to be confused with depression that commonly occurs with chronic pain arising from physical reasons)

Reproduced with permission from Merskey H, Bogduk N.[1]

*International Association for the Study of Pain (IASP) classification.

appreciate that psychiatric illness requires concomitant treatment to effectively treat the OFP.

5. *Normal oral structures mistakenly identified as physical disease.* Under the stress of the death of a friend or family member or the discovery of life-threatening disease in a close relative or friend, normal structures or sensations may be thought of as potential signs of disease.

6. *Disrupted oral functions.* The mouth serves as a means to obtain food, a modulator for producing speech, and a part of facial expression in interpersonal communication; it also features prominently in sexual encounters. It is not surprising that a limitation of oral function due to oral sensory abnormality can lead to a strong emotional reaction.

7. *Imagined or symbolic functions traditionally assigned to the mouth that may be threatened.* Unsupported by facts of physiology and anatomy, these functions of the mouth feature prominently in our language and thoughts and may be perceived by the patient as being threatened.

The extent to which these traditional images exist in the thoughts of patients with oral disease is largely undocumented and could probably be revealed only by psychoanalysis. However, comments patients make in regard to their oral symptoms during regular diagnostic interviews suggest that such symbolism is a common accompaniment of oral disease. It is important that the clinician recognize these psychological interactions because it may allow him or her to distinguish complaints that are essentially psychological in nature from those that are more directly related to altered physiologic states; the treatment of one is quite different from the treatment of the other, and simultaneous treatment of both problems may be needed. It is an error to consider the patient who uses symbolic images in relating oral problems to be necessarily psychologically abnormal even when the images appear to be somewhat bizarre and overly graphic.[146] It is likely that oral symbolism is normally well developed in most minds, and concern about oral pain and discomfort simply allows patients to be somewhat less reserved about expressing their thoughts than they might usually be. The following metaphors are examples: the "mouthpiece of the mind" (a source of pleasant, virtuous, complimentary, and encouraging statements as well as smiles, laughs, and blessings, versus an invective tight-lipped mouth); an "organ of perception" (the ability to distinguish pleasurable from noxious foods and by extension, pleasurable from unhappy aspects of life); and a "source of pleasure" (the mouth can provide kisses or caresses or can mark an aggressive hostile personality).

If the clinician suspects a psychological cause for OFP, it is important to keep the following in mind:

1. However sophisticated the diagnostic procedures used, no diagnosis is final, and time may often reveal a previously unrecognized organic problem underlying the patient's symptoms.

2. The diagnostic procedures used should be as exhaustive as possible, even in the presence of major psychological dysfunction.

3. Psychological and psychogenic pains cannot be clearly distinguished from pain that has an obvious organic cause; psychological factors are a component of all painful experiences.

4. Pain associated with overwhelming psychological dysfunction (psychogenic pain) is as real to the patient as is pain from an obvious organic cause and cannot be dismissed as something that is "just in the patient's head."

5. A diagnosis of psychological pain should be confirmed by psychiatric evaluation of the patient.

Importance of Follow-up and Repeated Examination and Testing: Of prime importance in the management of patients with unexplained oral symptoms is the recognition that an identification of the cause of the symptoms may come only with time. Several studies of chronic oral sensory complaints have shown that with time, as many as one-half of patients with unexplained OFP were found to have specific pathologic diagnoses that explained their symptoms (provided that repeated examinations and diagnostic tests were continued beyond the initial period of consultation).[136,137]

The success of referral clinics in managing problems of this type derives partly from a program of continued surveillance of the patient by a coordinated group of consultants[137,147] and partly from the availability of sophisticated diagnostic equipment. With time, small lesions such as tumors in the nasopharynx, parotid gland, infratemporal fossa, and cranium that can impinge on oral sensory and motor nerves increase in size and become apparent through the development of other abnormalities. Systemic neurologic diseases such as multiple sclerosis[148] develop from a prodromal stage, in which only unusual oral symptoms are present, to a stage in which a variety of tests will reveal the presence of disease and explain the patient's oral symptoms. The literature contains numerous references to patients whose oral symptoms remained unexplained for varied periods of time until further growth of a tumor revealed the focus of the patient's symptoms.[125,149–159] Included among these reports are many descriptions of tumors of the parotid gland, infratemporal space, and cranial cavity that initially mimicked the symptoms of a TMD. Such reports emphasize the need for continuous awareness of such possibilities.[158] Newer imaging techniques may reveal such lesions and are important tools in the management of undiagnosed chronic OFP.[152,160–162]

▼ DIAGNOSIS AND MANAGEMENT OF SPECIFIC OROFACIAL PAIN DISORDERS

Facial Neuralgias

The classic neuralgias that affect the craniofacial region are a unique group of neurologic disorders involving the cranial nerves and are characterized by (a) brief episodes of shooting, often electric shock–like pain along the course of the affected nerve branch; (b) trigger zones on the skin or mucosa that precipitate painful attacks when touched; and (c) pain-free periods between attacks and refractory periods immediately after an attack, during which a new episode cannot be triggered. These clinical characteristics differ from neuropathic pain, which tends to be constant and has a burning quality without the presence of trigger zones. Neuropathic pain most often results from disorders that involve the spinal nerves whereas involvement of the cranial nerves may result in either chronic neuropathic pain or the classic brief episodes of shooting pain. Whether a lesion involving a cranial nerve causes constant neuropathic pain or brief episodes of shooting pain depends on both the nature of the underlying disorder and the position of the lesion along the course of the nerve. For example, tumors involving the trigeminal nerve between the pontine angle in the posterior cranial fossa and the ganglion in the middle cranial fossa will usually result in the lacinating pain of trigeminal neuralgia whereas more peripheral lesions will usually result in neuropathic pain. The major craniofacial neuralgias include trigeminal neuralgia, glossopharyngeal neuralgia, and occipital neuralgia. Geniculate neuralgia involving the sensory portion of CN VII is a similar but rare disorder. Postherpetic neuralgia and post-traumatic neuralgia are common causes of neuropathic pain.

TRIGEMINAL NEURALGIA

Trigeminal neuralgia (TN), also called tic douloureux, is the most common of the cranial neuralgias and chiefly affects individuals older than 50 years of age. When younger individuals are involved, suspicion of a detectable underlying lesion such as a tumor, an aneurysm, or multiple sclerosis must be increased.

Etiology and Pathogenesis.   The cause of the majority of cases of TN remains controversial, but approximately 10% of cases have detectable underlying pathology such as a tumor of the cerebellar pontine angle, a demyelinating plaque of multiple sclerosis, or a vascular malformation. The most frequent tumor is a meningioma of the posterior cranial fossa. The remainder of cases of TN are classified as idiopathic. Several theories exist regarding the etiology of TN.

The most widely accepted theory is that a majority of cases of TN are caused by an atherosclerotic blood vessel (usually the superior cerebellar artery) pressing on and grooving the root of the trigeminal nerve. This pressure results in focal demyelinization and hyperexcitability of nerve fibers, which will then fire in response to light touch, resulting in brief episodes of intense pain.[163]

Evidence for this theory includes the observation that neurosurgery that removes the pressure of the vessel from the nerve root by use of a microvascular decompression procedure eliminates the pain in a majority of cases. In a recent study of 1,185 patients who had microvascular decompression surgery for TN that did not respond to drug therapy, 70% of the patients were pain free 10 years after the surgery.[164] Additional evidence for this theory was obtained from a study using tomographic magnetic resonance imaging (MRI), which showed that contact between a blood vessel and the trigeminal nerve root was much greater on the affected side.[165]

Evidence against this theory includes the finding by neurosurgeons that manipulation of the area of the nerve root may eliminate the painful episodes even when an atherosclerotic vessel is not pressing on the nerve root. Other investigators believe that a major factor in the etiology of TN is a degeneration of the ganglion rather than the nerve root.[166]

Clinical Features.   The majority of patients with TN present with characteristic clinical features, which include episodes of intense shooting stabbing pain that lasts for a few seconds and then completely disappears. The pain characteristically has an electric shock–like quality and is unilateral except in a small percentage of cases. The maxillary branch is the branch that is most commonly affected, followed by the mandibular branch and (rarely) the ophthalmic branch. Involvement of more than one branch occurs in some cases.

Pain in TN is precipitated by light touch on a "trigger zone" present on the skin or mucosa within the distribution of the involved nerve branch. Common sites for trigger zones include the nasolabial fold and the corner of the lip. Shaving, showering, eating, speaking, or even exposure to wind can trigger a painful episode, and patients often protect the trigger zone with their hand or an article of clothing. Intraoral trigger zones can confuse the diagnosis by suggesting a dental disorder, and TN patients often first consult a dentist for evaluation. The stabbing pain can mimic the pain of a cracked tooth, but the two disorders can be distinguished by determining whether placing food in the mouth without chewing or whether gently touching the soft tissue around the trigger zone will precipitate pain. TN pain will be triggered by touching the soft tissue whereas pressure on the tooth is required to cause pain from a cracked tooth. Just after an attack, there is a refractory period when touching the trigger zone will not precipitate pain. The number of attacks may vary from one or two per day to several per minute. Patients with severe TN may be severely disabled by attacks that are triggered by speaking or other mouth movements.

Diagnosis.   The diagnosis of TN is usually based on the history of shooting pain along a branch of the trigeminal nerve, precipitated by touching a trigger zone, and possibly examination that demonstrates the shooting pain. A routine cranial nerve examination will be normal in patients with idiopathic TN, but sensory and/or motor changes may be evident in patients with underlying tumors or other CNS pathology. Local anesthetic blocks, which temporarily eliminate the trigger zone, may also be helpful in diagnosis. Since approximately 10% of TN cases are caused by detectable underlying pathology, enhanced MRI of the brain is indicated to rule out tumors, multiple sclerosis, and vascular malformations.

Management. Initial therapy for TN should consist of trials of drugs that are effective in eliminating the painful attacks. Anticonvulsant drugs are most frequently used and are most effective. Carbamazepine is the most commonly used drug and is an effective therapy for greater than 85% of newly diagnosed cases of TN. The drug is administered in slowly increasing doses until pain relief has been achieved. Skin reactions, including generalized erythema multiforme, are serious side effects. Patients receiving carbamazepine must have periodic hematologic laboratory evaluations because serious life-threatening blood dyscrasias occur in rare cases. Monitoring of hepatic and renal function is also recommended. Patients who do not respond to carbamazepine alone may obtain relief from baclofen or by combining carbamazepine with baclofen.[167] Gabapentin, a newer anticonvulsant that has fewer serious side effects than carbamazepine, is effective in some patients but does not appear to be as reliable as carbamazepine. Other drugs that are effective for some patients include phenytoin, lamotrigine, and pimozide.[168] Since TN may have temporary or permanent spontaneous remissions, drug therapy should be slowly withdrawn if a patient remains pain free for 3 months.

Clinicians treating TN must be aware that drug therapy often becomes less effective over time and that progressively higher doses may be required for pain control. In cases in which drug therapy is ineffective or in which the patient is unable to tolerate the side effects of drugs after trials of several agents, surgical therapy is indicated. A number of surgical procedures that result in temporary or permanent remission of the painful attacks have been described. These include procedures performed on the peripheral portion of the nerve, where it exits the jaw; at the gasserian ganglion; and on the brainstem, at the posterior cranial fossa. Peripheral surgery includes cryosurgery on the trigeminal nerve branch that triggers the painful attacks. This procedure is most frequently performed at the mental nerve for cases involving the third division and at the infraorbital nerve for cases involving the second division. The potential effectiveness of this procedure can be evaluated prior to surgery by determining whether a long-acting local anesthetic eliminates the pain during the duration of anesthesia. This procedure is usually effective for 12 to 18 months, at which time it must be repeated or another form of therapy must be instituted.

The most commonly performed procedure at the level of the gasserian ganglion is percutaneous radiofrequency thermocoagulation[169] although some clinicians continue to advocate glycerol block at the ganglion[170] or compression of the ganglion by balloon microcompression.[171] An infrequent but severe surgical complication is anesthesia dolorosa, which is numbness combined with severe intractable pain. The most extensively studied surgical procedure is microvascular decompression of the nerve root at the brainstem. In a report of 1,185 patients who were observed for 1 to 6 years, 70% of the patients experienced long-term relief of symptoms.[172] It should be noted that 30% of the patients experienced a recurrence of symptoms and required a second procedure or alternative therapy. Complications were rare but included stroke, facial numbness, and facial weakness.

In summary, therapy for TN presently includes a variety of both medical and surgical approaches, each of which is effective for some patients. Drug therapy including trials of several drugs or combinations of drugs should be attempted before surgery is recommended. When surgery is necessary, the patient should be carefully counseled regarding the advantages and disadvantages of the available surgical procedures. Clinicians should also remember that since spontaneous remissions are a feature of TN, procedures resulting in temporary relief might be all that is necessary for some patients.

GLOSSOPHARYNGEAL NEURALGIA

Glossopharyngeal neuralgia is a rare condition that is associated with paroxysmal pain that is similar to, though less intense than, the pain of TN. The location of the trigger zone and pain sensation follows the distribution of the glossopharyngeal nerve, namely, the pharynx, posterior tongue, ear, and infra-auricular retromandibular area. Pain is triggered by stimulating the pharyngeal mucosa during chewing, talking, and swallowing. The pain can be easily confused with that of geniculate neuralgia (because of the common ear symptoms) or with that of TMDs (because of pain following jaw movement).

Glossopharyngeal neuralgia may occur with TN, and when this occurs, a search for a common central lesion is essential. Glossopharyngeal neuralgia also may be associated with vagal symptoms, such as syncope and arrhythmia, owing to the close anatomic proximity of the two nerves. The application of a topical anesthetic to the pharyngeal mucosa eliminates glossopharyngeal nerve pain and can aid in distinguishing it from the pain of other neuralgias. The most common causes of glossopharyngeal neuralgia are intracranial or extracranial tumors and vascular abnormalities that compress CN IX. Treatment is similar to that for TN, with a good response to carbamazepine and baclofen. Refractory cases are treated surgically by intracranial or extracranial section of CN IX, microvascular decompression in the posterior cranial fossa, or (more recently) by percutaneous radiofrequency thermocoagulation of the nerve at the jugular foramen.[173]

NERVOUS INTERMEDIUS (GENICULATE) NEURALGIA

Nervous intermedius (geniculate) neuralgia is an uncommon paroxysmal neuralgia of CN VII, characterized by pain in the ear and (less frequently) the anterior tongue or soft palate. The location of pain matches the sensory distribution of this nerve (ie, the external auditory canal and a small area on the soft palate and the posterior auricular region). Pain may be provoked by the stimulation of trigger zones within the ipsilateral distribution of the nerve. The pain is not as sharp or intense as in TN, and there is often some degree of facial paralysis, indicating the simultaneous involvement of the motor root. Geniculate neuralgia commonly results from herpes zoster of the geniculate ganglion and nervus intermedius of CN VII,[174] a condition referred to as Ramsay Hunt syndrome.[175] Viral vesicles may be observed in the ear canal or on the tympanic membrane. The symptoms result from inflammatory neural degeneration, and a short course (2 to 3 weeks) of high-dose steroid therapy is beneficial.[174] Acyclovir significantly reduces the duration of the pain. Patients with geniculate neuralgia are also treated with carbamazepine and antidepressants. Patients who do not respond to these medications may undergo surgery to section the nervus intermedius.

OCCIPITAL NEURALGIA

Occipital neuralgia is a rare neuralgia in the distribution of the sensory branches of the cervical plexus (most commonly unilateral in the neck and occipital region). The most common causes (in descending order of frequency) are trauma, neoplasms, infections, and aneurysms involving the affected nerve(s). Palpation below the superior nuchal line may reveal an exquisitely tender spot. Treatment has included corticosteroids, neurolysis, avulsion, and blocking the nerve with a local anesthetic.[176]

POSTHERPETIC NEURALGIA

Etiology and Pathogenesis. Herpes zoster (shingles), described in detail in Chapter 2 is caused by the reactivation of latent varicella-zoster virus infection that results in both pain and vesicular lesions along the course of the affected nerve. Approximately 15 to 20% of cases of herpes zoster involve the trigeminal nerve although the majority of these cases affect the ophthalmic division of the fifth nerve, resulting in pain and lesions in the region of the eyes and forehead. Herpes zoster of the maxillary and mandibular divisions is a cause of facial and oral pain as well as of lesions. In a majority of cases, the pain of herpes zoster resolves within a month after the lesions heal. Pain that persists longer than a month is classified as postherpetic neuralgia (PHN) although some authors do not make the diagnosis of PHN until the pain has persisted for longer than 3 or even 6 months.[177] PHN may occur at any age, but the major risk factor is increasing age. Few individuals younger than 30 years of age experience PHN whereas more than 25% of individuals older than 55 years of age and two-thirds of patients older than over 70 years of age will suffer from PHN after an episode of herpes zoster.[178] Elderly patients also have an increased risk of experiencing severe pain for an extended period of time.[179] The pain and numbness of PHN results from a combination of both central and peripheral mechanisms. The varicella-zoster virus injures the peripheral nerve by demyelination, wallerian degeneration, and sclerosis,[180] but changes in the CNS, including atrophy of dorsal horn cells in the spinal cord, have also been associated with PHN.[181] This combination of peripheral and central injury results in the spontaneous discharge of neurons and an exaggerated painful response to nonpainful stimuli.[180]

Clinical Manifestations. Patients with PHN experience persistent pain, paresthesia, hyperesthesia, and allodynia months to years after the zoster lesions have healed. The pain is often accompanied by a sensory deficit, and there is a correlation between the degree of sensory deficit and the severity of pain.[182]

Management. Many treatment options are available for the management of PHN, and the method chosen should depend on the severity of the symptoms as well as the general medical status of the patient. Treatment includes topical and systemic, drug therapy and surgery.

Topical therapy includes the use of topical anesthetic agents, such as lidocaine, or analgesics, particularly capsaicin. Lidocaine used either topically or injected gives short-term relief from severe pain.[183] Combinations of topical anesthetics such as EMLA Cream (AstraZeneca) have also been reported as helpful.[184] Capsaicin, an extract of hot chili peppers that depletes the neurotransmitter substance P when used topically, has been shown to be helpful in reducing the pain of PHN, but the side effect of a burning sensation at the site of application limits its usefulness for many patients.

The use of tricyclic antidepressants such as amitriptyline, nortriptyline, doxepin, and desiprimine is a well-established method of reducing the chronic burning pain that is characteristic of PHN.[185–188] Because a significant number of elderly patients cannot tolerate the sedative or cardiovascular side effects associated with tricyclic antidepressants, the use of other drugs, particularly gabapentin, has been advocated. In one controlled clinical trial, the use of gabapentin reduced pain by more than 30% and also improved sleep and overall quality of life.[189] Patients who undergo episodes of shooting pain may experience relief through the use of anticonvulsant drugs, such as carbamazepine or phenytoin.[188]

When medical therapy has been ineffective in managing intractable pain, nerve blocks or surgery at the level of the peripheral nerve or dorsal root have been effective for some patients. The best therapy for PHN is prevention. There is evidence that the use of antiviral drugs, particularly famciclovir, along with a short course of systemic corticosteroids during the acute phase of the disease may decrease the incidence and severity of PHN.[190] Although investigators agree that the use of antivirals and corticosteroids decreases acute pain and accelerates the healing of lesions, further controlled trials are necessary before the long-term benefits of using antivirals and corticosteroids are known.[191] The use of tricyclic antidepressants during the acute phase of herpes zoster has been advocated as an effective method of decreasing PHN.[192]

POST-TRAUMATIC NEUROPATHIC PAIN

Etiology and Pathogenesis. Trigeminal nerve injuries may result from facial trauma or from surgical procedures, such as the removal of impacted third molars, the placement of dental implants, the removal of cysts or tumors of the jaws, genioplasties, or osteotomies. In some individuals, nerve injury results only in numbness whereas others experience pain that may be either spontaneous or triggered by a stimulus. The pain associated with nerve injury often has a burning quality due to spontaneous activity in nociceptor C fibers.[193] Minor nerve injuries (classified as neurapraxia) do not result in axonal degeneration but may cause temporary symptoms of paresthesia for a few hours or days. More serious nerve damage (classified as axonotmesis) results in the degeneration of neural fibers although the nerve trunk remains intact. These injuries cause symptoms for several months but have a good prognosis for recovery after axonal regeneration is complete. Total nerve section (neurotmesis) frequently causes permanent nerve damage, resulting in anesthesia and/or dysesthesia.[194] Central sensitization probably plays a role in the symptoms of neuropathy.

Clinical Manifestations. The pain associated with peripheral nerve injury may be persistent or may occur only in response to a stimulus such as light touch. Patients with nerve damage may experience anesthesia (loss in sensation), paresthesia (a feeling of "pins and needles"), allodynia (pain caused by a stimulus that is normally not painful), or hyperalgesia (an exaggerated response to a mildly painful stimulus).

Management. Treatment of neuropathic pain may be surgical, nonsurgical, or a combination of both, depending on the nature of the injury and the severity of the pain. Systemic corticosteroids are considered helpful in decreasing the incidence and severity of traumatic neuropathies when administered within the first week after a nerve injury. Steroids used after this initial period are of little value. The most frequently used medications for the management of neuropathic pain include tricyclic antidepressants (TCAs) and gabapentin.

TCAs such as amitriptyline, doxepin, and nortriptyline have been extensively studied and widely used to treat neuropathic pain, including traumatic neuropathies of the trigeminal nerve.[195] The TCAs can be used alone; in severe intractable cases, they potentiate the effect of narcotic analgesics. The clinician prescribing TCAs must be aware of potential serious side effects in patients with cardiac arrhythmias or glaucoma and must be able to help the patient manage common side effects that include drowsiness, weight gain from increased appetite, and dry mouth.

Gabapentin, an anticonvulsant drug approved for the treatment of epilepsy, has been used with increasing frequency to treat a variety of neuropathic pain syndromes, including diabetic neuropathy and PHN. The low incidence of serious side effects has encouraged widespread use of this drug. A controlled clinical trial that compared the effectiveness of gabapentin with that of the TCA amitriptyline demonstrated that both were equally effective in controlling neuropathic pain associated with diabetic neuropathy.[196,197]

Topical capsaicin may also be effective in controlling pain and is especially useful for patients who are unable to tolerate the side effects of systemic therapy.

Complex Regional Pain Syndrome 1 (Reflex Sympathetic Dystrophy)

The terms "complex regional pain syndrome type 1" (CRPS-1) and "reflex sympathetic dystrophy" (RSD) are used to describe a poorly understood syndrome that consists of localized pain, motor and sweat abnormalities, and trophic changes in the soft tissues of the muscles and skin.

ETIOLOGY AND PATHOGENESIS

The constellation of signs and symptoms associated with CRPS is believed to result from changes after trauma that couples sensory nerve fibers to sympathetic stimuli. Evidence for the existence of CRPS includes studies that show that surgical or drug-induced blockades of the sympathetic nervous system relieve the symptoms. In a new taxonomy included in the classification of chronic pain, CRPS-1 is used in place of RSD, and CRPS-2 replaces causalgia, which is a pain syndrome resulting from a major nerve injury. RSD has rarely been described as involving the trigeminal nerve distribution, and the role of the sympathetic nervous system in chronic facial pain is unknown. One study of chronic facial pain patients who also had evidence of autonomic dysfunction described a subset of patients who improved after a stellate ganglion block, suggesting a possible role for the sympathetic nervous system.[198] There are also case reports of facial pain resolving after sympathectomy.[199]

CLINICAL MANIFESTATIONS

The most constant symptom of CRPS is spontaneous chronic burning pain and tenderness, frequently accompanied by motor dysfunction, sweating, and cutaneous atrophy. The involved skin may also be edematous and erythematous as a result of changes in blood flow, and the underlying bone is commonly demineralized. Allodynia and hyperesthesia are common symptoms, and movement exacerbates the pain. This syndrome most commonly involves the extremities distal to an injury. The existence of this disorder in the head and facial region is controversial.

TREATMENT

The recommended therapy for CRPS involves a multidisciplinary approach that includes physical therapy, nerve blocks, and drug therapy. Blockades of regional sympathetic ganglia or regional intravenous blockades with guanethidine, reserpine, or phenoxybenzamine combined with a local anesthetic have been reported as successful[200] and are used in anesthesia pain clinics. Bisphosphonates such as alendronate or pamidronate have decreased pain in some RSD patients when used intravenously. It is unclear whether these drugs are helpful because of their effect on bone or because of anti-inflammatory properties.[201]

Atypical Odontalgia (Atypical Facial Pain)

A classification that includes the diagnoses of atypical odontalgia (AO) and atypical facial pain (AFP) is controversial, and many workers in the field of facial pain believe that these terms should be discarded because they are often used either as catchalls to denote patients who have not been adequately evaluated or because they imply that the pain is purely psychological in origin. Some classification systems, including the IHS system, use the term "facial pain not fulfilling other criteria" to describe patients in this category. The disputed terms are still commonly used in clinical practice, however, since there exists a group of individuals who (1) have a chronic facial pain syndrome with characteristic clinical features, (2) have been thoroughly investigated, and (3) do not fall into any other diagnostic categories. The term "atypical odontalgia" is used in this context when the pain is confined to the teeth or gingivae whereas the term "atypical facial pain" is used when other parts of the face are involved.

ETIOLOGY AND PATHOGENESIS

There are several theories regarding the etiology of AO and AFP. One theory considers AO and AFP to be a form of de-afferentation or phantom tooth pain. This theory is supported by the high percentage of patients with these disorders who report that the symptoms began after a dental procedure such as endodontic therapy or an extraction. Others have theorized that AO is a form of vascular, neuropathic, or sympathetically maintained pain. Other studies support the concept that at least some of the patients in this category have a strong psychogenic component to their symptoms and that depressive, somatization, and conversion disorders have been described as major factors in some patients. It is frequently difficult to accurately study the psychological aspects of a chronic pain syndrome since anxiety and depression are part of the clinical picture of all patients with chronic pain.

There is often strong disagreement between facial pain experts who stress the biologic basis of AO and AFP and others who stress the emotional basis, but the etiology remains unknown at this time. It is likely that there are subgroups of patients who fall into the category of AO and AFP, some of whom have a strong component of de-afferentation pain while others have a psychological basis for similar symptoms. It is also possible that a combination of both neuropathic and psychological mechanisms are important in the etiology of this presently poorly understood facial pain syndrome.

CLINICAL MANIFESTATIONS

The major manifestation of AO and AFP is a constant dull aching pain without an apparent cause that can be detected by examination or laboratory studies. AO occurs most frequently in women in the fourth and fifth decades of life, and most studies report that women make up more than 80% of the patients. The pain is described as a constant dull ache, instead of the brief and severe attacks of pain that are characteristic of TN. There are no trigger zones, and lancinating pains are rare. The patient frequently reports that the onset of pain coincided with a dental procedure such as oral surgery or an endodontic or restorative procedure. Patients also report seeking multiple dental procedures to treat the pain; these procedures may result in temporary relief, but the pain characteristically returns in days or weeks. Other patients will give a history of sinus procedures or of receiving trials of multiple medications, including antibiotics, corticosteroids, decongestants, or anticonvulsant drugs. The pain may remain in one area or may migrate, either spontaneously or after a surgical procedure. Symptoms may remain unilateral, cross the midline in some cases, or involve both the maxilla and mandible.

A thorough history and examination including evaluation of the cranial nerves, oropharynx, and teeth must be performed to rule out dental, neurologic, or nasopharyngeal disease. Examination of the masticatory muscles should also be performed to eliminate pain secondary to undetected muscle dysfunction. Laboratory tests should be carried out when indicated by the history and examination. Patients with AO or AFP have completely normal radiographic and clinical laboratory studies.

MANAGEMENT

Once the diagnosis has been made and other pathologies have been eliminated, it is important that the symptoms are taken seriously and are not dismissed as imaginary. Patients should be counseled regarding the nature of AO and reassured that they do not have an undetected life-threatening disease and that they can be helped without invasive procedures. When indicated, consultation with other specialists such as otolaryngologists, neurologists, or psychiatrists may be helpful. TCAs such as amitriptyline, nortriptyline, and doxepin, given in low to moderate doses, are often effective in reducing or (in some cases) eliminating the pain. Other recommended drugs include gabapentin and clonazepam. Some clinicians report benefit from topical desensitization with capsaicin, topical anesthetics, or topical doxepin.

Burning Mouth Syndrome (Glossodynia)

Burning sensations accompany many inflammatory or ulcerative diseases of the oral mucosa, but the term "burning mouth syndrome" (BMS) is reserved for describing oral burning that has no detectable cause. The burning symptoms in patients with BMS do not follow anatomic pathways, there are no mucosal lesions or known neurologic disorders to explain the symptoms, and there are no characteristic laboratory abnormalities.

ETIOLOGY AND PATHOGENESIS

The cause of BMS remains unknown, but a number of factors have been suspected, including hormonal and allergic disorders, salivary gland hypofunction, chronic low-grade trauma, and psychiatric abnormalities. The increased incidence of BMS in women after menopause has led investigators to suspect an association with hormonal changes, but there is little evidence that women with BMS have more hormonal abnormalities than matched controls who do not have BMS. Studies of estrogen replacement therapy used to treat BMS have yielded mixed results, and few investigators recommend hormone replacement as a primary therapy for BMS in patients who do not require it for other reasons.

Allergic reactions have also been suspected, but there is no evidence to support the hypothesis that BMS is the result of allergic reactions to food, oral hygiene products, or dental materials. A contact allergy can affect the oral mucosa and result in burning sensations, but inflammatory, lichenoid, or ulcerative lesions are present in cases of contact allergy and absent in BMS patients. It was theorized that BMS is related to decreased salivary gland function, but most studies have shown no clear-cut association between BMS and decreased salivary flow rates.[202] Changes in taste have been reported in over 60% of patients with BMS, and BMS patients have been shown to have different thresholds of taste perception than matched controls.[203] Dysgeusia (particularly an abnormally bitter taste) has been reported by 60% of BMS patients.[204] This association has led to a concept that BMS may be a defect in sensory peripheral neural mechanisms.[202]

BMS has been associated with psychological disorders in many studies. Depression is frequently associated with BMS, and in some studies, close to one-third of BMS patients have significant depression scores although, as with any chronic pain disorder, it is unclear if depression is the cause or the effect of the symptoms.[205–207] It is likely that some cases of BMS have a strong psychological component, but other factors, such as chronic low-grade trauma resulting from parafunctional oral habits (eg, rubbing the tongue across the teeth or pressing it on the palate), are also likely to play a role.

CLINICAL MANIFESTATIONS

Women experience symptoms of BMS seven times more frequently than men.[208] When questioned, 10 to 15% of postmenopausal women are found to have a history of oral burning sensations, and these symptoms are most prevalent 3 to 12 years after menopause.[209] The tongue is the most common site of involvement, but the lips and palate are also frequently involved. The burning can be either intermittent or constant, but eating, drinking, or placing candy or chewing gum in the mouth characteristically relieves the symptoms. This contrasts with the increased oral burning noted during eating that occurs in patients with lesions or neuralgias affecting the oral mucosa. Patients presenting with BMS are often apprehensive and admit to being generally anxious or "high-strung." They may also have symptoms that suggest depression, such as decreased appetite, insomnia, and a loss of interest in daily activities.

Other causes of burning symptoms of the oral mucosa must be eliminated by examination and laboratory studies before the diagnosis of BMS can be made. Patients with unilateral symptoms should have a thorough evaluation of the trigeminal and other cranial nerves to eliminate a neurologic source of pain. A careful clinical examination for oral lesions resulting from candidiasis, lichen planus, or other mucosal diseases should be performed. Patients complaining of a combination of xerostomia and burning should be evaluated for the possibility of a salivary gland disorder, particularly if the mucosa appears to be dry and the patient has difficulty swallowing dry foods without sipping liquids. When indicated, laboratory tests should be carried out to detect undiagnosed diabetic neuropathy, anemia, or deficiencies of iron, folate, or vitamin B_{12}.

TREATMENT

Once the diagnosis of BMS has been made by eliminating the possibility of detectable lesions or underlying medical disorders, the patient should be reassured of the benign nature of the symptoms. Counseling the patient in regard to the nature of BMS is helpful in management, particularly because many patients will have had multiple clinical evaluations without an explanation for the symptoms. Counseling and reassurance may be adequate management for individuals with mild burning sensations, but patients with symptoms that are more severe often require drug therapy. The drug therapies that have been found to be the most helpful are low doses of TCAs, such as amitriptyline and doxepin, or clonazepam (a benzodiazepine derivative). It should be stressed to the patient that these drugs are being used not to manage psychiatric illness, but for their well-documented analgesic effect. Clinicians prescribing these drugs should be familiar with potential serious and annoying side effects.

Burning of the tongue that results from parafunctional oral habits may be relieved with the use of a splint covering the teeth and/or the palate.

Vascular Pain

Pain originating from vascular structures may cause facial pain that can be misdiagnosed and mistaken for other oral disorders, including toothache or TMD. This section discusses the major pain disorders of vascular etiology that have prominent orofacial signs and symptoms.

CRANIAL ARTERITIS

Cranial arteritis (temporal arteritis, giant cell arteritis) is an inflammatory disorder involving the medium-sized branches of the carotid arteries. The temporal artery is the most commonly involved branch. The blood vessel abnormality may be localized to the head and face or may be part of the generalized disease, polymyalgia rheumatica.

Etiology and Pathogenesis. Both cranial arteritis and polymyalgia rheumatica are caused by immune abnormalities that affect cytokines and T lymphocytes, resulting in inflammatory infiltrates in the walls of arteries. This infiltrate is characterized by the formation of multinucleated giant cells. The underlying trigger of the inflammatory response is unknown.

Clinical Manifestations. Cranial arteritis most frequently affects adults above the age of 50 years. Patients have a throbbing headache accompanied by generalized symptoms including fever, malaise, and loss of appetite. Patients with polymyalgia rheumatica will have accompanying joint and muscle pain. Examination of the involved temporal artery reveals a thickened pulsating vessel. Since the mandibular and lingual arteries may be involved, a throbbing pain in the jaw or tongue may be an early sign or even a presenting sign. A serious complication in untreated patients is ischemia of the eye, which may lead to progressive loss of vision or sudden blindness. These visual manifestations may be prevented by early diagnosis and prompt therapy.

Laboratory abnormalities include an elevated erythrocyte sedimentation rate (ESR) and anemia. Abnormal C-reactive protein may also be an important early finding. The most definitive diagnostic test is a biopsy specimen (from the involved temporal artery) that demonstrates the characteristic inflammatory infiltrate. Since the entire vessel is not involved, an adequate specimen must be taken to detect the changes. A negative biopsy result does not rule out temporal arteritis, and the diagnosis should continue to be considered in patients over 50 years of age who have chronic pounding head or orofacial pain and an elevated ESR.[210]

Treatment. Individuals with cranial arteritis should be treated with systemic corticosteroids as soon as the diagnosis is made. The initial dose ranges between 40 to 60 mg of prednisone per day, and the steroid is tapered once the signs of the disease are controlled. The ESR may be used to help monitor disease status. Patients are maintained on systemic steroids for 1 to 2 years after symptoms resolve. Steroids may be supplemented by adjuvant therapy with immunosuppressive drugs, such as cyclophosphamide, to reduce the complications of long-term corticosteroid therapy. Immediate steroid therapy should be initiated if visual symptoms are present.

CLUSTER HEADACHE

Cluster headache (CH) is a distinct pain syndrome characterized by episodes of severe unilateral head pain occuring chiefly around the eye and accompanied by a number of autonomic signs. The term "cluster" is used because individuals who are susceptible to CH experience multiple headaches per day for 4 to 6 weeks and then may be without pain for months or even years.

Etiology and Pathogenesis. There are several theories regarding the etiology of CH and its characteristic combination of both severe localized pain and autonomic symptoms. Some investigators postulate that a CH attack originates in the hypothalamus, which stimulates both the trigeminal and vascular systems in the brain.[211] Others believe that the pain originates peripherally in the cavernous sinus since sympathetic, parasympathetic, and sensory fibers from the first division of the trigeminal nerve are present and because organic lesions of the cavernous sinus can result in symptoms that resemble CH.[212]

Clinical Manifestations. Eighty percent of patients with CH are men. The attacks are sudden, unilateral, and stabbing, causing patients to pace, cry out, or even strike objects. Some patients exhibit violent behavior during attacks. This contrasts with the behavior of migraine patients, who lie down in a dark room and try to sleep. Individuals with CH frequently describe the pain as a hot metal rod in or around the eye. The symptoms most commonly affect the area supplied by the first division of the trigeminal nerve, but second-division symptoms may also occur, causing patients to consult a dentist to rule out an odontogenic etiology. Unnecessary extractions of maxillary teeth are often performed before a correct diagnosis is made. The severe painful episodes begin without an aura and become excruciating within a few minutes. Each attack lasts from 15 minutes to 2 hours and recurs several times daily. A majority of the painful episodes occur at night, often waking the patient from sleep. The pain is

associated with autonomic symptoms, particularly nasal congestion and tearing. Sweating of the face, ptosis, increased salivation, and edema of the eyelid are also common signs. During a cluster period, ingestion of alcohol or use of nitroglycerin will provoke an attack.

Treatment. An acute attack of CH can be aborted by breathing 100% oxygen, and CH patients may keep an oxygen canister at bedside to use at the first sign of an attack. Injection of sumatriptan or sublingual or inhaled ergotamine may also be effective therapy. Several drug protocols are recommended for preventing CH during active periods. Lithium is effective therapy for those who can tolerate the side effects, and patients who are using long-term lithium must be monitored for renal toxicity. Other drugs that are useful for preventing attacks include ergotamine, prophylactic prednisone, and calcium channel blockers. Methysergide is also effective therapy, but pulmonary or cardiac fibrosis are potential side effects, particularly during prolonged use.

CHRONIC PAROXYSMAL HEMICRANIA

Chronic paroxysmal hemicrania (CPH) is believed to be a form of CH that occurs predominantly in women between the ages of 30 to 40 years. The episodes of pain tend be shorter, but attacks of 5 to 20 minutes' duration can occur up to 30 times daily. Initially, episodes of CPH occur with a periodicity similar to that of CH; however, CPH symptoms tend to become chronic over time. CPH responds dramatically to therapy with indomethacin, which stops the attacks within 1 to 2 days. CPH will recur if indomethacin is discontinued.

MIGRAINE

Until recently, headaches were believed to be either vascular or muscular in origin, but studies performed in the past decade have indicated that many patients with frequent or chronic headaches have a mixture of both vascular and muscular pain and that headaches are frequently somewhere on a continuum between being purely vascular and purely muscular. Migraine is the most common of the vascular headaches, which may occasionally also cause pain of the face and jaws. It may be triggered by foods such as nuts, chocolate, and red wine; stress; sleep deprivation; or hunger. Migraine is more common in women.

Etiology and Pathogenesis. The classic theory is that migraine is caused by vasoconstriction of intracranial vessels (which causes the neurologic symptoms), followed by vasodilation (which results in pounding headache). Newer research techniques suggest a series of factors, including the triggering of neurons in the midbrain that activate the trigeminal nerve system in the medulla, resulting in the release of neuropeptides such as substance P. These neurotransmitters activate receptors on the cerebral vessel walls, causing vasodilation and vasoconstriction. There are several major types of migraine: classic, common, basilar, and facial migraine (also referred to as carotidynia).

Clinical Manifestations.   Classic migraine starts with a prodromal aura that is usually visual but that may also be sensory or motor. The visual aura that commonly precedes classic migraine includes flashing lights or a localized area of depressed vision (scotoma). Sensitivity to light, hemianesthesia, aphasia, or other neurologic symptoms may also be part of the aura, which commonly lasts from 20 to 30 minutes. The aura is followed by an increasingly severe unilateral throbbing headache that is frequently accompanied by nausea and vomiting. The patient characteristically lies down in a dark room and tries to fall asleep. Headaches characteristically last for hours up to 2 or 3 days.

Common migraine is not preceded by an aura, but patients may experience irritability or other mood changes. The pain of common migraine resembles the pain of classic migraine and is usually unilateral, pounding, and associated with sensitivity to light and noise. Nausea and vomiting are also common.

Basilar migraine is most common in young women. The symptoms are primarily neurologic and include aphasia, temporary blindness, vertigo, confusion, and ataxia. These symptoms may be accompanied by an occipital headache. Facial migraine (carotidynia) causes a throbbing and/or sticking pain in the neck or jaw. The pain is associated with involvement of branches of the carotid artery rather than the cerebral vessels.[213] The symptoms of facial migraine usually begin in individuals who are 30 to 50 years of age. Patients often seek dental consultation, but unlike the pain of a toothache, facial migraine pain is not continuous but lasts minutes to hours and recurs several times per week. Examination of the neck will reveal tenderness of the carotid artery. Face and jaw pain may be the only manifestation of migraine, or it may be an occasional pain in patients who usually experience classic or common migraine.[214]

Treatment.   Patients with migraine should be carefully assessed to determine common food triggers. Attempts to minimize reactions to the stress of everyday living by using relaxation techniques may also be helpful to some patients. Drug therapy may be used either prophylactically to prevent attacks in patients who experience frequent headaches or acutely at the first sign of an attack. Drugs that are useful in aborting migraine include ergotamine and sumatriptan, which can be given orally, nasally, rectally or parenterally. These drugs must be used cautiously since they may cause hypertension and other cardiovascular complications. Drugs that are used to prevent migraine include propranolol, verapimil, and TCAs.[215] Methysergide or monoamine oxidase inhibitors such as phenelzine can be used to manage difficult cases that do not respond to safer drugs.

▼ REFERENCES

1. Merskey H, Bogduk N, editors. Classification of chronic pain, Task Force on Taxonomy, International Association for the Study of Pain. 2nd ed. Seattle: IASP Press: 1994. p. 210–3.

2. Keefe F, Jacobs M, Underwood-Gordon L. NIH workshop summary: biobehavioral pain research: a multi-institute assessment of cross-cutting issues and research needs. Clin J Pain 1997;13:91–103.

3. Kaplan H, Saddock B. Synopsis of psychiatry. 8th ed. Baltimore: Williams & Wilkins; 1998.

4. Kandel E, James H, Jessell T. Principles of neural science. 3rd ed. Norwalk (CN): Appleton and Lange; 1991. p. 703.

5. Sessle B. Neurobiology of facial and dental pain. In: Sarnat B, Laskin D, editors. The temporomandibular joint. A biological basis for clinical practice. Philadelphia: W.B. Saunders; 1992. p. 124–42.

6. Gobel S, Hockfield S, Rudal M. Anatomical similarities between medullary and spinal dorsal horns. In: Oro-facial sensory and motor functions. Tokyo: Quintessence; 1981. p. 211–23.

7. Gobel S, Bennett GJ, Allan B. Synaptic connectivity of substantia gelatinosa neurons with reference to potential termination sites of descending axons. In: Sjolund B, Bjorkland A, editors. Brain stem control of spinal mechanisms. Elsevier; 1982. p. 135–58.

8. Turk D, Rudy T. Toward a comprehensive assessment of chronic pain patients. Behav Res Ther 1987;25:237–49.

9. Seymour R. The use of pain scales in assessing the efficacy of analgesics in post–operative dental pain. Eur J Clin Pharmacol 1982;23:441–4.

10. Varni J, Thompson K, Hanson V. The Varni-Thompson pediatric pain questionnaire. I. Chronic musculoskeletal pain in juvenile rheumatoid arthritis. Pain 1987;28:27–38.

11. Melzack R. The McGill Pain Questionnaire: major properties and scoring methods. Pain 1975;1:277–99.

12. Grushka M, Sessle B. Application of the McGill Pain Questionnaire for the differentiation of toothache pain. Pain 1984;19:49–57.

13. Melzack R, Terrence C, Fromm G, Amsel R. Trigeminal neuralgia and atypical facial pain: use of the McGill Pain Questionnaire for discrimination and diagnosis. Pain 1986;27:297–302.

14. Keefe F, Holzberg A, Beaupre P. Contributions of pain behavior assessment and pain assessment to the development of pain clinics. In: Cohen M, Campbell N, editors. Pain treatment centers at a crossroads: a practical and conceptual reappraisal. Seattle: IASP Press; 1996. p. 79–100.

15. Dorland's illustrated medical dictionary. 28th ed. Philadelphia: W.B. Saunders Co.; 1994.

16. Turk D, Rudy T. The robustness of an empirically derived taxonomy of chronic pain patients. Pain 1990;43:27–35.

17. Rudy T, Turk DC, Zaki HS, Curtin HD. An empirical taxometric alternative to traditional classification of temporomandibular disorders. Pain 1989;36:311–20.

18. Kerns R, Turk D, Rudy T. The West Haven-Yale Multidimensional Pain Inventory (WHYMPI). Pain 1985;23:345–6.

19. Turk D, Rudy T. Classification logic and strategies in chronic pain. In: Turk D, Melzack R, editors. Handbook of pain assessment. New York: Guilford Press; 1992.

20. Dworkin S, LeResche L. Research diagnostic criteria for temporomandibular disorders: review, criteria, examinations, and specifications, critique. J Craniomandib Disord 1992;6:301–55.

21. Von Korff M, Ormel J, Keefe FJ, Dworkin SF. Grading the severity of chronic pain. Pain 1992;50:133–49.

22. Derogatis L. SCL-90-R: administration, scoring and procedures manual - II for the revised version. Towson (MD): Clinical Psychometric Research; 1983.

23. Bonica J. The management of pain. Philadelphia: Lea & Febiger; 1953.

24. Fordyce W. Pain and suffering: a reappraisal. Am Psychol 1988;43:276–83.

25. Sternbach R. Psychological factors in pain. In: Bonica J, Albe-Fessard D, editors. Advances in pain research and therapy. New York: Raven Press; 1976.

26. Melzak R, Wall P. Pain mechanisms: a new theory. Science 1965;150:971–9.

27. Coderre TJ, Katz J, Vaccarino AL, Melzack R. Contribution of central neuroplasticity to pathological pain: review of clinical and experimental evidence. Pain 1993;52:259–85.

28. Woolf C. A new strategy for the treatment of inflammatory pain: prevention or elimination of central sensitization. Drugs 1994;47 Suppl 5:1–9.

29. Devor M. Pain mechanisms and pain syndromes. In: Campbell J, editor. Pain 1996 — an updated review. Seattle: IASP Press; p. 103–12.

30. Fordyce W. Behavioral methods for chronic pain and illness. St. Louis: Mosby; 1976.

31. Keefe F. Behavioral measurement of pain. In: Chapman C, Loeser J, editors. Advances in pain research and therapy. New York: Raven Press; 1989.

32. Craig K. Emotional aspects of pain. In: Wall P, Melzack R, editors. Textbook of pain. London: Churchill Livingstone; 1994. p. 261–74.

33. Jensen MP, Turner JA, Romano JM, Karoly P. Coping with chronic pain: a critical review of the literature. Pain 1991;47:249–83.

34. Caudill M. Clinical implications of the NIH Technology and Assessment Conference addressing behavioral treatment of chronic pain. IASP Newsl 1998;March/April:3–7.

35. Gamsa A. Is emotional disturbance a precipitator or a consequence of chronic pain? Pain 1990;42:183–95.

36. Turk D. Strategies for classifying chronic orofacial pain patients. Anesth Prog 1990;37:155–60.

37. Roberts A, Sternbach R, Polich J. Behavioral management of chronic pain and excess disability: long-term follow-up of an outpatient program. Clin J Pain 1993;9:41–8.

38. Moore M, Berk S, Nypaver A. Chronic pain: inpatient treatment with small group effects. Arch Phys Med Rehabil 1984;65:356–61.

39. Tollison C, Kriegel M, Downie G. Chronic low back pain: results of treatment at the pain therapy center. South Med J 1985;78:1291–5.

40. Flor H, Fydrich T, Turk D. Efficacy of multidisciplinary pain treatment centers: a meta-analytic review. Pain 1992;49:221–30.

41. Turk D. Efficacy of multidisciplinary pain centers in the treatment of chronic pain. In: Cohen M, Campbell J, editors. Pain treatment centers at a crossroads: a practical and conceptual reappraisal. Seattle: IASP Press; 1996. p. 257–73.

42. National Institutes of Health. Integration of behavioral and relaxation approaches into the treatment of chronic pain and insomnia. NIH Technol Assess Statement 1995; October 16–18:1–34.

43. Laska E, Sunshine A, Mueller F, et al. Caffeine as an analgesic adjuvant. JAMA 1984;251:1711–8.

44. Piletta P, Porchet H, Dayer P. Central analgesic effects of acetaminophen but not of aspirin. Clin Pharmacol Ther 1991;49:350–4.

45. Coyle N, Cherny N, Portnoy R. Pharmacological management of cancer pain. In: McGuire D, Yarbro C, Ferrell B, editors. Cancer pain management. Boston: Jones & Bartlett Publishers; 1995. p. 89–130.

46. Society AP. Principles of analgesic use in the treatment of acute pain and cancer pain. 3rd ed. Skokie (IL): American Pain Society; 1992.

47. McCaffery M, Pasero C. Pain, clinical manual. 2nd ed. St. Louis: Mosby, Inc.; 1999.

48. Koch M, Dezi A, Ferrario F, Capurso I. Prevention of non-steroidal anti-inflammatory drug-induced gastrointestinal mucosal injury: a meta-analysis of randomised controlled clinical trials. Arch Intern Med 1996;11:2321–32.

49. Henry D, Lim LL, Garcia Rodriguez LA, et al. Variability in risk of gastrointestinal complications with individual non-steroidal anti-inflammatory drugs: results of a collaborative meta–analysis. BMJ 1996;312:1563–6.

50. Insel P. Analgesic-antipyretic and antiinflammatory agents and drugs employed in the treatment of gout. In: Hardman J, Limbird L, editors. Goodman & Gilman's the pharmacological basis of therapeutics. New York: McGraw-Hill; 1996. p. 617–55.

51. Rang H, Dale MM, Ritter JM, Gardner P. Pharmacology. New York: Churchill Livingstone; 1995.

52. Portenoy R. Opioid therapy for chronic nonmalignant pain. Pain Res Manage 1996;1:17–28.

53. Fromm G, Terrence C. Medical treatment of trigeminal neuralgia. In: Fromm G, editor. The medical and surgical treatment of trigeminal neuralgia. New York: Futura; p. 61–70.

54. Feinmann C. Psychogenic facial pain: presentation and treatment. J Psychosm Res 1983;27(5):403–10.

55. Sharav Y, Singer E, Schmidt E, et al. The analgesic effect of amitriptyline on chronic facial pain. Pain 1987;31:199–209.

56. Onghena P, Houdenhove BV. Antidepressant-induced analgesia in chronic non-malignant pain: a meta-analysis of 39 placebo-controlled studies. Pain 1992:49:205–19.

57. McQuay H, Carroll D, Jadad AR, et al.. Anticonvulsant drugs for management of pain: a systematic review. BMJ 1995;311(7012):1047–52.

58. Imamura Y, Bennett G. Felbamate relieves several abnormal pain sensations in rats with experimental peripheral neuropathy. J Pharm Exp Ther 1995;275:177–82.

59. Nakamura-Craig M, Follenfant R. Effect of lamatrogine in the acute and chronic hyperalgesia induced by PGE2 and in the chronic hyperalgesia in rats with streptozotocin-induced diabetes. Pain 1995;63:33–7.

60. Rosenberg J, Harrell C, Ristic H, et al. The effect of gabapentin on neuropathic pain. Clin J Pain 1997;13:251–5.

61. Rosner H, Rubin L. Gabapentin adjunctive therapy in neuropathic pain states. Clin J Pain 1996;12:56–8.

62. McLean M. Gabapentin. Epilepsia 1995;36 Suppl:S73–86.

63. Buetefisch C, Gutierrez M. Choreoathetotic movements: a possible side effect of gabapentin. Neurology 1996;46:851–2.

64. Kalso E, Tramér MR, McQuay HJ, Moore RA. Systemic local anaesthetic type drugs in chronic pain: a qualitative systematic review. Eur J Pain 1998;2:3–14.

65. Ziegler D, Lynch SA, Muir J, et al. Transdermal clonidine versus placebo in painful diabetic neuropathy. Pain 1992; 48:403–8.

66. Harkins S, et al. Administration of clonazepam in the treatment of TMD and associated myofascial pain: a double-blind pilot study. J Craniomandib Disord 1991;5:179–86.

67. Russell IJ, Fletcher EM, Michalek JE, et al. Treatment of primary fibrositis/fibromyalgia syndrome with ibuprofen and alprazolam. Arthritis Rheum 1991;34:552–60.

68. Rowbotham M. Topical analgesic agents. In: Fields H, Leibeskind J, editors. Pharmacological approaches to the treatment of chronic pain: new concepts and critical issues. Seattle: IASP Press; p. 211–27.

69. Dray A. Mechanism of action of capsaicin-like molecules on sensory neurons. Life Sci 1992;51:1759–65.

70. Maggi, C. Therapeutic potential of capsaicin-like molecules: studies in animals and humans. Life Sci 1992;51:1777–81.

71. Pfaffenrath V, Rath M, Pollman W, Keeser W. Atypical facial pain—application of the IHS criteria in a clinical sample. Cephalalgia 1993;13 Suppl 12:84–8.

72. Levitt S, Lundeen T, McKinney M. The TMJ scale manual. Durham (NC): Pain Resource Center; 1987.

73. Moore RA, Tramér MR, Carroll D, et al. Quantitative systematic review of topically applied non-steroidal anti-inflammatory drugs

74. Fricton J, Nelson A, Monsein M. IMPATH: microcomputer assessment of behavioral and psychosocial factors in craniomandibular disorders. Cranio 1987;5:372–81.

75. LeResche L, Von Korff M. Research diagnostic criteria part II. J Craniomandib Disord 1992;6:327–34.

76. Olesen J. Classification and diagnostic criteria for headache disorders, cranial neuralgias and facial pain. Cephalalgia 1988; 8 Suppl 7:61–72.

77. Okeson J, editor. Orofacial pain: guidelines for assessment, diagnosis, and management. Chicago: Quintessence Publishing Co, Inc.; 1996.

78. Frazier C, Russell E. Neuralgia of the face: an analysis of 754 cases with relation to pain and other sensory phenomena before and after operation. Arch Neurol Psychiatr 1924;11:557–63.

79. Truelove E, et al. Orofacial pain. In: Millard H, Mason D, editors. 2nd world workshop on oral medicine. Ann Arbor: University of Michigan Continuing Dental Education: 1995.

80. McNeill C, editor. Temporomandibular disorders, guidelines for classification, assessment, and management. Chicago: Quintessence; 1993.

81. Committee on Headache Classification. International Headache Society. Classification and diagnosis criteria for headache disorders, cranial neuralgias, and facial pain. Cephalalgia 1988;8:1–96.

82. Marbach J. Phantom tooth pain. J Endodont 1978;4:362–71.

83. Lynch M, Elgeneidy A. The role of sympathetic activity in neuropathic orofacial pain. J Orofac Pain 1996;10:297–305.

84. American Psychiatric Association. Diagnostic and statistical manual of mental disorders. 4th ed. American Psychiatric Association; Washington (DC): 1994.

85. Bouquot J, Roberts AM, Person P, Christian J. Neuralgia-inducing cavitational osteonecrosis (NICO). Oral Surg Oral Med Oral Pathol 1992;73:307–19.

86. Donlon W. Invited commentary on neuralgia-inducing cavitational osteonecrosis. Oral Surg Oral Med Oral Pathol 1992;73:319–20.

87. Aghabeigi B, Feinmann C, Glover C, et al. Tyramine conjugation deficit in patients with chronic idiopathic temporomandibular joint and orofacial pain. Pain 1993;54(2):159–63.

88. Haque MF, Aghabeigi B, Wasil M, et al. Oxygen free radicals in idiopathic facial pain. Bangladesh Med Res Council Bull 1994;20(3):104–16.

89. Bouckoms AJ, Sweet WH, Poletti C, et al. Monoamines in the brain cerebrospinal fluid of facial pain patients. Anesth Prog 1993;39(6):201–8.

90. Verdugo R, Ochoa J. Placebo response in chronic causalgiform, 'neuropathic' pain patients: study and review. Pain Rev 1994;1:33–46.

91. Zuniga J, Meyer RA, Gregg JM, et al. The accuracy of clinical neurosensory testing for nerve injury diagnosis. J Oral Maxillofac Surg 1998;56:2–8.

92. Schnaetler J, Hopper C. Intracranial tumours presenting as facial pain. Br Dent J 1989;166:80–3.

93. Loeser J. Mitigating the dangers of pursuing cure. In: Cohen M, Campbell J, editors. Pain treatment at a crossroads: a practical and conceptual reappraisal. Seattle: IASP Press; 1996.

94. Travell J, Rinzler S. The myofascial genesis of pain. Postgrad Med 1952;11:425–34.

95. Mense S. Referral of muscle pain: new aspects. J Am Pain Soc 1994;3:1–9.

96. Sessle B, Hu JW, Amano N, Zhong G. Convergence of cutaneous, tooth pulp, visceral, neck and muscle afferents onto nociceptive neurons in trigeminal subnucleus caudalis (medullary dorsal horn) and its implications for referred pain. Pain 1986;27:219–35.

97. Ohrbach R, Gale E. Pressure pain thresholds, clinical assessment, and differential diagnosis: reliability and validity in patients with myogenic pain. Pain 1989;39:157–69.

98. Johnstone D, McCormick J. The feasibility of palpating the lateral pterygoid muscle. J Prosthet Dent 1980;44:318.

99. Thomas C, Okeson J. Evaluation of lateral pterygoid muscle symptoms using a common palpation technique and a method of functional manipulation. Cranio 1987;5:125–9.

100. Okeson, J. Management of temporomandibular disorders and occlusion. St. Louis: Mosby-Year Book, Inc.; 1998. p. 253–6.

101. Bradley L, Haile JM, Jaworski T. Assessment of psychological status using interviews and self-report instruments. In: Turk D, Melzack R, editors. Handbook of pain assessment. New York: Guilford Press; 1992. p. 193–213.

102. Brody D. Physician recognition of behavioral, psychological, and social aspects of medical care. Arch Intern Med 1980;140:1286–9.

103. Nielsen A, Williams T. Depression in ambulatory medical patients: prevalence by self-report questionnaire and recognition by nonpsychiatric physicians. Arch Gen Psychiatry 1980;37:999–1004.

104. Oakley M, McCreary CP, Flack VF, et al. Dentists' ability to detect psychological problems in patients with temporomandibular disorders and chronic pain. J Am Dent Assoc 1989;118:727–30.

105. Steer RA, Cavalieri TA, Leonard DA, Beck TA. Use of the Beck depression inventory for primary care to screen for major depressive disorders. Gen Hosp Psychiatry 1999;21:106–11.

106. Hyler S, Skodal AE, Oldham JM, et al. Validity of the Personality Diagnostic Questionnaire – Revised: a replication in an out patient sample. Compr Psychiatry 1992;38:73–7.

107. Goldberg D. Use of the general health questionnaire in clinical work. Medical Journal Clinical Research 1986;293:1188–9.

108. Gale E, Dixon D. A simplified psychologic questionnaire as a treatment planning aid for patients with temporomandibular joint disorders. J Prosthet Dent 1989;61:235–8.

109. Oakley M, et al. Screening for psychological problems in temporomandibular disorder patients. J Orofac Pain 1993;7:143–9.

110. Hathaway S, et al. Minnesota Multiphasic Personality Inventory-2: manual for administration. Minneapolis: University of Minneapolis Press; 1989.

111. Pincus T, Callanhan LF, Bradley LA, et al. Elevated MMPI scores for hypochondriasis, depression, and hysteria in patients with rheumatoid arthritis reflect disease rather than psychological status. Arthritis Rheum 1986;29:1456–66.

112. Moore JE, McFall ME, Kivlahan DR, Capestany F. Risk of misinterpretation of MMPI schizophrenia scale elevations in chronic pain patients. Pain 1988;32:207–13.

113. Naliboff B, Cohen M, Yellin A. Does the MMPI differentiate chronic illness from chronic pain. Pain 1982;13:333–41.

114. Bradley L, Prokop CK, Margolis R, Gentry WD. Multivariate analysis of the MMPI profiles of low back pain patients. J Behav Med 1978;1:253–72.

115. Bradley L, Heide LVD. Pain related correlates of MMPI profile subgroups among back pain patents. Health Psychol 1984;3:157–74.

116. Rugh J, Woods B, Dahlstrom L. Temporomandibular disorders: assessment of psychological factors. Adv Dent Res 1993;7:127–36.

117. Millon T, Green C, Meagher R. Millon behavioral health inventory manual. 3rd ed. Minneapolis: National Computer Systems; 1983.

118. Pilowsky I, Spence N. Illness behavior syndromes associated with intractable pain. Pain 1976;2:61–71.

119. Blasberg B, Remick R, Miles J. The psychiatric referral in dentistry: indications and mechanics. Oral Surg Oral Med Oral Pathol 1983;56:368–71.

120. Merrill RL. Orofacial pain mechanisms and their clinical application. Dent Clin North Am 1997;41(2):167–88.

121. Sethna N, Berde C. Diagnostic nerve blocks: caveats and pitfalls in interpretation. IASP Newsl 1995 May/June:3–5.

122. Verdugo R, Ochoa J. "Sympathetically maintained pain." I. Phentolamine block questions the concept. Neurology 1994;44:1003–10.

123. Verdugo R, Campero M, Ochoa J. Phentolamine sympathetic block in painful polyneuropathies. II. Further questioning of the concept of "sympathetically maintained pain." Neurology 1994;44:1010–4.

124. Dodick D. Headache as a symptom of ominous disease. Postgrad Med 1997;101:46–62.

125. Fernandez JM, Mederer S, Alvarez-Sabin J, et al. Hemifacial spasm associated with Paget's disease of bone: good response to calcitonin. Neurology 1991;41:1322.

126. Gergely J. Monostotic Paget's disease of the mandible. Oral Surg Oral Med Oral Pathol 1990;70:805.

127. Iwasaki Y, Kinoshita M, Ikeda K, et al. Thyroid function in patients with chronic headache. Int J Neurosci 1991;57:263–7.

128. Arm R, Brightman V. Multiple myeloma manifesting as atypical facial pain. In: Annual meeting of the American Academy of Oral Pathologists. New Orleans (LA): American Academy of Oral Pathologists; 1974.

129. Hjorting-Hansen E, Bertram U. Oral aspects of pernicious anemia. Br Dent J 1968;125:266.

130. Vazquez-Cruz J, Traboulssi H, Rodriguez-de la Serna A, et al. A prospective study of chronic or recurrent headache in systemic lupus erythematosus. Headache 1990;30:232–5.

131. McCarthy G, Skillings J. Jaw and other orofacial pain in patients receiving vincristine for the treatment of cancer. Oral Surg Oral Med Oral Pathol 1992;74:299–304.

132. Lamey PJ, Hammond A, Allam BF, MacIntosh WB. Vitamin status of patients with burning mouth syndrome and the response to replacement therapy. Br Dent J 1986;160:81.

133. Jacobs A, Cavill I. The oral lesions of iron deficiency anemia: pyridoxine and riboflavine status. Br J Haematol 1968;14:291.

134. Brightman, V. Disordered oral sensation and appetite. In: Kare M, Maller O, editors. Chemical senses and nutrition. New York: Academic Press; 1977.

135. Hampf G. Dilemma in treatment of patients suffering from orofacial dysaesthesia. Int J Oral Maxillofac Surg 1987;16:397.

136. Smith G, Monson R, Ray D. Patients with multiple unexplained symptoms: their characteristics, functional health and health care utilization. Arch Intern Med 1986;146:69.

137. Knutsson K, Hasselgren G, Nilner M, Petersson A. Craniomandibular disorders in chronic orofacial pain patients. J Craniomandib Disord 1989;3:15–9.

138. Feinman C, Harris M. Psychogenic facial pain. Part I: The clinical presentation: Part II: Management and prognosis. Br Dent J 1984;156:165.

139. Vickers ER, Cousins MJ, Walker S, Chisholm K. Analysis of 50 patients with atypical odontalgia. Oral Surg Oral Med Oral Pathol Oral Radiol Endod 1998;85:24–32.

140. Graff-Radford S, Solberg W. Atypical odontalgia. J Craniomandrib Disord 1992;6:260–6.

141. Mechanic D. The concept of illness behavior. J Chronic Dis 1962;15:189.

142. Campbell J. Illness is a point of view: the development of children's concepts of illness. Child Dev 1975;49:92.

143. Craig K. Modeling and social learning factors in chronic pain. In: Bonica J, Lindblom U, Iggo A, editors. Proceedings of the Third World Congress on Pain. Advances in pain research and therapy. New York: Raven; 1981.

144. Merskey H. Psychiatry and pain. In: Sternback R, editor. The psychology of pain. New York: Raven; 1986.

145. Harness D, Rome H. Psychological and behavioral aspects of chronic facial pain. Otolaryngol Clin North Am 1989;22:1073.

146. Delaney J. Atypical facial pain as a defense against psychosis. Am J Psychiatry 1976;133:1151.

147. Hampf G, Aalberg V, Sunden B. Experiences with a facial pain unit. J Craniomandib Disord 1990;4:267.

148. Cohen L. Disturbance of taste as a symptom of multiple sclerosis. Br J Oral Surg 1965;2:184.

149. Thomas J, Waltz A. Neurological manifestations of nasopharyngeal malignant tumors. JAMA 1965;192:95.

150. Grace E, North A. Temporomandibular joint dysfunction and orofacial pain caused by parotid gland malignancy. J Am Dent Assoc 1988;116:348.

151. Penarrocha Diago M, Bagan Sebastian JV, Alfaro Giner A, Escrig Orenga V, et al. Mental nerve neuropathy in systemic cancer. Oral Surg Oral Med Oral Pathol 1990;69:48–51.

152. Schreiber A, Kinney L, Salman R. Large-cell lymphoma of the infratemporal fossa presenting as myofascial pain. J Craniomandib Disord 1991;5:286.

153. Keith D, Glyman M. Infratemporal space pathosis mimicking TMJ disorders. J Am Dent Assoc 1991;122(11):59.

154. German D. A case report: acoustic neuroma confused with TMD. J Am Dent Assoc 1991;122(12):59.

155. Malins T, Farrow A. Facial pain due to occult parotid adenoid cystic carcinoma. J Oral Maxillfac Surg 1991;49:1127.

156. Monaghan A, McKinlay K. An intracranial tumor causing dental pain. Br Dent J 1991;171:249.

157. Zappia J, Wolf G, McClatchey K. Signet-ring adenocarcinoma metastatic to the maxillary sinus. Oral Surg Oral Med Oral Pathol 1992;73:89.

158. Levitt S, Spiegel E, Claypoole W. The TMJ scale and undetected brain tumors in patients with temporomandibular disorders. Cranio 1991;9:152.

159. Schoenen J, Broux R, Moonen G. Unilateral facial pain as the first symptom of lung cancer: are there diagnostic clues? Cephalalgia 1991;12:178.

160. Reskin A. Imaging aspects of new approaches to the differential diagnosis of chronic orofacial pain. In: Lipton JA, Bryant PS, editors. New approaches to the differential diagnosis of chronic orofacial pain. Proceedings of the Research Workshop on Chronic Orofacial Pain sponsored by National Institute of Dental Research, April 1989. Anesth Prog 1990;37:127.

161. Brixen K, Hansen HH, Mosekilde L, Halaburt H. SPECT bone scintigraphy in assessment of Paget's disease. Acta Radiol 1990;31:549–50.

162. King J, Caldarelli D, Petasnick J. Denta scan: a new diagnostic method for evaluation of mandibular and maxillary pathology. Laryngoscope 1992;102:378.

163. Rappaport ZH, Devor M. Trigeminal neuralgia: the role of self-sustaining discharge in the trigeminal ganglion. Pain 1994;56:127–38.

164. Barker FG, Jannetta PJ, Bissonette DJ, et al. The long-term outcome of microvascular decompression for trigeminal neuralgia. N Engl J Med 1996;334:1077–83.

165. Meaney JF, Eldridge PR, Dunn LT, et al. Demonstration of neurovascular compression in trigeminal neuralgia with magnetic resonance imaging: comparison with surgical findings in 52 consecutive operative cases. J Neurosurg 1995;83:799–805.

166. Wall PD, Devor M. Sensory afferent impulses originate from dorsal root ganglia as well as from the periphery in normal and nerve injured rats. Pain 1983;17:321.

167. Fromm GH, Terrence CF, Chattha AS. Baclofen in the treatment of trigeminal neuralgia: double-blind study and long-term follow-up. Ann Neurol 1984;15:240–4.

168. Lunardi G, Leandri M, Albano C, et al. Clinical effectiveness of lamotrigine and plasma levels in essential and symptomatic trigeminal neuralgia. Neurol 1998;50:1192.

169. Sweet WH, Wepsic JG. Controlled thermocoagulation of trigeminal ganglion and rootlets for differential destruction of pain fibers. I. Trigeminal neuralgia. J Neurosurg 1974;40:143–56.

170. Jessop J. Treatment for trigeminal neuralgia: choice of procedures is wide [letter]. BMJ 1997;314:519–20.

171. Mullan S, Lichtor T. Percutaneous microcompression of the trigeminal ganglion for trigeminal neuralgia. J Neurosurg 1983;59:1007–12.

172. Barker FG II, Jannetta PJ, Bissonette DJ, et al. The long-term outcome of microvascular decompression for trigeminal neuralgia. N Engl J Med 1996;334:1077–83.

173. Arias MA. Percutaneous radiofrequency thermocoagulation with low temperature in the treatment of glossopharyngeal nerve. Surg Neurol 1986;25:94.

174. Robillard RB, Hilsinger RL, Adour KK. Ramsay Hunt facial paralysis: clinical analysis of 185 patients. Otolaryngol Head Neck Surg 1986;95:292.

175. Hunt JR. Herpetic inflammation of the geniculate ganglion: a new syndrome and its aural complications. Arch Otol 1907;36:371.

176. Murali R. Neurosurgical considerations in headache. In: Jacobson AL, Donlon WC, editors. Headache and facial pain. New York: Raven Press; 1990. p. 245.

177. Brown GR. Herpes zoster: correlation of age, sex, distribution, neuralgia, and associated disorders. South Med J 1976;69:576–8.

178. Ragozzino MW, Melton LJ III, Kurland LT, Chu CP. Population-based study of herpes zoster and its sequelae. Medicine 1982;61:310–6.

179. Balfour HH Jr. Varicella zoster virus infections in immunocompromised hosts: a review of the natural history and management. Am J Med 1988;85:68–73.

180. Kost RG, Straus SE. Drug therapy: postherpetic neuralgia — pathogenesis, treatment, and prevention. N Engl J Med 1996;335:32–42.

181. Watson CPN, Deck JH, Morshead C, et al. Post-herpetic neuralgia: further post-mortem studies of cases with and without pain. Pain 1991;44:105–17.

182. Nurmikko T, Bowsher D. Somatosensory findings in postherpetic neuralgia. J Neurol Neurosurg Psychiatry 1990;53:135–41.

183. Rowbotham MC, Davies PS, Fields HL. Topical lidocaine gel relieves postherpetic neuralgia. Ann Neurol 1995;37:246–53.

184. Stow PJ, Glynn CJ, Minor B. EMLA cream in the treatment of post-herpetic neuralgia: efficacy and pharmacokinetic profile. Pain 1989;39:301–5.

185. Max MB, Schafer SC, Curnane M, et al. Amitriptyline, but not lorazepam, relieves postherpetic neuralgia. Neurology 1988;38:1427–32.

186. Kishore-Kumar R, Max MB, Schafer SC, et al. Desipramine relieves postherpetic neuralgia. Clin Pharmacol Ther 1990;47:305–12.

187. Watson CP, Vernich L, Chipman M, Reed K. Nortriptyline versus amitriptyline in postherpetic neuralgia: a randomized trial. Neurology 1998;51:166–71.

188. Swerdlow M. Anticonvulsant drugs and chronic pain. Clin Neuropharmacol 1984;7:51–82.

189. Rowbatham M, Harden N, Stacey B, et al. Gabapentin for the treatment of postherpetic neuralgia: a randomized controlled trial. JAMA 1998;280:1837–42.

190. Dworkin RH, Boon RJ, Griffin DR, Phung D. Postherpetic neuralgia: impact of famciclovir, age, rash severity, and acute pain in herpes zoster patients. J Infect Dis 1998;178 Suppl 1:S76–80.

191. Choo PW, Galil K, Donahue JG, Walker AM. Risk factors for postherpetic neuralgia. Arch Intern Med 1997;157:1217–24.

192. Bowsher D. The management of postherpetic neuralgia. Postgrad Med J 1997;73:623–9.

193. Woolf CJ, Mannion RJ. Neuropathic pain: aetiology, symptoms, mechanisms and management. Lancet 1999;353:1959–64.

194. LaBanc JP. Classification of nerve injuries. Oral Maxillofac Surg Clin N Am 1992;4:285–96.

195. Gregg JM. Abnormal responses to trigeminal nerve injuries. Oral Maxillofac Surg Clin N Am 1992;4:339–51.

196. Morello CM, Leckband SG, Stoner CP, et al. Randomized double-blind study comparing the efficacy of gabapentin with

amitriptyline on diabetic neuropathic pain. Arch Intern Med 1999;159:1931–7.

197. Rosenberg JM, Harrell C, Ristic H. The effect of gabapentin on neuropathic pain. Clin J Pain 1997;13:251–5.

198. Lynch ME, Elgeneidy AK. The role of sympathetic activity in neuropathic orofacial pain. J Orofac Pain 1996;10:297–305.

199. Saxen MA, Campbell RL. An unusual case of sympathetically maintained facial pain complicated by telangiectasia. Oral Surg Oral Med Oral Pathol 1995;79:455–8.

200. Malik V, Inchoisa MA, Mustafa K. Intravenous regional phenoxybenzamine in the treatment of reflex sympathetic dystrophy. Anesthesia 1998;88:823–7.

201. Schott GD. Bisphosphonates for pain relief in reflex sympathetic dystrophy. Lancet 1997;350:1117–8.

202. Ship JA, Grushka M, Lipton JA, et al. Burning mouth syndrome: an update. J Am Dent Assoc 1995;126:843–53.

203. Grushka M, Sessle BJ. Taste impairment in burning mouth syndrome. Gerodontics 1988;4:256–8.

204. Grushka M, Sessle BJ, Howley TP. Taste dysfunction in burning mouth syndrome. Chem Senses 1986;11:485–98.

205. Meresky LS, van der Bilj P, Gird I. Burning mouth syndrome: evaluation of multiple factors among 85 patients. Oral Surg Oral Med Oral Pathol 1993;75:303–7.

206. Bergdahl J, Anneroth G, Perris H. Personality characteristics of subjects with resistant burning mouth syndrome. Acta Odontol Scand 1995;53:7–11.

207. Rojo L, Silverstri FJ, Bagan JV, et al. Psychiatric morbidity in burning mouth syndrome. Oral Surg Oral Med Oral Pathol 1993;75:308–11.

208. Lamey PJ. Burning mouth syndrome. Dermatol Clin 1996;2:339–54.

209. Grushka M. Clinical features of burning mouth syndrome. Oral Surg Oral Med Oral Pathol 1987;63:30–6.

210. Duhaut P, Pinede L, Bornet H, et al. Biopsy proven and biopsy negative temporal arteritis: differences in clinical spectrum at the onset of the disease. Ann Rheum Dis 1999;58:335–41.

211. May A, Kaube H, Buecheel C, et al. Experimental cranial pain elicited by capsaicin: a PET-study. Pain 1998;74:61–6.

212. Goadsby PJ, Edvinsson L. Human in vivo evidence for trigeminovascular activation in cluster headache. Neuropeptide changes and effects of acute attacks therapies. Brain 1994;117:427–34.

213. Emmanuelli JL, Gutierrez JR, Chiossone JA, Chiossone E. Carotidynia: a frequently overlooked or misdiagnosed syndrome. Ear Nose Throat J 1998;77:462–4.

214. Wesselmann U, Reich SG. The dynias. Semin Neurol 1996;16:63–74.

215. Welsh KMA. Drug therapy of migraines. N Engl J Med 1993;329:1476.

▼ SUGGESTED READINGS

McCaffery M, Pasero C. Pain, a clinical manual. 2nd ed. St. Louis: Mosby, Inc.; 1999.

Caudill MA. Managing pain before it manages you. New York: The Guildford Press; 1995.

Davis M, Robbins E, Eshelman M. The relaxation and stress reduction workbook. 4th ed. Oakland: New Harbinger Publications, Inc.; 1995.

Wilson-Pauwels L, Akesson E, Stewart P. Cranial nerves: anatomy and clinical comments. Toronto: BC Decker Inc; 1988.

Gilman S, Newman S. Essentials of clinical neuroanatomy and neurophysiology. 9th ed. Philadelphia: C.A. Davis Company; 1996.

12

DISEASES OF THE RESPIRATORY TRACT

MARK LEPORE, MD

ROBERT ANOLIK, MD

MICHAEL GLICK, DMD

Respiratory infections are commonly encountered among dental patients. Commonalities between chemotherapeutic options and the anatomic proximity with the oral cavity lead to much interplay between oral and respiratory infections. There is a growing body of literature pointing to a direct association between oral pathogens and respiratory diseases. Recent studies have reported on oral bacteria as causative pathogens in respiratory diseases and conditions associated with significant morbidity and mortality. Furthermore, some respiratory illnesses (such as asthma) may have an effect on orofacial morphology or even on the dentition. This chapter discusses the more common respiratory illnesses and explores the relationship between these conditions and oral health.

▼ UPPER-AIRWAY INFECTIONS

There are several major oral health concerns for patients with upper respiratory infections. These concerns are about infectious matters, such as the possible transmission of pathogens from patients to health care workers and such as re-infection with causative pathogens through fomites such as toothbrushes and removable oral acrylic appliances. Furthermore, antibiotic resistance may develop because of the use of similar types of medications for upper respiratory infections and odontogenic infections. Lastly, oral mucosal changes (such as dryness due to decongestants and mouth breathing) and increased susceptibility to oral candidiasis in patients using long-term glucocorticosteroid inhalers may be noticed.

Viral Upper Respiratory Infections

The most common cause of acute respiratory illness is viral infection, which occurs more commonly in children than in adults. Rhinoviruses account for the majority of upper-respiratory infections in adults.[1] These are ribonucleic acid (RNA) viruses, which preferentially infect the respiratory tree. At least 100 antigenically distinct subtypes have been isolated. Rhinoviruses are most commonly transmitted by close person-to-person contact and by respiratory droplets. Shedding can occur from nasopharyngeal secretions for up to 3 weeks, but 7 days or less is more typical. In addition to rhinoviruses, several other viruses, including *Coronavirus*, influenza virus, parainfluenza virus, adenovirus, *Enterovirus*, coxsackievirus, and respiratory syncytial virus, have also been implicated as causative agents. Infection by these viruses occurs more commonly during the winter months in temperate climates.

PATHOPHYSIOLOGY

Viral particles can lodge in either the upper or lower respiratory tract. The particles invade the respiratory epithelium, and viral replication ensues shortly thereafter. The typical incubation period for *Rhinovirus* is 2 to 5 days.[2] During this time, active and specific immune responses are triggered, and mechanisms for viral clearance are enhanced. The period of communicability tends to correlate with the duration of clinical symptoms.

CLINICAL AND LABORATORY FINDINGS

Signs and symptoms of upper-respiratory-tract infections are somewhat variable and are dependent on the sites of inoculation.[3] Common symptoms include rhinorrhea, nasal congestion, and oropharyngeal irritation. Nasal secretions can be serous or purulent. Other symptoms that may be present include cough, fever, malaise, fatigue, headache, and myalgia.[4] A complete blood count (CBC) with differential shows an increase in mononuclear cells, lymphocytes, and monocytes ("right shift").

Laboratory tests are typically not required in the diagnosis of upper respiratory infections. Viruses can be isolated by culture or determined by rapid diagnostic assays. However, these tests are rarely clinically warranted.

DIAGNOSIS

The diagnosis is made on the basis of medical history as well as confirmatory physical findings. Diagnoses that should be excluded include acute bacterial rhinosinusitis, allergic rhinitis, and group A streptococcal pharyngitis.

MANAGEMENT

The treatment of upper respiratory infections is symptomatic as most are self-limited. Analgesics can be used for sore throat and myalgias. Antipyretics can be used in febrile patients, and anticholinergic agents may be helpful in reducing rhinorrhea. Oral or topical decongestants, such as the sympathomimetic amines, are an effective means of decreasing nasal congestion. Adequate hydration is also important in homeostasis, especially during febrile illnesses.

Antimicrobial agents have no role in the treatment of acute viral upper respiratory infections.[5] Presumptive treatment with antibiotics to prevent bacterial superinfection is not recommended.[6] The excessive use of antibiotics can result in the development of drug-resistant bacteria.[7]

PROGNOSIS

As most patients recover in 5 to 10 days, the prognosis is excellent. However, upper respiratory infections can put patients at risk for exacerbations of asthma, acute bacterial sinusitis, and otitis media; that is especially so in predisposed patients such as children and such as patients with an incompetent immune system.

ORAL HEALTH CONSIDERATIONS

The most common oral manifestation of upper respiratory viral infections is the presence of small round erythematous macular lesions on the soft palate. These lesions may be caused directly by the viral infection, or they may represent a response of lymphoid tissue. Individuals with excessive lingual tonsillar tissue also experience enlargement of these foci of lymphoid tissue, particularly at the lateral borders at the base of the tongue.

Treatment of upper respiratory infections with decongestants may cause decreased salivary flow, and patients may experience oral dryness (see Chapter 9 for a discussion of the treatment of oral dryness).

Although there has been some discussion in the dental literature in regard to a relationship between dentofacial morphology and mouth breathing, this association has not been verified in prospective longitudinal studies.[8]

Allergic Rhinitis and Conjunctivitis

Allergic rhinitis is a chronic recurrent inflammatory disorder of the nasal mucosa. Similarly, allergic conjunctivitis is an inflammatory disorder involving the conjunctiva. When both conditions occur, the term "allergic rhinoconjunctivitis" is used. The basis of the inflammation is an allergic hypersensitivity (type I hypersensitivity) to environmental triggers. Allergic rhinoconjunctivitis can be seasonal or perennial. Typical seasonal triggers include grass, tree, and weed pollens. Common perennial triggers include dust mites, animal dander, and mold spores.

Allergic rhinitis is the most prevalent chronic medical disorder. More than 35 million Americans are affected. Allergic rhinitis is associated with a significant health care cost burden, and more than $2 billion (US) are spent annually in the United States on medication for this condition alone. In addition, allergic rhinitis accounts for more than 2 million lost school days per year and more than 3 million lost workdays per year.[9]

PATHOPHYSIOLOGY

Patients with allergic rhinoconjunctivitis have a genetically predetermined susceptibility to allergic hypersensitivity reactions (atopy). Prior to the allergic response, an initial phase of sensitization is required. This sensitization phase is dependent on exposure to a specific allergen and on recognition of the allergen by the immune system. The end result of the sensitization phase is the production of specific immunoglobulin E (IgE) antibody and the binding of this specific IgE to the surface of tissue mast cells and blood basophils. Surface IgE can bind to the same allergens upon re-exposure. Once bound by surface IgE, subsequent IgE cross-linking will occur, which triggers degranulation of the mast cell and the release of mast cell mediators. This is the early-phase allergic reaction. Histamine is the primary preformed mediator released by mast cells, and it contributes to the clinical symptoms of sneezing, pruritus, and rhinorrhea. Mast cells also release cytokines that permit amplification and feedback of the allergic response. These cytokines cause an influx of other inflammatory cells, including eosinophils, resulting in the late-phase allergic reaction. Eosinophils produce many proinflammatory mediators that contribute to chronic allergic inflammation and to the symptom of nasal congestion.

CLINICAL AND LABORATORY FINDINGS

The symptoms of allergic rhinoconjunctivitis can vary from patient to patient and depend on the specific allergens to which the patient is sensitized. Conjunctival symptoms may include pruritus, lacrimation, crusting, and burning. Nasal symptoms may include sneezing, pruritus, clear rhinorrhea, and nasal congestion. Other symptoms can occur, such as postnasal drainage with throat irritation, pruritus of the palate and ear canals, and fatigue.

The clinical signs of allergic rhinoconjunctivitis include injection of the conjunctiva with or without "cobblestoning"; prominent infraorbital creases (Dennie-Morgan folds/pleats), swelling, and darkening ("allergic shiners"), a transverse nasal crease; and frequent upwards rubbing of the tip of the nose (the allergic "salute"). Direct examination of the nasal mucosa reveals significant edema and a pale blue coloration of the turbinates. A copious clear rhinorrhea is often present. Nasal polyps may also be visible. Postnasal drainage or oropharyngeal cobblestoning might be identified upon examination of the oropharynx. A high-arched palate, protrusion of the tongue, and overbite may be seen.

Laboratory investigations are usually kept to a minimum. Patients with allergic rhinitis might have elevated levels of serum IgE and an elevated total eosinophil count. These findings are not, however, sensitive nor specific indicators of atopy. Microscopic examination of nasal secretions often demonstrates significant numbers of eosinophils. The radioallergosorbent test (RAST) is a method of testing for specific allergic sensitivities that is based on circulating levels of specific IgE. Specific IgE levels are determined by using serum samples and are quantified by using radioactive markers. Although the RAST is somewhat less reliable than skin testing (see below), it is a useful test in certain situations (such as pregnancy or severe chronic skin disorders, including atopic dermatitis).

CLASSIFICATION

There is no universal classification system for allergic rhinoconjunctivitis. Many authors make the distinction between perennial and seasonal illness, with the former being caused mainly by indoor allergens and the latter being triggered primarily by outdoor allergens. Perennial allergic rhinitis sufferers might benefit more from specific environmental control measures than would seasonal allergic rhinitis sufferers.

DIAGNOSIS

The diagnosis of allergic rhinoconjunctivitis is usually apparent, based on history and physical examination. Patients present with a history suggestive of allergic sensitivity, recurrent symptoms with specific exposures, or predictable exacerbations during certain times of the year. Symptoms that have recurred for 2 or more years during the same season are very suggestive of seasonal allergic disease. Alternatively, the history might indicate a pattern of worsening symptoms while the patient is at home, with improvement while the patient is at work or on vacation; this pattern is highly suggestive of perennial allergic disease with indoor triggers. The presence of the characteristic physical findings described above would confirm the presence of allergic rhinoconjunctivitis.

The preferred method of testing for allergic sensitivities is skin testing, which is performed with epicutaneous (prick/scratch) tests, often followed by intradermal testing. Prick skin testing is the type most widely used. With prick testing, a small amount of purified allergen is inoculated through the epidermis only (ie, epicutaneously) with a pricking device. Positive (histamine) and negative (albumin-saline) controls are used for comparison. Reactions are measured at 15 minutes, and positive reactions indicate prior allergen sensitization. Tests that yield negative results may be repeated intradermally to increase the sensitivity of the testing. All tests with positive results need to be interpreted carefully, with attention to each patient's history and physical findings.

MANAGEMENT

Three general treatment modalities are used in the treatment of allergic rhinoconjunctivitis: allergen avoidance, pharmacotherapy (medication), and immunotherapy (allergy injections).[10] The best treatment is avoidance of the offending allergen. This requires the accurate identification of the allergens implicated and a thorough knowledge of effective interventions that can minimize or eliminate the exposure. Complete avoidance is rarely possible.

Pharmacotherapy is often recommended for patients with incomplete responses to allergen avoidance and for patients who are unable to avoid exposures. Many treatment options are available. For patients with prominent sneezing, pruritus, or rhinorrhea, antihistamines are an excellent treatment option. Second-generation nonsedating antihistamines such as loratadine and fexofenadine are now available. These medications deliver excellent antihistaminic activity with few side effects.[11] Oral decongestants (sympathomimetic amines) can be added to oral antihistamines to relieve nasal congestion and obstruction. Combination medications are available in once-daily and twice-daily dosage forms for ease of administration. For patients with daily nasal symptoms or severe symptoms that are not relieved with antihistamine-decongestants, topical anti-inflammatory agents for the nasal mucosa are available. These medications include cromolyn sodium and topical corticosteroid sprays. The benefits of topical corticosteroids include once-daily dosing, superior efficacy (when compared to cromolyn sodium), and relief of the total symptom complex.

Immunotherapy is an effective means of treatment for patients with allergic rhinoconjunctivitis. Numerous studies have shown the efficacy of long-term allergen immunotherapy in inducing prolonged clinical and immunologic tolerance.[12] Immunotherapy is available for a variety of airborne allergens, including grass, tree, and weed pollens; dust mites; animal dander; and mold spores. Excellent candidates for immunotherapy include those patients who are unable to avoid exposures, patients with suboptimal responses to pharmacotherapy, patients who prefer to avoid the long-term use of medications, and women who are contemplating pregnancy.

PROGNOSIS

Although allergic rhinoconjunctivitis is not a life-threatening disorder, it does have a significant impact on the patient's quality of life. With proper allergy care, most patients can lead normal lives with an excellent quality of life.

ORAL HEALTH CONSIDERATIONS

The use of decongestants and first-generation antihistamines may be associated with oral dryness. There may also be an increased incidence of oral candidiasis in long-term users of topical corticosteroid-containing sprays.

Otitis Media

Otitis media is inflammation of the middle-ear space and tissues. It is the most common illness that occurs in children who are 8 years of age or younger. Approximately 70% of children experience at least one episode of otitis media by age 3 years; of these, approximately one-third experience three or more episodes in this same time interval.

Otitis media can be subdivided into acute otitis media, recurrent otitis media, otitis media with effusion, and chronic suppurative otitis media. The underlying problem in all types of otitis media is dysfunction of the eustachian tube. A poorly functioning eustachian tube does not ventilate the middle-ear space sufficiently. This lack of proper ventilation results in pressure changes in the middle ear and subsequent fluid accumulation. The fluid frequently becomes infected, resulting in acute otitis media. The most common infectious causes are viruses, *Streptococcus pneumoniae, Haemophilus influenzae,* and *Moraxella catarrhalis.*[1] In infants younger than 6 weeks of age, other bacteria, including *Staphylococcus aureus, Escherichia coli, Klebsiella,* and *Enterobacter,* have also been implicated.

PATHOPHYSIOLOGY

There are several factors that influence the pathogenesis of otitis media. Nasopharyngeal colonization with large numbers of pathogenic viruses and bacteria such as *Streptococcus pneumoniae, Haemophilus influenzae,* or *Moraxella catarrhalis*

can increase the risk of otitis media. The likelihood of aspiration of these nasopharyngeal pathogens can be increased by nasal congestion or obstruction, negative pressure in the middle-ear space, acute viral upper respiratory infections, and exposure to tobacco smoke.[13] For infants, breast-feeding can decrease the risk of otitis media whereas impaired immune responsiveness can increase this risk.

Under normal circumstances, the eustachian tube acts to ventilate the tympanomastoid air cell system during the act of swallowing. Any process that impairs normal eustachian tube function can lead to negative pressure in the middle-ear space. Transient impairments of eustachian tube function are seen in conditions that cause nasopharyngeal mucosal edema and obstruction of the eustachian tube orifice, such as allergic rhinitis and viral upper respiratory infections. Chronic eustachian tube obstruction can be seen with several conditions, including cleft palate and nasopharyngeal masses. Aspiration of nasopharyngeal pathogens can then occur due to negative pressure in the middle-ear space, with subsequent infection by these pathogens. This leads to the clinical manifestations of otitis media.

CLINICAL AND LABORATORY FINDINGS

The most common symptoms in acute otitis media are fever and otalgia. Other symptoms include irritability, anorexia, and vomiting. Parents may note their child pulling or tugging at one or both ears. Symptoms of a viral upper respiratory infection might also be present, preceding the development of otitis media. On physical examination, the tympanic membrane may appear erythematous and bulging, suggesting inflammation of the middle ear. Other otoscopic findings include a loss of landmarks and decreased mobility of the tympanic membrane as seen by pneumatic otoscopy.

In otitis media with effusion, patients often complain of "clogged" ears and "popping." Otoscopic examination reveals serous middle-ear fluid, and air-fluid levels may be present. The mobility of the tympanic membrane is usually diminished, and mild to moderate conductive hearing loss may be demonstrated. In chronic suppurative otitis media, otorrhea is present and can be visualized either from a tympanic-membrane perforation or from surgically placed tympanostomy tubes.

Investigations that can aid the diagnosis or management of otitis media include tympanometry and myringotomy with aspiration. Tympanometry is a technique that measures the compliance of the tympanic membrane by using an electroacoustic impedance bridge. Decreased compliance of the tympanic membrane indicates a middle-ear effusion. Myringotomy with aspiration can be useful in situations when culture of the middle ear fluid is needed, such as with immunocompromised hosts or with patients who have persistent effusions despite medical management.

CLASSIFICATION

Acute otitis media is defined as middle-ear inflammation with an infectious etiology and a rapid onset of signs and symptoms. Otitis media with effusion is defined as a middle-ear effusion (often asymptomatic) that can be either residual (3 to 16 weeks following acute otitis media) or persistent (lasting more than 16 weeks). Recurrent otitis media is defined as three new episodes of acute otitis media in 6 months' time or four new episodes in a 12-month period. Chronic suppurative otitis media is defined as persistent otorrhea lasting longer than 6 weeks.

DIAGNOSIS

The diagnosis of otitis media is made on the basis of history and physical examination. The most useful tool for diagnosing otitis media is pneumatic otoscopy, which allows the clinician not only to visualize the tympanic membrane but also to assess its mobility. As stated above, an immobile tympanic membrane probably represents the presence of middle-ear fluid, and (in the context of a confirmatory medical history) the diagnosis of otitis media is made in such a case.

MANAGEMENT

Antibiotics are the treatment of choice for acute otitis media.[14] Initial antibiotic therapy is directed towards the most common middle-ear pathogens. Common choices include amoxicillin, trimethoprim plus sulfisoxazole, and erythromycin plus sulfisoxazole. In recalcitrant cases, treatment is directed towards β-lactamase–producing organisms and antibiotic-resistant strains of *Streptococcus pneumoniae*. Common choices include second- and third-generation cephalosporins, clarithromycin, and amoxicillin plus clavulanate (amoxicillin/clavulanate). The duration of therapy varies from 5 to 14 days.[15]

Insertion of tympanostomy tubes is indicated when a patient experiences more than six acute otitis media episodes during a 6-month period or has recurrent otitis media superimposed on otitis media with persistent effusion. Persistent bilateral effusions for longer than 4 months are also an indication for tympanostomy tubes.[16] Adenoidectomy as an adjunctive therapy can be considered in children older than 3 years of age. A trial of antibiotic prophylaxis is commonly carried out prior to surgical consultation.[17]

The management of chronic suppurative otitis media often includes parenteral antibiotics to cover infection by *Pseudomonas* spp and anaerobic bacteria. However, medical therapy is ineffective when a cholesteatoma (a mass filled with cellular debris and cholesterol crystals) is present.

PROGNOSIS

Although treatment with antibiotics is the norm, up to 81% of patients achieve resolution of acute otitis media without antibiotic treatment. Therefore, the prognosis for acute otitis media is excellent. However, complications can occur, more commonly in patients younger than 1 year of age. The most common complication is conductive hearing loss related to persistent effusions. Serious complications, including mastoiditis, cholesteatoma, labyrinthitis, extradural or subdural abscesses, meningitis, brain abscess, and lateral sinus thrombosis, are uncommon.[18]

ORAL HEALTH CONSIDERATIONS

Many children with recurrent otitis media are treated frequently (and sometimes for extensive periods) with various antibiotics. Included in the antibiotic armamentarium are medications that are also used for odontogenic infections. Oral health care providers need to be aware of what type of antibiotics the patient has taken within the previous 4 to 6 months, to avoid giving the patient an antibiotic to which resistance has already developed. Furthermore, the extended use of antibiotics may result in the development of oral candidiasis.

Sinusitis

Sinusitis is defined as an inflammation of the epithelial lining of the paranasal sinuses. The inflammation of these tissues causes mucosal edema and an increase in mucosal secretions. The most common trigger is an acute upper respiratory infection although other causes (such as exacerbations of allergic rhinitis, dental infections or manipulations, and direct trauma) can be implicated. If blockage of sinus drainage occurs, retained secretions can promote bacterial growth and subsequent acute bacterial sinusitis.

Acute sinusitis is a very common disorder, affecting more than 31 million Americans per year. This accounts for more than 18 million office visits to primary care physicians per year and for 124 million lost days from work each year. Chronic sinusitis is also very common.[19]

PATHOPHYSIOLOGY

The paranasal sinuses are air-filled cavities that are lined with pseudostratified columnar respiratory epithelium. The epithelium is ciliated, which facilitates the clearance of mucosal secretions. The frontal, maxillary, and ethmoid sinuses drain into an area known as the ostiomeatal complex. Rhythmic ciliary movement and the clearance of secretions can be impaired by several factors, including viral upper respiratory infections, allergic inflammation, and exposure to tobacco smoke and other irritants. In addition, foreign bodies (accidental or surgical) or a severely deviated nasal septum can cause obstruction. If blockage of the sinus ostia or obstruction of the ostiomeatal complex occurs, stasis of sinus secretions will allow pooling in the sinus cavities, which facilitates bacterial growth.

The most common organisms found in acute sinusitis are *Streptococcus pneumoniae, Haemophilus influenzae,* and *Moraxella catarrhalis.* In approximately 8 to 10% of cases of acute sinusitis, *Bacteroides* spp and *Staphylococcus aureus* are causative. Organisms that are commonly associated with chronic sinusitis are anaerobic bacteria such as *Bacteroides* spp, *Fusobacterium* spp, *Streptococcus, Veillonella,* and *Corynebacterium* spp. Sinusitis due to a fungal infection can rarely occur, usually in immunocompromised patients and in patients who are unresponsive to antibiotics.[20]

CLINICAL AND LABORATORY FINDINGS

The symptoms of acute sinusitis include facial pain, tenderness, and headache localized to the affected region. Sinusitis affecting the sphenoid sinuses or posterior ethmoid sinuses can cause headache or pain in the occipital region. Other symptoms that are commonly described include purulent nasal discharge, fever, malaise, and postnasal drainage with fetid breath. Occasionally, there may be toothache or pain with mastication. Patients with chronic sinusitis often present with other symptoms that are often vague and poorly localized. Chronic rhinorrhea, postnasal drainage, nasal congestion, sore throat, facial "fullness," and anosmia are common complaints.

Physical examination reveals sinus tenderness and purulent nasal drainage. On occasion, erythema and swelling of the overlying skin may be evident. The nasal mucosa will appear edematous and erythematous, and nasal polyps might be visible.

Although not often needed, plain-film sinus radiography can be helpful in the diagnosis of acute maxillary or frontal sinusitis. Poor visualization of the ethmoid sinuses and limited visualization of the sphenoid sinuses affect the usefulness of this type of radiography. Plain-film radiography is not helpful for establishing osteomeatal complex disease.[21] Computed tomography (CT) is the study of choice for documenting chronic sinusitis with underlying disease of the osteomeatal complex and is superior to magnetic resonance imaging (MRI) for the identification of bony abnormalities. CT can also accurately assess polyps, reactive osteitis, mucosal thickening, and fungal sinusitis.[22]

CLASSIFICATION

Sinusitis is classified as either acute or chronic, based on the duration of the inflammation and underlying infection. Patients with persistent symptoms for 3 to 8 weeks or longer are considered to have chronic disease.

DIAGNOSIS

The diagnosis of acute sinusitis is made on the basis of history and physical examination. As previously noted, radiologic evaluations might be helpful in certain situations. Patients with recurrent disease need to be evaluated for underlying factors that can predispose to sinusitis. Allergy evaluation for allergic rhinitis is often helpful. Other predisposing factors such as tobacco smoke exposure, immunodeficiency, and septal deviation should be considered.[23]

CT usually aids the diagnosis of chronic sinusitis. Evaluation of the osteomeatal complex is crucial in the management of these patients. In addition, rhinoscopy may be helpful for direct visualization of sinus ostia.

MANAGEMENT

Initial medical treatment consists of antibiotics to cover the suspected pathogens, along with topical or oral decongestants to facilitate sinus drainage. First-line antibiotics such as amoxicillin are often effective although second-generation cephalosporins, clarithromycin, and amoxicillin plus clavulanate can be helpful in resistant cases. Many patients who also have underlying allergic rhinitis may benefit from the addition of a topical nasal corticosteroid (many are available). Treatment courses often last 2 to 3 weeks. Acute frontal or sphenoid sinusitis is very serious because of the potential for intracranial complications. Intravenous antibiotics are indicated, and surgical intervention is considered, based on the condition's response to medical management.[24]

The management of chronic sinusitis involves antibiotics of a broader spectrum, and a prolonged treatment course may be required.[25] Topical corticosteroids or short courses of oral corticosteroids may help reduce the swelling and/or obstruction of the osteomeatal complex.[26] Avoidance of exacerbating factors such as allergens or tobacco smoke should be emphasized. Patients with histories suggestive of allergy should undergo a thorough allergy evaluation.

Patients who have chronic sinusitis with evidence of disease of the osteomeatal complex who fail medical management often require surgical intervention. Functional endoscopic sinus surgery involves the removal of the osteomeatal obstruction through an intranasal approach. This procedure can be performed with either local or general anesthesia and without an external incision. The recovery time from this procedure is short, and morbidity is generally low.

PROGNOSIS

Patients treated for acute sinusitis usually recover without sequelae. Children with sinusitis, particularly ethmoid and maxillary sinusitis, are at risk for periorbital or orbital cellulitis. Periorbital cellulitis is most often treated with intravenous antibiotics. Orbital cellulitis, on the other hand, requires prompt surgical intervention to prevent involvement of the globe or intracranial structures.

Frontal sinusitis can extend through the anterior wall and present as Pott's puffy tumor. Sinusitis can also spread intracranially and result in abscess or meningitis. These complications, although uncommon, are more likely to occur in male adolescent patients.

Patients with chronic sinusitis are more likely to require a prolonged recovery period, with a resultant decrease in quality of life. Chronic medication use can lead to side effects or other complications, such as rhinitis medicamentosa from prolonged use of topical decongestants. Surgical intervention and underlying-factor assessment will often reverse the chronic process, leading to an improvement in quality of life.

ORAL HEALTH CONSIDERATIONS

Patients with sinus infections who present with a complaint of a toothache are commonly encountered in a dental office. The oral health care professional evaluating the patient must be able to differentiate between an odontogenic infection and sinus pain. On history, sinus infections usually present with pain involving more than one tooth in the same maxillary quadrant whereas a toothache usually involves only a single tooth. Ruling out odontogenic infections by a dental examination and appropriate periapical radiography strengthens a diagnosis.

Chronic sinus infections are often accompanied by mouth breathing. This condition is associated with oral dryness and (in longtime sufferers) increased susceptibility to oral conditions such as gingivitis.[27]

As with other conditions for which the prolonged use of antibiotics is prescribed, the potential development of bacterial resistance needs to be considered. Switching to a different class of antibiotics to treat an odontogenic infection is preferable to increasing the dosage of an antibiotic that the patient has recently taken for another condition.

The use of decongestants may be associated with oral dryness, which may need to be addressed.

Laryngitis and Laryngotracheobronchitis

The upper airway is the site of infection and inflammation during the course of a common cold, but respiratory viruses can attack any portion of the respiratory tree. Laryngitis is defined as an inflammation of the larynx, usually because of a viral infection. Laryngotracheobronchitis (also termed viral croup) is an inflammation (also due to a viral illness) involving the larynx, trachea, and large bronchi. Although these illnesses have distinct presenting features, both result from a similar infectious process and the reactive inflammation that follows. Laryngitis can present at any age although it is more common among the adult population.[28] In contrast, laryngotracheobronchitis is an illness seen primarily in young children and has a peak incidence in the second and third years of life. These infections are most common during the fall and winter months, when respiratory viruses are more prevalent.

The viruses most commonly implicated in laryngitis are the coxsackieviruses, adenoviruses, and herpes simplex virus. The viruses most commonly associated with laryngotracheobronchitis are parainfluenza virus, respiratory syncytial virus, influenza virus, and adenovirus.[29]

Acute laryngitis can also result from excessive or unusual use of the vocal cords or from irritation due to tobacco smoking.

PATHOPHYSIOLOGY

The underlying infectious process is quite similar to that seen in viral infections of the upper respiratory tract (see above). After infection of the respiratory epithelium occurs, an inflammatory response consisting of mononuclear cells and polymorphonuclear leukocytes is mounted. As a result, vascular congestion and edema develop. Denudation of areas of respiratory epithelium can result. In addition to edema, spasm of laryngeal muscles can occur. Because the inflammatory process is triggered by viral infection, the disease processes are usually self-limited.

CLINICAL AND LABORATORY FINDINGS

Patients with laryngitis usually have an antecedent viral upper respiratory infection. Complaints of fever and sore throat are common. The most common manifestation of laryngitis is hoarseness, with weak or faint speech.[30] Cough is somewhat variable in presentation and is more likely when the lower respiratory tract is involved.

Children presenting with viral croup commonly have an antecedent upper respiratory infection, which may include fever. Shortly thereafter, a barking cough and intermittent stridor develop. Stridor at rest, retractions, and cyanosis can occur in children with severer inflammation. Neck radiography will demonstrate subglottic narrowing (a finding termed "steeple sign") on an anteroposterior view.

CLASSIFICATION

There is no universal classification system for these illnesses. The anatomic site most affected describes these diseases.

DIAGNOSIS

The diagnosis of laryngitis is based on the suggestive history. There are no specific findings on physical examination or laboratory tests although the presence of hoarseness is suggestive. The differential diagnosis includes other causes of laryngeal edema, including obstruction of venous or lymphatic drainage from masses or other lesions, decreased plasma oncotic pressure from protein loss or malnutrition, increased capillary permeability, myxedema of hypothyroidism, and hereditary angioedema. Carcinoma of the larynx can also present with hoarseness.

The diagnosis of laryngotracheobronchitis is usually apparent and is based on a suggestive history, with radiography confirming the clinical impression. With children, it is important to rule out other causes of stridor, including foreign body aspiration, acute bacterial epiglottitis, and retropharyngeal abscess.[31]

MANAGEMENT

Most cases of laryngitis are mild and self-limited, so only supportive care need be prescribed. The use of oral corticosteroids in severe or prolonged cases can be considered although their routine use is controversial.[32]

Treatment of laryngotracheobronchitis is also supportive. Cool-mist therapy and hydration are usually sufficient treatment. Hospitalization is usually indicated for patients with stridor at rest. Although somewhat controversial, a short course of oral or parenteral corticosteroids can reduce inflammation and help hasten recovery.[33,34] Nebulized racemic epinephrine has been shown to temporarily relieve airway obstruction although rebound airway edema is common.[35] The uncommon patient with impending respiratory failure requires endotracheal intubation or tracheotomy if intubation fails.

PROGNOSIS

As with viral upper respiratory infections, most cases of laryngitis and laryngotracheobronchitis are self-limited and require minimal medical intervention. Recovery within a few days to a week is the rule. In some cases, laryngotracheobronchitis can reoccur although the factors influencing this are not well understood.

Pharyngitis and Tonsillitis

Inflammation of the tonsils and pharynx is almost always associated with infection, either viral or bacterial. More than 90% of cases of sore throat are related to viral infections. These infections can be associated with fever, rhinorrhea, and cough.

The major viral etiologies are Epstein-Barr virus, coxsackievirus A, adenovirus, *Rhinovirus*, and measles virus.[36]

The most common bacterial cause of acute tonsillopharyngitis is group A beta-hemolytic *Streptococcus* (GABHS) infection, specifically *Streptococcus pyogenes* infection. Proper diagnosis and treatment of this infection is extremely important in order to prevent disease sequelae, namely, acute rheumatic fever and glomerulonephritis. Less common bacterial causes include *Corynebacterium diphtheriae*, *Neisseria gonorrhoeae*, *Chlamydia*, and *Mycoplasma pneumoniae*.

Chronic mouth breathing, chronic postnasal drainage, and inflammation due to irritant exposure can also cause pharyngitis and tonsillitis.

PATHOPHYSIOLOGY

Streptococcal infections are spread through direct contact with respiratory secretions. Transmission is often facilitated in areas where close contact occurs, such as schools and day care centers. The incubation period is 2 to 5 days.

CLINICAL AND LABORATORY FINDINGS

Sore throat is the predominant symptom. Associated clinical findings are based on the infectious etiology. Patients with Epstein-Barr virus infections develop infectious mononucleosis, a disease characterized by exudative tonsillopharyngitis, lymphadenopathy, fever, and fatigue. Physical examination can reveal hepatosplenomegaly. Common laboratory findings include leukocytosis with more than 20% atypical lymphocytes on blood smear. Blood chemistries may reveal elevated liver enzymes.

Infection with coxsackievirus can cause several distinct illnesses, each associated with tonsillopharyngitis. Herpangina is a disease that is characterized by ulcers that are 2 to 3 mm in size and located on the anterior tonsillar pillars and possibly the uvula and soft palate. Hand-foot-and-mouth disease is characterized by ulcers on the tongue and oral mucosa, in association with vesicles found on the palms and/or soles. Small yellow-white nodules on the anterior tonsillar pillars characterize lymphonodular pharyngitis; these nodules do not ulcerate.

Pharyngoconjunctival fever is a disorder characterized by exudative tonsillopharyngitis, conjunctivitis, and fever. Infection is due to an adenovirus.

Measles is a disease with a prodromal phase that is characterized by symptoms of upper respiratory infection, tonsillopharyngitis, and small white lesions with erythematous bases on the buccal mucosa and inner aspect of the lower lip (Koplik's spots). These lesions are pathognomonic of early measles infection.

Streptococcal pharyngitis is characterized by exudative tonsillitis and fever. Physical examination often reveals a beefy red uvula, cervical adenitis, and oral petechiae. Laboratory evaluation should include a throat culture for group A *Streptococcus*.[37]

CLASSIFICATION

Pharyngotonsillitis is classified on the basis of etiology and clinical presentation (see above).

DIAGNOSIS

Diagnosis is based on a history of sore throat and is established by appropriate physical findings and results of a throat culture (see above). A rapid antigen detection test is available for diagnosing streptococcal pharyngitis. The test has a high specificity (95%+) but a low sensitivity (60 to 95%). Therefore, negative results should be confirmed by throat culture.

Antistreptolysin O titers rise about 150 U within 2 weeks of acute infection. These titers are useful for documenting recent streptococcal infections, especially in the course of acute rheumatic fever.

MANAGEMENT

The viral causes of tonsillopharyngitis are treated symptomatically. Gargle solutions, analgesics, and antipyretics are often helpful. The course is always self-limited.[5]

Acute streptococcal pharyngitis is treated with a 10-day course of oral penicillin V or erythromycin (for penicillin-sensitive individuals). Alternatives include an intramuscular injection of benzathine penicillin G or oral cephalosporins. Failure rates for penicillin vary from 6 to 23%, so an additional antibiotic course may be necessary.[37]

PROGNOSIS

The prognosis for viral tonsillopharyngitis is very good as the infections are self-limited. Late sequelae from group A streptococcal tonsillitis can be avoided by prompt diagnosis and treatment.[38] Other complications due to streptococcal tonsillitis are uncommon but include cervical adenitis, peritonsillar abscesses, otitis media, cellulitis, and septicemia.

ORAL HEALTH CONSIDERATIONS

The association between GABHS infection and the development of severe complications, such as rheumatic fever and its associated heart condition, is well known. Although failure to successfully treat GABHS infections was more common in the pre-penicillin era, there are some concerns today regarding re-infection in cases in which penicillin is unable to eradicate the organism. One study found a significant association between the persistence of GABHS on toothbrushes and removable orthodontic appliances and the recovery of GABHS in the oropharynx of symptomatic patients after 10 days of treatment with penicillin.[39] Interestingly, when toothbrushes were rinsed with sterile water, organisms could not be cultured beyond 3 days whereas nonrinsed toothbrushes harbored GABHS for up to 15 days. Thus, patients with GABHS infections should be instructed to thoroughly clean their toothbrushes and removable acrylic appliances daily. It is also advisable to change to a new toothbrush after the acute stage of any oropharyngeal infections.

▼ LOWER-AIRWAY INFECTIONS

The association between oral health and respiratory diseases has recently received renewed attention. Several articles have suggested that dental plaque may be a reservoir for respiratory pathogens involved in pneumonia and chronic obstructive pulmonary disease.[40–45] Although this may not be a critical problem for ambulatory healthy individuals, deteriorating oral health may be a major factor for both morbidity and mortality among institutionalized elderly persons, as well as for patients in critical care units.

Acute Bronchitis

Acute bronchitis is an inflammatory process of the large airways (trachea and bronchi) or what is commonly termed the lower respiratory tract. In patients who are otherwise healthy and without underlying pulmonary disease, bronchitis is most commonly caused by a viral infection.[46] The viruses most commonly implicated are *Rhinovirus, Coronavirus*, influenza virus, parainfluenza virus, and adenovirus. Acute bronchitis due to bacterial infection is less common and is seen more commonly in patients who have chronic lung disease.[47] The most common cause in this group is *Streptococcus pneumoniae*. Infection with *Haemophilus influenzae* is common in patients with chronic obstructive pulmonary disease (COPD). Other causes of acute bacterial bronchitis include *Mycoplasma pneumoniae, Chlamydia pneumoniae, Bordetella pertussis*, and *Legionella* spp.[48] *Staphylococcus* and gram-negative bacteria are common causes of bronchitis among hospitalized individuals.

PATHOPHYSIOLOGY

The pathophysiology of acute bronchitis is similar to that of other respiratory tract infections. Following infection of the mucosal cells, congestion of the respiratory mucosa develops. Inflammation causes an increase in secretory activity, resulting in increased sputum production. Polymorphonuclear leukocytes infiltrate the bronchial walls and lumen. Desquamation of the ciliated epithelium may occur, and spasm of bronchial smooth muscle is common.

CLINICAL AND LABORATORY FINDINGS

Acute viral bronchitis usually presents with a viral prodrome consisting of fever, malaise, myalgias, headache, and weakness. Upper-respiratory-tract symptoms that may include sore throat and rhinorrhea usually follow. As the illness progresses, lower tract symptoms develop, with a prominent nonproductive cough. Chest discomfort may occur; this usually worsens with persistent coughing bouts.[49] Other symptoms, such as dyspnea and respiratory distress, are variably present. Physical examination may reveal wheezing. The presentation may closely resemble an acute asthma exacerbation. Symptoms gradually resolve over a period of 1 to 2 weeks. Patients with underlying chronic lung disease might also experience respiratory compromise, with a significant impairment in pulmonary function.

The presentation of acute bacterial bronchitis is very similar to that of bacterial pneumonia (see below). Symptoms may include fever, dyspnea, productive cough with purulent sputum, and chest pain. Bacterial bronchitis can be differentiated from pneumonia by the lack of significant findings on chest radiography.

CLASSIFICATION

Although there is no universal classification scheme, acute bronchitis can be differentiated on the basis of etiology. Viral bronchitis presents differently than bacterial bronchitis, as described above.

DIAGNOSIS

Diagnosis of acute bronchitis is based on a suggestive history and a physical examination. Neither blood cell counts nor sputum analyses are particularly diagnostic in otherwise healthy patients. Chest radiography may be helpful in distinguishing bacterial bronchitis from pneumonia. Patients with recurrent bouts of acute bronchitis should be evaluated for possible asthma. This evaluation would include pulmonary function testing.

Patients with persistent symptoms in the course of presumed viral bronchitis should be evaluated to determine possible underlying etiologies. Sputum culture might prove useful in these circumstances.[50]

MANAGEMENT

Viral bronchitis can be managed with supportive care only as most individuals who are otherwise healthy recover without specific treatment.[7] If significant airway obstruction or hyperreactivity is present, inhaled bronchodilators such as albuterol can be useful. Cough suppressants such as codeine can also be used for patients whose coughing interferes with sleep.

The treatment of bacterial bronchitis includes antibiotics. Amoxicillin is an excellent first-line agent although macrolide antibiotics can be used for patients with penicillin allergy. Second-generation cephalosporins and amoxicillin/clavulanate are good second-line agents for patients with suspected infection due to β-lactamase–producing organisms. Inhaled bronchodilators are also helpful in cases with a bronchospastic component.

PROGNOSIS

Acute bronchitis carries an excellent prognosis for patients who are without underlying pulmonary disease, and recovery without sequelae is the norm. However, for patients with chronic lung disease and respiratory compromise, bronchitis can be quite serious and may often lead to hospitalization and respiratory failure. In other high-risk individuals, such as those with human immunodeficiency virus (HIV) infection or other immunodeficiencies, acute bronchitis may lead to the development of bronchiectasis.

ORAL HEALTH CONSIDERATIONS

Resistance to antibiotics may develop rapidly and last for 10 to 14 days.[51] Thus, patients who are taking amoxicillin for acute bronchitis should be prescribed another type of antibiotic, (such as clindamycin or a cephalosporin) when an antibiotic is needed for an odontogenic infection.

Pneumonia

Pneumonia is defined pathologically as an infection and a subsequent inflammation involving the lung parenchyma. Both viruses and bacteria are causes, and the presentation is dependent on the causative organism. There are an estimated 2.5 million cases of pneumonia each year. These cases can be broadly classified as either community acquired or nosocomial. Nosocomial infections are infections that are acquired in a hospital or health care facility and often affect debilitated or chronically ill individuals. Community-acquired infections can affect all persons but are more commonly seen in otherwise healthy individuals.

The most common bacterial cause of community-acquired pneumonia is *Streptococcus pneumoniae*, followed by *Haemophilus influenzae*. *Staphylococcus aureus* and gram-negative bacteria are common causes of nosocomial pneumonia. Pneumonia due to *Klebsiella pneumoniae* is seen in predominantly older patients and in those with a history of alcoholism. Atypical organisms commonly associated with pneumonia include *Mycoplasma pneumoniae*, *Legionella*, and *Chlamydia*.[48] The atypical organisms cause a pneumonia that differs in clinical presentation from that caused by the aforementioned bacteria (see below). Pneumonia can also be caused by viruses; by fungi such as *Candida*, *Histoplasma*, *Cryptococcus*, and *Aspergillus*; and by protozoa such as *Pneumocystis carinii* (seen in immunocompromised hosts), *Nocardia*, and *Mycobacterium tuberculosis*. Infection with these organisms can often be differentiated by chest radiography.

PATHOPHYSIOLOGY

The pathophysiology of pneumonia is dependent on the causative infectious organism. In bacterial pneumonia caused by *Streptococcus pneumoniae*, for example, the bacteria first enter the alveolar spaces after inhalation. Once inside the alveoli, the bacteria rapidly multiply, and extensive edema develops. The bacteria cause a vigorous inflammatory response, which includes an influx of polymorphonuclear leukocytes. In addition, capillary leakage is pronounced. As the inflammatory process continues, the polymorphonuclear leukocytes are replaced by macrophages. Subsequent deposition of fibrin ensues as the infection is controlled, and the inflammatory response resolves.[52]

Atypical infections of the lung (ie, viral, mycoplasmal, etc.) are interstitial processes. The organisms are first inhaled into the alveolar spaces. The organisms then infect the type I pneumocytes directly. As these pneumocytes lose their structural integrity and necrosis ensues, alveolar edema begins. Type II pneumocytes proliferate and line the alveoli, and an exudative cellular debris accumulates. An interstitial inflammatory response is mounted, primarily by mononuclear leukocytes. This process can occasionally progress to interstitial fibrosis although resolution is the norm.

CLINICAL AND LABORATORY FINDINGS

Pneumonia due to community-acquired bacterial infection (*Pneumococcus*) typically presents acutely, with a rapid onset of symptoms. A prodrome similar to that seen with acute infections of the upper respiratory tract is unusual. Common symptoms include fever, pleuritic chest pain, and coughing that produces purulent sputum.[49] Chills and rigors are also common. Pneumonia due to *Haemophilus influenzae*, which is seen more commonly in patients with COPD or alcoholism, presents with fever, cough, and malaise. Chest pain and rigors are less common.

Nosocomial pneumonia due to *Staphylococcus* or gram-negative bacteria is usually associated with a prodrome due to an antecedent viral upper respiratory infection. Symptoms of pneumonia, including cough and fever, develop several days after the onset of the upper respiratory symptoms.

Physical examination demonstrates crackles (rales) in the affected lung fields. Decreased breath sounds and dullness to percussion might also be noted. Signs of respiratory distress may be present in severely affected individuals.

As many as 25% of all cases of community-acquired pneumonia are considered atypical. Symptoms usually develop over 3 to 4 days and initially consist of low-grade fever, malaise, a nonproductive cough, and headache. Sputum production, if present, is usually minimal. Findings on physical examination of the chest are usually unremarkable, with only scattered rhonchi. Infection due to *Mycoplasma* is common among younger patients. This organism is commonly spread to other family members. The onset of symptoms is gradual, and symptoms often include pharyngitis. Evidence of bullous disease of the tympanic membranes (bullous myringitis) is highly suggestive of mycoplasmal infection. Pneumonias due to viral causes have a similar presentation but can have a more rapid onset. Influenza virus is the most common viral etiology.

Infection with *Legionella* spp (legionnaires' disease) begins with a prodrome consisting of fever and malaise and progresses rapidly to an acute phase of high fever, rigors, pleuritic chest pain, gastrointestinal complaints, and confusion. The cough is typically nonproductive and is only variably present. Elevated liver enzymes and proteinuria indicate renal and hepatic involvement. Hypoxia can also develop and can rapidly progress. Legionnaires' disease was first described at an American Legion convention in Philadelphia in 1976. The causative organisms have a predilection for moist areas such as air-conditioning ducts and cooling towers. The infection tends to occur more commonly among middle-aged men with a history of tobacco smoking.

CLASSIFICATION

Pneumonia is initially classified on clinical presentation as either bacterial or atypical. Different classifications based on radiologic or pathologic manifestations are less commonly used.

DIAGNOSIS

When a patient with probable pneumonia is being evaluated, the possible causative organism will be suggested by (1) the clinical presentation and course of the illness, (2) the degree of immunocompetency of the patient, (3) the presence or absence of underlying lung disease, and (4) the place of acquisition (hospital or community). Ultimately, the goal is rapid diagnosis to establish an etiology so that appropriate antimicrobial therapy can be initiated. Sputum analysis is the most important tool for diagnosis and management. Spontaneously coughed or induced sputum should be immediately analyzed by Gram's stain. This will allow identification of the likely etiology and thus a more directed antibiotic therapy. Gram-positive cocci in pairs (diplococci) are suggestive of pneumococcal infection. Gram-positive cocci in clusters suggest infection with *Staphylococcus aureus*. Gram-negative pleomorphic rods are typical of *Haemophilus influenzae*, whereas *Klebsiella* is identified by its short plump gram-negative-rod appearance. Numerous polymorphonuclear leukocytes are also often seen.

Culture of sputum samples is used to help identify the causative organism. Routine culture can identify *Streptococcus pneumoniae*, *Haemophilus influenzae*, *Staphylococcus aureus*, and gram-negative rods. Specialized culturing techniques are needed to identify *Legionella*, *Mycobacterium*, *Nocardia*, *Mycoplasma*, and fungi. Tissue cultures are used to identify viruses and *Chlamydia*. Other cultures, such as blood and pleural fluid cultures, can be analyzed. Blood cultures are done routinely because many organisms are identified in this manner.[53] For example, blood cultures are positive in 35% of patients with pneumococcal disease and in 15% of those with *Klebsiella* infection.

Chest radiography can be a valuable tool in the evaluation of the patient with pneumonia. The radiologic presentation is dependent on the infectious etiology and the underlying medical condition of the patient. A pattern of lobar consolidation and air bronchograms is seen most commonly in cases of pneumococcal pneumonia. The lower lobes and right middle lobe are most commonly involved. A pattern of patchy non-homogenous infiltrates, pleural effusion, and cavitary lesions are common with staphylococcal pneumonia. *Klebsiella* pneumonia typically involves multiple lobes and can also be associated with effusion and cavitation. Viral or atypical organisms usually present with an interstitial infiltrative pattern or patchy segmental infiltrates. Organisms such as *Nocardia*, *Mycobacterium*, and fungi often cause nodular or cavitary lesions, which are demonstrable on chest radiography. Rapid accumulation of pleural fluid or empyema is seen most often with bacterial infection. Pneumococcal pneumonia is associated with pleural effusion in 10 to 15% of cases.

The presence of cold agglutinins is suggestive of *Mycoplasma* infection. Cold agglutinins are antibodies (produced in response to *Mycoplasma* infection) that agglutinate red blood cells upon cold exposure. Titers reach maximal levels in 3 to 4 weeks but can be detected 1 week after the onset of disease. These antibodies can be found in 60 to 70% of patients with *Mycoplasma* pneumonia but are not specific to this disease.

Legionella pneumonia is diagnosed either by culture of the organisms, using specialized media, or by direct fluorescent antibody staining of sputum.

MANAGEMENT

Empiric treatment is started immediately upon diagnosis of pneumonia. When a pneumococcal infection is suspected, treatment with penicillin is effective although penicillin resistance has emerged in several areas of the world.[54] Alternatives include the cephalosporins and macrolide antibiotics. Symptoms begin to improve within 1 to 2 days although chest radiograph abnormalities may persist for months. Treatment for *Haemophilus influenzae* pneumonia includes second-generation cephalosporins or ampicillin/clavulanate. Clarithromycin or quinolone antibiotics are alternatives.[55]

Erythromycin is the antibiotic of choice for pneumonia caused by *Legionella* or *Mycoplasma*. Alternatives include the quinolone antibiotics or clarithromycin.

Nonspecific treatment for patients with pneumonia includes aggressive hydration to aid in sputum clearance. Chest physiotherapy is advocated by many clinicians although evidence of efficacy is lacking. If hypoxia is present, supplemental oxygen is given.[56]

A pneumococcal vaccine is available for active immunization against pneumococcal disease. The vaccine is effective for preventing disease from 85% of pneumococcal serotypes. It is effective for adults and for children older than 2 years of age and is recommended for high-risk individuals, such as those with asplenia and all individuals over the age of 65 years.

PROGNOSIS

Mortality due to community-acquired pneumonia is low. The risk of mortality is higher for older patients, patients with underlying pulmonary disease, patients with immunodeficiency (ie, asplenia), and patients with positive blood cultures. Most deaths occur within 5 days of the onset of disease.

Mortality due to staphylococcal pneumonia is high, and patients who do recover often have residual pulmonary abnormalities. Mortality due to atypical pneumonia is low, with the exception of *Legionella* pneumonia, which has a 15% mortality rate if left untreated.

ORAL HEALTH CONSIDERATIONS

The aspiration of salivary secretions containing oral bacteria into the lower respiratory tract can cause pneumonia. Numerous periodontally associated oral anaerobes and facultative species have been isolated from infected pulmonary fluids.[57] Although most reports suggest increased susceptibility to the development of nosocomial pneumonia from periodontal pathogens, other oral bacteria (such as *Streptococcus viridans*) have been implicated in community-acquired pneumonia.[58] Colonization of dental plaque and oral mucosa with respiratory pathogens is more prevalent among patients in medical intensive care units (ICUs).[42] Furthermore, the amount of dental plaque among ICU patients has been shown to increase over time, resulting in the occurrence of nosocomial pneumonia with pathogens isolated from the dental plaque.[44] However, prerinsing with a 0.12% chlorhexidine gluconate mouth rinse may significantly reduce the mortality of nosocomial pneumonia in ICU patients.[59]

Elderly individuals residing in nursing homes have an increased prevalence of poor oral health, including increased plaque retention.[60] Studies have evaluated the occurrence of pneumonia in cohorts of elderly individuals who were receiving and not receiving oral care. In one such study, the relative risk of developing pneumonia increased 67% in the group without access to oral health interventions, compared with individuals who had access to oral care.[61] This data support the benefit of increased awareness and increased oral health interventions in hospitalized and institutionalized individuals. More intervention studies are needed to assess the impact of oral pathogens on the incidence of pneumonia, but at present, there is ample evidence that poor oral health status is a risk indicator for the development of pneumonia.

Bronchiolitis

Bronchiolitis is a disease that affects children under the age of 2 years; it is most common among infants aged 2 to 12 months. It is characterized by inflammation of the lower respiratory tract, with the bronchioles being most affected. The inflammatory response is secondary to an infectious trigger, usually respiratory syncytial virus (RSV).[62] Other organisms associated with bronchiolitis are parainfluenza virus, influenza virus, adenovirus, and *Mycoplasma pneumoniae*.[63]

PATHOPHYSIOLOGY

Infection of the bronchioles leads to a marked inflammatory response with a prominent mononuclear cell infiltrate. This inflammatory response results in mucosal edema with cellular debris, mucosal thickening, and mucous hypersecretion and plugging. Bronchiolar spasm is an occasional feature. Due to these changes, the lumina of the bronchioles are critically narrowed, leading to areas of microatelectasis and emphysema. Respiratory compromise is common, with decreased blood oxygen saturation, hypercarbia, respiratory acidosis, and in severe cases, respiratory failure.

CLINICAL AND LABORATORY FINDINGS

Infants first develop signs and symptoms of an infection of the upper respiratory tract, with low-grade fever, profuse clear rhinorrhea, and cough. Signs of infection in the lower respiratory tract soon follow, including tachypnea, retractions, wheezing, and (on occasion) cyanosis. Crackles can be audible, and thoracic hyper-resonance can be noted on percussion. Associated findings can include conjunctivitis, otitis media, and pharyngitis.

Chest radiography shows peribronchial cuffing, flattening of the diaphragms, hyperinflation, and increased lung markings.

Laboratory studies reveal a mild leukocytosis with a prominence of polymorphonuclear leukocytes ("left shift").

CLASSIFICATION

Bronchiolitis can be classified by the causative agent, as is the case with acute bronchitis.

DIAGNOSIS

The diagnosis is clinical, based on history and physical examination. The etiology can be determined (and the diagnosis confirmed) by performing a nasopharyngeal culture for RSV

and other respiratory viruses. Rapid viral diagnostic assays are also available.

The differential diagnosis includes other causes of wheezing and respiratory distress in this age group, such as asthma, heart failure due to congenital heart disease, and cystic fibrosis.

MANAGEMENT

Infants are usually managed in cool-mist oxygen tents, where continuous oxygen administration can be given. Due to an increase in insensible water losses, hydration must be ensured. Aerosolized bronchodilators are often used although their routine use is not recommended. Oral or parenteral corticosteroids are often used although validation of their efficacy through clinical trials is lacking.

Antiviral therapy with ribavirin is recommended for infants with severe disease, congenital heart disease, or underlying pulmonary disease. Ribavirin is delivered by aerosol on a semicontinuous basis for up to 1 week.[64]

Mechanical ventilation is required in the infant with respiratory failure. Very young infants (less than 1 month of age) are at risk for apnea due to RSV infection, so close observation is required.

Anti-RSV immunoglobulin preparations are available for passive immunization against RSV. These preparations are currently recommended for high-risk patient populations. A vaccine is under development for the prevention of RSV-related disease.[65]

PROGNOSIS

Although mortality due to bronchiolitis is not uncommon, most patients recover without sequelae. A subset of patients develop recurrent bronchospasm following RSV bronchiolitis. It is not known whether or not this represents a risk factor for persistent asthma in later childhood.[66]

Asthma

Asthma is a chronic disease that affects the lower airways. It is characterized by recurrent and reversible airflow limitation due to an underlying inflammatory process. The etiology of asthma is unknown, but allergic sensitivity is seen in most patients with asthma.[4] Genetic factors play a role, but no single gene or combination of genes has yet been identified as causative.

In the United States, asthma affects more than 14 million people. Its onset is most commonly during childhood, and almost 5 million children are affected. Asthma mortality numbers 5,000 people per year. In addition, the care of asthmatic persons represents a significant economic and social burden, accounting for numerous hospitalization days and days missed from school and work. These trends do not appear to be declining despite advances in our understanding of asthma and despite new pharmacologic modalities.

PATHOPHYSIOLOGY

The clinical features of asthma are due to the underlying chronic inflammatory process. Although the etiology is not known, certain histopathologic features provide insights into the chronic process. Inflammatory infiltrates are rich in activated eosinophils and T helper lymphocytes, suggesting an allergic process. Degranulated mast cells are in close proximity to the affected airway, most likely representing allergen-mediated activation. The inflammatory cascade results in disruption of the integrity of the normal airway. There is destruction of the airway epithelium, bronchial smooth-muscle hypertrophy, sub-basement membrane collagen deposition, edema, and mucous plugging, all of which are demonstrable in vivo.

Airway inflammation has been characterized as acute, subacute, or chronic. The acute inflammatory state is due to the release of mediators from activated inflammatory cells that are resident in the airways (such as histamine release from degranulated mast cells). Subacute inflammation is characterized by early cellular infiltrates, most notably eosinophils, and the release of mediators with direct toxicity to airway epithelium. Chronic inflammation is characterized by persistent ongoing inflammation mediated by lymphocytes and eosinophils, with resultant damage and repair processes. This may lead to irreversible airway obstruction in a subset of patients with asthma.

Airflow limitation develops as a result of the airway inflammation. Several inter-related factors play a role, including mucous plugging, airway edema, bronchospasm and constriction, and airway remodeling due to basement membrane thickening and sub-basement membrane fibrosis. The signs and symptoms of asthma are the direct results of these processes.

Atopy is the strongest risk factor associated with the development of asthma. Persistent exposure to relevant allergens in a sensitized individual can lead to chronic allergic inflammation of the airways. Although atopy is seen more commonly in childhood-onset asthma, it can also play an important role in asthma in adults.

CLINICAL AND LABORATORY FINDINGS

The hallmark clinical features of asthma are recurrent reversible airflow limitation and airway hyper-responsiveness. These factors lead to the development of the signs and symptoms of asthma, which include intermittent wheezing, coughing, dyspnea, and chest tightness. Symptoms of asthma tend to worsen at night and in the early morning hours. In addition, well-defined triggers may precipitate asthma symptoms. These triggers include allergens, exercise, cold air, respiratory irritants, emotional extremes, and infections (especially viral infections). Symptoms can progress slowly over time, or they may develop abruptly.[2,67,68]

Historical points that suggest asthma are chronic coughing with nocturnal awakenings, dyspnea or chest tightness with exertion, recurrent "bronchitis" associated with infections of the upper respiratory tract, and wheezing that occurs on a seasonal basis. Physical examination of patients with mild disease often shows no abnormalities. However, common findings in patients with more severe disease include an increased antero-posterior chest diameter, a prolonged expiratory phase, wheezing, and diminished breath sounds. Digital clubbing is rarely seen. Concurrent allergic disease such as allergic rhinitis may be present. During acute exacerbations, patients may show signs of respiratory distress, with tachypnea, intercostal retractions, nasal flaring, and cyanosis.

Spirometry is the best tool available to aid in the diagnosis and management of asthma. Spirometry allows the measurement of lung capacity and airflows and can be performed during a routine office visit. The technique involves a maximal forced expiration following a maximal inspiration. The key measurements are the forced vital capacity (FVC), which is the amount of air expired during the forced expiration, and the forced expiratory volume in 1 second (FEV_1), which is the volume of air expired during the first second of expiration; FEV_1 is a measure of the rate at which air can be exhaled. Given the FEV_1 and the FEV_1/FVC ratio, an objective determination of airflow limitation is possible. Reversibility can be demonstrated after administration of a short-acting bronchodilator (such as albuterol) and a repeat spirometric measurement. In patients with normal baseline spirometry values, a demonstration of bronchial hyperresponsiveness is useful. This is performed by bronchoprovocation, using nonspecific triggers such as histamine or methacholine. When delivered by aerosol, these agents allow the determination of bronchial hyperreactivity by triggering a decrease in the FEV_1 immediately following inhalation.

Measurement of the peak expiratory flow rate (PEFR) can be a useful adjunct for diagnosis and management of asthma. Patients with asthma often demonstrate a diurnal variation of 20% or more, when early-morning values are compared to evening values. The PEFR is easy to determine, and durable metering devices are available at little cost. In addition, measurement of PEFRs can predict when asthma is worsening and is often used as an indicator of asthma severity in patients who require daily anti-inflammatory therapy.

Allergen skin testing is another valuable tool. This testing allows the accurate identification of allergic triggers, which can translate into more specific therapies such as allergen avoidance and immunotherapy (see "Allergic Rhinitis and Conjunctivitis," above). Chest radiography may be useful, especially as a means of excluding other diseases from the diagnosis.

CLASSIFICATION

Asthma is classified according to its severity. Although there is no universal classification scheme, the guidelines set forth by the National Asthma Education and Prevention Program (NAEPP) are the most widely used in the United States.[69] Asthma patients are classified as having mild-intermittent, mild-persistent, moderate-persistent, or severe-persistent disease. The categories are defined by both subjective (historical) and objective (spirometric) points. Treatment guidelines are based on the level of severity of the patient's disease, and the classification can therefore change over time.[70] Asthma may also be classified by the underlying trigger (eg, exercise-induced asthma and occupational asthma).

DIAGNOSIS

The diagnosis of asthma is made on the basis of a suggestive history, confirmatory physical findings, and the demonstration of reversible airflow limitation. This can be documented during hospitalization, by outpatient use of spirometry or PEFR determinations, or by clinical assessment after therapeutic trials.

The differential diagnosis of asthma includes other causes of chronic coughing and wheezing. The diseases that are usually considered are chronic rhinitis or sinusitis, cystic fibrosis, gastroesophageal reflux disease, airway narrowing due to compression (ie, masses), and COPD (chronic bronchitis). Factors favoring the diagnosis of asthma include intermittent symptoms with asymptomatic periods, complete or nearly complete reversibility with bronchodilators, the absence of digital clubbing, and a history of atopy.

MANAGEMENT

The goals of asthma management include the patient's having little or no chronic symptoms, few or no exacerbations, no hospitalizations, and minimal or no activity limitation. Ideal control would include no need for short-acting bronchodilators, normal PEFRs, no PEFR variability, and no adverse effects from controller medications. All patients with asthma, regardless of its severity, should have an asthma control plan to aid in understanding the underlying process and treatment options and to effectively treat asthma exacerbations. Regular monitoring of asthma is important; spirometry, PEFR measurement, and questionnaires are useful for this purpose. Avoidance control measures are regularly emphasized, focusing on allergen and irritant triggers. Treatment for concomitant diseases that may exacerbate asthma (such as allergic rhinitis, gastroesophageal reflux disease, and chronic sinusitis) should be instituted.[71]

Pharmacotherapy of asthma is based on the severity of disease. NAEPP guidelines provide written algorithms to aid in treatment plan development. Patients with mild-intermittent disease usually require short-acting bronchodilators on an as-needed basis. These medications (such as albuterol) are preferably administered by inhalation. Preparations are available in metered-dose inhalers, in dry-powder inhalers, and as solutions for a nebulizer. Patients with mild-persistent asthma require routine therapy for control of underlying airway inflammation. Inhaled corticosteroids are the most widely used and most effective asthma anti-inflammatory agents.[72] They have an excellent safety profile at conventional doses although high-dose therapy can put patients at risk for corticosteroid side effects. These medications have been used for decades in both children and adults without significant long-term side effects in most patients. However, a concern about growth suppression in children has mandated warning labels on all inhaled corticosteroids. The long-term consequences of this short-term growth suppression are yet to be determined. Alternative medications include the non-steroidal anti-inflammatory agents nedocromil and cromolyn. These medications have less potent anti-inflammatory effects and are therefore most helpful for patients with mild disease. Leukotriene receptor antagonists such as montelukast and zafirlukast have been

used successfully as monotherapy in patients with mild-persistent asthma. Although the role of leukotrienes in allergic inflammation is well known, the long-term benefit of these agents when used alone is yet to be determined.[73]

Patients with moderate and severe persistent disease require more intensive therapy. Long-acting bronchodilators such as salmeterol have been shown to have an additive effect when used with inhaled corticosteroids and are useful additions to inhaled-corticosteroid therapy. Leukotriene receptor antagonists also are often a helpful addition to inhaled corticosteroids. A minority of patients might require long-term corticosteroids; these patients are difficult to manage, but adequate symptom control while minimizing the dose is of paramount importance.[74]

Patients with allergic triggers may benefit from allergen immunotherapy. Many studies have now documented improvement from following a 3- to 5-year course of specific immunotherapy.[75] This is an excellent means of minimizing medications while maintaining control for many patients.

PROGNOSIS

Although asthma is not a curable disease, it is a controllable disease. Asthma education programs are extremely important in making early diagnosis and interventions possible. Despite an increase in our knowledge of the underlying pathophysiology, asthma mortality rates have not declined. With early diagnosis and a comprehensive management plan, patients with asthma can experience a normal life expectancy with good quality of life.

ORAL HEALTH CONSIDERATIONS

The main concern when treating any medically complex patient is to avoid exacerbation of the underlying condition. Several protocols suggesting appropriate procedures for dental treatment of asthmatic patients have been put forth.[76–79] However, few studies assessing the respiratory response of patients to dental care have been performed. One recent study indicated that although 15% of asthmatic pediatric patients will have a clinically significant decrease in lung function, no clinical parameter or historical data pertaining to asthma can predict this phenomenon.[80]

However, numerous dental products and materials, including toothpaste, fissure sealants, tooth enamel dust, and methyl methacrylate, have been associated with the exacerbation of asthma whereas other items (such as fluoride trays and cotton rolls) have been suggested as being so associated.[76,81–85]

There is still no consensus regarding the association between asthma and dentofacial morphology.[86,87] Although nasal respiratory obstruction resulting in mouth breathing has been implicated in the development of a long and tapered facial form, an increased lower facial height, and a narrow maxillary arch, this relationship has never been substantiated with unequivocal evidence.

Oral manifestations include candidiasis, decreased salivary flow, increased calculus, increased gingivitis, increased periodontal disease, increased incidence of caries, and adverse effects of orthodontic therapy.[88–92]

It is possible that prolonged use of β_2-agonists may cause reduced salivary flow, with a resulting increase in cariogenic bacteria and caries and an increased incidence of candidiasis.[93] The increased incidence of caries is further accelerated by the use of cariogenic carbohydrates and sugar-containing anti-asthmatic medications.[94]

Dental treatment for asthmatic patients needs to address the oral manifestations of this condition, as well as its potential underlying systemic complications. Elective dental procedures should be avoided in all but those whose asthma is well controlled. The type and frequency of asthmatic attacks, as well as the type of medications used by the patient, indicate the severity of the disease.

The following are considerations and recommendations for administering dental care to patients who have asthma:

1. Fluoride supplements should be instituted for all asthmatic patients, particular those taking β_2-agonists.
2. The patient should be instructed to rinse his or her mouth with water after using inhalers.
3. Oral hygiene should be reinforced to reduce the incidence of gingivitis and periodontitis.
4. Antifungal medications should be administered as needed, particularly in patients who are taking inhaled corticosteroids.
5. Steroid prophylaxis need to be used with patients who are taking long-term systemic corticosteroids (see Chapter X).
6. Use stress-reducing techniques. Conscious sedation should be performed with agents that are not associated with bronchoconstrictions, such as hydroxyzine. Barbiturates and narcotics should be avoided due to their potential to cause bronchospasm and reduce respiratory functions. Nitrous oxide can be used for all but patients with severe asthma as it may irritate the airways.[95]
7. Avoid dental materials that may precipitate an attack. Acrylic appliances should be cured prior to insertion. Dental materials without methyl methacrylate should be considered.
8. Schedule these patients' appointments for late morning or later in the day, to minimize the risk of an asthmatic attack.[96]
9. Have oxygen and bronchodilators available in case of an exacerbation of asthma.
10. There are no contraindications to the use of local anesthetics containing epinephrine, but preservatives such as sodium metabisulfite may contribute to asthma exacerbation in susceptible patients.[97] Nevertheless, interactions between epinephrine and β_2-agonists may result in a synergistic effect, producing increased blood pressure and arrhythmias.
11. Judicious use of rubber dams will prevent reduced breathing capability.
12. Care should be used in the positioning of suction tips as they may elicit a cough reflex.
13. Up to 10% of adult asthmatic patients have an allergy to aspirin and other nonsteroidal anti-inflammatory agents.[98] A careful history concerning the use of these type of drugs need to be elicited. Although the use of acetaminophen has been proposed as an alternative to the use of aspirin, recent data suggest caution because these type of drugs have also been associated with more severe asthma.[99]
14. Drug interactions with theophylline are common. Macrolide antibiotics may increase the level of theophylline whereas phenobarbitals may reduce the level. Furthermore, drugs such as tetracycline have been associated with more accentuated side effects when given together with theophylline.
15. During an acute asthmatic attack, discontinue the dental procedure, remove all intraoral devices, place the patient in a comfortable position, make sure the airway is opened, and administer a β_2-agonist and oxygen. If no improvement is noted, administer epinephrine subcutaneously (1:1,000 concentration, 0.01 mg/kg of body weight, up to a maximum of 0.3 mg) and alert emergency medical assistance.

Chronic Obstructive Pulmonary Disease

"Chronic obstructive pulmonary disease" is a term used to describe chronic and largely irreversible airway obstruction due to inflammation of the lower airways. Chronic bronchitis is COPD due to chronic bronchial inflammation. Chronic bronchitis is diagnosed on clinical criteria and is defined as coughing and sputum production for 3 or more months per year for at least 2 consecutive years. Emphysema is diagnosed by histopathology and is defined by enlarged air spaces and the loss of alveolar tissue. The hallmark features of COPD are dyspnea and hypoxemia.[100] Alveolar hypoventilation and diffusion impairment causes hypercarbia, which may result in pulmonary hypertension and cor pulmonale. COPD is almost always due to the smoking of tobacco although air pollution has also been implicated. A deficiency in the enzyme α_1-antitrypsin causes a syndrome of emphysema only. This enzyme is responsible for inhibiting the activity of trypsin and other proteases in the serum and tissues. The characteristic panlobular emphysematous changes that are seen in α_1-antitrypsin deficiency are related to the loss of alveolar walls. Tobacco smoking accelerates this process.

The clinical course of patients with COPD is quite varied. Most patients display some degree of progressive dyspnea, exercise intolerance, and fatigue. In addition, patients are susceptible to frequent exacerbations, usually caused by infections of the upper or lower respiratory tract. Most patients with COPD have little respiratory reserve. Therefore, any process that causes airway inflammation can lead to clinical deterioration.

PATHOPHYSIOLOGY

Many toxins in tobacco smoke can cause a vigorous inflammatory response. Acrolein, for example, causes impairment of both ciliary and macrophage activities. Nitrogen dioxide causes direct toxic damage to the respiratory epithelium. Hydrogen cyanide is responsible for the functional impairment of enzymes that are required for respiratory metabolism. Carbon monoxide causes a decrease in the oxygen-carrying capacity of red blood cells by associating with hemoglobin to form carboxyhemoglobin. Lastly, polycyclic hydrocarbons have been implicated as carcinogens.

Episodes of infection can precipitate exacerbations of chronic bronchitis. Patients with chronic bronchitis develop bacterial colonization of the tracheobronchial tree. It is not known, however, whether these bacteria are responsible for clinical deterioration. Infection due to *Mycoplasma* pneumonia or viruses is associated with exacerbation in up to one-third of patients with chronic bronchitis.

Histopathologically, patients with end-stage chronic bronchitis display an increased number of airway goblet cells, hypertrophy of mucus glands, squamous metaplasia of the airway epithelium, and mucosal edema. The airways are obstructed by mucous plugging and edema due to the ongoing inflammatory infiltrate. Mucous plugging and narrowing due to fibrosis is also seen in the smaller (2 to 3 mm) airways. Destruction of the alveolar walls leads to emphysematous changes.[101]

Hypoxemia is the result of the ventilation-perfusion mismatch that accompanies airway obstruction and emphysema. Portions of the lung that are not aerated due to obstruction cannot oxygenate the blood. This causes a decrease in overall oxygen concentrations. In addition, emphysema causes a decreased diffusion capacity because of a loss of air-space capillary units. Hypercarbia also develops and is often progressive and asymptomatic. Pulmonary hypertension can result from chronic hypoxia due to vasoconstriction of pulmonary vessels.

Patients with emphysema alone have less ventilation-perfusion mismatching early in the course of the disease; this is due to the loss of both air space and supplying blood vessels. Severe hypoxia, pulmonary hypertension, and cor pulmonale are not seen until late in the disease process. Emphysema manifests as loss of the elastic recoil of the lungs, making the lungs more compliant. The work of breathing is therefore not significantly increased. However, the decrease in recoil allows the easy collapse of the peripheral airways, leading to airway obstruction and airflow limitation.[102]

CLINICAL AND LABORATORY FINDINGS

Patients with chronic bronchitis present with dyspnea, cough, and sputum production. An increase in the production of often purulent sputum is a sign of exacerbation due to respiratory infection. Physical findings include diffuse wheezing, possibly associated with signs of respiratory distress including the use of accessory muscles of respiration (retractions) and tachypnea.[103] Liver enlargement due to congestion, ascites, and peripheral edema can develop as the disease progresses to pulmonary hypertension and cor pulmonale. This leads to the characteristic clinical patient presentation termed the "blue bloater."

Patients with emphysema present primarily with dyspnea. Patients can be adequately oxygenated in the early stages of the disease and thus can have fewer signs of hypoxia; the term "pink puffer" has been used to describe these patients. Physical findings include an increase in chest wall size. Wheezing is present to varying degrees.

Chest radiography may show evidence of an increase in lung compliance, with flattened diaphragms, hyperexpansion, and an increase in anteroposterior diameter. Spirometry will show evidence of airflow limitation, with decreases in the FEV_1 and the FEV_1/FVC ratio. Complete pulmonary function studies will also indicate an increase in residual volume (RV) and total lung capacity.[103] Pulmonary diffusion capacity will be decreased due to a loss of gas-exchanging units.

CLASSIFICATION

COPD is traditionally divided into two major categories: chronic bronchitis and emphysema. Airway obstruction in chronic bronchitis is due to bronchospasm, edema, and mucous plugging of the airways as a result of chronic inflammation. In emphysema, airway obstruction occurs because of the loss of lung elasticity and the resultant collapse of the airways. It is uncommon for patients to fit neatly into one category. Most patients have features of both emphysema and chronic bronchitis.

DIAGNOSIS

The diagnosis is suggested by the history and physical findings. Alternative diagnoses such as asthma, cystic fibrosis, and congestive heart failure should be considered. Complete pulmonary function tests are a valuable means of assessing airflow limitation and the reversibility of airway obstruction. For patients with more severe disease, assessment of oxygen status with pulse oximetry is a valuable office procedure. A determination of arterial blood gases is important for patients who are clinically deteriorating and for the management of hospitalized patients.[101] Chest radiography can be helpful, but it is often used only as an adjunct to the above diagnostic investigations.

MANAGEMENT

There are no curative treatments for chronic bronchitis and emphysema. Management focuses on maintaining quality of life and preventing exacerbations. Maintenance therapy includes trials of inhaled bronchodilators such as albuterol and ipratropium bromide. Theophylline products have also been used with some efficacy. Inhaled corticosteroids do not benefit all patients with COPD although some patients might experience some improvement.[104] A recent large multicenter study indicated that patients treated with inhaled corticosteroids did not show any significant slowing of the decline in lung function but did have fewer symptoms and improved sensitivity of the lungs to external stimuli.[105]

Chest physiotherapy has not been proven to be of value in the management of COPD.

During exacerbations, oxygen therapy is often required. Caution must be used when administering oxygen to patients with COPD as their ventilatory drive will often be diminished. This is the result of chronic retention of carbon dioxide and subsequent insensitivity to hypercarbia. As a result, patients with COPD are sensitive to increases in oxygen tension, which provides the major stimulus for respiratory drive. A partial pressure of arterial oxygen (PaO_2) of 55 to 60 mm Hg is often a reasonable goal to help reduce hypoxemia while maintaining respiratory drive. Oxygen therapy during sleep can also be a useful means of limiting hypoxemia and subsequent pulmonary hypertension.

Antibiotics are used during exacerbations of chronic bronchitis. Typical treatment includes 7 to 10 days of an oral broad-spectrum antibiotic, such as a second-generation cephalosporin. Although an underlying infectious etiology should be sought, clinical responses to antibiotic treatment do not always correlate with organisms isolated from sputum cultures.

Early inflammatory changes are visible in the bronchi of young smokers. Education about smoking risks is therefore imperative. Patients should be instructed that smoking cessation does lead to the resolution of symptoms and early-stage disease.

PROGNOSIS

The prognosis is poor for patients who are frequently symptomatic due to COPD. The 5-year mortality rate is approximately 50%, with most patients dying from respiratory failure. Two-thirds of patients who survive one bout of respiratory failure will die within 2 years.[106]

ORAL HEALTH CONSIDERATIONS

Several epidemiologic studies have suggested an association between oral infections and COPD.[41,45] Apart from the periodontal pathogens mentioned above, *Streptococcus viridans* has been shown to be the causative pathogen of exacerbation in 4% of individuals with COPD.[107] One prospective study suggested that oral colonization with respiratory pathogens in patients residing in a chronic care facility was significantly associated with COPD.[40] The relationship between oral pathogens and exacerbations of COPD clearly deserves serious consideration. It is essential that elderly individuals (particularly, institutionalized patients) receive adequate oral hygiene in order to minimize respiratory complications.

Drug interactions with theophylline may arise (see above), and a change of medications by the oral health care provider may be appropriate.

As mentioned above, increased oxygen tension may diminish respiratory function in patients with COPD. Extreme caution must be exercised when administering supplemental oxygen in emergencies.

Cystic Fibrosis

Cystic fibrosis (CF) is a genetic disorder characterized by hyperviscous secretions in the respiratory and gastrointestinal tracts. The sweat glands, hepatobiliary system, and reproductive organs are also affected. Thickened secretions affect the pancreas and intestinal tract, causing malabsorption and intestinal obstruction. In the lungs, viscid mucus causes airway obstruction, infection, and bronchiectasis. Pulmonary complications are the major factors affecting life expectancy in patients with CF. This section focuses on the pulmonary manifestations of CF.

Cystic fibrosis is an autosomal recessive inherited disease. The responsible gene, which codes for the cystic fibrosis transmembrane conductance regulator (CFTR), is located on chromosome 7. The incidence of CF among white people is approximately 1 in 2,000 to 3,000 births; the incidence is lower among those of other races.[108]

PATHOPHYSIOLOGY

The primary defect in the *CFTR* gene results in a defective chloride transport system in exocrine glands. As a result, mucous production occurs without sufficient water transport into the lumen. The resultant mucus is dry, thick, and tenacious and leads to inspissation in the affected glands and organs. In the airways, the viscid secretions impair mucociliary clearance and promote airway obstruction and bacterial colonization. Bacterial superinfection is common and can lead to respiratory compromise.

CLINICAL AND LABORATORY FINDINGS

Patients with CF may present in infancy with extrapulmonary manifestations such as meconium ileus or failure to thrive. Pulmonary manifestations include coughing, recurrent infections of the lower respiratory tract, and bronchospasm. Tachypnea and crackles can be found on physical examination. As the disease progresses, digital clubbing and bronchiectasis may become apparent.

Spirometry is a useful tool for documenting and monitoring airflow limitation. Airway obstruction tends to worsen with disease progression although some patients with CF have mild pulmonary disease.

A sweat test can be performed to confirm the diagnosis. The procedure involves the collection of sweat after stimulation with pilocarpine. Samples containing > 60 mEq/L chloride are considered positive. Patients with indeterminate values (40 to 60 mEq/L) can be further assessed by using tissue genotyping.

CLASSIFICATION

There is no universally accepted classification system for CF.

DIAGNOSIS

The diagnosis of CF is based on the presence of pulmonary or extrapulmonary symptoms, as described above. A sweat chloride test result of > 60 mEq/L confirms the diagnosis.

MANAGEMENT

Conventional treatment of CF has included antibiotics, bronchodilators, anti-inflammatory agents, chest physiotherapy with postural drainage, and mucolytic agents. In addition to oral and parenteral antibiotics, inhaled antibiotics are used to help minimize systemic effects.[109] The use of anti-inflammatory agents is controversial but may help minimize airway inflammation. Recombinant deoxyribonuclease therapy has been used, with some success, to minimize airway obstruction.[110]

PROGNOSIS

Although the mortality rate is high, CF patients often survive into early adulthood. The severity of lung disease often determines long-term survival. New treatment modalities that are being investigated to help prolong survival include lung transplantation and gene therapy.

ORAL HEALTH CONSIDERATIONS

It has been suggested that patients with CF may have the same type of dentofacial morphology as other mouth-breathing patients.[111] However, larger prospective studies are need to confirm this.

As with other patients with chronic lower respiratory infections, improved oral hygiene may minimize exacerbation of the underlying condition.

Pulmonary Embolism

Pulmonary embolism (PE) is defined as a blockage of a pulmonary arterial vessel due to a thromboembolic event. The embolus may originate anywhere, but it is usually due to a thrombosis in the lower extremities.[112] Risk factors for PE include prolonged immobilization (such as in a postoperative state), lower-extremity trauma, a history of deep-vein thromboses, and the use of estrogen-containing oral contraceptives (especially in association with tobacco smoking).[113]

PATHOPHYSIOLOGY

PE causes occlusion of pulmonary arterial vessels, which results in a ventilation-perfusion mismatch. Massive PE causes right-sided heart failure and is rapidly progressive. Local bronchoconstriction may occur due to factors released by platelets and mast cells at the sites of occlusion. Pulmonary hypertension due to vessel occlusion and arterial vasospasm is a common finding.

CLINICAL AND LABORATORY FINDINGS

Patients usually present with dyspnea. Other features that are variably present include chest pain, fever, diaphoresis, cough, hemoptysis, and syncope. Physical findings can include evidence of a lower-extremity deep-vein thrombosis, tachypnea, crackles or rub on lung auscultation, and heart murmur.

Measurements of arterial blood gases are helpful as patients may demonstrate a decrease in PaO_2 and partial pressure of arterial carbon dioxide ($PaCO_2$), with an increase in hydrogen ion concentration (pH). However, normal arterial blood gases do not rule out the possibility of PE. Chest radiography is often unhelpful but may reveal suggestive signs such as elevated diaphragms, pleural effusions, and pulmonary artery dilatation.

Ventilation-perfusion (V-Q) scanning is a noninvasive study that can exclude the diagnosis of PE; however, it is inadequate for establishing the diagnosis of PE. V-Q scanning uses radioactive tracers to measure ventilation and perfusion in different parts of the lung. An area that shows no perfusion but normal ventilation is suggestive of PE. Pulmonary arteriography is the "gold standard" study and is usually performed when the results of V-Q scanning are inconclusive.[114]

CLASSIFICATION

Four separate PE syndromes have been described: (1) massive PE, (2) PE with pulmonary infarction, (3) PE without infarction or cor pulmonale, and (4) organized emboli in central arteries. There is significant overlap among these syndromes.[115]

DIAGNOSIS

The diagnosis is made on the basis of history and physical findings. V-Q scanning should be performed in suspected cases, with pulmonary arteriography reserved for suspected cases with inconclusive V-Q scanning results.

MANAGEMENT

Fibrinolytic agents, such as streptokinase and urokinase, are effective for rapid lysis of emboli. Newer fibrinolytic agents include tissue-type plasminogen activator, single-chain urokinase-like plasminogen activator, and anistreplase. A heparin infusion is started, followed by long-term management with warfarin. Surgical embolectomy can be performed in unstable patients for whom anticoagulants are contraindicated. Patients with recurrent disease may be candidates for vena caval interruption by placement of a Greenfield vena caval filter.

PROGNOSIS

Although many patients with PE die before medical attention is received, the rate of mortality due to PE once adequate anticoagulation therapy is initiated is less than 5%.

ORAL HEALTH CONSIDERATIONS

The main concern in the provision of dental care for individuals with PE is the patient who is being managed with oral anticoagulants. As a general rule, dental care (including simple extractions) can safely be provided for patients with prothrombin times of up to 20 seconds or an international normalized ratio of 2.5. However, it is recommended that any dental care for these patients be coordinated with their primary medical care provider.

Pulmonary Neoplasm

Lung cancer is the leading cause of cancer deaths in both men and women. More than 100,000 people in the United States die each year due to lung cancer. Men and women who are over the age of 45 years and who have a long history of tobacco smoking are at highest risk.[116]

Squamous cell carcinomas account for one-third of all lung cancers. The neoplasm derives from bronchial epithelial cells that have undergone squamous metaplasia. This is a slow-growing neoplasm that invades the bronchi and leads to airway obstruction.

Small cell carcinomas account for approximately one-fourth of all lung cancers. These derive from neuroendocrine cells in the airways and metastasize rapidly. Most small cell tumors have metastasized prior to diagnosis.

Adenocarcinomas account for approximately one-third of all lung cancers. These neoplasms are of glandular origin and develop in a peripheral distribution. They grow more rapidly than squamous cell carcinomas and tend to invade the pleura. The bronchoalveolar tumor (a type of adenocarcinoma) is derived from bronchiolar or alveolar epithelium. This cancer is not associated with exposure to tobacco smoke.[117]

Large cell carcinomas, which account for most of the remaining lung cancers, include anaplastic and giant cell tumors. They are poorly differentiated tumors that resemble neither squamous cell carcinomas nor adenocarcinomas.

PATHOPHYSIOLOGY

Metaplasia of the respiratory epithelium occurs in response to injury, such as that induced by tobacco smoking. With continued injury, the cells become dysplastic, with the loss of differentiating features. Neoplastic change first occurs locally; invasive carcinoma usually follows shortly thereafter.[118]

CLINICAL AND LABORATORY FINDINGS

A chronic nonproductive cough is the most common symptom. Sputum production may occur, usually associated with obstructive lesions. Hemoptysis is present in up to 30% of patients.[119] Dyspnea is variably present. Facial edema, cyanosis, and orthopnea indicate the possibility of superior vena cava syndrome, caused by compression of the superior vena cava by tumor. The acute onset of hoarseness may signal tumor compression of the recurrent laryngeal nerve. Shoulder and forearm pain might suggest the presence of Pancoast's tumor, which is found in the apical region of the lungs below the pleura.

Metastatic and paraneoplastic effects are also common. The symptoms of metastasis depend on the sites involved and on the size of the tumor. The bones, the brain, and the liver are common sites of metastasis. Paraneoplastic effects include endocrine abnormalities that are due to tumors that secrete hormones such as antidiuretic hormone, adrenocorticotropic hormone, and parathyroid hormone–related peptides.[120]

CLASSIFICATION

The World Health Organization has differentiated pulmonary neoplasms into 12 distinct histologic types. The major clinical distinction is between small cell types and non-small-cell types; each type has different therapeutic implications. The four major pathologic categories are squamous cell carcinoma, small cell carcinoma, adenocarcinoma, and large cell carcinoma.

DIAGNOSIS

Diagnosis is suggested by history and physical examination. Chest radiography should be performed in suspected patients. Radiographs of symptomatic patients are normal 90% of the time. Computerized tomography is useful for patients who show no visible lesions on plain-film radiography. Sputum cytology may establish the diagnosis, even in the absence of an abnormal chest radiograph. Bronchoscopy is often performed to obtain a tissue diagnosis and to help localize the tumor.

MANAGEMENT

Surgical excision is the treatment of choice. Nonresectable tumors are difficult to treat because most are only minimally responsive to chemotherapy; the exception is small cell carcinoma, which may respond dramatically, especially if the disease is limited to one hemithorax. Radiation therapy is an important palliative measure, especially for patients with superior vena cava syndrome, brain metastases, or bone lesions.

PROGNOSIS

The 5-year survival rate for all patients with lung cancer is 8%. However, the 5-year survival rate for patients treated by resection is greater than 50%. For patients with small cell carcinoma confined to one hemithorax, a 1-year survival rate of 70% can be achieved with chemotherapy.

▼ REFERENCES

1. Pitkaranta A. Rhinoviruses: important respiratory pathogens. Ann Med 1998;30(6):529.
2. Mygind N, Gwaltney JM Jr, Winther B, Hendley JO. The common cold and asthma. Allergy 1999;54 Suppl 57:146..
3. Van Kempen M, Bachert C, Van Cauwenberge P. An update on the pathophysiology of rhinovirus upper respiratory tract infections. Rhinology 1999;37:97.
4. Schneider LC, Lester MR. Atopic diseases and upper respiratory infections. Curr Opin Pediatr 1999;11:475.
5. Dowell SF, Schwartz B, Phillips WR. Appropriate use of antibiotics for URIs in children: part II. Cough, pharyngitis and the common cold. The Pediatric URI Consensus Team. Am Fam Physician 1998;58:1335–42, 1345.
6. Temte JL, Shult PA, Kirk CJ, Amspaugh J. Effects of viral respiratory disease education and surveillance on antibiotic prescribing. Fam Med 1999;31:101.
7. Butler CC, Rollnick S, Kinnersley P, et al. Reducing antibiotics for respiratory tract symptoms in primary care: consolidating 'why' and considering 'how'. Br J Gen Pract 1998;48:1865.
8. Shanker S, Vig KWL, Beck FM, et al. Dentofacial morphology amd upper respiratory function in 8-10-year-old children. Clin Orthod Res 1999;2:19.
9. Welch MJ, Kemp JP. Allergy in children. Prim Care 1987;14:575.
10. Suonpaa J. Treatment of allergic rhinitis. Ann Med 1996;28:17.
11. Simons FE. Recent advances in H1-receptor antagonist treatment. J Allergy Clin Immunol 1990;86(6 Pt 2):995.
12. Bousquet J, Lockey R, Malling HJ, et al. Allergen immunotherapy: therapeutic vaccines for allergic diseases. A WHO position paper. J Allergy Clin Immunol 1998;102(4 Pt 1):558.
13. Ramilo O. Role of respiratory viruses in acute otitis media: implications for management. Pediatr Infect Dis J 1999;18:1125.
14. Dowell SF, Schwartz B, Phillips WR. Appropriate use of antibiotics for URIs in children: part I. Otitis media and acute sinusitis. The Pediatric URI Consensus Team. Am Fam Physician 1998;58:1113–8, 1123.
15. Blumer JL. Fundamental basis for rational therapeutics in acute otitis media. Pediatr Infect Dis J 1999;18:1130.
16. Maw R, Stewart I, Schilder A, Browning G. Surgical treatment of chronic otitis media with effusion. Int J Pediatr Otorhinolaryngol 1999;49 Suppl 1:S239.

17. Klein JO. Review of consensus reports on management of acute otitis media. Pediatr Infect Dis J 1999;18:1152.

18. Schilder AG. Assessment of complications of the condition and of the treatment of otitis media with effusion. Int J Pediatr Otorhinolaryngol 1999;49 Suppl 1:S247.

19. Maltinski G. Nasal disorders and sinusitis. Prim Care 1998;25:663.

20. Brook I. Microbiology and management of sinusitis. J Otolaryngol 1996;25:249.

21. Low DE, Desrosiers M, McSherry J, et al. A practical guide for the diagnosis and treatment of acute sinusitis. Can Med Assoc J 1997;156 Suppl 6:S1.

22. Wagner W. Changing diagnostic and treatment strategies for chronic sinusitis. Cleve Clin J Med 1996;63:396.

23. Fagnan LJ. Acute sinusitis: a cost-effective approach to diagnosis and treatment. Am Fam Physician 1998;58:1795–805.

24. Josephson GD, Gross CW. Diagnosis and management of acute and chronic sinusitis. Compr Ther 1997;23:708.

25. Sandler NA, Johns FR, Braun TW. Advances in the management of acute and chronic sinusitis. J Oral Maxillofac Surg 1996;54:1005.

26. Arjmand EM, Lusk RP. Management of recurrent and chronic sinusitis in children. Am J Otolaryngol 1995;16:367.

27. Wagaiyu EG, Ashley FP. Mouthbreathing, lip seal and upper lip coverage and their relationship with gingival inflammation in 11-14 year-old schoolchildren. J Clin Periodontol 1991;18:698.

28. Barrow HN, Vastola AP, Wang RC. Adult supraglottitis. Otolaryngol Head Neck Surg 1993;109(3 Pt 1):474.

29. Rosekrans JA . Viral croup: current diagnosis and treatment. Mayo Clin Proc 1998;73:1102.

30. Sataloff RT, Speigel JR, Hawkshaw M, Rosen DC. Gastroesophageal reflux laryngitis. Ear Nose Throat J 1993;72:113.

31. Kaditis AG, Wald ER. Viral croup: current diagnosis and treatment. Pediatr Infect Dis J 1998;17:827.

32. Klassen TP. Recent advances in the treatment of bronchiolitis and laryngitis. Pediatr Clin North Am 1997;44:249.

33. Orlicek SL. Management of acute laryngotracheo-bronchitis. Pediatr Infect Dis J 1998;17:1164.

34. Sitzman SJ, Fiechtner HB. Treatment of croup with glucocorticoids. Ann Pharmacother 1998;32:973.

35. Dawson K, Cooper D, Cooper P, et al. The management of acute laryngo-tracheo-bronchitis (croup): a consensus view. J Paediatr Child Health 1992;28:223.

36. Denny FW Jr. Tonsillopharyngitis. Pediatr Rev 1994;15:185.

37. Pichichero ME, Green JL, Francis AB, et al. Recurrent group A streptococcal tonsillopharyngitis. Pediatr Infect Dis J 1998;17:809.

38. Margileth AM, Thompson HC, Osborne CE. Management criteria, recording of performance, and peer review of tonsillopharyngitis. Am J Dis Child 1977;131:270.

39. Brook I, Gober AE. Persistence of group A beta-hemolytic streptococci in toothbrushes and removable orthodontic appliances following treatment of pharyngotonsillitis. Arch Otolaryngol Head Neck Surg 1998;124:993.

40. Russell SL, Boylan RJ, Kaslick RS, et al. Respiratory pathogen colonization of the dental plaque of institutional elders. Spec Care Dentist 1999;19:128.

41. Hayes C, Sparrow D, Cohen M, et al. The association between alveolar bone loss and pulmonary function: the VA Dental Longitudinal Study. Ann Periodontol 1998;3:257.

42. Scannapieco FA, Stewart EM, Mylotte JM. Colonization of dental plaque by respiratory pathogens in medical intensive care patients. Crit Care Med 1992;20:740.

43. Mojon P, Budtz-Jorgensen E, Michel JP, Limeback H. Oral health and history of respiratory tract infection in frail institutionalized elders. Gerodontology 1997;14:9.

44. Fourrier F, Duvivier B, Boutigny H, et al. Colonization of dental plaque: a source of nosocomial infections in intensive care unit patients. Crit Care Med 1998;26:301.

45. Scannapieco FA, Papandonatos GD, Dunford RG. Associations between oral conditions and respiratory disease in a national sample survey population. Ann Periodontol 1998;3:251.

46. Becker KL, Appling S. Acute bronchitis. Lippincotts Prim Care Pract 1998;2:643–6.

47. Hueston WJ, Mainous AG 3rd. Acute bronchitis. Am Fam Physician 1998;57:1270–6, 1281–2.

48. Andersen P. Pathogenesis of lower respiratory tract infections due to Chlamydia, Mycoplasma, Legionella and viruses. Thorax 1998;53:302.

49. Macfarlane J. Lower respiratory tract infection and pneumonia in the community. Semin Respir Infect 1999;14:151.

50. Reimer LG, Carroll K. Role of the microbiology laboratory in the diagnosis of lower respiratory tract infections. Clin Infect Dis 1998;26:742.

51. Leviner E, Tzukert AA, Benoliel R, et al. Development of resistant oral viridans streptococci after administration of prophylactic antibiotics: time management in the dental treatment of patients susceptible to infective endocarditis. Oral Surg Oral Med Oral Pathol 1987;64:417.

52. Ewig S. Community-acquired pneumonia: definition, epidemiology, and outcome. Semin Respir Infect 1999;14:94.

53. Bryan CS. Blood cultures for community-acquired pneumonia: no place to skimp. Chest 1999;116:1153.

54. Cross JT Jr, Campbell GD Jr. Drug-resistant pathogens in community- and hospital-acquired pneumonia. Clin Chest Med 1999;20:499.

55. Pozzi E . Community-acquired pneumonia. The ORIONE Board. Monaldi Arch Chest Dis 1999;54:337.

56. Woodhead M. Management of pneumonia in the outpatient setting. Semin Respir Infect 1998;13:8.

57. Scannapieco FA. Role of oral bacteria in respiratory infection. J Periodontol 1999;70:793.

58. Marrie TJ, Peeling RW, Fine MJ, et al. Ambulatory patients with community-acquired pneumonia: the frequency of atypical agents and clinical course. Am J Med 1996;101:508.

59. Deriso AJ II, Ladowski JS, Dillon TA, et al. Chlorhexidine gluconate 0.12% oral rinse reduces the incidence of total nosocomial respiratory infection and non-prophylactic systemic antibiotic use in patients undergoing heart surgery. Chest 1996;109:1556.

60. Simons D, Kidd EAM, Beighton D. Oral health of elderly occupants in residential homes. Lancet 1999;353:1761.

61. Yoneyama T, Yoshida M, Matsui T, Sasaki H. Oral care and pneumonia. Lancet 1999;354:515.

62. Epler GR. Bronchiolar disorders with airflow obstruction. Curr Opin Pulm Med 1996;2:134.

63. Penn CC, Liu C. Bronchiolitis following infection in adults and children. Clin Chest Med 1993;14:645.

64. Rodriguez WJ, Parrott RH. Ribavirin aerosol treatment of serious respiratory syncytial virus infection in infants. Infect Dis Clin North Am 1987;1:425.

65. DeVincenzo J. Prevention and treatment of respiratory syncytial virus infections (for advances in pediatric infectious diseases). Adv Pediatr Infect Dis 1997;13:1.

66. Ellis EF. Relationship between the allergic state and susceptibility to infectious airway disease. Pediatr Res 1977;11(3 Pt 2):227.

67. Peebles RS Jr, Hartert TV. Respiratory viruses and asthma. Curr Opin Pulm Med 2000;6:10.

68. Rusznak C, Devalia JL, Davies RJ. The impact of pollution on allergic disease. Allergy 1994;49(18 Suppl):21.

69. Creer TL, Winder JA, Tinkelman D. Guidelines for the diagnosis and management of asthma: accepting the challenge. J Asthma 1999;36:391.

70. Georgitis JW. The 1997 Asthma Management Guidelines and therapeutic issues relating to the treatment of asthma. National Heart, Lung, and Blood Institute. Chest 1999;115:210.

71. Kwong KY, Jones CA. Chronic asthma therapy. Pediatr Rev 1999;20:327.

72. Weltman JK. The use of inhaled corticosteroids in asthma. Allergy Asthma Proc 1999;20:255.

73. Martinez FD. Present and future treatment of asthma in infants and young children. J Allergy Clin Immunol 1999; 104(4 Pt 2):169.

74. Balfour-Lynn I. Difficult asthma: beyond the guidelines. Arch Dis Child 1999;80:201.

75. Abramson M, Puy R, Weiner J. Immunotherapy in asthma: an updated systematic review. Allergy 1999;54:1022.

76. Mungo RP, Kopel HM, Church JA. Pediatric dentistry and the child with asthma. Spec Care Dentist 1986;6:270.

77. Steinbacher DM, Glick M. Asthma: an update in oral health considerations. General Am Health Assoc 2001;132:1229–39.

78. Copp PE. The asthmatic dental and oral surgery patient. A review of management considerations. Ont Dent 1995;72(6):33–42.

79. Zhu JF, Hidalgo HA, Holmgreen WC, et al. Dental management of children with asthma. Pediatr Dent 1996;18:363.

80. Mathew T, Casamassimo PS, Wilson S, et al. Effect of dental treatment on the lung function of children with asthma. J Am Dent Assoc 1998;129:1120.

81. Spurlock BW, Dailey TM. Shortness of (fresh) breath: toothpaste-induced bronchospasm. N Engl J Med 1990;323:143.

82. Subiza J, Subiza JL, Valdivieso R, et al. Toothpaste flavor-induced asthma. J Allergy Clin Immunol 1992;90:1004.

83. Hallstrom U. Adverse reaction to a fissure sealant: report of a case. ASDC J Dent Child 1993;60:143–6.

84. Housholder GT, Chan JT. Tooth enamel dust as an asthma stimulus: a case report. Oral Surg Oral Med Oral Pathol 1993;75:599.

85. Nayebzadeh A, Dufresne A. Evaluation of exposure to methyl methacrylate among dental laboratory technicians. Am Ind Hyg Assoc J 1999;60:625.

86. Vig KW. Nasal obstruction and facial growth: the strength of evidence for clinical assumptions. Am J Orthod Dentofacial Orthop 1998;113:603.

87. Yamada T, Tanne K, Miyamoto K, Yamauchi K. Influences of nasal respiratory obstruction on craniofacial growth in young Macaca fuscata monkeys. Am J Orthod Dentofacial Orthop 1997;111:38.

88. Laurikainen K, Kuusisto P. Comparison of the oral health status and salivary flow rate of asthmatic patients with those of nonasthmatic adults — results of a pilot study. Allergy 1998;53:316.

89. Lenander-Lumikari M, Laurikainen K, Kuusisto P, Vilja P. Stimulated salivary flow rate and composition in asthmatic and non-asthmatic adults. Arch Oral Biol 1998;43:151.

90. Kankaala TM, Virtanen JI, Larmas MA. Timing of first fillings in the primary dentition and permanent first molars of asthmatic children. Acta Odontol Scand 1998;56:20.

91. McDerra EJC, Pollard MA, Curzon MEJ. The dental status of asthmatic British school children. Pediatr Dent 1998;20:281.

92. McNab S, Battistutta D, Taverne A, Symons AL. External apical root resorption of posterior teeth in asthmatics after orthodontic treatment. J Orthod Dentofacial Orthop 1999;116:545.

93. Ryberg M, Moller C, Ericson T. Saliva composition and caries development in asthmatic patients treated with beta 2-adrenoceptor agonists: a 4-year follow-up study. Scand J Dent Res 1991;99:212.

94. Storhaug K. Caries experience in disabled pre-school children. Acta Odontol Scand 1985;43:241.

95. Malamed SF. Medical emergencies in the dental office. 5th ed. St. Louis (MO): Year Book Medical Publishers; 2000.

96. Turner-Warwick M. Epidemiology of nocturnal asthma. Am J Med 1988;85(Suppl 1B):6

97. Seng GF, Gay BJ. Dangers of sulfites in dental local anesthetic solutions: warning and recommendations. J Am Dent Assoc 1986;113:769.

98. Israel E, Fischer AR, Rosenberg MA, et al. The pivotal role of 5-lipoxygenase products in the reaction of aspirin-sensitive asthmatics to aspirin. Am Rev Respir Dis 1993;148:1447.

99. Shaheen SO, Sterne JA, Songhurst CE, Burney PG. Frequent paracetamol use and asthma in adults. Thorax 2000; 55(4):266–70.

100. Clausen JL. The diagnosis of emphysema, chronic bronchitis, and asthma. Clin Chest Med 1990;11:405.

101. Martinez FJ. Diagnosing chronic obstructive pulmonary disease. The importance of differentiating asthma, emphysema, and chronic bronchitis. Postgrad Med 1998;103:112–7, 121–2, 125.

102. Thurlbeck WM. Pathophysiology of chronic obstructive pulmonary disease. Clin Chest Med 1990;11:389.

103. Jeffery PK. Differences and similarities between chronic obstructive pulmonary disease and asthma. Clin Exp Allergy 1999;29 Suppl 2:14.

104. Make B. COPD: management and rehabilitation. Am Fam Physician 1991;43:1315.

105. The Lung Health Study Research Group. Effect of inhaled triamcinolone on the decline in pulmonary function in chronic obstructive pulmonary disease. N Engl J Med 2000;343:1902.

106. Hodgkin JE. Prognosis in chronic obstructive pulmonary disease. Clin Chest Med 1990;11:555.

107. Torres A, Dorca J, Zalacain R, et al. Community-acquired pneumonia in chronic obstructive pulmonary disease: a Spanish multicenter study. Am J Respir Crit Care Med 1996;154:1456.

108. Passero MA. Cystic fibrosis. Med Health R I 1999;82:164.

109. Campbell PW 3rd, Saiman L. Use of aerosolized antibiotics in patients with cystic fibrosis. Chest 1999;116:775.

110. Rubin BK. Emerging therapies for cystic fibrosis lung disease. Chest 1999;115:1120.

111. Hellsing E, Brattstrom V, Strandvik B. Craniofacial morphology in children with cystic fibrosis. Eur J Orthod 1992;14:147.

112. Davidson BL. Controversies in pulmonary embolism and deep venous thrombosis. Am Fam Physician 1999;60:1969.

113. Fennerty T. Thromboembolic disease: the new risk factors explained. Practitioner 1999;243:402, 405–8, 410.

114. Saro G, Campo JF, Hernandez MJ, et al. Diagnostic approach to patients with suspected pulmonary embolism: a report from the real world. Postgrad Med J 1999;75:285.

115. Girard P, Musset D, Parent F, et al. High prevalence of detectable deep venous thrombosis in patients with acute pulmonary embolism. Chest 1999;116:903.

116. Mizushima Y, Yokoyama A, Ito M, et al. Lung carcinoma in patients age younger than 30 years. Cancer 1999;85:1730.

117. Lee KS, Kim Y, Han J, et al. Bronchioloalveolar carcinoma: clinical, histopathologic, and radiologic findings. Radiographics 1997;17:1345.

118. Fong KM, Sekido Y, Minna JD. Molecular pathogenesis of lung cancer. J Thorac Cardiovasc Surg 1999;118:1136.

119. Colby TV. Malignancies in the lung and pleura mimicking benign processes. Semin Diagn Pathol 1995;12:30.

120. Sellars RE, Zimmerman PV. Lung cancer. Med J Aust 1997;167:99–104.

13

▼

DISEASES OF THE CARDIOVASCULAR SYSTEM

FRANK E. SILVESTRY, MD

MICHAEL GLICK, DMD

ELIZABETH A. TARKA, MD

IRVING M. HERLING, MD

Cardiovascular disease (CVD) is the leading cause of death in the world and accounts for well over one million deaths each year in the United States. Of the more than two million deaths in the United States in 1998, CVD was listed as the primary or contributing cause in 70% of cases.[1] According to the Centers of Disease Control and Prevention (CDC) and the National Health and Nutrition Examination Survey III, the probability at birth of dying from CVD is 47%, compared to 22% from cancer, 2% from diabetes, and less than 1% from human immunodeficiency virus (HIV) disease. The largest proportion of this high mortality is attributed to coronary artery disease (CAD) or coronary heart disease (CHD), which was the primary contributing cause of death in 459,841 Americans in 1998.[1]

CVD includes hypertension, coronary artery disease (CAD), congestive heart failure (CHF), congenital cardiovascular defects, and stroke. The prevalence of these entities in the United States surpasses 60 million cases (Table 13-1). Although these diseases are associated with a high mortality, the associated morbidity affects all walks of life and has a great impact on the quality of life of affected individuals. This chapter presents a brief overview of common cardiovascular conditions and their implications for the practice of dental medicine.

▼ HYPERTENSION

General Description and Incidence

About 20% of the entire US population has hypertension at any one time, and many will develop it as they age (Table 13-2). This sobering statistic translates into more than 50,000,000 Americans with high blood pressure (BP). However, although the majority of individuals are aware of their elevated BP, only an estimated 23 to 27% of hypertensive patients are being treated and have achieved normotensive control.[2,3]

Hypertension is defined as having systolic blood pressure (SBP) ≥ 140 mm Hg or diastolic blood pressure (DBP) ≥ 90 mm Hg or as having to use antihypertensive medications. Approximately every 5 years, the National Heart, Lung and

TABLE 13-1 Prevalence of Cardiovascular Disease in the United States

Type of Cardiovascular Disease	No. of Patients
High blood pressure	50,000,000
Coronary artery disease	12,400,000
Myocardial infarction	7,300,000
Angina pectoris	6,400,000
Stroke	4,500,000
Congenital cardiovascular disease	1,000,000
Congestive heart failure	4,700,000
Total	60,800,000

Reproduced with permission from American Heart Association.[1]

TABLE 13-2 Prevalence of Hypertension by Age (United States)

Age group (yr)	Percentage of Individuals with Hypertension		
	Men	Women	Total
18–24	4.6	0.7	2.6
25–34	8.4	2.4	5.4
35–44	16.0	10.2	13.0
45–54	30.0	25.2	27.6
55–64	44.2	43.2	43.7
65–74	55.8	62.7	59.6
≥75	60.5	76.2	70.3
Total	23.5	23.3	23.4

Reproduced with permission of Wolz M, Culter J, Roccella EJ, et al. Statement from the National High Blood Pressure Education Program: prevalence of hypertension. Am J Hypertens 2000;13:103.

Blood Institute (NHLBI), through its Joint National Committee on Prevention, Detection, Evaluation, and Treatment of High Blood Pressure, puts forth recommendations for the treatment of high BP. Its sixth and latest recommendation (JNC VI) was published in 1997.[3,4] This document defined cardiovascular risk stratification and treatment strategies and also re-defined BP classifications for adults (Tables 13-3 to 13-6). The purpose of these guidelines was to reduce the morbidity and mortality associated with high BP and hypertension as several clinical trials have suggested that the lowering of BP reduces the risk of end-organ disease.[5,6]

TABLE 13-3 Cardiovascular Risk Factors in Hypertensive Patients

Major risk factors
  Smoking
  Dyslipidemia
  Diabetes mellitus
  Age > 60 yr
  Male sex
  Postmenopause
  Family history of cardiovascular disease (women aged < 65 yr, men aged < 55 yr)

Target organ damage/clinical cardiovascular disease
  Heart diseases
    Left ventricular hypertrophy
    Angina/prior myocardial infarct
    Prior coronary revascularization
    Heart failure
  Stroke or transient ischemic attack
  Nephropathy
  Peripheral arterial disease
  Retinopathy

Reproduced with permission from National High Blood Pressure Education Program.[4]

TABLE 13-4   Cardiovascular Risk Stratification

Risk Group	Risk Factors and Disease
A	No risk factors No target organ disease/clinical CVD
B	At least one risk factor No target organ disease/clinical CVD
C	Target organ disease/clinical CVD and/or diabetes, with or without other risk factors

Reproduced with permission of National High Blood Pressure Education Program.[4]

CVD = cardiovascular disease.

Etiology

Hypertension is classified as primary (or essential) and secondary. Ninety-five percent of all hypertension is of unknown cause. The use of new molecular biologic tools will likely serve to better delineate some of the basic mechanisms of primary hypertension. There are many secondary causes, but these account for only 5 to 10% of patients with hypertension. These include renal disorders such as renal parenchymal disease, renovascular disease, renin-producing tumors, and primary sodium retention. Endocrinologic disturbances that may result in hypertension include thyroid disease, adrenal disorders, carcinoid, and exogenous hormones. Remaining causes include aortic coarctation, complications of pregnancy (such as pre-eclampsia), neurologic causes, acute stress, alcohol ingestion, nicotine use, increased intravascular volume, and the use of drugs such as cyclosporine or tacrolimus.

Risk Factor Modification

Hypertension is a well-recognized risk factor for CAD. With improved control of BP, there has been a steady decrease in mortality from CHD and an even greater decrease in mortality from stroke. It is important to realize that hypertension is a chronic disease with long-term sequelae. Therefore, treatment focuses on prevention to reduce complications that eventually affect target organs (mainly the brain, heart, kidneys, eyes, and peripheral arteries). Complications of hypertension include cerebral hemorrhage, left ventricular hypertrophy,

TABLE 13-6   Classification of Blood Pressure in Adults

Category*	SBP and/or DBP (mm Hg)
Optimal[†]	< 120 and < 80
Normal	< 130 and < 85
High-normal	130–139 or 85–89
Hypertension[‡]	
Stage 1	140–159 or 90–99
Stage 2	160–179 or 100–109
Stage 3	≥180 or ≥110

Reproduced with permission from National High Blood Pressure Education Program.[4]

DBP = diastolic blood pressure; SBP = systolic blood pressure.

*When SBP and DBP fall into different categories, the higher category should be used.

[†]Optimal blood pressure with respect to cardiovascular risk is < 120/80; however, unusually low readings should be evaluated for clinical significance.

[‡]Based on the average of two or more readings taken at each of two or more visits after an initial screening visit.

CHF, renal insufficiency, aortic dissection, and atherosclerotic disease of various vascular beds.

Diagnosis

Because hypertension is usually asymptomatic for many years, many patients are undiagnosed, and many hypertensive patients present with only a mild elevation in BP. The diagnosis of hypertension is made only after an elevated BP has been recorded on multiple BP readings. Stage 1 hypertension refers to an SBP of 140 to 159 mm Hg or a DBP of 90 to 99 mm Hg. Stage 2 hypertension is defined as an SBP of 160 to 179 mm Hg or a DBP of 100 to 109 mm Hg, and stage 3 hypertension is found when the SBP is ≥ 180 mm Hg and the DBP is ≥ 110 mm Hg (see Table 13-6). The BP level as well as other clinical factors determines the severity of hypertension. These other factors include certain demographic features (age, sex, race), the extent of the vascular damage induced by the high BP (ie, target organ involvement), and the presence of other risk factors for premature CVD (see Tables 13-3 and 13-4).

TABLE 13-5   Cardiovascular Treatment Strategies

Blood Pressure Stages (SBP/DBP [mm Hg])	Treatment Strategies		
	Risk Group A	Risk Group B	Risk Group C
High-normal (130–139/85–89)	Lifestyle modification	Lifestyle modification	Drug therapy;* lifestyle modification
1 (140–159/90–99)	Lifestyle modification (up to 12 mo)	Lifestyle modification (up to 6 mo)[†]	Drug therapy; lifestyle modification
2, 3 (≥160/≥100)	Drug therapy; lifestyle modification	Drug therapy; lifestyle modification	Drug therapy; lifestyle modification

Reproduced with permission from National High Blood Pressure Education Program.[4]

DBP = diastolic blood pressure; SBP = systolic blood pressure.

*For heart failure, renal insufficiency, or diabetes.

[†]For those with multiple risk factors, clinicians should consider drugs as initial therapy plus lifestyle modification.

The three main goals of the medical evaluation of patients with hypertension are to identify treatable (secondary) or curable causes, to assess the impact of persistently elevated BP on target organs, and to estimate the patient's overall risk profile for the development of premature CVD.

A routine history and physical examination should be performed. The history should focus on the duration of the hypertension and any prior treatment. Asking the patient, "How long have you had high blood pressure?" may be misleading as in many cases the patient often will not have had a BP measurement for many years prior to the discovery of hypertension. Symptoms of organ dysfunction, lifestyle habits, diet, and psychosocial factors should be included.

PHYSICAL EXAMINATION

The main goals of the physical examination are to look for signs of end-organ damage (such as retinopathy) and to find evidence of a cause of secondary hypertension. Thus, the peripheral pulses should be palpated, and the abdomen should be ausculted for a renal artery bruit that would indicate renovascular hypertension. The presence of an upper-abdominal diastolic bruit that localizes toward one side is highly suggestive of renal artery stenosis. The physical examination should include a fundoscopic assessment.

LABORATORY AND ADDITIONAL TESTING

The only laboratory procedures that should be routinely performed are hematocrit, urinalysis, routine blood chemistries (glucose, creatinine, electrolytes), and a fasting lipid profile consisting of total and high-density lipoprotein (HDL) cholesterol and triglycerides. Twelve-lead electrocardiography should also be performed. Additional tests, outlined below, may be indicated in certain clinical settings.

Echocardiography. Echocardiography is a more sensitive method of detecting left ventricular hypertrophy than is routine electrocardiography, and limited echocardiography offers a less expensive alternative to a complete echocardiographic examination when the sole question is whether the patient has left ventricular hypertrophy (LVH). LVH is an independent predictor of mortality in patients with hypertension. This hypertrophy of the ventricle initially results in the impairment of left ventricular diastolic function and, if progressive, may impair the systolic function of the ventricle, thus diminishing its capacity to perform its normal function of pumping the blood out of the heart through the aortic valve and into the aorta. This increase in left ventricular mass may result in increased myocardial oxygen demand, which can result in myocardial ischemia and ultimately myocardial fibrosis with CHF.

Thus, the main indication for echocardiography is possible end-organ damage (in this case, damage to the heart) in a patient with borderline BP values. Echocardiography may also identify patients who would not be treated on the basis of clinical criteria alone.

Ambulatory Blood Pressure Monitoring. Ambulatory BP monitoring is capable of identifying patients with "white-coat hypertension" and also ensures the adequacy of therapy in the outpatient setting. However, at the present, many insurers do not reimburse for this procedure. As a result, the main indication for ambulatory BP monitoring is persistent hypertension in the office setting but normal BP readings in the ambulatory setting.

The term "white-coat hypertension" is used to describe a phenomenon in which individuals present with persistent elevated BP in a clinical setting but present with non-elevated BP in an ambulatory setting. The relationship between white-coat hypertension and the development of essential hypertension has not been thoroughly elucidated, but it is estimated that about 20% of mild hypertensive individuals may present with white-coat hypertension. Since BP readings in the ambulatory BP setting reflect BP throughout the day, an accurate ambulatory measure would theoretically better predict end-organ damage than would occasional clinical or office BP readings; yet, it is not clear if white-coat hypertension is associated with end-organ damage.[7]

Plasma Renin Activity Testing. Although plasma renin activity testing may provide prognostic information, it is usually performed only in patients with possible low-renin forms of hypertension, such as primary hyperaldosteronism. Unexplained hypokalemia is the primary clinical clue to this disorder, and its presence should prompt further diagnostic testing.

Radiologic Testing. Radiographic testing for renovascular disease is indicated only for patients whose history is suggestive and in whom a corrective procedure will be performed if significant renal artery stenosis is detected. Intra-arterial digital subtraction angiography has historically been the initial test when the history is highly suggestive; however, spiral computed tomography (CT) and magnetic resonance imaging (MRI) are becoming the standard screening tests when renovascular hypertension is strongly suspected. Renal ultrasonography is often used in a hypertensive patient with a family history of polycystic kidney disease.

Assessment of Cardiovascular Risk

Numerous aspects contribute to the detrimental association between hypertension and CVD.[8] Most studies have shown a strong correlation between long-term sustained elevated BP and the subsequent development of CVD. Recent prospective longitudinal studies suggest that BP that is even slightly elevated above normal is associated with increased mortality.[9] The underlying causes include the promotion of atherosclerosis and thrombogenesis, reduced coronary vasodilatory reserve, and left ventricular hypertrophy.[10–15]

The incidence of CVD increases stepwise with increasing BP. Studies have indicated that the risk of a cardiac event increases by 1.6 times in men and 2.5 times in women when BP increases from an optimal level (< 120/80 mm Hg) to a high normal level (130 to 139/85 to 89 mm Hg).[16] As is well defined by data from the Framingham Heart Study, a number of other risk factors interact with hypertension to affect the overall risk status of the individual patient.[11,17] These include hypercholesterolemia, diabetes mellitus, and smoking. Increased age of the patient may suggest a more detrimental effect conferred by an elevated systolic rather than diastolic pressure.[18] The presence or absence of other risk factors can influence the decision of whether to institute antihypertensive medications in a patient with borderline values.

Management

The treatment of hypertension is among the leading indications for the use of drugs in the United States. A large number of agents exist, including diuretics, β-blockers, calcium channel blockers, angiotensin-converting enzyme inhibitors (ACEIs), angiotensin II receptor blockers, direct vasodilators, and centrally acting agents (Table 13-7). Each of the antihypertensive agents is roughly equally effective, producing a good antihypertensive response in 40 to 60% of cases. Thus, the choice among the different antihypertensive drugs is not generally made on the basis of efficacy. There is, however, wide interpatient variability as many patients will respond well to one drug but not to another. The identification of the particular drug class to which a patient is more likely to respond is therefore one major criterion used in the choice of an antihypertensive agent.

The results of an increasing number of trials suggest that at the same level of BP control, most antihypertensive drugs provide similar degrees of cardiovascular protection. As an example, several recent major antihypertension drug trials found little overall difference in outcome between older (eg, diuretics and β-blockers) and newer (eg, ACEIs and calcium channel blockers) antihypertensive drugs.[19,20] However, there is some evidence that the use of particular agents may be associated with specific positive outcomes in specific clinical settings. For example, in the Heart Outcomes Prevention Evaluation (HOPE) study, a cardiovascular benefit from angiotensin-converting enzyme inhibition with ramipril was demonstrated in patients who were at high risk for CVD.[21] High risk was defined as either evidence of vascular disease (including CHD, stroke, peripheral vascular disease) or diabetes and at least one other coronary risk factor. In this trial, the primary end point was any cardiovascular event (cardiovascular death, myocardial infarction, or stroke). Most of the patients were on other cardioprotective medications, including aspirin, β-blockers, and lipid-lowering agents.

Patient compliance is another important aspect of choosing an antihypertensive agent. Inexpensive once-a-day preparations with few side effects are often desired. As above, the specific antihypertensive agent chosen for a patient may also depend on comorbid diseases. For example, β-blocker therapy is an excellent choice for patients who have CAD and hypertension. An ACEI is usually first-line therapy for a diabetic patient with microalbuminuria since ACEIs retard the progression of diabetic nephropathy. Although the use of diuretics has been decreasing over the past 10 years, diuretics are still among the most frequently prescribed medica-

tions for treating hypertension, probably because they are well tolerated and are inexpensive.

The role of education and the importance of patient contact are paramount in successfully treating hypertension. Self-recorded measurements and ambulatory BP monitoring aid in the physician's titration of medications and monitoring of the 24-hour duration of action of antihypertensive agents. The monitoring of BP by oral health care providers will therefore support the overall medical care of their hypertensive patients.

At present, there is no consensus on optimal initial drug therapy for hypertension as four of the major classes of antihypertensive drugs (diuretics, β-blockers, calcium channel blockers, and ACEIs) appear to provide equal benefit at the same degree of BP control.[22] Many physicians recommend either low-dose therapy (to maximize efficacy in relation to side effects) or "sequential monotherapy." A patient who is relatively unresponsive to one drug has almost a 50% likelihood of becoming normotensive on a second drug. This regimen of trying to find the one drug to which the patient is most responsive should minimize side effects and maximize patient compliance while being as effective as combination therapy.

The Systolic Hypertension in the Elderly Program (SHEP) trial showed that in older patients with systolic hypertension, low-dose thiazide therapy effectively lowered BP and led to a reduction in cardiovascular events as compared to placebo treatment.[23] In a more recent study, therapy based on a long-acting dihydropyridine calcium channel blocker provided protection almost identical to that previously noted with diuretic-based therapy.[24]

In those with uncomplicated hypertension, beginning with a low dose of a thiazide diuretic (eg, 12.5 to 25 mg of hydrochlorothiazide) has the advantages of very low cost and low risk of metabolic complications such as hypokalemia, lipid abnormalities, and hyperuricemia. If low-dose thiazide monotherapy is ineffective, an ACEI, a β-blocker, or a calcium channel blocker can be sequentially substituted. A calcium channel blocker is likely to be most effective in African American patients. A report suggesting that calcium channel blockers may increase the risk of myocardial infarction in hypertensive patients has not been confirmed in studies with long-acting dihydropyridines; the appropriate use of these drugs should therefore not be curtailed.[25] However, given the preliminary evidence that the patient who is unresponsive to a diuretic may also have a similar response to a calcium channel blocker, an ACEI or a β-blocker may be the preferred second-line agent.

Managing hypertensive patients who are undergoing surgery poses unique problems because they have an increased risk of perioperative mortality. However, the administration of antihypertensive therapy reduces this risk, and patients taking medications prior to surgery should thus be continued on therapy until surgery. Intravenous preparations are used during surgery and during the postoperative period, while the patient is on a nothing-by-mouth (NPO) order.

TABLE 13-7   Common Oral Hypertensive Medications

Drug	Trade Name	Side Effects
Diuretics		Increased cholesterol and glucose levels; oral dryness
Chlorthalidone	Hygroton	
Hydrochlorothiazide (HCTZ)	Hydrodiuril, Microzide, Esidrix	
Indapamide	Lozol	
Metolazone	Mykrox, Zaroxolyn	
Loop diuretics		
Bumetanide	Bumex	
Ethacrynic acid	Edecrin	
Furosemide	Lasix	
Torsemide	Demadrex	
Potassium-sparing agents		
Amiloride	Midamor	
Amiloride and HCTZ	Moduretic	
Spironolactone	Aldactone	
Spironolactone and HCTZ	Aldactizide	
Triamterene	Dyrenium	
Triamterene and HCTZ	Dyazide	
Adrenergic inhibitors		Postural hypertension; nasal congestion; sedation; bradycardia; oral dryness; oral ulcerations
Peripheral agents		
Guanadrel	Hylorel	
Guanethedine monosulfate	Ismelin	
Reserpine	Serpasil	
Central α-agonists		
Clonidine	Catapres	
Guanabenz acetate	Wytensin	
Guanfacine	Tenex	
Methyldopa	Aldomet	
α–Blockers		
Doxazosin mesylate	Cardura	
Prazosin	Minipress	
Terazosin	Hytrin	
β-Blockers		
Acebutolol	Sectral	
Atenolol	Tenormin	
Betaxolol	Kerlone	
Bisoprolol fumarate	Zebeta	
Carteolol hydrochloride	Cartrol	
Metoprolol tartrate	Lopressor	
Metoprolol succinate	Torpol-XL	
Nadolol	Corgard	
Penbutolol sulfate	Levatol	
Pindolol	Visken	
Propranolol hydrochloride	Inderal, Inderal LA	
Timolol maleate	Blocadren	
Combined α- and β-blockers		
Carvedilol	Coreg	
Labetalol hydrochloride	Normodyne, Trandate	
Direct vasodilators		Headaches; tachycardia
Hydralazine hydrochloride	Apresoline	
Minoxiil		

Continued

TABLE 13-7   Common Oral Hypertensive Medications (Continued)

Drug	Trade Name	Side Effects
Calcium antagonists		Gingival overgrowth
Nondihydropyridines		
Diltiazem hydrochloride	Cardizem SR, Cardizem CD, Dilactor XR, Tiazac	
Mibefradil dihydrochloride	Posicor	
Dihydropyridines		
Amlodipine besylate	Norvasc	
Felodipine	Plendil	
Isradipine	DynaCirc, DynaCirc CR	
Nicardipine	Cardene SR	
Nifedipine	Procardia XL, Adalat CC	
Nisoldipine	Sular	
ACE inhibitors		Cough; loss of taste; lichenoid reactions of the oral mucosa
Benazepril	Lotensin	
Captopril	Capoten	
Enalapril	Vasotec	
Fosinopril	Monopril	
Lisinopril	Prinivil, Zestril	
Moexipril	Univasc	
Perindopril	Aceon	
Quinapril	Accupril	
Ramipril	Altace	
Trandolapril	Mavik	
Angiotensin II receptor blockers		
Candesartan	Atacand	
Losartan potassium	Cozaar	
Valsartan	Diovan	
Irbesartan	Avapro	

ACE = angiotensin-converting enzyme.

Prognosis

Treatment of hypertension is important because it reduces overall mortality. An analysis of the Framingham Heart Study cohort showed that improved control of hypertension contributed to the decline in mortality from CVD over the past 30 years.[26] In randomized controlled trials, antihypertensive pharmacotherapy appears to have its predominant effect on stroke mortality.[27]

Oral Health Considerations

It is clear that patients with high BP are at increased risk for adverse advents in a dental setting when target organ disease is present. However, the absence of target organ disease does not mitigate a careful evaluation and treatment of patients within safe and appropriate parameters of care. Based on the medical model for assessment, risk stratification, and treatment of patients with hypertension, dental guidelines can be proposed[28] (Table 13-8). These guidelines do not release the dental practitioner from good clinical judgment, and they should be used in accordance with the dental provider's knowledge, training, and experience.

Oral health care providers also need to be aware of medications that (1) may have systemic side effects that are of importance to the provision of care, (2) interact with medications used during dental care, and (3) cause intraoral changes (see Table 13-7).

▼ CORONARY ARTERY DISEASE

General Description and Incidence

Coronary artery disease (CAD) accounts for approximately 30 to 50% of all cases of CVD. It is estimated that 12,400,000 Americans alive today have already suffered a myocardial infarction (MI) or experienced angina pectoris (chest pain).[1] Atherosclerosis, the most common cause of CAD, results from a wide variety of pathologic processes that interact with and disrupt the vascular endothelium. The result is plaque formation, with the compromise of effective arterial luminal area. In the coronary circulation, this process may cause a chronic reduction in coronary blood flow and ensuing myocardial ischemia or it may cause acute plaque rupture,

TABLE 13-8   Blood Pressure Measurement in the Dental Setting

Routine BP measurements
   Measure and record at initial visit
   Recheck:
      Every 2 years for patients with BP < 130/85
      Every year for patients with BP of 130–139/85–89
      Every visit for patients with BP ≥ 140/90
      Every visit for patients with diagnosed hypertension

Before initiating dental care:
   Assess presence of hypertension
   Determine presence of target organ disease
   After checking BP, determine treatment modifications

Dental treatment for patients with elevated BP
   Asymptomatic, BP < 159/99, no target organ disease
      No dental modifications needed
      Can safely be treated in a dental outpatient setting
   Asymptomatic, BP = 160–179/100–109, no history of target organ disease
      Assessment on individual basis with regard to type of dental procedure
   BP ≥ 180/110, no history of target organ disease
      No elective dental care
   Target organ disease or poorly controlled DM
      Elective dental care only when BP is controlled, preferably < 140/90

BP = blood pressure; DM = diabetes mellitus.

with intracoronary thrombus formation and subsequent MI. Atherosclerosis may affect any vascular bed, including the coronary, cerebral, renal, mesenteric, and peripheral vascular systems. When end-organ blood flow is compromised, the resulting ischemia can cause subsequent organ dysfunction.

Etiology

Atherosclerosis is responsible for almost all cases of CAD. This insidious process begins with a fatty streak, first seen in early adolescence; these lesions progress into plaques in early adulthood and may result in thrombotic occlusions and coronary events in middle age and later life. Other lipid metabolism abnormalities, systemic hypertension, diabetes mellitus, and cigarette smoking contribute to the total atherosclerotic plaque burden although these factors differ in their impact on CAD in clinical subgroups. For example, diabetes and a low HDL cholesterol/total cholesterol ratio have a greater impact in women, cigarette smoking has more of an impact in men, and SBP and isolated systolic hypertension are major risk factors at all ages and in either sex.

Risk Factors

Risk factor assessment is useful as a guide to therapy for dyslipidemia, hypertension, and diabetes; multivariable prediction rules can be used to help estimate risks for subsequent coronary disease events. An emerging model uses the risk of cardiovascular events over a 10- to 20-year period as a basis for initiating risk factor–modifying therapy for lipids.[29]

Based on the increased risk conferred by the various CAD risk factors, concepts of "normal" have continued to evolve from "usual" or "average" to more biologically optimal values associated with long-term freedom from disease. As a result, acceptable BP, blood sugar, and lipid values have been continually revised downward in the past 20 years.[4,30,31]

LIPIDS

The total cholesterol concentration in serum is a major and clear-cut risk factor for CHD. In the Multiple Risk Factor Intervention Trial of more than 350,000 middle-aged American men, the risk of CHD progressively increased with higher values of serum total cholesterol.[32] Recent data emphasize the advantages in knowing the concentrations of lipid subfractions, such as low-density lipoprotein (LDL) and HDL, in addition to total cholesterol.[31] Conversely, the concentration of serum HDL cholesterol is inversely associated with CHD incidence, consistent with its suggested role in reverse cholesterol transport.[33] Data from the Framingham Heart Study suggest that the risk for MI increases by about 25% for every 5 mg/dL decrement below median values for men and women.[34]

The HDL cholesterol/total cholesterol ratio represents a simple and efficient way to estimate coronary disease risk. Data from the Lipid Research Clinics and the Framingham Heart Study show that among men, a ratio result of ≥ 6.4 identified a group that was at a 2 to 14% percent greater risk than that predicted from serum total or LDL cholesterol; among women, a ratio of ≥ 5.6 or more identified a group as at a 25 to 45% greater risk than that predicted from serum total or LDL cholesterol.[35] In contrast, serum total or LDL cholesterol did not add an independent predictive value to the ratio.

Recommendations for lipid evaluation and therapy in adults were formulated by an expert committee of the National Cholesterol Education Program (NCEP) and were revised in 2001 as the ATP III. Stepped care for abnormal lipid levels consider individuals' overall risk factor burden and their 20-year risk of cardiovascular events. Treatment includes the dietary restriction of fat and cholesterol and recommends medications when certain LDL cholesterol levels are exceeded despite dietary interventions and other lifestyle modifications (Table 13-9).

A number of clinical trials, including the Scandinavian Simvastatin Survival Study trial, the Cholesterol and Recurrent Events (CARE) trial, and the West of Scotland Coronary Prevention Study trial, have shown that reductions in total and LDL cholesterol levels through the use of 3-hydroxy-3-methylglutaryl coenzyme A (HMG CoA) reductase enzyme inhibitors reduce coronary events and mortality when given for primary and secondary prevention.[36–39]

HYPERTENSION

Hypertension and LVH are well-established risk factors for adverse cardiovascular outcomes, including CHD morbidity and mortality, stroke, CHF, and sudden death. SBP is as powerful a coronary risk factor as DBP, and isolated systolic hypertension is now established as a major hazard for CHD and stroke, especially in the elderly population.[18,40]

However, while controlled trials have demonstrated clear benefits with BP reduction in terms of stroke and heart failure risk, they have not consistently demonstrated a benefit in coronary events, particularly in patients with mild degrees of hypertension. The increased coronary risk associated with hypertension is primarily seen in subgroups that have other

TABLE 13-9   Common Cholesterol-Lowering Medications

Drug	Trade Name	Side Effects
HMG CoA reductase inhibitors (statins)*		Myopathy; increased liver transaminases
Atorvastatin	Lipitor	
Fluvastatin	Leschol	
Lovastatin	Mevacor	
Pravastatin	Pravachol	
Simvastatin	Zocor	
Bile acid sequestrants		Decreased absorption of other drugs
Cholestyramine	—	
Colestipol	—	
Colesevelam	Welchol	
Nicotinic acid		Flushing; hyperglycemia; upper-GI distress; hepatotoxicity
Crystalline nicotinic acid	—	
Sustained-release nicotinic acid	—	
Extended-release nicotinic acid	Niaspan	
Fibric acid derivatives		Dyspepsia; upper-GI distress; myopathy
Gemfibrozil	Lopid	
Fenofibrate	Tricor	
Clofibrate	—	

GI = gastrointestinal; HMG CoA = 3-hydroxy-3-methylglutaryl coenzyme A.

*Avoid use with macrolide antibiotics.

risk factors or underlying target organ damage, and individuals in these subgroups derive the greatest benefit from antihypertensive therapy. The recommendations of the Sixth Joint National Committee on Prevention, Detection, Evaluation, and Treatment of High Blood Pressure provide guidelines for therapy according to stratification based on BP level and the presence or absence of underlying target organ disease.[4]

GLUCOSE INTOLERANCE AND DIABETES MELLITUS

Insulin resistance, hyperinsulinemia, and glucose intolerance all appear to promote atherosclerosis. In the Framingham Heart Study, diabetes, impaired glucose tolerance, and high normal levels of glycosylated hemoglobin were powerful contributors to atherosclerotic cardiovascular events, particularly in women.[41,42]

As diabetic individuals have a greater number of additional atherogenic risk factors (including hypertension, hypertriglyceridemia, increased cholesterol-to-HDL ratio, and elevated levels of plasma fibrinogen) than do nondiabetic individuals, the CHD risk for diabetic persons varies greatly with the severity of these risk factors. Thus, aggressive treatment of these additional risk factors may help reduce cardiovascular events in diabetic patients. For example, there is increasing evidence of the value of aggressive BP control in diabetic patients.[43] JNC VI and recent guidelines published by the NCEP help to provide goals for aggressive risk factor modification in diabetic patients.[4,31]

CIGARETTE SMOKING

Cigarette smoking is an important and potentially reversible risk factor for CHD and CHD events such as MI. For both men and women, the risk increases with increasing tobacco consumption.[44] For example, in one study, the risk of MI was sixfold increased for women and threefold increased for men who smoked at least 20 cigarettes per day, compared to nonsmoking control patients.[45] Conversely, the risk of recurrent infarction in a study of smokers who had had an MI was reduced by 50% within 1 year of smoking cessation and normalized to levels similar to those of nonsmokers within 2 years.[46] This benefit of smoking cessation is independent of the prior duration of smoking or the amount of smoking in the past.

ESTROGEN DEFICIENCY

The incidence of CHD in women increases after menopause, an effect that is thought to be secondary to low serum levels of estrogen. Accordingly, hormone replacement with low-dose exogenous estrogens appears to provide a protective effect against initial cardiovascular events such as MI.[47,48]

LIFESTYLE AND DIETARY FACTORS

Dietary factors such as a high-calorie, high-fat, and high-cholesterol diet contribute to the development of other risk factors, such as obesity, hyperlipidemia, and diabetes, that predispose to CHD. Conversely, a diet that emphasizes fruit and vegetables, as well as one associated with an increased intake of dietary fiber, is associated with a decreased risk of CAD.[49] Weight gain and obesity directly worsen the major cardiovascular risk factors whereas weight loss appears to improve them.[50] Epidemiologic data indicate that the moderate intake of alcohol has a cardioprotective effect.[51–53] Elevation of serum HDL levels appears to be the primary mechanism by which alcohol imparts this benefit. It should be stressed that the benefits of alcohol apply only to moderate consumption and is not seen in those who "abuse" alcohol. Furthermore, the protective effects of alcohol are not seen in regard to the risks of hemorrhagic stroke, death due to trauma, or cancer, all of which may be increased in individuals who consume greater amounts of alcohol.

EXERCISE

Even a moderate degree of exercise appears to have a protective effect against CHD and all-cause mortality.[54] In one study of middle-aged men, participation in moderately vigorous physical activity was associated with a 23% lower risk of death than that associated with a less active lifestyle, and this improvement in survival was equivalent and additive to other lifestyle measures such as smoking cessation, hypertension control, and weight control.[55] Mechanisms that could account for the benefits of exercise include elevated serum HDL cholesterol levels, reduced blood pressure, weight loss, and a lower incidence of insulin resistance.

OBESITY

As stated above, obesity is associated with the development of a number of risk factors for CHD, including systemic hypertension, impaired glucose metabolism, insulin resistance, hypertriglyceridemia, reduced HDL cholesterol, and elevated fibrinogen. Data from the Framingham Heart Study, the Nurses' Health Study, and other studies have shown the risk of developing CHD that is associated with obesity.[56–58] The distribution of body fat appears to be an important determinant as patients with abdominal (central) obesity are at greatest risk for subsequent CHD.[59] Patients with central obesity, elevated levels of serum triglycerides and (to a lesser degree) LDL cholesterol, low HDL cholesterol, insulin resistance, and hypertension are classified as having atherogenic dyslipidemia (metabolic syndrome).[60] This syndrome is more difficult to treat and is associated with a worse prognosis than is an isolated increased LDL level.[61]

VITAMINS AND HOMOCYSTEINE

Multiple studies have now linked elevated serum levels of homocysteine with increased risk of CHD. For example, in the Physicians' Health Study of almost 15,000 male physicians who were without prior CHD events, those with homocysteine levels that were above the 95th percentile had a threefold increase in the risk of MI when compared to those in the lower 90th percentile.[62] Elevated homocysteine may be associated with reduced levels and intake of folate and vitamin B_{12}, as was shown in older subjects from the Framingham Heart Study.[63] Dietary supplementation with high levels of vitamins such as folate, vitamin B_{12}, and pyridoxine has been demonstrated to reduce serum homocysteine levels, but whether this translates into improved CHD end points is an active area of investigation.[64]

PLASMA FIBRINOGEN

Plasma fibrinogen levels have recently been shown to be predictors of CVD, and there is a linear relationship between fibrinogen and other cardiovascular risk factors, including age, smoking, diabetes, body mass index, total and LDL cholesterol, and triglycerides.[65] Data from the Framingham Offspring Study suggest that the measurement of fibrinogen is a useful screening tool for identifying individuals who are at increased thrombotic risk and therefore at increased risk of CVD.[66]

ANTIOXIDANTS

The oxidation of LDL particles is an integral part of the atherosclerotic process; this suggests that antioxidant therapy may reduce the incidence of CVD. Antioxidant vitamins such as vitamin E, vitamin C, and β-carotene have been studied in smaller clinical trials, with earlier studies demonstrating benefit only for vitamin E.[67] Despite this early data, the HOPE trial demonstrated that vitamin E use was associated with no protective effect on cardiovascular end points; therefore, its routine administration cannot be recommended at this time.[68]

ENDOTHELIAL DYSFUNCTION

Endothelial dysfunction appears to be an early step in the atherosclerotic process and may result from dyslipidemia, hypertension, and diabetes. Recent studies have suggested that coronary artery endothelial dysfunction predicts the long-term progression of atherosclerosis and an increased incidence of cardiovascular events.[69]

RISK FACTOR MODIFICATION

When atherosclerosis is identified, the immediate goals are to relieve symptoms and to improve organ perfusion. Aggressive risk factor modification to retard or prevent ongoing atherosclerosis is among the most important parts of long-term management. Smoking cessation, meticulous control of hypertension and diabetes, weight management, and aggressive lipid-lowering therapy should all be advised. Recently, lipid-lowering therapy with HMG CoA reductase inhibitors has been shown to reduce mortality in patients with CAD, even when total cholesterol and LDL are only modestly elevated.[37,70] A low-fat low-calorie diet may result in improved serum lipid levels as well as improved weight management, and a cardiovascular exercise program may result in reduced morbidity and mortality from CHD.[71,72]

Diagnosis

The diagnosis of CAD is usually suspected from the clinical presentation. A history of exertional or resting symptoms including (but not limited to) chest tightness, jaw discomfort, left arm pain, dyspnea, or epigastric distress should raise the suspicion of CAD. Many patients deny "chest pain" per se, but the clinician should recognize subtle symptoms (such as dyspnea, diaphoresis, or epigastric distress) that may limit activity. Some patients with CAD have no symptoms that are identified during careful questioning but have "silent ischemia" that is demonstrated by noninvasive testing such as exercise testing or ambulatory electrocardiography.[73] Careful attention should be directed to the risk factor profile for CAD since the probability of atherosclerosis is increased in these individuals.[8,74]

Diagnostic testing begins with baseline 12-lead electrocardiography. Unfortunately, this is neither sensitive nor specific for the presence of CAD or prior MI. The presence of Q waves on the electrocardiogram(ECG) may suggest prior MI although these are not invariably present, and often only nonspecific changes of the ST segments are observed in patients with chronic CAD. Even a normal ECG does not exclude the presence of severe or even life-threatening CAD. Exercise stress testing, often combined with nuclear or echocardiographic imaging modalities, remains the mainstay of a noninvasive diagnosis.[75] Exercise testing with electrocardiographic monitoring is associated with a relatively low sensitivity and specificity for the detection of CAD and should be performed only if the resting ECG is normal. Myocardial perfusion imaging with agents such as thallium 201 and technetium 99m sestamibi is used to assess coronary perfusion at rest and with physical stress. Since the uptake of these agents into the myocardium is an active process, ischemic or infarcted cells exhibit a reduced or absent uptake. A 70 to 80% stenosis of a coronary artery typically is associated with decreased myocardial perfusion on the stress images but with normal myocardial perfusion at rest. This reversible defect is the perfusion pattern associated with stress-induced myocardial ischemia. A fixed defect demonstrates reduced myocardial perfusion both at rest and on exercise. This abnormality usually implies (1) prior MI without viable tissue or (2) severe resting ischemia due to high-grade coronary stenosis with inadequate collateral blood flow. Stress echocardiography detects myocardial ischemia by demonstrating regional differences in left ventricular contractile function during stress. If there is an isolated lesion in the coronary arterial bed, the segmental wall motion abnormality will typically correlate to the distribution of a coronary artery. Ischemic myocardial tissue exhibits both diastolic and systolic dysfunction; the latter is more easily identified on two-dimensional echocardiographic images following exercise or pharmacologic stress with agents such as dobutamine. Both myocardial perfusion imaging and stress echocardiography offer much greater sensitivity and specificity than does exercise electrocardiography alone, and they provide important prognostic information as well. The sensitivity of either modality has been reported as between 85 and 90%, and specificity has been reported to be as high as 90%, but each modality has distinct advantages and disadvantages. Stress echocardiography may offer higher specificity, allows concomitant evaluation of cardiac anatomy and function, and is less expensive than perfusion imaging. Up to 5 to 10% of referred patients will have technically inadequate resting images and will require a perfusion imaging study for diagnostic accuracy. Stress perfusion imaging offers a higher technical success rate, higher sensitivity for the detection of single-vessel CAD, and better accuracy when multiple resting left ventricular (LV) wall motion abnormalities are present.[76,77] Coronary angiography is often needed to define the anatomy and to assist in planning an appropriate management strategy for selected intermediate- to high-risk patients.

Management

The management of CAD depends on a number of clinical factors, including the extent and severity of ischemia, exercise capacity, prognosis based on exercise testing, overall LV function, and associated comorbidities such as diabetes mellitus. Patients with a small ischemic burden, normal exercise tolerance, and normal LV function may be safely treated with pharmacologic therapy. The front line of modern medical therapy includes the selected use of aspirin, β-blockers, ACEIs, and HMG CoA reductase inhibitors. These agents have been shown to reduce the incidence of subsequent MI and death.[77,78] Nitrates and calcium channel blockers may be added to the primary agents to relieve symptoms of ischemia in selected patients. Percutaneous coronary intervention (PCI) with percutaneous transluminal coronary angioplasty (PTCA) and intracoronary stenting relieves symptoms of chronic ischemia, improves mortality when used acutely in patients with myocardial infarction, and improves regional or global LV function, specifically in patients with single-vessel or multivessel CAD.[79,80] Patients with complex multivessel CAD may not be completely revascularized with PCI because of technical limitations of the procedure and commonly require PCI with adjunct medical therapy or surgical revascularization. Early randomized trials in the 1970s, comparing then-current medical therapy to bypass surgery, demonstrated that patients with reduced LV function and severe ischemia, often associated with left main or multivessel CAD, are often best served by coronary artery bypass graft (CABG) surgery.[81–84] More recently, certain subgroups of patients, such as those with diabetes mellitus, have been shown to have improved mortality when treated with surgery as compared to treatment by PCI.[85]

Prognosis

Recent improvements in pharmacologic therapy, PCI, and surgical technique have resulted in significant improvements in morbidity and mortality in patients with CAD. Risk factor modification is a critical element of the therapy and may result in improved prognosis as well. Despite these improvements, over one million Americans die each year of CAD.

Acute Coronary Syndromes

The sudden rupture of an atherosclerotic plaque, with ensuing intracoronary thrombus formation that acutely reduces coronary blood flow, causes the acute coronary syndromes.[86,87] This results in myocardial ischemia and subsequent infarction if there is a prolonged and severe reduction in blood flow. Acute coronary syndromes represent a continuous spectrum of disease ranging from unstable angina to non-Q-wave myocardial infarction to acute Q-wave myocardial infarction.

If the intraluminal thrombus following acute plaque rupture is not completely occlusive, the corresponding clinical presentation is that of unstable angina (USA).[88] There is a sudden change in anginal pattern relating to the frequency or duration of the symptoms. In some cases, the patient may present with symptoms at rest. With a greater degree of obstruction of the epicardial coronary arterial lumen, a non-Q-wave myocardial infarction (NQWMI) may develop. This presents with pro-longed symptoms of resting ischemia, typically *without* ST-segment elevation or the development of pathologic Q waves. These electrocardiographic findings are both signs of a larger and more extensive MI. Electrocardiography in a NQWMI patient may show resting ST-segment depression or deep symmetric T-wave inversions, consistent with severe ischemia. If a large epicardial coronary artery becomes obstructed for a relatively long duration of time, a larger myocardial infarct results, and the electrocardiographic findings will be ST-segment elevation and the subsequent development of pathologic Q waves.

DIAGNOSIS OF ACUTE UNSTABLE CORONARY SYNDROMES

The diagnosis of an acute coronary syndrome is usually made on the basis of clinical data. The patient's history suggests a change in anginal pattern or prolonged intense ischemic symptoms at rest. Acutely, the electrocardiography is important to risk-stratify the patient and to make decisions regarding treatment. A normal ECG does not exclude the presence of acute myocardial infarction (AMI). If the MI is located in the posterior wall of the left ventricle, it will typically not be well represented on the standard 12-lead ECG. Resting ST-segment depression or T-wave inversions in the distribution of an epicardial coronary artery often accompanies USA or NQWMI; however, ST-segment elevation is the hallmark of an acute Q-wave (or transmural) infarct. Patients presenting with a history of USA or AMI and have a left bundle branch block pattern on the 12-lead ECG are usually treated expectantly for Q-wave myocardial infarction (QWMI), given the difficulty of interpreting the ST segments when this conduction delay is present.

Levels of serum cardiac enzymes, such as creatine phosphokinase (CPK) and the more cardiac-specific CPK MB fraction, can be used to establish myocardial injury and infarction. It is important to remember that these levels do not rise significantly until 8 to 12 hours following an MI. Recently, newer cardiac markers such as troponin T and troponin I have been used to risk-stratify patients with cardiac injury or infarction.[89] These markers are both more sensitive and more specific for cardiac-muscle injury. The serum levels become elevated approximately 4 to 8 hours after the acute insult and persist for 5 to 7 days following the event. As both markers can be normal in the early phases of USA or acute MI, neither CPK nor troponin is significantly useful in the *acute* management of patients with the unstable coronary syndromes. Patients with USA and positive troponin T or I have been shown to have an increased risk of recurrent cardiac events.[90,91] These patients are typically treated more aggressively and are referred for diagnostic and therapeutic cardiac catheterization.

THERAPY FOR UNSTABLE CORONARY SYNDROMES

The treatment of the unstable coronary syndromes is the relief of myocardial ischemia and the institution of pharmacologic therapy targeting the underlying thrombotic mechanism.[92] Aspirin should be promptly administered to inhibit platelet

function. The selective use of β-blockers may relieve ischemia by lowering heart rate and BP, which subsequently decreases myocardial oxygen demand (MVO_2). β-Blockers are also antiarrhythmic agents and reduce the risk of malignant ventricular arrhythmias. β-Blockers should not be administered to those with heart failure, bradycardia, heart block, or severe bronchospasm. Sublingual or intravenous nitroglycerin results in venodilation with a resultant decrease in LV preload and MVO_2, thereby reducing myocardial ischemia. They may also contribute to reducing ischemia by their action as epicardial coronary vasodilators as well.

Antithrombotic therapy with intravenous unfractionated or low-molecular-weight heparin and newer agents such as the platelet IIb/IIIa inhibitors (ie, tirofiban and abciximab) results in improved coronary blood flow and reduced myocardial infarct size. Procedural outcomes are improved when these agents are used during angioplasty and stenting (see Table 13-10 for a list of these agents).

In patients who have MI with ST-segment elevation, thrombolytic therapy with agents such as streptokinase, tissue plasminogen activator, and reteplase have all been shown to improve coronary blood flow and to reduce mortality from MI.[93,94] This benefit has not been demonstrated in patients with USA or NQWMI. As an alternative to thrombolytic therapy, percutaneous revascularization with balloon angioplasty and stenting may be performed acutely to improve coronary blood flow and reduce myocardial infarct size. Registry data have shown primary angioplasty in patients with QWMI to be slightly superior to thrombolytic therapy when it is completed within 1 to 2 hours of clinical presentation.[95–97] If a patient with QWMI presents to a center that lacks the ability to perform primary angioplasty, thrombolytic therapy is then the treatment of choice. Transferring the patient to a PTCA facility may result in an unacceptable

TABLE 13-10 Common Antiplatelet and Antithrombin Medications

Drug	Trade Name
Antiplatelet medications	
Aspirin	—
Ticlopidine	Ticlid
Clopidogrel	Plavix
Glycoprotein IIb/IIIa receptor antagonists	
Abciximab	ReoPro
Eptifibatide	Integrilin
Tirofiban	Aggrastat
Antithrombin medications	
Indirect thrombin inhibitors	
Unfractionated heparin	Heparin
Low-molecular-weight heparin	Enoxaparin
Direct thrombin inhibitors	
Lepirudin	Hirudin
Dicumarols	
Warfarin	Coumadin

delay in the restoration of myocardial blood flow. Certain subgroups of patients, including those in cardiogenic shock due to massive AMI, may not derive as great a benefit from thrombolytic therapy.[98–100] Transfer to a facility capable of PTCA and bypass surgery may be preferred for this selected patient population. Support with inotropic agents such as dobutamine or milrinone or with an intra-aortic balloon pump may be necessary in hemodynamically compromised patients while awaiting more definitive therapy.

Oral Health Considerations

Several considerations need to be addressed when treating dental patients with CAD. The primary concern for the dental provider is to prevent the recurrence of ischemia or infarction. The risk for such an event to take place is determined by numerous factors, including the underlying type of CAD (ie, stable angina, USA, or MI). Furthermore, there is a temporal relationship between recurrences of ischemic events, which influences the risk for subsequent acute episodes. Impaired hemostasis due to medication may also require dental modifications. Lastly, side effects from cardiac drugs may cause oral changes, and drug interactions with medications used for dental care may occur.

GENERAL PRECAUTIONS REGARDING DENTAL PROCEDURES

It is highly recommended that all dental providers treating patients who have a history of ischemic heart disease be versed in advanced cardiac life support (ACLS) or at least basic cardiac life support (BCLS). The use of a pulse oximeter to determine the level of oxygenation and the availability of an automatic external defibrillator should also be considered.

As with all patients, the determination of vital signs prior to dental care is essential. Blood pressure and pulse rate and rhythm should be recorded, and any abnormal findings should be addressed.

Patients with CAD are at increased risk of demand-related ischemia with increased heart rate and BP, as well as for plaque rupture and acute unstable coronary syndromes. Anxiety can increase the heart rate and BP and can provoke angina or ischemia.[101] Fortunately, this risk is low during outpatient dental procedures. Protocols to reduce the anxiety of the patient should be employed according to the level of anticipated stress. Premedication with antianxiety medications and inhalation nitrous oxide is commonly used.

Numerous studies have indicated the influence of circadian variation on the triggering of acute coronary events.[102] Most such events occur between 6:00 am and noon. It has been proposed that sympathetic nervous system activation and an increased coagulative state may be precipitating factors.[103] Medications designed to prevent these events, such as β-blockers, aspirin, and antihypertensives, should be continued. Dental care should therefore be provided in the late morning or the early afternoon.

Elective procedures, especially those requiring general anesthesia, should be avoided for at least 4 weeks following an AMI as there is a small increased risk of recurrent events.[104] Limited data indicate that the acute risk of administering local anesthesia for dental procedures 3 weeks after an uncomplicated AMI is very low; however, consultation with the patient's primary physician or cardiologist prior to dental therapy is recommended.

ANTICOAGULATION THERAPY AND DENTAL CARE

Patients with CAD require the use of aspirin. Additional antiplatelet agents such as clopidogrel or ticlopidine are instituted immediately after coronary artery stenting (see Table 13-10). The combination of acetylsalicylic acid (ASA) and clopidogrel is usually continued for 4 weeks after stent implantation, to prevent subacute thrombosis. Daily aspirin is continued at the conclusion of 4 weeks. These agents may increase the risk of bleeding when used in combination. Data that address the risks of bleeding from dental extractions in patients who use these newer antiplatelet agents are limited. Although a bleeding time may be used to assess a patient's ability to form an initial clot after a dental procedure, this diagnostic test has not been shown to have a good correlation with impaired intraoral hemostasis unless bleeding time is significantly longer than 15 to 20 minutes.[105]

Dental care for patients who are on anticoagulation therapy has been discussed in numerous dental and medical publications, and various protocols have been put forth.[106] The debate surrounding the decision on how to manage a patient's anticoagulation therapy when invasive dental procedures are to be performed centers on the potential risk for excessive bleeding after the procedures if anticoagulation therapy is not altered versus the risk of the patient's experiencing a thromboembolic event if the anticoagulation therapy is changed.[107] Authors have suggested a wide range of alternatives, including discontinuing all anticoagulation therapy before invasive procedures, changing the anticoagulation regimen, and making no changes. Ultimately, the core of the problem of developing a uniform protocol for anticoagulated patients is the ability to quantify risk, using parameters that can be applied to the majority of patients. Several relevant issues need to be considered, including the underlying medical condition requiring anticoagulation therapy, the type of medication used to achieve anticoagulation, the level of anticoagulation, the timing of dental care, and the cost and convenience to the patient.

Anticoagulant therapy is used both to treat and to prevent thromboembolism, and different types of medications are used to achieve anticoagulation, based on the patient's underlying medical condition. Dental providers treating ambulatory patients in an outpatient setting will almost exclusively treat patients who are using anticoagulation therapy for prophylactic purposes. Medical conditions for which prophylactic anticoagulation therapy is instituted include (but are not limited to) atrial fibrillation (with and without concomitant systemic embolism), valvular heart disease, the presence of prosthetic heart valves, ischemic heart disease, cerebrovascular accidents, pulmonary embolism, and deep-vein thrombosis.

Two major types of medications are used for anticoagulation: drugs with antiplatelet activity and drugs with antithrombin activity.

The most common antiplatelet drug is aspirin, which is used chronically in very low doses to prevent cardiovascular and cerebrovascular events. Aspirin will irreversibly decrease platelet aggregation and consequently increase the bleeding time. Most patients will take between 40 to 325 mg of aspirin once per day, and at this dosage, the antiplatelet effect will have little impact on bleeding after oral surgical procedures.[108] If the patient has other underlying medical conditions that predispose to impaired hemostasis (such as uremia or liver disease), takes other anticoagulants (including nonaspirin nonsteroidal anti-inflammatory drugs [NSAIDs]), or abuses alcohol, aspirin should be discontinued 3 to 7 days prior to surgery.[109]

If emergency surgery needs to be performed and the patient's bleeding time is higher than 15 to 20 minutes, 1-desamino-8-D-arginine vasopressin (DDAVP) can be instituted to improve hemostasis.[110] DDAVP is administered parenterally at 0.3 µg per kilogram of body weight, with a maximum dose of 20 to 24 µg within 1 hour of surgery. A nasal spray containing 1.5 mg of DDAVP per milliliter can be given in a dose of 300 mg per kilogram. There have been no studies indicating the need to discontinue or alter anticoagulation therapy prior to minor oral surgical procedures for patients taking other types of antiplatelet medications (see Table 13-10 for a list of antiplatelet medications).

The most commonly used antithrombin medications are the dicumarols (eg, warfarin), which inhibit the biosynthesis of vitamin K–dependent coagulation proteins (factors II [prothrombin], VII, IX, and X). The full therapeutic effect of warfarin is reached after 48 to 72 hours and will last for 36 to 72 hours if the drug is discontinued. The efficacy of warfarin therapy is monitored by the prothrombin time (PT) or (as PT has been shown to vary depending on the source and brand of thromboplastin as well as the type of instrumentation used to perform the test) the international normalized ratio (INR). The INR is calculated on the basis of the international sensitivity index (ISI) of the specific thromboplastin used in the test (see Chapter 17 for more information on PT, INR, and normal hemostatic values). The therapeutic level of the INR is dependent on the underlying condition but is usually kept at a range of from 2.0 to 4.5. For an accurate assessment of an individual's anticoagulation status, an INR calculation should be performed within 24 hours of surgery. There is little indication that anticoagulation therapy should be discontinued before minor oral surgical procedures when the patient's INR is < 3.0.[107,111] This conclusion is based on the minimal increase of intraoral bleeding tendency at this level of anticoagulation and on the ease with which it is possible to stop most intraoral bleeding with local measures.

Three different protocols can be used to treat patients with significantly elevated INR. In the first protocol, warfarin is not discontinued. This minimizes adverse thromboembolic events but increases the risk for excessive bleeding after surgery. If localized antihemostatic measures are inadequate to stop bleeding after surgery, vitamin K injections and antifibrinolytic mouth rinses can be instituted.[112]

With the second protocol, warfarin therapy is discontinued, and the patient is not placed on any alternative anticoagulation therapy. In order to diminish the anticoagulative effect of warfarin, the medication must be discontinued 2 to 3 days before surgery. It will take an additional 2 to 3 days after surgery to regain the therapeutic effect of the medication. During this time, the patient is at an increased risk for developing a thromboembolic event but will not exhibit increased bleeding tendencies after surgery. The patients who are at a considerably increased risk for adverse events are those who have been placed on anticoagulation regimens requiring high-intensity therapy, such as patients with prosthetic heart valves or recent deep-vein thrombosis.

In the third protocol, warfarin therapy is discontinued, and the patient is placed on an alternative anticoagulation therapy. This protocol has both advantages and disadvantages. The greatest advantage is that the patient's risk for developing thromboembolic events is minimized. As a rule, however, the patient will be admitted to a hospital, will have their oral anticoagulation (warfarin) therapy discontinued, and will be administered vitamin K and started on parenteral (heparin) therapy. Heparin is continued until approximately 6 hours before surgery and is continued after surgery in combination with oral anticoagulation therapy until a desirable INR has been reached. This is both a time-consuming and costly course of action. The advantages of using heparin are its short half-life of 4 to 6 hours and the availability of an antidote, protamine sulfate, that has an immediate effect. Protamine sulfate should be administered by slow intravenous infusion over a period of at least 10 minutes, with a dose of 1 mg/100 U (or approximately 1.6 mg per milligram of heparin). The disadvantage of using heparin is heparin's potential to induce thrombocytopenia.[113] An alternative to using standard heparin is to have the patient self-administer a subcutaneous injection of low-molecular-weight heparin.[114]

There are also limited data addressing the risk from dental procedures performed following coronary stenting.[115] It is prudent to wait approximately 1 month after the procedure, to allow endothelialization of the stent to decrease the risk of subacute thrombosis, and to discontinue additional antiplatelet agents. As endothelialization is considered complete approximately 4 weeks after stent placement, any dental care rendered within this period should be accompanied by antibiotic prophylaxis according to the American Heart Association's protocol for the prevention of subacute bacterial endocarditis.[116]

Considerations for dental patients who have undergone coronary artery bypass grafting are similar to those who have had a stent procedure. In addition, due to the surgical procedure involved, such patients may be in significant pain when sitting in a dental chair, even several weeks after their heart surgery. Elective dental care should therefore be postponed until the patient can sit comfortable in the dental chair.

▼ VALVULAR HEART DISEASE

Mitral Valve Disease

Mitral valve disease may occur in many forms, including mitral valve prolapse (MVP), mitral regurgitation (MR), and mitral stenosis. In addition to the hemodynamic alterations that are present in patients with these conditions, there are additional issues with regard to the prevention of bacterial endocarditis.

DEFINITION AND INCIDENCE

Mitral valve prolapse typically occurs as a result of myxomatous degeneration of the mitral leaflets and supporting apparatus. This results in abnormal movement or prolapse of the mitral leaflets posteriorly toward the left atrium during mechanical systole. Thus, there is abnormal coaptation of the valve with varying degrees of mitral regurgitation. MVP has been reported in 2.4% of the Framingham Heart Study population and in up to 4 to 5% of the general population.[117] A small percentage of those with MVP have significant MR and ensuing LV volume overload. Acute chordal rupture within the subvalvular apparatus can occur, and this leads to the rapid development of a flail mitral leaflet with acute MR. Rarely, mitral prolapse can be accompanied by malignant dysrhythmias such as ventricular tachycardia or fibrillation. Typically, more benign atrial dysrhythmias are seen and manifest clinically as palpitations. MVP syndrome is characterized by the clinical and echocardiographic findings of MVP, but patients additionally exhibit increased sympathetic autonomic activity and an enhanced sense of cardiac perception. Patients often complain of atypical chest pain or palpitations, and this generates a sense of anxiety regarding their cardiac situation. Often patients are diagnosed as having MVP with a similar symptom complex, but the rigorous clinical and echocardiographic criteria for its diagnosis are not strictly applied.[118]

Mitral regurgitation occurs as a result of a wide variety of abnormalities of the mitral leaflets.[119] These abnormalities have various causes, including myxomatous degeneration and leaflet prolapse, rheumatic heart disease, endocarditis, and use of anorectic agents such as fenfluramine and phentermine (fen-phen).[120–122] Another mechanism of MR is secondary to dilation of the annulus in patients with dilated cardiomyopathy, along with displacement of papillary-muscle geometry secondary to LV dilation. Regardless of the mechanism, if MR is left untreated, the final common end point is significant LV volume overload, with subsequent eccentric hypertrophy of the left ventricle and resultant heart failure.

Mitral stenosis most often occurs as a result of rheumatic heart disease (RHD) or a congenital process. In RHD, there is characteristic thickening and fusion of the mitral commissures as well as thickening and calcification of the leaflets and subvalvular apparatus. This results in a restriction to LV inflow, subsequent left atrial hypertension and enlargement, atrial arrhythmias, and secondary pulmonary hypertension.

The clinical diagnosis of mitral disease requires a careful history suggesting a previously heard heart murmur, exertional or resting dyspnea, or symptoms of heart failure such as orthopnea, paroxysmal nocturnal dyspnea, or peripheral edema. Auscultatory findings include a midsystolic click in MVP, a holosystolic murmur in MR, and an opening snap and diastolic rumble in mitral stenosis. Ancillary findings such as pulmonary or peripheral edema may be present as well.

Transthoracic echocardiography (TTE) remains the mainstay of noninvasive diagnosis in the vast majority of patients with mitral valve disease, and Doppler techniques are extremely useful in establishing the severity of stenosis or regurgitation.[123] Transesophageal echocardiography (TEE) is occasionally needed to further define the mechanism of mitral regurgitation or stenosis and to better assess the severity of the hemodynamic lesion;[124] this is instrumental in planning appropriate surgical therapy. TEE offers improved image quality due to the proximity of the transducer to the mitral valve and left atrium, which allows much greater anatomic definition of the mitral apparatus than can be attained with TTE. It is also widely used to help guide intraoperative management in patients who are referred for valve repair or replacement. Recently, exercise stress echocardiography has been used to evaluate the LV contractile response to exercise in patients with MR, which can predict the LV contractile decompensation earlier, thereby allowing better timing of operative intervention.[125] Cardiac catheterization has a limited role in the diagnosis of mitral valve disease and is primarily reserved for those patients who are referred for cardiac surgery.[126]

TREATMENT OF MITRAL VALVULAR DISEASE

The American College of Cardiology and the American Heart Association have recently published guidelines for treating valvular heart disease that are based on the strength of the currently available evidence in the medical literature.[127] MVP with relatively minor degrees of MR can be observed with serial clinical and echocardiographic examinations to screen for worsening degrees of regurgitation. Antibiotic prophylaxis for infective endocarditis is indicated for patients with MVP and significant MR. Symptomatic patients with significant degrees of MR or mitral stenosis are typically referred for operative or other mechanical intervention. Asymptomatic patients with MR can be observed with serial clinical and echocardiographic examinations. The development of symptoms or an increase in LV diastolic dimension with eventual systolic decompensation are important factors in determining the timing of surgical intervention. Unfortunately, ideal criteria for proceeding to intervention prior to irreversible LV enlargement and contractile decompensation do not exist. MR can be treated by either repair of the mitral valve or replacement with a mechanical or biologic prosthesis. Mitral repair is usually accomplished with the resection of the prolapsing or flail segment of the mitral leaflets and the placement of an annuloplasty ring to decrease mitral annular dimension in order to improve mitral coaptation. More complicated mitral repair is possible and includes the resection and transposition of the chordal structures. If significant fibrosis or calcification of the mitral valve is present, replacement with either a biologic or mechanical prosthesis may be necessary. Mitral stenosis can be treated with mitral percutaneous balloon valvuloplasty (PBV) or mitral replacement. PBV may be the initial treatment of choice in carefully selected patients although many will require repeat PBV or valve replacement over time. Patients with highly calcified valves or those with significant degrees of MR that accompanies mitral stenosis are typically referred for valve replacement.

Aortic Valve Disease

The three major causes of aortic stenosis (AS) are congenital, rheumatic, and senile calcific valve disease. The leaflet excursion is restricted, and a pressure gradient develops from the left ventricle to the aorta, causing subsequent LV pressure overload. This leads to concentric hypertrophy of the left ventricle. The natural history of untreated AS is eventual LV failure due to afterload mismatch.

Aortic regurgitation (AR) results from a wide variety of processes that directly affect the aortic leaflets, including congenital abnormalities, rheumatic disease, infective endocarditis, senile calcific valve degeneration, and the use of anorexigens.[128] Additionally, abnormalities of the aortic root such as aneurysm or aortic dissection may dilate or disrupt the aortic annulus, resulting in malcoaptation and regurgitation. AR imposes an acute or chronic volume load to the left ventricle, with subsequent eccentric hypertrophy, LV enlargement (cor bovinum), and eventual LV contractile failure if the regurgitation is not corrected.

DIAGNOSIS

The clinical diagnosis of aortic valve disease requires a careful history suggesting a previously heard heart murmur, exertional or resting dyspnea, or symptoms of heart failure such as orthopnea, paroxysmal nocturnal dyspnea, or peripheral edema. Severe AR may produce angina due to impaired coronary filling, which results from a decrease in aortic diastolic pressure and an increase in LV diastolic pressure.

The auscultatory findings of AS include a harsh systolic crescendo-decrescendo murmur and a diminished or absent aortic component of the second heart sound. Congenital AS may be accompanied by an ejection click in the early stages because the valve remains relatively pliable. AR is manifest on physical examination by a diastolic murmur heard best at the right upper sternal border when the patient is sitting upright with breath held after exhalation. Pulmonary or peripheral edema may also be clinically evident. Chronic AR often yields findings of a hyperdynamic circulation with bounding or "water hammer" pulses, head bobbing (titubation), "to-and-fro" murmurs heard in the femoral arteries, and Quincke's pulse (visible in the nail beds). Acute AR may present with heart failure and acute pulmonary edema, without the characteristic murmur of AR. Because of early closure of the mitral valve with acute severe AR, the only auscultatory finding may be a soft or absent first sound (S_1).

TTE remains the mainstay of noninvasive diagnosis in the vast majority of patients with aortic valve disease. Doppler techniques are useful in establishing the severity of stenosis or regurgitation.[129–131]

TEE may be needed to define the mechanism of AR or AS, to evaluate the aortic root and ascending aorta, and to investigate the possibility of endocarditis. It is also used to guide intraoperative management in patients who are referred for valve replacement.[132,133] As in cases of MR, exercise stress echocardiography can be used to evaluate the LV contractile response to exercise in patients with AR.[125] The ability to predict the LV contractile decompensation earlier allows optimal timing of operative intervention. A role exists for cardiac catheterization in the diagnosis of aortic valve disease as well; it is primarily reserved for both evaluating the possibility of CAD and determining the need for surgical revascularization in patients who are being considered for cardiac surgery. Hemodynamic data obtained by cardiac catheterization are used to corroborate Doppler-derived measures of aortic valve area and pressure gradients.

TREATMENT OF AORTIC VALVULAR DISEASE

Antibiotic prophylaxis for infective endocarditis is indicated for patients with acquired aortic valve disease. Aortic disease with relatively minor degrees of stenosis or regurgitation can be observed clinically, with serial clinical and echocardiographic examinations to monitor progression. In cases of AS, the severity of AS as well as the development of symptoms determines the timing of surgery. Both retrospective and prospective studies have demonstrated that the risk of sudden death is low in asymptomatic patients with even a severe degree of stenosis.[134] Although largely unproved, some have suggested that asymptomatic patients should undergo operative intervention if they have critical AS (aortic valve area < 0.6 cm^2 and a mean gradient > 50 mm Hg on Doppler echocardiography) or if they have severe AS and are found to have significant ventricular arrhythmia or myocardial ischemia, progressive decline in systolic function, or a rapid increase in the aortic jet velocity (> 0.3 m/s), as measured by Doppler echocardiography, over 1 year.[135]

In patients with AR, the key factors to observe are the development of symptoms and a worsening of LV enlargement, resulting in systolic decompensation.[127] This typically occurs in the late or decompensated stages of LV volume overload. Symptomatic patients with significant degrees of AR or AS are typically referred for operative or other mechanical intervention. Unfortunately, as with MR, ideal criteria for proceeding to operative intervention prior to irreversible LV enlargement and contractile decompensation do not exist. Severe AR or AS is usually treated with aortic valve replacement with either a mechanical or biologic valve prosthesis. AS can be treated with PBV; however, minimal hemodynamic improvements post procedure and rapid restenosis rates limit the usefulness of this procedure in AS cases. It is usually reserved for patients who are not operative candidates but who require end-stage symptomatic palliation or temporary hemodynamic improvements to tolerate additional noncardiac surgery or to overcome acute illness.

Prosthetic Heart Valves

There are numerous types and models of prosthetic heart valves, each with their own characteristics. These valves are either mechanical or bioprosthetic. The mechanical valves, which are classified according to their structure, include the caged-ball (Starr-Edwards) valve, the single tilting-disk (Björk-Shiley) valve, and bileaflet tilting-disk valves (ie, St. Jude, Edwards-MIRA). Bioprosthetic valves are either (1) heterografts made from porcine or bovine tissue or (2) homografts from preserved human aortic valves. Patients with mechanical valves are placed on anticoagulation therapy (typically warfarin) to prevent thromboembolism, according to the type of their replacement valve. The thrombogenic potential is high for caged-ball valves, moderate for single tilting-disk valves, and low for bileaflet tilting-disk valves. In patients with mechanical valves, the risk of systemic embolization is approximately 4% per patient per year without anticoagulation, 2.2% with aspirin therapy, and 0.7 to 1.0% with warfarin therapy.[136] Patients with mitral valve prostheses are at approximately twice the risk of those with aortic valve prostheses.[137] The risk of thromboembolism is highest in the period following placement of the valve and decreases over time as the valve becomes endothelialized. Bioprosthetic valves have a lower thrombogenic potential and do not need to be accompanied by long-term anticoagulation therapy. The recommended anticoagulation therapy for each type of prosthetic valve is summarized in Table 13-11. It is important that although these recommendations serve as broad guidelines, the level of chronic anticoagulation should be individualized and based on the location, type, and number of prosthetic valves, as well as the patient's age and comorbidities. Thus, the intensity of anticoagulation is determined by weighing the patient's risk of thromboembolic events against the risk of adverse anticoagulation consequences.

Prosthetic heart valves increase the risk for infectious endocarditis, which typically manifests as fever and as other systemic symptoms.[138] Although endocarditis within 60 days of surgery typically is caused by non-oral bacteria, the cause of endocarditis that occurs 60 days after valve surgery is similar to that of native-valve endocarditis.

Oral Health Considerations

Antibiotic prophylaxis should be considered for all patients with valvular heart disease. The American Heart Association (AHA) issues guidelines based on analysis of the relevant literature regarding the risk of endocarditis, results of prophylactic studies in animals, and results of retrospective analyses in humans (Tables 13-12 and 13-13).[139] Oral and dental procedures for which antibiotic prophylaxis is recommended are listed in Table 13-14. These guidelines serve as an aid to practitioners but are not intended as a standard of care or a substitute for clinical judgment. According to AHA guidelines, antibiotic prophylaxis should be administered to patients who have undergone mitral or aortic valve repair or replacement, patients with a prior history of infective endocarditis, and patients with mitral or aortic regurgitation or stenosis. Patients with MVP should receive prophylaxis only if there is valvular regurgitation or thickening of the mitral leaflets. Patients with MVP who do not have valvular regurgitation or thickening of the leaflets do not require antibiotic prophylaxis as the incidence of endocarditis among them is identical to that in the general population.

The risk for thromboembolism increases for patients with prosthetic heart valves if anticoagulation therapy is discontinued.[140] It is therefore prudent to continue anticoagulation therapy in patients who require intensive high INR levels (see Table 13-11 and the above discussion on anticoagulation therapy and dental care).

TABLE 13-11 Anticoagulation Therapy for Patients with Prosthetic Heart Valves

Risk of Thromboembolism	Type of Valve	Recommended INR	Antiplatelet Therapy
Low	Mechanical		
	More than one prosthesis	4.0–4.9	Not indicated
	Caged-ball	4.0–4.9	Not indicated
	Single tilted-disk	3.0–3.9	Not indicated
	Bileaflet tilted-disk	2.5–2.9	Not indicated
	Bioprosthetic		
	Heterograft	2.0–3.0 (1st 3 mo)	ASA, 325 mg/d
	Homograft	Not indicated	Not indicated
High*	Mechanical	3.0–4.5	ASA, 80–160 mg/d
	Bioprosthetic		
	Heterograft	2.0–3.0	Not indicated
	Homograft	2.0–3.0	Not indicated

Reproduced with permission from Vongpatanasin W, Hillis LD, Lange RA. Prosthetic heart valves. N Engl J Med 1996;335:407.

ASA = acetylsalicylic acid; INR = international normalized ratio.

*High risk patients are those with a history of atrial fibrillation, previous systemic embolism, left ventricular thrombus, or severe left ventricular dysfunction.

TABLE 13-12   Cardiac Conditions Associated with Endocarditis

Endocarditis Prophylaxis Recommended	Endocarditis Prophylaxis Not Recommended
Prosthetic heart valves (bioprosthetic or homograft valve)	Isolated secundum atrial septal defect
Previous bacterial endocarditis	Surgical repair of atrial septal, ventricular septal defect, or patent ductus arteriosus (without residua beyond 6 mo)
Complex cyanotic congenital heart disease (eg, single ventricle states, transposition of the great arteries, tetralogy of Fallot)	Previous coronary artery bypass graft surgery performed more than 6 weeks prior to treatment
Surgically constructed systemic pulmonary shunts or conduits	
Most other congenital cardiac malformations*	Mitral valve prolapse without valvular regurgitation
Acquired valvular dysfunction (eg, rheumatic heart disease)*	Physiologic, functional, or innocent heart murmurs
Hypertrophic cardiomyopathy*	Previous Kawasaki disease or rheumatic fever without valvular dysfunction
Mitral valve prolapse with valvular regurgitation and/or thickened leaflets*	Cardiac pacemakers and implanted defibrillators

Reproduced with permission from Dajani AS et al.[139]

*Moderate-risk category.

▼ HEART FAILURE

Definition and Incidence

Heart failure represents a clinical syndrome that is due to a wide variety of heterogeneous etiologies.[141,142] Broadly defined, heart failure is the inability of the cardiovascular system to meet the demands of the end organs. Heart failure may result from abnormal contractile function (systolic dysfunction) or impaired relaxation (diastolic dysfunction). Diastolic dysfunction is defined as clinical heart failure syndrome with normal LV systolic function on cardiac testing.[143,144] In many series, it represents the most common type of heart failure encountered in the general population. Several common causes of diastolic dysfunction are hypertension, coronary artery disease with ischemic or infarcted segments of the myocardium, idiopathic dilated cardiomyopathy, or alcoholic cardiomyopathy (Table 13-15).

Diagnosis

Dyspnea, orthopnea, and paroxysmal nocturnal dyspnea are classic symptoms, but nonspecific complaints such as chest discomfort, fatigue, palpitations, dizziness, and syncope are not uncommon. The onset of symptoms may be insidious, and symptoms may present for medical attention only when an acute decompensation occurs. For example, a patient with asymptomatic LV dysfunction develops atrial fibrillation and is unable to increase his cardiac output. Asymptomatic patients are often diagnosed when routine testing is performed for other reasons and reveals abnormalities on ECGs, chest radiographs, or echocardiograms.

The physical-examination findings in cases of heart failure syndrome are numerous. A relative decrease in SBP (due to reduced cardiac output) and an increase in DPB (due to peripheral vasoconstriction) result in a decrease in pulse pressure. Cardiac percussion and palpation reveal an enlarged

TABLE 13-13   Standard Regimens for Antibiotic Prophylaxis to Minimize Risk of Bacterial Endocarditis after Oral Procedures

Patient Category	Oral Medications	Non-Oral Medications*
Adults, not allergic to penicillin	2.0 g amoxicillin 1 h before procedure	2.0 g ampicillin IM or IV within 30 min before procedure
Adults, penicillin allergic	600 mg clindamycin 1 h before procedure or 2.0 g cephalexin 1 hour before procedure or 500 mg azithromycin or clarithromycin 1 h before procedure	600 mg clindamycin IV within 30 min before procedure or 1.0 g cefazolin IM or IV within 30 min before procedure
Children, not allergic to penicillin	50 mg/kg amoxicillin 1 h before procedure[†]	50 mg/kg ampicillin IM or IV within 30 min before procedure[†]
Children, penicillin allergic	20 mg/kg clindamycin 1 h before procedure or 50 mg/kg cephalexin or cefadroxil 1 h before procedure or 15 mg/kg azithromycin or clarithromycin 1 h before procedure	20 mg/kg IV clindamycin within 30 min prior to procedure or 25 mg/kg IM or IV cefazolin 30 min before procedure

Reproduced with permission from Dajani AS et al.[139]

IM = intramuscularly; IV = intravenously.

*For patients who are unable to take oral medications.

[†]The total pediatric dose calculated by weight should not exceed the adult dose.

TABLE 13-14   Oral Procedures and Need for Antibiotic Prophylaxis to Minimize Risk of Bacterial Endocarditis

Oral Procedures Requiring Antibiotic Prophylaxis	Oral Procedures Not Requiring Prophylaxis*
Extractions	Operative and prosthodontic procedures with or without retraction cord (including restoration of decayed teeth and replacement of missing teeth)
Periodontal procedures including surgery, subgingival placements of antibiotic fibers or strips, scaling, and root planning	Local anesthetic injections (nonintraligamentary)
Placement of subgingival antibiotic fibers or strips	Intracanal endodontic procedures (including post placement and buildup)
Implant placement	Placement of removable prosthodontic or orthdontic appliances
Tooth reimplantation	Orthodontic appliance adjustment
Placement of orthodontic bands (not brackets)	Impression taking
Endodontic instrumentation (beyond the apex) or surgery	Exfoliation of primary teeth
Intraligamentary injections	Oral radiography
Prophylactic cleaning of teeth where bleeding is anticipated	Fluoride treatments
Other procedures in which significant bleeding is anticipated	Placement of rubber dams
	Postoperative suture removal

Reproduced with permission from Dajani AS et al.[139]

*Clinical judgment may indicate antibiotic prophylaxis with any procedure that may result in significant bleeding.

heart with a laterally displaced and diffuse apical impulse. Auscultation can reveal an apical holosystolic murmur of mitral regurgitation and the lower parasternal murmur of tricuspid regurgitation. Third and fourth heart sounds can be heard, signifying evidence of systolic and diastolic dysfunction. Rales signify pulmonary congestion secondary to elevated left atrial and LV end-diastolic pressures. Jugular venous distention, peripheral edema, and hepatomegaly signify evidence of elevated right-heart pressures and right ventricular dysfunction. Other findings on physical examination may include cool extremities with decreased pulses, generalized cachexia, muscle atrophy, and weakness due to chronic heart failure.

Chest radiography may demonstrate cardiac enlargement, pulmonary congestion, and pleural effusions. The ECG is frequently abnormal in a nonspecific manner and may be the only indication of heart disease in asymptomatic patients.

TABLE 13-15   Heart Failure Etiologies

Coronary artery disease (ischemic cardiomyopathy)

Hypertension

Cardiomyopathy

   Idiopathic dilated cardiomyopathy
   Hypertrophic cardiomyopathy
   Alcohol
   Diabetes
   Viruses (coxsackie virus, *Enterovirus*, HIV)
   Infiltrative disorders (amyloidosis, hemochromatosis, sarcoidosis)
   Toxins (chemotherapeutic agents)
   Metabolic disorders (hypothyroidism)

Valvular heart disease

Pericardial disease

Incessant tachyarrhythmia

High output states (thyrotoxicosis, AV fistula, thiamine deficiency)

AV = atrioventricular; HIV = human immunodeficiency virus.

Electrocardiography may reveal prolonged repolarization (ie, Q–T interval), and nonspecific ST and T-wave changes. Conduction disturbances such as degrees of atrioventricular block, bundle branch block, and hemiblocks are also seen. Criteria for LV hypertrophy with a repolarization abnormality may suggest hypertension as an etiology. Electrocardiography may also reveal evidence of arrhythmias such as atrial fibrillation and atrial flutter as well as premature atrial or ventricular contractions. Supraventricular tachyarrhythmias and unsustained ventricular tachycardia are also associated with heart failure, as is the development of ventricular fibrillation with sudden cardiac death.

TTE is the most useful noninvasive diagnostic tool for the evaluation of a patient with heart failure.[145] It has become the study of choice in the initial and ongoing evaluation of most forms of heart failure. In addition, TTE provides information not only on overall heart size and function but also on valvular structure and function, wall motion and thickness, LV mass, and the presence of pericardial disease. Doppler-derived hemodynamic measurements accurately predict the severity of valvular regurgitation seen in heart failure and give a noninvasive estimation of pulmonary artery pressures. Doppler techniques may also be used to evaluate LV diastolic abnormalities, which are frequently present in those with heart failure.

Nuclear imaging techniques such as perfusion imaging with thallium 201 and technetium 99m sestamibi, radionuclide ventriculography and multiple gated acquisition scanning, and positron emission tomography (PET) scanning may be useful in evaluating cardiac size and function and in screening for coronary disease as a cause of heart failure. However, because of the inability of these tests to answer important etiologic questions with absolute certainty and their inherent use of radiation, these tests are often unnecessary in the routine evaluation of patients with heart failure.

Cardiac catheterization (with measurement of intracardiac pressures and cardiac output), along with coronary angiography, is useful in evaluating the etiology of heart failure. The most common cause of heart failure and cardiomyopathy is CAD. Typical findings at catheterization in cases of heart failure include elevated LV end-diastolic, wedge, pulmonary artery, and right-heart pressures; increased LV size with decreased overall function; and MR. Regional wall motion abnormalities may be seen in either ischemic or dilated cardiomyopathy but are usually less prominent in patients who do not have ischemic heart disease.

Therapy

The treatment of heart failure must be individualized to the etiology of the heart failure and to the patient. Patients with ischemic heart disease and heart failure should be evaluated for ischemia as well as viable but hibernating myocardium that would improve systolic and diastolic performance with revascularization.[146–148] Patients with alcoholic cardiomyopathy should be advised to abstain from alcohol, in addition to the usual therapeutic options, as this often leads to an improvement in LV performance.[149] Hypertension should be aggressively treated with pharmacologic intervention and dietary measures. For patients with primary systolic dysfunction, ACEIs are the mainstays of oral drug therapy. These agents have clearly been shown to decrease mortality and to prolong survival. They also delay onset and reduce the symptoms of heart failure in patients with LV systolic dysfunction. When ACEIs cannot be tolerated, angiotensin receptor antagonists or the combination of hydralazine and nitrate derivatives may be substituted. Digoxin is effective in reducing morbidity and hospitalizations but has little effect on overall mortality. Loop diuretics are useful in controlling congestive symptoms but have not been shown to affect mortality. Conversely, the RALES trial found that spironolactone improves survival in patients with advanced CHF.[150] Additionally, data exist to support the use of "triple therapy" with ACEIs, digoxin, and diuretics in preference to ACEIs used alone.[151] Recent data suggest a mortality benefit as well as improved functional capacity from the use of β-blockers in patients with compensated heart failure and LV systolic dysfunction.[152–154] Doses should be initiated at low levels and slowly titrated up over weeks to months. Symptoms of heart failure may initially worsen, and other medication doses may need to be adjusted during the initial stages of β-blocker therapy.[155]

Anticoagulation with warfarin (Coumadin) in patients with LV dysfunction has been shown to reduce morbidity and mortality from cardioembolic events that develop secondary to chamber enlargement and stasis of blood; however, the risks of bleeding need to be considered.[156] Anticoagulation therapy is likely to be most beneficial for patients with atrial fibrillation or atrial flutter or for patients in sinus rhythm with a LV ejection fraction of less than 20%.

For those patients who remain symptomatic, intravenous therapy with diuretics and inotropes may need to be initiated. Some patients respond well to this treatment, and oral therapy can subsequently be resumed rapidly; other patients require long-term intravenous therapy. For the subset of patients who cannot be successfully weaned from intravenous treatment and who do not have other significant morbidities, cardiac transplantation is another therapeutic option.

Oral Health Considerations

For well-compensated patients with heart failure, no special dental modifications are necessary unless the underlying causes for the heart failure require modifications. However, when patients suffer from uncompensated CHF, it is prudent to inquire about the patient's ability to be placed in supine position because lying down flat in a dental chair my cause severe dyspnea in such patients.

▼ ARRHYTHMIA

Definition and Incidence

Abnormalities of cardiac rhythm can be broadly defined as any deviation from the normal cardiac pacemaker and conduction mechanism. Tachyarrhythmias occur as a result of increased automaticity of cardiac pacemaker cells' re-entry or triggered activity and are defined as any abnormal heart rhythm with a rate > 100 bpm. Bradyarrhythmias occur as a result of sinoatrial node dysfunction and conduction block at any level of the conduction tissues, including the atrioventricular node, His-Purkinje system, or distal branches of the left and right bundles. Bradyarrhythmias are associated with heart rates of < 60 bpm. Both tachyarrhythmias and bradyarrhythmias may be hemodynamically well tolerated in patients with normal cardiac function, or they may result in cardiovascular collapse if cardiac output is significantly compromised.

Supraventricular Tachycardia

Re-entrant supraventricular rhythms such as atrioventricular nodal re-entrant tachycardia (AVNRT) occur commonly in the absence of structural heart disease and are usually well tolerated from a hemodynamic standpoint. AVNRT is the most common etiology, and the atrioventricular (AV) node is functionally dissociated into two discrete electrical pathways.[157,158] These pathways have different refractory periods and conduction velocities, which are both prerequisites for re-entry. AVNRT also requires a fortuitously timed premature atrial or ventricular impulse and therefore may be observed in settings where there is increased atrial ectopy due to anxiety or other types of sympathetic stimulation.[159] Interrupting conduction within the re-entrant circuit in the AV node can terminate AVNRT. Therefore, vagal maneuvers (such as Valsalva's maneuver) or drugs that act on the AV node (such as adenosine, β-blockers, and diltiazem or verapamil) are particularly effective in terminating AVNRT. Recently, radiofrequency ablation (RFA) with modification of the normally quiescent slow pathway in the AV node has been used to interrupt the re-entrant circuit, thereby preventing the perpetuation of the tachycardia.[160] Patients with frequent symptomatic episodes, who experience presyncope or frank syncope, or who do not wish or cannot tolerate medication therapy may be referred for this procedure.

Wolff-Parkinson-White (WPW) syndrome is characterized by the presence of an accessory pathway that enables conduction from atria to ventricles outside the normal conduction system.[161] This produces AV re-entrant tachycardia, a narrow complex tachycardia with retrograde P waves on the surface ECG following each QRS complex. The surface ECG of a patient with WPW syndrome is characterized by a short P–R interval and the slurred onset of the QRS complex (called a delta wave), representing atrial-to-ventricular conduction via the accessory pathway. This may result in either orthodromic or antidromic AV re-entrant tachycardia, depending on whether the re-entrant rhythm conducts antegrade or retrograde through the AV node, or rapidly conducted atrial fibrillation with an increased ventricular response due to the rapid conduction of the accessory pathway. This may precipitate ventricular fibrillation if not promptly terminated with electrical cardioversion or intravenous procainamide.

Atrial Fibrillation

Atrial fibrillation is a common dysrhythmia and occurs both with and without structural heart disease.[162] It represents rapid and chaotic atrial activity with an irregular and rapid ventricular response. Atrial fibrillation (AF) can be classified as valvular as it frequently accompanies mitral stenosis or regurgitation. Nonvalvular AF may accompany a structurally normal heart (lone AF), hypertensive heart disease, cardiomyopathy, and a

TABLE 13-16   Etiologies of Atrial Fibrillation

Hypertension

Rheumatic valvular disease

Coronary artery disease (including acute MI and ischemic cardiomyopathy)

Atrial septal defects

Hypertrophic cardiomyopathy

Congenital heart disease (Ebstein's disease, patent ductus arteriosus, tetralogy of Fallot)

Dilated cardiomyopathy

Alcoholic cardiomyopathy

Holiday heart syndrome

Pulmonary embolism

Pericardial disease

Chronic obstructive lung disease, cor pulmonale

Peripartum cardiomyopathy

Sleep apnea

Thyrotoxicosis

Autonomic dysfunction

Postcardiac surgery and transplantation

Noncardiac surgery (thoracic and esophageal)

Medications (theophylline, caffeine, digitalis)

Familial

Pheochromocytoma

MI = myocardial infarction.

wide variety of other clinical conditions (Table 13-16). In a case of AF, the chaotic atrial activity results in ineffective atrial contraction and in stasis of blood within the LA and LAA. This stasis may lead to thrombus formation and may increase the risk of embolic events, including cerebral and peripheral embolization. Embolic stroke occurs in 1.6 to 5.3% of patients per year, and the risks increase with increasing age, comorbidities, and CVD.[163] Frequently, younger patients with brief episodes of paroxysmal AF are treated with antiplatelet drugs such as ASA because the risk of stroke is low; however, anticoagulation with warfarin is typically used in older patients who have other comorbidities and for whom the risk of thromboembolic events is significantly increased.[164] A number of trials have shown that warfarin use is associated with a 45 to 82% reduction in the risk of stroke in patients with chronic AF.[164,165]

A wide variety of strategies have been used in the attempt to restore and maintain normal sinus rhythm, including β-blocker drugs, antiarrhythmic therapy, and electrical cardioversion.[166] Historically, chemical or electrical cardioversion has been performed after at least 3 to 4 weeks of anticoagulation with warfarin as this has been shown to reduce the risk of thromboembolism. TEE can be used to facilitate earlier cardioversion by evaluating the LA and LAA for thrombus.[167]

Whether antiarrhythmic drugs should be used to maintain sinus rhythm is controversial. Earlier studies revealed an increased risk of death due to proarrhythmia with quinidine therapy. However, more limited data exist on the use of newer agents such as amiodarone, sotalol, and propafenone. However, even the newer agents are not always effective and are associated with side effects, including the risk of proarrhythmia. Newer investigational approaches include surgical or percutaneous catheter ablation of focal AF, transcatheter internal cardioversion, and the insertion of an implantable atrial defibrillator. However, the long-term safety and efficacy of these approaches have not been determined.

Dental protocols for patients with AF have been proposed. These protocols specifically address the underlying cause of AF and the subsequent need for antibiotic prophylaxis, the need to alter dental care on the basis of the patient's anticoagulation therapy, and the use of anxiety-reducing strategies.[168]

Ventricular Tachycardia and Fibrillation

Ventricular tachycardia (VT) and ventricular fibrillation (VF) typically occur in patients with structural heart disease of the left ventricle, such as those with CAD, various forms of dilated cardiomyopathy, and hypertrophic cardiomyopathy. Rarely, VT may occur as an idiopathic event in an individual with a structurally normal heart or may originate in the right ventricle as in the case of arrhythmogenic right ventricular dysplasia. VF may occur in the setting of acute ischemia and infarction, in dilated and hypertrophic cardiomyopathy, and as a result of a variety of drug and electrolyte effects. VT may occur as a sustained event or as a nonsustained event. Nonsustained VT is a marker of increased risk of sudden cardiac death in patients with coronary disease who have suffered an MI and have reduced LV function. Sustained VT in the setting of CAD typically occurs as a result of re-entry within an infarcted segment of the left ventricle.[169]

Patients with VT are often treated with electrophysiologically guided antiarrhythmic drug therapy. An implantable cardiac defibrillator is placed if the arrhythmia is not suppressible in the electrophysiology laboratory with appropriate antiarrhythmic therapy. The treatment of VF largely depends on the underlying cause. Acute coronary revascularization is performed in those patients who have myocardial ischemia and infarction, followed by appropriate electrophysiologic guided therapy for those with structurally abnormal hearts. Torsade de pointe is a unique form of polymorphic VT that may result from a lengthening of the Q–T interval because of drugs, electrolyte disturbances, or congenital long QT syndrome.

▼ PERMANENT PACEMAKERS

Permanent cardiac pacing is used in a wide variety of cardiac conditions, including symptomatic heart block and bradycardia, brady-tachy syndrome, carotid hypersensitivity, neurocardiogenic syncope, heart failure, and hypertrophic cardiomyopathy. Single (typically ventricular) or dual chamber (atrial and ventricular) models are typically employed. Guidelines for the implantation of cardiac pacemakers have been established by the American College of Cardiology and the American Heart Association joint task force on the basis of available evidence in the medical literature.[170]

▼ REFERENCES

1. American Heart Association. 2001 Heart and stroke statistical update. Dallas (TX): American Heart Association; 2000.

2. Hyman DJ, Pavlik VN. Characteristics of patients with uncontrolled hypertension in the United States. N Engl J Med 2001;345:479.

3. Report of the Joint National Committee on Prevention, Detection, Evaluation and Treatment of High Blood Pressure (JNC VI). Arch Intern Med 1997;157:2413.

4. National High Blood Pressure Education Program. The Sixth Report of the Joint National Committee on Prevention, Detection, Evaluation, and Treatment of High Blood Pressure. Bethesda (MD): National Institutes of Health/National Heart, Lung, and Blood Institute. 1997 Nov. NIH Publication No. 98-4080.

5. Psaty BM, Smith NL, Siscovick DS, et al. Health outcomes associated with antihypertensive therapies used as first-line agents. A systematic review and meta-analysis. JAMA 1997;277:739.

6. Perreault S, Dorais M, Coupal L, et al. Impact of treating hyperlipidemia or hypertension to reduce the risk of death from coronary artery disease. Can Med Assoc J 1999;160:1449.

7. Cavallini MC, Roman MJ, Pickering TG, et al. Is white coat hypertension associated with arterial disease or left ventricular hypertrophy? Hypertension 1995;26:413.

8. Glick M. Screening for risk factors for cardiovascular disease: a review for oral health care providers. J Am Dent Assoc 2002;133:291–300.

9. Katsuyuki M, Daviglus ML, Dyer AR, et al. Relationship of blood pressure to 25-year mortality due to coronary heart disease, cardiovascular diseases, and all causes in young adult men: the Chicago Heart Association Detection Project in Industry. Arch Intern Med 2001;161:1501.

10. Sun P, Dwyer KM, Merz C, et al. Blood pressure, LDL cholesterol, and intima-media thickness: a test of the "response to injury" hypothesis of atherosclerosis. Arterioscler Thromb Vasc Biol 2000;20:2005.

11. Poli KA, Tofler GH, Larson MG, et al. Association of blood pressure with fibrinolytic potential in the Framingham Offspring population. Circulation 2000;101:264.

12. Sechi LA, Zingaro L, Catena C, et al. Relationship of fibrinogen levels and hemostatic abnormalities with organ damage in hypertension. Hypertension 2000;36:978.

13. Lip GYH, Blann AD, Jones AF, et al. Relation of endothelium, thrombogenesis, and hemorheology in systemic hypertension to ethnicity and left ventricular hypertrophy. Am J Cardiol 1997;80:1566.

14. Lip GYH. Target organ damage and the prothrombotic state in hypertension. Hypertension 2000;36:975.

15. Vogt M, Strauer BE. Systolic ventricular dysfunction and heart failure due to coronary microangiopathy in hypertensive heart disease. Am J Cardiol 1995;76:48D.

16. Vasan RS, Larson MG, Kannel WB, Levy D. Evolution of hypertension from non-hypertensive blood pressure levels: rates of progression in The Framingham Heart Study. J Am Coll Cardiol 2000;35:292A.

17. Grundy SM, Balady GJ, Criqui MH, et al. Primary prevention of coronary heart disease: guidance from Framingham: a statement for healthcare professionals from the AHA Task Force on Risk Reduction. Circulation 1998;97:1876.

18. Izzo JL, Levy D, Black HR. Importance of systolic blood pressure in older Americans. Hypertension 2000;35:1021.

19. Hansson L, Lindholm LH, Niskanen L, et al, for the Captopril Prevention Project (CAPPP) study group. Effect of angiotensin-converting-enzyme inhibition compared with conventional therapy on cardiovascular morbidity and mortality in hypertension: the Captopril Prevention Project (CAPPP) randomised trial. Lancet 1999;353:611.

20. Hansson L, Hedner T, Lung-Johansen P, et al, for the NORDIL Study Group. Randomised trial of effects of calcium antagonists compared with diuretics and beta-blockers on cardiovascular morbidity and mortality in hypertension: the Nordic Diltiazem (NORDIL) study. Lancet 2000;356:359.

21. Heart Outcomes Prevention Evaluation Study Investigators. Effect of an angiotensin-converting-enzyme inhibitor, ramipril, on cardiovascular events in high-risk persons. N Engl J Med 2000;342:145.

22. Moser M. National recommendations for the pharmacological treatment of hypertension: should they be revised? Arch Intern Med 1999;159:1403.

23. SHEP Cooperative Research Group. Prevention of stroke by hypertensive drug treatment in older persons with isolated systolic hypertension: final results of the Systolic Hypertension in the Elderly Program (SHEP). JAMA 1991;265:3255.

24. Staessen JA, Fagard R, Thijs L, et al. Randomised double-blind comparison of placebo and active treatment for older patients with isolated systolic hypertension. The Systolic Hypertension in Europe (Syst-Eur) Trial Investigators. Lancet 1997;350:757.

25. Silvestry FE, Sutton MGS. Sustained-release calcium channel antagonists in cardiovascular disease. Eur Heart J 1998;19 Suppl I:8–14.

26. Sytkowski PA, D'Agostino RB, Belanger AJ, et al. Secular trends in long-term sustained hypertension, long-term treatment and cardiovascular mortality. The Framingham Heart Study 1950 to 1990. Circulation 1996;93:697.

27. Kaplan NM. Hypertension in the population at large. In: Clinical hypertension. 7th ed. Baltimore (MD): Williams & Wilkins; 1998.

28. Glick M. New guidelines for prevention, detection, evaluation and treatment of high blood pressure. J Am Dent Assoc 1998;129:1588.

29. Navas-Nacher EL, Colangelo L, Beam C, et al. Risk factors for coronary heart disease in men 18 to 39 years of age. Ann Intern Med 2001;134:433.

30. Anonymous. Report of the Expert Committee on the Diagnosis and Classification of Diabetes Mellitus. Diabetes Care 2001;24 (Suppl 1):S5.

31. The Third Report of the National Cholesterol Education Program (NCEP) Expert Panel on Detection, Evaluation, and Treatment of High Blood Cholesterol in Adults (Adult Treatment Panel III). Bethesda (MD): NCEP/National Heart, Lung, and Blood Institute/National Institutes of Health. 2001.

32. Multiple Risk Factor Intervention Trial Research Group. Risk factor changes and mortality results. JAMA 1982;248:1465.

33. Tall AR. An overview of reverse cholesterol transport. Eur Heart J 1998;19 Suppl A:A31.

34. Wilson PW. Established risk factors and coronary artery disease: The Framingham Study. Am J Hypertens 1994;7:7S.

35. Kinosian B, Glick H, Garland, G. Cholesterol and coronary heart disease: predicting risks by levels and ratios. Ann Intern Med 1994;121:641.

36. Scandinavian Simvastatin Survival Study Group. Baseline serum cholesterol and treament effect in the Scandinavian Simvastatin Survival Study (4S). Lancet 1995;345:1274.

37. Scandinavian Simvastatin Survival Study Group. Randomized trial of cholesterol lowering in 4,444 patients with coronary heart disease: the Scandinavian Simvastatin Survival Study (4S). Lancet 1994;344:1383.

38. Sacks FM, Pfeffer MA, Moyé LA, et al. The effect of pravastatin on coronary events after myocardial infarction in patients with average cholesterol levels. N Engl J Med 1996;335:1001.

39. Sheperd J, Cobbe SM, Ford I, et al. Prevention of coronary heart disease with pravastatin in men with hypercholesterolemia. N Engl J Med 1995;333:1301.

40. Stamler J, Stamler R, Neaton JD. Blood pressure, systolic and diastolic, and cardiovascular risks: U.S. population data. Arch Intern Med 1993;153:598.

41. Kannel WB, McGee DL. Diabetes and cardiovascular risk factors: The Framingham Study. Circulation 1979;59:8.

42. Kannel WB, McGee DL. Diabetes and glucose tolerance as risk factors for cardiovascular disease: The Framingham Study. Diabetes Care 1979;2:120.

43. Basta E, Bakris G. Choices and goals in the treatment of the diabetic hypertensive patient. Curr Hypertens Rep 2001;3:387–91.

44. Njolstad I, Arnesen E, Lund-Larsen PG. Smoking, serum lipids, blood pressure, and sex differences in myocardial infarction. A 12-year follow-up of the Finnmark Study. Circulation 1996;93:450.

45. Prescott E, Hippe M, Schnohr P, et al. Smoking and the risk of myocardial infarction in women and men: longitudinal population study. BMJ 1998;316:1043.

46. Willhemsson C, Elmfeldt D, Vedim JA, et al. Smoking and myocardial infarction. Lancet 1975;1:415.

47. Barrett-Connor EL, Bush TL. Estrogen and coronary heart disease in women. JAMA 1991;265:1861.

48. Stampfer MJ, Colditz GA, Willett WC, et al. Postmenopausal estrogen therapy and cardiovascular disease: ten-year follow-up from the Nurses' Health Study. N Engl J Med 1991;325:756.

49. Wolk A, Manson JE, Stampfer MJ, et al. Long-term intake of dietary fiber and decreased risk of coronary heart disease among women. JAMA 1999;281:1998.

50. Eckel RH. Obesity in heart disease. Circulation 1997;96:3248.

51. Fuchs CS, Stampfer MJ, Colditz GA, et al. Alcohol consumption and mortality among women. N Engl J Med 1995; 332:1245.

52. Rimm EB, Giovannucci EL, Willett WC, et al. Prospective study of alcohol consumption and risk of coronary disease in men. Lancet 1991;338:464.

53. Mukamal KJ, Jadhav PP, D'Agostino RB, et al. Alcohol consumption and hemostatic factors: analysis of the Framingham offspring cohort. Circulation 2001;104:1367.

54. US Department of Health and Human Services. Physical activity and health: a report of the Surgeon General. Atlanta (GA): Department of Health and Human Services, Centers for Disease Control and Prevention, National Center for Disease Prevention and Health Promotion; 1996.

55. Sandvik L, Erikssen J, Thaulow E, et al. Physical fitness as a predictor of mortality among healthy, middle-aged Norwegian men. N Engl J Med 1993;328:533.

56. Hubert HB, Feinleib M, McNamara PM, et al. Obesity as an independent risk factor for cardiovascular disease: a 26-year follow-up of participants in the Framingham Heart Study. Circulation 1983;67:968.

57. Manson JE, Colditz GA, Stampfer MJ, et al. A prospective study of obesity and risk of coronary heart disease in women. N Engl J Med 1990;322:882.

58. Krauss RM, Winston M. Obesity: impact on cardiovascular disease. Circulation 1998;98:1472.

59. Rimm EB, Stampfer MJ, Giovannucci E, et al. Body size and fat distribution as predictors of coronary heart disease among middle-aged and older US men. Am J Epidemiol 1995;141:1117.

60. Grundy SM. Atherogenic dyslipidemia: lipoprotein abnormalities and implications for therapy. Am J Cardiol 1995;75:45B.

61. Jeppesen J, Hein HO, Suadicani P, et al. Relation of high TG-low HDL cholesterol and LDL cholesterol to the incidence of ischemic heart disease: an 8-year follow-up in the Copenhagen Male Study. Arterioscler Thromb Vasc Biol 1997;17:1114.

62. Stampfer MJ, Malinow MR, Willett WC, et al. A prospective study of plasma homocysteine and risk of myocardial infarction in US physicians. JAMA 1992;268:877.

63. Jacques PF, Selhub J, Bostom AG, et al. The effect of folic acid fortification on plasma folate and total homocysteine concentrations. N Engl J Med 1999;340:1449.

64. Clark R, Collins R. Can dietary supplement with folic acid or vitamin B_6 reduce cardiovascular risk? Design of trials to test the homocysteine hypothesis of vascular disease. J Cardiovasc Risk 1998;5:249.

65. Cremer P, Nagel D, Mann H, et al. Ten-year follow-up results from the Goettingen Risk, Incidence and Prevalence Study (GRIPS). I. Risk factors for myocardial infarction in a cohort of 5790 men. Atherosclerosis 1997;129:221.

66. Stec JJ, Silbershatz H, Ofler GH, et al. Association of fibrinogen with cardiovascular risk factors and cardiovascular disease in the Framingham offspring population. Circulation 2000;102:1634.

67. Stephens NG, Parsons A, Schofield PM, et al. Randomised control trial of vitamin E in patients with coronary disease: Cambridge Heart Antioxidant Study (CHAOS). Lancet 1996;347:781–6.

68. Heart Outcomes Prevention Evaluation Study Investigators. Vitamin E supplementation and cardiovascular events in high-risk patients. N Engl J Med 2000;342:154.

69. Suwaidi JA, Hamasaki S, Higano ST, et al. Long-term follow-up of patients with mild coronary artery disease and endothelial dysfunction. Circulation 2000;101:948.

70. Prevention of cardiovascular events and death with pravastatin in patients with coronary heart disease and a broad range of initial cholesterol levels. The Long-Term Intervention with Pravastatin in Ischaemic Disease (LIPID) Study Group. N Engl J Med 1998;339:1349.

71. Paffenberger RS Jr, Hyde RT, Wing AL, et al. The association of changes in physical-activity level and other lifestyle characteristics with mortality among men. N Engl J Med 1993;328:538.

72. Ekelund LG, Haskell WL, Johnson JL, et al. Physical fitness a predictor of cardiovascular mortality in asymptomatic North American men: The Lipid Research Clinics Mortality Follow up Study. N Engl J Med 1988;319:1379.

73. Smith SC Jr, Amsterdam E, Balady GJ, et al. Prevention Conference V: tests for silent and inducible ischemia. Circulation 2000;101:12.

74. Grundy SM, Bazzarre T, Cleeman J, et al. Prevention Conference V: medical office assessment. Circulation 2000;101:3.

75. Mayo Clinic Cardiovascular Working Group on Stress Testing. Cardiovascular stress testing: a description of the various types of stress tests and indications for their use. Mayo Clin Proc 1996;71:43.

76. San Roman JA, Vilacosta I, Castillo JA, et al. Selection of the optimal stress test for the diagnosis of coronary artery disease. Heart 1998;80:370.

77. Gibbons RJ, Chatterjee K, Daley J, et al. ACC/AHA/ACP-ASIM guidelines for the management of patients with chronic stable angina. A report of the American College of Cardiology/ American Heart Association Task Force on Practice Guidelines (Committee on Management of Patients with Chronic Stable Angina). J Am Coll Cardiol 1999;33:2092.

78. Collaborative overview of randomised trials of antiplatelet therapy. I. Prevention of death, myocardial infarction, and stroke by prolonged antiplatelet therapy in various categories of patients. BMJ 1994;304:81–106.

79. Bittl JA. Medical progress: advances in coronary angioplasty. N Engl J Med 1996;335:1290.

80. Gandhi MM, Dawkins KD. Fortnightly review: intracoronary stents. BMJ 1999;318:650.

81. Kaiser GC. CABG: lessons learned from the randomized trials. Ann Thorac Surg 1986;42:3.

82. Caracciolo EA, Davis KB, Sopko G, et al. Comparison of surgical and medical group survival in patients with left main equivalent coronary artery disease. Long-term CASS experience. Circulation 1995;91:2335.

83. Myers WO, Schaff HV, Gersh BJ, et al. Improved survival of surgically treated patients with triple vessel coronary artery disease and severe angina pectoris. A report from the Coronary Artery Surgery Study (CASS) registry. J Thorac Cardiovasc Surg 1989;97:487.

84. Yusuf S, Zucker D, Peduzzi P, et al. Effect of coronary artery bypass graft surgery on survival: overview of 10-year results from randomized trials by the Coronary Artery Bypass Surgery Trialists Collaboration. Lancet 1994;344:563.

85. Brooks MM, Jones RH, Bach RG, et al. Predictors of mortality and mortality from cardiac causes in the Bypass Angioplasty Revascularization Investigation (BARI) randomized trial and registry. Circulation 2000;101:2682.

86. Willerson JT, Golino P, Eidt J, et al. Specific platelet mediators and unstable coronary lesions. Circulation 1989;80:198.

87. MacIsaac AI, Thomas JD, Topol EJ. Toward the quiescent coronary plaque. J Am Coll Cardiol 1993;22:1228.

88. Yeghiazarians Y, Braunstein JB, Askari A, et al. Medical progress: unstable angina pectoris. N Engl J Med 2000;342:101.

89. Hamm CW, Ravkilde J, Gerhardt W, et al. The prognostic value of serum troponin T in unstable angina. N Engl J Med 1992;327:146.

90. Luescher MS, Thygesen K, Ravkilde J, et al. Applicability of cardiac troponin T and I for early risk stratification in unstable coronary disease. Circulation 1997;96:2578.

91. Hamm CW, Goldman BU, Heeschen C, et al. Emergency room triage of patients with acute chest pain by means of rapid testing for cardiac troponin T or I. N Engl J Med 1997;337:1648.

92. Reeder GS. Contemporary diagnosis and management of unstable angina. Mayo Clin Proc 2000;75:953.

93. The thrombolysis in myocardial infarction (TIMI) trial: phase I findings. N Engl J Med 1985;312:932.

94. Chesebro JH, Knatterud G, Roberts R, et al. Thrombolysis in myocardial infarction (TIMI) trial, phase I: a comparison between intravenous tissue plasminogen activator and intravenous streptokinase. Circulation 1987;76:142.

95. Agati L, Voci P, Hickle P, et al. Tissue-type plasminogen activator therapy versus primary coronary angioplasty: impact on myocardial tissue perfusion and regional function 1 month after uncomplicated myocardial infarction. J Am Coll Cardiol 1998;31:338.

96. Grines CL, Browne KF, Marco J, et al. A comparison of immediate angioplasty with thrombolytic therapy for acute myocardial infarction. N Engl J Med 1993;328:673.

97. The Global Use of Strategies to Open Occluded Coronary Arteries in Acute Coronary Syndromes (GUSTO 2B) Angioplasty Substudy Investigators. A clinical trial comparing angioplasty with tissue plasminogen activator for acute myocardial infarction. N Engl J Med 1997;336:1621.

98. TIMI Research Group. Immediate vs. delayed catheterization and angioplasty following thrombolytic therapy for acute myocardial infarction. JAMA 1988;260:2849.

99. Second International Study of Infarct Survival Collaborative Group. Randomised trial of intravenous streptokinase, oral aspirin, both, or neither among 171,817 cases of suspected acute myocardial infarction: ISIS-2. Lancet 1988;2:349.

100. GUSTO Investigators. An international randomized trial comparing four thrombolytic strategies for acute myocardial infarction. N Engl J Med 1993;329:673.

101. Krantz DS, Kop WJ, Santiago HT, et al. Mental stress as a trigger for myocardial ischemia and infarction. Cardiol Clin 1996;14:271.

102. Muller JE. Circadian variation and triggering of acute coronary events. Am Heart J 1999;137:S1.

103. Muller JE, Kaufman PG, Luepker RV, et al. Mechanisms precipitating acute cardiac events: review and recommendations of an NHLBI workshop. Circulation 1997;96:3233.

104. Roberts HW, Mitnitsky EF. Cardiac risk stratification for post-myocardial infarction dental patients. Oral Surg Oral Med Oral Pathol Oral Radiol Endod 2001;91:676.

105. DeRossi SS, Glick M. Bleeding time: an unreliable predictor of clinical hemostasis. J Oral Maxillofac Surg 1996;54:1119.

106. Herman WW, Konzelman JL, Sutley SH. Current perspectives on dental patients receiving coumadin anticoagulant therapy. J Am Dent Assoc 1997;128:327.

107. Whal MJ. Myths of dental surgery in patients receiving anticoagulant therapy. J Am Dent Assoc 2000;131:77.

108. Ardekian L, Gaspar R, Peled M, et al. Does low-dose aspirin therapy complicate oral surgery procedures? J Am Med Assoc 2000;131:331.

109. Conti CR. Aspirin and elective surgical procedures. Clin Cardiol 1992;15:709.

110. Beck KH, Mohr P, Bleckmann U, et al. Desmopressin effect on acetylsalicylic acid impaired platelet function. Semin Thromb Hemost 1995;21 Suppl 2:32.

111. Cambell JH, Alvarado F, Murray RA. Anticoagulation and minor oral surgery: should the anticoagulation regimen be altered? J Oral Maxillofac Surg 2000;58:131.

112. Blinder D, Manor Y, Martinowitz U, et al. Dental extractions in patients maintained on continued oral anticoagulant: comparison of local hemostatic modalities. Oral Surg Oral Med Oral Pathol Oral Radiol Endod 1999;88:137.

113. Warkentin TE, Levine MN, Hirsch J, et al. Heparin induced thrombocytopenia in patients treated with low molecular weight heparin or unfractionated heparin. N Engl J Med 1995;332:1330.

114. Todd DW, Roman A. Outpatient use of low-molecular weight heparin in an anticoagulated patient requiring oral surgery: case report. J Oral Maxillofac Surg 2001;59:1090.

115. Roberts HW, Redding SW. Coronary artery stents: review and patient-management recommendations. J Am Dent Assoc 2000;131:797.

116. Farb A, Sangiorgi G, Carter AJ, et al. Pathology of acute and chronic coronary stenting in humans. Circulation 1999;99:44.

117. Freed LA, Levy D, Levine RA, et al. Prevalence and clinical outcome of mitral-valve prolapse. N Engl J Med 1999;341:1.

118. Nishimura RA, McGoon MD, Shub C, et al. Echocardiographically documented mitral valve prolapse. N Engl J Med 1985;313:1305.

119. Otto CM. Evaluation and management of chronic mitral regurgitation. N Engl J Med 2001;345:740.

120. Burger AJ, Charlamb MJ, Singh S, et al. Low risk of significant echocardiographic valvulopathy in patients treated with anorectic drugs. Int J Cardiol 2001;79:159.

121. Cannistra LB, Gaasch WH. Appetite-suppressing drugs and valvular heart disease. Cardiol Rev 1999;7:356.

122. Connolly HM, Crary JL, McGoon MD, et al. Valvular heart disease associated with fenfluramine-phentermine. N Engl J Med 1997;337:581.

123. Cheitlin MD, Alpert JS, Armstrong WF, et al. ACC/AHA Guidelines for the clinical application of echocardiography. A report of the American College of Cardiology/American Heart Association Task Force on practical guidelines (Committee on Clinical Application of Echocardiography). Circulation 1997;95:1686.

124. Enriquez-Sarano M, Freeman WK, Tribouilloy CM, et al. Functional anatomy of mitral regurgitation: accuracy and outcome implications of transesophageal echocardiography. J Am Coll Cardiol 1999;34:1129.

125. Schwammenthal E, Vered Z, Rabinowitz B, et al. Stress echocardiography beyond coronary artery disease. Eur Heart J 1997;18 Suppl D:D130.

126. Silvestry FE, Kolansky D. Assessment of mitral valvular regurgitation. Cardiac Catheterization 1997;1:25.

127. Bonow RO, Carabello B, de Leon AC Jr, et al. Guidelines for the management of patients with valvular heart disease: a report of the American College of Cardiology/American Heart Association Task Force on Practice Guidelines (Committee on Management of Patients with Valvular Heart Disease). J Am Coll Cardiol 1998;32:1486.

128. Gardin JM, Schumacher D, Constantine G, et al. Valvular abnormalities and cardiovascular status following exposure to dexfenfluramine or phentermine/fenfluramine. JAMA 2000;283:1703.

129. Yeager M, Yock PG, Popp RL. Comparison of Doppler-derived pressure gradient to that determined at cardiac catheterization in adults with aortic valve stenosis: implications for management. Am J Cardiol 1986;57:644.

130. Teague SM, Heinsimer JA, Anderson JL, et al. Quantification of aortic regurgitation utilizing continuous wave Doppler ultrasound. J Am Coll Cardiol 1986;8:592.

131. Perry GJ, Helmcke F, Nanda NC, et al. Evaluation of aortic insufficiency by Doppler color flow mapping. J Am Coll Cardiol 1987;9:952.

132. Smith MD, Harrison MR, Pinton R, et al. Regurgitant jet size by transesophageal compared with transthoracic Doppler color flow imaging. Circulation 1991;83:79.

133. Sutton DC, Cahalan MK. Intraoperative assessment of left ventricular function with transesophageal echocardiography. Cardiol Clin 1993;11:389.

134. Pellikka PA, Nishimura RA, Bailly KR, et al. The natural history of adults with asymptomatic, hemodynamically significant aortic stenosis. J Am Coll Cardiol 1990;15:1012.

135. Rosenhek R, Binder T, Porenta G, et al. Predictors of outcome in severe, asymptomatic aortic stenosis. N Engl J Med 2000;343:611.

136. Cannegeister SC, Rosendaal FR, Wintzen AR, et al. Optimal oral anticoagulant therapy in patients with mechanical heart valves. N Engl J Med 1995;333:11.

137. Cannegeister SC, Rosendaal FR, Briet, E. Thromboembolic and bleeding complications in patients with mechanical heart valve prostheses. Circulation 1994;89:635.

138. Grover FL, Cohen DJ, Oprian C, et al. Determinants of the occurrence of and survival from prosthetic valve endocarditis: experience of the Veterans Affairs Cooperative Study on Valvular Heart Disease. J Thorac Cardiovasc Surg 1994;108:207.

139. Dajani AS, Taubert KA, Wilson W, et al. Prevention of bacterial endocarditis. Recommendations by the American Heart Association. JAMA 1997;277:1794.

140. Eckman MH, Beshansky JR, Durand-Zaleski I, et al. Anticoagulation for noncardiac procedures in patients with prosthetic heart valves: does the risk mean high cost? JAMA 1990;263:1513.

141. Lloyd-Jones DM. The risk of congestive heart failure: sobering lessons from the Framingham Heart Study. Curr Cardiol Rep 2001;3:184–90.

142. McMurray JJ, Stewart S. Epidemiology, aetiology, and prognosis of heart failure. Heart 2000;83:596.

143. Vasan RS, Benjamin EJ, Levy D. Congestive heart failure associated with normal left ventricular systolic function. Arch Intern Med 1996;156:146.

144. Gillespie ND, McNeil G, Pringle T, et al. Cross sectional study of contribution of clinical assessment and simple cardiac investigations in patients admitted with acute dyspnea. BMJ 1997;314:936.

145. Senni M, Rodeheffer RJ, Tribouilloy CM, et al. Use of echocardiography in the management of congestive heart failure in the community. J Am Coll Cardiol 1999;33:164.

146. Bonow R. The hibernating myocardium: implications for management of congestive heart failure. Am J Cardiol 1995;75:17A.

147. Braunwald E, Rutherford JD. Reversible ischemic left ventricular dysfunction: evidence for the "hibernating myocardium." J Am Coll Cardiol 1986;8:1467.

148. Rahimtoola S. From coronary artery disease to heart failure: role of the hibernating myocardium. Am J Cardiol 1995;75:16E.

149. Demakis JG, Proskey A, Rahimtoola SH, et al. The natural course of alcoholic cardiomyopathy. Ann Intern Med 1974;80:293.

150. Pitt B, Zannad F, Remme WJ, et al. The Effect of spironolactone on morbidity and mortality in patients with severe heart failure. N Engl J Med 1999;341:709.

151. Young JB, Gheorghiade M, Uretsky BF, et al. Superiority of "triple" drug therapy in heart failure: insights from the PROVED and RADIANCE trials. J Am Coll Cardiol 1998;32:686.

152. Packer M, Bristow MR, Cohn JN, et al, for the US Carvedilol Heart Failure Study Group. The effect of carvedilol on morbidity and mortality in patients with chronic heart failure. N Engl J Med 1996;334:1349.

153. Pfeffer MA, Stevenson LW. Beta-adrenergic blockers and survival in heart failure [editorial]. N Engl J Med 1996;334:1396.

154. Doughty RN, MacMahon S, Sharpe N. Beta-blockers in heart failure: promising or proved? J Am Coll Cardiol 1994;23:814.

155. Eichhorn EJ, Bristow MR. Practical guidelines for initiation of beta-adrenergic blockade in patients with chronic heart failure. Am J Cardiol 1997;79:794.

156. Al-Khadra AS, Salem DN, Rand WM, et al. Warfarin anticoagulation and survival: a cohort analysis from the Studies of Left Ventricular Dysfunction. J Am Coll Cardiol 1998;31:749.

157. Denes P, Wu D, Dhingra RC, et al. Dual atrioventricular nodal pathways. A common electrophysiologic response. Br Heart J 1975;37:1069–76.

158. Denes P, Wu D, Dhingra RC, et al. Demonstration of dual AV nodal pathways in patients with paroxysmal supraventricular tachycardia. Circulation 1973;48:549.

159. Denes P, Wu D, Amat-Y-Leon F, et al. The determinants of atrioventricular nodal reentrance with premature atrial stimulation in patients with dual AV nodal pathways. Circulation 1977;56:253.

160. Lee Ma, Morady F, Kadish A, et al. Catheter modification of the atrioventricular junction with radiofrequency energy for control of atrioventricular reentry tachycardia. Circulation 1991;83:827.

161. Wellens HJJ. Electrophysiologic properties of the accessory pathway in Wolff-Parkinson-White syndrome. In: Wellens HJJ, Lie KI, Janse MJ, editors. Conduction system of the heart: structure, function, and clinical implication. Leiden: Stenfert Krose BV; 1976. p. 567.

162. The National Heart, Lung and Blood Institute Working Group on Atrial Fibrillation. Atrial fibrillation: current understandings and research imperatives. J Am Coll Cardiol 1993;22:1830.

163. Wolf PA, Kannel WB, McGee DL, et al. Duration of atrial fibrillation and imminence of stroke: The Framingham study. Stroke 1983;14:664.

164. Atrial Fibrillation Investigators. Risk factors for stroke and efficacy of antithrombotic therapy in atrial fibrillation. Analysis of pooled data from five randomized controlled trials. Arch Intern Med 1994;154:1449.

165. Ezekowitz MD, Levine JA. Preventing stroke in patients with atrial fibrillation. JAMA 1999;281:1830.

166. Fuster V, Ryden LE, Asinger RW, et al. American College of Cardiology/American Heart Association/European Society of Cardiology Board. ACC/AHA/ESC guidelines for the management of patients with atrial fibrillation: executive summary. A Report of the American College of Cardiology/American Heart Association Task Force on Practice Guidelines and the European Society of Cardiology Committee for Practice Guidelines and Policy Conferences (Committee to Develop Guidelines for the Management of Patients With Atrial Fibrillation): developed in Collaboration With the North American Society of Pacing and Electrophysiology. J Am Coll Cardiol 2001;38:1231.

167. Manning WJ, Silverman DI, Keighley CS, et al. Transesophageal echocardiographically facilitated early cardioversion from atrial fibrillation using short-term anticoagulation: final results of a prospective 4.5 year study. J Am Coll Cardiol 1995;25:1354.

168. Muzyka BC. Atrial fibrillation and its relationship to dental care. J Am Dent Assoc 1999;130:1080.

169. Josephson ME, Marchlinski FE, Buxton AE, et al. Electrophysiologic basis for sustained ventricular tachycardia: the role of reentry. In: Josephson ME, Wellens HJJ, editors. Tachycardias: mechanisms, diagnosis, treatment. Philadelphia: Lea & Febiger; 1984. p. 305.

170. Gregoratos G, Cheitlin MD, Conill A, et al. ACC/AHA Guidelines for implantation of cardiac pacemakers and antiarrhythmia devices: executive summary. A report of the American College of Cardiology/American Heart Association Task Force on Practice Guidelines (Committee on Pacemaker Implantation). Circulation 1998;97:1325.

14

DISEASES OF THE GASTROINTESTINAL TRACT

MICHAEL A. SIEGEL, DDS, MS
JED J. JACOBSON, DDS, MS, MPH
ROBERT J. BRAUN, DDS, MS

▼ DISEASES OF THE UPPER DIGESTIVE
TRACT
Gastroesophageal Reflux Disease
Hiatal Hernia

▼ DISEASES OF THE LOWER DIGESTIVE
TRACT
Disorders of the Stomach
Disorders of the Intestines

▼ DISEASES OF THE HEPATOBILIARY
SYSTEM
Jaundice
Alcoholic Hepatitis
Drug-Induced Hepatotoxicity
Liver Cirrhosis

▼ GASTROINTESTINAL SYNDROMES
Eating Disorders: Anorexia and Bulimia
Gardner's Syndrome
Plummer-Vinson Syndrome
Peutz-Jeghers Syndrome
Cowden's Syndrome

In this chapter, diseases of the gastrointestinal tract that primarily affect areas other than the oral cavity are discussed. This chapter is not intended to be a complete review of all diseases affecting the gastrointestinal tract; rather, emphasis is on the medical aspects, the dentist's role as a primary health care provider in screening for undiagnosed conditions, and the dentist's role in monitoring patient compliance with recommended medical therapy for gastrointestinal conditions that are likely to be encountered in the general practice of dentistry. Dental health care workers are expected to recognize, diagnose, and treat oral conditions associated with gastrointestinal diseases, as well as provide dental care for afflicted individuals. To provide safe and appropriate dental care, dentists are typically concerned with the proper diagnosis of oral manifestations of gastrointestinal disorders, homeostasis, risk of infection, drug actions and interactions, the patient's ability to withstand the stress and trauma of dental procedures, and proper medical referral (when necessary). These dental management issues are therefore discussed, where appropriate, for each gastrointestinal disorder.

Both dentists and gastroenterologists have their primary focus within the alimentary canal. The common embryogenesis of the oral cavity and gastrointestinal tract is occasionally reinforced for the clinician when he or she finds heterotopic gastric mucosal cysts in the oral mucous membranes or on the tongue.[1,2] However, in addition to these relatively rare anomalies, the paths of gastroenterologists and dentists cross quite frequently in clinical practice. The digestive tract is a long muscular tube that moves food and accumulated secretions from the mouth to the anus. As ingested food is slowly propelled through this tract, the gut assimilates calories and nutrients that are essential for the establishment and maintenance of normal bodily functions. Protein, fats, carbohydrates, vitamins, minerals, water, and orally ingested drugs (prescription and nonprescription) are digested in this tract. This digestive process depends on the hydrolysis of large nonabsorbable molecules into smaller absorbable molecules through secreted enzymes and the absorption of substances through the epithelial lining of the digestive tract. From there, digested substances are transported by blood vessels and lymphatic channels through the body. The remaining contents of undigested food, typically cellulose fiber, are excreted out of the digestive tract through the rectum and anus. The digestion and absorption of nutrient materials depend on: (1) an optimal hydrogen ion concentration (pH) in the gut; (2) the presence of conjugated bile salts; (3) adequate concentrations of enzymes to split fats, proteins, and carbohydrates; and (4) adequate intestinal mobility.

Some of the foods entering the blood from the digestive tract can be used by cells without being altered. However, the majority of the absorbed food passes to special organs, where it is changed into new substances that are needed by cells. One such special organ is the liver, where this intermediate metabolism takes place. Additionally, the gastrointestinal tract is a primary route for drug administration, absorption, biotransformation, detoxification, and excretion. Many dental patients require drug therapy in which pharmacokinetic parameters may be altered by gastrointestinal and hepatobiliary dysfunction. Consequently, oral health care providers must have a comprehensive understanding of the gastrointestinal system and of how normal and abnormal function may affect the oral health care of patients.

The digestive system is composed of the esophagus, stomach, small intestine, and large intestine. Each of these components performs specific functions as ingested substances move through the different anatomic areas. Additionally, the exocrine functions of the pancreas, liver, and gall bladder combine to complete the assimilation of dietary calories and nutrients.

This chapter is organized such that disorders are presented under the following anatomic divisions: esophagus, stomach, small intestine, large intestine, and hepatobiliary tree. A final section on gastrointestinal syndromes introduces disorders the affect both the oral cavity and the gastrointestinal tract but that are not primarily oral or gastrointestinal in etiology.

▼ DISEASES OF THE UPPER DIGESTIVE TRACT

Gastroesophageal Reflux Disease

MEDICAL ASPECTS

Gastroesophageal reflux disease (GERD) is one of the most commonly occurring diseases affecting the upper gastrointestinal tract. The incidence of GERD is increasing in the developed world; upwards of 10% of the population experience heartburn daily. Symptoms can range from mild to severe. There is no difference between the percentage of men and the percentage of women that are affected by GERD. GERD is a disease which has a significant effect on one's activities of daily living as well as an economic effect on individuals and society.

During gastroesophageal reflux, gastric contents (chyme) passively move up from the stomach into the esophagus. While this can occur normally, it may be attributed to GERD if it is associated with symptoms. GERD is often considered a syndrome because it can present with a wide variety of symptoms. Patients may experience mild symptoms with an esophagus that appears to be clinically normal or they may have severe symptoms with surface abnormalities that can be detected with an endoscope. A presumptive diagnosis of GERD may be made for any symptomatic condition that is the result of gastric contents moving into the esophagus. Functional bowel disease is a syndrome with similar symptoms and may mimic GERD; it is often misdiagnosed as GERD.

Heartburn is the cardinal symptom of GERD and is defined as a sensation of burning or heat that spreads upward from the epigastrium to the neck.[3] Although symptoms of GERD can be quite varied, they are primarily symptoms that are associated with the sequelae of mucosal injury. These resultant injuries include esophagitis, esophageal ulceration, stricture, and dysplasia. Chest pain is another important symptom that is related to disorders of the esophagus. Chest pain can mimic the symptoms of an acute cardiovascular disorder and is often the impetus for patients seeking medical care. Dysphagia is also a common presenting complaint that may serve to prompt the dentist to refer the patient to the patient's physician. Several studies have shown that a number of airway problems that were previously thought to be idiopathic, such as laryngitis, chronic cough, hoarseness, and asthma, are in fact the result of microaspiration of refluxate into the airway.[4,5] Alternatively, these symptoms may also arise from disorders of the upper or lower respiratory tracts. GERD complications include premalignant and malignant conditions of the esophagus.

Barrett's esophagus is a variant of GERD in which normal squamous epithelium is replaced by columnar epithelium.[6] Patients with this phenomenon show an increased incidence of adenocarcinoma. This condition may increase the incidence of carcinoma by as much as 10%. A protective effect for adenocarcinoma may result if *Helicobacter pylori* is present.

In one study, esophageal *H. pylori* infection was found in only 8 (5%) of 160 patients with Barrett's esophagus or Barrett's adenocarcinoma. *Helicobacter pylori* organisms in the esophagus were found only on nonintestinalized mucosa. All patients with esophageal *H. pylori* infection and an antral biopsy had antral *H. pylori* infection. Gastric antral *H. pylori* infection was significantly less prevalent in patients in the Barrett's esophagus study group (15 of 91 patients [16.5%]) than in the non-Barrett's esophagus control group (67 of 214 patients [31.3%]). Patients from the control group with an endoscopic diagnosis of duodenal ulcer, gastric ulcer, gastritis, or duodenitis had a significantly higher prevalence of infection when compared with the Barrett's esophagus group. There was no difference in the prevalence of infection in patients in the Barrett's esophagus group and in patients with reflux esophagitis, hiatal hernia, no endoscopic abnormality, or any other diagnosis. This study concluded that esophageal *H. pylori* infection is uncommon in patients with Barrett's esophagus, dysplasia, or adenocarcinoma and may be restricted to non-intestinalized columnar epithelium. Gastric *H. pylori* infection may have a protective effect for the development of Barrett's esophagus.[7]

The relaxation of the lower esophageal sphincter for the purpose of relieving pressure in the stomach (from gas and the ingestion of food) is called the "burp" mechanism. This phenomenon is a normal process and occurs only when a person is in an erect posture; gastric contents are thereby prevented from flowing into the esophagus and possibly being aspirated. The gastroesophageal junction, which prevents the regurgitation (retrograde or upward flow) of gastric contents, is composed of an internal lower esophageal sphincter. External pressure on the junction by the diaphragm also assists in this function. When this barrier fails, gastric contents may make their way into the esophagus and cause symptoms. The cause of lower-esophageal sphincter incompetence is unknown; however, it does not appear to be mechanical. Hiatal hernia was historically recognized as a cause of GERD, but there is no correlation between sphincter pressure and the presence of a hiatal hernia, which leads to the widely accepted position that GERD is not caused by hiatal hernia. Surgery, scleroderma, and drugs such as anticholinergics, cardiac vasoconstrictors, and nicotine can also cause an incompetent sphincter. Estrogen/progesterone combinations used in contraceptives and during pregnancy also have been shown to decrease sphincter pressures.

Symptoms occur when refluxate proceeds through the junction. The severity of the symptoms depends on the amount of acid in the refluxate, the speed with which the esophagus can clear the refluxate, and the presence of buffering agents such as swallowed saliva. An insufficient amount of alkaline fluid prohibits the esophagus from properly buffering the acid that has moved up from the stomach. Patients who smoke, take certain drugs, have had head and neck radiation, or suffer from diseases such a Sjögren's syndrome often do not produce enough saliva to protect the esophagus from the acid in the refluxate. Increased abdominal pressure as a result of obesity, pregnancy, or a large meal may predispose patients to gastric content reflux. Moving into or out of various positions (eg, lying down too soon after eating) will also promote reflux.

MEDICAL MANAGEMENT

Significant success in preventing or reducing the symptoms of GERD is seen with lifestyle modification. Weight loss reduces the pressure difference between the abdomen and the thorax, thereby reducing reflux. Smoking cessation will increase the production of saliva and therefore counteract the symptoms of GERD. Fatty meals slow down gastric emptying and produce distention and reflux. An increase in the fat content of meals may be an important factor in explaining the increase of reflux in the Western world in recent years. Eating large meals and reclining too soon after meals also predisposes to reflux disease. Sleeping with the head of the bed elevated may help empty the esophagus of any refluxate and may prevent symptoms.

Since the mid-1970s, H_2 receptor antagonists have been used to treat GERD and ulcer disease. In patients with GERD, H_2 receptor antagonists improve the symptoms of heartburn and regurgitation and heal mild to moderate esophagitis. Symptoms have been eliminated in up to 50% of patients by twice-a-day prescription dosages of H_2 receptor antagonists. Approximately 50% of patients require higher or more frequent doses to promote the healing of esophagitis. Only about 25% of patients will remain in remission while taking these agents only.

Proton pump inhibitors (PPIs) such as omeprazole and (more recently) lansoprazole have been found to heal erosive esophagitis more efficaciously than do H_2 receptor antagonists. PPIs provide not only symptomatic relief but also resolution of signs, including those that involve significant ulcers and/or esophageal damage.[8] Studies have shown that PPI therapy can provide complete endoscopic mucosal healing of esophagitis at 6 to 8 weeks in 75 to 100% of cases. Daily PPI treatment provides the best long-term reduction of symptoms for patients with moderate to severe esophagitis. Remission for as long as 5 years has been seen.

Promotility drugs are effective in the treatment of mild to moderately symptomatic GERD. These drugs increase lower-esophageal sphincter pressure (which helps decrease acid reflux) and improve the movement of food from the stomach. They decrease heartburn symptoms, especially at night, by improving the clearance of acid from the esophagus. Cisapride is the most effective of the promotility agents.[8]

During the last decade, a significant change has been seen in the role of surgery for the treatment of GERD. Once relatively rare and reserved for patients who had failed every form of medical treatment, antireflux operations are now common and are considered part of the regular armamentarium by those who treat this disease.[9] Patients with a good initial response to medical therapy but who have severe functional and anatomic abnormalities of the gastroesophageal junction are the ones who are most commonly treated with surgery.

ORAL HEALTH CONSIDERATIONS

Patients who experience gastric reflux disease complain of dysgeusia (foul taste), dental sensitivity, erosion and/or pulpitis. Dental sensitivity is generally due to the erosion of enamel by gastric acid. Erosion leads to dentin sensitivity and, at times, irreversible pulpal involvement. Patients who exhibit signs of reflux disease must be medically evaluated and referred appropriately. Patients who have a diagnosis of GERD may need to be treated in a semisupine position and premedicated with H_2 receptor antagonists or antacids. Any medications that may cause nausea (such as narcotic analgesics) should be prescribed judiciously because of the increased likelihood of regurgitation and possible aspiration. Mild baking soda mouth rinses (one-half teaspoon of sodium bicarbonate in 8 ounces of water) may be rinsed and expectorated to minimize dysgeusia due to acid reflux. Topical fluoride applications via a custom-made occlusive tray will ensure optimal dental mineralization.

H_2 receptor antagonists may cause central nervous system (CNS) effects in a continuum from fatigue and lethargy to confusion, delirium, and seizures. These effects are dose dependent; thus, they may be seen more commonly in elderly persons or in those with impaired kidney or liver function. Patients who are taking cimetidine may experience a toxic reaction to lidocaine if injected intravascularly. Cimetidine also has been shown to inhibit the absorption (and therefore, the blood concentration) of the systemic antifungal drug ketaconazole. Soft-tissue changes such as esophageal fibrosis and stricture may complicate intubation if the patient requires general anesthesia. Oral mucosal changes are minimal; however, erythema and mucosal atrophy may be present as a result of the exposure of tissues to acid.

Hiatal Hernia

MEDICAL ASPECTS

The esophagus passes through the diaphragmatic hiatus and into the stomach just inferior to the diaphragm. The hiatus causes an anatomic narrowing of the opening into the stomach and thus helps prevent reflux of stomach contents into the esophagus. Some patients have a weakened or enlarged hiatus, perhaps due to hereditary factors. It may also may be caused by obesity, exercising (eg, weight lifting), or chronic straining when passing stools. When a weakened or enlarged hiatus occurs, a portion of the stomach herniates into the chest cavity through this enlarged hole, resulting in a hiatal hernia. Hiatal hernias are quite common; occurrence rates of between 20 and 60% have been reported in the medical literature.[3] The incidence of hiatal hernia increases with age although the condition is also seen in infants and children. Because the diaphragm separates the thorax from the abdomen, symptoms of hiatal hernia often include chest pain, which may radiate in patterns similar to those of myocardial infarction pain. If the hiatal hernia is small, there may be no symptoms. On the other hand, if the area of the hiatus is very weak, the function of preventing reflux may be compromised, resulting in the entry of acidic digestive juices into the esophagus.

Hiatal hernias are classified into three major types.[3] The sliding type is the most common hiatal hernia. In this type, the herniated portion of the stomach slides back and forth through the diaphragm into the chest. These hernias are normally small and often present with minimal (if any) symptoms. In the fixed type of hiatal hernia, the upper part of the stomach is fixed through the diaphragm into the chest. There may be few symptoms with this type as well. However, the potential for problems in the esophagus increases. The complicated type is the most serious and least common form of hiatal hernia. This form includes a variety of herniation patterns of the stomach, including those in which the entire stomach moves into the chest. The likelihood of significant medical problems with this type is high; its treatment requires surgery.

Infants with hiatal hernia usually regurgitate bloodstained food and may also have difficulty in breathing and swallowing. Adult patients with hiatal hernia may experience chronic acid reflux into the esophagus. Chronic gastrointestinal reflux can erode the esophageal lining, causing bleeding, which may lead to anemia. Additionally, chronic esophageal inflammation may produce scarring, resulting in esophageal narrowing. This narrowing causes dysphagia, and because food does not pass easily into the stomach, patients experience an uncomfortable feeling of fullness or "bloating." Adults typically present with heartburn that is exacerbated when bending forward or lying down. The pain may spread to the jaw and down the arms, similar to an attack of angina pectoris. Other symptoms include hiccups, a dry cough, and an increase in the contractile force of the heart. In contrast to abdominal hernias, hiatal hernias have no outward physical signs. Diagnosis is made through a combination of endoscopy and contrast radiography.

MEDICAL MANAGEMENT

Defects present at birth may sometimes correct themselves. Until this occurs, however, the infant should sleep in a crib with the head raised and be given an altered diet consisting of food that has a thicker-than-normal consistency. With adults, anything that will increase abdominal pressure and cause reflux, such as bending, abdominal exercises, and tight belts and girdles, should be avoided. Because obesity increases intra-abdominal pressure, weight loss may be recommended to relieve symptoms. Sleeping with the head elevated will also prevent the symptoms of hiatal hernia. Antacids help relieve heartburn by neutralizing stomach acids. H_2 receptor antagonists are effective in inhibiting the action of histamine on parietal cells, which reduces the production of gastric acids.[8] Patients should also eat smaller and more frequent meals and should have their main meal at lunchtime. This should be followed by a light supper, with nothing being consumed within 2 to 3 hours of bedtime. Foods and habits that increase the reflux of acid should be avoided or significantly reduced. These foods or habits include nicotine (tobacco products), alcohol, caffeine, chocolate, fatty foods, and peppermint or spearmint oil flavorings.

Drug therapy usually allows patients to avoid all symptoms of hiatal hernia without significant inconvenience. The disadvantage to this approach is that many patients object to taking daily medications for the rest of their lives or find the process too onerous to carry out. When conservative medical measures fail to control the condition, the hernia is surgically corrected. However, surginal correction is complex, and nonsurgical remedies are preferable.[10,11]

Surgery is currently considered to be a treatment of last resort, and some authors argue that surgery is never indicated for a hiatal hernia. Surgical access is gained either through the chest or through the abdomen. These approaches carry high risks of operative and perioperative morbidity. Recent surgical advances have made it possible to do the repair laparoscopically.[10]

ORAL HEALTH CONSIDERATIONS

If a hiatal hernia is treated with medications that cause xerostomia (dry mouth), the dose or drug type may need to be altered by the patient's physician. Various treatment modalities for dry mouth (such as artificial saliva, alcohol-free mouthwashes, or increased fluid intake) may need to be prescribed. Class V caries or root caries are sequelae of dry mouth, even in patients who have been relatively free of caries prior to developing the disease. If reflux into the oral cavity is present, oral manifestations that are the same as those of GERD are seen (see "Gastroesophageal Reflux Disease," above).

▼ DISEASES OF THE LOWER DIGESTIVE TRACT

Disorders of the Stomach

The stomach serves primarily as a secretory organ and as a reservoir. The stomach secretes acid, mucus, pepsinogen, and intrinsic factor. The secreted hydrochloric acid is essential for killing swallowed bacteria while the mucus helps to coat and lubricate the stomach's lining epithelium, in order to propel the ingested contents through the digestive system. Pepsinogen is a proteolytic enzyme that helps digest protein and intrinsic factor, a glycoprotein that permits the adequate absorption of dietary vitamin B_{12}. The stomach collects food that is often ingested in bursts, then slowly empties the chyme (the semifluid mass of partly digested food) into the duodenum over time.

PEPTIC ULCER DISEASE

Peptic ulcer disease is a common benign (nonmalignant) ulceration of the epithelial lining of the stomach (gastric ulcer) or duodenum (duodenal ulcer). When patients or physicians refer to ulcers or ulcer disease, they are usually referring to a duodenal or gastric ulcer. About 6% of patients attending a dentist office will have peptic ulcer disease.[12,13] Since peptic ulcer disease includes both gastric (stomach) ulcers and duodenal ulcers, a general discussion of peptic ulcer disease is presented first, followed by specific information on gastric and duodenal ulcers, under the corresponding anatomic region.

Peptic ulcer disease represents a serious medical problem largely because of its frequency; there are approximately 500,000 new cases and 4,000,000 recurrences each year in the United States. The estimated annual direct cost for treatment of patients with ulcer disease is approximately $8 billion to $10 billion (US). It is likely that the enlarging geriatric population in the United States, coupled with the increasing use of nonsteroidal anti-inflammatory drugs (NSAIDs) that have inherent damaging effects on the gastroduodenal mucosa, will contribute to the costs of this disease.[14,15]

Data indicate that the lifetime prevalence of peptic ulcers ranges from 11 to 14% for men and 8 to 11% for women. The 1-year point prevalence of active gastric and duodenal ulcers in the United States is about 1.8%.[12–15] Genetic factors appear to play a role in the pathogenesis of ulcers. The concordance for peptic ulcers among identical twins is approximately 50%.

In first-degree relatives of ulcer patients, the lifetime prevalence of developing ulcers is about threefold greater than that in the general population.[12–15]

Within the last decade, it has become accepted that gastric ulcers primarily result from altered mucosal defenses whereas duodenal ulcers are associated with increased acid production. It has become clear that *Helicobacter pylori* plays a vital role in peptic ulcer development in both sites. A complex relationship exits between host defense mechanisms, the presence of elevated acid, pepsin levels, and *H. pylori*. The incidence of duodenal ulcers also increases in cigarette smokers, patients with chronic renal disease, and alcoholics. *Helicobacter pylori* is observed in the gastric mucosa in 90 to 100% of patients with duodenal ulcers and 70 to 90% of patients with gastric ulcers. Consequently, it has been proposed that the bacteria may be the cause of both the gastritis and the reduced mucosal resistance that leads to ulcer formation in the stomach.[13] It is noteworthy that healing of peptic ulcers of either the stomach or duodenum is usually facilitated by specific antimicrobial treatment and by the elimination of this bacterium.[14]

Many patients with duodenal ulcers have demonstrable hyperacidity, and it is thought that this is the dominant factor in the development of ulcer disease. Concomitant inflammation and infection with *H. pylori* are noted in the gastric antrum in more than 80% of cases of duodenal ulcers. In gastric ulcers, however, the relative importance of the two major factors of acid amounts and mucosal resistance is reversed. Typically, the concentration of gastric acid is normal or reduced, and prior injury (mucosal) from other causes appears to be a prerequisite for the development of gastric ulcers. Most patients with the disease have recurrent pain and consult their physician periodically for relief of symptoms and to preventi recurrence. About 10 to 20% of these patients have a life-threatening complication (ie, hemorrhage, perforation, or obstruction).[12,13,15] Failure to recognize and manage these patients properly on these occasions can have grave consequences. Since about 6% of the patients attending a dental office will have a peptic ulcer, it is essential that dentists (1) recognize the morbidity associated with peptic ulcers and the symptoms associated with undiagnosed or poorly managed peptic ulcer disease and (2) make a referral to the primary care physician or gastroenterologist when these symptoms are recognized.

It is important to discuss gastric and duodenal ulcers separately because each has implications for dentists and the patients they treat. As this chapter is organized anatomically, gastric ulcer disease is discussed first, and duodenal ulcer disease is discussed later, under "Disorders of the Intestines."

MEDICAL ASPECTS OF GASTRIC ULCER DISEASE

Gastric ulcers are only one-tenth to one-fourth as frequent as duodenal ulcers. They are also more common in lower socioeconomic groups. Gastric ulcers occur more often after 50 years of age and are seen at a male-to-female ratio of 3:1. Gastric ulcers are generally of more concern because approximately 3 to 8% of gastric ulcers represent malignant ulceration of the gastric mucosa.[12–16] Therefore, accurate diagnosis requires multiple biopsies and brush specimens for cytologic examination. These additional diagnostic tests are often performed by a gastroenterologist. In general, the diagnostic procedures are the same as those performed in cases of duodenal ulcers, except that the diagnosis is more urgent and that additional diagnostic studies other than gastroscopy are warranted. It is essential to ascertain gastric acidity levels with ulcers of the stomach because a stomach ulcer in the presence of histamine-fast achlorhydria has a very high chance of being a malignant ulcer rather than a peptic ulcer.

Patients with gastric ulcers often present with epigastric pain radiating to the back. In contrast to the symptoms of duodenal ulcers, the pain is aggravated by food. The management and the treatment of gastric ulcers are similar to those of duodenal ulcers, except that gastric ulcers are usually diagnosed and treated more vigorously, and follow-up studies to document the healing process are essential for gastric ulcers. Nevertheless, the standard medical treatment of gastric ulcers involves antacid compounds, antibiotics to eradicate *H. pylori*, H_2 blocking agents, and other protective drugs. Additional information about peptic ulcer disease and management in the dental office is presented in the following section on duodenal ulcers.

Disorders of the Intestines

The small intestine comprises the duodenum, jejunum, and ileum. The duodenum is the principal site of digestion and absorption. When chyme enters the duodenum, it stimulates the pancreas to secrete sodium bicarbonate (to neutralize the gastric acid) and to secrete digestive enzymes for normal digestion of food. Additionally, chyme in the duodenum stimulates the gall bladder to discharge stored bile through the common bile duct. Vitamin B_{12} in the presence of intrinsic factor is absorbed in the distal small intestine (ileum). The bile acids that promote fat absorption in the duodenum are themselves also reabsorbed in the small bowel, returned to the liver, and resecreted into the bile. The motor activity of the small intestine propels the chyme forward to the large intestine. The major role of the large intestine is to receive the ileal effluent, absorb most of the water and salt, and thus produce solid feces.

DUODENAL ULCER DISEASE

Medical Aspects.   A duodenal ulcer represents a break through the mucosa into the submucosa or deeper. The base of the ulcer is necrotic tissue consisting of pus and fibrin. When the ulcer erodes into an adjacent blood vessel, there is hemorrhage. If erosion continues through the serous outer layer of the duodenum, adjacent organs or perforation into the peritoneal cavity occurs. When conditions are favorable the ulcer heals, with granulation tissue and new epithelium. If the ulcer is present for prolonged periods, it becomes associated with scar tissue and possible deformity.

The incidence of duodenal ulcer is thought to be declining, but it is still a common disorder developing in about 10% of the US population. Of all peptic ulcers, 80 to 85% are duode-

nal, and duodenal ulcers occur at a male-to-female ratio of 4:1. The most common primary cause is *Helicobacter pylori* infection, but NSAID use also can be an associated etiologic factor. Less commonly, factors such as stress, exogenous steroids, parathyroid disease, malignant carcinoid, cirrhosis, gastrinoma of the pancreas (Zollinger-Ellison disease), polycythema vera, and chronic lung disease have been associated with duodenal ulcers.[12–16] The ulceration is usually located in the first part of the duodenum because the acidic chyme ordinarily becomes alkaline after pancreatic secretions enter the intestines in the second part of the duodenum.

The most common symptom of an uncomplicated ulcer is epigastric pain. The pain is often perceived as a burning or gnawing sensation sometimes associated with nausea and vomiting and usually occurs when the stomach is empty or when not enough of a meal remains in the stomach to adequately buffer the acid stimulated by the meal. Therefore, the pain often begins 1 or more hours after eating and when the patient is asleep. The pain is characteristically relieved within a few minutes by buffering or diluting the gastric acid with ingestion of an antacid, milk, food, or even water. Once an individual has had a duodenal ulcer, the chance of recurrence is high. Frequently, these attacks will occur with a change of season, especially in spring or autumn. When an ulcer perforates and hemorrhages, the patient often vomits gross blood or (when the blood interacts with acid) material that appears as coffee grounds. Also, the stools can appear black or tarlike or may sometimes contain gross blood. The blood loss can lead to iron deficiency anemia, and if the blood loss is acute, the patient may be weak, light-headed, and short of breath.[15]

Physical examination is usually of little use in the diagnosis of duodenal ulcers. The early diagnostic cues are based on the history of a periodic pain pattern. Duodenal ulcers usually feel better postprandially, and the pain of gastric ulcers is frequently exacerbated by meals. The mainstay of the diagnosis of a duodenal ulcer is an upper-gastrointestinal radiologic examination, which will demonstrate the presence of an ulcer in up to 85% of patients. In this procedure, the patient swallows a barium salt that outlines the lumen and mucosal surface of the gastrointestinal tract and thereby demonstrates any disruption of the mucosal surface. Endoscopy is an acceptable and sometimes preferable means of diagnosis. If the ulceration is too superficial to be detected by a gastrointestinal radiologic examination or if a gastric ulcer with the possibility of malignancy is suspected, endoscopy is recommended.[16] The presence of *H. pylori* can be demonstrated by biopsy if endoscopy is used. Serologic tests and tests that detect the presence of labeled carbon dioxide in the breath after oral administration of labeled urea are available.[13]

In cases of Zollinger-Ellison syndrome caused by a gastrinoma of the pancreas, specific determination of the etiology is necessary because this disease is treatable and is particularly severe, causing multiple ulcers and debilitating diarrhea. The tumor of Zollinger-Ellison syndrome secretes gastrin, a potent acid producer, and the diagnosis is made on the basis of extremely high levels of gastric acid and elevated levels of serum gastrin.[15] The usual laboratory tests include a complete blood count for detecting anemia and leukocytosis, an examination of the stool for occult blood, and a serum calcium test for detecting an occasional elevation from an associated hyperparathyroidism or endocrine tumors with Zollinger-Ellison syndrome.

Management.   In the absence of complications such as massive bleeding, obstruction due to scarring, and perforation, medical rather than surgical treatment is preferred. Obviously, foods that cause discomfort to the patient should be avoided. Substances or drugs that have potent acidogenic properties with little ability to neutralize acid should be avoided; among these are alcohol, tobacco, aspirin, and NSAIDs. If NSAIDs cannot be avoided, the patient also should be treated with misoprostol. Attempts to eradicate *H. pylori* are necessary in all patients with a peptic ulcer in which the organism can be demonstrated. Bismuth, metronidazole, amoxicillin, and tetracycline have been shown to be effective.[12–16]

In addition to the drugs used to eliminate *H. pylori*, medical treatment involves the following six other classes of drugs: (1) sedatives to reduce mental stress if anxiety is thought to be etiologic; (2) antacids to neutralize acid; (3) drugs that act by covering and protecting the ulcer; (4) anticholinergic drugs to decrease the production of acid by the gastric mucosa; (5) histamine H_2 receptor antagonists (cimetidine, famotidine, nizatidine, or ranitidine), which block the action of histamine on the gastric parietal cells, thus reducing food-stimulated acid secretion up to 75%; and (6) omeprazole, which also suppresses gastric acid secretion but which has a different mechanism of action from that of anticholinergics or H_2 receptor antagonists. Antacids and dietary changes are the mainstays of therapy. Anticholinergics are sometimes prescribed, particularly for reducing acid production at night. However, limited effectiveness and side effects such as mouth dryness make anticholinergics less attractive than histamine H_2 receptor antagonists. In most patients, the pain is controlled within 1 week, and most ulcers heal by the sixth week. Intractable symptoms or complicated duodenal ulcers may require surgery.[12,15]

Oral Health Considerations.   If a patient presents with symptoms of epigastric pain, as described previously, the dentist should refer this person to the primary care physician for diagnostic work-up. Oral manifestations of peptic ulcer disease are rare unless there is anemia from gastrointestinal bleeding or persistent regurgitation of gastric acid as a result of pyloric stenosis leading to dental erosion, typically of the palatal aspect of the maxillary teeth. Vascular malformations of the lip have been reported and range from a very small macule to a large venous pool.[17,18]

The dentist will often see patients with a history of peptic ulcer disease. To prevent the aggravation of the disease in these patients, the avoidance of actions that increase the production of acid is essential. Thus, lengthy dental procedures should be avoided or spread out over shorter appointments to minimize

stress. Also, dentists should avoid administering drugs that exacerbate ulceration and cause gastrointestinal distress, such as aspirin and other NSAIDs; acetaminophen products are preferable and are recommended. A patient who reacts to dental procedures in a particularly stressful way may be a candidate for sedation. Dentists should be aware that patients who are taking anticholinergic drugs often present with dry mouth. This may be particularly problematic for denture wearers. Denture adhesives and artificial saliva may aid in the retention of these prostheses. There is an increased risk of dental caries if hyposalivation is prolonged and if the patient places sugar-containing items into the mouth in an effort to stimulate saliva flow or uses sugar-ladened antacid lozenges. Therefore, artificial saliva and/or chewing sugarless gum to stimulate salivary flow may help prevent dental caries. Informing the patient of this side effect of anticholinergic drugs and stressing proper diet and oral hygiene are critical for these patients. Additionally, because many antacids contain calcium, magnesium, and aluminum salts that bind antibiotics such as erythromycin and tetracycline, the dentist should be aware that administration of one of these drugs within an hour of antacid therapy may decrease the absorption of the antibiotic by 75 to 85%. Consequently, antibiotics should be taken 2 hours before or 2 hours after ingestion of antacids. Exogenous steroid administration is likely to exacerbate the ulcer because of the increased production of acid caused by the steroid and should be avoided. Although it is generally good policy to prescribe penicillin V instead of penicillin G (because of the destruction of penicillin G by gastric acid), it is essential with patients who have peptic ulcers.

Before extensive oral surgical or periodontal procedures are undertaken, it may be prudent to determine the patient's red blood cell count, hemoglobin, hematocrit, and platelet count. If the patient has a history of ulcer perforation and subsequent hemorrhage, blood loss can result in anemia. Consequently, the associated risks of performing surgery on an anemic patient will be encountered. Delayed healing, risk of bacterial infection (particularly with anaerobic bacteria, due to tissue hypoxia), and grave side effects of respiratory depression by narcotic analgesics enhanced by a state of anemia are examples of such associated risks. Lastly, cimetidine and rantidine, drugs commonly prescribed for duodenal ulcer patients, have occasionally been associated with thrombocytopenia.

INFLAMMATORY BOWEL DISEASE

Inflammatory bowel disease (IBD) is a general classification of inflammatory processes that affect the large and small intestines. Ulcerative colitis and Crohn's disease together make up inflammatory bowel disease. Since many other intestinal diseases with known etiologies also have an inflammatory basis, it has been suggested that Crohn's disease and ulcerative colitis should more appropriately be designated as idiopathic inflammatory bowel disease. Ulcerative colitis involves the mucosa and submucosa of the colon. Crohn's disease or regional enteritis is an inflammatory condition involving all layers of the gut.

The precise etiology and pathogenesis of ulcerative colitis and Crohn's disease are unknown, and the two diseases share many features. Accordingly, the diagnostic separation of these two disorders often depends on the results of the radiographic, endoscopic, and histologic examinations. The two conditions are presented separately in this chapter since the management and prognosis of each may be different.

The medical and dental literature is replete with articles describing extra-abdominal and oral signs of inflammatory bowel diseases, including pyostomatitis vegetans, aphthous ulcerations, cobblestone appearance of the oral mucosa, oral epithelial tags and folds, gingivitis, persistent lip swelling, lichenoid mucosal reactions, granulomatous inflammation of minor salivary gland ducts, candidiasis, and angular cheilitis.[19–29] Recent dental literature has focused on the oral status of IBD patients with regard to their caries rate, salivary antimicrobial proteins, and infections of bacterial and fungal origins.[30–35] In fact, it is accepted that oral manifestations of IBD may precede the onset of intestinal radiographic lesions by as much as 1 year or more.[24,36] Both diseases are of interest to the dentist because of their associated oral findings and the impact of their medical management (particularly the use of corticosteroids) on dental management.

Once IBD is established, patients suffer episodic acute attacks that become superimposed on chronic disease. As a result, the patient is likely to suffer from disabling disease for decades. The annual incidence of IBD in the United States ranges from 3.9 to 10 new cases per 100,000 persons. Incidence rates for both diseases are higher in urban areas than in rural areas. Crohn's disease occurs less frequently than ulcerative colitis, but both are slightly on the rise.[12,13,15,16]

Overall, both diseases show three peak incidence rates. The first and highest peak occurs between the ages of 20 and 24 years, the second at ages 40 to 44 years, and the third at ages 60 to 64 years. By the age 60 years, the incidence of ulcerative colitis far exceeds that of Crohn's disease. Northern European and English women appear to have a 30% increased risk of developing ulcerative colitis or Crohn's disease. IBD more frequently affects Caucasians, and Ashkenazi Jews, especially those originating in Middle Europe, Poland, or Russia, exhibit a particularly high IBD risk.[12,13,15,16]

ULCERATIVE COLITIS

Medical Aspects. The inflammation in ulcerative colitis may affect all or part of the large intestine. Macroscopically, the mucosa may have a granular appearance if the disease is mild. When fulminant, the disease may include stripping of the mucosa, with areas of sloughing, ulceration, and bleeding. Ulcerative colitis remains a disease of unknown etiology. Despite intense interest in possible bacterial, viral, immunologic, and psychological factors, there has been no firm etiology established. Although much has been written about psychological factors associated with IBD, most gastroenterologists no longer accept the idea that the disease is primarily a psychiatric disorder. Rather, the frequent psychi-

atric problems experienced by patients are a result of the disease, not the cause of it. The most likely explanation of the evidence involves an autoimmune reaction, with sensitization and destruction of the colonic mucosa in the setting of abnormal immunologic regulation. As the superficial mucosal lesions enlarge, they may be perpetuated by secondary bacterial invasion.[12,13,15,16]

The hallmark of ulcerative colitis is rectal bleeding and diarrhea. The frequency of bowel movements and the amount of blood present reflect the activity of the disease. Typically, the diarrhea is severe, possibly five to eight bowel movements in 24 hours. Patients usually complain of pain that is in both abdominal quadrants and that is crampy in nature and exacerbated prior to bowel movement. Along with the change in the pattern of bowel movements, the patient may have nocturnal diarrhea. Extraintestinal manifestations may be prominent. Erythema nodosum, characterized by red swollen nodules that are usually on the thighs and legs, may be present. Eye changes such as episcleritis, uveitis, corneal ulcers, and retinitis may cause pain and photophobia. Joint symptoms occur in up to 20% of patients with the disease, usually affecting the ankles, knees, and wrists. Perhaps the most pernicious complication of ulcerative colitis is liver disease. Although the other extraintestinal manifestations usually undergo remission with control of the colon inflammation, liver disease may continue, and the dentist must recognize this risk.[12,13,15,16] Anemia is commonly associated with ulcerative colitis. It is most likely caused by blood loss and is typically a microcytic hypochromic anemia of iron deficiency. Leukocytosis occurs in active disease and is usually associated with intra-abdominal abcess. Electrolyte imbalances, hypoalbuminemia, and low serum magnesium and potassium levels may occur because of the severe diarrhea.[12,13,15,16]

Diagnosis and Treatment. Diagnosis of ulcerative colitis is made on the basis of careful history, physical examination, gastrointestinal radiography, and endoscopy, which involves direct visualization of the intestinal mucosa. Most important is the sigmoidoscopic examination, which usually reveals the characteristic picture of multiple tiny mucosal ulcers covered by blood and pus. Lacking any specific markers, the diagnosis of ulcerative colitis is essentially one of exclusion.[15]

The therapy for ulcerative colitis is aimed at reducing the inflammation and correcting the effects of the disease. Sulfazalazine is used to initiate and maintain a remission in ulcerative colitis. Its active moiety, 5-aminocsalicylate, has a direct anti-inflammatory effect on intestinal tissues without altering the colon flora. Corticosteroids and corticotropin (adrenocorticotropic hormone [ACTH]) are used in patients who have not responded satisfactorily to sulfazalazine. They are administered in high doses (eg, 40 to 60 mg of oral prednisone daily initially, then maintenance doses of 10 to 20 mg of prednisone daily). Immunosuppressive agents such as azathioprine, cyclosporine, and mercaptopurine are being used, with varying results. Because of the risk of hematologic suppression and superinfection in patients taking these medications, they are reserved for patients who have not responded to traditional medical therapy. Approximately 15 to 20% of patients will receive surgery for intractable disease. Proctocolectomy combined with ileostomy is a curative procedure for ulcerative colitis. With the new disposable ileostomy equipment available today, most patients can look forward to an active lifestyle and normal life expectancy.[12,15]

Oral Health Considerations. Due to the symptoms of severe frequent diarrhea and abdominal pain or cramping, it is unlikely that a patient will be seeking routine dental care with undiagnosed ulcerative colitis. Nonetheless, should an undiagnosed patient attend a dental office for care, then the risks associated with anemia (such as delayed healing, an increased risk of infection, the side effects of narcotic analgesics, and depression of respiration) collectively contraindicate surgical treatment until the disease is under control. Obviously, following a history and a thorough examination, signs and symptoms of ulcerative colitis and/or anemia would warrant a referral to the patient's primary care physician. More likely is the situation of a diagnosed and medically managed patient attending a dental office for routine or episodic oral health care. The following section addresses those issues a dentist must be knowledgeable about when treating patients who have ulcerative colitis.

The oral changes that occur in ulcerative colitis cases are nonspecific and uncommon, with an incidence of less than 8%. Aphthous stomatitis of the major and minor variety has been reported in patients with active ulcerative colitis. There is nothing unique about these lesions, and it has been suggested that their appearance is coincidental.[18] However, they may result from nutritional deficiencies of iron, folic acid, and vitamin B_{12} due to poor absorption in the gut and/or blood loss directly related to the ulcerative colitis. In addition, antiinflammatory medications such as the 5-aminosalicylates, which often represent the mainstay of therapy for IBD patients and which are excreted in saliva, are known to cause aphthous ulcers and RAU in some patients.[37–39] In patients who are prone to develop aphthous ulcers, the appearance of a new crop of oral ulcers often heralds a flare-up of the bowel disease. Other nonspecific forms of ulceration associated with skin lesions have been reported. Pyoderma gangrenosum may occur in the form of deep ulcers that sometimes ulcerate through the tonsillar pillar.[18]

Pyostomatitis vegetans, a purulent inflammation of the mouth, may also occur. These oral lesions are characterized by deep-tissue vegetating or proliferative lesions that undergo ulceration and then suppuration. As the lesions disappear with a total colectomy, it is speculated that these manifestations are due to the effects of circulating immunocomplexes induced by antigens that are derived from the gut lumen or the damaged colonic mucosa.[20] Lastly, ulcerative colitis patients also can develop hairy leukoplakia, a lesion more commonly associated with acquired immunodeficiency syndrome (AIDS).[40] This lesion probably serves as a marker of severe immunosuppression and may result from the use of corticosteroids or other immunosuppressive agents. Medical management for ulcera-

tive colitis may necessitate alterations of dental therapy or special precautions. Sulfasalazine interferes with folate metabolism, and supplemental folic acid may be needed, especially if a macrocytic anemia is revealed in a complete blood count.

Many side effects are associated with the use of corticosteroids and ACTH. The development of hypertension and diabetes are serious side effects for patients who are taking these two drugs and the dentist must be aware of this. Obtaining a blood pressure reading and obtaining a blood glucose measurement by finger prick in the office and/or consultation with the treating physician to understand the patient's current medical status is critical. Long-term corticosteroid therapy may cause osteoporosis and vertebral compression fractures; thus, carefully positioning the patient in the dental chair and encouraging the patient to take dietary calcium supplements may help prevent fractures. Long-term use of steroids can also result in adrenal suppression. Major operative procedures can precipitate adrenal insufficiency if the steroid doses are not adjusted properly. Patients undergoing surgery require increased doses of steroids before and after the procedure because their own adrenal response to stress is blunted. Patients who were formerly on steroid therapy may also experience adrenal suppression. For example, 20 mg of prednisone daily for 7 to 10 days can cause adrenal suppression, and adrenal activity may not return to normal for 9 to 12 months. Clearly, consultation with the patient's physician is warranted prior to surgical procedures. The details of steroid dosage adjustment for various dental procedures are described on pages XX to XX.

Chronic bleeding can be associated with ulcerative colitis. Prior to dental procedures, blood studies that include hemoglobin, hematocrit, and a red blood cell count should be undertaken to rule out the presence of anemia. Further, patients on immunosuppressive agents such as azathioprine might be expected to have changes in white and red blood cell counts, and total and differential white blood cell counts should be ascertained before embarking on surgical procedures. Patients who have extensive bowel surgery may suffer from malabsorption of vitamin K, vitamin B_{12}, and folic acid. Again, before any surgical procedures are completed, these patients should be evaluated for both macrocytic and microcytic anemia and bleeding disorders from insufficient levels of vitamin K (fibrin clot formation). Clotting factors II, VII, IX, and X are all dependent on Vitamin K. Thus, a prothrombin time and a partial thromboplastin time should be obtained. Alternatively, an international normalized ratio (INR) will also provide critical information about the patient's ability to form a blood clot.

Finally, patients taking the immunosuppressive agent azathioprine may suffer from additional side effects that impact dental management. Suppression of the liver can be expected, and liver function tests should be completed in those patients who will receive dentist-prescribed medications that are metabolized in the liver. Typically, patients taking an immunosuppressive agent like azathioprine are monitored by their primary care physician with liver function tests. Consequently, consultation with the patient's physician will help the dentist determine the patient's liver function. Obviously, toxic doses of the same drugs may be reached if reduced drug metabolism is not taken into consideration.

CROHN'S DISEASE

Medical Aspects.   Crohn's disease is an inflammatory disease of the small or large intestine. The inflammation involves all the layers of the gut. Gross examination may reveal mucosal ulceration (aphthous ulcers within the mucosa that appear normal, deep ulcers within areas of swollen mucosa, or long linear serpiginous ulcers). Recent epidemiologic evidence suggests that there are two forms of Crohn's disease: a nonperforating form that tends to recur slowly and a perforating or aggressive form that evolves more rapidly. Patients with the aggressive perforating type are more prone to develop fistulae and abscesses whereas the more indolent nonperforating type tends to lead to stenotic obstruction.[12,13,15,16] With the involvement of either the colon or small intestine, microscopic examination reveals inflammatory infiltrate in all layers of affected bowel, with plasma cells and lymphocytes predominating in the lamina propria.

Crohn's disease shares many epidemiologic features with ulcerative colitis. There has been a steady rise in the incidence and prevalence of Crohn's disease, but no clear correlation exists between the increased incidence and environmental or lifestyle changes. Crohn's disease affects all ages and both sexes and occurs most frequently in urban women aged 20 to 39 years. The prevalence of Crohn's disease among first-degree relatives is 21 times higher than that among nonrelatives. Evidence for familial association in Crohn's disease includes increased incidence in Jewish populations, strong familial aggregation, and increased concordance among monozygotic twins or triplets.[12,13,15,16]

The cause and evolution of Crohn's disease are unknown. The single strongest risk factor for Crohn's disease, overpowering any influences of diet, smoking, stress, or hygiene, is having a relative with the disease. The fact that first-degree relatives of Crohn's disease patients exhibit increased intestinal permeability supports the theory of an inheritable permeability defect in Crohn's disease. This abnormal intestinal barrier could result in the increased uptake of injurious materials and/or enhanced immune reaction to intestinal antigens. Other theories have included vascular disease, lymphatic obstruction, and emotional stress. Whatever the process, tiny erosions of the overlying normal mucosal lymphoid tissues coalesce to form small aphthous ulcers and more diffuse ulceration of the mucosa eventually. With progression, there is marked hyperplasia of the lymphoid tissue extending through the wall, fibrosis and muscular hypertrophy leading to constrictures, and inflammatory tracts. Granulomas are present in about 50% of patients.[12,13,15,16]

The clinical presentation of Crohn's disease depends on the extent of inflammation and on the site of intestinal involvement. The usual presentation is that of a young person in the late teens or twenties who has been ill for an indefinite period and whose disease suddenly worsens. The history often reveals intermittent episodes of abdominal distress, fever, and crampy abdominal pain accompanied by loose stools. Although bleeding is a prominent feature of ulcerative colitis, it is rare in cases of small-bowel Crohn's disease.[15]

Inflammation of the small intestine may impair its absorption of vital nutrients. Calcium, iron, and folate are absorbed in the duodenum, and their decreased absorption due to inflammation can lead to deficiencies. Disease in the terminal ileum may interfere with the absorption of bile salts and vitamin B_{12}. Inflammation of the small or large intestines may impair the absorption of fat, fat-soluble vitamins, salt, water, protein, and iron.

The absorptive function of the small bowel is more likely to be altered in patients with Crohn's disease than in those with ulcerative colitis. Electrolyte abnormalities and low albumin levels commonly occur in cases of severe diarrhea. Anemia, usually resulting from an iron or folate deficiency, also may be present. Leukocytosis may be present; counts of $> 15,000/cm^3$ are suggestive of abscess or perforation.

The signs and symptoms of Crohn's disease are often more subtle than those associated with ulcerative colitis, frequently delaying the diagnosis. However, the diagnosis can usually be made on the basis of a careful history, physical examination, and diagnostic testing. The most reliable and sensitive method for differentiating between ulcerative colitis and Crohn's disease is a colonoscopy with endoscopically directed colonic biopsies. The following features distinguish Crohn's disease from ulcerative colitis: (1) involvement of the small intestine or the upper part of the alimentary canal; (2) segmental disease of the colon, with "skip" areas of normal rectum; (3) the appearance of fissures or sinus tracts; and (4) the presence of well-formed sarcoid-type granulomas.[12,13,15,16]

In the case of ulcerative colitis, the signs and symptoms of disease are rather dramatic, and it is unlikely that a patient would attend a dentist's office with undiagnosed disease. The probabilities are greater that someone with undiagnosed Crohn's disease could visit the dentist. Consequently, a thorough history and examination may uncover signs and symptoms of this inflammatory bowel disease, in which case a referral to the primary care physician is warranted. The associated risks of proceeding with dental care in a patient with undiagnosed Crohn's disease are essentially the same as those described for patients with ulcerative colitis. Anemias, vitamin K–dependent blood clotting disorders, and general nutritional deficiencies may occur if the diagnosis and treatment of Crohn's disease is delayed.

Oral Health Considerations.   Oral lesions, both symptomatic and asymptomatic, affect 6 to 20% of Crohn's disease patients. Most oral manifestations of Crohn's disease occur in patients with active intestinal disease, and their presence frequently correlates with disease activity. Recurrent aphthous ulcers are the most common oral manifestation of Crohn's disease.[18,25] It is not clear whether these oral manifestations are true expressions of Crohn's disease, pre-existing and/or co-incidental findings, direct results of medical treatment, or manifestations of an associated problem such as anemia. Certainly, pyostomatitis vegetans, cobblestone mucosal architecture, and minor salivary gland duct pathology represent granulomatous changes that constitute the hallmark of Crohn's disease. Biopsy specimens of these multiple small nonhealing aphthous ulcers reveal granulomatous inflammation. Less often, Crohn's disease patients develop diffuse swelling of the lips and face, inflammatory hyperplasias of the oral mucosa with a cobblestone pattern, indurated polypoid taglike lesions in the vestibule and retromolar pad area, and persistent deep linear ulcerations with hyperplastic margins. Granulomatous lesions have also been observed in the salivary glands, where they may cause rupture of the ducts and localized mucocele formation. Numerous medications, including anti-inflammatory and sulfa-containing preparations that are commonly used to manage IBD patients, have been reported to cause oral lichenoid drug reactions.[41,42] Superinfection with *Candida albicans* is often associated with IBD and may represent a primary manifestation of the disorder, a reaction to the bacteriostatic effect of sulfasalazine, or an impaired ability of neutrophils to kill this granuloma-provoking organism.[43] Of interest is the possibility that oral lesions may precede the radiologic changes of the disease by up to 1 year. This underscores the sometimes subtle signs and symptoms of Crohn's disease and the possibility that a dentist may encounter a patient with undiagnosed Crohn's disease. Frequently, patients will complain of pain associated with ulcerative lesions in the oral cavity. Palliative rinses, ointment, and topical steroids may be helpful. There appears to be an increased risk of dental caries that is probably related to dietary changes in patients with IBD.[31] The causes of the dental caries and increased incidence of bacterial and fungal infections are multifactorial but appear to be related to either the patient's altered immune status or diet.[30–35]

Oral effects of malabsorption may also be seen. Pallor, angular cheilitis, and glossitis, all oral manifestations of anemia, may occur, particularly in undiagnosed or poorly controlled disease. Nutritional deficiencies that are directly related to the section of the bowel affected by the disease can occur. Malnutrition is often a problem, and monitoring the patient's compliance with dietary supplementation is essential.[18,25]

As with ulcerative colitis, the medical management of a patient with Crohn's disease may alter his or her dental management. (See page 397 for a description of dental management in patients with ulcerative colitis.) The following description of dental management is applicable to patients with a diagnosis of IBD. The underlying assumption of this management is that patients with IBD are at increased risk for the development of oral infections, including dental caries. Consequently, dental management of patients with IBD should include the following:

1. Frequent preventive and routine dental care to monitor oral health and to prevent the destruction of hard and soft tissue. If the patient is taking a systemic corticosteroid, monitoring of blood pressure and evaluation of blood glucose is necessary.

2. Evaluation of hypothalamic-pituitary-adrenocortical function, to determine the patient's ability to undergo extensive dental procedures.

3. Diagnosis of oral inflammatory, infectious, or granulomatous lesions (including performance of a biopsy if necessary).

4. Treatment of oral manifestations of IBD, particularly symptomatic lesions. Palliative rinses and topical steroid therapy (fluocinonide 0.05%) may be helpful. Topical steroid therapy should be short-term and monitored because of the side effect of mucosal atrophy and systemic absorption.

5. Consultation with the patient's physician to completely comprehend the medical management of the patient. In particular, knowledge of the effects, side effects, and drug interactions of any medications the patient is taking is essential.

Depending on the results of the consultation with the patient's physician, the following laboratory studies may be indicated before surgical procedures are performed:

1. Complete blood count (red and white blood cells)
2. Hematocrit
3. Hemoglobin test
4. Platelet count
5. Coagulation studies (INR, prothrombin time, and partial thromboplastin time)
6. Liver function test
7. Blood glucose test

Clearly, coordination and collaboration with the patient's primary care physician is essential.

ANTIBIOTIC-INDUCED DIARRHEA AND PSEUDOMEMBRANOUS ENTEROCOLITIS

Medical Aspects. In patients who are receiving antibiotic therapy, diarrhea may occur as a result of an alteration of the colonic flora. Often, this condition is mild and subsides when antibiotic therapy is discontinued. Occasionally, a severe disease results, with the development of a thick mucosal exudate that has the appearance of a membrane and that is termed psuedomembranous enterocolitis. This condition is extremely serious and demands aggressive treatment. Practically all antibiotics can be associated with this condition. Patients who are debilitated or who have renal failure seem to be at a higher risk of contracting the disease. Recent studies have shown a major role for *Clostridium difficile* in the pathogenesis of antibiotic-produced pseudomembranous enterocolitis. Infections with *C. difficile* account for 10 to 25% of cases of antibiotic-associated diarrhea and virtually all cases of antibiotic-associated psuedomembranous colitis.[44]

The type of antibiotic and the route of its administration influence disease incidence. More cases occur when the drug is given orally than when it is administered parenterally. Clindamycin, ampicillin, and the cephalosporins are most commonly associated with antibiotic-associated pseudomembranous colitis, but virtually any antibiotic may produce this disorder. However, pseudomembranous colitis is not known to follow a single dose of clindamycin, amoxicillin, or the cephalosporins, all of which are now recommended for antibiotic prophylaxis of infective endocarditis and late prosthetic joint infections. Presumably, the normal colonic flora is inhibited when antibiotics are administered, allowing *C. difficile* to proliferate and produce a cytopathic toxin. The precise mechanism is not known but probably involves both the cytotoxic and vasoconstrictive effects of toxins. The timing is highly variable, with some cases appearing after a single dose and about one-third of cases occurring after the medicine is stopped. About 1 to 3 of 100,000 individuals who take antimicrobial agents develop *C. difficile* colitis.[15,44] Diarrhea is present in all cases and is associated with colitis and hemorrhage in 20% of cases. Bowel movements may occur every 15 to 20 minutes. The patient may be febrile and may have lost considerable fluid, electrolytes, and protein. Sigmoidoscopy may reveal mild or severe inflammation, along with yellow raised membranous plaques of exudate. Stool cultures may demonstrate *C. difficile* or may be tested for the enterotoxin.[12,13,15,16]

Pseudomembranous colitis is a life-threatening disease, and individuals must be treated aggressively with fluids and electrolyte replacement. Vancomycin, given orally in dosages of 125 to 500 mg four times daily for 10 to 14 days, is effective in eliminating *C. difficile* infection. Metronidazole, in doses of 250 mg to 500 mg three times daily, is also effective and is less expensive.[12,13,15,16]

Oral Health Considerations.   The primary role of the dentist is to recognize the signs and symptoms of antibiotic-associated diarrhea and pseudomembranous colitis in patients who either are taking an antibiotic or have a recent history of an antibiotic regimen. Cessation of the antibiotic and prompt referral to the patient's physician is necessary for definitive diagnosis.

▼ DISEASES OF THE HEPATOBILIARY SYSTEM

In this section, the liver, biliary tract, and pancreas are considered together due to their interrelated functions with regard to the digestive system. The liver dominates this group of structures in size and multiplicity of roles. Consequently, the majority of this section focuses on liver disease and dental management in patients with disease or dysfunction.

The liver serves as the major locus of synthetic, catabolic, and detoxifying activities in the body. The intermediary metabolism of all foodstuffs occurs here. The liver is essential in the excretion of heme pigments, and it participates in the immune response. Impairment of the hepatocyte will interfere with the liver's ability to synthesize and store glycogen, a major source of glucose. Should glycogen stores be depleted, liver gluconeogenesis from amino acids is initiated to maintain glucose levels. Lipids are metabolized in the liver to form cholesterol and triglycerides. Cholesterol is the major building block of cell membranes, steroids, and bile salts. Bile salts are essen-

tial in the absorption of fat in the small intestine. Proteins, albumin, and clotting factors are synthesized and stored in the liver; specifically, clotting factors I, II, V, VII, IX, and X are synthesized in the liver. Since some of the clotting factors are also dependent on vitamin K (eg, II, VII, IX, and X), coagulopathy can occur from hepatocyte dysfunction and/or vitamin K malabsorption due to biliary problems. The metabolism of drugs is principally performed by the cytochrome P-450 microsomal enzyme system in the hepatocyte. Local anesthetics, analgesics, sedatives, antibiotics, and antifungals are all metabolized in the liver. Consequently, cautious use of these drugs in a person with liver dysfunction is essential. Lastly, the liver inactivates or metabolizes hormones such as insulin, aldosterone, antidiuretic hormone, estrogens, and androgens. Clearly, liver dysfunction can express itself through multiple signs and symptoms. Liver disease commonly manifests itself through jaundice, and the disease process can lead to liver failure and cirrhosis.[45-47] Accordingly, jaundice and cirrhosis are considered separately, below.

Jaundice

Jaundice (or icterus), which is a sign rather than a disease, results from excess bilirubin in the circulation and the accumulation of bilirubin in the tissues. Jaundice is a yellow discoloration most often seen in the skin, in mucous membranes, and in the sclera of the eye. This excess bile pigment may be caused by (1) excess production of bilirubin by hemolysis of red blood cells (hemolytic jaundice); (2) obstruction in the biliary tree, preventing the excretion of bilirubin (obstructive jaundice); or (3) liver parenchymal disease (hepatocellular jaundice). Each of these three processes are briefly reviewed in this section, and the role of the dentist is discussed with regard to dental management.

HEMOLYTIC JAUNDICE

Hemolytic jaundice is not a gastrointestinal disease. Hemolytic anemias are the most common cause of this disorder, so it is critical that one understands the implications of hemolytic jaundice. Excessive destruction of erythrocytes will lead to mild hyperbilirubinemia. This excess destruction is often due to an inherent abnormality in the cells (eg, sickle cell disease, hereditary sphenocytosis, thalassemia, and glucose-6-phosphate-dehydrogenase deficiency). Additionally, drugs and poisonous agents (eg, nitrobenzene, toluene, and phenacetin) as well as acquired immune disease (eg, systemic lupus erythematosus) can lead to hemolytic jaundice. Even with a thorough history and examination, it would be difficult for a dentist to make a diagnosis of hemolytic jaundice with only a presenting sign of jaundice. Referral to the patient's primary care physician is necessary to elucidate the source of the excess pigmentation of the tissues. Medical diagnosis of jaundice by a hemolytic process is based on laboratory studies demonstrating the presence of anemia with a high reticulocyte count, a decreased level of serum haptoglobins, and elevated serum bilirubin. The specific cause of the increased hemolysis of red blood cells is determined by studies such as hemoglobin electrophoresis, erythrocyte fragility studies, and Coombs' test for antibodies to red cells. Typically, once a proper diagnosis is made and the underlying disorder (excessive hemolysis) is controlled, the jaundice resolves as the liver functions normally to remove bilirubin. Since the liver has enormous reserve capacity, the dentist should anticipate little to no residual damage to the liver unless liver function tests indicate otherwise.[46]

OBSTRUCTIVE JAUNDICE (CHOLESTASIS)

As its name implies, this form of jaundice is caused by a partial or complete stoppage in bile flow. The causes of this disorder are obstructions of the extrahepatic biliary tree and those associated with intrahepatic abnormalities. In either case, the flow of bile through the liver and out of the common bile duct can be impeded, resulting in an increase in bilirubin in the tissues. Gallstones and malignancies are the causes of most cases of extrahepatic cholestasis. Tumors of the pancreatic head are the most common malignant cause of extrahepatic cholestasis, and adenocarcinoma is the most frequent. The causes of intrahepatic cholestasis include neoplasms (eg, metastatic carcinomas, lymphomas), toxic drugs and chemicals (eg, phalloidin, the toxic component of mushrooms), hepatitis, IBD, and metabolic derangements.[46]

Again, the dentist's primary function is recognition of the clinical signs of jaundice and timely referral to a primary care physician for appropriate diagnosis and treatment. Once successful disease management is achieved, routine dental care can continue. Consultation with the patient's physician to ascertain the patient's liver function and ability to undergo dental treatment is necessary. Oral surgical procedures in the jaundiced patient should be deferred whenever possible. The main danger in surgery on the patient with obstructive jaundice is excessive bleeding resulting from vitamin K malabsorption. If surgery is essential, vitamin K should be given parenterally at a dose of 10 mg daily for several days. General anesthesia in a severely jaundiced patient can lead to renal failure.

HEPATOCELLULAR JAUNDICE

Hepatocellular jaundice can be caused by hepatitis and cirrhosis. Alcoholic hepatitis and drug-induced hepatotoxicity is discussed in this section, along with cirrhosis.

Alcoholic Hepatitis

MEDICAL ASPECTS

"Alcoholic hepatitis" is a term used to describe the clinical presentation of alcoholic patients with jaundice. Alcoholic hepatitis is a form of toxin-induced liver disease that runs a wide clinical spectrum from subclinical disease to cirrhosis and fulminant hepatic failure. Excessive use of alcohol remains the most important cause of cirrhosis in the Western world and a leading cause of death and mortality during midlife. Although alcoholic hepatitis is somewhat dose related, the variability and extent of injury is remarkable. Clearly, it is a matter not only of how much alcohol is ingested but by whom. Ingestion of at least 40 to 60 g of ethanol per day for more than 15 years

is necessary for development of alcoholic cirrhosis; this is equal to about six 12-ounce beers per day, 4 glasses of wine, or three 2-ounce shots of whisky. Hepatocyte injury from alcohol develops predominantly as a consequence of the direct cellular toxicity of acetaldehyde, the major metabolite of alcohol. However, there are important contributions from the associated nutritional deficiencies that often accompany alcoholism. There is compelling evidence that the tendency to alcoholism is inherited. Only 1 in 12 alcoholics develops evidence of severe liver injury. Genetic variation in the metabolism of ethanol may explain the higher prevalence of alcoholic liver injury in some populations. Clinicians from around the world are generally convinced that females are at greater risk of developing alcohol-induced liver disease than are males. The reasons for this observation remain obscure. However, women have lower levels of alcohol dehydrogenase (essential for metabolizing alcohol into acetaldehyde) in the gut; consequently, more alcohol reaches the liver.[47]

Due to the large number of individuals who have only mild symptoms, the true incidence of alcoholic hepatitis can only be estimated. In a US study involving veterans with liver disease who underwent liver biopsy, approximately 35% of subjects had changes consistent with alcoholic hepatitis. There have been numerous efforts to identify cofactors that may affect the progression of alcohol-induced injury. Nutrition, genetics, cytokines, hepatitis B and C, and therapeutic drugs all have been implicated. However, the evidence to date is only suggestive.[47]

There is a broad spectrum of clinical manifestations of alcoholic liver disease. Often, there is little correlation and sometimes considerable disassociation between the apparent severity of injury as based on clinical findings and as based on evidence found on liver biopsy. Alcoholic hepatitis is often found superimposed on cirrhosis that is already established. Alcoholic hepatitis is considered to be at least partially reversible. The earliest indication of alcoholic liver disease is an enlarged liver. The patient may also exhibit signs of both acute hepatitis (jaundice, fever, anorexia, and malaise) and more chronic liver disease, which may include spider angiomas, gynecomastia, jaundice, ascites, and ethanol intoxication.[46,47]

The clinical problems associated with alcoholic hepatitis reflect the disordered metabolism and circulation in the liver. Jaundice reflects the inability of the hepatocyte to conjugate and excrete bilirubin, and bleeding is secondary to decreased synthesis of clotting factors by the hepatocytes. Also, there can be an associated thrombocytopenia in cases of alcoholic jaundice. Mental confusion results from failure of the liver cells to metabolize and excrete toxins such as ammonia. Spider angiomas and gynecomastia result from elevated levels of estrogen, which is normally metabolized by hepatocytes.[46,47]

Alcoholic hepatitis requires consideration in the case of any patient who has a history of regular alcohol use. Confirmation of the diagnosis and assessment of the extent of injury is best done by performing a liver biopsy. There are no biochemical tests that have proven to be sufficiently helpful in establishing a diagnosis of alcohol-induced injury. Even with a liver biopsy, one can only guess the extent of reversible injury. However, the severity of alcoholic hepatitis can be objectively measured by using the laboratory criteria of prothrombin time and bilirubin. This measure is called a Maddrey discriminate function or Child-Pugh classification. Values of > 32 in this measure indicate severe disease and poor prognosis with significant mortality.[47]

Abstinence is the mainstay of the treatment of alcoholic hepatitis. However, this is difficult to achieve. Nutritional support for the malnourished patient is also important. Although medications such as corticosteroids, anabolic steroids, propylthiouracil, colchicine, and insulin/glucagon show promise, there is insufficient evidence to support their general use. In those patients with alcoholic hepatitis without liver cirrhosis, the disease is reversible.[47]

ORAL HEALTH CONSIDERATIONS

The oral lesions that may be seen in patients with alcoholic hepatitis are primarily related to dysfunction of the hepatocyte. Jaundice (yellow pigmentation) may be observed on the mucosa and may be accompanied by cutaneous and scleral jaundice. Jaundice usually occurs when total serum bilirubin reaches levels $\geq$ 3 mg/dL. There may be extraoral and/or intraoral petechiae and eccyhmoses, gingival crevicular hemorrhage due to the deficient clotting factors associated with dysfunctioning hepatocytes, and thrombocytopenia associated with alcohol. Additional oral findings can include manifestations of malnutrition such as vitamin deficiencies and anemia. Consequently, pallor, angular cheilitis, and glossitis may be exhibited as expressions of related problems. Additionally, the sweet ketone breath, indicative of liver gluconeogenesis, should raise the suspicion of hepatotoxicity. The presentation of the above clinical signs, as well as a history or symptoms suggestive of alcohol abuse, should warrant a referral to the patient's primary care physician for evaluation. Liver impairment would necessitate specific dental management procedures before proceeding with dental treatment.[45]

Obviously, elective dental treatment should not be carried out in a patient who has ingested a large amount of alcohol. Conversely, routine dental treatment of a patient with a history of alcoholic liver disease is not contraindicated unless there is significant cirrhosis. Cirrhotic changes due to alcoholism are not reversible whereas noncirrhotic changes generally are. Consequently, the dentist must determine the functioning level of the liver through consultation with the patient's physician and through appropriate liver function tests. To obtain the appropriate information from the physician, the dentist must be familiar with the laboratory tests used in evaluating the patient's status.[45,47]

Drug-Induced Hepatotoxicity

MEDICAL ASPECTS

Drug-induced liver disease can mimic any acute or chronic liver disease. Patients may present with fulminant hepatic failure from an intrinsic hepatotoxin such as acetaminophen or may simply have had an abnormal liver function test result on a laboratory screening panel. Ingested drugs are absorbed into the portal circulation and pass through the liver en route to distant sites of action. The liver is responsible for the conversion of lipid-soluble drugs, which are difficult to excrete, into polar soluble metabolites that are easily excreted through the kidneys. This solubilization and detoxification may paradoxically produce toxic intermediates. Fortunately, death from drug-induced hepatic injury is uncommon. Nevertheless, the dentist's role in recognizing the potential for drug-induced hepatotoxicity from drugs prescribed by the dentist, other medications (either prescribed or over-the-counter) being taken by the patient, and drug interactions is critical. Herbal and other alternative (nontraditional) drugs, which are increasing in popularity, have been reported to elicit hepatocellular toxicity as well.[46]

Drugs may be conjugated, oxidized, or reduced through the cytochrome P-450 system. This system can be induced by the long-term use of alcohol, barbiturates, or other drugs. With some hepatotoxic drugs, the relative activity of the cytochrome P-450 system is crucial; a drug that exerts its toxic actions through the generation of cytochrome P-450 metabolites may be relatively more toxic in a patient who uses alcohol or other agents that are capable of inducing cytochrome P-450. An example is the enhanced toxicity of acetaminophen in chronic alcoholics.[46,47]

Most drug reactions occur in one of two general patterns: dose-dependent drug toxicity and idiosyncratic drug reaction. In dose-dependent drug toxicity, a particular agent may be expected to produce hepatic injury in virtually all persons who take a large enough dose. A classic example of this type of toxicity is associated with acetaminophen. Toxicity usually occurs with weeks or months of use, is usually reversible, and recurs at approximately the same dose if stopped and then re-introduced.[46]

Idiosyncratic drug reactions occur at an unpredictable dose, recur at lower doses if stopped and re-introduced, and are occasionally associated with features suggesting involvement of the immune system. Sulfanomides and phenytoin are examples of drugs associated with this type of drug-induced hepatotoxicity. Because of the nature of the reaction, a small dose is as likely to produce a serious reaction as is a full therapeutic dose. Consequently, death may occur upon rechallenge, even at low doses. Idiosyncratic hypersensitivity reactions make up the most common type of drug-induced hepatotoxicity.[46]

Regardless of the mechanism involved, drug-induced hepatotoxicity can result in hepatocellular injury, cholestatic drug reactions, abnormal lipid storage, cirrhosis, and vascular injury. Hepatocellular injury and cholestatic drug reactions account for the majority of drug reactions encountered in dentistry. Hepatocellular injury is the most commonly recognized drug-induced injury, with acetaminophen toxicity probably being the most frequent risk in the practice of dentistry. Nonetheless, there are many categories of drugs that are known to have demonstrated hepatotoxicity that are not covered in this chapter.

ORAL HEALTH CONSIDERATIONS

As stated previously, drug-induced liver disease can present as any acute or chronic disorder. Also, since idiosyncratic reactions often have an immunoallergic basis, the patient can present not only with jaundice and other features of chronic liver disease but also with fever, dermatitis, arthralgias, and eosinophilia. Regardless of clinical presentation, referral to the patient's primary care physician is necessary should the dentist suspect drug-induced hepatotoxicity. It is simplistic to recommend that, since any drug may produce hepatotoxicity, the drug in question should be stopped. Rather, consultation with the physician is necessary to weigh the relative risks of stopping or changing therapy. Fortunately, most of the drugs that dentists might use or prescribe that are known to be hepatotoxic have safe and effective alternatives, and stopping the most likely offending drug is a prudent course of action. Nonetheless, coordination of dental therapy and medical therapy is critical. For example, the alternative agent in the case of NSAID toxicity would be a drug from a different subclass. However, after starting the alternative agent, the patient should be followed for at least 4 to 8 weeks with biochemical tests in order to ensure that the original drug reaction has resolved.

Since many drugs produce idiosyncratic drug toxicity, there is no way to predict or prevent such reactions. A patient who experiences an abrupt episode of hepatocellular injury should be considered to have an idiosyncratic drug reaction and should not be challenged again. For patients who take drugs associated with dose-dependent drug reactions, the obvious precaution is to keep the dose to a minimum. Since it is possible to take a toxic dose of acetaminophen without greatly exceeding the recommended doses, patients with chronic pain should be warned of the potential toxicity of acetaminophen. Also, patients who are taking large doses of acetaminophen should be advised to avoid alcohol and to ensure adequate nutrition.

Because most drug reactions are hepatocellular and may lead to hepatocyte failure and death, patients with a history of drug-induced hepatotoxicity should be evaluated with serial liver function tests. There may be cell death to the extent that drug metabolism and homeostasis are affected and that the patient's ability to undergo dental care is significantly affected. (See page XX for a complete description of dental management of patients with dysfunctional liver status.)

Liver Cirrhosis

MEDICAL ASPECTS

Cirrhosis is neither a single process nor a single disease; rather, it is the end result of a variety of conditions that produce chronic inflammatory change and liver cell injury. The progressive scarring leads to abnormal fibrosis and nodular regeneration. Cirrhosis is a leading cause of death in the United States, and over 45% of these deaths are alcohol related.[46,47]

Symptoms are the result of hepatocellular dysfunction, portal hypertension, or a combination of the two conditions. The most common symptoms include malaise, weakness, dyspepsia, anorexia, and nausea. One-third of the patients complain of abdominal pain, and 30 to 78% of patients present with ascites. Approximately 65% of cirrhotic individuals are jaundiced at presentation. Increased pigmentation, particularly on overexposed surfaces, is seen in hemochromatosis whereas xanthomas are suggestive of biliary cirrhosis. Less frequently seen are nonspecific findings of clubbing, cyanosis, and spider angiomas.[46,47]

The medical management of liver cirrhosis is dependent on the underlying etiology. The main objective is to prevent further injury to the liver. Discontinuation of alcohol and other toxins is essential. Some patients may benefit from taking corticosteroids and other immunosuppressive agents such as methotrexate. Phlebotomy to deplete iron stores and deferoxamine is used as an iron-chelating agent in patients with hemochromatosis. Liver transplantation is reserved for irreversible progressive liver disease.[46,47]

ORAL HEALTH CONSIDERATIONS

Oral findings may be associated with vitamin deficiencies and anemia; these findings include angular cheilitis, glossitis, and mucosal pallor. Yellow pigmentation may be observed on the oral mucosa and may be accompanied by scleral and cutaneous jaundice. Salivary gland dysfunction secondary to Sjögren's syndrome may be associated with primary biliary cirrhosis. Pigmentation of the oral mucosa is only rarely observed in cases of hemochromatosis.

The dental patient who presents with a history of liver cirrhosis deserves special attention. First, patients with cirrhosis may have significant hemostatic defects, both because of an inability to synthesize clotting factors and because of secondary thrombocytopenia. These deficits can be overcome with replacement with fresh frozen plasma and platelets. Therefore, laboratory evaluation prior to any surgical or periodontal procedures should be directed at bleeding parameters; specifically, complete blood count, prothrombin time or INR, partial thromboplastin time, platelet count, and bleeding time values should be obtained.[45]

Second, the ability to detoxify substances is also compromised in patients with hepatic insufficiency, and drugs and toxins may accumulate. Patients may become encephalopathic due to an ammonia buildup from the incomplete detoxification of nitrogenous wastes. Patients with encephalopathy are likely to be taking neomycin or lactulose. The use of sedatives and tranquilizers should be avoided in patients with a history of taking encephalopathy narcotics. Additionally, there may be an induction of liver enzymes, leading to a need for increased dosages of certain medications. Consequently, consultation with the patient's physician is essential to the proper management of the dental patient with liver cirrhosis. The patient with ascites may not be able to fully recline in the dental chair because of increased pressure on abdominal vessels. Lastly, liver transplantation patients who are on immunosuppressive therapy should be monitored for systemic infection of oropharyngeal origin, oral viral infection (herpes simplex virus, *Cytomegalovirus*), and oral ulcers of unknown origin.

▼ GASTROINTESTINAL SYNDROMES

Eating Disorders: Anorexia and Bulimia

MEDICAL ASPECTS AND DIAGNOSIS

The two most common eating disorders are anorexia nervosa and bulimia.[48] A variety of specialists, including psychiatrists, psychologists, dentists, internists, clinical social workers, nurses, and dietitians, must provide the treatment of eating disorders.[49] Anorexia involves individuals who intentionally starve themselves when they are already underweight. People suffering from this disorder have an intense fear of becoming fat, even when they are extremely underweight (defined as body weight that is 15% or more below the recommended levels). Those who suffer from anorexia are unable to perceive their physical appearance accurately.

In contrast to those with anorexia, persons with bulimia nervosa consume large amounts of food during "binge" episodes in which they feel out of control of their eating. Bulimic individuals are also not as successful in dieting as are those with anorexia. They may successfully diet for a short time, but they often again lose the ability to restrict food intake, often as a result of some emotional trauma. They then try to prevent weight gain after such episodes by vomiting, using laxatives or diuretics, dieting, and/or exercising aggressively. Persons with bulimia, like those with anorexia, are very dissatisfied with their body shape and weight, and their self-esteem is unduly influenced by their appearance. To be diagnosed with bulimia nervosa, an individual must engage in bingeing and purging at least twice a week for 3 months; exhibit a feeling of lack of control over eating; regularly use self-induced vomiting, laxatives, or diuretics to prevent weight gain; and exhibit a persistent excessive concern with body shape and weight.

The diagnosis of anorexia or bulimia is not always clear. For example, some anorexic persons may binge and purge whereas some bulimic persons may restrict food intake and overcompensate for overeating by exercising. If an individual eats through bingeing but is 15% or more below recommended weight, then anorexia nervosa is the appropriate diagnosis.

Both of these disorders seem to be most prevalent in industrialized societies, particularly where thinness is espoused as the ideal. Anorexia usually develops in adolescence, between the ages of 14 and 18 years, whereas bulimia is more likely to develop in the late teens or early twenties. It is estimated that anorexia occurs in about 0.5% of adolescent girls and that bulimia occurs in about 1 to 2% of adolescent girls. However, 5 to 10% of young women may exhibit less severe signs and symptoms of these diseases. The National Center for Health Statistics estimates that about 9,000 people admitted to hospitals were diagnosed with bulimia in 1994 (the latest year for which statistics are available) and that about 8,000 were diagnosed with anorexia. Studies indicate that by their first year of college, 4.5 to 18% of women and 0.4% of men have a history of bulimia and that as many as 1 in 100 females between the ages of 12 and 18 years have anorexia.

Anorexia and bulimia are both considered psychiatric disorders with physical complications.[50] Before diagnosing either of these eating disorders, other possible causes of significant changes in weight or appetite (eg, tumors, immunodeficiency, malabsorption, and alcohol) must be ruled out. Symptoms of eating disorders can also be primary signs of depression and schizophrenia. Eating disorders can be differentiated from these other disorders by the presence of a distorted body image and preoccupation with losing weight. Because patients may develop a good rapport with their dentists, dentists may be the first health care providers to sense that a diagnosis of an eating disorder is appropriate.

While many people with an eating disorder recover fully, relapse is common and may occur months or even years after treatment. An estimated 5 to 10% of anorexic patients will die from the disorder; their deaths most commonly result from starvation, suicide, or electrolyte imbalance.

ORAL HEALTH CONSIDERATIONS

The cardinal oral manifestation of eating disorders is severe erosion of the enamel on the lingual surfaces of the maxillary teeth. Acids from chronic vomiting are the cause.[51,52] Examination of the patient's fingernails may disclose abnormalities related to the use of fingers to initiate purging. Mandibular teeth may be affected but not as severely as the maxillary teeth. Parotid enlargement may develop as a sequela of starvation. Rarely does one observe soft-tissue changes of the oral mucosa because of trauma from gastric acids.

The dentist should be aware of a possible eating disorder when these symptoms are encountered and should take steps to arrange for referral to other practitioners.[53] Support of the patient both physically, by treatment of tooth desensitization and esthetics, and psychologically, by demonstrating a caring and compassionate attitude, is a part of the dental practitioner's treatment responsibility to these patients.

Gardner's Syndrome

Gardner's syndrome consists of intestinal polyposis (which represents premalignant lesions) and multiple impacted supernumerary (extra) teeth. This disorder is inherited as an autosomal dominant trait, and few patients afflicted with this syndrome reach the age of 50 years without surgical intervention.[54] In a young patient with a family history of Gardner's syndrome, dental radiography (such as pantomography) can provide the earliest indication of the presence of this disease process.[55]

Plummer-Vinson Syndrome

Plummer-Vinson syndrome, originally described as "hysterical dysphagia," is noted primarily in women in the fourth and fifth decades of life. The hallmark of this disorder is dysphagia resulting from esophageal stricture, causing many patients to have a fear of choking.[56] Patients may present with a lemon-tinted pallor and with dryness of the skin, spoon-shaped fingernails, koilonychia, and splenomegaly. The oral manifestations are the result of an iron deficiency anemia. Oral findings include atrophic glossitis with erythema or fissuring, angular cheilitis, thinning of the vermilion borders of the lips, and leukoplakia of the tongue. Inspection of the oral mucous membranes will disclose atrophy and hyperkeratinization. These oral changes are similar to those encountered in the pharynx and esophagus. Carcinoma of the upper alimentary tract has been reported in 10 to 30% of patients.[57] Thorough oral, pharyngeal, and esophageal examinations are mandatory to ensure that carcinoma is not present. Artificial saliva may reduce the sensation (and thereby, the fear) of choking.

Peutz-Jeghers Syndrome

Peutz-Jeghers syndrome is characterized by multiple intestinal polyps throughout the gastrointestinal tract but primarily in the small intestine. Malignancies in the gastrointestinal tract and elsewhere in the body have been reported in approximately 10% of patients with this syndrome. Pigmentation (present from birth) of the face, lips, and oral cavity is a hallmark of this syndrome.[58] Interestingly, the facial pigmentation fades later in life although the intraoral mucosal pigmentation persists. No specific oral treatment is necessary.

Cowden's Syndrome

Cowden's syndrome (multiple hamartoma and neoplasia syndrome) is an autosomal dominant disease characterized chiefly by facial trichilemmomas, gastrointestinal polyps, breast and thyroid neoplasms, and oral abnormalities. Cowden's syndrome is considered to be a cutaneous marker of internal malignancies.[59] Pebbly papilloma-like lesions and multiple fibromas may be found widely distributed throughout the oral cavity.[60]

▼ REFERENCES

1. Lipsett J, Sparnon AL, Byard RW, et al. Embryogenesis of enterocystomas-enteric duplication cysts of the tongue. Oral Surg Oral Med Oral Pathol 1993;75:626–30.

2. Gorlin RJ, Jirasek JE. Oral cysts containing gastric or intestinal mucosa: unusual embryologic accident or heterotopia. J Oral Surg 1970;28:9–11.

3. Wyngaarden JB, Smith LH. Cecil textbook of medicine. 16th ed. Philadelphia (PA): W.B. Saunders; 1982;16(1):1370–82.

4. DeMeester SR, Campos GM, DeMeester TR, et al. The impact of an antireflux procedure on intestinal metaplasia of the cardia. Ann Surg 1998;228:547–56.

5. Richter JE. Typical and atypical presentation of gastroesophageal reflux disease. Gastroenterol Clin North Am 1996;25(1):75–102.

6. Richter JE. Short segment Barrett's esophagus: the need for standardization of the definition and of endoscopic criteria. J Gastrointest Surg 1993;93:1033–6.

7. Sampliner RE. Practice guidelines on the diagnosis, surveillance, and therapy of Barrett's esophagus. The Practice Parameters Committee of the American College of Gastroenterology. Am J Gastroenterol 1998;93:1028–32.

8. Yagiela JA, Neidle EA, Dowd FJ. Pharmacology and theraputics for dentistry. 4th ed. St. Louis (MO): Mosby; 1998;449–52.

9. Spechler SJ. Comparison of medical and surgical therapy for complicated gastroesophageal reflux disease in veterans. The Department of Veterans Affairs Gastroesophageal Reflux Disease Study Group.N Engl J Med 1992;326(12):786–92.

10. Spivak H, Farrell TM, Trus TL, et al. Laparoscopic fundoplication for dysphagia and peptic esophageal stricture. J Gastrointest Surg 1998;2(6):555–60.

11. Patti MG, De Pinto M, de Bellis M, et al. Comparison of laparoscopic total and partial fundoplication for gastroesophageal reflux. J Gastrointest Surg 1997;1(4):309–15.

12. Achkar E, Farmer RG, Flesher B, editors. Clinical gastroenterology. 2nd ed. Philadelphia: Lea and Febiger; 1992.

13. Ming SC, Goldman H, editors. Pathology of the gastrointestinal tract. 2nd ed. Baltimore: Williams and Wilkins; 1998.

14. National Institutes of Health Consensus Development Panel statement. *Helicobacter pylori* in peptic ulcer disease. JAMA 1994;272:65–9.

15. Yamada T, editor. Textbook of gastroenterology. Vol. 1. 2nd ed. Philadelphia: J.B. Lippincott; 1995.

16. Fenoglio-Preiser CM, Noffsinger AE, Lantz PE, et al. Gastrointestinal pathology. 2nd ed. Philadelphia: Lippincott-Raven; 1999.

17. Gius JA, Boyle DE, Castle DD, et al. Vascular formations of the lip and peptic ulcer. JAMA 1963;133:725–9.

18. Siegel MA, Jacobson JJ. Inflammatory bowel diseases and the oral cavity. Oral Surg Oral Med Oral Pathol Oral Radiol Endod 1999;87:12–4.

19. Chan SWY, Scully C, Prime SS, et al. Pyostomatitis vegetans: oral manifestation of ulcerative colitis. Oral Surg Oral Med Oral Pathol 1991;72:689–92.

20. Calobrisi SD, Mutasim DF, McDonald JS. Pyostomatitis vegetans associated with ulcerative colitis: temporary clearance with fluocinonide gel and complete remission after colectomy. Oral Surg Oral Med Oral Pathol Oral Radiol Endod 1995;79:452–4.

21. Healy CM, Farthing PM, Williams DM, et al. Pyostomatitis vegetans and associated systemic disease: a review and two case reports. Oral Surg Oral Med Oral Pathol 1994;78:323–8.

22. Ficarra G, Cicchi P, Amorosi A, et al. Oral Crohn's disease and pyostomatitis vegetans: an unusual association. Oral Surg Oral Med Oral Pathol 1993;75:220–4.

23. Hansen LS, Silverman S Jr, Daniels TE. The differential diagnosis of pyostomatitis vegetans and its relation to bowel disease. Oral Surg Oral Med Oral Pathol 1983;55:363–73.

24. Ghandour K, Moneim I. Oral Crohn's disease with late intestinal manifestations. Oral Surg Oral Med Oral Pathol 1991; 72:565–7.

25. Halme L, Meurman JH, Laine P, et al. Oral findings in patients with active or inactive Crohn's disease. Oral Surg Oral Med Oral Pathol 1993;76:175–81.

26. Ward CS, Dunphy EP, Jagoe WS, et al. Crohn's disease limited to the mouth and anus. J Clin Gastroenterol 1985;7:516–21.

27. Plauth M, Jenss J, Meyle J. Oral manifestations of Crohn's disease: an analysis of 79 cases. J Clin Gastroenterol 1991; 13:29–37.

28. Kano Y, Shiohara T, Yagita A, et al. Erythema nodosum, lichen planus and lichen nitidus in Crohn's disease: report of a case and analysis of T-cell receptor V gene expression in the cutaneous and intestinal lesions. Dermatology 1995;190:59–63.

29. Schnitt SJ, Antonioli DA, Jaffe B, et al. Granulomatous inflammation of minor salivary gland ducts: a new oral manifestation of Crohn's disease. Hum Pathol 1987;18:405–7.

30. Bevenius J. Caries risk in patients with Crohn's disease: a pilot study. Oral Surg Oral Med Oral Pathol 1988;65:304–7.

31. Rooney TP. Dental caries prevalence in patients with Crohn's disease. Oral Surg Oral Med Oral Pathol 1984;57:623–4.

32. Sundh B, Emilson CG. Salivary and microbial conditions and dental health in patients with Crohn's disease: a 3-year study. Oral Surg Oral Med Oral Pathol 1989;67:286–90.

33. Sundh B, Johansson I, Emilson GC, et al. Salivary antimicrobial proteins in patients with Crohn's disease. Oral Surg Oral Med Oral Pathol 1993;76:564–9.

34. Meurman JH, Halme L, Laine P, et al. Gingival and dental status, salivary acidogenic bacteria, and yeast counts of patients with active or inactive Crohn's disease. Oral Surg Oral Med Oral Pathol 1994;77:465–8.

35. Malins TJ, Wilson A, Ward-Booth RP. Recurrent buccal space abscesses: a complication of Crohn's disease. Oral Surg Oral Med Oral Pathol 1991;72:19–21.

36. Siegel MA. Oral manifestations of gastrointestinal disease: diagnosis and treatment. In: Bayless TM, editor. Current therapy in gastroenterology and liver disease. Burlington (ON), Canada: B.C. Decker; 1989. p. 1–5.

37. Siegel MA, Balciunas BA. Medication can cause severe ulcerations. J Am Dent Assoc 1991;122:75–7.

38. Physicians Desk Reference. 55th ed. Montvale: Medical Economics; 2001.

39. Dhote R, Bergmann JF, Leglise P, et al. Orocecal transit time in humans assessed by sulfapyridine appearance in saliva after sulfasalazine intake. Clin Pharmacol Ther 1995;57:461–70.

40. Fluckiger R, Laifer G, Itin P, et al. Oral hairy leukoplakia in a patient with ulcerative colitis. Gastroenterology 1994; 106(2):503–8.

41. Van Dis ML, Parks ET. Prevalence of oral lichen planus in patients with diabetes mellitus. Oral Surg Oral Med Oral Pathol Oral Radiol Endod 1995;79:696–700.

42. Vincent SD, Fotos PG, Baker KA, Williams TP. Oral lichen planus: the clinical, historical, and therapeutic features of 100 cases. Oral Surg Oral Med Oral Pathol 1990;70:165–71.

43. Curran FT, Youngs DJ, Allan RN. Candidacidal activity of Crohn's disease neutrophils. Gut 1991;32:55–60.

44. Gilbert DN. Clostridial infections. In: Stein JH, editor. Internal medicine. St. Louis: Mosby-Year Book; 1994. p. 2096–101.

45. Glick M. Medical considerations for dental care of patients with alcohol-related liver disease. J Am Dent Assoc 1997;128(8):61–70.

46. Wu GY, Isreal J, editors. Diseases of the liver and the bile ducts: diagnosis and treatment in current clinical practice. Totowa (NJ): Humona Press, Inc.; 1998.

47. Hall P, editor. Alcoholic liver disease pathology and pathogenesis. London: Edward Arnold; 1995.

48. Ruff JC, Koch MO, Perkins S. Bulimia: dentomedical complications. Gen Dent 1992;40(1):22–5.

49. Stege P, Visco-Dangler L, Rye L. Amorexia nervosa: review including oral and dental manifestations. J Am Dent Assoc 1982;104(5):648–52.

50. Chatoor I. Feeding and eating disorders of infancy and early childhood. In: Kaplan HI, Sadock BJ, editors. Comprehensive textbook of psychiatry. 7th ed. Baltimore (MD): Williams & Wilkins; 2000. p. 2704–10.

51. Shaw BM. Orthodontic/prosthetic treatment of enamel erosion resulting from bulimia: a case report. J Am Dent Assoc 1994;125(2):188–90.

52. Tylenda CA, Roberts MW, Elin RJ, et al. Bulimia nervosa: its effects on salivary chemistry. J Am Dent Assoc 1991; 122(7):37–41.

53. Montgomery MT, Ritvo J, Weiner K. Eating disorders: phenominology, identification and dental intervention. Gen Dent 1988;36(6):485–8.

54. Katz JO, Chilvarquer LW, Terezhalmy GT. Gardner's syndrome: report of a case. J Oral Med 1987;42:211–5.

55. Arendt DM, Frost R, Whitt JC, Palomboro J. Multiple radiopaque masses in the jaws. J Am Dent Assoc 1989; 118(3):349–51.

56. Hoffman RM, Jaffe PE. Plummer-Vinson syndrome: a case report and literature review. Arch Intern Med 1995; 155(18):2008–11.

57. Chen TS, Chen PS. Rise and fall of the Plummer-Vinson syndrome. J Gastroenterol Hepatol 1994;9(6):654–8.

58. Wescott WB, Correll RW. Oral and perioral pigmented macules in a patient with gastric and intestinal polyposis. J Am Dent Assoc 1984;108(3):385–6.

59. Mignogna MD, Lo Muzio L, Ruocco V, Bucci E. Early diagnosis of multiple hamartoma and neoplasia syndrome (Cowden syndrome): the role of the dentist. Oral Surg Oral Med Oral Pathol Oral Radiol Endod 1995;79(3):295–9.

60. Porter S, Cawson R, Scully C, Eveson J. Multiple hamartoma syndrome presenting with oral lesions. Oral Surg Oral Med Oral Pathol Oral Radiol Endod 1996;82(3):295–301.

15

▼

RENAL DISEASE

SCOTT S. DEROSSI, DMD
S. GARY COHEN, DMD

▼ KIDNEY STRUCTURE AND FUNCTION

▼ FLUIDS, ELECTROLYTES, AND pH HOMEOSTASIS

▼ DIAGNOSTIC PROCEDURES IN RENAL DISEASE
Serum Chemistry
Urinalysis
Creatinine Clearance Test
Intravenous Pyelography
Renal Ultrasonography
Computed Tomography and Magnetic Resonance Imaging
Biopsy

▼ RENAL FAILURE
Acute Renal Failure
Chronic Renal Failure

▼ MANIFESTATIONS OF RENAL DISEASE: UREMIC SYNDROME
Biochemical Disturbances
Gastrointestinal Symptoms
Neurologic Signs and Symptoms
Hematologic Problems
Calcium and Skeletal Disorders (Renal Osteodystrophy)
Cardiovascular Manifestations
Respiratory Symptoms
Immunologic Changes
Oral Manifestations

▼ MEDICAL MANAGEMENT OF CHRONIC RENAL FAILURE
Conservative Therapy
Renal Replacement Therapy

▼ ORAL HEALTH CONSIDERATIONS
Acute Renal Failure Patients
Chronic Renal Failure and End-Stage Renal Disease Patients

Diseases of the kidney are a major cause of morbidity and mortality in the United States, affecting close to nine million Americans. The kidneys are vital organs for maintaining a stable internal environment (homeostasis). The kidneys have many functions, including regulating the acid-base and fluid-electrolyte balances of the body by filtering blood, selectively reabsorbing water and electrolytes, and excreting urine. In addition, the kidneys excrete metabolic waste products, including urea, creatinine, and uric acid, as well as foreign chemicals. Apart from these regulatory and excretory functions, the kidneys have a vital endocrine function, secreting renin, the active form of vitamin D, and erythropoietin. These hormones are important in maintaining blood pressure, calcium metabolism, and the synthesis of erythrocytes, respectively.

Disorders of the kidneys can be classified into the following diseases or stages: disorders of hydrogen ion concentration (pH) and electrolytes, acute renal failure, chronic renal failure, and end-stage renal failure or uremic syndrome. Approximately 1 of 20 hospitalized patients develops acute renal failure, most often related to trauma of surgery. Death from acute renal failure occurs in 30 to 80% of patients, depending on their underlying medical conditions. Almost 1 in 10,000 persons develops end-stage renal failure annually while mortality related to chronic renal failure accounts for more than 50,000 deaths each year in the United States. Oral health care professionals are frequently challenged to meet the dental needs of medically complex patients. This chapter reviews the etiology and pathophysiology of renal disorders and reviews considerations for the provision of dental care.

▼ KIDNEY STRUCTURE AND FUNCTION

The human kidneys are bean-shaped organs located in the retroperitoneum at the level of the waist. Each adult kidney weighs approximately 160 g and measures 10 to 15 cm in length. Coronal sectioning of the kidney reveals two distinct regions: an outer region, or cortex, and an inner region known as the medulla (Figure 15-1, A). Structures that are located at the corticomedullary junction extend into the kidney hilum and are called papillae. Each papilla is enclosed by a minor calyx that collectively communicates with the major calyces to form the renal pelvis. The renal pelvis collects urine flowing from the papillae and passes it to the bladder via the ureters. Vascular flow to the kidneys is provided by the renal artery, which branches directly from the aorta. This artery subdivides into segmental branches to perfuse the upper, middle, and lower regions of the kidney. Further subdivisions account for the arteriole-capillary-venous network, or vas recta. The venous drainage of the kidney is provided by a series of veins leading to the renal vein and ultimately to the inferior vena cava.

The kidney's functional unit is the nephron (see Figure 15-1, B), and each kidney is made up of approximately one million nephrons. Each nephron consists of Bowman's capsule, which surrounds the glomerular capillary bed; the proximal convoluted tubule; the loop of Henle; and the distal convoluted tubule, which empties into the collecting ducts. The glomerulus is a unique network of capillaries that is suspended between afferent and efferent arterioles enclosed within Bowman's capsule and that serves as a filtering funnel for waste. The filtrate drains from the glomerulus into the tubule, which alters the concentration along its length by various processes to form urine. The glomerulus funnels ultrafiltrate to the remaining portion of the nephron, or renal tubule. Following filtration, the second step of urine formation is the selective reabsorption of filtered substances, which occurs along the length of the tubule via active and passive transport processes.

Each day, the kidneys excrete approximately 1.5 to 2.5 L of urine. Although the removal of toxic and waste products from the blood remains their major role, the kidneys are also essential for the production of hormones such as vitamin D and erythropoietin and for the modulation of salt and water excretion. The major functions of the kidney are summarized in Table 15-1.

Once destroyed, nephrons do not regenerate. However, the kidney compensates for the loss of nephrons by hypertrophy of the remaining functioning units. This theory, often referred to as the intact nephron hypothesis, maintains that

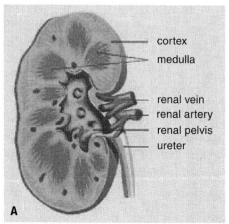

A

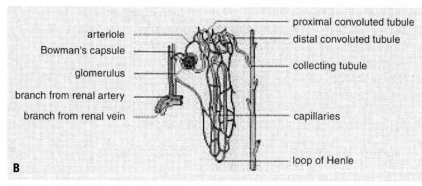

B

FIGURE 15-1 **A,** Structure of the kidney. **B,** Nephron.

TABLE 15-1 Major Functions of the Kidneys

Non-excretory functions

  Degradation of polypeptide hormones

    Insulin

    Glucagon

    Parahormone

    Prolactin

    Growth hormone

    Antidiuretic hormone

    Gastrin

    Vasoactive intestinal polypeptide

  Synthesis and activation of hormones

    Erythropoietin (stimulates erythrocyte production by bone marrow)

    Prostaglandins (vasodilators that act locally to prevent renal ischemia)

    Renin (important in regulation of blood pressure)

    $1,25(OH_2)D_3$ (final hydroxylation of vitamin D to its most potent form)

Excretory functions

  Excretion of nitrogenous end products of protein metabolism (eg, creatinine, uric acid, urea)

  Maintenance of ECF volume and blood pressure by altering Na^+ excretion

  Maintenance of plasma electrolyte concentration within normal range

  Maintenance of plasma osmolality by altering water excretion

  Maintenance of plasma pH by eliminating excess H^+ and regenerating HCO_3^-

  Provision of route of excretion for most drugs

$1,25(OH_2)D_3$ = 1,25-dihydroxyvitamin D_3; ECF = extracellular fluid; H^+ = hydrogen; HCO_3^- = bicarbonate; Na^+ = sodium; pH = hydrogen ion concentration.

diseased nephrons are totally destroyed. Normal renal function can be maintained until approximately 50% of the nephrons per kidney are destroyed, at which point abnormal laboratory values and changes in the clinical course occur. This hypothesis is most useful in explaining the orderly pattern of functional adaptation in progressive renal failure.

▼ FLUIDS, ELECTROLYTES, AND pH HOMEOSTASIS

With advancing nephron destruction, water and electrolyte regulation becomes increasingly more difficult. Adaptations to sudden shifts in intake occur slowly, resulting in wide swings in water and solute concentrations. The first clinical sign of diminished renal function is a decreased ability to concentrate the urine (isosthenuria). As a result of this inability to conserve water, dehydration ensues. With early renal insufficiency, sodium is also lost in the urine. This loss is often independent of the amount of water lost. As renal disease progresses, volume overload leading to hypertension and congestive heart failure can be serious sequelae. When glomerular filtration becomes markedly diminished, the distal tubule can no longer secrete sufficient potassium, leading to hyperkalemia.

In a healthy body, the acid-base balance is maintained via buffers, breathing, and the amounts of acid or alkaline wastes in the urine; this is because the daily load of endogenous acid is excreted into the urine with buffering compunds such as phosphates. As the glomerular filtration rate (GFR) progressively decreases, the tubular excretory capacity for positive hydrogen (H^+) ions is overwhelmed because renal ammonia production becomes inadequate. In its early phases, the resultant acidosis usually has a normal anion gap. As the kidney deteriorates, metabolically derived acids accumulate, leading to an increase in the anion gap. Clinically, this metabolic acidosis is manifested as anorexia, nausea, fatigue, weakness, and Kussmaul's respiration (a deep gasping respiration similar to that observed in patients with diabetic ketoacidosis).

▼ DIAGNOSTIC PROCEDURES IN RENAL DISEASE

Serum Chemistry

In the presence of renal dysfunction, changes in homeostasis are reflected in serum chemistry. Sodium, chloride, blood urea nitrogen (BUN), glucose, creatinine, carbon dioxide, potassium, phosphate, and calcium levels provide a useful tool to evaluate the degree of renal impairment and disease progression. Serum creatinine and BUN are often important markers to the GFR. Both of these products are nitrogenous waste products of protein metabolism that are normally excreted in the urine, but they may increase to toxic levels in the presence of renal dysfunction. A characteristic profile of changes occurs with advancing renal dysfunction, including elevations in serum creatinine, BUN, and phosphate, compared to low levels of serum calcium. Laboratory findings commonly seen in renal disease are summarized in Table 15-2.

Urinalysis

The most important aspects of urine examination in patients with renal disease include the detection of protein or blood in the urine, determination of the specific gravity or osmolality, and microscopic examination. The hallmarks of renal dysfunction detected by urinalysis are hematuria and proteinuria. Hematuria (the presence of blood in the urine) can result from bleeding anywhere in the urinary tract. Rarely, hematuria is a sign of clinically significant renal disease. Microscopic hematuria in patients less than 40 years of age is almost always benign, and further work-up is rarely indicated. Occasionally, significant underlying disease such as a neoplasm or proliferative glomerulonephritis can cause hematuria. However, the accompanying active sediment of proteins and red blood cell casts makes the diagnosis relatively straightforward. In older people, hematuria warrants further evaluation, including urologic studies to rule out prostatic hypertrophy and neoplasia, urine cultures to rule out infection, urine cytology, and advanced renal studies (such as an intravenous pyelography) to rule out intrinsic abnormalities.

TABLE 15-2   Laboratory Changes in Progressive Renal Disease

Laboratory Test	Normal Range	Level in Symptomatic Renal Failure
Glomerular filtration rate	100–150 mL/min	< 6–10 mL/min
Creatinine clearance	85–125 mL/min (female)	10–50 mL/min (moderate failure)
	97–140 mL/min (male)	< 10 mL/min (severe failure)
Serum creatinine	0.6–1.20 mg/dL	> 5 mg/dL
Blood urea nitrogen	8–18 mg/dL	> 50 mg/dL
Serum calcium	8.5–10.5 mg/dL	Depressed
Serum phosphate	2.5–4.5 mg/dL	Elevated
Serum potassium	3.8–5.0 mEq/L	Elevated

Proteinuria is probably the most sensitive sign of renal dysfunction. However, many benign conditions (including, exercise, stress, and fever) can produce elevated protein in the urine, or the proteinuria may be idiopathic. A 24-hour urine collection should be done for persistent proteinuria. The upper limit of normal urinary protein is 150 mg per day; patients who excrete > 3g of protein per day carry a diagnosis of nephrotic syndrome (discussed below).

Specific gravity is measured to determine the concentration of urine. In chronic renal disease, the kidney initially loses its ability to concentrate the urine, then loses its abilty to dilute the urine, resulting in a relatively fixed osmolality near the specific gravity of plasma. This occurs when 80% of the nephron mass has been destroyed.

Creatinine Clearance Test

The glomerular filtration rate assesses the amount of functioning renal tissue and can be calculated indirectly by the endogenous creatinine clearance test. Creatinine is a breakdown product of muscle, liberated from muscle tissue and excreted from the urine at a constant rate. This results in a steady plasma concentration of 0.7 to 1.5 mg/dL (often slightly higher in men because of increased muscle mass). Creatinine is 100% filtered by the glomerulus and is not reabsorbed by the tubule. Although a very small portion is secreted by the tubule, this test is an effective way to estimate the GFR. The creatinine clearance test is performed by collecting a 24-hour urine specimen and a blood sample in the same 24-hour period. In chronic renal failure and in some forms of acute disease, the GFR is decreased below the normal range of 100 to 150 mL/min. Advancing age also diminishes the GFR, by approximately 1 mL/min every year after age 30 years. The most accurate way to measure the GFR is by the inulin clearance test. However, this clinical test is infrequently used because it requires intravenous infusion at a constant rate and timed urine collection by catheterization.

Intravenous Pyelography

Intravenous pyelography (IVP) is the most commonly used and relied upon radiologic examination of the kidneys. Following the intravenous (IV) injection of a contrast medium, a plain-film abdominal radiograph is taken. Further films are exposed every minute for the first 5 minutes, followed by a film exposed at 15 minutes and a final film exposed at 45 minutes. Since various diseases of the kidney alter its ability to concentrate and excrete the dye, the extent of renal damage can be assessed. The location and distribution of the dye itself gives information regarding the position, size, and shape of the kidneys. This examination has limited application, particularly since in severely azotemic patients (whose BUN > 70 mg/dL), this test is deferred because there is sufficiently low glomerular filtration to prevent the excretion of the dye, rendering information about the kidney nondiagnostic.

Renal Ultrasonography

Ultrasonography of the kidneys finds its usefulness in the enhanced ability to distinguish solid tumors from fluid-filled cysts.[1] This diagnostic procedure uses high-frequency sound waves (ultrasound) directed at the kidneys to produce reflected waves or echoes from tissues of varying densities, thereby forming images (sonograms). Renal ultrasonography is particularly useful for patients with severe renal failure who are not candidates for IVP. It is most often indicated to determine kidney size, to view an obstruction, to evaluate renal transplants for abscesses or hematomas, and to localize the organ during percutaneous renal biopsy.

Computed Tomography and Magnetic Resonance Imaging

Computed tomography (CT) and magnetic resonance imaging (MRI) have limited application for imaging the kidney and associated areas of interest. Because CT is more expensive than conventional radiographic studies, its clinical application has been limited to the detection of retroperitoneal masses that are difficult to detect with other modalities. MRI gives the same information as renal CT but does not use ionizing radiation or require intravenous contrast media.

Biopsy

The development and growing use of renal biopsy has considerably advanced the knowledge of the natural history of kidney diseases. Percutaneous needle biopsy guided by ultrasonographic or radiographic reference is usually performed by nephrologists, with the patient in the supine position. Intrarenal and perirenal bleeding are common sequelae, with serious postprocedural bleeding and hematuria occuring in 5% of cases. Patients are placed on bed rest for 24 hours following the procedure while vital signs and abdominal changes are monitored.

▼ RENAL FAILURE

The classification of renal failure is based on two criteria: the onset (acute versus chronic failure) and the location that precipitates nephron destruction (prerenal, renal or instrinsic, and postrenal failure). Chronic renal failure is a slow, irreversible, and progressive process that occurs over a period of years whereas acute renal failure develops over a period of days or weeks. The distinction between acute and chronic disease is important; acute disease is usually reversible if managed appropriately whereas chronic renal failure is a progressive and irreversible process that leads to death in the absence of medical intervention. In both cases, the kidneys lose their normal ability to maintain the normal composition and volume of bodily fluids. Although the terminal functional disabilities of the acute and chronic diseases are similar, acute renal failure has some unique aspects that warrant its separate discussion.

Acute Renal Failure

Acute renal failure (ARF) is a clinical syndrome characterized by a rapid decline in kidney function over a period of days to weeks, leading to severe azotemia (the building up of nitrogenous waste products in the blood). It is very common in hospitalized patients; ARF occurs in up to 5% of all admitted patients and in as many as 30% of patients admitted to intensive care units. Medications, surgery, pregnancy-related complications, and trauma are the most common causes of ARF. Unlike patients who undergo chronic renal failure, patients who develop ARF usually have a normal baseline renal function; yet, mortality from ARF (even with medical intervention including dialysis) can reach 80%, demonstrating the critical illness of these patients.[2] The clinical course of acute renal failure most often progresses through three stages: oliguria (urine volume < 400 mL per day), diuresis (high urine volume output > 400 mL per day), and ultimately, recovery.[3] The causes of ARF are often divided into three diagnostic categories: prerenal failure, postrenal failure, and acute intrinsic renal failure.

PRERENAL FAILURE

Prerenal failure, defined as any condition that compromises renal function without permanent physical injury to the kidney, is the most common cause of hospital-acquired renal failure. This condition, often referred to as prerenal azotemia, results from reversible changes in renal blood flow and is the most common cause of acute renal failure, accounting for more than 50% of cases.[4] Some etiologic factors commonly associated with prerenal failure include volume depletion, cardiovascular diseases that result in diminished cardiac output, and changes in fluid volume distribution that are associated with sepsis and burns.[5]

POSTRENAL FAILURE

Postrenal causes of failure are less common (< 5% of patients) than prerenal causes. Postrenal failure refers to conditions that obstruct the flow of urine from the kidneys at any level of the urinary tract and that subsequently decrease the GFR. Postrenal failure can cause almost total anuria with complete obstruction or polyuria. Renal ultrasonography often shows a dilated collecting system (hydronephrosis). Most commonly, obstruction results from prostatic enlargement (benign hypertrophy or malignant neoplasia) or cervical cancer. It is usually seen in older men as a result of the enlargement of the prostate gland. Although postrenal failure is the least common cause of acute renal failure, it remains the most treatable.

ACUTE INTRINSIC RENAL FAILURE

Glomerular disease, vascular disease, and tubulointerstitial disease comprise the three major causes of acute intrinsic renal failure and describe the sites of pathology. Glomerulonephritis is an uncommon cause of acute renal failure and usually follows a more subacute or chronic course. However, when fulminant enough to cause acute failure, it is associated with active urinary sediment. Prominent clinical and laboratory findings include hypertension, proteinuria, hematuria, and red blood cell casts. Postinfectious, membranoproliferative, and rapidly progressive glomerulonephritis, as well as glomerulonephritis associated with endocarditis and infections of the vascular access, are the most common glomerular diseases to cause a sudden renal deterioration. The pathogenesis of glomerulonephritis appears to be related to the immunocomplex and complement-mediated damage of the kidney.[6]

Vascular occlusive processes such as renal arterial or venous thromboses are also causes of acute intrinsic renal failure. The clinical presentation is archetypal, consisting of a triad of severe and sudden lower back pain, severe oliguria, and macroscopic hematuria. By far, the most common causes of acute intrinsic failure are tubulointerstitial disorders (> 75% of cases), including interstitial nephritis and acute tubular necrosis (ATN). Infiltrative diseases (such as lymphoma or sarcoidosis), infections (such as syphilis and toxoplasmosis), and medications are the leading causes of interstitial nephritis. With drug-induced interstitial nephritis, there are accompanying systemic signs of a hypersensitivity reaction, and the presence of eosinophils is a common finding in the urine. Although renal function returns to normal with the discontinuation of the offending drug, recovery may be hastened with corticosteroid therapy.[7] ATN is a renal lesion that forms in response to prolonged ischemia or exposure to a nephrotoxin.[8] ATN remains more of a clinical diagnosis of exclusion than a pathologic diagnosis. The period of renal failure associated with ATN can range from weeks to months, and the major complications of this transient failure are infections, imbalances in fluid and electrolytes, and uremia. Serum levels of BUN and creatinine peak, plateau, and slowly fall, accompanied by a return of renal function over 10 to 14 days in most cases.[9]

Sudden renal failure in hospitalized patients is often very apparent from either oliguria or a rise in BUN and creatinine levels. However, renal dysfunction in the outpatient population is often more subtle. A patient can present to the dental office with vague complaints of lethargy and fatigue or entirely without symptoms. These patients can often go undiagnosed but for abnormal results on routine urinalysis, the most common test for screening for renal disease.[10,11]

Chronic Renal Failure

Chronic renal failure (CRF) can be caused by many diseases that devastate the nephron mass of the kidneys. Most of these conditions involve diffuse bilateral destruction of the renal parenchyma. Some renal conditions affect the glomerulus (glomerulonephritis), others involve the renal tubules (polycystic kidney disease or pyelonephritis), while others interfere with blood perfusion to the renal parenchyma (nephrosclerosis). Ultimately, nephron destruction ensues in all cases unless this process is interrupted. The United States Renal Data System has generated statistics showing that the most common primary diagnosis for CRF or end-stage renal disease (ESRD) patients is diabetes mellitus, followed by hypertension, glomerulonephritis, and others (Table 15-3). Despite the varying causes, the clinical features of CRF are always remarkably similar because the common denominator remains nephron destruction.

The prognosis of the patient with renal disease has improved significantly during the last two decades. The improvement of antimicrobial therapy to combat increased susceptibility to infection, along with advances in dialysis and transplantation techniques, has provided patients with the opportunity for survival in the face of a complete loss of renal function. However, despite these advances, the current annual mortality rate for patients with ESRD in the United States is approximately 24%.

CLINICAL PROGRESSION

The clinical course of CRF is divided into three progressive stages: (1) diminished renal reserve, (2) renal insufficiency, and (3) end-stage renal failure or uremia.

TABLE 15-3 Etiology of End-Stage Renal Disease

Disorder	Percentage of New Dialysis Patients
Diabetes mellitus	44.4
Hypertension	26.6
Glomerulonephritis	12.2
Interstitial nephritis, pyelonephritis, and polycystic kidney disease	7.2
Other disorders	9.6

Reproduced with permission from United States Renal Data System 1999 Annual Report. http://www.usrds.org.

Diminished renal reserve is characterized by normal serum creatinine and BUN levels. There are no symptoms or prominent biochemical disturbances. Renal impairment may be detected only when severe demands are being placed on the kidneys or by sophisticated testing of the GFR. The second clinical stage, renal insufficiency, occurs when the GFR drops to 25% of normal (> 75% of functional kidney tissue has then been destroyed). As nephron destruction progresses, the GFR falls, and the BUN level rises. Among the consequences are (usually) mild azotemia, nocturia, polyuria, and an impaired ability to concentrate urine. The third and final stage of chronic renal failure is end-stage renal failure or uremia. With continued destruction of nephrons (destruction of > 90% of nephron mass), frank renal disease follows, with associated polyuria. The GFR is 10% of normal, and creatinine clearance may be 5 to 10 mL/min or less. Sharp increases in serum creatinine and BUN are seen in response to small decrements in the GFR. At this point, patients experience severe symptoms as their kidneys cannot maintain fluid and electrolyte homeostasis. The complex biochemical changes, including anemia, hypocalcemia, hyperphosphatemia, and metabolic acidosis, along with vast systemic symptoms, a patient experiences, has been termed "uremic syndrome." Without renal replacement therapy, death is a certain consequence.[12]

ETIOLOGY AND PATHOGENESIS

The progression of the varied renal diseases, culminating in chronic renal failure, ranges from a few months to 30 to 40 years. The most common causes of renal failure are summarized in Table 15-3. Currently, diabetes and hypertension account for 44.4% and 26.6%, respectively, of the total cases of ESRD. Glomerulonephritis is the third most common cause of ESRD (12.2% of cases). Interstitial nephritis, pyelonephritis, and polycystic kidney disease account for 7.2% of cases. The remaining 9.6% of the causes of ESRD include systemic lupus erythematosus (SLE) and relatively uncommon conditions such as obstructive uropathy.

Age, race, gender, and family history have been identified as risk factors for the development of ESRD.[13] The average age of a newly diagnosed patient with ESRD is 61.1 years, and 53.1% of ESRD patients are male. White people, including Hispanics, account for 63.5% of ESRD patients; black people account for 28.7% of ESRD patients, and people of Asian ancestry make up 2.9%. Family history is a risk factor for diabetes and hypertension, both of which adversely affect the kidneys and therefore constitute a risk for developing ESRD. Recent evidence suggests that smoking is a major renal risk factor, increasing the risk of nephropathy and doubling the rate of progression to end-stage disease.[14]

Glomerulonephritis. Glomerulonephritis represents a heterogeneous group of diseases of varying etiology and pathogenesis that produce irreversible impairment of renal function. This is often initiated by an attack of acute glomerulonephritis of streptococcal or nonstreptococcal origin. Glomerulonephritis also may enter the chronic stage from a nephrotic syndrome. The most typical examples of this are idiopathic membranous glomerulonephritis and membranoproliferative glomerulonephritis.[15] In most cases, the patients present with the features of CRF and hypertension or with a chance proteinuria that has progressed to chronic nephritis over a period of years.

Chronic glomerulonephritis is usually insidious in onset. The course is very slow but is steadily progressive, leading to renal failure and uremia in up to 30 years. It is thought to be a disorder of immunologic origin. The continuous nature of the immunologic injury is shown by the recurrence of disease in kidneys that have been transplanted to patients with some type of glomerulonephritis, even after their own kidneys had been removed.[16]

Nephrotic Syndrome. Nephrotic syndrome is the clinical manifestation of any glomerular lesion that causes an excess of more than 3 g of protein excretion in the urine per day. Nephrotic syndrome is caused by multiple diseases, all of which enhance the permeability of the glomerulus to plasma proteins. Excessive protein excretion leads to a decline of plasma osmotic pressure, with consequent edema and serosal effusions. The differential diagnosis of nephrotic syndrome is vast but includes sickle cell anemia, diabetes mellitus, multiple myeloma, SLE, and membranous glomerulonephritis. Bacterial infections secondary to hypogammaglobulinemia have been described as a cause of death in children with nephrotic syndrome.

Pyelonephritis. Pyelonephritis refers to the effects of bacterial infection in the kidney, with Escherichia coli being the most frequent cause of infection.[17] Pyelonephritis may present in an acute form with active pyogenic infection or in a chronic form in which the principal manifestations are caused by an injury sustained during a preceding infection. The chronic form of bacterial pyelonephritis can be further subdivided into reactive and inactive forms, and one or both kidneys may be affected.

Any lesion that produces an obstruction of the urinary tract can predispose to active pyelonephritis. Pyelonephritis also may occur as part of a generalized sepsis as seen in patients with bacterial endocarditis or staphylococcal septicemia.

The clinical picture of acute pyelonephritis is often characteristic, consisting of a sudden rise in body temperature (to 38.9° to 40.6°C), shaking chills, aching pain in one or both costovertebral areas or flanks, and symptoms of bladder inflammation. Microscopic evaluation of the urine reveals large numbers of bacteria and a polymorphonuclear leukocytosis. There are no signs of impaired renal function or acute hypertension as is sometimes seen in patients with acute glomerulonephritis. Patients with chronic active pyelonephritis often suffer from recurrent episodes of acute pyelonephritis or may have persistent smoldering infections that gradually result in end-stage renal failure secondary to destruction from the scarring of renal parenchyma. This process may continue for many years. The inability to conserve sodium (a feature in any patient with impaired renal function) is more pronounced in patients with pyelonephritis than in those with glomerulonephritis. This "salt-losing" defect may be pronounced and may dominate the clinical picture.

Polycystic Renal Disease. Polycystic kidney disease exhibits autosomal dominant inheritance.[18] Most patients present with microscopic or gross hematuria, abdominal or flank pain, and recurrent urinary tract infections. The disease causes renal insufficiency in 50% of individuals by age 70 years.[19] Clinically, these patients have large palpable kidneys, and the diagnosis is confirmed via renal ultrasonography, CT, or IVP. Most patients develop hypertension during the course of their disease, and more than one-half of patients are hypertensive at the time of presentation. Although no preventive therapies have proven to be effective, treating the hypertension with angiotensin-converting enzyme inhibitors may help to slow the progression of polycystic disease. Another form of polycystic kidney disease is an acquired reactive process that is seen in over 50% of patients treated by hemodialysis or peritoneal dialysis for longer than 3 years. The development of adenocarcinomas is seen in approximately 5% of these multiple cysts throughout the remnant kidneys.

Hypertensive Nephrosclerosis. The association between the kidneys and hypertension is recognized, yet the primary disease often is not. Hypertension may be the primary disorder damaging the kidneys, but conversely, severe chronic renal failure may lead to hypertension or perpetuate it through changes in sodium and water excretion and/or in the renin-angiotensin system.[20] Hypertension remains one of the leading causes of chronic renal failure, especially in nonwhite populations. (See Chapter 13, "Diseases of the Cardiovascular System," for detailed discussion of hypertension.) The heart, brain, eyes, and kidneys comprise the four major target organs of hypertension. Long-standing hypertension leads to fibrosis and sclerosis of the arterioles in these organs and throughout the body. Benign nephrosclerosis results from arteriosclerotic changes due to long-standing hypertension. It is the direct result of ischemia caused by narrowing of the lumina of the intrarenal vascular supply. The progressive closing of the arteries and arterioles leads to atrophy of the tubules and destruction of the glomerulus. "Malignant nephrosclerosis" refers to the structural changes that are associated with the malignant phase of essential hypertension.

Connective-Tissue Disorders. Renal diseases are very prevalent among patients with connective-tissue disorders, commonly referred to as collagen vascular diseases. Approximately two-thirds of patients with SLE and scleroderma or progressive systemic sclerosis (PSS) have clinical evidence of renal involvement. In rheumatoid arthritis, the prevalence of renal involvement is considerably less and is often related to complications of treatment with gold salts or D-penicillamine).

End-stage renal failure occurs in 25% of patients with SLE. Lupus nephritis, caused by circulating immunocomplexes that become trapped in the glomerular basement membrane, produces a clinical picture similar to that of acute glomerular nephritis or nephrotic syndrome.[21] PSS is characterized by the progressive sclerosis of the skin and viscera, including the kidneys and their vasculature, leading to changes resembling the nephrosclerosis seen in patients with long-standing hypertension.

Metabolic Disorders. The most common metabolic disorders that may lead to CRF include diabetes mellitus (DM), amyloidosis, gout, and primary hyperparathyroidism. By far, diabetes mellitus is one of the most important causes of CRF and accounts for nearly one-half of new ESRD patients (data from US Renal Data System, 1999). The type of diabetes the patient has affects the probability that the patient will develop ESRD. It has been estimated that about 50% of patients with type 1 DM develop ESRD within 15 to 25 years after the onset of diabetes, compared to 6% for patients with type 2 DM. The term "diabetic nephropathy" refers to the various changes that affect the structure and function of the kidneys in the presence of diabetes. Glomerulosclerosis is the most characteristic lesion of diabetic nephropathy. Other lesions include chronic tubulointerstitial nephritis, papillary necrosis, and ischemia. The natural progression of diabetic nephropathy follows five stages, beginning with early functional changes (stage 1) and progressing through early structural changes (stage 2), incipient nephropathy (stage 3), clinical diabetic nephropathy (stage 4), and finally, progressive renal insufficiency or failure (stage 5). The final stage is characterized by azotemia (elevated BUN and serum creatinine) resulting from a rapid decline in the GFR and leading to ESRD.

Toxic Nephropathy. The kidney is particularly exposed to the toxic effects of chemicals and drugs because it is an obligatory route of excretion for most drugs and because of its large vascular perfusion.[22] There are medications and other agents (referred to as "classic" nephrotoxins) whose use leads directly to renal failure. However, abuse of nonsteroidal anti-inflammatory drugs (NSAIDs) can also result in CRF. The renal protective effects of prostaglandins are inhibited by NSAIDs. Currently, abuse of analgesics accounts for 1 to 2% of all ESRD cases in the United States.

▼ MANIFESTATIONS OF RENAL DISEASE: UREMIC SYNDROME

Two groups of symptoms are present in patients with uremic syndrome: symptoms related to altered regulatory and excretory functions (fluid volume, electrolyte abnormalities, acid-base imbalance, accumulation of nitrogenous waste, and anemia) and a group of clinical symptoms affecting the cardiovascular, gastrointestinal, hematologic, and other systems (Table 15-4).

Biochemical Disturbances

Metabolic acidosis is a common biochemical disturbance experienced by patients with renal failure. As kidney function fails, excretion of hydrogen (H^+) ions diminishes, leading to systemic acidosis that results in a lower plasma pH and bicarbonate (HCO_3^-) concentration. Ammonium (NH_4^+) excretion, decreased because of reduced nephron mass, is the most important factor in the kidney's ability to eliminate H^+ and regenerate HCO_3^-. These patients often suffer from a moderate acidosis (serum bicarbonate level stabilized at 18 to 20 mEq/L). The symptoms of anorexia, lethargy, and nausea frequently observed in patients with uremia may be due partly to this metabolic acidosis. Kussmaul's breathing, a symptom caused by acidosis, is a deep sighing respiration aimed at increasing carbon dioxide excretion and reducing the metabolic acidosis. Disturbances in potassium balance are serious sequelae of renal dysfunction since only a narrow plasma concentration (normal = 3.5 to 5.5 mEq/L) is compatible with life. Because 90% of the daily intake of potassium is excreted in the urine, hypokalemia is common with the polyuria of early CRF. However, as kidney function continues to deteriorate, hyperkalemia ensues. Fatal dysrythmias or cardiac standstill will occur when the potassium level reaches 7 to 8 mEq/L. The normally functioning kidney allows great flexibility, excreting and conserving sodium in response to changing intake. Patients with CRF lose this adaptability, and small fluctuations often have serious consequences. Initially, patients experience osmotic diuresis and excess sodium excretion because of the polyuria. Sodium loss is more common in those conditions that are likely to affect the tubules (polycystic kidney disease and pyelonephritis). When oliguria develops in end-stage renal failure, sodium retention invariably occurs, resulting in edema, hypertension, and congestive heart failure.

Gastrointestinal Symptoms

The gastrointestinal system, particularly the esophagus, stomach, duodenum, and pancreas, show a myriad of symptoms in cases of uremic syndrome. The more common symptoms are often the first signs of the disease and include nausea, vomiting, and anorexia. Gastrointestinal inflammations such as gastritis, duodenitis, and esophagitis are common in late renal failure and can affect the entire gastrointestinal tract. Mucosal ulceration in the stomach, small intestine, and large intestine may hemmorhage, resulting in lowered blood pressure and a resultant lowered GFR. Digestion of hemorrhagic blood may lead to a rapid increase in BUN.[23]

Neurologic Signs and Symptoms

Some of the early signs and symptoms of CRF are related to changes in the neurologic system.[24] Both central and peripheral nervous systems are involved, with diverse consequences. The degree of cerebral disturbance roughly parallels the degree of azotemia. The patient's electroencephalogram becomes abnormal, with changes that are commensurate with metabolic encephalopathy. As the disease progresses, asterixis and myoclonic jerks may become evident; central nervous system

TABLE 15-4 Systemic Disturbances in Renal Disease (Uremic Syndrome)

Body System	Manifestations
Gastrointestinal	Nausea, vomiting, anorexia, ammoniacal taste and smell, stomatitis, parotitis, esophagitis, gastritis, gastrointestinal bleeding
Neuromuscular	Headache, peripheral neuropathy, paralysis, myoclonic jerks, seizures, asterixis
Hematologic-immunologic	Normocytic and normochromic anemia, coagulation defect, increased susceptibility to infection, decreased erythropoietin production, lymphocytopenia
Endocrine-metabolic	Renal osteodystrophy (osteomalacia, osteoporosis, osteosclerosis), secondary hyperparathyroidism, impaired growth and development, loss of libido and sexual function, amenorrhea
Cardiovascular	Arterial hypertension, congestive heart failure, cardiomyopathy, pericarditis, arrhythmias
Dermatologic	Pallor, hyperpigmentation, ecchymosis, uremic frost, pruritus, reddish brown distal nail beds

irritability and eventual seizures may occur. Seizures also can occur secondary to hypertensive encephalopathy, electrolyte disturbances (such as hyponatremia), and alkalosis, which induces hypocalcemia.

Along with neurologic hyperirritability, peripheral neuropathy is commonly present as a result of a disturbance of the conduction mechanism rather than a quantitative loss of nerve fiber. The clinical picture is dominated by sensory symptoms and signs. Impairment of vibratory sense and loss of deep tendon reflexes are the earliest, most frequent, and most constant findings. The predominant patient complaint is paresthesia or "burning feet" that may progress to eventual muscle weakness, atrophy, and finally, paralysis; there is a tendency toward increasing incidence with decreasing renal function. This predominantly affects the lower extremities but can affect the upper extremities as well. Rarely, facial, oral, and paraoral regions also can be affected. Severe uremic neuropathy is less commonly seen today because dialysis or transplantation is usually performed before uremic symptoms become prolonged or severe. Renal replacement therapy may halt the progress of peripheral neuropathy, but once these changes occur, sensory changes are poorly reversible while motor changes are considered irreversible.

The treatment of renal failure also may lead to the development of neurologic abnormalities in the form of dialysis disequilibrium, often seen during the first or second dialysis treatments and characterized by headache, nausea, and irritability that can progress to seizures, coma, and death.

Hematologic Problems

Patients with chronic renal dysfunction will often have hematologic problems, most commonly anemia and increased bleeding. The anemia associated with renal disease is a function of decreased erythropoiesis in the bone marrow and is usually normocytic and normochromic. It is not uncommon for these patients to have hematocrit levels in the 20 to 35% range (normal levels are 42 to 54% in males and 37 to 47% in females). The pathogenesis of the anemia is multifactorial, with nutritional deficiencies, iron metabolism abnormalities, and circulating uremic toxins that inhibit erythropoiesis all playing a role. The major factor, however, is the inability of the

diseased kidney to produce erythropoietin, which stimulates (through a feedback mechanism) the bone marrow to produce red blood cells. Hypertension, retention of waste products, and altered body fluid pH and electrolyte composition create a suboptimal environment for living cells; therefore, an accelerated destruction of red blood cells contributes to the anemia. Another cause of anemia in many dialysis patients is the frequent blood sampling and loss of blood in hemodialysis tubing and coils.

These patients may also have a microcytic hypochromic anemia that is usually caused by aluminum ion overload or deficiencies in iron stores. The former occurs from aluminum-containing medications, often given as phosphate-binding agents to control hyperphosphatemia. Aluminum also can be found in domestic tap water supplies or in nondealuminized dialysis water. This form of anemia is treated by chelation with desferoxamine.[25]

Interestingly, these patients tolerate their anemia quite well. Whole-blood transfusions are usually unnecessary, with the exception of cases of significant surgical blood loss or when the patient exhibits severe symptoms of anemia. These symptoms and signs of anemia may include pallor, tachycardia, systolic ejection murmur, a widened pulse pressure, and angina pectoris (in patients with underlying coronary artery disease). Transfusions may further suppress the production of red blood cells. The risk of hepatitis B and C, human immunodeficiency virus (HIV) infection, and other bloodborne infections is increased with the number of transfusions although blood screening techniques continue to minimize these risks.

Recombinant human erythropoietin (epoetin alfa [Epogen, Procrit]) corrects the anemia of ESRD and eliminates the need for transfusions in virtually all patients.[26] A dosage of 50 to 150 U/kg of body weight IV three times a week produces an increase in hematocrit of approximately 0.01 to 0.02 per day.[27–29] During early therapy, iron deficiency will develop in most patients. It is therefore initially essential to monitor the body's iron stores monthly.[30] With all patients, except those with transfusional iron overloads, prophylactic supplementation with ferrous sulfate (325 mg up to three times daily) is recommended.[31,32] Onset or exacerbation of hypertension has been observed as a possible complication of recombinant human erythropoietin therapy for the anemia of ESRD.[33] This effect is attributed to an overly rapid rise in the hematocrit level in the accompanying increased hemoglobin, blood viscosity, and renal cell mass.[34]

Bleeding may be a significant problem in patients with end-stage renal failure, and it has been attributed to increased prostacycline activity, increased capillary fragility, and a deficiency in platelet factor 3. The bleeding risk in renal failure results from an acquired qualitative platelet defect secondary to uremic toxins that decrease platelet adhesiveness. In addition, the low hematocrit levels commonly found in uremic patients negatively influence the rheologic component of platelet–vessel wall interactions. Platelet defects secondary to uremia is best remedied by dialysis but is also treated successfully by cryoprecipitate or 1-deamino-8-D-arginine vasopressin (DDAVP).[35] Platelet numbers affect bleeding, and mechanical trauma to the platelets during dialysis can cause a decrease of up to 17% in the platelet count. In addition to lowered platelet counts (which are usually not clinically significant) and qualitative platelet defects, the effects of medications on platelets contribute to bleeding episodes.

During dialysis, patients are given heparin to facilitate blood exchange and to maintain access patency. However, since the effects of heparinization during dialysis last only approximately 3 to 4 hours after infusion, the risk of excessive clinical bleeding because of anticoagulation is minimal in dentistry.[36] Some patients have a tendency to be hypercoagulable; for these patients, a regimen of warfarin sodium (Coumadin) therapy may be instituted to maintain a continuous anticoagulated state and to ensure shunt patency.

Calcium and Skeletal Disorders (Renal Osteodystrophy)

"Renal osteodystrophy" refers to the skeletal changes that result from chronic renal disease and that are caused by disorders in calcium and phosphorus metabolism, abnormal vitamin D metabolism, and increased parathyroid activity. In early renal failure, intestinal absorption of calcium is reduced because the kidneys are unable to convert vitamin D into its active form. Upon exposure to sunlight, 7-dehydroxycholesterol in the skin is converted to cholecalciferol (vitamin D_3) and is subsequently metabolized in the liver to a more biologically active form, 25-hydroxycholecalciferol (25-HCC). Further conversion to either 1,25-dihydroxycholecalciferol (1,25-DHCC) or 21,25-dihydroxycholecalciferol (21,25-DHCC) then occurs in the kidney parenchyma.

When the serum calcium level is high, 25-HCC is metabolized to 21,25-DHCC; conversely, a hypocalcemic state initiates the conversion of 25-HCC to 1,25-DHCC. This form is the most biologically active for absorbing calcium from the digestive tract. Impaired absorption of calcium because of defective kidney function and the corresponding retention of phosphate cause a decrease in the serum calcium level. This hypocalcemia is associated with a compensatory hyperactivity of the parathyroid glands (parathyroid hormone production) that increases the urinary excretion of phosphates,

decreases urinary calcium excretion, and augments the release of calcium from bone.

The most frequently observed changes associated with compensatory hyperparathyroidism (HPTH) are those that involve the skeletal system. These changes can appear before and during treatment with hemodialysis. Although it is a life-saving therapy, hemodialysis unfortunately fails to perform vital metabolic or endocrine functions and does not correct the crucial calcium-phosphate imbalance. In some cases, renal osteodystrophy becomes worse during hemodialysis. Some of the changes that are accelerated are bone remodeling, osteomalacia, osteitis fibrosa cystica (a rarefying osteitis with fibrous degeneration and cystic spaces that result from hyperfunction of the parathyroid glands), and osteosclerosis.[37]

The bone lesions are usually in the digits, the clavicle, and the acromioclavicular joint. Other lesions that can be seen are mottling of the skull, erosion of the distal clavicle and margins of the symphysis pubis, rib fractures, and necrosis of the femoral head.[38] The manifestations of metabolic renal osteodystrophy of the jaws include bone demineralization, decreased trabeculation, a "ground-glass" appearance, loss of lamina dura, radiolucent giant cell lesions, and metastatic soft-tissue calcifications.

In children, the predominant lesion is osteomalacia (a deficiency or absence of osteoid mineralization), which is associated with bone softening that leads to deformities of the ribs, pelvis, and femoral neck (renal rickets). Early stages of renal osteodystrophy may be detected histologically or biochemically without the presence of definitive radiographic changes because dependable radiographic evidence of bone disease appears only after 30% of bone mineral contents have been lost.

Osteodystrophy patients are placed on protein-restricted diets and phosphate binders (calcium carbonate or calcium acetate) to keep the serum phosphorus within the normal range (between 3.5 and 5.0 mg/dL). They also are given vitamin D supplements (such as 1,25-DHCC). If these measures fail, a parathyroidectomy may be performed, whereby two or more of the four glands are removed, leaving residual parathyroid hormone–secreting tissue.[39]

Most recently, a new form of renal bone disease termed adynamic bone disease has emerged as the most frequent finding on bone biopsy of patients who are on dialysis. The etiology of this new condition is not fully understood, but relatively low levels of intact serum parathyroid hormone are often associated with this disorder and may play a role in its pathogenesis.[40]

Cardiovascular Manifestations

Hypertension and congestive heart failure are common manifestations of uremic syndrome. Alterations in sodium and water retention account for 90% of cases of hypertension in CRF patients.[41] The association of circulatory overload and hypertension caused by disturbances in sodium and water balance contributes to an increased prevalence of congestive heart failure. In addition, retinopathy and encephalopathy can result from severe hypertension. Because of the early initiation of dialysis, the once frequent complication of pericarditis resulting from metabolic cardiotoxins is rarely seen.[42]

Respiratory Symptoms

Kussmaul's respirations (the deep sighing breathing seen in response to metabolic acidosis) is seen with uremia. Initially, however, dyspnea on exertion is a more frequent and often overlooked complaint in patients with progressing disease. The other respiratory complications, pneumonitis and "uremic lung," result from pulmonary edema associated with fluid and sodium retention and/or congestive heart failure.

Immunologic Changes

The significant morbidity experienced by patients with renal failure can be attributed to their altered host defenses. Uremic patients appear to be in a state of reduced immunocapacity, the cause of which is thought to be a combination of uremic toxemia and ensuing protein and caloric malnutrition compounded by protein-restricted diets. Uremic plasma contains nondialyzable factors that suppress lymphocyte responses that are manifested at the cellular and humoral levels, such as granulocyte dysfunction, suppressed cell-mediated immunity, and diminished ability to produce antibodies.[43] In addition, impaired or disrupted mucocutaneous barriers decrease protection from environmental pathogens. Together, these impairments place uremic patients at a high risk of infection, which is a common cause of morbidity and mortality.

Oral Manifestations

With impaired renal function, a decreased GFR, and the accumulation and retention of various products of renal failure, the oral cavity may show a variety of changes as the body progresses through an azotemic to a uremic state (Table 15-5). The general dentist should be able to recognize these oral symptoms as part of the patient's systemic disease and not as an isolated occurrence. In studies of renal patients, up to 90% were found to have oral symptoms of uremia. Some of the presenting signs were an ammonia-like taste and smell, stomatitis, gingivitis, decreased salivary flow, xerostomia, and parotitis.

As renal failure develops, one of the early symptoms may be a bad taste and odor in the mouth, particularly in the morning. This uremic fetor, an ammoniacal odor, is typical of any uremic patient and is caused by the high concentration of urea in the saliva and its subsequent breakdown to ammonia. Salivary urea levels correlate well with the BUN levels, but no fixed linear relationship exists. An acute rise in the BUN level may result in uremic stomatitis, which may appear as an erythemopultaceous form characterized by red mucosa covered with a thick exudate and a pseudomembrane or as an ulcerative form characterized by frank ulcerations with redness and a pultaceous coat. In all reported cases, intraoral changes have been related to BUN levels > 150 mg/dL and disappear spontaneously when medical treatment results in a lowered BUN level. Although its exact cause is uncertain, uremic stomatitis can be regarded as a chemical burn or as a general loss of tissue resistance and inability to withstand normal and traumatic influences. White plaques called "uremic frost" and occasionally found on the skin can rarely be found intraorally. This uremic frost results from residual urea crystals left on the epithelial surfaces after

TABLE 15-5 Oral and Radiographic Manifestations of Renal Disease and Dialysis

Oral manifestations
  Enlarged (asymptomatic) salivary glands
  Decreased salivary flow
  Dry mouth
  Odor of urea on breath
  Metallic taste
  Increased calculus formation
  Low caries rate
  Enamel hypoplasia
  Dark brown stains on crowns
    Extrinsic (secondary to liquid ferrous sulfate therapy)
    Intrinsic (secondary to tetracycline staining)
  Dental malocclusions
  Pale mucosa with diminished color demarcation between attached gingiva and alveolar mucosa
  Low-grade gingival inflammation
  Petechiae and ecchymosis
  Bleeding from gingiva
  Prolonged bleeding
  Candidal infections
  Burning and tenderness of mucosa
  Erosive glossitis
  Tooth erosion (secondary to regurgitation associated with dialysis)
  Dehiscence of wounds
Radiographic manifestations
  Demineralization of bone
  Loss of bony trabeculation
  Ground-glass appearance
  Loss of lamina dura
  Giant cell lesions, "brown tumors"
  Socket sclerosis
  Pulpal narrowing and calcification
  Tooth mobility
  Arterial and oral calcifications

perspiration evaporates or as a result of decreased salivary flow. A more common oral finding is significant xerostomia, probably caused by a combination of direct involvement of the salivary glands, chemical inflammation, dehydration, and mouth breathing (Kussmaul's respiration). Salivary adenitis can occasionally be seen. Another finding associated with increased salivary urea nitrogen, particularly in children, is a low caries activity. This is observed despite a high sugar intake and poor oral hygiene, suggesting an increased neutralizing capacity of the urea arising from ureal hydrolysis. With the increased availability and improved techniques of dialysis and transplantation, many of the oral manifestations of uremia and renal failure are less commonly observed.

Other oral manifestations of renal disease are related to renal osteodystrophy (RO) or secondary HPTH. These manifestations usually become evident late in the course of the disease. The classic signs of RO in the mandible and maxilla are bone demineralization, loss of trabeculation, ground-glass appearance, total or partial loss of lamina dura, giant cell lesions or brown tumors, and metastatic calcifications (Figure 15-2). These changes appear most frequently in the mandibular molar region superior to the mandibular canal. The rar-

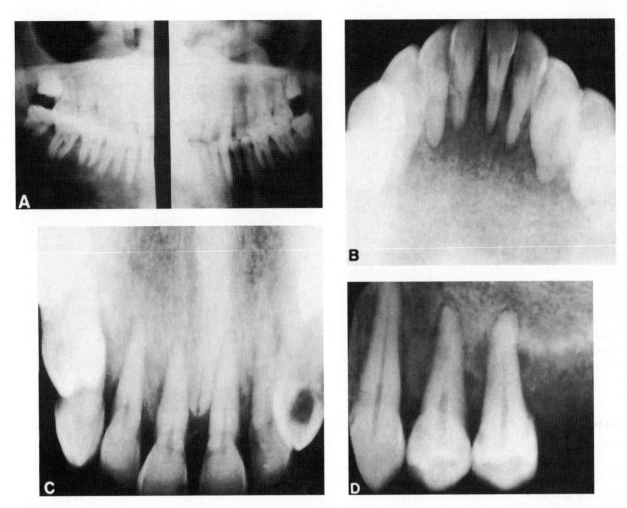

FIGURE 15-2 **A,** Panoramic image showing trabecular changes. Also note erupted lower third molars without fully developed root formations. **B,** Mandibular anterior loss of trabeculation. **C,** Maxillary anterior loss of trabeculation. **D,** Loss of lamina dura.

efaction in the mandible and maxilla is secondary to generalized osteoporosis. The finer trabeculae disappear later, leaving a coarser pattern. Small lytic lesions that histologically prove to be giant cell or brown tumors may occur.

The compact bone of the jaws may become thinned and eventually disappear. This may be evident as loss of the lower border of the mandible, the cortical margins of the inferior dental canal and floor of the antrum, and lamina dura. Studies have shown that the finding of decreasing thickness of cortical bone at the angle of the mandible correlates well with the degree of RO. Spontaneous and pathologic fractures may occur with the thinning of these areas of compact bone and may complicate dental extractions.

While the skeleton may undergo decalcification, fully developed teeth are not directly affected; however, in the presence of significant skeletal decalcification, the teeth will appear more radiopaque. The loss of lamina dura is neither pathognomonic for nor a consistent sign of HPTH. A similar loss of lamina dura also may be seen in Paget's disease, osteomalacia, fibrous dysplasia, sprue, and Cushing's and Addison's diseases. Various studies indicate changes in lamina dura in only 40 to 50% of known HPTH patients.

The radiolucent lesions of HPTH are called "brown tumors" because they contain areas of old hemorrhage and appear brown on clinical inspection. As these tumors increase in size, the resultant expansion may involve the cortex. Although the tumor rarely breaks through the periosteum, gingival swelling may occur. The brown tumor lesion contains an abundance of multinucleated giant cells, fibroblasts, and hemosiderin. This histologic appearance is also consistent with central giant cell tumor and giant cell reparative granuloma. Associated bone changes consist of a generalized osteitis fibrosa, with patches of osteoclastic resorption on all bone surfaces. This is replaced by a vascular connective tissue that represents an abortive formation of coarse-fibered woven bone. This histologic picture also may be seen in fibrous dysplasia, giant cell reparative granuloma, osteomalacia, and Paget's disease.

Other clinical manifestations of RO include tooth mobility, malocclusion, and metastatic soft-tissue calcifications. Increasing mobility and drifting of teeth with no apparent pathologic periodontal pocket formation may be seen. Periapical radiolucencies and root resorption also may be associated with this gradual loosening of the dentition. The teeth may be painful to percussion and mastication, and positive thermal and electric pulp test responses often will be elicited. Splinting is a useful adjunct to prevent pain and further drifting, and the splint should be maintained until adequate treatment of the HPTH results in bone remineralization. Malocclusion may result from the advanced mobility and drifting of the dentition. Extreme demineralization and collapse of the temporomandibular and paratemporomandibular bones may also produce a malocclusion.

Metastatic calcification can occur, particularly when the calcium-phosphate solubility product (Ca × P) is > 70. In normal subjects, a relationship exists between plasma calcium and inorganic phosphate. When expressed in terms of total calcium and inorganic phosphate (both as milligrams per deciliter), the ion product or calcium-phosphate solubility product (Ca × P) is normally an average of 35. A rise in the calcium-phosphate ion product in the extracellular fluid may cause metastatic calcifications because of the precipitation of calcium phosphate crystals into the soft tissues, such as the sclera, corner of the eye, subcutaneous tissue, skeletal and cardiac muscle, and blood vessels. This also may occur in the oral and associated paraoral soft tissues. These calcifications are often visible radiographically.

Abnormal bone repair after extraction, termed "socket sclerosis" and radiographically characterized by a lack of lamina dura resorption and by the deposition of sclerotic bone in the confines of the lamina dura, has been reported in patients with renal disease although it is not unique to them (Figure 15-3).

Enamel hypoplasia (a white or brownish discoloration) is frequently seen in patients whose renal disease started at a young age. The location of the hypoplastic enamel on the permanent teeth corresponds to the age of onset of advanced renal failure. Prolonged corticosteroid administration also may contribute to this deficiency (Figure 15-4). Another frequent dental finding is pulpal narrowing and calcifications. In some patients who are on dialysis, severe tooth erosion as a result of the nausea and extensive vomiting that often follows dialysis treatment may be seen. Because of the platelet changes with renal disease itself and with dialysis therapy, gingival bleeding may be a common patient complaint.

▼ MEDICAL MANAGEMENT OF CHRONIC RENAL FAILURE

The treatment of CRF is often divided into (1) conservative therapy aimed at delaying progressive renal dysfunction and (2) renal replacement therapy, instituted when conservative measures are no longer effective in sustaining life.

Conservative Therapy

Once the extent of renal impairment is established and reversible causes are excluded, medical management is devoted to the elimination of symptoms and the prevention of further deterioration.[44] Conservative measures are initiated when the patient becomes azotemic. Initial conservative therapy is directed towards managing diet, fluid, electrolytes, and calcium-phosphate balance and toward the prevention and treatment of complications.[45] Dietary modifications are initiated with the onset of uremic symptoms. Dietary regulation of pro-

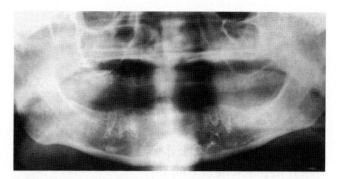

FIGURE 15-3 Panoramic radiograph of extraction sites representative of socket sclerosis. Teeth were extracted 6 years before the radiograph and 2 years before diagnosis of end-stage renal disease.

tein (20 to 40 g per day) may improve acidosis, azotemia, and nausea. The restriction of protein not only reduces BUN levels but reduces potassium and phosphate intake and hydrogen ion production. Also, a low-protein intake reduces the excretory load of the kidney, thereby reducing glomerular hyperfiltration, intraglomerular pressure, and secondary injury of nephrons.[46,47] This restricted diet is often supplemented with multivitamins specific to the needs of the renal patient. Despite difficulties with hypertension, edema, and weight gain, salt and fluid excess and depletion must be avoided. For patients with early renal insufficiency, prevention of hyperphosphatemia by limiting the intake of phosphate-containing foods and by supplementing the diet with calcium carbonate (which prevents intestinal absorption) may potentially minimize the sequelae of uremic osteodystrophy.[48]

Recently, a practical clinical approach to the management of patients with CRF, using the acronym BEANS, has gained popularity. To temper renal dysfunction, attenuate uremic complications, and prepare patients for renal replacement therapy, medical care providers should "take care of the BEANS," as follows.[49] *Blood pressure* should be maintained in a target range lower than 130/85 mm Hg. (Toward this end, the use of angiotensin-converting enzyme inhibitors, because of their renal protective effects, has gained favor with many clin-

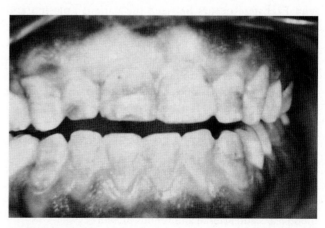

FIGURE 15-4 Enamel hypoplasia and tetracycline stains in a young patient with end-stage renal disease.

icians.) Hemoglobin levels should be maintained at 10 to 12 g/dL with *Erythropoietin. A*ccess for dialysis should be created when the serum creatinine reaches > 4.0 mg/dL or the GFR falls to < 20 mL/min. Close monitoring of *Nutritional status* is important to avoid protein malnutrition, correct metabolic acidosis, prevent and treat hyperphosphatemia, administer vitamin supplements, and guide the initiatiation of dialysis therapy. *Specialty evaluation by a nephrologist should be insti-*tuted when serum creatinine is > 3.0 mg/dL.

Renal Replacement Therapy

For patients with ESRD, dialysis has significantly decreased the mortality of this once invariably fatal disease. Long-term maintenance dialysis therapy has been a reality since 1961. In 1964, there were fewer than 300 patients in the United States receiving dialysis. Because of amendments to the Social Security Act in 1972 and the extension of Medicare benefits in 1973, dialysis therapy was made available to virtually everybody who developed ESRD. Although access to treatment is of less concern today, discrepancies between the morbidity and mortality rates of for-profit and not-for-profit dialysis centers remain a source of controversy.[50,51] Today, approximately 260,000 people are given treatments in more than 3,000 dialysis facilities in the United States.

There are no clear guidelines for determining when renal replacement therapy should begin. Most nephrologists base their decisions on the individual patient's ability to work full-time, the presence of peripheral neuropathy, and the presence of other signs of clinical deterioration. Serum creatinine levels of > 6 mg/dL in males (4 mg/dL in females) and a GFR < 4 mL/min are the laboratory thresholds that are often used to indicate the need for dialysis therapy.

There are two major techniques of dialysis: hemodialysis and peritoneal dialysis. Each follows the same basic principle of diffusion of solutes and water from the plasma to the dialysis solution in response to a concentration or pressure gradient.

HEMODIALYSIS

Hemodialysis is the removal of nitrogenous and toxic products of metabolism from the blood by means of a hemodialyzer system. Exchange occurs between the patient's plasma and dialysate (the electrolyte composition of which mimics that of extracellular fluid) across a semipermeable membrane that allows uremic toxins to diffuse out of the plasma while retaining the formed elements and protein composition of blood (Figure 15-5). Dialysis does not provide the same degree of health as normal renal function provides, because there is no resorptive capability in the dialysis membrane; therefore, valuable nutrients are lost, and potentially toxic molecules are retained. The usual dialysis system consists of a dialyzer, dialysate production unit, roller blood pump, heparin infusion pump, and various devices to monitor the conductivity, temperature, flow rate, and pressure of dialysate and to detect blood leaks and arterial and venous pressures.[52]

Dialysis therapy can be delivered to the patient in outpatient dialysis centers, where trained personnel administer ther-apy on a regular basis, or in the home, where family members trained in dialysis techniques assist the patient in dialysis therapy. It has been shown that patients who undergo dialysis at home fare better psychologically, have a better quality of life, and have lower rates of morbidity and mortality than hospital dialysis patients.[53,54] Unfortunately, home dialysis may not be applicable for all patients because it is more difficult and requires a high degree of motivation.

The frequency and duration of dialysis treatments are related to body size, residual renal function, protein intake, and tolerance to fluid removal. The typical patient undergoes hemodialysis three times per week, with each treatment lasting approximately 3 to 4 hours on standard dialysis units and slightly less time on high-efficiency or high-flux dialysis units. During treatments and for varying amounts of time afterward, anticoagulants are administered by regional or systemic methods.

Vascular access for hemodialysis can be created by a shunt or external cannula system or by an arteriovenous fistula; the fistula is preferred for long-term treatment. The classic construction is a side-to-side anastomosis between the radial artery and the cephalic vein at the forearm. In patients with very thin veins, it can be technically impossible to create a direct arteriovenous fistula, and in some patients, fistulae have clotted in both arms, resulting in a demand for other forms of vascular access (sometimes the thigh is used as a site). A great advance in access capability was the introduction of subcutaneous artificial arteriovenous grafts, beginning with Gore-Tex heterografts (W.L. Gore, Flagstaff, Ariz.). Fistulae are now constructed between arteries and veins by means of saphenous vein, autografts, polytetrafluoroethylene (PTFE) grafts, Dacron, and other prosthetic conduits. Hemodialysis is performed by direct cannulation of these grafts or vascular anastomoses[55,56] (Figure 15-6). There is an increasing trend toward the use of indwelling central venous catheters for maintenance hemodialysis.[57]

Despite optimal dialysis, these patients remain chronically ill with hematologic, metabolic, neurologic, and cardiovascular problems that are more or less permanent. Growth alterations may be seen in very young renal disease patients, particularly if they are maintained on hemodialysis. This growth deficiency has been attributed to the poor caloric intake of these patients and to the uremic state.[58] Dietary supplements have produced accelerated growth spurts, and successful kidney transplantation may restore a normal growth rate.[59] The major determining factor is the bone age. For patients older than 12 years of age, it is doubtful that significant growth would be attained.

PERITONEAL DIALYSIS

Peritoneal dialysis accounts for only 10% of dialysis treatments. During peritoneal dialysis, access to the body is achieved via a catheter through the abdominal wall into the peritoneum. One to two liters of dialysate is placed in the peritoneal cavity and is allowed to remain for varying intervals of time. Substances diffuse across the semipermeable peritoneal

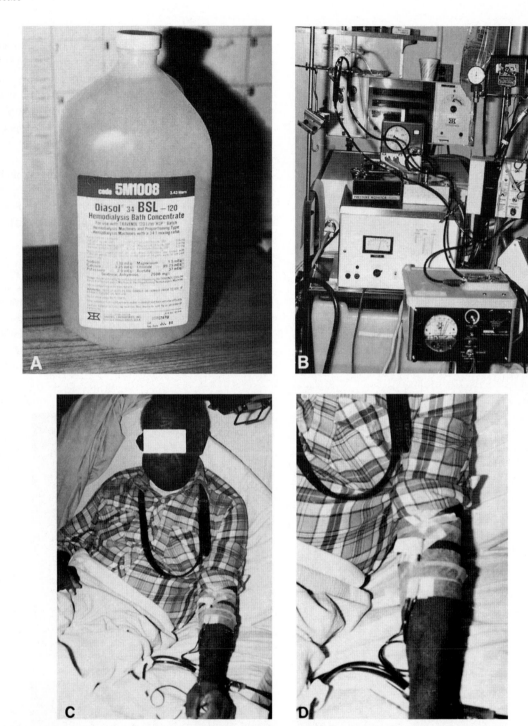

FIGURE 15-5 **A,** Dialysate. **B,** Dialysis unit. **C,** Patient receiving dialysis. **D,** Close-up of access.

membrane into the dialysate. Compared to the membranes used for hemodialysis, the peritoneal membrane has greater permeability for high-molecular-weight species. The Tenckhoff silastic catheter has made peritoneal puncture for each dialysis unnecessary. The Tenckhoff catheter is a permanent intraperitoneal catheter that has two polyester felt cuffs into which tissue growth occurs. If used with a sterile technique, it permits virtually infection-free long-term access to the peritoneum (Figure 15-7).

Several regimens can be used with peritoneal dialysis. In one, chronic ambulatory peritoneal dialysis (CAPD), 2 L of dialysis fluid is instilled into the peritoneal cavity, allowed to remain for 30 minutes, and then drained out. This is repeated every 8 to 12 hours, 5 to 7 days per week. A popular variation of this is continuous cyclic peritoneal dialysis (CCPD), in which 2 L of dialysate is exchanged every 6 to 8 hours around the clock, 7 days per week.[60]

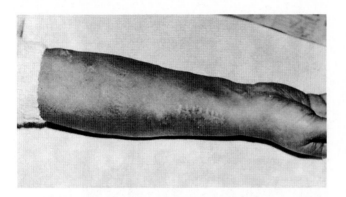

FIGURE 15-6 Vascular access site in arm.

Two of the benefits of peritoneal dialysis are that heparinization is unnecessary and that there is no risk of air embolism and blood leaks. It also allows a great deal of personal freedom; for this reason, is often used as the primary therapy or as a temporary measure. These features, along with its simplicity, make peritoneal dialysis safe for patients who are

at risk when hemodialysis is used (eg, the young, elderly patients, those with high-risk coronary and cerebral vascular disease, and those with vascular access problems).[61] Some of the problems encountered with peritoneal dialysis are pain, intra-abdominal hemorrhage, bowel infarction, inadequate drainage, leakage, and peritonitis (approximately 70% of which is caused by a single gram-positive microorganism that is indigenous to the patient's skin or upper respiratory tract and that infects the peritoneal cavity).[62]

Today, renal transplantation is the treatment of choice for patients with irreversible kidney failure. However, the use of transplantation is limited by organ availability. (Renal transplantation and its specific dental management considerations are discussed in Chapter ##.)

OTHER APPROACHES TO SOLUTE REMOVAL

Many patients continue to have various disturbances in metabolic functions despite optimal dialysis, maintaining uremic metabolites (eg, urea, creatinine, and phosphate) at nearly normal levels. These observations have led investigators to postulate that uremic toxins of a molecular weight between that of urea (< 500 Da) and that of plasma proteins (> 50,000

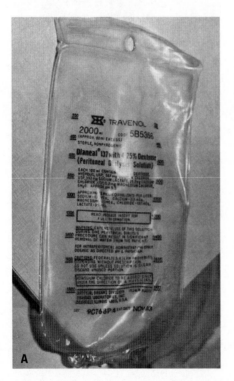

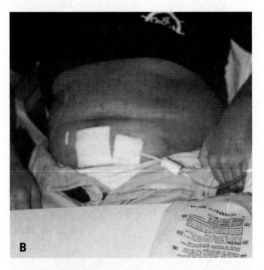

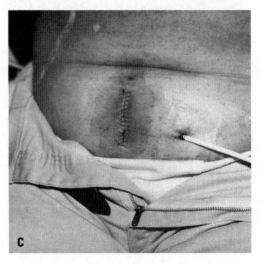

FIGURE 15-7 **A,** Dialysate for chronic ambulatory peritoneal dialysis. **B,** Close-up of patient receiving dialysis. **C,** Close-up of peritoneal access.

Da), effectively unfiltered by dialysis, account for these clinical abnormalities. This theory, termed the middle molecular hypothesis, has led to the development of two techniques: hemofiltration (HF) and absorbent therapy. Hemofiltration is based on the principle of convection instead of diffusion and is based on the physiologic function of the glomerulus.[63] In HF, the standard dialysis technique is modified by sequentially prediluting the blood with an electrolyte solution that is similar to plasma and subsequently "ultrafiltering" it under high hydraulic pressures. This technique is more efficient than dialysis in removing solutes in the middle molecular range and results in patients who feel well and have little hemodynamic instability. Adjunctive techniques used with maintenance dialysis or for patients with significant residual renal function (a GFR of 5 to 10 mL/min) include the use of absorbent materials for solute removal. These absorbents may be used through direct action on the bloodstream (hemoperfusion), through regeneration of dialysate (REDY sorbent hemodialysis), or indirectly, through introduction into the gut.

In hemoperfusion, membrane-encapsulated activated charcoal is the absorbent whereas REDY sorbent dialysis systems use an enzyme sorbent cartridge for reprocessing dialysate. The REDY systems are widely used for patients who require specialized treatment and for home dialysis. A technique that uses the oral ingestion of absorbents such as activated charcoal is in its infancy although a similar technique using aluminum hydroxides is used conventionally for controlling phosphate levels.

▼ ORAL HEALTH CONSIDERATIONS

For the purposes of dental management, patients with renal disease can be categorized into two groups: patients with acute renal failure and patients with chronic progressing renal failure or end-stage renal failure who are undergoing dialysis.

Acute Renal Failure Patients

Acute renal failure (ARF) is most commonly observed in young healthy adults after injury to the renal tubules as a result of toxic agents, severe necrotizing glomerular disease, or complications of surgery, including hemorrhage and transfusion. Patients with ARF are not candidates for elective dental care, and some patients with ARF require the institution of dialysis therapy. In such cases, elective dental care should be deferred until the patient makes a complete renal recovery. Peritoneal dialysis generally poses no contraindications to dental treatment. The exceptions are in times of acute peritoneal infections, when elective care should be postponed.

Chronic Renal Failure and End-Stage Renal Disease Patients

Many patients with chronic renal disease have poor oral health. The results of a study assessing the dental needs of hemodialysis patients showed that 64% of these patients needed dental treatment and that the majority of these patients were not aware of the possible complications of den-

tal neglect while on hemodialysis.[64] In addition to the more common reasons for not receiving routine dental treatment, these patients have limited access to dental care because many general dentists are reluctant to treat patients with severe systemic diseases. Because most dialysis centers refer their patients to general practitioners for most forms of treatment, it is important that more general dentists become familiar with the management problems associated with patients with ESRD who are undergoing dialysis.

Excessive bleeding and anemia are the two major hematologic conditions that most commonly affect patients with uremia and renal failure. Bleeding tendencies in these patients are attributed to a combination of qualitative and quantitative platelet defects, increased prostacycline activity, intrinsic coagulation defects, and capillary fragility. This hemorrhagic tendency can be magnified in the presence of uremia. Hemorrhagic episodes in the gingiva are not uncommon. Ulcerations and purpural or petechial lesions may be noted throughout the oral mucosa. Bruising after trauma is common, and hematoma formation should be expected after alveolectomy or periodontal surgery. Adjunctive hemostatic measures should be considered for patients who are at risk. DDAVP, the synthetic analogue of the antidiuretic hormone vasopressin, has been shown to be effective in the short-term management of bleeding in patients with renal failure. The effects of conjugated estrogen, used for longer-term hemostasis, commonly last for up to 2 weeks, compared to a few hours for DDAVP. Tranexamic acid (an antifibrinolytic agent) administered in the form of a mouthrinse or soaked gauze significantly reduces operative and postoperative bleeding. Meticulous surgical technique, primary closure, and local hemostatic aides such as microfibrillar collagen and oxidized regenerated cellulose should be used as the standards of care. Although rare, hemorrhagic effusions into the temporomandibular-joint space presenting as pain and swelling have been reported in a patient who was on dialysis and warfarin sodium therapy.

The timing of dental care for the patient who is undergoing dialysis has long been a source of discussion in the literature. Since dialysis will return hydration, serum electrolytes, urea nitrogen, and creatinine toward normal levels, arguments have been made for treating patients in a dental setting on the day of dialysis treatment. This argument is countered by the facts that patients often do not feel well immediately after undergoing dialysis and that they are heparinized. Ideally, elective dental procedures, as well as extractions and other surgery, should be done early in the dialysis cycle. At this point, the blood is free of uremic toxins, and the patient is far enough removed from dialysis to allow sufficient time after surgery for clotting before the next cycle and re-heparinization. Also, it is less likely that the patient will have a clotting defect that is due to uremia-related platelet dysfunction, which develops because of retained urea metabolites. A platelet count and complete blood count are important guides for the dental practitioner with regard to the management of bleeding tendencies and anemic conditions. However, since patients are physically and emotionally exhausted and do not feel well following dialysis treatments, elective dental procedures should be scheduled on nondialysis days, when patients are more likely to tolerate care.

Apart from serving as a potential site for infection, the arteriovenous site should never be jeopardized. The arm with the patent vascular access should be identified and noted on the patient's chart with instructions to avoid both intramuscular and intravenous injection of medication into this arm; nor should the access site be used as an injection site. The blood flow through the arm should not be impeded by requiring the patient to assume a cramped position or by using that arm to measure blood pressure. When the access site is located in a leg, the patient should avoid sitting for long periods. Obstructing venous drainage by compression at the groin or behind the knee must be avoided, especially because it tends to occur normally when the patient is in the sitting position. Such patients should be permitted to walk about for a few minutes every hour during a lengthy dental procedure.

Susceptibilty to infection is a serious concern for patients with uremia or ESRD who are undergoing hemodialysis.[65] These patients have an increased susceptibility to bacterial infections that results from altered cellular immunity secondary to the effects of uremic toxins combined with malnutrition from protein-restricted diets. Oral diseases and dental manipulation create bacteremias that may lead to significant morbidity and potential mortality in patients with renal failure who are undergoing hemodialysis. A majority of septicemic infections have been attributed to the vascular access site, but oral diseases such as periodontal disease, pulpal infection, and oral ulcerations, along with dental treatment, may provide microorganisms a convenient portal of entry the circulatory system.[66] Therefore, every effort should be made to eliminate potential sources of infection. Meticulous oral hygiene, including good home care, frequent oral health maintenance, and routine use of antifungal and antimicrobial oral rinses may reduce the risk of dentally induced infections.

Infective endocarditis is a serious concern in hemodialysis patients. Sepsis and bacterial endarteritis occur from infections at the access site by organisms seeded through punctures. Infective endocarditis has been reported in patients with access site grafts on hemodialysis after receiving dental treatment. The incidence of infective endocarditis in patients undergoing hemodialysis is 2.7%. In those patients with a history of vascular access site infection, the incidence increases to 9.0%. *Streptococcus viridans* accounts for almost one-third of the cases of infective endocarditis whereas staphylococcal organisms such as *Staphylococcus epidermidis* and *Staphylococcus aureus* account for the majority of cases. The cause of endocarditis in these patients is debatable but seems to be related to a combination of vascular access and intrinsic cardiaovalvular pathology. The presence of an arteriovenous shunt or synthetic graft (fistula) sutured in place increases the risk for infective colonization at the suture lines or at the surface discrepancies between normal arterial intima and the so-called prosthetic pseudointima. These sites may provide a nidus for intravascular lodgment of bacteria, leading to the persistence of an otherwise transient bacteremia (such as one resulting from dental manipulation), with subsequent endarteritis, embolization, and possible endocardial infection.[67] A period of high susceptibility to infection is usually seen within the first 3 months after implantation (risk is highest in the first 3 weeks), after which there is a gradual decline in risk. This reduced risk is possibly caused by an "insulating effect" of the developing pseudointima and endothelialization.

Endocarditis infection is more likely to affect previously abnormal cardiac valves; yet, there is a high incidence of endocarditis in hemodialysis patients with no previously demonstrated valvulopathy. A possible explanation may lie in the theory that changes in fluid volume with uremia and hemodialysis may affect blood flow through the heart and cardiac function, creating mechanical stresses on the valves that play a role in the development of infective endocarditis. Therefore, according to the American Heart Association's protocol for prevention of infective endocarditis, antimicrobial premedication should be used routinely prior to appropriate dental procedures.

The choice of antibiotic depends on many variables but is primarily based on the type of microorganisms that have been cultured at the site of manipulation. In patients who were reported to have acquired infective endocarditis after dental treatment, either viridans streptococci or *Enterococcus* spp were the causative agents. This indicates a prophylactic regimen of either (1) amoxicillin or clindamycin or (2) a broad-spectrum antibiotic such as oral clarithromycin (as recommended by the American Heart Association) or IV vancomycin in patients with hypersensitivity to penicillin or clindamycin. Limited insurance reimbursement for vancomycin infusion may limit many patients' access to this therapy.

Because these patients are exposed to a large number of blood tranfusions and exchanges and also because of their renal failure–related immune dysfunction, they are at greater risk of hepatotropic viral infections (such as hepatitis B and C), HIV infection, and tuberculosis. Many patients with renal disease may have viral hepatitis without clinical manifestations. In these patients, the disease tends to run a chronic and persistently active (although subclinical) course. With the advent of prophylactic immunoglobulin and the hepatitis B vaccine, the number of dialysis unit outbreaks of hepatitis has decreased; however, the dialysis patient should still be considered to be in a high-risk group. The prevalence of hepatitis C virus (HCV) infection in dialysis patients ranges from 3.9 to 71%.[68,69] Patients undergoing dialysis should be encouraged to undergo periodic testing for hepatitis infectivity and for HIV antibody. Hemodialysis patients with accompanying conditions such as HIV disease, viral hepatitis (and associated liver dysfunction), and tuberculosis (TB) have complicating issues that affect the provision of dental care. CRF patients who are on hemodialysis have been reported to be at increased risk of developing tuberculosis.[70] (The dental management of patients with HIV infection, TB, and viral hepatitis is discussed in Chapter 20.)

TABLE 15-6 Drug Therapy for Renal Disease

Drug	Normal	Adjustments for Renal Failure Moderate (GFR = 10–50 mL/min)	Severe (GFR < 10 mL/min)
Antifungal agents			
Amphotericin	q 24 h	Unchanged	Unchanged
Fluconazole	q 24 h	Unchanged	Unchanged
Miconazole	q 8 h	Unchanged	Unchanged
Aminoglycosides			
Gentamicin	q 8 h	q 12–24 h	Avoid if possible
Tobramycin	q 8 h	q 8–24 h	Avoid if possible
Streptomycin	q 12 h	Avoid if possible	Avoid if possible
Other antimicrobials			
Penicillin G	q 6–8 h	q 8–12 h	q 12–18 h
Penicillin V	q 6 h	q 6 h	q 6 h
Erythromycin	q 6 h	Unchanged	Unchanged
Ampicillin	q 6 h	q 6–12 h	q 12–16 h
Amoxicillin	q 8 h	q 8–12 h	q 12–16 h
Cephalothin	q 6 h	Unchanged	q 8–12 h
Carbenicillin	q 4 h	q 8–12 h	Avoid if possible
Clindamycin	q 8 h	q 8 h	q 8 h
Metronidazole	q 8 h	q 8 h	q 12–16 h
Vancomycin	q 6 h	q 72–240 h	q 240 h
Tetracycline	q 6 h	q 6 h	q 6 h
Doxycycline	q 12–24 h	q 12–24 h	q 12–24 h
Analgesics			
Acetaminophen	q 4 h	q 6 h	q 8 h
Acetylsalicylic acid	q 4 h	q 4–6 h	Avoid
Ketorolac	q 6 h	Avoid	Avoid
Phenacetin	q 6 h	Avoid	Avoid
Ibuprofen	q 6 h	Avoid	Avoid
Local anesthetics	Unchanged	Unchanged	Unchanged
Narcotics			
Codeine	q 4 h	Unchanged	Unchanged
Meperidine (Demerol)	q 4 h	Unchanged	Unchanged
Morphine	q 4 h	Unchanged	Unchanged
Pentazocine (Talwin)	q 4–6 h	Unchanged	Unchanged
Propoxyphene (Darvon)	q 4 h	Unchanged	Unchanged
Naloxone (Narcan)	Bolus	Unchanged	Unchanged
Sedatives, hypnotics, barbiturates, and tranquilizers			
Chlordiazepoxide (Librium)	q 6–8 h	Unchanged	Unchanged
Diazepam (Valium)	q 8 h	Unchanged	Unchanged
Flurazepam (Dalmane)	q 24 h	Unchanged	Unchanged
Meprobamate (Miltown)	q 6 h	q 9–12 h	q 12–18 h
Methaqualone (Quaalude)	q 8 h	Unchanged	Unchanged
Amitriptyline (Elavil)	q 8 h	Unchanged	Unchanged
Secobarbital	q 8 h	Unchanged	Unchanged
Phenobarbital	q 8 h	Unchanged	Unchanged
Pentobarbital	q 8 h	Unchanged	Unchanged
Antihistamines			
Chlorpheniramine (Chlortrimeton)	q 4–6 h	Unchanged	Unchanged
Diphenhydramine (Benadryl)	q 6 h	q 6–9 h	q 9–12 h
Corticosteroids			
Cortisone	q 8 h	Unchanged	Unchanged
Hydrocortisone	q 8 h	Unchanged	Unchanged
Prednisone	q 8 h	Unchanged	Unchanged
Neurologic agents			
Phenytoin (Dilantin)	q 8 h	Unchanged	Unchanged
Lidocaine	—	Unchanged	Unchanged

GFR = glomerular filtration rate.

As a result of changes in fluid volume, sodium retention, and the presence of vascular access, these patients are commonly affected by a host of cardiovascular conditions. Often, hypertension, postdialysis hypotension, congestive heart failure, and pulmonary hypertension can be seen in patients who are undergoing hemodialysis.[71] Hypertension in the presence of ESRD can lead to accelerated atherosclerosis. Although the medical management of these patients includes the aggressive use of antihypertensive agents, the dental practitioner should obtain blood pressure readings at every visit, prior to and during procedures. Avoiding excessive stress in the dental chair is important to minimize intraoperative elevations of systolic pressure. The use of sedative premedication should be considered for patients who are to undergo stressful procedures. Hypotension resulting from fluid depletion is a common complication of hemodialysis and occurs in up to 30% of dialysis sessions. Cerebrovascular accidents, angina, fatal dysrhythmias, and myocardial infarction are less common but serious sequelae of hemodialysis and most commonly present during or immediately following dialysis. Therefore, elective dental care should be performed on nondialysis days, when the patients are best able to tolerate treatment.

Pharmacotherapeutics are a serious concern for dentists treating patients who have renal disease. Most drugs are excreted at least partially by the kidney, and renal function affects drug bioavailability, the volume of drug distribution, drug metabolism, and the rate of drug elimination. The dentist can obviate problems of drug reactions and further renal damage by following simple principles related to drug administration and by altering dosage schedules according to the amount of residual renal function. Many ordinarily safe drugs must not be administered to the uremic patient, and many others must be prescribed over longer intervals (Table 15-6). The plasma half-lives of medications that are normally eliminated in the urine are often prolonged in renal failure and are effectively reduced by dialysis. Even drugs that are metabolized by the liver can lead to increased toxicity because the diseased kidneys fail to excrete them effectively. Theoretically, a 50% decrease in creatinine clearance corresponds to a twofold increase in the elimination half-life of any medication excreted fully by the kidneys. For drugs that are partially excreted by the kidneys, the change in plasma half-life is proportionally less. For most drugs, it is proper to give a loading dose similar to that given to patients without renal disease; this provides a clinically desirable blood concentration that can be sustained by the necessary dosage adjustments. Whenever reliable blood drug level measurements are available, they can be used to monitor therapy. In the absence of precise blood levels, the best guide to therapy is carefully obtained data on biologic half-lives of drugs in humans with varying degrees of renal failure.

Certain drugs are themselves nephrotoxic and should be avoided. Particular medications may be metabolized to acid

TABLE 15-7 Drugs to Limit or Avoid When Treating Dialysis Patients

Indication	Drug
Magnesium content	Antacids (Maalox, milk of magnesia) Laxatives
Potassium content	IV fluids Salt substitutes Massive penicillin therapy (1.7 mEq/million U)
Sodium content	Carbenicillin (4.7 mEq/g) Alka Seltzer (23 mEq tablet) IV fluid
Acidifying effects	Ascorbic acid Ammonium chloride (in cough syrup) Nonsteroidal anti-inflammatory agents
Catabolic effects	Tetracyclines Steroids
Nephrotoxicity	Phenacetin Ketorolac Cephalosporins*
Alkalosis effect	Absorbed antacids Carbenicillin (large doses) Penicillin (large doses)

*Long term, especially when combined with gentamicin.

TABLE 15-8 Summary of Dental Considerations and Management of the Patient with Renal Disease

Before treatment
 Determine dialysis schedule and treat on day after dialysis.
 Consult with patient's nephrologist for recent laboratory tests and discussion of antibiotic prophylaxis.
 Identify arm with vascular access and type; notate in chart and avoid taking blood pressure measurement/injection of medication on this arm.
 Evaluate patient for hypertension/hypotension.
 Institute preoperative hemostatic aids (DDAVP, conjugated estrogen) when appropriate.
 Determine underlying cause of renal failure (underlying disease may affect provision of care).
 Obtain routine annual dental radiographs to establish presence and follow manifestations of renal osteodystrophy.
 Consider routine serology for HBV, HCV, and HIV antibody.
 Consider antibiotic prophylaxis when appropriate.
 Consider sedative premedication for patients with hypertension.
During treatment
 Perform a thorough history and physical examination for presence of oral manifestations.
 Aggressively eliminate potential sources of infection/bacteremia.
 Use adjunctive hemostatic aids during oral/periodontal surgical procedures.
 Maintain patient in a comfortable uncramped position in the dental chair.
 Allow patient to walk or stand intermittently during long procedures.
After treatment
 Use postsurgical hemostatic agents.
 Encourage meticulous home care.
 Institute therapy for xerostomia when appropriate.
 Consider use of postoperative antibiotics for traumatic procedures.
 Avoid use of respiratory-depressant drugs in presence of severe anemia.
 Adjust dosages of postoperative medications according to extent of renal failure.
 Ensure routine recall maintenance.

DDAVP = 1-deamino-8-D-arginine vasopressin; HBV = hepatitis B virus; HCV = hepatitis C virus; HIV = human immunodeficiency virus.

and nitrogenous waste or may stimulate tissue catabolism. NSAIDs may induce sodium retention, impair the action of diuretics, prevent aldosterone production, affect renal artery perfusion, and cause acidosis. Tetracyclines and steroids are antianabolic, increasing urea nitrogen to approximately twice the baseline levels. Other drugs, such as phenacetin, are nephrotoxic and put added strain on an already damaged kidney (Table 15-7). The challenge for dentists in prescribing medications is to maintain a therapeutic regimen within a narrow range, avoiding subtherapeutic dosing and toxicity.

The safety of a fluoridated community water supply for patients undergoing hemodialysis has been questioned in regard to whether such water is a contributing factor to the incidence of renal osteodystrophy, fluoride toxicity, and fluorosis. There is no satisfactory evidence that the fluoride content of fluoridated drinking water is harmful to patients with severe renal disease. Dialysis patients, however, should receive dialysates that are water-purified and deionized. No studies have reported on the dental use of topical fluoride in patients with renal disease or on any related problems. If a patient with renal disease needs fluoride supplements for caries control (particularly because of diminished salivary flow), the preferred route should be fluoride rinses until more definitive studies are carried out.

▼ REFERENCES

1. O'Neill WC. Sonographic evaluation of renal failure. Am J Kidney Dis 2000;35(6):1021–38.
2. Thadhani R, Pascual M, Bonventre JV. Acute renal failure. N Engl J Med 1996;334:1448–60.
3. Racusen LC. Pathology of acute renal failure: structure/function correlations. Adv Ren Replace Ther 1997;4(2 Suppl 1):3–16.
4. Dishart MK, Kellum JA. An evaluation of pharmacological strategies for the prevention and treatment of acute renal failure. Drugs 2000;59(1);79–91.
5. Wardle EN. Acute renal failure and multiorgan failure. Nephrol Dial Transplant 1994;9 Suppl 4:104–7.
6. Kashtan CE. Glomerular disease. Semin Nephrol 1999; 19:353–63.
7. Meyers CM. New insights into the pathogesesis of interstitial nephritis. Curr Opin Nephrol Hyperten 1999;8:287–92.
8. Lieberthal W, Nigam SK. Acute renal failure. II. Experimental models of acute renal failure: imperfect but indispensible. Am J Physiol Renal Physiol 2000;278(1):F1–12.
9. Bennett WM. Drug-related renal dysfunction in the elderly. Geriatr Nephrol Urol 1999;(1):21–5.
10. Jungers P. Screening for renal insufficiency: is it worth while? Is it feasible? Nephrol Dial Transplant 1999;14:2083–4.
11. Rahman M, Smith MC. Chronic renal insufficiency: a diagnostic and therapeutic approach. Arch Intern Med 1998;158:1743–52.
12. Vleming LJ, Brujlin JA, van Es LA. The pathogenesis of progressive renal failure. Neth J Med 1999;54:114–28.
13. Schelling JR, Zarif L, Sehgal A, et al. Genetic susceptibility to end-stage renal disease. Curr Opin Nephrol Hypertens 1999;8(4):465–72.
14. Orth SR. Smoking—a renal risk factor. Nephron 2000;86(1):12–26.
15. Levin A. Management of membranoproliferative glomerulonephritis: evidence-based recommendations. Kidney Int Suppl 1999;70:S41–6.
16. Couser WG. Glomerulonephritis. Lancet 1999;353:1509–15.
17. Roberts JA. Etiology and pathophysiology of pyelonephritis. Am J Kidney Dis 1991;17:1–9.
18. Avner ED, Woychik RP, Dell KM, Sweeney WE. Cellular pathophysiology of cystic kidney disease: insight into future therapies. Int J Dev Biol 1999;43(5 Spec No):457–61.
19. Wilson PD, Guay-Woodford L. Pathophysiology and clinical management of polycystic kidney disease in women. Semin Nephrol 1999;19:123–32.
20. Townsend RR, Cirigliano M. Hypertension in renal failure. Dis Mon 1998;44(6):243–53.
21. Cameron JS. Lupus nephritis. J Am Soc Nephrol 1999; 10(2):413–24.
22. Bennett WM. Drug nephrotoxicity: an overview. Ren Fail 1997;19(2):221–4.
23. Etemad B. Gastrointestinal complications of renal failure. Gastroenterol Clin North Am 1998;27:875–92.
24. Levy NB. Psychiatric considerations in the primary medical care of the patient with renal failure. Adv Ren Replace Ther 2000;7(3):231–8.
25. Von Bonodorff M, Sipila R, Pikanen E. Correction of hemodialysis-associated anemia by deferoxamine. Scand J Urol Nephrol 1990;131 Suppl:49–54.
26. Van-Damme-Lombaerts R, Herman J. Erythropoietin treatment in children with renal failure. Pediatr Nephrol 1999;13(2):148–52.
27. Mann JF. What are the short-term and long-term consequences of anaemia in CRF. Nephrol Dial Transplant 1999;14 Suppl 2:29–36.
28. Levin A. How should anemia be managed in pre-dialysis patients? Nephrol Dial Transplant 1999;14 Suppl 2:66–74.
29. Cameron JS. European best practice guidelines for the management of anaemia in patients with chronic renal failure. Nephrol Dial Transplant 1999;14 Suppl 2:61–5.
30. Nissenson AR. Achieving target hematocrit in dialysis patients: new concepts in iron management. Am J Kidney Dis 1997; 30(6):907–11.
31. Cameron JS. Towards the millenium: a history of renal anemia and optimal use of erythropoietin. Nephrol Dial Transplant 1999;14 Suppl 2:10–21.
32. Nissenson AR, Strobos J. Iron deficiency in patients with renal failure. Kidney Int Suppl 1999;69:S18–21.
33. Ligtenberg G. Regulation of blood pressure in chronic renal failure: determinants of hypertension and dialyisis-related hypertension. Neth J Med 1999;55(1):13–8.
34. Leypoldt JK, Lindsay RM. Hemodynamic monitoring during hemodialysis. Adv Ren Replace Ther 1999;6(3):233–42.
35. Bonomini M, Sirolli V, Stuard S, Settefrati N. Interactions between platelets and leukocytes. Artif Organs 1999;23(1):23–8.
36. Ziccardi VB, Saini J, Demas PN, Braun TW. Management of the oral and maxillofacial surgery patient with end-stage renal disease. J Oral Maxillofac Surg 1992;50:1207–12.
37. Sakhaee K, Gonzalez GB. Update on renal osteodystrophy: pathogenesis and clinical management. Am J Med Sci 1999;317(4):251–60.
38. Kurokawa K, Fukagawa M. Introduction to renal osteodystrophy: calcium metabolism in health and uremia. Am J Med Sci 1999;317(6):255–7.

39. Drueke TB. Medical management of secondary hyperparathyroidism in uremia. Am J Med Sci 1999;317(6):383–9.

40. Mucsi I, Herc G. Relative hypoparathyroidism and adynamic bone disease. Am J Med Sci 1999;317(6):405–9.

41. Shemin D, Dworkin LD. Sodium balance in renal failure. Curr Opin Nephrol Hypertens 1997 Mar;6(2):128–32.

42. Woolfson RG. Renal disease and the heart. Hosp Med 1999;60(2):85–9.

43. Heinzelman M, Mercer-Jones MA, Passmore JC. Neutrophils and renal failure. Am J Kidney Dis 1999;34(2):384–99.

44. Smith PS. Management of end-stage renal disease in children. Ann Pharmacother 1998;32(9):929–39.

45. Hood VL, Gennari FJ. End-stage renal disease. Measures to prevent it or slow its progression. Postgrad Med 1996;100(5):163–6,171–6.

46. Burgess E. Conservative treatment to slow deterioration of renal function: evidence based recommendations. Kidney Int Suppl 1999;70:S17–25.

47. McQuiston B. Current topics in renal nutrition. J Ren Nutr 1999;9(3):172–4.

48. Hruska KA. New insights related to aging and renal osteodystrophy. Geriatr Nephrol Urol 1999;9:49–56.

49. McCarthy JT. A practical approach to the management of patients with chronic renal failure. Mayo Clin Proc 1999;74:269–73.

50. Ledebo I, Ronco C, Schindler R, et al. Progress in dialysis technology — clinical benefit vs. increased complexity and risk. Report on the Dialysis Opinion Symposium at the ERA-EDTA Congress, 7 June 1998, Rimini. Nephrol Dial Transplant 1999;14:2101–5.

51. Ledebo I, Lamiere N, Charra B, et al. Improving the outcome of dialysis — opinion vs scientific evidence. Nephrol Dial Transplant 2000;15(9):1310–6.

52. Mallick NP, Gokal R. Haemodialysis. Lancet 1999;353:737–42.

53. Berkoben M, Schwab S. Dialysis or transplantation: fitting the treatment to the patient. Ann Rev Med 1999;50:193–205.

54. Berkoben M. Patient mortality in chronic dialysis: comparisons between hemodialysis and peritoneal dialysis. Curr Opin Nephrol Hypertens 1999;8(6):681–3.

55. Hakim R, Himmelfarb J. Hemodialysis access failure: a call to action. Kidney Int 1998;54(4)1029–40.

56. Burkhart HM, Cikrit DF. Arteriovenous fistulae for hemodialysis. Semin Vasc Surg 1997;10(3):162–5.

57. Swartz RD, Boyer CL, Messana JM. Central venous catheters for maintenance hemodialysis: a cautionary approach. Adv Ren Replace Ther 1997;4(3):275–84.

58. Cano N. Haemodialysis and peritoneal dialysis: metabolic alterations and nutritional status. Curr Opin Clin Nutr Metab Care 1999;2:329–33.

59. Makoff R. Vitamin replacement therapy in renal failure patients. Miner Electrolyte Metab 1999;25(4–6):349–51.

60. Locatelli AJ, Marcos GM, Gomez MG, et al. Comparing peritonitis in continuous ambulatory peritoneal dialysis versus automated peritoneal dialysis patients. Adv Perit Dial 1999;15:193–6.

61. Gokal R, Mallick NP. Peritoneal dialysis. Lancet 1999;353(9155):823–8.

62. Locatelli A, Marcos G, Gomez M. Adequacy in peritoneal dialysis: a true challenge. Int J Artif Organs 1999;22:123–4.

63. Ledebo I. On-line hemodialfiltration: technique and therapy. Adv Ren Replace Ther 1999;6(2):195–208.

64. Naugle K, Darby ML, Bauman DB, et al. The oral health of individuals on renal dialysis. Ann Periodontol 1998;3:197–205.

65. DeRossi SS, Glick M. Dental considerations for the patient with renal disease receiving hemodialysis. J Am Dent Assoc 1996;127:211–9.

66. Naylor GD, Hall EH, Terezhalmy GT. The patient with chronic renal failure who is undergoing dialysis or renal transplantation: another consideration for antimicrobial prophylaxis. Oral Surg Oral Med Oral Pathol 1988;65:116–21.

67. McCarthy JT, Steckelberg JM. Infective endocarditis in patients receiving long-term hemodialysis. Mayo Clin Proc 2000;75(10):1008–14.

68. Wreghitt TG. Blood-borne viral infections in dialysis units — a review. Rev Med Virol 1999;9:101–9.

69. Pereira BJ. Hepatitis C virus infection in dialysis: a continuing problem. Artif Organs 1999;23:51–60.

70. Al Shohaib S. Tuberculosis in chronic renal failure in Jeddah. J Infect 2000;40(2):150–3.

71. Maggiore Q, Pizzarelli F, Dattolo P, et al. Cardiovascular stability during hemodialysis, hemofiltration, and hemodialfiltration. Nephrol Dial Transplant 2000;15 Suppl 1:68–73.

16

HEMATOLOGIC DISEASES

SCOTT S. DeROSSI, DMD
ADI GARFUNKEL, DDS
MARTIN S. GREENBERG, DDS

▼ THE PROCESS OF HEMATOPOIESIS

Hematopoiesis is the formation of cellular components of the blood from a small population of pluripotential stem cells, which are formed in embryonic life and persist thereafter through self-regeneration. When stimulated by hematopoietic growth factors such as cytokines, these precursor cells give rise to progenitor cells committed to development along specific pathways. These progenitor cells, through a series of divisions and maturational changes, give rise to myeloid or lymphoid mature cells in the circulating blood. The earliest recognizable erythroid progenitors are the burst-forming units–erythroid (BFU-E) and the less primitive colony-forming units–erythroid (CFU-E). Erythropoietin, produced by the kidney, circulates to the bone marrow, where it stimulates the erythroid progenitor cells to differentiate and mature into erythrocytes.[1]

▼ RED BLOOD CELL DISORDERS

Polycythemia

Polycythemia may be defined as an abnormal increase in the erythrocyte count in the peripheral blood, usually accompanied by an increase in hemoglobin and hematocrit. Polycythemia is divided into absolute erythrocytosis (a true increase in red-cell mass) and relative erythrocytosis (the red-cell mass is normal, but the plasma volume is reduced). Relative polycythemia is caused by the loss of tissue and intravascular fluid, which may be the result of such diverse conditions as diabetic ketoacidosis, postsurgical dehydration, prolonged vomiting or diarrhea, or rapid diuresis secondary to treatment for congestive heart failure. In relative polycythemia, the hemoglobin rarely rises more than 25%, and there are no appreciable oral changes.

Three main groups of polycythemia are recognized: primary proliferative polycythemia (polycythemia rubra vera), secondary polycythemia resulting from changes in erythropoietin concentration, and apparent polycythemia. The latter condition lacks a true increase in red-cell mass.[2]

POLYCYTHEMIA VERA

Polycythemia vera (PV) is a myeloproliferative disorder characterized by excessive proliferation of erythroid elements along with granulocytic and megakaryocytic cells; it usually begins after 50 years of age. The etiology of PV is unknown; however, it is likely a result of acquired genetic changes in the stem cell leading to disturbances of normal cellular growth.

The red blood cell (RBC) volume increases to an erythrocyte count of 6 to 12 million/mm^3 with a hemoglobin concentration of 18 to 24 g/dL, leading to increased blood viscosity and thrombosis. Seventy percent of cases also have high white blood cell and platelet counts. Patients with PV develop episodes of thrombosis and hemorrhage in the later stages of the disease. Hyperuricemia and hyperuricosuria are seen in 40% of the cases at diagnosis. Serum iron and ferritin are low owing to excessive iron use, and the leukocyte alkaline phosphatase is elevated. Erythropoietin levels are decreased. PV may progress to myelofibrosis or acute myeloid leukemia in 5 to 50% of cases, with a median survival of 10 to 16 years.

A characteristic clinical picture of ruddy cyanosis is seen on the face and extremities, owing to the presence of deoxygenated blood in cutaneous vessels. Patients complain of headache, dizziness, tinnitus, fullness of the head and face, and pruritus. Splenomegaly is a common finding on physical examination. Frequently, coronary thrombosis is diagnosed, and complications known as "erythromelalgia" may manifest as paresthesias involving the cranial nerves.

Oral Manifestations.   A purplish red discoloration of the oral mucosa is visible on the tongue, cheeks, and lips. The gingivae are red and may bleed spontaneously. Petechiae and ecchymoses are observed in patients with platelet abnormalities. Varicosities in the ventral tongue, a frequent normal finding, are exaggerated in cases of polycythemia.

Treatment.   The major therapy for PV involves repeated phlebotomy. Patients with severe disease and elderly patients receive myelosuppressive agents to reduce the hematocrit to its upper limit of 50%. Alkylating agents and radioactive phosphorus (^{32}P) have been shown to increase the risk of leukemia and should be avoided. Chemotherapy with agents such as busulfan, chlorambucil, cyclophosphamide, and melphalan may also be beneficial. Hydroxyurea is now being widely used when myelosuppressive therapy is indicated because of the established leukemogenic potential of other agents. Treatment with hydroxyurea also decreases the thrombotic complications.

Oral and Dental Considerations.   Dental treatment presents a risk because of the possibility of bleeding or thrombosis.

Patients should have a complete blood count prior to treatment. To prevent complications, it is recommended that the hemoglobin be reduced below 16 g/dL and the hematocrit to below 47% as these are the thresholds at which medical management is instituted. Patients with this disease require special attention to local hemostasis. Preoperative myelosuppressive treatment should be considered prior to dental treatment when the blood counts are not controlled with phlebotomy alone.

SECONDARY POLYCYTHEMIA: ERYTHROCYTOSIS

Secondary polycythemia is due to an increase in erythropoietin production to compensate for hypoxia. This reactive erythrocytosis has been described in people who live at high altitudes with low atmospheric pressure and in people with chronic pulmonary disease, congenital heart disease (right-to-left shunt), and renal disease (hydronephrosis). Pheochromocytoma and other endocrine disorders also have been described as possible causes of erythrocytosis.

Secondary polycythemia also may occur with some tumors, particularly brain, renal, and lung carcinomas that produce an erythropoietin-like substance. The increased blood viscosity may lead to thrombosis or coagulation defects. When the elevated erythrocyte volume becomes dangerously high, it may be treated by phlebotomy to reduce viscosity.

APPARENT POLYCYTHEMIA

Apparent polycythemia, characterized by an increased hemoglobin concentration and packed-cell volume but normal RBC mass, is caused by a reduction in plasma volume. Apparent polycythemia most commonly affects middle-aged obese men with hypertension and a significant social history of smoking and high alcohol consumption. Some cases are associated with diuretic therapy. Treatment is usually geared toward the underlying disorder; however, more aggressive measures may be taken in patients with definite cardiovascular risks.[3]

Anemia

Anemia is present whenever there is a decrease in the normal amount of circulating hemoglobin. This reduction in hemoglobin may result from blood loss, as in common iron deficiency anemia; from increased destruction of red blood cells, as in the hemolytic anemias; from decreased production of red cells, as in pernicious and folic acid deficiency anemias; or from combinations of these three. When there is a combination of causes, one mechanism usually predominates.

Anemias also may be classified according to their pathophysiologic basis: size (microcytic, normocytic, or macrocytic) of the red cells or their hemoglobin concentration (hypochromic, normochromic). The term "hyperchromic" is seldom used, but it refers to a macrocytic cell with normal hemoglobin concentration that, because of its large size, has an increased hemoglobin content. General symptoms of all anemias include pallor of the skin, palpebral conjunctiva, and nail beds; dyspnea; and easy fatigability. The more common anemias or those with common oral manifestations are discussed in this chapter.

ANEMIA OWING TO BLOOD LOSS: IRON DEFICIENCY

Iron deficiency anemia (blood loss anemia, hypochromic microcytic anemia) is the most common of all anemias, affecting approximately 30% of the world's population and accounting for up to 500 million cases worldwide.[4] Iron deficiency anemia may result from chronic blood loss, such as occurs in menstrual or menopausal bleeding, parturition, bleeding hemorrhoids, or a bleeding malignant lesion or ulcer in the gastrointestinal tract. It also may develop in patients from a variety of causes that may decrease the rate of absorption of iron, such as subtotal or complete gastrectomy, or a habit of clay eating, or as part of malabsorption syndromes.[5]

An inadequate dietary intake of iron also may be responsible, but the diagnosis of iron deficiency caused by dietary insufficiency must be made with extreme caution. The body zealously guards its iron stores, and it has been estimated that the adult male can go up to a decade without iron intake before an iron deficiency anemia develops. Women normally lose about 50 mL of blood with each menstrual period and are thereby more likely to become anemic with an iron deficient diet. Chronic iron deficiency anemia is one of the typical findings in gastrointestinal malignancy and in certain forms of parasitic infections. The margin of iron balance (intake versus loss) is decreased in infants, growing children, and menstruating women.

In addition to the symptoms common to all anemias, patients with iron deficiency anemia also note a tendency of the nails to crack and split. Weakness and dyspnea may be present for some time before the development of other clinical signs or symptoms of anemia.

Oral Manifestations. The major oral sign of iron deficiency anemia is pallor of the mucosa. In addition, the oral epithelial cells become atrophic, with loss of normal keratinization. The tongue may become smooth due to atrophy of the filiform and fungiform papillae, and glossodynia can be a presenting or associated symptom. In long-standing cases, esophageal strictures or webs can develop, resulting in dysphagia. Recent clinical investigation has shown lingual signs and symptoms to be much less common than was previously believed.

Histologic examination of the tongue mucosa shows a reduction in epithelial thickness, with a reduction in the number of cells in spite of an increase in the progenitor cell layer. The cell size is decreased in the maturation layers (in males), and the nucleocytoplasmic ratio is higher than normal. Lingual mucosal atrophy may occur in the absence of other overt clinical findings.

Diagnosis. Diagnosis is based on a lowered hemoglobin in routine blood counts; on a peripheral smear, the cells are microcytic and hypochromic. When the anemia is well developed, the mean corpuscular hemoglobin, the mean corpuscular hemoglobin concentration, and the mean corpuscular volume are decreased. Whenever the hemoglobin value is less than 11 g/dL, it is of definite clinical significance. The patient with iron deficiency anemia will have low serum iron concentrations and a high serum iron-binding capacity; serum ferritin levels are markedly reduced.[6] There is a characteristic absence of stainable iron in the bone marrow, which is an early finding in the disease. The physician must perform a thorough search for the source of bleeding, including using radiologic surveys of the gastrointestinal tract, sigmoidoscopy, a gynecologic examination, and a complete menstrual and dietary history.

Dental Considerations. Dental patients presenting with symptoms of anemia or oral signs suggestive of this condition should have a complete blood count (CBC) with differential. If significantly lowered hemoglobin values are obtained, the patient should be referred to his or her physician for a more thorough medical history, laboratory diagnosis, and treatment. Elective oral surgical or periodontal procedures should not be performed on patients with marked anemia because of the potential for increased bleeding and impaired wound healing. When hemoglobin levels fall below 10 g/dL, the low oxygen tension affects the rheologic interactions between the cellular components of blood, mainly platelets and endothelium, decreasing their ability to clot effectively. General anesthesia should not be administered unless the hemoglobin is at least 10 g/dL. The patient should never be treated with iron until the cause of the microcytic hypochromic anemia is found and corrected or until a thorough search for the cause has proved fruitless.

Treatment. The diagnosis of iron deficiency anemia is made either by demonstration of an iron deficient state or by evaluation of the response to therapeutic iron replacement. The single most important aspect of treatment is identification of the cause, especially a source of occult blood loss.[7]

Plummer-Vinson Syndrome. First described by Plummer and Vinson, this syndrome is characterized by dysphagia and a microcytic hypochromic anemia. A smooth and sore tongue, dry mouth, spoon-shaped nails, and angular stomatitis are common findings. There is atrophy of the tongue papillae, but it is less severe than in pernicious anemia. There are atrophic changes in the oral mucosa, the pharynx, the upper esophagus, and the vulva. These tissues are dry, inelastic, and glazed in appearance. In addition, general symptoms include listlessness, pallor, ankle edema, and dyspnea, all related to the anemia.

Many patients with this syndrome are edentulous, having lost their teeth early in life. Complaints of a sore mouth and an inability to wear dentures are frequent. In addition, patients with Plummer-Vinson syndrome often complain of a "spasm in the throat" or of "food sticking in the throat." The dysphagia, which represents an important feature of this condition, appears to be the result of muscular degeneration in the esophagus, and stenoses or webs of the esophageal mucosa.

The diagnosis of this syndrome can be made on the basis of the history and hematologic findings. The esophageal lesions are demonstrable radiologically (barium swallow) or by esophagoscopy. Relative degrees of achlorhydria are usually present. Because many of the symptoms in this syndrome are similar to those observed in vitamin B complex deficiency and simple hypochromic anemias, these conditions should be treated. A variable and apparently unpredictable response to therapy can be expected. At times, the dysphagia improves following iron therapy.

Plummer-Vinson syndrome is potentially serious because pharyngeal and intraoral carcinoma are more common in these patients. Patients with symptoms of this syndrome should be followed up at short intervals and checked for the development of lesions that raise the suspicion of malignancy.

ANEMIA OWING TO HEMOLYSIS

The hemolytic anemias result from decreased survival of erythrocytes, either episodically or continuously, resulting from intracorpuscular defects in the erythrocytes (often hereditary) or from extracorpuscular factors. Some of the more common causes are summarized in Table 16-1.

The bone marrow has the capacity to increase production of erythrocytes by up to eightfold in response to reduced erythrocyte survival, and considerable hemolysis can take place before anemia results. This mechanism is overcome when the RBC survival is extremely short or when the ability of the marrow to compensate is impaired. Similarly, a small amount of hemolysis can take place without resulting in jaundice because of the normal liver's ability to excrete increased amounts of bilirubin.

Diagnosis.   Laboratory findings common to all hemolytic anemias are decreased hemoglobin, increased reticulocytes (young red cells released into the circulation as a result of the marrow's producing more red cells to compensate for the excessive destruction), and increases in serum bilirubin, mostly

TABLE 16-1   Common Causes of Hemolytic Anemia

Extracorpuscular factors
  Overwhelming infections and toxins
  Cardiac valvular prostheses
  Hypersplenism
  Rh factor incompatibility (hemolytic disease of newborn, erythroblastosis fetalis)
  Chronic liver disease
  Autoimmune hemolytic disease (eg, as in systemic lupus erythematosus)
  Transfusion reactions

Intracorpuscular defects
  Abnormal shape of the erythrocytes
    Hereditary spherocytosis
    Hereditary elliptocytosis

  Paroxysmal nocturnal hemoglobinuria

  Erythrocyte enzyme deficiencies
    Glucose-6-phosphate dehydrogenase deficiency
    Pyruvate kinase deficiency

  Abnormal hemoglobins (hemoglobinopathies)
    Sickle cell anemia and sickle cell trait
    Thalassemia
    Other hemoglobinopathies (eg, hemoglobin C and F)

  Erythrocyte defects associated with other disease
    CGL
    Folic acid and vitamin B_{12} deficiency anemias

in the indirect (unconjugated, prehepatic) fraction. Other diagnostic tests that may be useful in certain of the hemolytic anemias are outlined below.

To measure red cell survival time, a small amount of the patient's red cells may be tagged with radioactive chromium (^{51}Cr) and re-injected. If the hemolysis is caused by an extracorpuscular factor, a compatible donor's red cells, similarly tagged and injected into the patient, should disappear as quickly as the patient's own red cells. If the hemolysis is caused by intracorpuscular defects, the compatible donor's red cells should survive longer than do the patient's red cells when injected into the veins of the patient.

Most hemolytic anemias are accompanied by a decrease in the serum haptoglobins, which are globulins with a marked affinity to bind hemoglobin. When hemoglobin is released into the blood by hemolysis, it is quickly bound by haptoglobins, and the haptoglobin-hemoglobin complex is rapidly removed from the circulation by the reticuloendothelial system, thus resulting in a lowered serum haptoglobin level.

Although the hemolytic anemias are usually characterized by normocytic normochromic morphology on a blood smear with normal red cell indices, the cells in hereditary spherocytosis and hereditary elliptocytosis may exhibit an abnormal spheric or elliptic shape. This may be more apparent in wet preparations than in dried smears.

The cells in hereditary spherocytosis show increased hemolysis (osmotic fragility) in hypotonic solutions. The Coombs test is useful in demonstrating antibodies to the erythrocytes. The direct Coombs test demonstrates incomplete antibodies attached to the erythrocytes, which require a substance such as antihuman globulin to produce hemolysis. The indirect Coombs test detects antibodies to the red cells, which are present in the patient's serum, usually immunoglobulin IgG1 and IgG3, both of which activate complement.

Hemoglobin electrophoresis is a verstile and broadly effective procedure for the detection of pathologic hemoglobin proteins.

Oral Manifestations.   There are certain oral and physical findings that are common to all hemolytic anemias. When sufficient hemolysis has taken place to produce anemia, pallor results. This is most easily observed in the nail beds and palpebral conjunctiva. Pallor of the oral mucosa—especially evident in the soft palate, tongue, and sublingual tissues—also is observable as the anemia progresses. In contrast to the anemias produced by bleeding or by factor deficiencies, the hemolytic anemias produce jaundice caused by the hyperbilirubinemia secondary to erythrocyte destruction. This is best seen in the sclera, but the skin, soft palate, and tissues of the floor of the mouth also become icteric as the serum bilirubin increases. The erythroid elements of the bone marrow are hyperplastic in an attempt to compensate for the anemia. This hyperplasia produces a characteristic appearance on the dental radiograph. Because of the enlargement of the medullary spaces, the trabeculae become more prominent, creating increased bone radiolucency with prominent lamellar striations.

Paroxysmal Nocturnal Hemoglobinuria. This intracorpuscular defect is an acquired clonal stem cell disorder that results in abnormal sensitivity of the RBC membrane to lysis by complement.[8] Lymphocytes are not affected. Patients present with variable degrees of anemia, mild granulocytopenia, and thrombocytopenia. Complications include venous thromboses, hemoglobinuria, and hemosiderinuria. Patients complain of back pain, abdominal pain, and headaches that result from ischemia. This diagnosis should be suspected in confusing cases of hemolytic anemia or pancytopenia. Diagnosis is made by tests that demonstrate the increased sensitivity of the erythrocytes to complement, such as the sucrose hemolysis test. Most patients with this rare disease survive for less than 10 years, owing to complications of thrombosis or renal failure. Treatment with corticosteroids or androgens brings some degree of improvement in the anemia. Blood transfusions are necessary prior to surgical intervention, and some patients are treated with anticoagulants.

Glucose-6-Phosphate Dehydrogenase Deficiency. Glucose-6-phosphate dehydrogenase (G6PD) deficiency is a hereditary enzyme defect that causes episodic hemolysis because of a reduced capacity of RBCs to deal with oxidative stresses. Patients with an enzymatic defect, such as the one found in the hexose monophosphate shunt, do not maintain the required level of reduced glutathione in their RBCs. As a result, hemoglobin sulfhydryl groups and the cell membranes themselves are oxidized, leading to hemoglobin precipitation in the cell and eventual cell lysis. This X-linked hereditary deficiency is the most common metabolic disorder of the RBCs. More than 400 variants of the enzyme have been described.

Anemia is the most frequent sign of this deficiency because the erythrocyte is the most sensitive cell to the oxidative processes. The highest incidence of G6PD deficiency has been found among people of Mediterranean and African descent.

In the G6PD deficient erythrocyte, the denatured hemoglobin with stromal proteins forms particles, called Heinz bodies, as a result of an oxidative process. These cells circulate with difficulty through the spleen and liver and are removed from the circulation, resulting in hemolytic anemia. No treatment is necessary except avoidance of known oxidant drugs such as dapsone.[9]

Dental Considerations. The severity of anemia and its correction should be evaluated before major dental interventions because the decline in hemoglobin can reach 3 to 4 g/dL during hemolytic episodes. Blood transfusions may be used prior to dental treatment in severe cases. Drugs that might induce hemolysis, such as dapsone, sulfasalazine, and phenacetin, should be avoided. Analgesics and antibiotics can be given safely in therapeutic doses, provided special attention is given to the written recommendations of the manufacturer.

The hemolytic episodes are self-limited, and most patients with drug- or infection-induced hemolysis recover fully following treatment.

Hemoglobinopathies. The hemoglobinopathies, exemplified by sickle cell disease and thalassemia, are caused by defects in the globin portion of the hemoglobin molecule. These defects render the erythrocyte containing the abnormal hemoglobin more susceptible to hemolysis. A normal hemoglobin molecule consists of two pairs of amino acid chains, the α and β chains. This normal hemoglobin, hemoglobin A, may be represented by the formula $\alpha_2^A\beta_2^A$, indicating that there are two α and two β chains. In the hemoglobinopathies, abnormal hemoglobins are produced either in the form of abnormal chains (eg, γ, δ) or of small alterations in the α or β chain. Fetal hemoglobin, normal in the fetus but abnormal if persisting into adult life, is designated hemoglobin F and is represented by the formula $\alpha_2^A\gamma_2^F$, indicating that it differs from hemoglobin A in that the β chains are replaced by two γ chains. Sickle cell disease involves a single amino acid abnormality: the glutamic acid normally found in position 6 of the β chain is replaced by valine. Thus, the formula for hemoglobin S is $\alpha_2^A\beta_2^A 6$ valine.

More than 30 different hemoglobins have been identified. Identification is made possible by the use of serum electrophoresis. Many of the abnormal hemoglobins show slower or faster electrophoretic mobility than does hemoglobin A. Specific identification of the exact biochemical abnormality depends on more sophisticated analysis of the molecule. At present, the specific molecular abnormality in many of the hemoglobinopathies has not been identified.

Sickle Cell Disease. In sickle cell disease, an autosomal recessive disorder, an abnormality in the β chain of hemoglobin is present in which valine is substituted for the normal glutamic acid residue on position 6. This relatively minor biochemical change results in profound undesirable physical characteristics in the hemoglobin. In the presence of either a lowered blood oxygen tension or an increased blood pH, the hemoglobin forms a sickle-shaped crystal (a tactoid) within the erythrocyte. This sickling of the erythrocyte leads to stasis and hemolysis of the red cells, especially in end-capillary circulation. The stasis then results in an even lower oxygen tension, an increased pH, and further sickling. The disease is hereditary and may manifest itself as the sickle cell trait or as sickle cell anemia.

In sickle cell anemia, 75 to 100% of the hemoglobin is S hemoglobin S, and the remainder is hemoglobin F; in sickle cell trait, only 20 to 45% of the hemoglobin is hemoglobin S, and the rest is normal hemoglobin A. In sickle cell trait (heterozygous), only one of the β chains is thought to be abnormal, whereas in sickle cell anemia (homozygous), both β chains are abnormal.

Patients with sickle cell trait an estimated 9% of African Americans are not anemic and have no symptoms of their disease unless they are placed in situations where there is abnormally low oxygen, such as in an unpressurized airplane or under injudicious administration of general anesthesia. On the other hand, patients with sickle cell anemia (approximately 0.15% of the African descent population), usually exhibit marked clinical manifestations.

CLINICAL MANIFESTATIONS.   Patients with sickle cell anemia show marked underdevelopment and often die before 40 years of age. The clinical manifestations are the results of the basic anemia and hemolytic process (jaundice, pallor, and cardiac failure) or of necrosis following stasis of blood and vaso-occlusion. This latter phenomenon is manifested by splenic infarction, chronic leg ulcers, priapism, cerebral vascular thromboses ("strokes"), and painful attacks of abdominal and bone pain (pain crises). The long bones may present radiodense sclerotic areas as a residual of small infarcts.

Aplastic crises sometimes develop from infection, hypersensitivity reactions, or unknown causes. In these aplastic crises, the patient becomes acutely ill, red cell production virtually stops, and the hemoglobin drops precipitously. It has been suggested that folic acid deficiency may develop in these patients because of the increased demand for folic acid as a result of increased erythropoiesis. The folic acid deficiency may play a part in the genesis of the aplastic crisis.

ORAL MANIFESTATIONS.   Other than the jaundice and pallor of the oral mucosa, patients often show delayed eruption and hypoplasia of the dentition secondary to their general underdevelopment. Because of the chronic increased erythropoietic activity and marrow hyperplasia, which are attempts to compensate for the hemolysis, increased radiolucency resulting from the decreased number of trabeculae is seen on dental radiographs. This change is noted especially in the alveolar bone between the roots of the teeth, where the trabeculae may appear as horizontal rows, creating a ladderlike effect (Figure 16-1). By contrast, the lamina dura appears dense and distinct. In skull films, the diploë is thickened, and the trabeculae are coarse and tend to run perpendicular to the inner and outer tables, giving a radiographic appearance of "hair on end" (Figure 16-2). The teeth do not present undue mobility. Areas of sclerosis or increased radiopacity represent areas of past thromboses with subsequent bony infarction.

Patients with sickle cell anemia are particularly prone to developing osteomyelitis, probably because of hypovascularity of the bone marrow secondary to thromboses. Inasmuch as the initial radiographic changes in vascular thrombosis and osteomyelitis are quite similar, confusion often results in the differential diagnosis of these two conditions, and other supporting data must be used to differentiate the two.

Hays study of the nuclear characteristics of the buccal mucosa cells in sickle cell anemia showed that, in those who were folate deficient, there was an increased number of cells with enlarged nuclei. This is not a surprising finding because it also is found in patients who have generalized megaloblastic changes, as in those with pernicious anemia or folic acid deficiency anemia.

Patients presenting with temporary anesthesia of the mental nerve, thought to be secondary to vascular occlusion involving the nerve's blood supply, have been reported.

DIAGNOSIS.   A smear of peripheral blood usually shows normochromic normocytic cells. Sickling does not often occur until the oxygen tension is lowered. To this end, a special preparation was formerly used for diagnosis: fresh blood was sealed in a small chamber of a microscopic slide with sodium metabisulfite (a reducing agent) for 1 hour and then observed for sickling. Hemoglobin electrophoresis is less expensive, more accurate, and more definitive in the diagnosis of sickle cell disease as it detects hemoglobin S.[10]

TREATMENT.   There is no treatment for sickle cell disease other than symptomatic treatment. Antibiotics should be used early in the treatment of infection, and analgesic drugs should be used if necessary but with caution to prevent

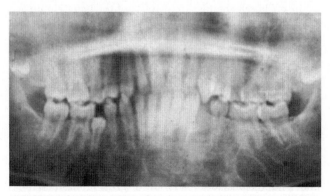

FIGURE 16-1   Radiograph of a patient with sickle cell anemia, demonstrating horizontal trabeculation creating a ladderlike effect. (Courtesy of Dr. Eisa Mozaffari, Philadelphia, PA).

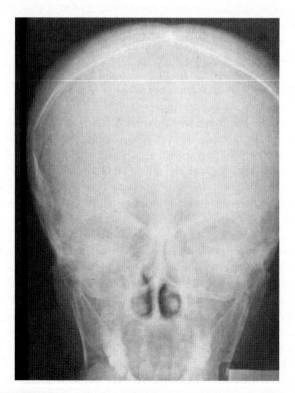

FIGURE 16-2   Lateral skull film demonstrating thinned cortex with wavy lines, called "hair on end." (Courtesy of Dr. Eisa Mozaffari, Philadelphia, PA).

iatrogenic addiction. Neither splenectomy nor antianemic drugs (except possibly folic acid) are of any value. Transfusions are avoided unless the patient has an aplastic crisis with a resulting extremely low hemoglobin level, because the transfusion effects are transitory, and the patients tend to develop antibodies, making it difficult to find suitable donors for future transfusions. Also there is an ever-present risk of hepatitis transmission with transfusions, and because these patients do not lose the iron portion of the hemoglobin molecule, transfusion can result in iron overload and eventual hemosiderosis.

Many physicians routinely use folic acid dietary supplements for patients with sickle cell anemia, increasing levels to therapeutic doses to treat an aplastic crisis. There is no good evidence that folic acid treatment increases the blood hemoglobin level.

Cytotoxic agents such as hydroxyurea have been shown to increase hemoglobin F and reduce the frequency of painful episodes; they are indicated in patients whose quality of life is disrupted by frequent painful episodes. Allogeneic stem cell transplantation is being studied as a possible curative option for severely affected young patients.[11]

DENTAL CONSIDERATIONS.   Elective dental procedures involving the soft tissues should not be performed in patients with poorly controlled disease unless absolutely necessary because of increased risk of complications secondary to chronic anemia and delayed wound healing. Elimination of oral sources of infection should be instituted since infection can precipitate an aplastic crisis. General anesthesia should be used with caution in patients with sickle cell trait or sickle cell anemia; when used, it is imperative to avoid episodes of hypoxia because cerebral or myocardial thrombosis can result.

Thalassemias.   The thalassemias are a group of congenital disorders characterized by a deficient synthesis of either the α or the β chains of globin in the hemoglobin molecule. As a result, the red blood cells are microcytic and hypochromic with an aberrant morphology. Thalassemias are often considered among the hypoproliferative anemias, the hemolytic anemias, and the anemias related to abnormal hemoglobin.

In α-thalassemia (deficient or reduced α chain) intracellular inclusions, Heinz bodies are formed by the precipitation of the α chains that accumulate in excess following the impaired chain production. In the most severe form of this disease, the fetus's red blood cells contain hemoglobin composed of γ chains only. This condition is incompatible with life, due to the hemoglobin's lack of oxygen-carrying capacity. Clinical signs in α-thalassemia depend on the severity of the α-chain production deficiency.

β-Globin synthesis is impaired in β-thalassemia with mutations in the sequences of the β-globin gene, leading to errors in the splicing of messenger ribonucleic acid (mRNA). In some cases, reduced amounts of β chains are produced (β^+-thalassemia); in others, no normal β chains are produced (β^o-thalassemia).

Affected individuals are either heterozygotes, homozygotes, or double heterozygotes for the β-chain genes. The heterozygous individual has the β-thalassemia trait; the homozygous state is known as β-thalassemia major or Cooley's anemia. The frequency of the disease approaches 0.1% in the Mediterranean basin, the Middle East, Africa, Asia, and the South Pacific. In India and Thailand, it is particularly prevalent.

Reduced erythropoiesis and hemolysis are characteristic of the disease as a result of an imbalance in β-chain production. In the major type, there is a relative excess of β chains that eventually aggregate and form inclusion bodies. Due to this defect, the RBCs that show abnormalities in membrane permeability are entrapped and removed from circulation by phagocytosis or lysis. As a compensatory process, an erythropoietic stimulus follows, causing an expansion of the red cell compartments of the marrow and extramedullary hematopoiesis. Another compensatory process increases the synthesis of γ chains that are able to combine with the free α chains and form a stable tetramer (fetal hemoglobin). This minimizes the severity of the clinical manifestations.

Clinical signs are minimal in β-thalassemia minor (β-thalassemia trait); most of the affected individuals are never diagnosed and have only a mild, clinically insignificant mycrocytic anemia. No treatment is needed, but genetic counseling should be offered and the opportunity for prenatal diagnosis discussed with at-risk couples.

β-thalassemia major or Cooley's anemia is the most severe congenital hemolytic anemia.[12] At 4 to 6 months of life, with the change from fetal XX chain to adult XX chain hemoglobin production, the first clinical manifestations appear. The hematocrit decreases to less than 20, the degree of anemia can reach a hemoglobin level of 2 to 3 g/dL, and the hemolysis is extensive, as is the iron overload. Growth and development in children is slow. In adolescence, secondary sex characteristics are delayed. The skin color becomes ashen-gray due to the combination of pallor, jaundice, and hemosiderosis. Patients also present with cardiomegaly, hepatomegaly, and splenomegaly.

DIAGNOSIS.   Hemolytic anemia with hypochromic microcytic red blood cells that vary in size and shape is characteristic of thalassemia major. The hemoglobin electrophoresis shows increased amounts of fetal hemoglobin and variable amounts of normal adult hemoglobin. In patients homozygous for β^o-thalassemia, there is no detectable hemoglobin A. Prenatal diagnosis of thalassemia is facilitated by deoxyribonucleic acid (DNA) analysis of amniotic fluid cells, and it plays an important role in genetic counseling.

TREATMENT.   Patients with mild thalassemia (α trait or β minor) are clinically normal and require no treatment. In other cases, the patient's survival depends on blood transfusions. Prevention of a hemoglobin concentration decrease to under 10 g/dL improves the chances of normal development and survival into adulthood. This hypertransfusion treatment results in iron overload with hemosiderosis and iron deposition in all body tissues. As a result, patients may develop abnormalities in cardiac, endocrine, and hepatic functions, with cardiac insufficiency, diabetes, pituitary hypofunction, and a possible bleeding tendency due to liver disease.

If regular blood transfusions are given to children with thalassemia to maintain the hemoglobin level between 10 and 14 g/dL, the children develop normally, without the marked skeletal changes. Some patients with thalassemia undergo splenectomy in an attempt to prolong RBC survival. Folic acid supplement also seems to be of some benefit. The iron overload is treated with continuous injections of a chelator, deferiprone, which mobilizes and excretes the excess iron. Hematopoietic stem cell transplantation constitutes a future hope for the treatment of thalassemia.[13]

ORAL MANIFESTATIONS. Bimaxillary protrusion and other occlusal abnormalities are frequent in thalassemia major cases. Dental and facial abnormalities include poor spacing of teeth, a marked opened bite, prominent malar bones, and a saddle nose. In addition, the pneumatization of the maxillary sinuses is delayed. As a result of these skeletal changes, the upper lip is retracted, giving the child a "chipmunk facies."

The radiographic changes seen in the jaws include generalized rarefaction of the alveolar bone, thinning of cortical bone, enlarged marrow spaces, and coarse trabeculae, which are similar to the changes observed in sickle cell disease patients. In the parietal bones, the thin cortex covering the coarse vertical trabeculae and the enlarged diploë produce a "hair on end" picture (see Figure 16-2).

Cranial nerve palsies have been described in thalassemia due to the extramedullary hematopoiesis resulting in pressure on the nerves.

In β-thalassemia major, there is no correlation between the chronologic, skeletal, and dental developmental age. The skeletal retardation increases with age due to hypoxia from severe anemia, endocrine hypofunction secondary to iron deposition, or the toxic action of iron enzyme systems leading to tissue injury.

The dentin and enamel are indicators of iron deposition, and deciduous and permanent teeth of patients with thalassemia contain up to five times the iron concentration measured in normal patients. The high concentration of iron explains the discoloration of teeth in patients with β-thalassemia major.

DENTAL MANAGEMENT. As in any patient with a chronic anemia, poor healing may ensue after surgical dental procedures. The possibility always exists of exacerbating the symptoms of cerebral or cardiac hypoxia if substantial bleeding occurs in a patient who is already anemic. Surgery has been used successfully to treat the facial deformities.

ANEMIA OWING TO DECREASED PRODUCTION OF RED CELLS

Megaloblastic Anemias. The term "megaloblastic anemia" is used to describe a group of disorders characterized by a distinct morphologic pattern in hemapoietic cells. These cells have small immature nuclei and large mature cytoplasms. Microscopically, this nuclear-cytoplasmic asynchrony is described as "megaloblastic." This group of disorders chiefly affects cells with rapid turnover. In addition to the hematopoi-

etic cells, epithelial cells, gastrointestinal mucosa, and oral mucosa are involved. Deficiencies of vitamin B_{12} (cobalamine) or folic acid are the major causes of megaloblastic anemia.[14]

Vitamin B_{12} (Cobalamine) Deficiency/Pernicious Anemia. The development of a vitamin B_{12} deficiency is a slow process and is most frequently due to impaired absorption rather than dietary deficiency. Conditions that can lead to cobalamine deficiency include pernicious anemia, gastrectomy, small-bowel bacterial overgrowth, diverticulosis, blind intestinal loops, scleroderma, tapeworm, tropical sprue, alcoholism, and medications such as neomycin and colchicine. The major manifestations are anemia, gastrointestinal disorders, and neurologic complications.

The most common form of vitamin B_{12} deficiency is pernicious anemia, which is due to atrophy of the gastric mucosa resulting in a lack of intrinsic factor secretion. Intrinsic factor acts by binding to the vitamin B_{12} molecule, forming a complex that crosses the ileal mucosa and protects the vitamin from proteolysis. The disease can be the result of an autoimmune reaction to either the gastric parietal cells or intrinsic factor and is often seen in connection with other autoimmune diseases such as Graves' disease.

ORAL MANIFESTATIONS. Glossitis and glossodynia are the classic oral symptoms of pernicious anemia (Figure 16-3). The tongue is "beefy red" and inflamed, with small erythematous areas on the tip and margins. There is a loss of filiform papillae, and, in advanced disease, the papillary atrophy involves the entire tongue surface together with a loss of the normal muscle tone. The erythematous macular lesions also can involve the buccal and labial mucosa.[15] Patients may complain of dysphagia and taste aberrations. Discomfort described by denture wearers who have pernicious anemia is probably due to the weakened mucosal tissues. Although the "burning mouth" sensation diagnosed in pernicious anemia can be due to a neuropathy, other causes of oral burning, including candidiasis, should be considered.

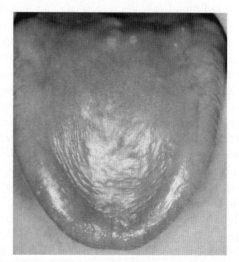

FIGURE 16-3 Atrophic glossitis in a patient with vitamin B_{12} deficiency. (Courtesy of Dr. Thomas P. Sollecito, University of Pennsylvania School of Dental Medicine, Philadelphia, PA)

Oral mucosa biopsy results from patients with pernicious anemia show epithelial atrophy, enlarged basal cell nuclei, increased mitoses in the basal epithelium, epithelial dysplasia, and a nonspecific infiltrate of lymphocytes, plasma cells, and polymorphonuclear leukocytes in the lamina propria.

Following treatment with vitamin B_{12}, the tongue undergoes complete healing with cessation of the symptoms and reversal of the morphologic alterations.

DIAGNOSIS. Pernicious anemia should be suspected in any anemic patient with neurologic symptoms. The first definitive clue that one is dealing with pernicious anemia, however, is the finding of macrocytic normochromic red cells on the blood smear. The mean corpuscular volume is increased, the mean corpuscular hemoglobin increased, and the mean corpuscular hemoglobin concentration normal. In addition, the shape of the red cells varies considerably, the platelets are abnormally large, and the neutrophils often are hypersegmented, having as many as six lobes to their nuclei instead of the usual three. A bone marrow examination will confirm these morphologic changes by revealing the presence of megaloblastic marrow changes. Because folic acid deficiency also may produce these hematologic changes, further studies are necessary to pinpoint vitamin B_{12} deficiency as the cause. A serum assay for vitamin B_{12} and folate should be performed using a microbiologic or radioisotope technique. Once vitamin B_{12} deficiency has been established, the cause of the deficiency must be determined. To diagnose pernicious anemia, the Schilling test is used.

In the Schilling test, the patient is given a measured small amount of radioactive vitamin B_{12} by mouth, followed shortly by a large flushing dose of parenteral nonradioactive vitamin B_{12}. Because the total dose of vitamin B_{12} far exceeds the renal threshold for this vitamin, the excess appears in the urine within the next 24 hours. The amount of radioactivity in the urine is proportional to the amount of the orally administered vitamin B_{12} that has been absorbed. The normal patient excretes 7 to 30% of the radioactive B_{12} in 24 hours, whereas the patient with pernicious anemia excretes no more than 3%. Further studies may be necessary to determine that intestinal disease is not responsible for the malabsorption, and these studies involve administration of a complex of radioactive B_{12} and intrinsic factor. The patient with pernicious anemia will exhibit normal absorption and urine excretion of vitamin B_{12}.

Serum antibodies to gastric parietal cells are found in 90% of the patients; antibodies to the intrinsic factor are found in 60%. These antibodies also have been found in saliva.[16,17]

TREATMENT. Management consists of administration of parenteral cyanocobalamin. Large oral doses may be used when intramuscular injection is contraindicated. This treatment corrects the hematologic changes but will only arrest, not correct, the neurologic changes. It should be given by the patient's physician and must be continued for the rest of the patient's life. Patients who have a history of being treated for anemia for "a while" with B_{12} shots, who no longer take the injections, and who are not anemic, almost certainly do not have pernicious anemia. Almost 100% of patients with pernicious anemia have a relapse within 6 months after discontinuation of B_{12} therapy.

Because the hematologic changes of pernicious anemia may be reversed by oral folic acid therapy without arrest of the neurologic changes, patients who are anemic should never be given folic acid therapy without the possibility of pernicious anemia first being ruled out. Folic acid removes a valuable diagnostic sign (low hemoglobin) and allows the neurologic changes, which are mostly irreversible even with B_{12} therapy, to progress. It is best when prescribing therapeutic vitamins to choose one without folic acid or to ensure that the hemoglobin is normal before instituting vitamin therapy.

Folic Acid Deficiency Anemia. Folic acid deficiency causes severe anemia but does not cause the neurologic abnormalities seen in pernicious anemia. Folate deficiency is prevalent in patients whose diet is devoid of leafy vegetables, such as alcoholics and drug abusers, and in patients with an increased requirement for folate, such as pregnant women and young children. Drugs used for cancer chemotherapy treatment, such as methotrexate, azathioprine, 6-mercaptopurine, 5-fluorouracil, and cytosine arabinoside, are known to cause folate deficiency by interfering with DNA synthesis.

Diagnosis is made by detection of hematologic changes (the same as those in pernicious anemia) with a normal Schilling test and serum vitamin B_{12} assays, but low serum assays of folic acid. Treatment of folic acid deficiency consists of oral folic acid tablets. Oral doses of 1 mg/d are adequate for most patients, and a 5 mg tablet suffices to treat even a patient with intestinal malabsorption.

Oral manifestations may include angular cheilitis and, with severe cases, ulcerative stomatitis and pharyngitis.

Aplastic Anemia. Aplastic anemia is a normochromic normocytic anemia caused by bone marrow failure. Although the cause is frequently unknown, approximately half of the cases are suspected to be caused by chemical substances (eg, paint solvents, benzol, chloramphenicol) or exposure to high levels of x-ray radiation. The term "anemia" is, in a sense, a misnomer since all three cellular elements of the marrow are often involved (pancytopenia).

Fanconi's anemia is an inherited aplastic anemia that manifests in early childhood. It is associated with brown skin pigmentation, hypoplasia of the kidney and spleen, absent or hypoplastic thumb or radius, microcephally, and mental and sexual retardation.

Dental Considerations. There are two major problems in the dental management of patients with aplastic anemia: infection and bleeding. Local infections and bacteremias originating in the oral region can have a fatal course. A thorough oral examination of teeth, periodontium, soft tissues, and salivary glands should be conducted once the diagnosis of aplastic anemia is established. Gingival bleeding can be reduced by the use of systemic antifibrinolytic agents, such as aminocaproic acid or tranexamic acid, as well as local hemostatic measures.

Tranexamic acid is given in a dosage of 20 mg/kg body weight four times a day starting 24 hours before oral procedures and continuing for 3 to 4 days afterward. Oral rinses with chlorhexidine 0.2% in an aqueous solution will reduce the amount of plaque and the number of microorganisms in the oral cavity. However, intramuscular injections and nerve block anesthesias are to be avoided because of the risk of thrombocytopenia and the bleeding tendency. Intraligamentary anesthesia can be used safely in these cases.

▼ WHITE BLOOD CELL DISORDERS

Leukocytes protect against foreign invaders such as fungi, bacteria, viruses, and parasites. Recent advances have expanded our understanding of the cellular and molecular basis of both normal and neoplastic leukocyte function. To understand leukocyte disease, several aspects of normal function must be appreciated. Leukocytes originate from pluripotent hematopoietic stem cells in either the bone marrow or lymphoid tissue; under various external influences and regulating mechanisms, including cytokines and matrix proteins, stem cells develop into progenitor cells of various lineages.[18] Granulocytes and monocytes are derived from the same stem cell precursors in the bone marrow, whereas lymphocytes originate in the lymph nodes. The majority of leukocytes are produced and stored in the bone marrow in several "pools." The mitotic pool consists of immature precursors, the maturing pool consist of white blood cells (WBCs) undergoing maturation, and the storage pool consists of functional WBCs that can be released when needed.

The three types of granulocytes are neutrophils, eosinophils, and basophils. Neutrophils are the most dominant of all circulating phagocytes. They provide the first line of defense against bacterial invasion of the mucous membranes and skin, and comprise greater than half of all leukocytes.[19] Three cellular functions must be intact for neutrophils to provide this protection against infection. They must respond to chemotactic stimuli and migrate to the site of tissue damage, they must be capable of phagocytosis, and they must destroy bacteria through enzymatic activity. The risk of infection is increased if insufficient numbers of neutrophils are present or if one of the three actions of neutrophils is not intact. Neutrophil function is aided by the presence of immunoglobulins, complement, and fibronectin, which help the neutrophils attach to the surface of microorganisms. If these pro-

teins are not present, neutrophil function decreases. The largest number of neutrophils (90%) can be found in the bone marrow. However, neutrophils are released into the circulation into two pools: circulating and marginal. Cells in the marginal pool adhere to vessel walls and are readily available to help fight invading organisms.

The function of the other granulocytes, eosinophils, and basophils is not as well understood. Eosinophils have a weak ability to phagocytize foreign substances and cannot kill bacteria. They function in immune-related antigen-antibody reactions, such as asthmatic attacks and allergic reactions. In addition, levels are increased in parasitic infections. Basophils migrate to tissues carrying heparin and histamine- and platelet-activating factors, and they act as mast cells in allergic reactions. Monocytes are immature cells when in the bloodstream, and they use the bloodstream briefly as a transportation system. Once in the tissues, they mature to macrophages, which have a number of vital functions, including processing antigens to initiate lymphocyte response; secretion of lysosome, complement components, and interleukin-1; and activation and mobilization of other leukocytes.

Lymphocytes are the primary cells involved in immunity. They appear to originate from pluripotential stem cells in the bone marrow and migrate to other lymphoid tissues, including lymph nodes, spleen, thymus, and mucosal surfaces of the gastrointestinal tract. There are two types of lymphocytes: thymus-dependent T lymphocytes and non-thymus-dependent B lymphocytes.[20] Both B and T lymphocytes are seen in the peripheral blood. A description of lymphocyte function is contained in Chapter 18, "Immunologic Diseases."

Peripheral blood contains approximately 4,000 to 11,000 WBCs per cubic millimeter. The hematology laboratory also reports the differential WBC count, which reports the proportion of cell types by percentages. When interpreting the differential WBC count, the clinician should not rely on the percentage to decide whether a cell type is increased or deficient because this number may be misleading. The clinician should determine the absolute number of each cell type by multiplying the total WBC count by the percentage. Automated laboratory systems count the cells directly. The absolute number is a more accurate reflection of disease because it maintains the relationship of the total to the differential count. The normal range of the absolute number of WBCs is summarized in Table 16-2.

In this chapter, diseases of granulocytes are described. (Lymphocyte disorders are described in Chapter 18,

---

TABLE 16-2   White Blood Cell Count with Differential

Cell	Percent	Number	High Count	Low Count
Neutrophils	50–70 (segments), 3–5 (bands)	3,000–7,000	Infection, drugs	Viral disease, drugs, agranulocytosis
Lymphocytes	20–40	1,000–3,500	Viral disease, mononucleosis	HIV, AIDS
Monocytes	0–7	0–700	Infection, SBE	—
Eosinophils	0–5	0–500	Parasitic disease, allergy	—
Basophils	0–1	0–100	—	—

AIDS = acquired immunodeficiency syndrome; HIV = human immunodeficiency virus; SBE = subacute bacterial endocarditis.

"Immunologic Diseases.") Diseases of granulocytes are divided into three major types: quantitative, qualitative, and myeloproliferative. Quantitative disorders result from an abnormal number of white cells, qualitative disorders result from poorly functioning cells, and myeloproliferative disease results from acquired clonal abnormalities of hematopoietic stem cells. The leukemias are the myeloproliferative diseases described in this chapter.

Quantitative Leukocyte Disorders

GRANULOCYTOSIS

Increases in the number of white blood cells may result from infection, tissue necrosis, allergic reactions, neoplastic diseases, inflammatory diseases, or any activity, such as stress or exercise, that increases epinephrine release. A persistent elevation of the WBC count with the absolute neutrophil count remaining above 30,000/mm^3 with a pronounced left shift and the presence of myelocytes, metamyelocytes, and band forms is called a "leukemoid reaction." In response to increased demand, an increased number of immature neutrophils called "bands" enter the circulation, a process called a "left shift." This reaction, often secondary to a severe viral infection, is distinguished from acute leukemia because, in leukemoid reactions, there is an orderly maturation and proliferation of all normal myeloid elements in the bone marrow.

GRANULOCYTOPENIA AND AGRANULOCYTOSIS

Granulocytopenia may occur alone or as part of a generalized suppression of the bone marrow also affecting the erythrocytes and platelets (aplastic anemia). A decrease in granulocytes chiefly results from a decrease in neutrophils, and most cases of granulocytopenia are known as neutropenia. The degree of neutropenia predicts the risk of serious bacterial infections.

Neutropenia is defined as an absolute neutrophil count of more than two standard deviations below a normal mean value. The normal absolute number of neutrophils in the peripheral blood is 3,000/mm^3 to 6,000/mm^3. Mild neutropenia occurs when 1,000/mm^3 to 2,000/mm^3 neutrophils are present, moderate neutropenia occurs when 500/mm^3 to 1,000/mm^3 neutrophils are present, and severe neutropenia occurs when fewer than 500/mm^3 neutrophils are present in the peripheral blood. The term "agranulocytosis" is used when no neutrophils are seen on a peripheral blood smear. Agranulocytosis is a serious condition characterized by an extremely low leukocyte count and the absence of neutrophils; it most often is caused by a drug or medication that interferes with cell formation or enhances cell destruction.

Neutropenia, like anemia, is not a disease but a sign of an underlying disorder; it has a wide range of underlying causes. Decreased production of neutrophils is associated with deficiencies of vitamin B$_{12}$ and folic acid. Certain infections decrease the number of neutrophils in the circulating blood because of increased migration of neutrophils into the tissues, sequestration of neutrophils, or the direct toxic effect of the microorganism and its toxins on the blood marrow. Infections with viruses, particularly hepatitis A and B viruses, parvovirus,

human immunodeficiency virus (HIV-1), and *Cytomegalovirus*, are associated with neutropenia. Overwhelming bacterial infection, particularly septicemia, can be accompanied by neutropenia because the cells are used at rapid rate to overcome the infection. Diseases causing sequestration of neutrophils include systemic lupus erythematosus and Felty's syndrome.[21] The most common cause of neutropenia is a drug reaction. A large number of drugs can cause neutropenia or aplastic anemia. Neutropenia secondary to a drug reaction results from either a toxic (ie, dose-related) or an idiosyncratic phenomenon. Toxic neutropenia occurs predictably in all people who take the offending drugs at sufficient doses for a sufficient time. These drugs interfere with DNA synthesis, protein synthesis, or mitosis. Drugs that cause toxic neutropenia include those used in cancer chemotherapy, benzene, and alcohol. Increasingly, more commonly used drugs, such as analgesics, antibiotics, and antihistamines, have been identified as potential causes of severe neutropenia or agranulocytosis. Neutropenia secondary to ionizing radiation also results from a direct toxic effect on the division of bone marrow cells.

Idiosyncratic reactions are not dose related and occur only in a small percentage of individuals taking the drug. Idiosyncratic drug reactions causing neutropenia are thought to be either an immunologic reaction affecting the bone marrow or an inherited inability to metabolize the drug properly. Drugs that have an increased risk of causing idiosyncratic neutropenia include phenothiazides, phenylbutazone, sulfonamides, and chloramphenicol.[22]

Clinical Manifestations. Along with feelings of general malaise (headache, discomfort, and muscle aches), the most common complication of neutropenia and agranulocytosis is infection.[20] The clinician must be aware that the localizing clinical signs of infection may be few or absent owing to a decreased inflammatory reaction. Swelling and pus will be minimal. The most common sign of infection in neutropenic patients is fever. Other common manifestations include mucosal ulcers, tachycardia, acute pharyngitis, and lymphadenopathy. Common sites of infection include the lungs, urinary tract, skin, rectum, and mouth. Acute bacterial infections are the most common and usually are caused by *Staphylococcus aureus* or gram-negative bacilli, such as *Klebsiella*, *Pseudomonas*, and *Proteus*.

Treatment. The cause of neutropenia must be determined. All drugs should be discontinued and the patient carefully observed for signs of infection. At the first sign of infection, cultures must be taken and the patient started on a regimen of combined often broad-spectrum antibiotics. A combination of antibiotics is commonly used because of the broad coverage against most organisms known to cause infection in neutropenic patients, such as those in *Staphylococcus* species and enteric gram-negative bacteria. Some medical centers use reverse isolation or sterile environments, such as laminar flow beds, to reduce the risk of infection. Third-generation cephalosporins such as ceftazidime are effective single-agent therapies.[23]

Patients with antibodies to neutrophils benefit from corticosteroids; those with neutropenia associated with Felty's syndrome, a disease in which neutrophils sequester in the spleen, benefit from splenectomy. Hematopoietic stem cell transplantation has been used to treat patients with severe aplastic anemia when a suitable donor is available. The myeloid growth factors granulocyte colony-stimulating factor (G-CSF) (filgrastim) and granulocyte-macrophage colony-stimulating factor (sargramostim) may be useful in shortening the duration of neutropenia associated with chemotherapy.[24]

Oral and Dental Considerations. The most common oral sign of neutropenia is ulceration of the oral mucosa (Figure 16-4). Neutropenic ulcers differ from other oral ulcers in that they usually lack surrounding inflammation and are characterized by necrosis. Because the bacteria are poorly opposed by neutrophils, the ulcers become large irregular deep lesions that are extremely painful. The necrotic tissue is often foul smelling, a characteristic of fusospirochetal organisms, although invasion by species of *Staphylococcus* or gram-negative bacilli is common.

Oral ulcers, advanced periodontal disease, pericoronitis, and pulpal infections in patients with severe neutropenia should be considered potentially life threatening because they can lead to bacteremia and septicemia. The infection must be cultured to determine the predominant organism, and the patient should be placed on the appropriate combination of parenteral broad-spectrum antibiotics. Topical application of antibacterial mouth rinses also may be helpful for ulcers. Also useful is an individualized soft splint made from a maxillary study cast that covers palatal lesions and carries medication in a well that continually bathes the oral ulcers. A combination of topical neomycin, bacitracin, and nystatin has been used to reduce the risk of severe infection. Chlorhexidine oral rinses are usually ordered, although their chronic use may be controversial because chlorhexidine use is accompanied by increased gram-negative rods in the oral flora.[25] The pain of the ulcers is reduced by the use of topical anesthetic mouth rinses. A solution containing 5% diphenhydramine hydrochloride mixed with magnesium hydroxide or kaolin with pectin is useful for this purpose. Dental treatment for neutropenic patients is discussed in detail in the section below entitled "Leukemia."

CYCLIC NEUTROPENIA

Cyclic neutropenia is a rare disorder that occurs secondary to a periodic failure of the stem cells in the bone marrow. This failure results from an abnormality in the regulation of bone marrow precursor cells or an inhibitor of neutrophils released from monocytes. It is characterized by transient severe neutropenia that occurs approximately every 21 days.[26] The nadir neutrophil count lasts 3 to 7 days and is occasionally associated with elevations in monocytes. One-third of cases are inherited as an autosomal dominant trait, and two-thirds arise spontaneously during the first few years of life. The disease is frequently present during infancy or childhood,

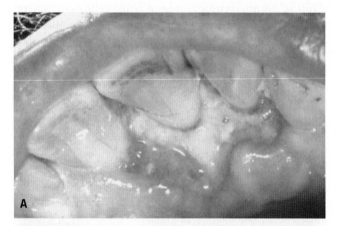

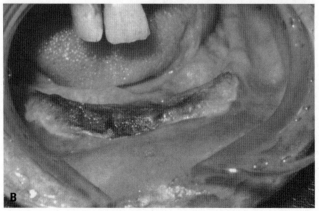

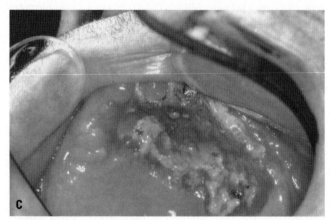

FIGURE 16-4 Oral ulcers in patients with severe neutropenia involving the palate (**A** and **B**) and the alveolar ridge (**C**).

although there is an adult-onset form of the disease, and both sexes appear to be equally affected. The patient is healthy between neutropenic episodes, but at regular intervals the absolute neutrophil count falls quickly below 500/mm³; in some patients, the neutrophil count falls to 0. Normal hematopoiesis is not constant in the bone marrow of patients with cyclic neutropenia, causing fluctuations in marrow platelet and erythrocyte precursors and granulocytes.

Clinical Manifestations.   The major signs and symptoms of cyclic neutropenia are related to infection occurring during neutropenic episodes.[27] The most common signs are fever, stomatitis, pharyngitis, and skin abscesses. The severity of the infections is related to the severity of the neutropenia. Some patients with severe periodic neutropenia experience few infections owing to a compensatory increase in monocytes, which act as phagocytes to prevent the spread of bacterial infection. Less frequently, patients experience lung and urinary tract infections and rectal and vaginal ulcers. Life expectancy is good for patients who receive careful monitoring.

Treatment.   The universally accepted treatment for most cases of cyclic neutropenia is careful monitoring of the patient for infection during neutropenic periods and vigorous early management of infection. In some patients, use of corticosteroids, adrenocorticotropin, or testosterone modulates the sharp reduction in marrow function. Unfortunately, these drugs are not successful for all patients. The use of granulocyte colony-stimulating factor (G-CSF) has been employed to boost neutrophil levels. Unlike with congenital agranulocytosis, G-CSF therapy in cyclic neutropenia is not associated with the development of acute myeloid leukemia or myelodyplasia.[28]

Oral and Dental Considerations.   Oral lesions are common in cyclic neutropenia and may be the major clinical manifestation of the disease. The two most common oral manifestations are oral mucosal ulcers and periodontal disease. The oral ulcers recur with each new bout of neutropenia and resemble the large deep scarring ulcers seen in major aphthous stomatitis. The periodontal manifestations range from marginal gingivitis to rapidly advancing periodontal bone loss caused by bacterial infection of the dental supporting structures (Figures 16-5 and 16-6). In patients with major aphthous ulcers or generalized rapidly advancing periodontal disease that cannot be

explained by local factors alone, cyclic neutropenia should be ruled out as a possible cause. Suspicion of cyclic neutropenia should be particularly high when either of these oral diseases is seen in children.

Clinicians must remember that a single WBC count is not a sufficient test to rule out the diagnosis of cyclic neutropenia because the examination may be performed as the peripheral neutrophils are being replenished. A series of three total and differential WBC counts per week for 4 to 6 weeks is necessary to rule out this disease. Patients with known cyclic neutropenia require frequent dental treatment to minimize advancing periodontal disease. Routine treatment should be confined to the periods when the absolute neutrophil count is above 2,000/mm³. A white cell count taken the day of a dental procedure is a wise precaution because the neutrophil count can change rapidly. Oral hygiene must be carefully maintained, and patients should be recalled for oral hygiene every 2 to 3 months. The use of colony-stimulating factor has reduced oral ulcers and periodontal disease in these patients.

Qualitative Leukocyte Disorders

CHÉDIAK-HIGASHI SYNDROME

First described just more than 30 years ago, Chédiak-Higashi syndrome is a rare autosomal recessive defect characterized by oculocutaneous albinism, progressive neurologic abnormalities, and large blue-grey granules in the cytoplasms of neutrophils, eosinophils, basophils, and platelets. Abnormal granules also have been observed in renal tubular cells, nerve cells, and fibroblasts. The abnormal granules seen in all blood granulocytes result in neutrophils with decreased chemotactic and bactericidal ability, although phagocytosis remains intact. The abnormality in bactericidal activity is thought to be caused by an inefficient use of lysosomal enzymes resulting from a mutation in the lysosomal trafficking regulator, or *LYST* gene.[29] This leads to defective T-cell signaling and the potential for an associated lymphoproliferative syndrome.[30] Patients develop severe neutropenia as a result of ineffective granulopoiesis, and most die in childhood from infections or advanced lymphoproliferative syndrome.

Clinical Manifestations.   Hypopigmentation resulting from the pigment dilution is noted in skin and hair during infancy. The hair will have gray streaks. Neuropathy and ataxis are prominent features in some patients. The degranulation defect

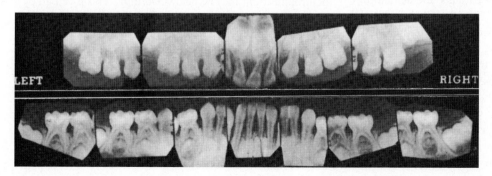

FIGURE 16-5 Full-mouth radiographs of a 4-year-old boy with cyclic neutropenia, showing resorption of the alveolar and supporting bone. (Reproduced with permission from Cohen DW, Morris AL. J Periodontol;32:159.)

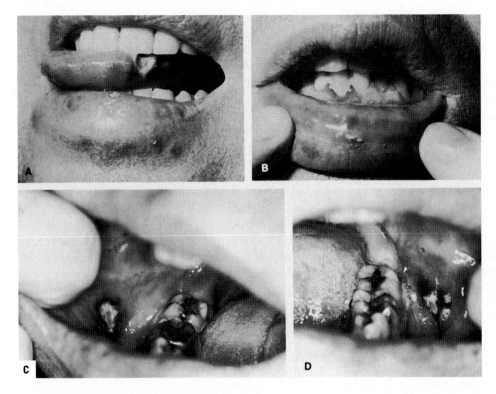

FIGURE 16-6 Lesions of cyclic neutropenia on second day of attack (**A,** tongue; **B,** lip and gingival margins; **C** and **D,** cheek lesions). (Reproduced with permission from Levy EJ, Schetman D. Arch Dermatol;84:432.)

of neutrophils causes recurrent bacterial infections of the skin and respiratory tract, chiefly by gram-positive organisms, such as *Staphylococcus aureus* and β-hemolytic *Streptococcus*. This differs from the infections seen in patients who are neutropenic from leukemia or cancer chemotherapy, in whom gram-negative bacilli cause the majority of infections. Patients usually die of recurrent infections before the age of 10 years. Patients who survive the recurrent infections experience an accelerated phase of the disease that resembles lymphoma. The lymph nodes, spleen, liver, and bone marrow become infiltrated with lymphohistiocytic cells. Diagnosis of Chédiak-Higashi syndrome is based on the pathognomonic giant blue-gray granules seen in the cytoplasm of granulocytes when examining a peripheral blood smear.

Treatment.   Medical management of Chédiak-Higashi syndrome in infants centers on rigorous treatment of infections as soon as they occur. Because gram-positive organisms cause a majority of infections, the infections respond well to antibiotics. Treatment of neutrophils with ascorbate has enhanced the function of neutrophils in some patients, and hematopoietic stem cell transplantation (HSCT) has been helpful in others. Approximately 50% of these patients are cured by HSCT when it is applied early in the course of the disease. Chemotherapy has been used to treat the accelerated lymphoproliferative phase of the disease.

Oral and Dental Considerations.   Gingival and periodontal disease are common findings in patients with Chédiak-Higashi syndrome, and early loss of teeth owing to periodontal disease and caries is frequently reported in the literature.[31]

CHRONIC IDIOPATHIC NEUTROPENIA

Reports of long-standing severe neutropenia with few associated abnormalities have appeared in the literature under a variety of names, including familial neutropenia, chronic benign neutropenia, chronic neutropenia, and hypoplastic neutropenia. Chronic idiopathic neutropenia (CIN) refers to neutropenias whose characteristics do not fit into other categories. The etiology of this group of disorders is unknown, but it is characterized by a decreased production of neutrophils in the bone marrow. Some patients have antineutrophil antibodies detectable in the serum and comprise a subset of patients with so-called chronic immunoneutropenia. The bone marrow of patients with CIN shows a normal number of immature cells but a decreased number of mature neutrophils. This phenomenon has been called "maturation arrest," but the reason for this problem is unclear. Increased margination of neutrophils has been noted in some cases.

Clinical Manifestations.   Many patients with CIN are asymptomatic and are free from infections, even though their absolute neutrophil count may be below 500/mm³. This is caused by a compensatory monocytosis, which accounts for a normal number of phagocytes present at the site of a tissue injury.

A minority of patients experience recurrent bacterial infections, but these are rarely life threatening. The most common infections are recurring upper respiratory tract infections, otitis media, bronchitis, and furunculosis. Oral ulcers, periodontal disease, sinusitis, and perirectal infections also occur.

Treatment.   When managing CIN, the clinician must refrain from overtreating patients who are asymptomatic. G-CSF is now the therapy of choice for patients who have serious infections. Corticosteroids and cytotoxic agents have also been effective in increasing the neutrophil count.

Oral and Dental Considerations. There have been many isolated case reports of patients with CIN with oral signs and symptoms. The most distressing oral problem repeatedly reported in patients with CIN is severe rapidly advancing periodontal disease. The gingivae appear intensely red, despite the neutropenia, with granulomatous margins. Severe gingival recession is common, and early severe periodontal disease with advanced bone loss, mobility, denuded roots, and loss of teeth has been described. These patients may also report recurring oral ulcerations that may correspond to the neutrophil count (Figure 16-7).

The dental management of patients with CIN depends on their past history of infections. The dentist needs to remember that even a patient with CIN with severe neutropenia may not be highly susceptible to infection, owing to a compensatory monocytosis. If a patient with CIN has never experienced an infection, it would not be reasonable to take extraordinary precautions for routine dental procedures.

Leukemia

Leukemia, originally described by Virchow in 1874 as "white blood," is a malignancy affecting the WBCs of the bone marrow. This neoplastic process is characterized by differentiation and proliferation of malignantly transformed hematopoietic stem cells, leading to suppression of normal cells. The malignant cells replace and turn off the normal marrow elements, causing anemia, thrombocytopenia, and a deficiency of normally functioning leukocytes. In time, the leukemic cells infiltrate other body organs, destroying normal tissue. The most widely accepted classification system of leukemia is the French-American-British (FAB) classification. Although further subclassifications have been added, this system is a morphologic classification based on the differentiation and maturation of predominant leukemic cells in the bone marrow and on cytochemical analysis.

Leukemia is classified as either acute or chronic and by cell type. The etiology of leukemia, in most cases, is unknown (see below), but several factors that increase the risk of the disease are well established. Genetic factors play a role in some cases of leukemia, and families with a high incidence of the disease have been reported. Genetic disorders, such as Down, Klinefelter's, and Fanconi's syndromes, also are associated with an increased risk of leukemia. Familial leukemias are rare, but there seems to be a higher incidence of leukemia in siblings of affected children. Individuals with chromosomal abnormalities like those in Down syndrome have a 20-fold increased incidence of acute leukemia. Radiation in doses over 1 Gy is known to significantly increase the risk of leukemia. For example, a high incidence of leukemia was observed in survivors of atomic blasts as well as in early radiologists. Patients with a past history of radiotherapy also have an increased rate of leukemia.

Exposure to certain chemicals and drugs has been related to an increased risk of leukemia. Benzene has been related to leukemia incidence, and acute leukemia has been reported to occur after the use of the arthritis drug phenylbutazone and the antibiotic chloramphenicol. Patients treated with certain anticancer drugs have an increased risk of developing leukemia; particularly susceptible are patients treated for lymphoma with chemotherapy and radiation.

ACUTE LEUKEMIA

The acute leukemias are malignancies of hematopoietic progenitor cells, which consequently fail to mature and differentiate. They are divided into two major groups: acute lymphocytic leukemia (ALL) and acute myelogenous leukemia (AML) (Table 16-3). The common type of ALL, which comprises 65% of cases, is derived from B lymphocytes or their precursors. The T-cell type comprises 20% of cases, and 15% of ALLs are classified as null cell leukemia because they originate from the T or B cells.

In older patients, AML may be preceded by a preleukemic or myelodysplastic syndrome, with generalized bone marrow abnormalities affecting RBCs, leukocytes, and platelets. Leukemia preceded by these syndromes responds poorly to therapy.[32]

Clinical Manifestations. Acute leukemia can occur at any age, but ALL is commonly found in children, whereas AML occurs more frequently in adults.[33] The symptoms and signs of acute leukemia result from either bone marrow suppression or infiltration of leukemic cells into other organs and tissues. The bone marrow changes cause anemia, thrombocytopenia, and a decrease in normally functioning neutrophils. The anemia results in pallor, shortness of breath, and fatigue, which is the most common presenting symptom.

Thrombocytopenia causes spontaneous bleeding, such as petechiae, ecchymoses, epistaxis, melena, increased menstrual bleeding, and gingival bleeding, when the platelet count falls below 25,000/mm³. Approximately 50% of patients have some complaint of purpura or bleeding at the time of diagnosis.

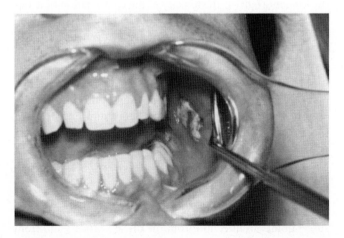

FIGURE 16-7 Ulcer of the buccal mucosa in a patient with chronic idiopathic neutropenia. The ulcer was infected with gram-negative enteric bacilli.

TABLE 16-3   Morphologic Subtypes of Acute Myelogenous Leukemia

Cell Line	Classification		Subtype	Incidence (%)
Myeloid	AML	M0	Acute myeloblastic leukemia; minimally differentiated	3–5
	AML	M1	Acute myeloblastic leukemia without maturation	15–20
	AML	M2	Acute myeloblastic leukemia with maturation	25–30
	APL	M3	Acute promyelocytic leukemia; hypergranular	5–10
	APL	M3v	Acute promyelocytic leukemia; variant, microgranular	20
Myeloid and monocytic	AMML	M4	Acute myelomonocytic leukemia	20–30
	AMML	M4e0	Acute myelomonocytic leukemia with eosinophilia	15–30
Monocytic	AML	M5a	Acute monoblastic leukemia; poorly differentiated	2–9
	AML	M5b	Acute monocytic leukemia; differentiated	—
Erythroid and myeloid	AEL	M6	Acute erythroleukemia	3–5
Megakaryocytic	—	M7	Acute megakaryocytic leukemia	3–12

Although most bleeding results from decreased numbers of platelets, disseminated intravascular coagulation (DIC) can result from substances released from leukemic cells that activate coagulation. These patients, who usually have promyelocytic leukemia, have the ironic combination of thrombosis and hemorrhage owing to depletion of coagulation factors.

Although leukemic patients often present with a greatly increased number of leukocytes, these leukemic cells do not function normally, resulting in defective migration, phagocytosis, or bactericidal action. Infection is therefore a frequent complication of the disease and is the most common cause of morbidity and mortality. Fever is an early sign of disease owing to recurrent infections of the lungs, urinary tract, skin, mouth, rectum, and upper respiratory tract. Infiltration of organs and tissues by leukemic cells causes lymphadenopathy, hepatomegaly, and splenomegaly. Cells may infiltrate the central nervous system or peripheral nerves, leading to cranial nerve palsy, paresthesia, anesthesia, and paralysis. Localized tumors consisting of leukemic cells are called "chloromas." The surface of these tumors turns green when exposed to light because of the presence of myeloperoxidase.

The diagnosis of acute leukemia is made with laboratory examination of the peripheral blood and bone marrow. The peripheral WBC count is usually elevated, but some cases present with normal or decreased counts. These cases are called subleukemic or aleukemic leukemia. In most cases, significant numbers of immature granulocytic or lymphocytic precursors or even stem cells are present in the peripheral blood, accompanied by a significant anemia and thrombocytopenia. Microscopic examination of a bone marrow aspirate finalizes the diagnosis.

Treatment.   The first step in treatment is to obtain complete remission, which is characterized by normal peripheral blood with resolution of cytopenias, normal marrow with normal blasts, and normal clinical status. This, however, is not synonymous with a cure, and the leukemia will return without additional therapy. Combination chemotherapy, including daunorubicin and cytarabine, is the treatment of choice for patients with acute leukemia. The cytotoxic drugs are used in doses that kill more than 99.9% of leukemic cells. Chemotherapy is divided into three stages: (1) induction, an intense myelosuppressing regimen of a combination of toxic drugs attempting to achieve remission; (2) consolidation, involving a second course of intensive therapy in an attempt to prevent relapse; and (3) maintenance chemotherapy using a lower dose of drugs, which may be continued periodically from months to years.

The chemotherapy used depends on the type of leukemia. The treatment of ALL in children is one of the dramatic success stories of the use of cancer chemotherapy. Previously, patients with ALL died within months of diagnosis, but now more than 90% of children achieve remission after induction and consolidation chemotherapy, and 50% of these remissions are prolonged enough to be considered cures. The term "remission" is used when the patient is asymptomatic, peripheral blood counts are normal, and fewer than 5% of cells in the marrow are blasts. A combination of drugs has been found to be more effective than a single agent.

The treatment of AML has not been as successful, and most patients die within a few years of diagnosis. A major reason for the high mortality is the toxicity of the combination of drugs used to treat AML. Cytogenetic studies have emerged as great predictors in AML survival. Favorable cytogenetics in AML include t(8;21), t(15;17), and inv(16)(p13;q22) and result in both short-term and long-term disease control.[34]

In addition to chemotherapy, treatment of acute leukemia includes supportive care during the severe bone marrow aplasia. The use of platelet transfusions has significantly reduced the mortality from hemorrhage. Packed red blood cells are widely used to decrease the signs and symptoms of anemia, and heparin is administered to patients with DIC to prevent thrombosis along with the malignant leukemic cells.

Infection, especially with bacteria and fungi, is the major cause of death in leukemic patients because of their increased susceptibility to infection from the disease process and from the bone marrow aplasia caused by toxic chemotherapy. Infections with gram-negative bacilli such as *Pseudomonas,*

Klebsiella, and *Proteus* are common, as are fungal infections with *Candida*, *Aspergillus*, and *Phycomycetes*. Early diagnosis and prompt treatment of infections of the urinary tract, respiratory tract, rectum, skin, and mouth are necessary. Generalized viral infections, especially with herpes simplex virus (HSV), varicella-zoster virus, and *Cytomegalovirus*, also are common complications (see Figure 16-6).

The transplantation of hemopoietic stem cells, previously known as "bone marrow transplantation," has been used to treat acute leukemia and other hematologic malignancies, genetic diseases of the immune and blood systems, and, more recently, solid tumors. The purpose of HSCT in leukemia is to eradicate all malignant cells and replace them with normal progenitor cells from the marrow. Stem cell transplantation in solid tumors, such as in breast cancer, is used to treat patients with extremely high doses of toxic chemotherapy, which would normally be fatal due to bone marrow failure.

Stem cell grafts may be syngeneic (from a genetically identical twin); allogeneic (from a donor who is genetically similar but not identical); or autologous (a portion of the patient's own marrow is removed prior to chemotherapy, screened, preserved, and reimplanted after therapy).

Stem cell transplantation is preceded by a combination of high-dose chemotherapy and, in some cases, total body radiation. The pluripotent stem cells engraft up to 4 weeks after transplantation, and during this period, the patient is highly susceptible to infection and hemorrhage and therefore must be carefully supported in medical centers that have skilled experienced oncology teams.

After engraftment, complications include acute and chronic graft-versus-host disease (GVHD) caused by T lymphocytes from the graft that destroy normal vital host tissues and organs. Acute GVHD occurs within the first 100 days after transplantation, causing mild to severe skin, liver, intestinal, and immunologic disease. Chronic GVHD begins more than 100 days after transplantation and resembles autoimmune diseases such as lupus and scleroderma. This complication frequently is treated successfully with immunosuppressives. Hematopoietic stem cell transplantation is discussed in further detail in Chapter 19.

CHRONIC LEUKEMIA

Chronic leukemias are characterized by the presence of large numbers of well-differentiated cells in the bone marrow, peripheral blood, and tissues and a prolonged clinical course even without therapy. This distinguishes chronic leukemia from acute leukemia, in which immature cells predominate, and the untreated clinical course leads to death in months. The two major types of chronic leukemia are chronic granulocytic leukemia (CGL, or chronic myelocytic leukemia [CML]) and chronic lymphocytic leukemia (CLL), which differ in natural history, clinical presentation, prognosis, and treatment.

Chronic Myelocytic Leukemia. CGL was the first type of leukemia identified by physicians in the 1840s, when macroscopic changes in the blood were noted in patients with splenomegaly. More commonly called CML, it is the form of leukemia most closely related to exposure to ionizing radiation and toxic chemicals. The disease is identified by genetic changes seen in the patient's chromosomes; 90% of CML patients have the Philadelphia chromosome, an acquired genetic defect resulting from translocation of genetic material from chromosome 22 to chromosome 9.[35] This chromosomal abnormality affects the hematopoietic stem cell and thus is present in the myeloid and some lymphoid cell lines. Another change is the depletion of leukocyte alkaline phosphatase. These two biochemical abnormalities are not present in the other forms of leukemia.

CML has two phases: chronic and blastic. During the chronic phase, large numbers of granulocytes are present in the bone marrow and peripheral blood, but the cells retain normal functions. It takes between 5 and 8 years after the formation of the first CML cell for clinical signs and symptoms to develop. The blastic phase, which takes place 2 to 4 years after diagnosis, is characterized by further malignant transformation to immature cells, which act similarly to cells in acute leukemia.[36]

Clinical Manifestations. CML occurs most frequently in patients between the ages of 30 and 50 years. No symptoms are noted by the patient during the first few years, and the disease may be discovered during a routine examination when splenomegaly or an elevated WBC count is noted. Early signs and symptoms are usually secondary to anemia or the packing of leukocytes into the spleen and bone marrow. The anemia causes weakness, fatigue, and dyspnea on exertion, while bone pain or abdominal pain in the upper left quadrant results from the spleen and bone marrow changes. As the disease progresses, thrombocytopenia can cause petechiae, ecchymoses, and hemorrhage.

Laboratory tests taken during this stage show a markedly elevated WBC count that may reach several hundred thousand leukocytes per cubic millimeter. The bone marrow is hypercellular. Diagnosis is confirmed by the presence of the Philadelphia chromosome in 90% of cases and the absence of leukocyte alkaline phosphatase. The patient often survives for years before the disease enters the blastic phase. Transformation of the blastic phase may occur suddenly or develop slowly over months. The symptoms caused by splenomegaly worsen, and other organs, particularly the liver, lymph nodes, and skin, become involved. Death occurs within months after the blastic phase begins.[37]

Treatment. Control of the chronic phase of CML is often successful. If the disease is discovered while the patient is asymptomatic, only careful monitoring is necessary. When symptoms begin, the most common treatment is the use of busulfan or other alkylating agents. The disease is controlled during the chronic phase with chemotherapy and radiation, but true remissions are rare unless bone marrow transplantation from a histocompatible donor is performed during the chronic phase. The blastic phase of the disease is refractory to treatment. Life may occasionally be prolonged by use of the chemotherapy protocols used in the treatment of acute leukemia.

Chronic Lymphocytic Leukemia. CLL results from a slowly progressing malignancy involving the lymphocytes. More than 90% of cases involve the B lymphocytes, which are responsible for immunoglobulin synthesis and antibody response, rather than T lymphocytes, which account for only 5% of cases.[38] The CLL B lymphocytes do not carry out their normal immunologic function and do not differentiate into normal immunoglobulin-producing plasma cells when exposed to antigen. One reason the disease progresses slowly is that, unlike the cells in other forms of leukemia, the CLL cells do not turn off normal marrow cells until late in the course of the disease. Occasional cases of T-lymphocytic CLL have been reported.

Clinical Manifestations. CLL occurs most frequently in males older than 40 years, with 60 years being the most common age of onset. As a result of the slow natural history, it is not uncommon for the disease to be detected incidentally by routine hematology before any signs or symptoms are apparent. The peripheral blood shows many small well-differentiated lymphocytes; hundreds of thousands, even millions, of cells per cubic millimeter may be present in the peripheral blood. The asymptomatic phase of the disease may last for years, but eventually signs and symptoms of infiltration of leukemic cells in the bone marrow, lymph nodes, or other tissues appear. Bone marrow infiltration causes anemia and thrombocytopenia, resulting in pallor, weakness, dyspnea, and purpura. Infiltration of other tissues causes lymphadenopathy, splenomegaly, hepatomegaly, and leukemic infiltrates of skin or mucosa. Cervical lymphadenopathy and tonsillar enlargement are frequent head and neck signs of CLL.

Patients with CLL exhibit some degree of hypogammaglobulinemia, with an increased susceptibility to bacterial infection. Infection with varicella-zoster virus also is common. Late in the disease, massive lymphadenopathy may cause intestinal or urethral obstruction and obstructive jaundice. Leukemic infiltrates result in skin masses, liver dysfunction, intestinal malabsorption, pulmonary obstruction, or compression of the central or peripheral nervous system. Abnormal immunoglobulins may cause hemolytic anemia or thrombocytopenia.

Treatment. Most oncologists do not treat asymptomatic CLL patients with chemotherapy because there is no convincing evidence that early treatment enhances survival. Indications for treatment include progressive fatigue, troublesome lymphadenopathy, or the development of anemia or thrombocytopenia. The standard treatment for CLL used to be chlorambucil; however, fludarabine has been shown to produce a higher response rate.[39]

Hairy cell leukemia is a distinct variant of CLL characterized by leukemic B lymphocytes with cytoplasmic projections and a striking 5:1 male predominance. Common signs and symptoms include splenomegaly, vasculitis, and erythema nodosum. The treatment of choice is cladribine. This nontoxic drug produces

benefit in 95% of cases and complete remission in more than 80%. Interferon and splenectomy are rarely used.[40]

ORAL AND DENTAL CONSIDERATIONS

Dentists in clinical practice and research have become increasingly interested in leukemia because the oral complications are common throughout the clinical course of the disease, dental management is complex, and the mouth is a potential source of morbidity and mortality.

Because oral signs and symptoms are common, the dentist may be the first clinician to suspect the disease. Head and neck signs result from leukemic infiltrates or marrow failure. These include cervical lymphadenopathy, oral bleeding, gingival infiltrates, oral infections, and oral ulcers.

Thrombocytopenia and anemia caused by marrow suppression from disease and chemotherapy result in pallor of the mucosa, petechiae, and ecchymoses, as well as gingival bleeding (Figures 16-8 and 16-9). The extent of gingival bleeding depends on the severity of the thrombocytopenia and the extent of local irritants. Spontaneous gingival bleeding is common when the platelet count falls below 20,000/mm^3; severe gingival bleeding may often be managed successfully with local treatment, reducing the need for platelet transfusions. The dentist should always weigh the risk of platelet transfusions against their benefit before recommending their use for treatment of oral bleeding. The risks of platelet transfusion include hepatitis, HIV infection, transfusion reactions, and the formation of antiplatelet antibodies, which reduce the usefulness of platelet transfusions during future hemorrhagic episodes. Oral hemorrhage also may result from DIC, causing hypofibrinogenemia.

Topical treatment to stop gingival bleeding should always include removal of obvious local irritants, and direct pressure. Helpful is the use of absorbable gelatin or collagen sponges, topical thrombin, or the placement of microfibrillar collagen held in place by packing or splints. Some have reported successful management of gingival bleeding with oral rinses of antifibrinolytic agents such as tranexamic acid or

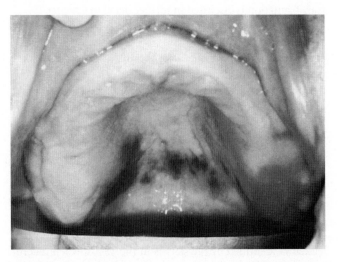

FIGURE 16-8 Ecchymosis of the palate in a patient with thrombocytopenia secondary to acute leukemia.

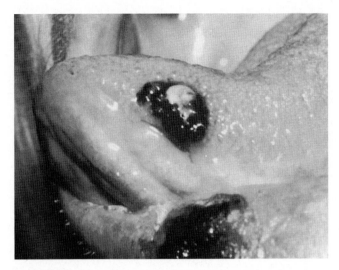

FIGURE 16-9 Hematoma of the tongue in a patient with thrombocytopenia secondary to acute leukemia.

ε-aminocaproic acid. If these local measures are not successful in stopping significant gingival hemorrhage, platelet transfusions are necessary.

Oral Ulcers. Oral mucosal ulcers are common findings in leukemic patients taking chemotherapy and are frequently caused by the direct effect of chemotherapeutic drugs on the oral mucosal cells. Lockhart and Sonis have reported that ulcers secondary to chemotherapy begin approximately 7 days following the start of treatment. Bacterial invasion secondary to severe neutropenia also plays a role in the formation of oral ulcers, and these lesions may be seen as an early sign of disease (see Figure 16-4). The ulcers are characteristically large, irregular, and foul smelling, and are surrounded by pale mucosa caused by anemia and a lack of normal inflammatory response.

The most common cause of oral ulcers in leukemic patients receiving chemotherapy is recurrent HSV infections. These infections involve the intraoral mucosa and the lips. The

lesions frequently begin with the classic cluster of vesicles typical of recurrent HSV and quickly spread, causing large ulcers that often have a raised white border (Figure 16-10). However, they can often appear atypical. In all patients receiving immunosuppressive doses of chemotherapy, HSV should be ruled out as a cause of oral ulcers with a cytology smear stained with fluorescent antibody to HSV antibody (direct fluorescent antibody) and a viral culture. The lesions respond well to parenteral acyclovir administered intravenously or by mouth, although acyclovir-resistant HSV strains have been reported.

The management of non-HSV oral ulcers in leukemic patients should prevent the spread of localized infection, minimize bacteremia, promote healing, and reduce pain. The ulcers in hospitalized leukemic patients taking chemotherapy may be infected with organisms not commonly associated with oral infection, particularly gram-negative enteric bacilli. Topical antibacterial treatment can be attempted with povidone-iodine solutions, bacitracin-neomycin ointments, or chlorhexidine rinses. Kaolin and pectin plus diphenhydramine oral rinses can be used to reduce pain. Other oral preparations containing sucralfate suspensions have been advocated for their ability to bind to and protect ulcers.

Oral Infections. Oral infection is a serious potentially fatal complication in neutropenic leukemic patients. Candidiasis is a common oral fungal infection, but infections with other fungi, such as *Histoplasma*, *Aspergillus*, or Phycomycetes, fungi, also may begin on the oral tissues. When these lesions are suspected, a biopsy specimen, a fine-needle aspiration, or a cytology smear must be obtained because a culture alone is not a reliable test for these organisms.

Diagnosis of dental infection, particularly periodontal and pericoronal infections, is difficult in neutropenic leukemic patients because normal inflammation is absent. The early diagnosis of oral infection is imperative because it has been demonstrated that oral flora is a significant source of potentially life-threatening infections with gram-positive and gram-negative bacilli. It is a dentist's obligation to carry out screening examinations and eliminate obvious sources of potential

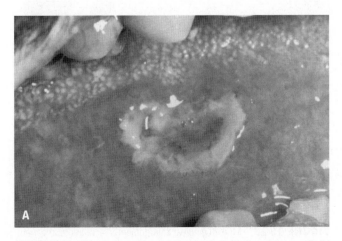
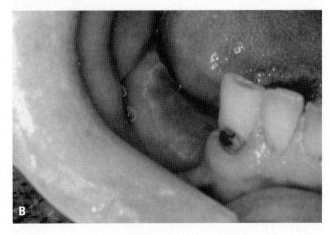

FIGURE 16-10 **A,** Secondary herpes simplex infection of tongue. **B,** Edentulous ridge in a patient receiving chemotherapy for treatment of acute leukemia.

acute infection or bacteremia before chemotherapy is instituted, although platelet transfusions and intravenous combinations of antibiotics may be required before dental treatment. With the newer broad-spectrum antibiotics now employed by hematology-oncology teams, the rate of infection and septicemia from odontogenic sources is unknown, but it may be less than previously reported.

Oral signs also may result from the presence of leukemic infiltrates. These are most frequently reported as gingival infiltrates in patients with myelomonocytic and monoblastic leukemia (M4,5) or acute promyelocytic leukemia (M3) (Figures 16-11, 16-12, and 16-13). Leukemic infiltrates involving the palate, alveolar bone, and dental pulp also have been reported. Leukemic infiltrates may cause oral signs and symptoms because of the involvement of the fifth and seventh cranial nerves. Disorders of the fifth and seventh cranial nerves also have been reported in leukemic patients as a result of the use of vincristine, a drug commonly used to treat ALL.

Children with ALL receive radiation to the cranium and chemotherapy to prevent a relapse of the disease in the brain. Craniofacial deformities and dental anomalies are common in patients who receive this therapy as children, particularly if given before age 5 years. The most common anomalies reported are deficient mandibular development, dental agenesis, arrested root development, microdontia, and enamel dysplasia.

Oral lesions are common complications of HSC transplant patients. Lesions occur in approximately 80% of patients with GVHD. Lichenoid lesions, including desquamative gingivitis, keratotic lesions, atrophy, and ulceration, may be present (Figure 16-14). The lesions appear clinically and histologically similar to lichen planus or discoid lupus. Patients with GVHD also develop xerostomia. Biopsy results of minor salivary glands of GVHD patients show changes compatible with those in Sjögren's syndrome.

▼ LYMPHOMA

The lymphomas are a group of malignant solid tumors involving cells of the lymphoreticular or immune system, such as B

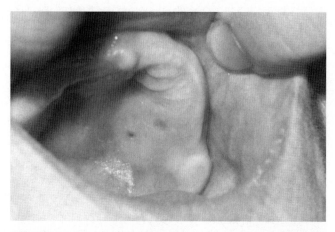

FIGURE 16-12   Palatal chloromas in a patient with acute myelogenous leukemia.

lymphocytes, T lymphocytes, and monocytes. The etiology is unknown, but identified risk factors include immunodeficiency states, viral infections, and chemical exposure. The initial tumor formation in lymphoma is in the secondary lymphatic tissues, where normal tissue is replaced by malignant lymphocytes. Lymphomas are divided into two major categories: Hodgkin's disease (HD) and non-Hodgkin's lymphoma (NHL). These diseases usually begin in the lymph nodes but may be first diagnosed in extranodal lymphoid tissue.

Hodgkin's Disease

Hodgkin's Disease (HD), a malignant lymphatic disease, was first described by British pathologist Thomas Hodgkin in 1832. The etiology remains unknown, but it is probably the culmination of diverse pathologic processes such as viral infections, environmental exposures, and a genetically determined host response.

HD used to be a uniformly fatal disease, but modern modes of diagnosis and treatment have given a newly diagnosed patient a more than 70% chance of cure. One reason for this advance is improved methods of classifying and staging

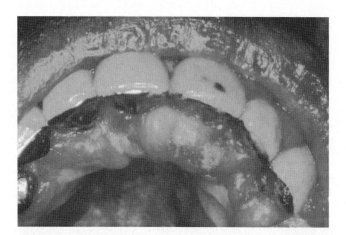

FIGURE 16-11   Gingival infiltrates in a patient with acute monomye logenous leukemia.

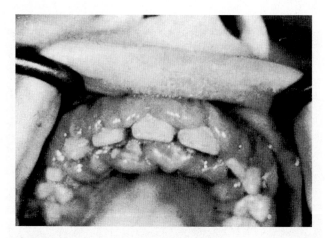

FIGURE 16-13   Marked gingival enlargement in a 12-year-old patient with monocytic leukemia.

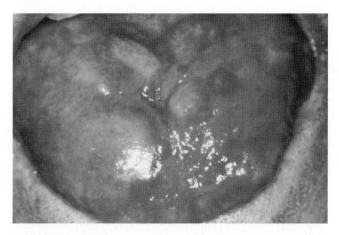

FIGURE 16-14 Tongue lesions of GVHD in a hemapoietic stem cell transplantation patient.

the disease; this improves the opportunity for the patient to be managed properly. Accurate classification of the disease clinically and histologically is essential because treatment is determined by stage. Staging must include lymph node biopsy, chest radiography, computed tomography scan of the abdomen and pelvis, bone marrow biopsy, and laboratory evaluation of liver, kidney, and bone. In selected cases, lymphography, exploratory laparotomy, radionuclide scans, and magnetic resonance imaging are indicated.

HD is classified histologically according to the Rye system, which lists four major subgroups: lymphocyte predominance type, nodular sclerosis type, mixed cellularity type, and lymphocyte depletion type. The lymphocyte predominance type has the best prognosis, and the lymphocyte depleted type has the worst. The disease also is staged clinically according to the criteria established at the Ann Arbor conference of 1971 and modified by Cotswolds (Table 16-4).[41] Stage I has the best prognosis, and stage IV has the worst. The presence or absence of significant systemic symptoms is indicated by the suffixes "A" (symptoms absent) or "B" (symptoms present). The suffix "E" indicates extralymphatic disease, and "X" indicates the presence of bulky disease.

TABLE 16-4   Staging of Hodgkin's Disease: Ann Arbor Staging Classification with Cotswolds Modification

Classification	Extent of Disease
Stage I	Involvement of one lymph node region or single extranodal site
Stage II	Involvement of multiple lymph node regions on the same side of the diaphragm
Stage III (1 and 2)	Involvement of lymph nodes on both sides of the diaphragm
Stage IV	Generalized involvement

Subclassifications include the following: A = no symptoms; B = fever, night sweats, >10% weight loss in prior 6 mo; X = bulky disease; E = involvement of single extranodal site; CS = clinical stage; PS = pathologic stage (determined by laparotomy).

Males have an increased incidence of HD (male-to-female ratio is 3:2), and the disease has two peaks of highest incidence. The first peak occurs during the second and third decades of life, and the second occurs after the fifth decade. Differences in clinical presentation in the two age groups have led some to speculate that these peaks may represent distinct disease entities.

CLINICAL MANIFESTATIONS

The most common presentation of HD is a painless enlargement of the lymph nodes in a patient without other symptoms of disease. The cervical lymph nodes are the initial sites of detection in more than 50% of cases. Early involvement of the axillary, inguinal, and mediastinal nodes also is common. Other patients may seek medical attention because of constitutional symptoms, such as fever, weight loss, pruritus, or night sweats. On examination, the involved peripheral nodes are nontender and feel rubbery. The presentation of asymptomatic enlarged lymph nodes is most common in younger patients with HD and is consistent with a histologic classification of lymphocyte predominance or nodular sclerosis. In older patients with increased risk of developing the lymphocyte depleted or mixed cellularity histologic pattern, systemic symptoms, such as malaise, fever, and night sweats, may precede noticeable lymphadenopathy.

As the disease progresses, signs and symptoms arise from pressure and obstruction caused by enlarging nodes. Enlarged mediastinal nodes cause dysphagia, whereas retroperitoneal nodes can cause ureteral obstruction. Further progression of the disease leads to invasion of the bone marrow, lungs, liver, bones, and spinal cord.

Characteristic clinical features of HD include the Pel-Ebstein fever, a cyclic spiking of high fever, and generalized severe pruritus of unknown etiology. Pruritus is a symptom seen most frequently in young women with HD. Many investigators of HD have demonstrated a defective functioning of T lymphocytes that results in a faulty delayed-type hypersensitivity reaction. Early in the course of HD, this immunodeficiency can be demonstrated by a decreased reaction to skin tests and prolonged survival of grafts from noncompatible donors. When the disease is generalized, the immunodeficiency leads to increased susceptibility to viral and fungal infections. Diagnosis of HD is always finalized by an adequate biopsy of enlarged lymphoid tissue. A needle biopsy does not provide sufficient tissue for this purpose. Demonstration of the characteristic Reed-Sternberg cells is diagnostic, but the nature of this cell's involvement is still controversial.

TREATMENT

The management of HD consists of radiotherapy, chemotherapy, or a combination of both, depending on the stage of the disease at time of diagnosis. Radiation therapy is used as initial treatment only for patients with low-risk stage IA and IIA disease. Currently, combination chemotherapy of doxorubicin, bleomycin, vincristine, and dacarbazine (ABVD) is used for most HD patients.[42] The combination of radiotherapy and chemotherapy is used for advanced disease, but it increases the chance of complications such as bone marrow aplasia and acute leukemia.[43] Five-year survival of patients with localized (IA or IIA) disease exceeds 80%, and the mean 5-year survival exceeds 50% for all stages of the disease.

Radiation commonly consists of 3,500 to 4,500 cGy delivered to the involved lymph node chain and contiguous areas. Three distinct radiation fields have been developed to treat HD: the mantle, para-aortic, and pelvic fields. The mantle field includes the submandibular region, neck, axillae, and mediastinum.

Non-Hodgkin's Lymphoma

The group of malignant disorders known as non-Hodgkin's lymphoma (NHL) arises from B or T lymphocytes. There are several classification systems in use for NHL. The disorders are variable in clinical presentation and course. The classification of the lymphomas is a controversial area undergoing evolution. The National Cancer Institute uses monoclonal-antibody immunophenotyping to characterize NHL according to biologic behavior. Low-grade NHL has a favorable prognosis, may respond to radiotherapy alone, and is localized in 10 to 25% of cases. Intermediate- and high-grade NHLs are treated with intensive chemotherapy regimens.

CLINICAL MANIFESTATIONS

The most common presentation of NHL is a painless persistent enlargement of the lymph nodes, but extranodal lesions occur more commonly than in HD, especially in the intermediate- and high-grade forms of the disease. NHL lesions may be detected in Waldeyer's ring, the gastrointestinal tract, the spleen, the skin, and bone marrow. NHL is more common in patients older than age 40 years but can occur at any age. In children, NHL may enter a leukemic phase, with malignant lymphocytes pouring into the peripheral blood. Signs and symptoms depend on the site of involvement and result from the pressure of enlarged lymph nodes or infiltration. Renal obstruction, neurologic impairment, liver or skin infiltration, and bone marrow involvement commonly occur during the course of the disease.

TREATMENT

Indolent lymphomas are usually not curable and are treated with palliative therapy. Within 1 to 3 years, the disease usually progresses and requires therapy. Radiation and chemotherapy are the most successful modes of treatment. Localized NHL is highly radiosensitive, so it is treated with 3,000 to 4,000 cGy to the involved area. Intensive combinations of chemotherapeutic drugs are the treatment of choice for intermediate- and high-grade NHL. The specific regimen used depends on the result of clinical staging and classification according to the Working Formulation of the National Cancer Institute. Cancer centers use several combinations of agents. Commonly used drug protocols include cyclophosphamide, vincristine, and prednisone (CVP); or cyclophosphamide, doxorubicin, vincristine, and prednisone (CHOP). A monoclonal antibody directed against the B-cell surface antigen CD20 has been shown to be effective for relapsed indolent lymphomas.[44] High-dose chemotherapy with autologous stem cell transplantation is the treatment of choice for patients with relapsed disease.

Burkitt's Lymphoma

During the 1950s, Denis Burkitt described rapidly growing jaw and abdominal lymphoid tumors in East African children. This neoplasm had a strict geographic distribution and occurred in zones where malaria was endemic. The tumor, named Burkitt's lymphoma (BL), is the human cancer most closely linked with a virus. Epstein-Barr virus is associated with 90% of African patients with BL, but this percentage is considerably lower for BL seen in other parts of the world. The reason for the association between BL and Epstein-Barr virus remains unknown. The virus may be a prime etiologic agent, a cocarcinogen, or just an innocent passenger. Since its original description by Burkitt, BL has been found in many countries outside Africa, including the United States. The primary tumor cell has been shown to be a poorly differentiated B lymphocyte.

CLINICAL MANIFESTATIONS

The African form of BL most frequently manifests itself as rapid-growing extranodal jaw tumors in young children, but it also may be first detected as an abdominal mass involving the kidneys or ovaries. Cases reported in the United States appear to follow a pattern that differs from the African disease. A majority of US cases involve abdominal lesions arising from Peyer's patches or mesenteric lymph nodes. The tumor expands rapidly and may double in size every 1 to 3 days, making it the fastest growing human cancer. This rapid growth nullifies the usefulness of the Ann Arbor classification used for other NHLs. BL patients are divided into two categories: small tumor burden and large tumor burden.

TREATMENT

BL lesions have a dramatic response to chemotherapy, particularly cyclophosphamide. The tumor also has been shown to be sensitive to methotrexate, vincristine, and cytarabine. Combinations of drugs have achieved remissions in more than 90% of patients. Half of the patients relapse but may respond to bone marrow transplantation. Surgical debulking of large localized jaw or abdominal tumors is beneficial prior to chemotherapy.

Oral and Dental Considerations

Asymptomatic enlargement of the cervical lymph node chains is a common early sign of lymphoma, and the dentist should play a significant role in early detection by routine examination of the neck. Suspicion of lymphoma should increase when lymphadenopathy appears without signs of infection, more than one lymph node chain is involved, or a lymph node of 1 cm or greater in diameter persists for more than 1 month. It is uncommon for primary lesions of HD to begin in an extranodal site, so primary jaw lesions are uncommon but have been reported. More commonly, dental complications result from radiotherapy or chemotherapy administered to children with HD during tooth development. These abnormalities include agenesis, hypoplasia, and blunted or thin roots. Extranodal primary NHL is reported more frequently. One common site for extranodal NHL is the lymphoid tissue of Waldeyer's ring; therefore, nontender enlargements of tonsillar tissue in adults should be referred for evaluation. NHL is more frequent in immunocompromised patients, including patients with acquired immunodeficiency syndrome (AIDS) and those receiving immunosuppressive drug therapy. NHL of the jaws and mouth, particularly the palate, has been reported by several authors. These palatal lesions have been described as slow-growing, painless, bluish, soft masses, and they have been confused with minor salivary gland tumors. Oral NHL also mimics inflammatory diseases and may present as a gingival mass, tongue mass, or intraosseous lesion. Isolated loose teeth, paresthesia of the face, and major salivary gland enlargement also may be presenting signs of NHL.

When lymphoma is included in the differential diagnosis of an oral lesion, a biopsy specimen which has not been traumatized should be taken from the center of the lesion and sent to an experienced pathologist. The pathologist should be informed of the possibility of lymphoma because NHL is easily confused with benign lymphoproliferative disorders. Special staining with Giemsa and periodic acid–Schiff and typing with immunohistochemistry are helpful in making the diagnosis of NHL. The use of these special studies has clarified the diagnosis of lesions that previously could not be properly classified. For example, midline lethal granuloma has recently been shown to be a form of NHL.

Oral lesions also have been described in patients with cutaneous T-cell lymphoma (mycosis fungoides). These lesions are often described as either indurated plaques with a red or white surface or ulcerated tumors. The most common site of involvement is the tongue and usually follow skin lesions.

▼ MULTIPLE MYELOMA

Multiple myeloma (MM) is a malignant neoplasm of plasma cells that is characterized by the production of pathologic M proteins, bone lesions, kidney disease, hyperviscosity, and hypercalcemia. Human leukocyte antigen studies suggest a genetic predisposition to the disease, which occurs equally in both sexes, most often in patients older than 50 years of age. Skeletal pain is the most common presenting symptom and is caused by bone lysis that may result either directly from accumulation of tumor cells or indirectly from osteoclast-activating factors secreted by the malignant myeloma cells. Approximately 80% of patients with MM have bone lesions, and pathologic fractures are a frequent complication. Often the disease is detected during radiologic examination for other purposes. The most common radiographic abnormality is the presence of "punched-out" radiolucent lesions (plasmacytomas), but generalized osteoporosis may occur in the absence of these discrete punched-out lesions (Figure 16-15).

Proliferation of abnormal plasma cells causes most of the manifestations of the disease. These plasma cells produce abnormal M proteins that are useful in the diagnosis of the disease due to their characteristic electrophoretic pattern but useless in functioning as normal antibodies. Hypogammaglobulinemia results in increased susceptibility to bacterial infections, particularly of the lungs and urinary tract.

Renal failure also is a common complication resulting from a combination of amyloidosis, hypercalcemia, and infiltration of malignant cells. Amyloid also may deposit in the heart, liver, nervous system, or other organs, interfering with normal function. Deposition of this amorphous protein under the skin or mucosa also is common. Clotting defects result from the abnormal myeloma (M) proteins coating platelets or interfering with the normal coagulation cascade.

Diagnosis is based on serum M proteins demonstrated with serum protein electrophoresis or immunoelectrophoresis, or on Bence Jones proteins, which are monoclonal immunoglobulin light chains detected in 24-hour urine specimens. Bone marrow biopsy results reveal atypical plasma cells.

Treatment

The alkylating agents, such as melphalan or cyclophosphamide, are the treatment of choice for patients with extensive bone lesions or rising levels of M proteins. Local symptomatic lesions are treated with radiotherapy. Average survival with treatment is 2 to 3 years, but with the introduction of newer chemotherapeutic agents, the time of survival is increasing; some patients have remissions of 6 years or more. A common cause of death is the myeloma kidney, caused by the accumulation of abnormal proteins in the renal tissue.[45]

Oral Manifestations

Approximately 5 to 30% of myeloma patients have jaw lesions, and accidental discovery of lesions in the jaws may be the first evidence of this disease. The patient may experience pain, swelling, numbness of the jaws, epulis formation, or unexplained mobility of the teeth. Skull lesions are more common than jaw lesions. Multiple radiolucent lesions of varying size, with ill-defined margins and a lack of circumferential osteosclerotic activity, should suggest this diagnosis (see Figure 16-15).

The mandible is more frequently involved in MM because of its greater content of marrow. Lesions are most common in the region of the angle of the jaw, where red marrow generally is present. In most instances, the lesions appear unassociated with the apices of the teeth. Extraosseous lesions also occur in a significant number of patients (Figure 16-16) although a majority of the lesions are asymptomatic.

Several authors have called attention to the development of oral amyloidosis as a complication of this disease. Tongue biopsy is an excellent method of diagnosis. Clinically, the tongue may be enlarged and studded with small garnet-colored enlargements, including nodes on the cheeks and lips. Amyloidosis occurs in 6 to 15% of patients with MM and may be detected in tissue specimens with use of a Congo red stain or electron microscopy. When a dentist is requested to take a biopsy specimen to detect amyloidosis, the specimen must include muscle tissue from the mucobuccal fold or tongue.

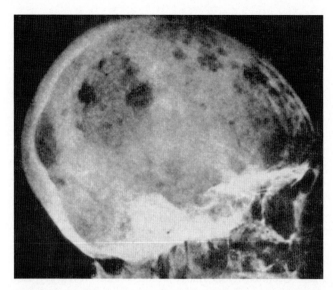

FIGURE 16-15 Radiograph of the skull discloses widely distributed lesions in multiple myeloma. (Reproduced with permission from Calman HI. Oral Surg. 5:1308.)

Dental Management

Hemorrhage and infection are the dentist's major concerns when treating a patient with MM. Bleeding may result from several causes, including thrombocytopenia, abnormal platelet function, abnormal coagulation, or hyperviscosity. If surgery is necessary, recent results of platelet count, bleeding time, prothrombin time, and partial thromboplastin time should be obtained. If hyperviscosity is present, excess bleeding may occur even if these tests are normal, and a hematology consultation should be considered.

The dentist also should determine whether the patient has an increased susceptibility to bacterial infection due to hyper-gammaglobulinemia, bone marrow failure, or complications of cancer chemotherapy. A consultation with the managing oncologist is indicated to determine whether there is evidence of renal failure or complications of hyperviscosity, such as heart or pulmonary failure.

▼ REFERENCES

1. Papayannopoulou T, Abkowitz J, D'Andrea A. Biology of erythropoiesis, erythroid differentiation and maturation. In: Hoffman R, Benz EJ, Shattil SJ, et al, editors. Hematology: basic principles and practice. 3rd ed. New York: Churchill Livingstone; 2000. p. 202.
2. Berlin NI. Polycythemia vera. Semin Hematol 1997;34:1–5.
3. Pearson TC. Apparent polycythemia. Blood Rev 1991;5:205–13.
4. Cook JD, Skikne BS, Baynes RD. Iron deficiency: the global perspective. Adv Exp Med Biol 1994;356:219–28.
5. Provan D. Mechanisms and management of iron deficinecy anemia. Br J Haematol 1999;105 Suppl 1:19–26.
6. Besa EL, Kim PW, Havran FL. Treatment of primary defective iron-reutilization syndrome: revisited. Ann Hematol 2000;79:465–8.
7. Lindenbaum J. An approach to anemias. In: Bennett JC, Plum F, editors. Cecil textbook of medicine. 20th ed. Philadelphia: WB Saunders Co.; 1996. p. 823.
8. Socie G, Mary JY, deGramont A, et al. Paroxysmal noncturnal hemoglobinuria: long-term follow up and prognostic factors. Lancet 1996;348:573–7.
9. Chang JG, Liu TC. Glucose-6-phosphate dehydrogenase deficiency. Crit Rev Oncol Hematol 1995;20:1–7.
10. Steinberg MH. Management of sickle cell disease. N Engl J Med 1999;340;1021–30.
11. Walters MC. Collaborative multicenter investigation of marrow transplantation for sickle cell disease: current results and future directions. Biol Blood Marrow Transplant 1997;3:310–5.
12. Clarke GM, Higgins TN. Laboratory investigation of hemoglobinopathies and thalassemias: review and update. Clin Chem 2000;46:1284–90.
13. Lucarelli G. Bone marrow transplantation in adult thalassemia patients. N Engl J Med 1999;93:1164–7.
14. Wickramasinghe SN. Morphology, biology, and biochemistry of cobalamin- and folate-deficient bone marrow cells. Ballieres Clin Haematol 1995;8:441–59.

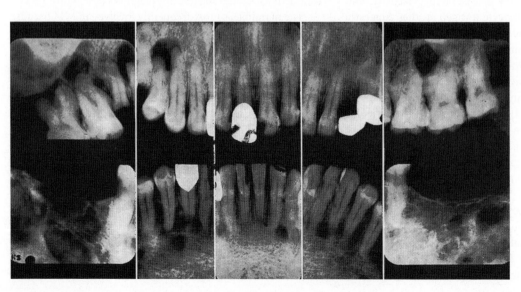

FIGURE 16-16 Intraoral radiographic series showing multiple involvement of the maxilla and the mandible in multiple myeloma. (Reproduced with permission from Calman HI. Oral Surg;5:1034.)

15. Greenberg MS. Clinical and histologic changes of the oral mucosa in pernicious anemia. Oral Surg Oral Med Oral Pathol 1981;52:38–42.

16. Waters HM, Dawson DW, Howarth JE, Geary CG. High incidence of type II autoantibodies in pernicious anemia. J Clin Pathol 1993;46:45–7.

17. Carmel R, Herbert V. Intrinsic factor antibody in saliva of a patient with pernicious anemia. Lancet 1967;1:80–1.

18. Ogawa M. Differentiation and proliferation of hematopoietic stem cells. Blood 1993;81:2844–53.

19. Malech HL, Gallin JI. Current concepts: neutrophils in human disease. N Engl J Med 1987;317:687–94.

20. Stock W, Hoffman R. White blood cells 1: non-malignant disorders. Lancet 2000;355:1351–7.

21. Shastri KA, Logue GM. Autoimmune neutropenia. Blood 1993;81:1984–95.

22. Stroncek DF. Drug-induced immune neutropenia. Tranfus Med Rev 1993;7:268–74.

23. Welte K, Dale D. Pathophysiology and treatment of severe chronic neutropenia. Ann Hematol 1996;72:158–65.

24. Freedman MH. Safety of long-term administration of granulocyte colony-stimulating factor for severe neutropenia. Curr Opin Hematol 1997;4:217–24.

25. Wahlin YB. Effects of chlorhexidine mouthrinse on oral health in patients with acute leukemia. Oral Surg 1989;68:279–87.

26. Palmer SE, Stephens K, Dale DC. Genetics, phenotype, and natural history of autosomal dominant cyclic hematopoiesis. Am J Med Genet 1996;66:413–22.

27. Freifeld AG, Pizzo PA. The outpatient management of febrile neutropenia in cancer patients. Oncology 1996;10:599–612.

28. Golub TR, Barker GF, Stegmaier K, Gilliland DG. The TEL gene contributes to the pathogenesis of myeloid and lymphoid leukemias by diverse molecular genetic mechanisms. Curr Top Microbiol Immunol 1997;220:67–79.

29. Misumi DJ, Nagle DL, McGrail SH. The physical and genetic map surrounding the LYST gene on mouse chromosome 13. Genomics 1997;40:147–50.

30. Barrat FJ, LeDeist F, Bankerrov M, et al. Defective CTLA-4 cycling pathway in Chédiak-Higashi syndrome: a possible mechanism for deregulation of T lymphocyte activation. Proc Natl Acad Sci U S A 1999;96:8645–50.

31. Shibutani T, Gen K, Shibata M, et al. Long-term follow up of periodontitis in a patient with Chédiak-Higashi syndrome. A case report. J Periodontol 2000;71:1024–8.

32. Heaney ML. Myelodysplasias. N Engl J Med 1999;340:1649–60.

33. Lowenberg B, Downing JR, Burnett HA. Acute myeloid leukemia. N Engl J Med 1999;341:1051–62.

34. Grimwade D. The importance of diagnostic cytogenetics on outcome in AML: analysis of 1612 patients entered into the MRC AML 10 Trial. Blood 1998;92:2322–33.

35. Kurzrock R, Gutterman JU, Talpaz M. The molecular genetics of Philadelphia chromosome positive leukemias. N Engl J Med 1988;319:990–8.

36. Sawyers CL. Chronic myeloid leukemia. N Engl J Med 1999;340:1330–40.

37. Faderl S, Talpaz M, Estrov Z, et al. The biology of chronic myeloid leukemia. N Engl J Med 1999;341:164–72.

38. Cheson BD, Bennet JM, Grever M, et al. National Cancer Institute–sponsored working group guidelines for chronic-lymphocytic leukemia: revised guidelines for diagnosis and treatment. Blood 1996;87:4990–7.

39. Robertson LE, Huh YO, Butler JJ. Response assessment in chronic lymphocytic leukemia after fludarabine plus prednisone: clinical, pathologic, immunophenotypic and molecular analysis. Blood 1992;80:29–36.

40. Saven A. Long-term follow up of patients with hairy cell leukemia after cladribine treatment. Blood 1998;92:1918–26.

41. Lister TA, Crowther D. Staging for Hodgkin's disease. Semin Oncol 1990;17:696–703.

42. Andre M. Comparison of high-dose therapy and autologous stem-cell transplantation with conventional therapy for Hodgkin's disease induction failures: a case-control study. J Clin Oncol 1999;17:222–9.

43. Aisenberg AC. Problems in Hodgkin's disease management. Blood 1999;93:761–9.

44. Mclaughlin P. Rituximab chimeric anti-CD20 monoclonal antibody therapy for relapsed indolent lymphomas: half of patients respond to a four-dose treatment program. J Clin Oncol 1998;16:2825–33.

45. Bataille R. Multiple myeloma. N Engl J Med 1997; 336:1657–64.

17

BLEEDING AND CLOTTING DISORDERS

LAUREN L. PATTON, DDS

Dental health care workers are increasingly called upon to provide quality dental care to individuals whose bleeding and clotting mechanisms have been altered by inherited or acquired diseases. This provides an opportunity for the dentist who is trained in the recognition of oral and systemic signs of altered hemostasis to assist in the diagnosis of the underlying condition. A number of dental procedures result in the risk of bleeding that can have serious consequences, such as severe hemorrhage or possibly death, for the patient with a bleeding disorder. Safe dental care may require consultation with the patient's physician, systemic management, and dental treatment modifications.

Of the inherited coagulopathies, von Willebrand's disease (vWD) is the most common. It results from deficiency of von Willebrand's factor (vWF) and affects about 0.8 to 1% of the population.[1] Hemophilia A, caused by coagulation factor (F) VIII deficiency, is the next most common, followed by hemophilia B, a F IX deficiency. The age-adjusted prevalence of hemophilia in six surveillance states in 1994 was 13.4 cases in 100,000 males (10.5 for hemophilia A and 2.9 for hemophilia B).[2] Application to the US population resulted in an estimated national prevalence of 13,320 cases of hemophilia A and 3,640 cases of hemophilia B, with an incidence rate of 1 per 5,032 live male births. Hemophilia A was predominant, accounting for 79% of all hemophiliacs, and prevalence of disease severity was 43% severe (< 1% F VIII), 26% moderate (1–5% F VIII), and 31% with mild (6–30% F VIII) disease.[2]

Acquired coagulation disorders can result from drug actions or side effects, or underlying systemic disease. A stratified household sample of 4,163 community residents aged 65 years or older living in a five-county area of North Carolina revealed 51.7% to be taking one or more medications (aspirin, warfarin, dipyridamole, nonsteroidal anti-inflammatory drugs

[NSAIDs], or heparin) with the potential to alter hemostasis.[3] The use of coumarin anticoagulants is increasing as a result of their demonstrated effectiveness in the treatment of atrial fibrillation and venous thromboembolism, and control of thrombosis in the presence of a mechanical heart valve.[4]

▼ PATHOPHYSIOLOGY

Basic Mechanisms of Hemostasis and Their Interactions

Interaction of several basic mechanisms produces normal hemostasis. For clarity and understanding, these are presented separately. Hemostasis can be divided into four general phases: the vascular phase; the platelet phase; the coagulation cascade phase, consisting of intrinsic, extrinsic, and common pathways; and the fibrinolytic phase. The first three phases are the principal mechanisms that stop the loss of blood following vascular injury. Briefly, when vessel integrity is disrupted, platelets are activated, adhere to the site of injury, and form a platelet plug that reduces or temporarily arrests blood loss.[5] The exposure of collagen and activation of platelets also initiates the coagulation cascade, which leads to fibrin formation and the generation of an insoluble fibrin clot that strengthens the platelet plug.[5] Fibrinolysis is the major means of disposing of fibrin after its hemostatic function has been fulfilled, and it can be considered the rate-limiting step in clotting. It leads to fibrin degradation by the proteolytic enzyme plasmin. As seen in Figure 17-1, multiple processes occur either simultaneously or in rapid sequence, such that, following almost immediate vascular contraction, platelets begin to aggregate at the wound site. The coagulation cascade is underway within 10 to 20 seconds of injury, an initial hemostatic plug is formed in 1 to 3 minutes, and fibrin has been generated and added to stabilize the clot by 5 to 10 minutes.

Vascular Phase

After tissue injury, there is an immediate reflex vasoconstriction that may alone be hemostatic in small vessels. Reactants such as serotonin, histamine, prostaglandins, and other materials are vasoactive and produce vasoconstriction of the microvascular bed in the area of the injury.

Platelet Phase

When circulating platelets are exposed to damaged vascular surfaces (in the presence of functionally normal vWF, endothelial cells, collagen or collagen-like materials, basement membrane, elastin, microfibrils, and other cellular debris), platelets are activated to experience physical and chemical changes.[6] These changes produce an environment that causes the platelets to undergo the aggregation-and-release phenomenon and form the primary vascular plug that reduces blood loss from small blood vessels and capillaries. These platelet plugs adhere to exposed basement membranes. As this reaction is occurring, the release reaction is underway, involving the intracellular release of active

components for further platelet aggregation as well as promotion of the clotting mechanism. Adenosine diphosphate (ADP) is a potent nucleotide that activates and recruits other platelets in the area, immensely adding to the size of the plug. Platelet factor 3 (PF3) is the intracellular phospholipid that activates F X and subsequently results in the conversion of prothrombin to thrombin. Additionally, the platelet plug, intermixed with fibrin and cellular components such as red and white cells, contracts to further reduce blood loss and to seal the vascular bed.

Coagulation Phase

The generation of thrombin and fibrin the end product of the third phase of hemostasis, the coagulation phase. This process involves multiple proteins, many of which are synthesized by the liver (fibrinogen, prothrombin, Fs V, VII, IX, X, XI, XII, and XIII) and are vitamin K dependent (Fs II, VII, IX, and X). The process of coagulation essentially involves three separate pathways. It initially proceeds by two separate pathways (intrinsic and extrinsic) that converge by activating a third (common) pathway.

The blood clotting mechanism is the most studied unit; it was outlined originally in 1903 by Markowitz as the prothrombin-to-thrombin and fibrinogen-to-fibrin conversion system. In 1964, the "cascade" or "waterfall" theory was proposed.[7,8] It offered a useful device for understanding this complex system and its control, as well as the clinically important associated laboratory tests.

Figure 17-2 depicts the sequence of interactions between the various clotting factors following injury of tissue. The scheme of reaction is a bioamplification, in which a precursor is altered to an active form, which, in turn, activates the next precursor in the sequence. Beginning with an undetectable biochemical reaction, the coagulation mechanism results in a final explosive change of a liquid to a gel. The major steps involve the conversion of a precursor protein to an "activated" form, which activates another precursor protein, and so on down the cascade. The coagulation of blood also requires the presence of both calcium ions and phospholipid (or a phospholipid-containing membrane fragment derived from blood platelets).

The intrinsic pathway is initiated when F XII is activated by surface contact (eg, with collagen or subendothelium), and it involves the interaction of F XII and F XI. The next step of intrinsic coagulation, the activation of F IX to F XIa, requires a divalent cation.[9] Once activated, F IXa forms a complex with F VIII, in a reaction that requires the presence of both calcium ions and phospholipid, which, in turn, converts F X to an activated form— F Xa.

The extrinsic pathway is initiated by the release of tissue thromboplastin, also called tissue factor, and does not require contact activation. Tissue thromboplastin binds to F VII in the presence of calcium, and this complex is capable of activating Fs IX and X, linking the intrinsic and extrinsic pathways.

It is the activation of X that begins the common pathway. Once activated, F Xa converts prothrombin to thrombin in a reaction similar to the activation of F X by F IXa. The

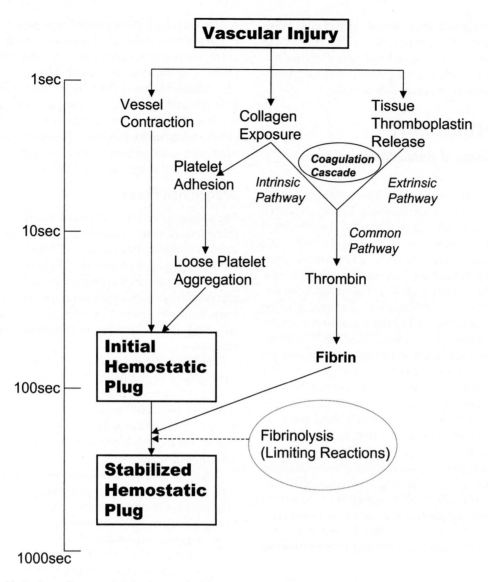

FIGURE 17-1 Mechanisms of hemostasis following vascular injury.

activation of prothrombin by F Xa requires the presence of calcium ions and phospholipid as well as F V, a plasma protein cofactor.[10] Once formed, thrombin converts fibrinogen, a soluble plasma protein, to insoluble fibrin. Fibrin polymerizes to form a gel, stabilizing the platelet plug. Finally, F XIII, which has been converted to an activated form by thrombin,[11] produces covalent cross-links between the fibrin molecules that strengthen the clot and make it more resistant to lysis by plasmin. Individuals deficient in this clotting factor experience poor wound healing.[12]

Fibrinolytic Phase

The fourth phase of hemostasis is fibrinolysis; this is considered the major means of disposing of fibrin after its hemostatic function has been fulfilled. Once the microvascular bed is sealed and primary hemostasis is complete, the secondary hemostasis pathway has already commenced in parallel. As the monomeric fibrin is cross-linked with the aid of F XIII (fibrin-

stabilizing factor), the propagation of the formed clot is limited by several interactions.[12] One of these limiting systems is the fibrinolytic system (Figure 17-3). Kallikrein, which is an intrinsic activator of plasminogen, is generated when prekallikrein is bound to kininogen, thereby becoming a substrate for F XIIa. Tissue plasminogen activator (TPA) is released from the endothelial cells and converts plasminogen to plasmin that degrades fibrinogen and fibrin into fibrin degradation products (FDPs). TPA is a proteolytic enzyme that is nonspecific and also degrades Fs VIII and V. Regulation of this system is controlled tightly by plasminogen activator inhibitor that limits TPA, and by α_2-antiplasmin that restricts plasmin. TPA has been used with great success in therapeutic doses to lyse thrombi in individuals with thromboembolic disorders associated with myocardial infarction.[13] Effectiveness of this drug is limited to the first 6 hours post infarction.

Extended function of the fibrinolytic system is realized during wound healing. As the wound is revascularized and

Coagulation Cascade

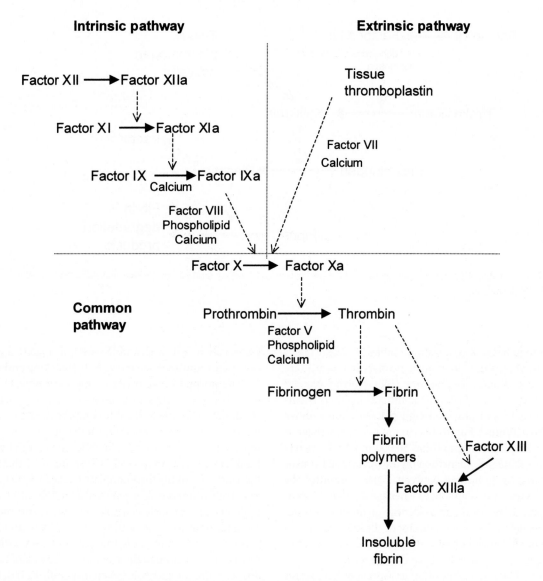

FIGURE 17-2 The coagulation cascade. *Solid arrow* (⟶) indicates conversion; *broken arrow* (- - ➤) indicates catalytic action.

the capillary beds extend into the fibrin clot, the way for plasmin to remove the cross-linked fibrin is paved by the release of TPA. Without this unique system, wound healing would be impossible. While the fibrinolytic system limits the coagulation process as described above, other systems function to limit the extent of the microvascular thrombosis in the area of injury. Antithrombin III is a potent inhibitor directed at thrombin.

▼ CLINICAL AND LABORATORY FINDINGS

Clinical Manifestations

Clinical manifestations of bleeding disorders can involve various systems, depending on the extent and type of disease.

Individuals with mild disease may present with no clinical signs, whereas individuals with severe coagulopathies may have definite stigmata. When skin and mucosa are involved, individuals may present with petechiae, ecchymoses, spider angiomas, hematomas, or jaundice. Deep dissecting hematomas and hemarthroses of major joints may affect severe hemophiliacs and result in disability or death. Disorders of platelet quantity may result in hepatosplenomegaly, spontaneous gingival bleeding, and risk of hemorrhagic stroke. Table 17-1 illustrates clinical features that distinguish coagulation disorders from platelet or vascular disorders.

Clinical Laboratory Tests

There are a variety of common and less common laboratory tests that help to identify deficiency of required elements or dys-

Fibrinolytic System

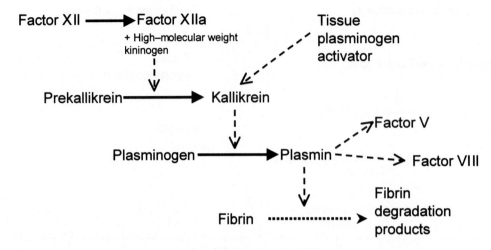

FIGURE 17-3 The fibrinolytic system. *Thin solid arrow* (——▶) indicates conversion; *broken arrow* (--▶) indicates catalytic actions; *dotted arrow* (·····▶) indicates degradation.

function of the phases of coagulation (Tables 17-2 and 17-3). The two clinical tests used to evaluate primary hemostasis are the platelet count and bleeding time (BT). Normal platelet counts are 150,000 to 450,000/mm³. Spontaneous clinical hemorrhage is usually not observed with platelet counts above 10,000 to 20,000/mm³. Surgical or traumatic hemorrhage is more likely with platelet counts below 50,000/mm³. BT is determined from a standardized incision on the forearm. BT is usually considered to be normal between 1 and 6 minutes (by modified Ivy's test) and is prolonged when greater than 15 minutes. The skin BT test, thought to identify qualitative or functional platelet defects, is a poor indicator of clinically significant bleeding at other sites, and its use as a predictive screening test for oral surgical procedures has been discouraged.[14]

Tests to evaluate the status of other aspects of hemostasis include prothrombin time (PT)/international normalized ratio (INR), activated partial thromboplastin time (aPTT), thrombin time (TT), FDPs, specific coagulation factor assays

(especially Fs VII, VIII, and IX and fibrinogen), and coagulation factor inhibitor screening tests (blocking antibodies).

The normal range of PT is approximately 11 to 13 seconds. Because of individual laboratory reagent variability and the desire to be able to reliably compare the PT from one laboratory to that from another, the PT test is now commonly reported with its INR.[15,16] The INR, introduced by the World Health Organization in 1983, is the ratio of PT that adjusts for the sensitivity of the thromboplastin reagents, such that a normal coagulation profile is reported as an INR of 1.0.[17] This test evaluates the extrinsic coagulation system and measures the presence or absence of clotting Fs I, II, V, VII, and X. Its most common use is to measure the effects of coumarin anticoagulants and reduction of the vitamin K–dependent Fs II, VII, IX, and X. Since the extrinsic system uses only Fs I, II, VII, and X, it does not measure the reduction of Fs VIII or IX, which characterizes hemophilias A and B. Additionally, the PT is used to measure the metabolic aspects of protein synthesis in the liver.

TABLE 17-1 Clinical Features of Bleeding Disorders

Feature	Vascular or Platelet Disorders	Coagulation Disorders
Bleeding from superficial cuts and scratches	Persistent, often perfuse	Minimal
Delayed bleeding	Rare	Common
Spontaneous gingival bleeding	Characteristic	Rare
Petechiae	Characteristic	Rare
Ecchymoses	Characteristic, usually small and multiple	Characteristic, usually large and solitary
Epistaxis	Common	Common
Deep dissecting hematomas	Rare	Characteristic
Hemarthroses	Rare	Characteristic

TABLE 17-2 Laboratory Tests for Assessing Hemostasis

Test	Normal Range
Platelet count	150,000 to 450,000/mm^3
Bleeding time	< 7 min (by simplate); 1–6 min (modified Ivy's test)
Prothrombin time/international normalized ratio	Control ± 1 s (eg, PT: 11–13 s/INR 1.0)
Activated partial thromboplastin time	Comparable to control (eg, 15–35 s)
Thrombin time	Control ± 3 s (eg, 9–13 s)
Fibrin degradation products	< 10 µg/dL
Fibrinogen assay	200–400 mg/dL
von Willebrand's antigen	60–150% vWF activity
Coagulation factor assays (eg, F VIII assay)	60–100% F VIII activity
Coagulation factor inhibitor assays (eg, Bethesda inhibitor assay for F VIII)	0.0 Bethesda inhibitor units

F = factor; INR = international normalized ratio; PT = prothrombin time; vWF = von Willebrand's factor.

The aPTT is considered normal if the control aPTT and the test aPTT are within 10 seconds of each other. Control aPTT times are usually 15 to 35 seconds. Normal ranges depend on the manufacturer's limits; each supplier varies slightly. The unactivated PTT was originally described by Langdell and associates in 1953 as a simple one-stage assay for measuring F VIII.[18] Now it is used to evaluate the intrinsic cascade and

TABLE 17-3 Results of Hemostatic Screening Tests for Selected Bleeding Disorders

	Screening Laboratory Test			
Bleeding Disorder	Platelet Count	PT/INR	aPTT	BT
Thrombocytopenia Leukemia	↓	N	N	↑
F VIII, IX, XI deficiency Heparin anticoagulation	N	N	↑	N
F II, V, X deficiency Vitamin K deficiency Intestinal malabsorption	N	↑	↑	N
F VII deficiency Coumarin anticoagulation Liver disease	N	↑	N	N
von Willebrand's disease	N, ↓	N	N, ↑	↑
DIC Severe liver disease	↓	↑	↑	↑
F XIII deficiency	N	N	N	N
Vascular wall defect	N	N	N	↑

aPTT = activated partial thromboplastin time; BT = bleeding time; DIC = disseminated intravascular coagulation; INR = international normalized ratio; N = normal; PT = prothrombin time; ↑ = increased; ↓ = decreased.

measure the functional levels of Fs VIII, IX, XI, and XII. Since the addition of the activator (a rare earth), the test no longer measures Fs XI and XII. As a screening test, the aPTT is prolonged only when the factor levels in the intrinsic and common pathways are less than about 30%. It is altered in hemophilias A and B and with the use of the anticoagulant heparin.

The TT is used specifically to test the ability to form the initial clot from fibrinogen and is considered normal in the range of 9 to 13 seconds. Additionally, it is used to measure the presence of heparin, FDPs, or other paraproteins that inhibit conversion of fibrinogen to fibrin. Fibrinogen can also be specifically assayed and should be present at a level of 200 to 400 mg/dL.

FDPs are measured using a specific latex agglutination system to evaluate the presence of the D dimer of fibrinogen and/or fibrin above normal levels. Such presence indicates that intravascular lysis has taken place or is occurring. This state can result from primary fibrinolytic disorders or disseminated intravascular coagulation (DIC). DIC is a catastrophic state that may result from massive trauma, extensive and terminal metastatic cancer, or fulminant viral or bacterial infections. DIC is rarely seen in the practice of dentistry, but it can occur.

To further identify factor deficiencies and their level of severity, specific activity levels of factors can be measured. Normal factor activity is usually in the 60 to 150% range. Inhibitor screening tests are essential when sufficient factor concentrate to correct the factor deficiency under normal conditions fails to control bleeding. To identify the specific type of von Willebrand's disease (types I–III and platelet type), additional studies such as the ristocetin cofactor, ristocetin-induced platelet aggregation studies, and monomer studies are helpful.

The tourniquet test for capillary fragility, which assesses the Rumpel-Leede phenomenon, is useful for identifying disorders of vascular wall integrity or platelet disorders. Stasis is produced by inflating a sphygmomanometer cuff around the arm in the usual manner to a pressure halfway between systolic and diastolic levels. This moderate degree of stasis is maintained for 5 minutes. At 2 minutes following cuff deflation and removal, a 2.5 cm diameter region (size of a quarter) of skin on the volar surface of the arm at 4 cm distal to the antecubital fossa is observed for petechial hemorrhages. Normally petechiae in men do not exceed five, and in women and children they do not exceed 10.

▼ CLASSIFICATION OF BLEEDING DISORDERS

Vessel Wall Disorders

Vessel wall disorders can result in hemorrhagic features. Bleeding is usually mild and confined to the skin, mucosa, and gingiva. Vascular purpura can result from damage to capillary endothelium, from abnormalities in the vascular subendothelial matrix or extravascular connective tissue bed, or from abnormal vessel formation. The pathogenesis of bleeding is not well defined in many conditions, and the capillary fragility test is the only test to demonstrate abnormal results.

Scurvy, resulting from dietary deficiency of water-soluble vitamin C, is found primarily in regions of urban poverty, among either infants on nonsupplemented processed milk formulas, elderly who cook for themselves, or adults with alcohol or drug dependencies.[19,20] Many of the hemorrhagic features of scurvy result from defects in collagen synthesis. Vitamin C is necessary for the synthesis of hydroxyproline, an essential constituent of collagen. One of the first clinical signs is petechial hemorrhages at the hair follicles and purpura on the back of the lower extremities that coalesce to form ecchymoses. Hemorrhage can occur in the muscles, joints, nail beds, and gingival tissues. Gingival involvement may include swelling, friability, bleeding, secondary infection, and loosening of teeth.[20] Scurvy results when dietary vitamin C falls below 10 mg/d. Implementation of a diet rich in vitamin C and administration of 1 g/d of vitamin C supplements provides rapid resolution.

Cushing's syndrome, resulting from excessive exogenous or endogenous corticosteroid intake or production, leads to general protein wasting and atrophy of supporting connective tissue around blood vessels. Patients may show skin bleeding or easy bruising. Aging causes similar perivascular connective-tissue atrophy and lack of skin mobility. Tears in small blood vessels can result in irregularly shaped purpuric areas on arms and hands, called purpura senilis. Other metabolic or inflammatory disorders resulting in purpura include Schönlein-Henoch or anaphylactoid purpura, hyperglobulinemic purpura, Waldenström's macroglobulinemia, multiple myeloma, amyloidosis, and cryoglobulinemia.

Ehlers-Danlos syndrome is an inherited disorder of connective-tissue matrix, generally resulting in fragile skin blood vessels and easy bruising. It is characterized by hyperelasticity of the skin and hypermobile joints. Eleven subtypes have been identified with unique biochemical defects and varying clinical features.[21] Type I is the classic form, with soft velvety hyperextensible skin, easy bruising and scarring, hypermobile joints, varicose veins, and prematurity. Type VIII has skin findings similar to those in type I, with easy bruising following minor trauma, and is characterized by early-onset periodontal disease with loss of permanent dentition.[22] Children with type VII syndrome may present with microdontia and collagen-related dentinal structural defects in primary teeth, in addition to bleeding after tooth brushing.[23] Other oral findings include fragility of the oral mucosa, gingiva, and teeth, as well as hypermobility of the temporomandibular joint, and stunted teeth and pulp stones on dental radiographs.[24,25]

Rendu-Osler-Weber syndrome, also called hereditary hemorrhagic telangiectasia, is a group of autosomal dominant disorders with abnormal telangiectatic capillaries, frequent episodes of nasal and gastrointestinal bleeding, and associated brain and pulmonary lesions.[26,27] Perioral and intraoral angiomatous nodules or telangiectases are common with progressive disease, involving areas of the lips, tongue, and palate that may bleed with manipulation during dental procedures.[28] Diagnosis is facilitated by the history and the observation of multiple nonpulsating vascular lesions, where arterioles connect to venules representing small arteriovenous malformations. These lesions blanch in response to applied pressure, unlike petechiae or ecchymoses. Mucocutaneous lesions may bleed profusely with minor trauma or, occasionally, spontaneously.[29] Persistently bleeding lesions may be treated with cryotherapy, laser ablation, electrocoagulation, or resection.[30] Blood replacement and iron therapy may be necessary following dental extractions in involved areas.[29]

Platelet Disorders

Platelet disorders may be divided into two categories by etiology—congenital and acquired—and into two additional categories by type—thrombocytopenias and thrombocytopathies (Table 17-4). Thrombocytopenias occur when platelet quantity is reduced and are caused by one of three mechanisms: decreased production in the bone marrow, increased sequestration in the spleen, or accelerated destruction. Thrombocytopathies, or qualitative platelet disorders, may result from defects in any of the three critical platelet reactions: adhesion, aggregation, or granule release. Dysfunctional platelet mechanisms may occur in isolated disorders or in conjunction with dysfunctional coagulation mechanisms.

TABLE 17-4   Classification of Platelet Disorders

Congenital
    Thrombocytopenic—quantitative platelet deficiency
        May-Hegglin anomaly
        Wiskott-Aldrich syndrome
        Neonatal alloimmune thrombocytopenia

    Nonthrombocytopenic—qualitative or functional platelet defect
        Glanzmann's thrombasthenia
        Platelet-type von Willebrand's disease
        Bernard-Soulier syndrome

Acquired
    Thrombocytopenic—quantitative platelet deficiency
        Autoimmune or idiopathic thrombocytopenia purpura
        Thrombotic thrombocytopenia purpura
        Cytotoxic chemotherapy
        Drug-induced (eg, quinine, quinidine, gold salts, trimethoprim/
            sulfamethoxazole, rifampin)
        Leukemia
        Aplastic anemia
        Myelodysplasia
        Systemic lupus erythematosus
        Associated with infection: HIV, mononucleosis, malaria
        Disseminated intravascular coagulation

    Nonthrombocytopenic—qualitative or functional platelet defect
        Drug-induced (eg, by aspirin, NSAIDs, penicillin, cephalosporins)
        Uremia
        Alcohol dependency
        Liver disease
        Myeloma, myeloproliferative disorders, macroglobulinemia
        Acquired platelet-type von Willebrand's disease

HIV=human immunodeficiency virus; NSAIDs = nonsteroidal anti-inflammatory drugs.

CONGENITAL PLATELET DISORDERS

Congenital abnormalities of platelet function or production are rare. Glanzmann's thrombasthenia is a qualitative disorder characterized by a deficiency in the platelet membrane glycoproteins IIb and IIIa.[31–33] Clinical signs include bruising, epistaxis, gingival hemorrhage, and menorrhagia. Treatment of oral surgical bleeding involves platelet transfusion and use of antifibrinolytics and local hemostatic agents. Wiskott-Aldrich syndrome is characterized by cutaneous eczema (usually beginning on the face), thrombocytopenic purpura, and an increased susceptibility to infection due to an immunologic defect.[34] Oral manifestations include gingival bleeding and palatal petechiae. May-Hegglin anomaly is a rare hereditary condition characterized by the triad of thrombocytopenia, giant platelets, and inclusion bodies in leukocytes. Clinical features and the pathogenesis of bleeding in this disease are poorly defined.[35] Bernard-Soulier syndrome and platelet-type vWD also result from identified defects in platelet membrane glycoproteins.[36] Unlike the other types of vWD, the platelet type is rare and presents with less severe clinical bleeding.

ACQUIRED PLATELET DISORDERS

Two of the most commonly encountered platelet disorders, idiopathic or immune thrombocytopenia purpura (ITP) and thrombotic thrombocytopenia purpura (TTP), have clinical symptoms including petechiae and purpura over the chest, neck, and limbs—usually more severe on the lower extremities. Mucosal bleeding may occur in the oral cavity and gastrointestinal and genitourinary tracts.

ITP may be acute and self-limiting (2 to 6 weeks) in children. In adults, ITP is typically more indolent in its onset, and the course is persistent, often lasting many years, and may be characterized by recurrent exacerbations of disease. In severe cases of ITP, oral hematomas and hemorrhagic bullae may be the presenting clinical sign.[37,38] Most patients with chronic ITP are young women. Intracerebral hemorrhage, although rare, is the most common cause of death. ITP is assumed to be caused by accelerated antibody-mediated platelet consumption. The natural history and long-term prognosis of adults with chronic ITP remain incompletely defined.[39] ITP may be a component of other systemic diseases. Autoimmune thrombocytopenia associated with systemic lupus erythematosus is often of little consequence but may occasionally be severe and serious, requiring aggressive treatment.[40] Immune-mediated thrombocytopenia may occur in conjunction with HIV disease in approximately 15% of adults, being more common with advanced clinical disease and immune suppression, although less than 0.5% of patients have severe thrombocytopenia with platelet counts below 50,000/mm^3.[41]

TTP is an acute catastrophic disease that, until recently, was uniformly fatal. Causes include metastatic malignancy, pregnancy, mitomycin C, and high-dose chemotherapy. If untreated, it still carries a high mortality rate. In addition to thrombocytopenia, clinical presentation of TTP includes microangiopathic hemolytic anemia, fluctuating neurologic abnormalities, renal dysfunction, and occasional fever. Microvascular infarcts occur in gingival and other mucosal tissues in about 60% of the cases. These appear as platelet-rich thrombi. Serial studies of plasma samples from patients during episodes of TTP have often shown vWF multimer abnormalities.[42]

Thrombocytopenia may be a component of other hematologic disease such as myelodysplastic disorders,[43] aplastic anemia,[44] and leukemia.[45] Bone marrow suppression from cytotoxic chemotherapy can result in severe thrombocytopenia, requiring platelet transfusions for prevention of spontaneous hemorrhage. Thrombocytopenia and thrombocytopathy in liver disease are complicated by coagulation defects, as discussed below. Alcohol can, itself, induce thrombocytopenia.[46] The coagulopathy of renal disease consists of an acquired qualitative platelet defect resulting from uremia.[47]

Medications can also reduce absolute numbers of platelets or interfere with their function, resulting in postsurgical hemorrhage.[48–50] Drug-related platelet disorders are reversible within 7 to 10 days of discontinuation of the drug. Aspirin induces a functional defect in platelets detectable as prolongation of BT. It inactivates an enzyme called prostaglandin synthetase, resulting in inactivation of cyclo-oxygenase catalytic activity and decreasing biosynthesis of prostaglandin and thromboxanes that are needed to regulate interactions between platelets and the endothelium.[51] A single 100 mg dose of aspirin provides rapid complete inhibition of platelet cyclo-oxygenase activity and thromboxane production. Aspirin is commonly used as an inexpensive and effective antiplatelet therapy for thromboembolic protection. Antiplatelet therapy reduces the risk of death from cardiovascular causes by about one-sixth and the risk of nonfatal myocardial infarction and stroke by about one-third for patients with unstable angina or a history of myocardial infarction, transient ischemia, or stroke.[51] Most NSAIDs have similar, but less significant, antiplatelet effects compared with aspirin. The new NSAIDs that act as cyclo-oxygenase-2 inhibitors, rofecoxib (Vioxx, Merck and Co. Inc, Whitehouse Station, NJ) and celecoxib (Celebrex, Pfizer, New York, NY), generally do not inhibit platelet aggregation at indicated doses.

Coagulation Disorders

Coagulation disorders may be either congenital or acquired secondary to drugs or disease processes.

CONGENITAL COAGULOPATHIES

Inherited disorders of coagulation can result from deficiency of a number of factors (seen in Table 17-5) that are essential in the coagulation cascade or deficiency of vWF. Clinical bleeding can vary from mild to severe, depending on the specific clotting factor affected and the level of factor deficiency.

Hemophilia A. A deficiency of F VIII, the antihemophilic factor, is inherited as an X-linked recessive trait that affects males (hemizygous). The trait is carried in the female (heterozygous) without clinical evidence of the disease, although a few do manifest mild bleeding symptoms. Males with hemophilia transmit the affected gene to all their female

TABLE 17-5 Coagulation Factors

Factor (Name)	Coagulation Factor Affected		t½ (h)
	Intrinsic	Extrinsic	
XIII (fibrin-stabilizing factor)	*	*	336
XII (Hageman factor)	*		60
XI (plasma thromboplastin antecedent)	*		60
X (Stuart factor)	*	*	48
IX (Christmas factor)	*		18–24
VIII (antihemophilic factor)	*		8–12
VII (proconvertin)		*	4–6
V (proaccelerin)	*	*	32
IV (calcium)	*	*	—
III (tissue thromboplastin)		*	—
II (prothrombin)	*	*	72
I (fibrinogen)	*	*	96

t½ = half-life in hours

offspring, yet their sons are normal, and the effects skip a generation unless their wives were carriers and their daughters received the maternal affected X chromosome as well. Only 60 to 70% of families with newly diagnosed hemophiliacs report a family history of the disease, suggesting a high mutation rate. There is no racial predilection. Clinical symptoms and F VIII levels vary from pedigree to pedigree.[52] Severe clinical bleeding is seen when the F VIII level is less than 1% of normal. Severe hemorrhage leads to joint synovitis and hemophilic arthropathies, intramuscular bleeds, and pseudotumors (encapsulated hemorrhagic cyst). Retroperitoneal and central nervous system bleeds, occurring spontaneously or induced by minor trauma, can be life threatening. Moderate clinical bleeding is found when F VIII levels are 1 to 5% of normal. Only mild symptoms, such as prolonged bleeding following tooth extraction, surgical procedures, or severe trauma, occur if levels are between 6 and 50% of normal.

Hemophilia B. F IX (Christmas factor) deficiency is found in hemophilia B. The genetic background, factor levels, and clinical symptoms are similar to those in hemophilia A. The distinction was made only in the late 1940s between these two X-linked diseases. Concentrates used to treat F VIII and F IX deficiencies are specific for each state, and therefore a correct diagnosis must be made to ensure effective replacement therapy. Further discussion of the clinical management is presented later in this chapter. Circulating blocking antibodies or inhibitors to Fs VIII and IX may be seen in patients with these disorders. These inhibitors are specific for F VIII or F IX and render the patient refractory to the normal mode of treatment with concentrates. Catastrophic bleeding can occur, and only with supportive transfusions can the patient survive.

Factor XI Deficiency. Plasma thromboplastin antecedent deficiency is clinically a mild disorder seen in pedigrees of Jewish descent; it is transmitted as an autosomal dominant trait. Bleeding symptoms do occur but are usually mild. In the event of major surgery or trauma, hemorrhage can be controlled with infusions of fresh frozen plasma.

Factor XII Deficiency. Hageman factor deficiency is another rare disease that presents in the laboratory with prolonged PT and partial thromboplastin time (PTT). Clinical symptoms are nonexistent. Treatment is therefore contraindicated.

Factor X Deficiency. Stuart factor deficiency, also a rare bleeding diathesis, is inherited as an autosomal recessive trait. Clinical bleeding symptoms in the patient with levels less than 1% are similar to those seen in hemophilias A and B.

Factor V Deficiency. Proaccelerin deficiency, like F XI and F X deficiencies, is a rare autosomal recessive trait that presents with moderate to severe clinical symptoms. When compared with hemophilias A and B, this hemorrhagic diathesis is moderate, only occasionally resulting in soft-tissue hemorrhage, and only rarely presenting with hemarthrosis; it does not involve the devastating degenerative joint disease seen in severe hemophilias A and B.

Factors XIII and I Deficiencies. Fibrin-stabilizing deficiency and fibrinogen deficiency are very rare, and these diagnoses can be made only with extensive laboratory tests usually available only in tertiary-care medical centers. Both are autosomal recessive traits. Most dysfibrinogenemias result in no symptoms, others lead to moderate bleeding, and a few induce a hypercoagulable state. Factor XIII deficiency appears to have different forms of penetrance, and in some families appears only in the males.

Von Willebrand's Disease. vWD is a unique disorder that was described originally by Erik von Willebrand in 1926.[53] This disorder is usually transmitted as an autosomal dominant trait with varying penetrance. The defect is found in the F VIII protein complex. The clinical features of the disease are usually mild and include mucosal bleeding, soft tissue hemorrhage, menorrhagia in women, and rare hemarthrosis.[54] The common genetic profile suggests a heterozygous state, with both males and females affected. Normal plasma vWF level is 10 mg/L, with a half-life of 6 to 15 hours.

vWD is often classified into four basic types based on the separation of vWF multimers or subunits of varying molecular weights by electrophoresis.[55] Type I accounts for approximately 85% of occurrences, with all multimeric forms present in reduced concentrations. Type II is characterized by an absence of high-molecular-weight multimers and occurs in 10 to 15% of vWD patients. Rarely diagnosed is the homozygous individual with type III vWD (autosomal recessive inheritance), who has less than 1% F VIII, a long BT (> 15 minutes), and reduced levels (usually < 1%) of vWF. The fourth type is called pseudo- or platelet-type vWD, and it is a primary platelet disorder that mimics vWD. The increased platelet affinity for large multimers of vWF results primarily in mucocutaneous bleeding. Due to familial genetic variants, wide variations occur in the patient's laboratory profile over time; therefore, diagnosis may be difficult.[56] The uncovering of all of the biochemical, physiologic, and clinical manifestations of vWD has held experts at bay for many years. As early as 1968, acquired vWD was noted to occur as a rare complication of autoimmune or neoplastic disease, associated mostly with lymphoid or plasma cell proliferative disorders and having clinical manifestations that are similar to congenital vWD.[57]

ANTICOAGULANT-RELATED COAGULOPATHIES

Heparin.   Intentional anticoagulation is delivered acutely with heparin or as chronic oral therapy with coumarin drugs. Indications for heparin therapy include prophylaxis or treatment for venous thromboembolism, including prophylaxis in medical and surgical patients.[58] Heparin is a potent anticoagulant that binds with antithrombin III to dramatically inhibit activation of Fs IX, X, and XI, thereby reducing thrombin generation and fibrin formation. The major bleeding complications from heparin therapy are bleeding at surgical sites and bleeding into the retroperitoneum.

Heparin has a relatively short duration of action of 3 to 4 hours, so is typically used for acute anticoagulation, whereas chronic therapy is initiated with coumarin drugs. For acute anticoagulation, intravenous infusion of 1,000 units unfractionated heparin per hour, sometimes following a 5,000-unit bolus, is given to raise the aPTT to 1.5 to 2 times the pre-heparin aPTT. Alternatively, subcutaneous injections of 5,000 to 10,000 units of heparin are given every 12 hours. Newer biologically active low-molecular-weight heparins administered subcutaneously once or twice daily are less likely to result in thrombocytopenia and bleeding complications. Protamine sulfate can rapidly reverse the anticoagulant effects of heparin.

Coumarin.   Coumarin anticoagulants, which include warfarin and dicumarol (Coumadin, DuPont Pharmaceuticals, Wilmington, DE), are used for anticoagulation to prevent recurrent thrombotic phenomena (pulmonary embolism, venous thrombosis, stroke, myocardial infarction), to treat atrial fibrillation, and in conjunction with prosthetic heart valves.[59] They slow thrombin production and clot formation by blocking the action of vitamin K. Levels of vitamin K–dependent Fs II, VI, IX, and X (prothrombin complex proteins) are reduced. The anticoagulant effect of coumarin drugs may be reversed rapidly by infusion of fresh frozen plasma, or over the course of 12 to 24 hours by administration of vitamin K. PT/INR is used to monitor anticoagulation levels. Therapeutic ranges, depending on the indication for anticoagulation, vary from a PT of 18 to 30 seconds (INR of 1.5 to 4.0). Doses of 2.5 to 7.5 mg coumarin daily

typically are required to maintain adequate anticoagulation. Patients with paroxysmal atrial fibrillation and porcine heart valves require minimal anticoagulation (INR target 1.5–2.0), venous thrombosis is managed with intermediate-range coagulation (INR 2.0–3.0), whereas mechanical prosthetic heart valves and hypercoagulable states require more intense anticoagulation (INR target 3.0–4.0).

Coumarin therapy requires continual laboratory monitoring, typically every 2 to 8 weeks, as fluctuations can occur. It has a longer duration of action, with coagulant activity in blood decreased by 50% in 12 hours and 20% in 24 hours of therapy initiation. Coagulation returns to normal levels in approximately 2 to 4 days following discontinuation of coumarin drugs. Coumarin therapy can result in bleeding episodes that are sometimes fatal. Intramuscular injections are avoided in anticoagulated patients because of increased risk of intramuscular bleeding and hematoma formation. Coumarin drugs are particularly susceptible to drug interactions. Drugs that potentially increase coumarin potency (ie, elevate the INR) include metronidazole, penicillin, erythromycin, cephalosporins, tetracycline, fluconazole, ketoconazole, chloral hydrate, and propoxyphene; those that reduce its potency (ie, decrease the INR) include barbiturates, ascorbic acid, dicloxacillin, and nafcillin.[60] Additive hemostatic effect is seen when coumarin drugs are used in combination with aspirin or NSAIDs.

DISEASE-RELATED COAGULOPATHIES

Liver Disease.   Patients with liver disease may have a wide spectrum of hemostatic defects depending upon the extent of liver damage.[61] Owing to impaired protein synthesis, important factors and inhibitors of the clotting and the fibrinolytic systems are markedly reduced. Additionally, abnormal vitamin K–dependent factor and fibrinogen molecules have been encountered. Thrombocytopenia and thrombocytopathy are also common in severe liver disease. Acute or chronic hepatocellular disease may display decreased vitamin K–dependent factor levels, especially Fs II, VII, IX, and X and protein C, with other factors still being normal.

Vitamin K Deficiency.   Vitamin K is a fat-soluble vitamin that is absorbed in the small intestine and stored in the liver. It plays an important role in hemostasis. Vitamin K deficiency is associated with the production of poorly functioning vitamin K–dependent Fs II, VII, IX, and X.[62] Deficiency is rare but can result from inadequate dietary intake, intestinal malabsorption, or loss of storage sites due to hepatocellular disease. Biliary tract obstruction and long-term use of broad-spectrum antibiotics, particularly the cephalosporins, can cause vitamin K deficiency. Although there is a theoretic 30-day store of vitamin K in the liver, severe hemorrhage can result in acutely ill patients in 7 to 10 days. A rapid fall in F VII levels leads to an initial elevation in INR and a subsequent prolongation of aPTT. When vitamin K deficiency results in coagulopathy, supplemental vitamin K by injection restores the integrity of the clotting mechanism.

Disseminated Intravascular Coagulation. DIC is triggered by potent stimuli that activate both F XII and tissue factor to initially form microthrombi and emboli throughout the microvasculature.[63] Thrombosis results in rapid consumption of both coagulation factors and platelets, while also creating FDPs that have antihemostatic effects. The most frequent triggers for DIC are obstetric complications, metastatic cancer, massive trauma, and infection with sepsis. Clinical symptoms vary with disease stage and severity. Most patients have bleeding at skin and mucosal sites. Although it can be chronic and mild, acute DIC can produce massive hemorrhage and be life threatening.

Fibrinolytic Disorders

Disorders of the fibrinolytic system can lead to hemorrhage when clot breakdown is enhanced, or excessive clotting and thrombosis when clot breakdown mechanisms are retarded. Primary fibrinolysis typically results in bleeding and may be caused by a deficiency in α_2-plasmin inhibitor or plasminogen activator inhibitor. Laboratory coagulation tests are normal with the exception of decreased fibrinogen and increased FDP levels. Impaired clearance of TPA may contribute to prolonged bleeding in individuals with severe liver disease. As discussed above, deficiency of F XIII, a transglutaminase that stabilizes fibrin clots, is a rare inherited disorder that leads to hemorrhage. Patients with primary fibrinolysis are treated with fresh frozen plasma therapy and antifibrinolytics.

Differentiation must be made from the secondary fibrinolysis that accompanies DIC, a hypercoagulable state that predisposes individuals to thromboembolism. Dialysis patients with chronic renal failure show a fibrinolysis defect at the level of plasminogen activation.[64] Reduced fibrinolysis may be responsible, along with other factors, for the development of thrombosis, atherosclerosis, and their thrombotic complications. Activators of the fibrinolytic system (TPA, streptokinase, and urokinase) are frequently used to accelerate clot lysis in patients with acute thromboembolism, for example, to prevent continued tissue damage in myocardial infarction or treat thrombotic stroke.

▼ IDENTIFICATION OF THE DENTAL PATIENT WITH A BLEEDING DISORDER

Identification of the dental patient with or at risk for a bleeding disorder begins with a thorough review of the medical history.[65,66] Patient report of a family history of bleeding problems may help to identify inherited disorders of hemostasis. A patient's past history of bleeding following surgical procedures, including dental extractions, can help identify a risk. Surveying the patient for current medication use is important. Identification of medications with hemostatic effect, such as coumarin anticoagulants, heparin, aspirin, NSAIDs, and cytotoxic chemotherapy, is essential. Active medical conditions, including hepatitis or cirrhosis, renal disease, hematologic malignancy, and thrombocytopenia, may predispose to

bleeding problems. Additionally, a history of heavy alcohol intake is a risk factor for bleeding consequences.

A review-of-systems approach to the patient interview can identify symptoms suggestive of disordered hemostasis (see Table 17-1). Although the majority of patients with underlying bleeding disorders of mild to moderate severity may exhibit no symptoms, symptoms are common when disease is severe. Symptoms of hemorrhagic diatheses reported by patients may include frequent epistaxis, spontaneous gingival or oral mucosal bleeding, easy bruising, prolonged bleeding from superficial cuts, excessive menstrual flow, and hematuria. When the history and the review of systems suggest increased bleeding propensity, laboratory studies are warranted.

▼ MANAGEMENT

Management of the patient with a hemorrhagic disorder is aimed at correction of the reversible defect(s), prevention of hemorrhagic episodes, prompt control of bleeding when it occurs, and management of the sequelae of the disease and its therapy.

Platelet Disorders

Treatment modalities for platelet disorders are determined by the type of defect. The thrombocytopenias are primarily managed acutely with transfusions of platelets to maintain the minimum level of 10,000 to 20,000/mm^3 necessary to prevent spontaneous hemorrhage. Corticosteroids are indicated for ITP, with titration governed by the severity of hemorrhagic symptoms.[37,38] Splenectomy may be necessary in chronic ITP to prevent antiplatelet antibody production and sequestration and removal of antibody-labeled platelets.[38] Plasma exchange therapy combined with aspirin/dipyridamole or corticosteroids has recently lowered the mortality rate for patients with TTP over that previously obtained by treatment with fresh frozen plasma (FFP) infusions.[67,68] The thrombocytopenia of Wiskott-Aldrich syndrome may be managed with platelet transfusions, splenectomy, or bone marrow transplantation.[34]

Treatment of bleeding episodes in the patient with the congenital qualitative platelet defect of Glanzmann's thrombasthenia is usually not warranted unless hemorrhage is life threatening. Therapy has included periodic random platelet transfusions, which carry the risk of development of antiplatelet isoantibodies. Human leukocyte antigen (HLA)–matched platelets may be required after antibody development, to reduce the number of platelet transfusions needed for hemostasis. In the absence of satisfactorily compatible platelets, blood volume and constituents can be maintained with low-antigenicity blood products. Plasmapheresis to remove circulating isoantibodies is held in reserve for cases of severe thrombasthenia and life-threatening bleeding.

Hemophilias A and B

Therapy for hemophilias A and B is dependent upon the severity of disease, type and site of hemorrhage, and presence or absence of inhibitors. Commercially prepared Fs VIII and IX complex concentrates, desmopressin acetate, and, to a lesser extent, cryoprecipitate and FFP are replacement options (Tables 17-6 and 17-7). Since partially purified Fs VIII and IX complex concentrates prepared from pooled plasma were first used in the late 1960s and 1970s, multiple methods of manufacturing products with increased purity and reduced risk of viral transmission have been developed.[69,70] Current intermediate-purity products are prepared by heat or solvent/detergent treatment of the final product. In 1987, dry heat–treated concentrates constituted approximately 90% of the total F VIII concentrate consumption in the United States.[70]

High-purity F VIII products, manufactured using recombinant or monoclonal antibody purification techniques, are preferred today for their improved viral safety.[71] However, their cost of up to 10 times more than dry-heated concentrates can be financially restrictive for uninsured patients.[70] High-purity products generally cost over $1.00 (US) per unit. F VIII concentrates are dosed by units, with one unit of F VIII being equal to the amount present in 1 mL of pooled fresh normal plasma. The plasma level of F VIII is expressed as a percentage of normal. Since one unit of F VIII concentrate per kilogram of body weight raises the F VIII level by 2%, a 70 kg patient would require infusion of 3,500 units to raise his factor level from < 1% to 100%. A dose of 40 U/kg F VIII con-

centrate typically is used to raise the F VIII level to 80 to 100% for management of significant surgical or traumatic bleeding in a patient with severe hemophilia. Additional outpatient doses may be needed at 12-hour intervals, or continuous inpatient infusion may be established.

Highly purified recombinant and monoclonal F IX concentrates were developed in the late 1980s and early 1990s and are the treatment of choice for hemophilia B patients undergoing surgery.[72–74] F. IX complex concentrates (prothrombin complex concentrate [PCC]), which contain Fs II, VII, IX, and X, are also widely used at present for patients with hemophilia B. One unit of PCC or higher-purity F IX concentrates given by bolus per kilogram of body weight raises the F IX level by 1 to 1.5%. Thus, a dose of 60 U/kg of F IX concentrate typically is needed to raise the F IX level to 80 to 100% for management of severe bleeding episodes in a patient with a severe F IX deficiency. Repeat outpatient doses may be needed at 24-hour intervals. Properly supervised home therapy, in which patients self-treat with factor concentrates at the earliest evidence of bleeding, is a cost-effective method offered to educable and motivated patients by some medical centers.[75]

Currently, cryoprecipitate and FFP are rarely the treatment of choice for hemophilias A and B because of their disadvantages of potential viral transmission and the large volumes

TABLE 17-6   Principal Products for Systemic Management of Patients with Bleeding Disorders

Product	Description	Source	Common Indications
Platelets	"One pack" = 50 mL; raises count by 6,000	Blood bank	< 10,000 in nonbleeding individuals < 50,000 presurgical < 50,000 in actively bleeding individuals Nondestructive thrombocytopenia
Fresh frozen plasma	Unit = 150–250 mL 1 hour to thaw Contains Fs II, VII, IX, X, XI, XII, XIII and heat labile V and VII	Blood bank	Undiagnosed bleeding disorder with active bleeding Severe liver disease When transfusing > 10 units blood Immune globulin deficiency
Cryoprecipitate	Unit = 10–15 mL Contains Fs VIII, XIII, vWF and fibrinogen	Blood bank	Hemophilia A, von Willebrand's disease, when factor concentrates/DDAVP are unavailable Fibrinogen deficiency
F VIII concentrate (purified antihemophilic factor) *	Unit raises F VIII level by 2% Heat treated contains vWF Recombinant and monoclonal technologies are pure F VIII	Pharmacy	Hemophilia A, with active bleeding or presurgical; some cases of von Willebrand's disease
F IX concentrate (PCC)*	Unit raises F IX level by 1–1.5% Contains Fs II, VII, IX, and X Monoclonal F IX is only F IX	Pharmacy	Hemophilia B, with active bleeding or presurgical PCC used for hemophilia A with inhibitor
DDAVP	Synthetic analogue of antidiuretic hormone 0.3 µg/kg IV or SQ Intranasal application	Pharmacy	Active bleeding or presurgical for some patients with von Willebrand's disease, uremic bleeding, or liver disease
E-Aminocaproic acid	Antifibrinolytic 25% oral solution (250 mg/mL) Systemic: 75 mg/kg q6h	Pharmacy	Adjunct to support clot formation for any bleeding disorder
Tranexamic acid	Antifibrinolytic 4.8% mouth rinse—not available in US Systemic: 25 mg/kg q8h	Pharmacy	Adjunct to support clot formation for any bleeding disorder

F = factor; DDAVP = desmopressin acetate; PCC = prothrombin complex concentrate.

* see Table 17-7 for additional factor concentrate products.

TABLE 17-7   Coagulation Factor Concentrate Products

Product Category	Proprietary Name*	Manufacturer/ Distributor	Corporate Location
High purity F. VIII concentrates			
Monoclonal:	Hemofil-M	Baxter Healthcare Corp.	Deerfield, IL, USA
	Monoclate-P	Aventis-Behring	King of Prussia, PA, USA
Recombinant:	Kogenate	Bayer Corp.	Clayton, NC, USA
	Recombinate	Baxter Healthcare Corp.	Deerfield, IL, USA
	Helixate-FS	Aventis-Behring	King of Prussia, PA, USA
	Bioclate	Aventis-Behring	King of Prussia, PA, USA
	ReFacto	Wyeth Biopharma	Andover, MA, USA
Intermediate purity F. VIII concentrates			
Pasturized:	Humate-P	Aventis-Behring	King of Prussia, PA, USA
Solvent/Detergent:	Koate-DVI	Bayer Corp.	Clayton, NC, USA
	Alphanate	Alpha Therapeutic Corp.	Los Angeles, CA, USA
Porcine F. VIII concentrates	Hyate-C	Ipsen, Inc.	Milford, MA, USA
High purity F. IX concentrates			
Monoclonal:	AlphaNine-SD	Alpha Therapeutic Corp.	Los Angeles, CA, USA
	Mononine	Aventis-Behring	King of Prussia, PA, USA
Recombinant:	BeneFix	Wyeth Biopharma	Andover, MA, USA
Prothrombin complex concentrates (PCC)	Profilnine-SD	Alpha Therapeutic Corp.	Los Angeles, CA, USA
	Proplex-T	Baxter Healthcare Corp.	Deerfield, IL, USA
F. IX activated PCCs	FEIBA-VH	Baxter Healthcare Corp.	Deerfield, IL, USA
	Autoplex-T	Nabi	Boca Raton, FL, USA
F. VIIa concentrate			
Recombinant:	NovoSeven	Novo-Nordisk	Bagsvaerd, Denmark

F = factor; PCCs = prothrombin complex concentrates.

*Product availability changes periodically.

needed to raise factor levels adequately for hemostasis. Cryoprecipitate is the cold insoluble precipitate remaining after FFP is thawed at 4°C. A typical bag (1 unit) of cryoprecipitate contains about 80 units of F VIII and vWF, and 150 to 250 mg fibrinogen in a 10 to 15 mL volume. Cryoprecipitate has been used to treat selected patients with vWD and hemophilia A. FFP contains all coagulation factors in nearly normal concentrations and may aid hemorrhage control in a patient with mild hemophilia B. In the average-size patient, one unit of FFP raises F IX levels by 3%. Postoperative bleeding in mild to moderate F X deficiency can be managed with FFP, and PCCs may be held in reserve for severely deficient patients.[76]

Desmopressin acetate (DDAVP [1-deamino-8-D-arginine vasopressin]) provides adequate transient increases in coagulation factors in some patients with mild to moderate hemophilia A and type I vWD, avoiding the need for plasma concentrates.[77] This synthetic vasopressin analogue is now considered the treatment of choice for bleeding events in patients with these bleeding diatheses owing to its absence of viral risk and lower cost. DDAVP can be given at a dose of 0.3 μg/kg body weight by an intravenous or subcutaneous route prior to dental extractions or surgery, or to treat spontaneous or traumatic bleeding episodes.[78] It results in a mean increase of a two- to fivefold rise (range 1.5–20 times) in F VIII coagulant activity, vWF antigen, and ristocetin cofactor activity, with a plasma half-life of 5 to 8

hours for F VIII and 8 to 10 hours for vWF.[77] Intranasal spray application of DDAVP (Stimate, Aventis Behring, King of Prussia, PA) contains 1.5 mL of desmopressin per milliliter, with each 0.1 mL pump spray delivering a dose of 150 μg. Children require one nostril spray, and adults require two nostril sprays to achieve favorable response; correction of bleeding occurs in around 90% of patients with mild to moderate hemophilia A and type I vWD.[79] Time to peak levels is 30 to 60 minutes after intravenous injection and 90 to 120 minutes following subcutaneous or intranasal application.[77]

Unfortunately, DDAVP is ineffective in individuals with severe hemophilia A. A DDAVP trial or test dose response may be indicated prior to extensive surgery, to evaluate the level of drug effect on assayed F VIII activity in the individual patient. DDAVP, thought to stimulate endogenous release of F VIII and vWF from blood vessel endothelial cell storage sites, is hemostatically effective provided that adequate plasma concentrations are attained.[80] Prolonged use of DDAVP results in exhaustion of F VIII storage sites and diminished hemostatic effect; hence, antifibrinolytic agents are useful adjuncts to DDAVP therapy.

Complications of factor replacement therapy, in addition to allergic reactions, include viral disease transmission (hepatitis B and C, *Cytomegalovirus*, and human immunodeficiency virus [HIV]), thromboembolic disease, DIC, and development of antibodies to factor concentrates. Hepatitis B and non-A/non-B have been major causes of morbidity and mortality in the hemophiliac population, resulting in chronic active hepatitis and cirrhosis in a number of patients.[52] More recently, hepatitis C and HIV infection have become the most common transfusion-related infections in hemophiliacs. By the end of 1986, some centers reported that 80 to 90% of hemophiliacs treated with F VIII concentrates and around 50% of those who had received F IX concentrates were HIV seropositive.[81] Since 1986, with viral screening of donated plasma, there have been few transfusion-related HIV seroconversions.

Use of factor IX complex concentrate can result in thrombotic complications, such as deep venous thromboses, myocardial infarctions, pulmonary emboli, and DIC. Concurrent use of systemic antifibrinolytics with these products may increase the risks. DIC is believed to occur as a consequence of high levels of activated clotting factors, such as Fs VIIa, IXa, and Xa, that cannot adequately be cleared by the liver.

Development of a F VIII or F IX inhibitor is a serious complication. These pathologic circulating antibodies of the IgG class, which specifically neutralize F VIII or F IX procoagulant activity, arise as alloantibodies in some patients with hemophilia.[82] Inhibitors develop in at least 10 to 15% of patients with severe hemophilia A and less commonly in patients with hemophilia B.[83,84] Development is related to exposure to factor products and genetic predisposition.[82,83] Inhibitor level is quantified by the Bethesda inhibitor assay and is reported as Bethesda units (BU).

The inhibitor titer and responsiveness to further factor infusion (responder-type) dictate which factor replacement therapy should be used. Patients with inhibitors are classified according to titer level—low (< 10 BU/mL) or high (> 10 BU/mL)—and also by responder type.[84] Low responders typically maintain low titers with repeated factor concentrate exposure, whereas high responders show a brisk elevation in titer due to the amnestic response and are the most challenging to manage.[84,85] Patients with low inhibitor titers are usually low responders, and those with high titers are often high responders. Seventy-five percent of hemophilia A patients with inhibitors are high responders, whereas only 25% are low responders.[84]

For hemorrhages, hemophilia A patients with low-level low-responding inhibitors are treated with F VIII concentrates in doses sufficient to raise plasma F VIII levels to the therapeutic range. Critical hemorrhages in patients with high-responding inhibitors may be treated with large quantities of porcine F VIII; however, routine hemorrhages are often managed initially with PCCs, which provoke anamnesis in a few patients.[82] PCCs can bypass the F VIII inhibitor and are effective about 50% of the time.[86] Activated PCCs show slightly increased effectiveness (65–75%). Highly purified porcine F VIII product use can be advantageous in patients with less than 50 BU, since human F VIII inhibitors cross-react less frequently with porcine products.[82] However, because of the risk of hemostatic failure, surgery should be performed under coverage of F VIII.[87] Treatment of the patient with low-level

(< 10 BU) F IX inhibitors requires higher doses of F IX complex concentrates to achieve hemostasis. Developed in the early 1990s, recombinant F VIIa is a novel product that provides an alternative treatment option for patients with hemophilia A or B with inhibitors by enhancing the extrinsic pathway.[88] It has been proven to effectively control bleeding in patients with high-titer inhibitors.[89,90]

Several methods have demonstrated temporary removal of high-titer inhibitors in both hemophilia A and B. Exchange transfusion or plasmapheresis produces a rapid transient reduction in antibody level, with a rate of 40 mL plasma per kilogram decreasing levels by half.[91] Although laborious, it may be attempted in cases of critical hemorrhage as an adjunct to high-dose F VIII concentrate therapy. Antibody removal by extracorporeal adsorption of the plasma to protein A-Sepharose or a specific F IX–Sepharose in columns has also shown promise in hemophilias A and B.[92,93]

Von Willebrand's Disease

Therapy for vWD depends on the type of vWD and the severity of bleeding. Type I is treated preferentially with DDAVP as described above. Intermediate-purity F VIII concentrates, FFP, and cryoprecipitate are held in reserve for DDAVP nonresponders.[55] Types II and III require intermediate-purity F VIII concentrates, such as Humate-P or Koate-HS, or, rarely, cryoprecipitate or FFP. Bleeding episodes in patients with platelet-type vWD are usually controlled with platelet concentrate infusions. Other therapy is used for site-specific bleeding, such as estrogens or oral contraceptive agents for menorrhagia and local hemostatic agents and antifibrinolytics for dental procedures. Occasionally, circulating plasma inhibitors of vWF are observed in multiply transfused patients with severe disease. Cryoprecipitate infusion can cause transient neutralization of this inhibitor.[94]

Disease-Related Coagulopathies

Management of disease-related coagulopathies varies with hemostatic abnormality.

LIVER DISEASE

Hepatic disease that results in bleeding from deficient vitamin K–dependent clotting factors (Fs II, VII, IX, and X) may be reversed with vitamin K injections for 3 days, either intravenously or subcutaneously. However, infusion of FFP may be employed when more immediate hemorrhage control is necessary, such as prior to dental extractions.[95] Cirrhotic patients with moderate thrombocytopenia and functional platelet defects may benefit from DDAVP therapy.[96] Antifibrinolytic drugs, if used cautiously, have markedly reduced bleeding and thus reduced need for blood and blood product substitution.[61]

RENAL DISEASE

In uremic patients, dialysis remains the primary preventive and therapeutic modality used for control of bleeding, although it is not always immediately effective.[97] Hemodialysis and peritoneal dialysis appear to be equally efficacious in improving platelet function abnormalities and clinical bleeding in the uremic patient. The availability of cryoprecipitate[98] and DDAVP[99] offers alternative effective therapy for patients who require shortened bleeding times acutely in preparation for urgent surgery. Conjugated estrogen preparations[100] and recombinant erythropoietin[101] have also been shown to be beneficial for uremic patients with chronic abnormal bleeding.

DISSEMINATED INTRAVASCULAR COAGULATION

Although somewhat controversial, active DIC is usually treated initially with intravenous unfractionated heparin or subcutaneous low-molecular-weight heparin, to prevent thrombin from acting on fibrinogen, thereby preventing further clot formation.[102–104] It is important to expeditiously identify and institute therapy for the underlying triggering disease or condition if long-term survival is to be a possibility. The dentist may be called upon to provide a gingival or oral mucosal biopsy specimen for histopathologic examination to confirm the diagnosis of DIC by the presence of microthrombi in the vascular bed. Replacement of deficient coagulation factors with FFP and correction of the platelet deficiency with platelet transfusions may be necessary for improvement or prophylaxis of the hemorrhagic tendency of DIC prior to emergency surgical procedures. Elective surgery is deferred due to the volatility of the coagulation mechanism in these patients.

▼ PROGNOSIS

Prognosis for patients with bleeding disorders depends on appropriate diagnosis and the ability to prevent and manage acute bleeding episodes. Individuals with mild or manageable disease have a normal life expectancy, with morbidity relating to bleeding episode frequency and severity. Acute DIC carries the highest risk of death by exsanguination. Individuals with severe liver disease may succumb to rupture of esophageal varices. Severe thrombocytopenia and other severe coagulopathies carry a higher risk of hemorrhagic stroke.

Advances in the treatment of hemophilia, from the use of cryoprecipitate in the 1960s to the introduction of plasma-derived factor concentrates in the 1970s, have led to dramatic improvement in quality of life and raised the lifespan for hemophiliacs from 11 years in 1921 to 60 years in 1980.[105] Viral infections, such as hepatitis B, C, and G and HIV acquired from infected blood products, have altered the prognosis for some patients.[106–110] As discussed above, before effective virucidal methods were used in the manufacture of clotting-factor concentrates in 1985, hemophiliacs were at a very high risk of contracting bloodborne viruses from factor concentrates that exposed them to the plasma of thousands of donors. HIV seroprevalence increased to 60 to 75% of patients with hemophilia (85–90% with severe hemophilia), with HIV-associated opportunistic infections and neoplasms contributing substantially to the morbidity and mortality of hemophiliacs.[106,107,109] Oral mucosal diseases are common in hemophiliacs with HIV, particularly in those with advanced immunosuppression,[110,111] and are discussed in more detail in chapter ***. HIV protease

inhibitor–containing drug combinations that resulted in improved health of some HIV-infected patients in the late 1990s are showing significant clinical and laboratory benefits when used by HIV-infected hemophiliacs.[112] Co-infection with viral hepatitis remains a challenge for the next decade.

▼ ORAL HEALTH CONSIDERATIONS

Oral Findings

Platelet deficiency and vascular wall disorders result in extravasation of blood into connective and epithelial tissues of the skin and mucosa, creating small pinpoint hemorrhages, called petechiae, and larger patches, called ecchymoses. Platelet or coagulation disorders with severely altered hemostasis can result in spontaneous gingival bleeding, as may be seen in conjunction with hyperplastic hyperemic gingival enlargements in leukemic patients. Continuous oral bleeding over long periods of time fosters deposits of hemosiderin and other blood degradation products on the tooth surfaces, turning them brown. A variety of oral findings are illustrated in Figures 17-4 to 17-6.

Hemophiliacs may experience many episodes of oral bleeding over their lifetime. Sonis and Musselman[113] reported an average 29.1 bleeding events per year serious enough to require factor replacement in F VIII–deficient patients, of which 9% involved oral structures. Location of oral bleeds was as follows: labial frenum, 60%; tongue, 23%; buccal mucosa, 17%; and gingiva and palate, 0.5% (Figure 17-7). Bleeding occurrences were most frequent in patients with severe hemophilia, followed by moderate, and then mild hemophilia. They most often resulted from traumatic injury. Bleeding events may also be induced by poor oral hygiene practices and iatrogenic factors. Kaneda and colleagues[114] reported frequency of oral hemorrhage by location in individuals deficient of F VIII and F IX as follows: gingiva, 64%; dental pulp, 13%; tongue, 7.5%; lip, 7%; palate, 2%; and buccal mucosa, 1%. Many minor oral bleeds, such as those from the gingiva or dental pulp, can be controlled by local measures.

Hemarthrosis is a common complication in hemophiliacs' weight-bearing joints, yet it rarely occurs in the temporomandibular joint (TMJ). Two TMJ cases have been reported.[115,116] An acute TMJ hemarthrosis associated with F IX deficiency was resolved with factor replacement without aspiration;[115] a chronic hemophilic TMJ arthropathy required arthrotomy, arthroscopic adhesion lysis, factor replacement, splint therapy, and physical therapy in a patient with F XI deficiency.[116]

Evaluation of dental disease patterns in the patient population with bleeding disorders revealed a higher caries rate, a greater number of unrestored teeth,[117] and more severe periodontal disease[118] in individuals with severe hemophilia. The severity of dental disease in severe bleeders was attributed to a lack of proper oral hygiene and proper professional dental care.

Dental Management

Dental management required for patients with bleeding disorders depends on both the type and invasiveness of the den-

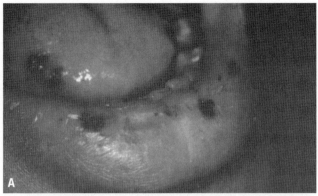

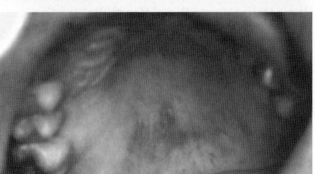

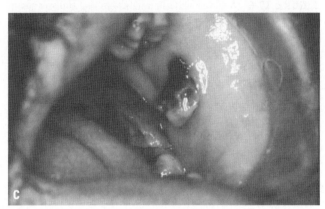

FIGURE 17-4   A 36-year-old male with idiopathic thrombocytopenia purpura and a platelet count of 5,000/mm³. Supportive platelet transfusions and immunoglobulin therapy were used to control bleeding. **A,** Labial and tongue ecchymoses; **B,** palatal ecchymoses; **C,** buccal ecchymoses and fibrinous clot.

tal procedure and the type and severity of the bleeding disorder. Thus, less modification is needed for patients with mild coagulopathies in preparation for dental procedures anticipated to have limited bleeding consequences. When significant bleeding is expected, the goal of management is to preoperatively restore the hemostatic system to an acceptable range, while supporting coagulation with adjunctive and/or local measures. For reversible coagulopathies, (eg, coumarin anticoagulation), it may be best to remove the causative agent or treat the primary illness or defect in order to allow the patient to return to a manageable bleeding risk for the dental treatment period. For irreversible coagulopathies, the missing or defective element may need to be replaced from an exogenous source to allow control of bleeding (eg, coagulation factor concentrate therapy for hemophilia). Assessment of the coagulopathy and delivery of appropriate therapy prior to dental procedures is best accomplished in consultation with a hematologist.

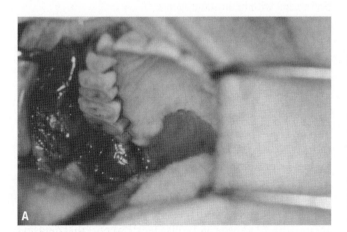

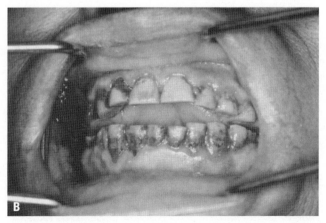

FIGURE 17-5   A 68-year-old female with acute myelogenous leukemia and a platelet count of 9,000/mm³. Platelet transfusion and ε-aminocaproic acid oral rinses were used to control bleeding. **A,** Buccal mucosa and palatal ecchymoses. **B,** Extrinsic stains on teeth from erythrocyte degradation following continual gingival oozing.

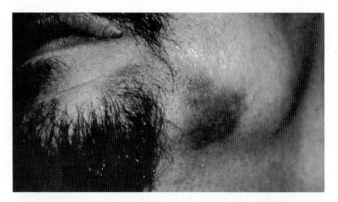

FIGURE 17-6 A 46-year-old male with severe liver cirrhosis due to hepatitis C infection. Shown is purpura of facial skin 1 week after full-mouth extractions.

Platelet Disorders

When medical management is unable to restore platelet counts to above the level of 50,000/mm³ required for surgical hemostasis, platelet transfusions may be required prior to dental extractions or other oral surgical procedures. The therapeutically expected increment in platelet count from infusion of one unit of platelets is approximately 10,000 to 12,000/mm³. Six units of platelets are commonly infused at a time. Patients who have received multiple transfusions may be refractory to random donor platelets as a result of alloimmunization. These individuals may require single-donor apheresis or leukocyte-reduced platelets. Local hemostatic measures are also important. The thrombasthenic patient needing dental extractions may be successfully treated with the use of hemostatic measures such as microfibrillar collagen and antifibrinolytic drugs.[32,33]

Since the antiplatelet activity of aspirin remains for the 8- to 10-day lifetime of the affected platelets, avoidance of aspirin is recommended for 1 to 2 weeks prior to extensive oral surgical procedures. Other NSAIDs have a similar but less pronounced antiplatelet effect. Adjunctive local hemostatic agents are useful in preventing postoperative oozing when aspirin

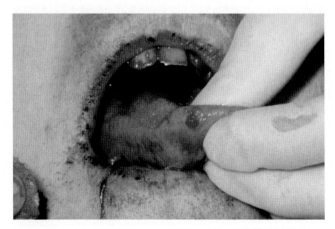

FIGURE 17-7 A 27-year-old male with type III von Willebrand's disease and a 2-week duration of bleeding from the tongue that reduced his hematocrit to 16%. Hemorrhage control was obtained with cryoprecipitate.

therapy is in use at the time of minor oral surgery. When extensive surgery is emergently indicated, DDAVP can be used to decrease the aspirin-induced prolongation of the BT or to treat aspirin-related postoperative oozing, often eliminating the need for platelet infusion.[119]

Chemotherapy-associated oral hemorrhages, most frequently related to thrombocytopenia, are best managed by transfusions of HLA-matched platelets and FFP, together with topically applied clot-promoting agents.[45] A pilot study suggests a possible benefit of DDAVP for the prevention or treatment of bleeding in patients with thrombocytopenia associated with hematologic malignancy.[120]

Hemophilias A and B and Von Willebrand's Disease

ORAL SURGICAL PROCEDURES

Oral surgical procedures have the greatest potential for hemorrhage of all dental procedures. Hemorrhagic problems after extractions have drastically declined over the last 20 years such that only an estimated 8% of hemophilic patients experience one or more delayed bleeding episodes.[121] Appropriate precautionary measures now allow surgery to be performed safely. To make certain that preoperative factor levels of at least 40 to 50% of normal activity have been obtained, transfusion recommendations generally aim for replacement of missing coagulation factors to levels of 50 to 100% when single-bolus infusion is used for outpatient treatment. This provides greater assurance of hemorrhage control, given the problems of possible failure of factor activity to rise as high as expected and variable plasma half-lives of 8 to 12 hours for F VIII and 18 to 24 hours for F IX. Additional postoperative factor maintenance may be indicated for extensive surgery. This can be accomplished by infusion of factor concentrates, DDAVP, cryoprecipitate, or FFP, depending on the patient's deficiency state. When postsurgical bleeding occurs due to fibrinolysis, it commonly starts 3 to 5 days after surgery and can usually be controlled by local measures and use of antifibrinolytics. Continual oozing from unstable fibrinous clots may require their removal and the repacking of the extraction socket with hemostatic agents.

Determination of factor replacement requirements for surgical hemostasis and selection of plasma product or drug therapy should be accomplished in consultation with the patient's hematologist. Canadian clinical practice guidelines[122] recommend replacement factor levels of 40 to 50% of F VIII (dose 20–25 U/kg) and F IX (dose 40–50 U/kg), used in conjunction with antifibrinolytics. Gingival or dental bleeding unresponsive to antifibrinolytics requires 20 to 30% clotting F VIII or F IX.[122] The level of factor activity required for hemostasis varies in relation to local factors. Higher hemostatic factor levels are needed for large wound cavities created by extraction of multiple or multirooted teeth, or when gingival inflammation, bleeding, tooth mobility, or apical lesions are present.[114] Kaneda and colleagues[114] report that deficient factor activity levels required for postextraction hemostasis varied from 3.5 to 25% for deciduous teeth and 5.5 to 20% for permanent teeth.[114]

Three methods of replacement therapy have been employed to maintain circulating factor levels above the 20% minimum necessary for hemostasis during surgical and healing phases. These include intermittent replacement therapy, continuous intravenous factor infusion therapy, and a single preoperative factor concentrate infusion combined with an antifibrinolytic mouthwash.[123] Factor VIII levels may be sufficiently raised by DDAVP in some patients with mild to moderate hemophilia A and vWD to allow dental extractions without transfusion.

Local hemostatic agents and techniques include pressure, surgical packs, vasoconstrictors, sutures, surgical stents, topical thrombin, and use of absorbable hemostatic materials. Although having no direct effect on hemostasis, primary wound closure aids patient comfort, decreases blood clot size, and protects clots from masticatory trauma and subsequent bleeding.[124] Sutures can also be used to stabilize and protect packing. Resorbable and nonresorbable suture materials have proven to be equally effective. Avitene (Davol Inc, Cranston, RI) or Helitene (Integra Life Sciences Plainsboro, NJ), a microfibrillar collagen fleece, aids hemostasis when placed against the bleeding bony surface of a well-cleansed extraction socket. It acts to attract platelets, causing the release phenomenon to trigger aggregation of platelets into thrombi in the interstices of the fibrous mass of the clot.[125] Topical Thrombin (Thrombogen; Johnson and Johnson,New Brunswick,NJ), which directly converts fibrinogen in the blood to fibrin, is an effective adjunct when applied directly to the wound or carried to the extraction site in a nonacidic medium on oxidized cellulose. Surgifoam (Ethicon Inc, Piscataway, NJ) is an absorbable gelatin sponge with intrinsic hemostatic properties. A collagen absorbable hemostat manufactured as a 3 × 4–inch sponge (INSTAT; Ethican Inc, Piscataway, NJ) or fabricated as a nonwoven pad is also a useful adjunct. Surgical acrylic stents may be useful if carefully fabricated to avoid traumatic irritation to the surgical site. Diet restriction to full liquids for the initial 24 to 48 hours, followed by intake of soft foods for 1 to 2 weeks, will further protect the clot by reducing the amount of chewing and resultant soft-tissue disturbances.

Antifibrinolytic drugs such as ε-aminocaproic acid[126] (EACA; Amicar; Xanodyne Pharmacal Inc, Florence, KY) and tranexamic acid (AMCA; Cyclokapron; Pharmacia Corp, Peapack, NJ) inhibit fibrinolysis by blocking the conversion of plasminogen to plasmin, resulting in clot stabilization. Postsurgical use of EACA has been shown to significantly reduce the quantity of factor required to control bleeding when used in conjunction with presurgical concentrate infusion sufficient to raise plasma F VIII and F IX levels to 50%.[123,127,128] A regimen of 50 mg/kg of body weight EACA given topically and systemically as a 25% (250 mg/mL) oral rinse every 6 hours for 7 to 10 days appears adequate as an adjunct. Tranexamic acid (4.8%) oral rinse was found to be 10 times more potent than was EACA in preventing postextraction bleeding in hemophiliacs, with fewer side effects, but it is not routinely available in the United States.[129,130] Systemic antifibrinolytic therapy can be given orally or intravenously as EACA 75 mg/kg (up to 4 g) every 6 hours or AMCA 25 mg/kg every 8 hours until bleeding stops.[122]

Fibrin sealants or fibrin glue has been used effectively in Europe since 1978 as an adjunct with adhesive and hemostatic effects to control bleeding at wound or surgical sites, but it is not available as a commercial product in the United States.[131] Its use has allowed reduction in factor concentrate replacement levels in hemophiliacs undergoing dental surgeries when used in combination with antifibrinolytics.[132–134] Use of fibrin glue does not obviate the need for factor concentration replacement in severe hemophiliacs.[133] In the United States, extemporaneous fibrin sealant can be made by combining cryoprecipitate with a combination of 10,000 units topical thrombin powder diluted in 10 mL saline and 10 mL calcium chloride. When dispensed over the wound simultaneously from separate syringes, the cryoprecipitate and calcium chloride precipitate almost instantaneously to form a clear gelatinous adhesive gel.

PAIN CONTROL

A variety of techniques are used to control pain in individuals with coagulopathies. An assessment of the patient's pain threshold and invasiveness of the dental procedure to be undertaken allows selection of an effective management approach. Some patients opt for treatment without anesthesia. Hypnosis,[135] intravenous sedation with diazepam, or nitrous oxide/oxygen analgesia, used as adjuncts to control anxiety, drastically reduce or totally eliminate the need for local anesthesia.[136] Intrapulpal anesthesia is safe and effective following access for pulp extirpation. Periodontal ligament and gingival papillary injections can be accomplished with little risk when delivered slowly with minimal volume.[137] Anesthetic solutions with vasoconstrictors such as epinephrine should be used when possible. In patients with mild disease, buccal, labial, and hard palatal infiltration can be attempted for maxillary teeth, with slow injection and local pressure to the injection site for 3 to 4 minutes.[136] If a hematoma develops, ice packs should be applied to the area to stimulate vasoconstriction, and emergency factor replacement should be administered in a hospital.

Block injections used in dentistry, including inferior alveolar, posterior superior alveolar, infraorbital, and (to a lesser extent) long buccal, require minimal coagulation factor levels of 20 to 30%. These injections place anesthetic solutions in highly vascularized loose connective tissue with no distinct boundaries, where formation of a dissecting hematoma is possible.[138] Webster and colleagues[117] reported development of hematomas in 8% of hemophilic patients not treated with prophylactic factor replacement prior to mandibular block injection.[117] Greater risk occurred with severe disease than with mild, and with hemophilia A than with B.[117] Extravasation of blood into the soft tissues of the oropharyngeal area in hemophiliacs can produce gross swelling, pain, dysphagia, respiratory obstruction, and grave risk of death from asphyxia[139–141] (Figure 17-7).

Dental treatment in the operating room under general anesthesia may be indicated when extensive procedures necessitate numerous expensive factor infusions, when patient cooperation or anxiety prohibits outpatient clinic or office treatment, or when the patient with an inhibitor has multiple treatment needs. Although oral endotracheal intubation provides access challenges for the dental operator, it is preferred over nasal endotracheal intubation, which carries the risk of inducing a nasal bleed that can be difficult to control. The use of aspirin and other NSAIDs for pain management are contraindicated in patients with bleeding disorders due to their inhibition of platelet function and potentiation of bleeding episodes. Intramuscular injections should also be avoided due to the risk of hematoma formation.

PREVENTIVE AND PERIODONTAL THERAPIES

Periodontal health is of critical importance for the hemophiliac for two principal reasons: (1) hyperemic gingiva contributes to spontaneous and induced gingival bleeding and (2) periodontitis is a leading cause of tooth morbidity, necessitating extraction. Individuals with bleeding diatheses are unusually prone to oral hygiene neglect due to fear of toothbrush-induced bleeding. On the contrary, oral physiotherapy can be accomplished without risk of significant bleeding. Periodontal probing and supragingival scaling and polishing can be done routinely. Careful subgingival scaling with fine scalers rarely warrants replacement therapy. Severely inflamed and swollen tissues are best treated initially with chlorhexidine oral rinses or by gross débridement with a cavitron or hand instruments to allow gingival shrinkage prior to deep scaling.[118] Deep subgingival scaling and root planing should be performed by quadrant to reduce gingival area exposed to potential bleeding. Locally applied pressure and post-treatment antifibrinolytic oral rinses are usually successful in controlling any protracted oozing.[142] Local block anesthesia required for scaling may necessitate raising factor levels to a minimum of 30% of normal prior to treatment.[143] Periodontal surgical procedures warrant elevating circulating factor levels to 50% and use of post-treatment antifibrinolytics. Periodontal packing material aids hemostasis and protects the surgical site; however, it may be dislodged by severe hemorrhage or subperiosteal hematoma formation.

RESTORATIVE AND PROSTHODONTIC THERAPY

General restorative and prosthodontic procedures do not result in significant hemorrhage. Rubber dam isolation is advised to minimize the risk of lacerating soft tissue in the operative field and to avoid creating ecchymoses and hematomas with high-speed evacuators or saliva ejectors. Care is required to select a tooth clamp that does not traumatize the gingiva. Matrices, wedges, and a hemostatic gingival retraction cord may be used with caution to protect soft tissues and improve visualization when subgingival extension of cavity preparation is necessary. Removable prosthetic appliances can be fabricated without complications. Denture trauma should be minimized by prompt and careful postinsertion adjustment.

ENDODONTIC THERAPY

Endodontic therapy is often the treatment of choice for a patient with a severe bleeding disorder, especially when an inhibitor is present because extraction carries a high risk of hemorrhage, and treatment is expensive. Generally, there are no contraindications to root canal therapy, provided instrumentation does not extend beyond the apex.[144] Filling beyond the apical seal also should be avoided. Application of epinephrine intrapulpally to the apical area is usually successful in providing hemostasis. Endodontic surgical procedures require the same factor replacement therapy as do oral surgical procedures.

PEDIATRIC DENTAL THERAPY

The pediatric dental patient occasionally presents with prolonged oozing from exfoliating primary teeth. Administration of factor concentrates and extraction of the deciduous tooth with curettage may be necessary for patient comfort and hemorrhage control. Moss[29] advocates extraction of mobile primary teeth using periodontal space anesthesia without factor replacement after 2 days of vigorous oral hygiene to reduce local inflammation. Hemorrhage control is obtained with gauze pressure, and seepage generally stops in 12 hours. Pulpotomies can be performed without excessive pulpal bleeding. Stainless steel crowns should be prepared to allow minimal removal of enamel at gingival areas.[145] Topical fluoride treatment and use of pit-and-fissure sealants are important noninvasive therapies to decrease the need for extensive restorative procedures.

ORTHODONTIC THERAPY

Orthodontic treatment can be provided with little modification. Care must be observed to avoid mucosal laceration by orthodontic bands, brackets, and wires. Bleeding from minor cuts usually responds to local pressure. Properly managed fixed orthodontic appliances are preferred over removable functional appliances for the patient with a high likelihood of bleeding from chronic tissue irritation. The use of extraoral force and shorter treatment duration further decrease the potential for bleeding complications.[146]

Patients on Anticoagulants

Management of the dental patient on anticoagulant therapy involves consideration of the degree of anticoagulation achieved as gauged by the PT/INR, the dental procedure planned, and the level of thromboembolic risk for the patient.[147] In general, higher INRs result in higher bleeding risk from surgical procedures. It is generally held that nonsurgical dental treatment can be successfully accomplished without alteration of the anticoagulant regimen, provided the PT/INR is not grossly above the therapeutic range and trauma is minimized.[148,149] Greater controversy exists over the management of anticoagulated patients for oral surgical procedures.[60,150] Preparation of the anticoagulated patient for surgical procedures depends on the extent of bleeding expected. No surgical treatment is recommended for those with an INR of > 3.5 to 4.0 without coumarin dose modification.[60,150] With an INR < 3.5 to 4.0, minor surgical procedures with minimal anticipated bleeding require local measures but no coumarin modification. At an INR of < 3.5 to 4.0, when moderate bleeding is expected (multiple extractions or removal of wisdom teeth), local measures should be used, and INR reduction should be considered. When significant bleeding is anticipated, as from full-mouth or full-arch extractions, local measures are combined with reduction of anticoagulation to an INR of < 2.0 to 3.0.[60,151] Extensive flap surgery or multiple bony extractions may require an INR of < 1.5.[60]

For surgical procedures, physician consultation is advised in order to determine the patient's most recent PT/INR level and the best treatment approach based on the patient's relative thromboembolic and hemorrhagic risks. When the likelihood of sudden thrombotic and embolic complications is small and hemorrhagic risk is high, coumarin therapy can be discontinued briefly at the time of surgery, with prompt re-institution postoperatively.[147,152,153] Coumarin's long half-life of 42 hours necessitates dose reduction or withdrawal 2 days prior to surgery in order to return the patient's PT/INR to an acceptable level for surgery.[147,154] For patients with moderate thromboembolic and hemorrhagic risks, coumarin therapy can be maintained in the therapeutic range with the use of local measures to control postsurgical oozing.[155,156]

High-risk cardiac patients undergoing high-bleeding-risk surgical procedures may be managed most safely with a combination heparin-coumarin method,[153] which allows maximal hemostasis with minimal nonanticoagulated time (14–18 hours for a 2-hour surgery, as opposed to 3–4 days with the coumarin discontinuation method). This technique, which requires hospitalization at additional cost, substitutes parenteral heparin, which has a 4-hour half-life, for coumarin. Coumarin is withheld 24 hours prior to admission. Heparin therapy, instituted on admission, is stopped 6 to 8 hours preoperatively. Surgery is accomplished when the PT/INR and aPTT are within the normal range. Coumarin is re-instituted on the night of the procedure and may require 2 to 4 days to effectively reduce the patient's procoagulant levels to a therapeutic range. Heparin is reinstituted 6 to 8 hours after surgery when an adequate clot has formed. Heparin reinstitution by bolus injection (typically a 5,000 U bolus) carries a greater risk of postoperative bleeding than does gradual re-infusion (typically 1,000 U/h).

Use of additional local hemostatic agents such as microfibrillar collagen, oxidized cellulose, or topical thrombin is recommended for anticoagulated patients. Fibrin sealant has been used successfully as an adjunct to control bleeding from oral surgical procedures in therapeutically anticoagulated patients with INRs from 1.0 to 5.0, with minimal bleeding complications.[157] In Europe, 4.8% tranexamic acid solution used as an antifibrinolytic mouthwash has proven effective in control of oral surgical bleeding in patients with INRs between 2.1 and 4.8.[158,159] Use of antifibrinolytics may have value in control of oral wound bleeding, thereby alleviating the need to reduce the oral anticoagulant dose.[160] Use of medications that interact with coumarin, altering its anticoagulant effectiveness as discussed above, is to be avoided.

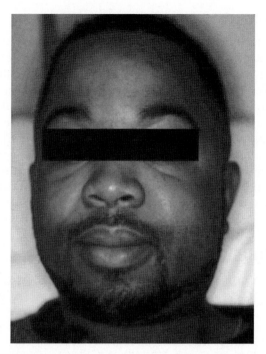

FIGURE 17-8 A 24-year-old male with severe hemophilia A and low-titer inhibitor, 3 days after inferior alveolar block–induced parapharyngeal hemorrhage. Patient presented with difficulty swallowing and pending airway compromise 8 hours after nerve block. Subsequent treatment with prothrombin complex concentrates over 3 days controlled the bleeding and began the resolution of facial swelling.

The shorter-acting anticoagulant heparin is administered by intravenous or subcutaneous route. The most common outpatient use of subcutaneous heparin is for the treatment of deep venous thrombophlebitis during pregnancy,[161] with the goal being regulation of the aPTT between 1.25 and 1.5 times control. In general, oral surgical procedures can be carried out without great risk of hemorrhage when local hemostatics are used in a patient receiving heparin subcutaneously; however, on consultation, the patient's physician may recommend withholding the scheduled injection immediately prior to the operation. Continuous intravenous heparin, with greater hemorrhagic potential than heparin delivered subcutaneously, is discontinued 6 to 8 hours prior to surgery to allow adequate surgical hemostasis. If a bleeding emergency arises, the action of heparin can be reversed by protamine sulfate.

Susceptibility to Infection

Susceptibility to infection among patients with congenital bleeding disorders is not a significant concern. Should a hematoma form as a result of an anesthetic injection or other dental trauma or spontaneously, use of a broad-spectrum antibiotic is indicated to prevent infection during resolution. If bleeding results from bone marrow suppressive systemic disease or chemotherapeutic drug use, antibiotics may be required to prevent infection from bacteremia-inducing dental procedures when production of mature functional neutrophils is substantially diminished (see "Leukemia" in Chapter 16).

Ability to Withstand Care

Patients with bleeding disorders, appropriately prepared preoperatively, are generally as able to withstand dental care as well as unaffected individuals. Consultation with the patient's physician is recommended for guidance on medical management required for higher-risk surgical dental procedures. Because of the expense of some medical management approaches to severe bleeding disorders (eg, coagulation factor replacement for severe hemophiliacs), the coumarin withdrawal–heparinization approach to extractions for patients at high risk of thrombosis, and the bleeding risk to the patient, long treatment sessions may be required to maximize treatment accomplishments while minimizing the risk and cost.

▼ REFERENCES

1. Rodeghiero F, Castaman G, Dini E. Epidemiological investigation of the prevalence of von Willebrand's disease. Blood 1987;692:454–9.
2. Soucie JM, Evatt B, Jackson D, et al. Occurrence of hemophilia in the United States. Am J Hematol 1998;59:288–94.
3. Lewis IK, Hanlon JT, Hobbins MJ, et al. Use of medications with potential oral adverse drug reactions in community-dwelling elderly. Spec Care Dent 1993;13:171–6.
4. Becker RC, Ansell J. Antithrombotic therapy: an abbreviated reference for clinicians. Arch Intern Med 1995;155:149–61.
5. Davie EW, Fujikawa K, Kisiel W. The coagulation cascade: initiation, maintenance, and regulation. Biochemistry 1991;30:10363–70.
6. Mustard JF, Packman MA. Factors influencing platelet function: adhesion, release, and aggregation. Pharmacol Rev 1970;22:97–187.
7. Davie EW, Ratnoff OD. Waterfall sequence for intrinsic blood clotting. Science 1964;145:1310–2.
8. MacFarlane RG. An enzyme cascade in the blood clotting mechanism and its function as a biochemical amplifier. Nature 1964;202:498–9.
9. Kingdon HS, Davie EW. Further studies on the activation of factor IX by activated factor XI. Thromb Diath Haemorrh (Stuttg) 1965;Suppl 17:15–22.
10. Bajaj SP, Butkowski RJ, Mann KG. Prothrombin fragments—Ca^{2+} binding and activation kinetics. J Biol Chem 1975;250:2150–6.
11. Lorand L. Fibrinoligase: the fibrin-stabilizing factor system of blood plasma. Ann N Y Acad Sci 1972;202:6–30.
12. Duckert F. Documentation of the plasma factor XIII deficiency in man. Ann N Y Acad Sci 1972;202:190–9.
13. Verstraete M, Bleifeld W, Brower RW, et al. Double-blind randomized trial of intravenous tissue-type plasminogen activator versus placebo in acute myocardial infarction. Lancet 1985;2:965–9.
14. De Rossi SS, Glick M. Bleeding time: an unreliable predictor of clinical hemostasis. J Oral Maxillofac Surg 1996;54:1119–20.
15. Meehan S, Schmidt MC, Mitchell PF. The international normalized ratio as a measure of anticoagulation: significance for the management of the dental outpatient. Spec Care Dent 1997;17:94–6.
16. Smith RE. The INR: a perspective. Semin Thromb Hemost 1997;23:547–9.
17. Stern R, Karlis V, Kinney L, et al. Using the international normalized ratio to standardize prothrombin time. J Am Dent Assoc 1997;128:1121–2.
18. Langdell RD, Wagner RH, Brinkhous KM. Effect of antihemophilic factor on one-stage clotting tests. J Lab Clin Med 1953;41:637–47.
19. Reuler JB, Broudy VC, Cooney TG. Adult scurvy. JAMA 1985;253:805–7.
20. Touyz LZ. Oral scurvy and periodontal disease. J Can Dent Assoc 1997;63:837–45.
21. De Paepe A. The Ehlers-Danlos syndrome: a heritable collagen disorder as cause of bleeding. Thromb Haemost 1996;75:379–86.
22. Nelson DL, King RA. Ehlers-Danlos syndrome type VIII. J Am Acad Dermatol 1981;5:297–303.
23. Ooshima T, Abe K, Kohno H, et al. Oral manifestations of Ehlers-Danlos syndrome type VII: histological examination of a primary tooth. Pediatr Dent 1990;12;102–6.
24. Barabas GM, Barabas AP. The Ehlers-Danlos syndrome. A report of the oral and haematological findings in nine cases. Br Dent J 1967;123:473–9.
25. Welbury RR. Ehlers-Danlos syndrome: historical review, report of two cases in one family and treatment needs. J Dent Child 1989;56:220–4.
26. Guttmacher AE, Marchuk DA, White RI Jr. Hereditary hemorrhagic telangiectasia. N Engl J Med 1995;333:918–24.
27. Haitjema T, Westermann CJ, Overtoom TT, et al. Hereditary hemorrhagic telangiectasia (Osler-Weber-Rendu disease): new insights in pathogenesis, complications, and treatment. Arch Intern Med 1996;156:714–9.
28. Christensen GJ. Nosebleeds may mean something much more serious: an introduction to HHT. J Am Dent Assoc 1998;129:635–7.
29. Moss SJ. Newer approaches to dental therapy. Ann N Y Acad Sci 1975;240:259–62.
30. Flint SR, Keith O, Scully C. Hereditary hemorrhagic telangiectasia: family study and review. Oral Surg Oral Med Oral Pathol 1988;66:440–4.
31. Bisch FC, Bowen KJ, Hanson BS, et al. Dental considerations for a Glanzmann's thrombasthenia patient: case report. J Periodontol 1996;67:536–40.
32. Perkin RF, White GC, Webster WP. Glanzmann's thrombasthenia. Report of two oral surgical cases using a new microfibrillar collagen preparation and EACA for hemostasis. Oral Surg Oral Med Oral Pathol 1979;47:36–9.
33. Jackson MR, MacPhee MJ, Drohan WN, et al. Fibrin sealant: current and potential clinical applications. Blood Coagul Fibrinolysis 1996;7:737–46.
34. Boraz RA. Dental considerations in the treatment of Wiskott-Aldrich syndrome: report of case. ASDC J Dent Child 1989;56:225–7.
35. Noris P, Spedini P, Belletti S, et al. Thrombocytopenia, giant platelets, and leukocyte inclusion bodies (May-Hegglin anomaly): clinical and laboratory findings. Am J Med 1998;104:355–60.
36. Clemetson KJ, Clemetson JM. Molecular abnormalities in Glanzmann's thrombasthenia, Bernard-Soulier syndrome, and platelet-type von Willebrand's disease. Curr Opin Hematol 1994;1:388–93.
37. James WD, Guirty CC, Grote WR. Acute thrombocytopenia purpura. Oral Surg Oral Med Oral Pathol 1984;57:149–51.

38. Fotos PG, Graham WL, Bowers DC, et al. Chronic autoimmune thrombocytopenia purpura. A 3-year case study. Oral Surg Oral Med Oral Pathol 1983;55:564–7.

39. George JN, Raskob GE. Idiopathic thrombocytopenic purpura: a concise summary of the pathophysiology and diagnosis in children and adults. Semin Hematol 1998;35:5–8.

40. Keeling DM, Isenberg DA. Haematological manifestations of systemic lupus erythematosus. Blood Rev 1993;7:199–207.

41. Patton LL. Hematologic abnormalities among HIV-infected patients. Associations of significance for dentistry. Oral Surg Oral Med Oral Pathol Oral Radiol Endod 1999;88:561–7.

42. Moake JL, Chow TW. Thrombotic thrombocytopenic purpura: understanding a disease no longer rare. Am J Med Sci 1998;316:105–19.

43. Heaney ML, Golde DW. Myelodysplasia. N Engl J Med 1999; 340:1649–60.

44. Valdez IH, Patton LL. Aplastic anemia: current concepts and dental management. Spec Care Dent 1990;10:185–9.

45. Dreizen S, McCredie KB, Keating MJ. Chemotherapy-associated oral hemorrhages in adults with acute leukemia. Oral Surg Oral Med Oral Pathol 1984;57:494–8.

46. Heiman JL. Alcohol-induced thrombocytopenia: review of the literature and report of case. J Am Dent Assoc 1972;85:1358–61.

47. Zachee P, Vermylen J, Boogaerts MA. Hematologic aspects of end-stage renal failure. Ann Hematol 1994;69:33–40.

48. George JN, Raskob GE, Shah SR. Drug-induced thrombocytopenia: a systematic review of published case reports. Ann Intern Med 1998;129:886–90.

49. Barak S, Shaked Y, Bar ZG, et al. Drug-induced post-surgical haemorrhage resulting from trimethoprim-sulphamethoxazole. A case report. Int J Oral Maxillofac Surg 1989;18:206–7.

50. Laskin JL. Oral hemorrhage after the use of quinidine: report of case. J Am Dent Assoc 1974;88:137–9.

51. Wood AJJ. Aspirin as an antiplatelet drug. N Engl J Med 1994;330:1287–94.

52. White GC II, Blatt PM, McMillan CW. Medical complications of hemophilia. South Med J 1980;73:155–60.

53. De Gopegui RR, Feldman BF. Von Willebrand's disease. Comp Haematol Int 1997;7:187–96.

54. Federici AB. Diagnosis of von Willebrand disease. Haemophilia 1998;4:654–60.

55. Johnson RS, Heldt LV, Keaton WM. Diagnosis and treatment of von Willebrand's disease. J Oral Maxillofac Surg 1987;45:608–12.

56. Batlle J, Torea J, Rendal E, et al. The problem of diagnosing von Willebrand's disease. J Intern Med 1997;740:121–8.

57. Tefferi A, Nichols WL. Acquired von Willebrand disease: concise review of occurrence, diagnosis, pathogenesis, and treatment. Am J Med 1997;103:536–40.

58. Hirsch J, Warkentin TE, Rasche R, et al. Heparin and low-molecular-weight heparin: mechanisms of action, pharmacokinetics, dosing considerations, monitoring, efficacy, and safety. Chest 1998;114:489–510S.

59. Hirsch J, Dalen JE, Anderson DR, et al. Oral anticoagulants: mechanism of action, clinical effectiveness, and optimal therapeutic range. Chest 1998;114:445–69S.

60. Herman WW, Konzelman JL Jr, Sutley SH. Current perspectives on dental patients receiving coumarin anticoagulant therapy. J Am Dent Assoc 1997;128:327–35.

61. Mammen EF. Coagulation defects in liver disease. Med Clin North Am 1994;78:545–54.

62. Shearer MJ. Vitamin K. Lancet 1995;345:229–34.

63. Levi M, Ten Cate H. Disseminated intravascular coagulation. N Engl J Med 1999;341:586–92.

64. Opatrny K Jr. Hemostasis disorders in chronic renal failure. Kidney Int Suppl 1997;62:S87–9.

65. Thomson PJ, Langton SG. Persistent haemorrhage following dental extractions in patients with liver disease: two cautionary tales. Br Dent J 1996;180:141–4.

66. Sallah S, Kato G. Evaluation of bleeding disorders. A detailed history and laboratory tests provide clues. Postgrad Med 1998;103:209–18.

67. Rock GA, Shumak KH, Buskard NA, et al. Comparison of plasma exchange with plasma infusion in the treatment of thrombotic thrombocytopenia purpura. N Engl J Med 1991;325:393–7.

68. Bell WR, Braine HG, Ness PM, et al. Improved survival in thrombotic thrombocytopenic purpura–hemolytic uremic syndrome. Clinical experience in 108 patients. N Engl J Med 1991;325:398–403.

69. Brinkhous KM, Shanbrom E, Roberts HR, et al. A new high-potency glycine-precipitated antihemophilia factor (AHF) concentrate. JAMA 1968;205:613–7.

70. Pierce GF, Lusher JM, Brownstein AP, et al. The use of purified clotting factor concentrates in hemophilia. Influence of viral safety, cost, and supply on therapy. JAMA 1989;261:3434–8.

71. Schwartz RS, Abildgaard CF, Aledort LM, et al. Human recombinant DNA-derived antihemophilic factor (factor VIII) in the treatment of hemophilia A. N Engl J Med 1990;323:1800–5.

72. White GC II, Beebe A, Nielsen B. Recombinant factor IX. Thromb Haemost 1997;78:261–5.

73. Goldsmith JC, Kasper CK, Blatt PM, et al. Coagulation factor IX: successful surgical experience with a purified factor IX concentrate. Am J Hematol 1992;40:210–5.

74. Djulbegovic B, Marasa M, Pesto A, et al. Safety and efficacy of purified factor IX concentrate and antifibrinolytic agents for dental extractions in hemophilia B. Am J Hematol 1996;51:168–70.

75. Levine PH. Efficacy of self-therapy in hemophilia. A study of 72 patients with hemophilia A and B. N Engl J Med 1974; 291:1381–4.

76. Eastman JR, Triplett DA, Nowakowski AR. Inherited factor X deficiency: presentation of a case with etiologic and treatment considerations. Oral Surg Oral Med Oral Pathol 1983; 56:461–6.

77. Mannucci PM. Desmopressin (DDAVP) in the treatment of bleeding disorders: the first 20 years. Blood 1997;90:2515–21.

78. Saulnier J, Marey A, Horellou M-H, et al. Evaluation of desmopressin for dental extractions in patients with hemostatic disorders. Oral Surg Oral Med Oral Pathol 1994;77:6–12.

79. Semeritis SV, Aledort LM. Desmopressin nasal spray for hemophilia A and type I von Willebrand disease. Ann Intern Med 1997;126:744–5.

80. Mannucci PM, Pareti FI, Ruggeri ZM, et al. 1-Deamino-8-arginine vasopressin: a new therapeutic approach to the management of haemophilia and von Willebrand's disease. Lancet 1977;I:869–72.

81. Ragni MV, Winkelstein A, Kingsley L, et al. 1986 update of HIV seroprevalence, seroconversion, AIDS incidence, and immunologic correlates of HIV infection in patients with hemophilia A and B. Blood 1987;70:786–90.

82. Kasper CK. Complications of hemophilia A treatment: factor VIII inhibitors. Ann N Y Acad Sci 1991;614:97–105.

83. Roberts HR, Cromartie R. Overview of inhibitors to factor VIII and IX. Prog Clin Biol Res 1984;150;1–18.

84. Aledort L. Inhibitors in hemophilia patients: current status and management. Am J Hematol 1994;47:208–17.

85. Durham TM, Hodges ED, Harper J, et al. Management of traumatic oral-facial injury in the hemophiliac patient with inhibitor: case report. Pediatr Dent 1993;15:282–7.

86. Lusher JM, Shapiro SS, Palasczk JE, et al. Efficacy of prothrombin-complex concentrates in hemophiliacs with antibodies to factor VIII. A multicenter therapeutic trial. N Engl J Med 1980;303:421–5.

87. Blatt PM, Pearsall AH, Givhan EG, et al. Haemostatic failure of prothrombin complex concentrates during elective dental procedure. Thromb Haemost 1980;42:1604–6.

88. Lusher J, Ingerslev J, Roberts H, et al. Clinical experience with recombinant factor VIIa. Blood Coagul Fibrinolysis 1998; 9:119–28.

89. McPherson J, Teague L, Lloyd J, et al. Experience with recombinant factor VIIa in Australia and New Zealand. Haemostasis 1996;26:109–17.

90. Ciavarella N, Schiavoni M, Valenzano E, et al. Use of recombinant factor VIIa (NovoSeven) in the treatment of two patients with type III von Willebrand's disease and an inhibitor against von Willebrand factor. Haemostasis 1996;26:150–4.

91. Francesconi M, Korninger C, Thaler E, et al. Plasmapheresis: its value in the management of patients with antibodies to factor VIII. Haemostasis 1982;11:79–86.

92. Nilsson IM, Sundqvist S-B, Freiburghaus C. Extracorporeal protein A–sepharose and specific affinity chromatography for removal of antibodies. Prog Clin Biol Res 1984;150:225–41.

93. Freiburghaus C, Berntorp E, Ekman M, et al. Immunoadsorption for removal of inhibitors: update on treatments in Malmo-Lund between 1980 and 1995. Haemophilia 1998; 4:16–20.

94. Stratton RD, Wagner RH, Webster WP, et al. Antibody nature of circulating inhibitor of plasma von Willebrand factor. Proc Natl Acad Sci U S A 1975;72:4167–71.

95. Spector I, Corn M, Ticktin HE. Effect of plasma transfusions on the prothrombin time and clotting factors in liver disease. N Engl J Med 1966;275:1032–7.

96. Mannucci PM. Desmopressin (DDAVP) for treatment of disorders of hemostasis. Prog Hemostat Thromb 1986;8:19–45.

97. Jubelirer SJ. Hemostatic abnormalities in renal disease. Am J Kidney Dis 1985;5:219–25.

98. Janson PA, Jubelirer SJ, Weinstein JM, et al. Treatment of the bleeding tendency in uremia with cryoprecipitate. N Engl J Med 1980;303:1318–22.

99. Mannucci PM, Remuzzi G, Pusineri F, et al. Deamino-8-D-arginine vasopressin shortens the bleeding time in uremia. N Engl J Med 1983;308:8–12.

100. Liu YK, Kosfeld RE, Marcum SG. Treatment of uraemic bleeding with conjugated oestrogen. Lancet 1984;2:887–90.

101. Moia M, Vizzotto L, Cattaneo M, et al. Improvement in the haemostatic defect of uraemia after treatment with recombinant human erythropoietin. Lancet 1987;2:1227–9.

102. Falace DA, Kelly DE. Disseminated intravascular coagulation and fibrinolysis as a cause of postextraction hemorrhage. Report of a case. Oral Surg Oral Med Oral Pathol 1976; 41:718–25.

103. Shikimori M, Oka T. Disseminated intravascular coagulation syndrome. Int J Oral Surg 1985;14:451–5.

104. De Jonge E, Levi M, Stoutenbeek CP, et al. Current drug treatment strategies for disseminated intravascular coagulation. Drugs 1998;55:767–77.

105. Larsson S. Life expectancy of Swedish haemophiliacs, 1831–1980. Br J Haematol 1985;59:593–602.

106. Telfer MC. Clinical spectrum of viral infections in hemophilic patients. Hematol Oncol Clin North Am 1992;6:1047–56.

107. Eyster M, Diamondstone L. Natural history of hepatitis C virus infection in multitransfused hemophiliacs: effect of coinfection with human immunodeficiency virus. The Multi-center Haemophilia Cohort Study. J Acquir Immun Defic Syndr 1993;6:602–10.

108. Wilde JT, Ahmed MM, Collingham KE, et al. Hepatitis G virus infection in patients with bleeding disorders. Br J Haematol 1997;99:285–8.

109. Lee CA, Sabin CA, Phillips AN, et al. Morbidity and mortality from transfusion-transmitted disease in haemophilia [letter]. Lancet 1995;345:1309.

110. Bolski E, Hunt R. The prevalence of AIDS-associated oral lesions in a cohort of patients with hemophilia. Oral Surg Oral Med Oral Pathol 1988;65:406–10.

111. Ficarra G, Chiodo M, Morfini M, et al. Oral lesions among HIV-infected hemophiliacs. A study of 54 patients. Haematologica 1994;79:148–53.

112. Merry C, McMahon C, Ryan M, et al. Successful use of protease inhibitors in HIV-infected haemophilia patients. Br J Haematol 1998;101:475–9.

113. Sonis AL, Musselman RJ. Oral bleeding in classic hemophilia. Oral Surg Oral Med Oral Pathol 1982;53:363–6.

114. Kaneda T, Shikimori I, Watanabe F, et al. The importance of local hemostatic procedures in dental extractions and oral mucosal bleeding of hemophiliac patients. Int J Oral Surg 1981;10:266–71.

115. Kaneda T, Nagayama M, Ohmori M, et al. Hemarthrosis of the temporomandibular joint in a patient with hemophilia B: report of case. J Oral Surg 1979;37:513–4.

116. Nishioka GJ, Van Sickels JE, Tilson HB. Hemophilic arthropathy of the temporomandibular joint: review of the literature, a case report, and discussion. Oral Surg Oral Med Oral Pathol 1988;65:145–50.

117. Webster WP, Roberts HR, Penick GD. Dental care of patients with hereditary disorders of blood coagulation. In: Ratnoff OD, editor. Treatment of hemorrhagic disorders. New York: Harper & Row; 1968. p. 93–110.

118. Webster WP, Courtney RM. Diagnosis and treatment of periodontal disease in the hemophiliac. In: Proceedings, Dental Hemophilia Institute, January, 1968. The National Hemophilia Foundation, U.S.A.

119. Kobrinsky NL, Israeles ED, Gerrard JM, et al. Shortening of bleeding time by 1-deamino-8-d-arginine vasopressin in various bleeding disorders. Lancet 1984;I:1145–8.

120. Castaman G, DiBona E, Schiavotto C, et al. Pilot study on the safety and efficacy of desmopressin for the treatment or prevention of bleeding in patients with hematologic malignancy. Haematologica 1997;82:584–7.

121. Vinckier F, Vermylen J. Dental extractions in hemophilia: reflections on 10 years' experience. Oral Surg Oral Med Oral Pathol 1985;59:6–9.

122. Association of Hemophilia Clinic Directors of Canada. Clinical practice guidelines. Hemophilia and von Willebrand's disease: 2. Management. Can Med Assoc J 1995;153:147–57.

123. Webster WP, McMillan CW, Lucas ON, et al. Dental management of the bleeder patient. A comparative review of replacement therapy. In: Ala F, Denson KWE, editors. Haemophilia. Amsterdam: Excerpta Medica; 1973. p. 33–7.

124. Stajcic Z, Baklaja R, Elezovic I, et al. Primary wound closure in haemophiliacs undergoing dental extractions. Int J Oral Maxillofac Surg 1989;18:14–6.

125. Evans BE. Local hemostatic agents (and techniques). Scand J Haematol 1984;33:417–22.

126. Lucas ON, Albert TW. Epsilon aminocaproic acid in hemophiliacs undergoing dental extractions: a concise review. Oral Surg Oral Med Oral Pathol 1981;51:115–20.

127. Walsh PN, Rizza CR, Matthews JM, et al. Epsilon-aminocaproic acid therapy for dental extractions in haemophilia and Christmas disease: a double blind controlled trial. Br J Haematol 1971;20:463–75.

128. Walsh PN, Rizza CR, Evans BE, et al. The therapeutic role of epsilon aminocaproic acid (EACA) for dental extractions in hemophiliacs. Ann N Y Acad Sci 1975;240:267–76.

129. Forbes CD, Barr RD, Reid G, et al. Tranexamic acid in control of haemorrhage after dental extraction in haemophilia and Christmas disease. Br Med J 1972;2:311–3.

130. Tavenner RWH. Use of tranexamic acid in control of haemorrhage after extraction of teeth in haemophilia and Christmas disease. Br Med J 1972;2:314–5.

131. Sugar AW. The management of dental extractions in cases of thrombasthenia complicated by the development of isoantibodies to donor platelets. Oral Surg Oral Med Oral Pathol 1979;48:116–9.

132. Rakocz M, Mazar A, Varon D, et al. Dental extractions in patients with bleeding disorders. The use of fibrin glue. Oral Surg Oral Med Oral Pathol 1993;75:280–2.

133. Martinowitz U, Schulman S. Fibrin sealant in surgery of patients with a hemorrhagic diathesis. Thromb Hemost 1995;74:486–92.

134. Martinowitz U, Schulman S, Horoszowski H, et al. Role of fibrin sealants in surgical procedures on patients with hemostatic disorders. Clin Orthop 1996;328:65–75.

135. Lucas ON. The use of hypnosis in hemophilia dental care. Ann N Y Acad Sci 1975;240:263–6.

136. Geffner I, Porteous JR. Haemorrhage and pain control in conservative dentistry for haemophiliacs. Br Dent J 1981;151:256–8.

137. Spuller RL. Use of the periodontal ligament injection in dental care of the patient with hemophilia-a clinical evaluation. Spec Care Dent 1988;8:28–9.

138. Nazif M. Local anesthesia for patients with hemophilia. J Dent Child 1970;37:79–84.

139. Archer WH, Zubrow HJ. Fatal hemorrhage following regional anesthesia for operative dentistry in a hemophiliac. Oral Surg Oral Med Oral Pathol 1954;7:464–70.

140. Leatherdale RAI. Respiratory obstruction in haemophilic patients. Br Med J 1960;II:1316–20.

141. Bogdan CJ, Strauss M, Ratnoff OD. Airway obstruction in hemophilia (factor VIII deficiency): a 28-year institutional review. Laryngoscope 1994;104:789–94.

142. Sindet-Pedersen S, Stenbjerg S, Ingerslev J. Control of gingival hemorrhage in hemophilic patients by inhibition of fibrinolysis with tranexamic acid. J Periodontal Res 1988; 23:72–4.

143. Michaelides PL. Outpatient management of periodontal patients with hemophilia. Int J Periodont Restorative Dent 1983;3:65–73.

144. Keila S, Kaufman A, Itckowitch D. Uncontrolled bleeding during endodontic treatment as the first symptoms for diagnosing von Willebrand's disease. Oral Surg Oral Med Oral Pathol 1990;69:243–6.

145. White GE. Medical review—factor VIII deficiency and pedodontics. J Pedodont 1979;3:176–92.

146. van Venrooy JR, Proffit WR. Orthodontic care for medically compromised patients: possibilities and limitations. J Am Dent Assoc 1985;111:262–6.

147. Mulligan R, Weitzel KG. Treatment management of the patient receiving anticoagulant drugs. J Am Dent Assoc 1988;117:479–83.

148. Rooney TP. General dentistry during continuous anticoagulation therapy. Oral Surg Oral Med Oral Pathol 1983;56:252–5.

149. Benoliel R, Leviner E, Katz J, et al. Dental treatment for patients on anticoagulant therapy: prothrombin time value—what difference does it make? Oral Surg Oral Med Oral Pathol 1986; 62:149–51.

150. Wahl MJ. Myths of dental surgery in patients receiving anticoagulant therapy. J Am Dent Assoc 2000;131:77–80.

151. Beirne OR, Koehler JR. Surgical management of patients on warfarin sodium. J Oral Maxillofac Surg 1996;54:1115–8.

152. Ziffer AM, Scopp IW, Beck J, et al. Profound bleeding after dental extractions during dicumarol therapy. N Engl J Med 1957;256:351–3.

153. Roser SM, Rosenbloom B. Continued anticoagulation in oral surgery procedures. Oral Surg Oral Med Oral Pathol 1975;40:448–57.

154. Mulligan R. Response to anticoagulant withdrawal. J Am Dent Assoc 1987;115:435–8.

155. Waldrep AC, McKelvey LE. Oral surgery for patients on anticoagulant therapy. J Oral Surg 1968;26:374–80.

156. Bailey BMW, Fordyce AM. Complications of dental extractions in patients receiving warfarin anticoagulant therapy. A controlled clinical trial. Br Dent J 1983;155:308–10.

157. Bodner L, Weinstein JM, Baumgartner AK. Efficacy of fibrin sealant in patients on various levels of oral anticoagulant undergoing oral surgery. Oral Surg Oral Med Oral Pathol Oral Radiol Endod 1998;86:421–4.

158. Ramstrom G, Sindet-Pedersen S, Hall G, et al. Prevention of postsurgical bleeding in oral surgery using tranexamic acid without dose modification of oral anticoagulants. J Oral Maxillofac Surg 1993;51:1211–6.

159. Sindet-Pedersen S, Ramstrom G, Bernvil S, et al. Hemostatic effect of tranexamic acid mouthwash in anticoagulant-treated patients undergoing oral surgery. N Engl J Med 1989;320:840–3.

160. Souto JC, Oliver A, Zuazu-Jausoro I, et al. Oral surgery in anticoagulated patients without reducing the dose of oral anticoagulant: a prospective randomized study. J Oral Maxillofac Surg 1996;54:27–32.

161. Belfiglio EJ. The heparinized dental patient. Gen Dent 1991;39:38–9.

18

▼

IMMUNOLOGIC DISEASES

KATHARINE N. CIARROCCA, DMD, MSED
MARTIN S. GREENBERG, DDS

▼ GENERAL PRINCIPLES OF IMMUNOLOGIC DISEASE

The science of immunology, once a small branch of microbiology, has grown into one of the principal sciences concerned with human disease. In recent years, the explosion of information in the field of immunology has both enhanced the understanding of disease processes and provided tools with which to investigate a continually growing number of clinical conditions. This wealth of knowledge has led to the development of better diagnostic tests and treatment specifically targeted to the disease process.

Concepts of disease are rapidly changing due to the ever-increasing information gained in immunologic research. A competent clinician must understand the basic concepts of modern immunology and how they relate to disease. Much of the current research dealing with dental caries, periodontal disease, and oral ulcers uses the techniques of immunology to investigate the etiology and treatment of these diseases. In this chapter, pertinent basic principles of clinical immunology are reviewed, diseases that involve the immune system are discussed, and the relationship of these diseases to oral mucosal disease is highlighted.

Immunity: Protection against Disease

The environment contains a large variety of microbial agents (viruses, bacteria, fungi, protozoa, and parasites) that can cause disease if they multiply unchecked. The function of the immune system is to distinguish these potentially infectious agents as foreign and to eliminate them from the body.

An immune response involves both the recognition of the foreign substance and the reaction that serves to eliminate it. This response can be divided into two functional systems: (1) the innate system, or first line of defense, and (2) the acquired or adaptive system, the specific response to each infectious agent, which eliminates the infection. These two systems work closely together to eliminate pathogens. The innate immune response is the immune defense system that lacks memory whereas the acquired immune defense is dependent on previous encounters with a pathogen. The unique characteristic of the acquired immune response is its high specificity for a particular pathogen. This specificity improves with each successive encounter with the same pathogen, thus creating a "memory" that enables the body to prevent the same infectious agent from causing disease later. The innate response, however, does not change with repeated exposure to a given infectious agent and therefore does not possess the same antigen-specific recognition.

INNATE IMMUNITY

The major constituents of innate immunity are the cellular components, represented by phagocytes; natural killer (NK) cells; and the molecular component, which includes the complement cascade and cytokines.

Phagocytic cells express surface glycoproteins and scavenger receptors that are used to recognize and engulf microbial organisms and foreign particles.[1] There are two types of phagocytes: mononuclear phagocytes or tissue macrophages and polymorphonuclear neutrophils.

Mononuclear phagocytic cells are derived from bone marrow stem cells, and their function is to engulf, internalize, and destroy particles. Monocytes are strategically placed where they will encounter foreign particles. In time, they migrate into the tissues, where they develop into tissue macrophages. Macrophages activate T lymphocytes by the secretion of interleukins and present foreign antigens to lymphocytes. Macrophages act together with large granular lymphocytes to mediate both the lysis of cells coated with antibody and NK cells.

Neutrophils constitute the majority of the blood leukocytes and develop from the same precursors as monocytes and macrophages. They are activated by bacterial products to phagocytize and kill bacteria. Phagocytosis is further increased by the opsonization of bacteria with immunoglobulins and complement products. Neutrophils are short-lived cells that engulf and destroy material and then die.

Natural killer cells account for 10 to 15% of blood lymphocytes and are designed to kill any cells that do not express self–major histocompatibility complex (MHC) antigens. They are predominantly confined to the blood and spleen. Their responsibility is to lyse virus-infected cells, foreign cells, or malignant cells, without the help of antibodies.[2]

The complement system uses a simple self- or non-self-discriminatory system: host tissues have cell surface molecules that inhibit the activation of complement, and microbial organisms lack these inhibitory molecules. The complement system has multiple functions, including the direct killing of microorganisms or tumor cells by lysis, the opsonization of microorganisms for phagocytosis, the chemotaxis and activation of leukocytes and mast cells, the processing of immunocomplexes, and the regulation of antibody production by B cells.

ACQUIRED IMMUNITY

Lymphocytes are central to all adaptive immune responses as they specifically recognize individual pathogens in host cells and/or in the tissue fluids or blood. Lymphocytes are derived from undifferentiated stem cell precursors that originate in the bone marrow. These stem cells differentiate into two distinct populations of lymphocytes, to form the two components of adaptive immunity. One population of lymphoid stem cells contacts the thymus and forms the thymus-dependent or T-cell system. Other cells contact the human equivalent of the bursa of Fabricius of birds, possibly the intestinal lymphoid tissue of Peyer's patches, to differentiate into the bursa or B-cell system.[3]

The diversity of these cells is extraordinary, and it has been estimated that B and T lymphocytes are capable of responding to 10 to 15 different antigens.

T-Cell System (Cell-Mediated Immunity). T cells populate the paracortical areas of lymph nodes and the white pulp of the spleen and constitute 70 to 80% of lymphocytes in the peripheral blood. T cells have a wide range of activities. One group interacts with B cells and helps them to divide, differentiate, and make antibody. Another group interacts with phagocytic cells to help them destroy pathogens they have engulfed. These two groups are the T helper cells. A third group of T lymphocytes, the cytotoxic T cells, recognizes cells infected by virus and destroys them. The T-cell system is responsible for cell-mediated immunity, which serves as the body's primary defense against viruses and fungi and which is also responsible for delayed hypersensitivity reactions.

The use of monoclonal antibodies has permitted the further subdivision of T lymphocytes by the detection of molecules present on the cell surface. T lymphocytes are classified as CD1 to CD8, according to cell surface molecules, with each cell differing in function and stage of development. The two T-cell types that are most important for clinicians to understand are the CD4 (T4) and CD8 (T8) cells. Cells with CD4 surface molecules (T4 lymphocytes) are important in directing the immune response by inducing the proliferation of both T8 lymphocytes and B lymphocytes. The CD4 molecule present on the T4 lymphocyte is the molecule used by human immunodeficiency virus (HIV) to penetrate and infect the cells. T8 lymphocytes (with CD8 surface molecules) suppress antibody synthesis and are cytotoxic to tumor cells and cells infected with viruses, fungi, or protozoa. They are also the cells that are active in graft rejection.

T lymphocytes perform many of their functions by releasing cytokines. Cytokines are proteinaceous mediators of cell-to-cell interaction and act as local hormones. Cytokines are produced by virtually all nucleated cells and are called lymphokines when produced by lymphocytes. Interleukins, colony-stimulating factors, and interferons are among the main types of cytokines. Interleukins are a large group of cytokines that are mainly involved in directing other cells to divide and differentiate. Colony-stimulating factors are involved in directing the division and differentiation of bone marrow stem cells and the precursors of blood leukocytes. Interferons are produced early in infection and are the first line of resistance to many viruses. Certain types of interferons and interleukins also play a role in B-cell stimulation and modulation.

B-cell System (Humoral Immunity).   The B cells populate the follicles around germinal centers of lymph nodes, spleen, and tonsils. B lymphocytes have immunoglobulin receptors on their surfaces. When these receptors combine with an antigen, they differentiate into plasma cells and produce antibodies, which are vital to the body's defense against bacterial infections and other toxic foreign substances. Five major classes of antibodies or immunoglobulins are now recognized: immunoglobulin (Ig) M, IgG, IgA, IgD, and IgE. Each of these immunoglobulins has different chemical and biologic properties.

IgM antibodies are macromolecules composed of five antibody monomers and are produced chiefly in the body's primary response to a foreign antigen. IgM also plays an important role in the activation of complement and in the formation of immunocomplexes. IgG constitutes 75% of the serum immunoglobulins and is the major component of the secondary antibody response. IgG is also the immunoglobulin that crosses the placenta, giving protection to the newborn. Four subgroups of IgG have been identified. IgA antibodies are found in blood in small amounts, but secretory IgA is the main antibody found in external secretions such as saliva, tears, and bile. Levels of secretory IgA in saliva may have an important role in protecting oral tissues against disease by preventing microorganisms from attaching to the mucosa. Dysfunction of the IgA system may help explain certain oral diseases, and in the future, the induction of specific salivary secretory IgA antibodies may protect patients from dental caries and periodontal disease. Low quantities of both IgD and IgE are found in normal human serum. IgD acts as a receptor for antigen on B lymphocytes; IgE binds to mast cells and basophils, triggering the release of histamine during allergic reactions such as anaphylaxis, hay fever, and asthma.

Immunologic Disease

The immune response, so necessary for protection against disease, can also cause disease or other undesirable consequences when it reacts against tissues. The immune system can fail in one of three ways:

IMMUNODEFICIENCY (INEFFECTIVE IMMUNE RESPONSE)
An immune response is comprised of a multitude of cells, cytokines, and reactions. If any one part of an individual's immune system is defective, the individual may not be able to fight infections adequately. Immunodeficiency may be hereditary, manifesting shortly after birth, or may be acquired as the result of viral (ie, HIV) infection or medication (ie, chemotherapy).

AUTOIMMUNITY (INAPPROPRIATE REACTION TO SELF)
A normally functioning immune system recognizes foreign antigens and reacts against them; it simultaneously recognizes its own tissues as self and mounts no reaction. If the system reacts against self-components, autoimmune disease occurs. The body produces antibodies against its own tissues and therefore causes damage. These autoantibodies play a significant role in the pathogenesis of diseases such as pemphigus, pemphigoid, and Hashimoto's thyroiditis.

Immunocomplex disease is a subdivision of autoimmune disorders. In these diseases, antigen-antibody complexes combine with complement to cause a nonspecific vasculitis. Systemic lupus erythematosus, glomerulonephritis, Behçet's syndrome, and erythema multiforme are examples of disorders in which immunocomplexes play a significant role.

Antibodies may also cause disease by blocking the receptor sites and preventing chemical agents that normally attach at those sites from functioning. Myasthenia gravis and insulin-resistant diabetes are caused by receptor sites blocked by antibodies.

HYPERSENSITIVITY (OVERACTIVE IMMUNE RESPONSE)
Occasionally, immune reactions are out of proportion to the damage caused by a pathogen, or the immune system produces a reaction to a harmless antigen, causing hypersensitivity reactions. The immediate (type I) reaction responsible for anaphylactic shock, angioedema, and hives is caused when IgE and antigens bind to basophils and mast cells, resulting in the release of chemical mediators such as histamine and platelet-activating factor. These substances contract smooth muscle and cause an accumulation of extravascular fluid by increasing vascular permeability. The delayed-type hypersensitivity reaction is mediated by a T-cell response rather than by antibodies and leads to granulomatous inflammation. Two examples of this reaction are inflammation resulting from a tuberculin test and contact allergy to a topical antigen. The immune nature of an allergic reaction is well accepted, but the relationship of the immune response to other diseases remains controversial.

Every immunologic disease can be classified with one of the above immune-system malfunctions. The remainder of the chapter discusses different examples of immunologic disorders and their impact on oral disease and dental treatment.

▼ PRIMARY IMMUNODEFICIENCIES

Primary immunodeficiencies are hereditary abnormalities characterized by an inborn defect of the immune system. These diseases may involve only the B-cell system, with a resultant deficiency of humoral antibodies, or only the T-cell system, with a deficiency of cellular immunity. Since B-cell function in humans is largely T-cell dependent, T-cell deficiency also results in humoral immunodeficiency. Therefore, T-cell deficiency can lead to a combined deficiency of both humoral and cell-mediated immunity. The following is a discussion of various illustrative primary immunodeficiencies. The oral manifestations of these deficiencies are discussed together at the end of the section.

Immunodeficiency Disease with Primary Defect in Humoral Immunity

X-LINKED AGAMMAGLOBULINEMIA

A hereditary disease of male children, X-linked agammaglobulinemia (XLA), or Bruton's agammaglobulinemia, occurs in 1 of 50,000 births and is caused by a defect in B-cell function. Symptoms begin at 6 months of age, when transplacentally acquired maternal antibodies have been metabolized. The infant's serum usually contains no IgA, IgM, IgD, or IgE and only small amounts of IgG (< 100 mg/dL).[4] Recent epidemiologic studies have shown that most children develop clinical problems during the first year of life but that as many as 21% first present clinically as late as 3 to 5 years.[5]

The primary defect in XLA is a lesion on the gene that regulates the production of immunoglobulin heavy chains. The affected individual lacks the ability to synthesize all classes of antibodies, including the secretory immunoglobulins, making the person considerably more susceptible to bacterial infections.[6] The disease gene for XLA was identified in 1993 as encoding Bruton tyrosine kinase (Btk).[7] The exact role of Btk in B-cell maturation is not yet understood, but defective Btk results in an inability to develop B cells from pre-B cells.[8]

Patients with XLA experience severe recurrent bacterial infections of the lungs, meninges, skin, and sinuses. The most common organisms involved in these infections are pneumococci, streptococci, staphylococci, and *Haemophilus influenzae*. Although recurrent sinopulmonary infection is the most common infection in patients with XLA, septicemia, septic arthritis, and osteomyelitis may be present in untreated children.[9] Untreated children also have an increased incidence of rheumatoid arthritis, dermatomyositis with neurologic involvement, lymphoma, and leukemia. The patient's ability to combat most viral and fungal infection is normal because of the intact T-cell system.

A diagnosis of XLA is determined by the presence of very little or no immunoglobulin and few or no B cells. Specific mutation detection or measurement of Btk activity can confirm the genetic cause in a patient without an X-linked family history.[10] Examination of patients with XLA will reveal hypoplasia of the lymph nodes, tonsils, and adenoids. Biopsy specimens of lymphoid tissue reveal a lack of germinal centers and plasma cells.

Even with careful therapy, the patient's life span is decreased because of repeated severe infections. Reductions in hospitalization and infection rates have been well documented in patients who receive high doses of intravenous immunoglobulin (> 400 mg/kg every 3 weeks).[11] Aggressive antimicrobial therapy is often needed as adjunctive care in spite of intravenous immunoglobulin replacement.

SELECTIVE IMMUNOGLOBULIN DEFICIENCIES

Selective immunoglobulin deficiencies are a group of disorders characterized by an abnormality of the B-cell antibody system that does not become clinically apparent until adulthood. Usually, only one or two immunoglobulin classes are deficient, which accounts for the relatively asymptomatic nature of the disease throughout childhood. There is evidence that patients with deficiencies of one immunoglobulin will compensate by the increased production of others. For this reason, selective immunoglobulin deficiencies have been difficult to detect.[12] Routine serum protein electrophoresis appears normal, and specific tests for immunoglobulin levels must be used in diagnosis.

The primary adult deficiencies rarely become apparent until the third decade of life. The most common symptoms include recurrent gram-positive bacterial infections, especially of the respiratory tract. The infections are severe in patients who lack all classes of immunoglobulins and are moderate to mild in patients with a selective immunoglobulin deficiency. Other organ systems commonly involved are the joints, gastrointestinal tract, and skin. Chronic compensatory hyperplasia of the lymphoid tissue may occur, causing these disorders to be confused with lymphomas.

IgA deficiency is the most common primary immunodeficiency, with an estimated 1 in 400 persons affected.[13] One in 700 Caucasians have the defect; however, it is rarely found in other ethnic groups. A majority of these patients are apparently clinically normal and have no specific signs or symptoms related to the deficiency and no obvious susceptibility to infection. The most common disorders related to selective IgA deficiency are chronic sinusitis, chronic pulmonary infection, and malabsorption syndromes. In addition, people with IgA deficiency tend to develop malignant disorders. Finally, autoimmune and collagen vascular diseases such as systemic lupus erythematosus and rheumatoid arthritis afflict people with IgA deficiency more frequently.[14] The reason for this is unclear, but it has been speculated that in the normal patient, secretory IgA blocks antigens that cause autoimmune diseases.

Approximately 20% of IgA-deficient individuals also lack subclasses of IgG, specifically IgG2 and IgG4. In humans, most antibodies to the capsular polysaccharides of pyogenic bacteria are in the IgG2 subclass; therefore, a deficiency in IgG2 alone also results in recurrent pyogenic infections. These class and subclass deficiencies result from a failure in terminal B-cell differentiation.

COMMON VARIABLE IMMUNODEFICIENCY

Individuals with common variable immunodeficiency (CVID) have acquired agammaglobulinemia, which becomes apparent in the second or third decade of life or later. As its genetic basis and cause remain unknown, CVID is a diagnosis of exclusion. It is clinically indistinguishable from the other primary B-cell disorders and shares features of hypogammaglobulinemia, recurrent pyogenic infections, and impaired antibody responses. Both males and females are equally affected. Most patients with CVID have B cells that are not fully mature and thus do not function properly. The cells are not defective, but they fail to receive proper signals from the T cells. T-cell defects have not been well-defined in CVID. Many patients develop autoimmune diseases (most prominently, pernicious anemia), but the reason for this is unknown.

Immunodeficiency Disease with Primary Defect in Cellular Immunity

DiGEORGE SYNDROME (VELOCARDIOFACIAL SYNDROME)

DiGeorge syndrome has recently been shown to be one of a group of disorders caused by a deletion on chromosome 22q11.[15] This genetic defect results in abnormal development of the facial and neural crest tissues, causing abnormal development of derivatives of the third and fourth pharyngeal pouches.

The result of this defect in embryonic growth are abnormalities of the thymus, the parathyroid glands, and the great vessels of the heart. The subsequent malfunction of these organs accounts for the respective features of DiGeorge syndrome: variable immunodeficiency, neonatal hypocalcemia secondary to hypoparathyroidism, and congenital cardiac defects. Abnormal ear, palatal (cleft palate), maxillary, and mandibular development define the characteristic facies of this disorder. These features include short palpebral fissures, a small mouth, and a prominent forehead.[16]

The immunodeficiency associated with DiGeorge syndrome becomes apparent during the first few months of life. Most patients have normal leukocyte function and normal humoral immunity but a nearly total lack of cellular immunity. As a result, patients have an increased susceptibility to infections with viruses and fungi. Infections with *Candida albicans* are especially prominent (Figure 18-1).

DiGeorge syndrome was important in the development of the concept of separate immune systems for humoral and cellular hypersensitivity because hypoplasia of the thymus produced impairment of only cellular immunity. The T-cell deficiency is variable, depending on how severely the thymus is affected. It is now believed that the thymus is completely absent in less than 5% of patients with 22q11 deletion syndrome, but maldescent of the thymus leads to an absence of thymus tissue in the mediastinum in most cases.[17] Partial DiGeorge syndrome exists with partial aplasia of the thymus and parathyroid glands.

Spontaneous improvement in the immunologic defect of DiGeorge syndrome has been described. Transplantation of fetal or postneonatal thymic tissue may restore immune function.

SEVERE COMBINED IMMUNODEFICIENCY

Severe combined immunodeficiency (SCID) (Swiss-type agammaglobulinemia) is a genetic disease that can be inherited as either a sex-linked or autosomal recessive trait that causes a variety of molecular defects.[18] Because over 50% of cases are caused by a genetic defect on the X chromosome, SCID is more common in male infants than in female infants (a ratio of 3:1). The remaining cases of SCID are due to recessive genes on other chromosomes; one-half of these patients have a genetic deficiency of adenosine deaminase or purine nucleoside phosphorylase. A deficiency of these purine degradation enzymes results in the accumulation of metabolites that are toxic to lymphoid stem cells. These patients have low peripheral lymphocyte counts, a severe deficiency of immunoglobulins, and a lack of cellular immunity.

The symptoms of this disease begin in the first few weeks of life and include bacterial, viral, and fungal infections. Localized or systemic candidiasis is common. Cutaneous granulomas may also occur.[19] Infants are also at risk for lethal graft-versus-host disease (GVHD) if given transfusions with nonirradiated blood products, and they can die of progressive infection if vaccinated with live organisms. The severity of these immunologic disorders has made them logical candidates for treatments such as bone marrow transplantation and gene replacement therapy. Gene therapy has shown limited success in individuals with adenosine deaminase deficiency. Early diagnosis and the availability of matched donors for bone marrow transplantation remain the most important factors in a hopeful prognosis for patients with this group of disorders.

Partial Combined Immunodeficiencies

ATAXIA TELANGIECTASIA

Ataxia telangiectasia (AT) is a disorder characterized by cerebellar ataxia, oculocutaneous telangiectasia, and immunodeficiency. The ataxia usually begins in infancy and is progressive. Telangiectasias of the skin and eyes become apparent between 3 and 6 years of age. Though not all patients with AT have immunodeficiency, AT is clinically manifested by recurrent and chronic sinopulmonary infections.

AT is inherited as an autosomal recessive trait. The AT gene (*ATM*), identified in 1995, encodes a protein involved in the repair of double-strand breaks in deoxyribonucleic acid (DNA).[20] Since radiosensitivity is a characteristic of AT in vitro, understanding the mechanism of action of *ATM* may provide additional information on radiation signaling in human cells; it may be possible to sensitize tumor cells to radiation and subsequently increase the therapeutic benefit of radiotherapy.[21] In addition, the *ATM* locus is a common event in some tumor types, suggesting a general role for *ATM* in cancer. Defective DNA repair mechanisms common to these patients may account for the high incidence of malignancies. The *ATM* gene, therefore, has the potential for wide-ranging roles such as detecting DNA damage, preventing genomic re-arrangements in malignancy, and preventing programmed cell death.

The immunologic abnormalities of AT include T-cell and B-cell deficiencies, causing both an abnormal cellular response and a deficiency of immunoglobulins. Due to a markedly hypoplastic thymus, the peripheral T-cell pool is frequently reduced in size. Although the number and class distribution of B lymphocytes are usually normal, about 70% of AT patients are serum IgA deficient and can also be deficient in IgG2 and IgG4.[9] These immunologic abnormalities may be the result of cells that exhibit chromosomal breaks (usually in chromosomes 7 and 14) at the sites of the T-cell receptor genes and the genes that encode the heavy chains of immunoglobulins.

Treatment for AT is limited to supportive care as no cure is available. Unless a severe IgG deficiency is present, therapy with gamma globulin is not indicated. Due to the highly variable incidence of infection, bone marrow transplantation is usually not advised.

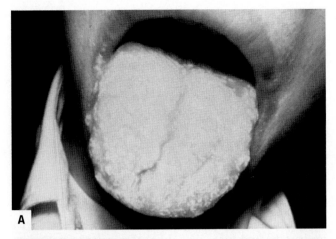

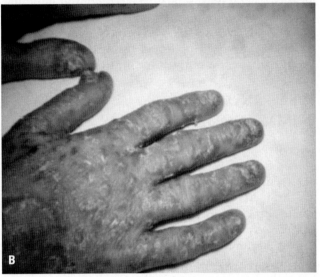

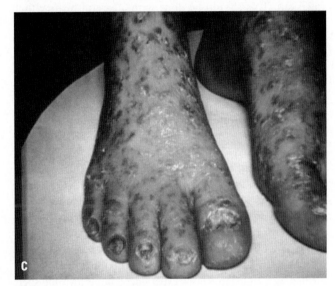

Figure 18-1 A, Chronic mucocutaneous candidiasis in patient with DiGeorge syndrome, with lesions of the tongue. **B,** Lesions of the same infection, on the hands. **C,** Lesions of the same infection, on the feet.

WISKOTT-ALDRICH SYNDROME

Wiskott-Aldrich syndrome (WAS) is an X-linked disorder characterized by lymphocytes and platelets that are faulty due to an altered cell surface glycoprotein they share. The classic clinical features include a microcytic thrombocytopenia, severe eczema, and pyogenic and opportunistic infections. The immunologic findings of WAS are a result of both T-cell defects and abnormal immunoglobulin levels. The T cells have a uniquely abnormal appearance due to a cytoskeletal defect. Moreover, the T cells are defective in function, and this malfunction becomes progressively worse. Impaired response to polysaccharide antigens, elevated serum IgA and IgE levels, normal levels of IgG, and decreased amounts of IgM are among the variable effects on humoral immunity.

In addition, the collaboration among immune cells is also faulty in patients with WAS. During the normal collaboration of T cells and B cells in antibody formation, the cytoskeleton of the T cells becomes polarized toward the B cells. This reorientation of T cells to B cells fails to occur in patients with Wiskott-Aldrich syndrome, most likely because of the cytoskeletal defect in the T cells. The end result is a poorly collaborated immune response.

Oral Manifestations

Patients with T-lymphocyte abnormalities have a higher incidence of oral disease than patients with B-lymphocyte disorders have. T-lymphocyte abnormalities lead to chronic fungal and viral infections, which are more likely to occur in the oral mucosa than are the bacterial infections seen in B-lymphocyte deficiencies.[22] A consistent oral sign noted in patients with T-cell diseases such as thymic hypoplasia or AT is chronic oral candidiasis. Herpes simplex virus infections are also common in patients with T-cell disease. The infections may be localized to the mouth but frequently become disseminated and are potentially lethal if not treated with antiviral medication.[23] Other oral signs seen with T-cell deficiencies include the dermal and mucosal telangiectases of AT. Congenital defects of the mouth and jaws (including cleft palate, micrognathia, bifid uvula, and short philtrum of the upper lip) have also been seen in patients with thymic hypoplasia. In patients with AT, hypotonia of facial muscles and atrophy of the skin gives rise to a characteristic dull expression; drooling can also be a problem.[24]

The major sign in patients with B-cell abnormalities is recurrent bacterial infections[25] that frequently involve the respiratory tract. The most common of these infections that comes to the attention of dentists is chronic maxillary sinusitis.

The weight of evidence indicates that patients with primary immunoglobulin deficiencies do not have an increase in dental caries or periodontal disease.[26,27] Although oral ulceration has been occasionally described in patients with CVID and IgA deficiency, it is not a characteristic finding.[28] Neutropenia and neutrophil dysfunction syndromes commonly cause oral ulcers, but immunoglobulin deficiencies do not.

Factors other than primary immunodeficiency may cause candidiasis and maxillary sinusitis, but for patients with these infections who are not successfully treated by antibiotic or antifungal therapy or who have a history of other recurring infections, immunodeficiency should be ruled out. This should be done with a careful history that includes past episodes of pneumonia, recurrent otitis media, autoimmune disease, severe asthma, malabsorption syndrome, and pyoderma.

Laboratory studies should be performed when the history suggests immunodeficiency. With rare exceptions, a deficiency of humoral immunity is accompanied by diminished serum concentration of one or more classes of immunoglobulin. Laboratory studies to rule out B-lymphocyte dysfunction should include a quantitation of the major immunoglobulins, using immunodiffusion techniques. In questionable cases, the clinical immunologist will test the patient's ability to synthesize specific antibodies after immunization with standard antigens. Estimation of numbers of circulating B lymphocytes has also been of great value in determining the pathogenesis of certain types of immunodeficiency.

Screening for T-lymphocyte dysfunction must be performed by a clinician who is experienced in performing such tests. Normal levels of serum immunoglobulins and antibody responsiveness are reliable indices of intact T-helper-cell function. T-cell function can be measured directly by delayed hypersensitivity skin testing, using a variety of antigens such as purified protein derivative (PPD) of tuberculin, *Candida*, and *Trichophyton*. Negative reactions to these antigens suggest a defect of cellular (T-cell) immunity. Laboratory studies that are used to check T-cell activity include lymphocyte proliferation, T-cell subset quantification, and T-cell cytotoxicity assays.

Dental Management

Dental treatment for patients with primary immunodeficiency must minimize the chances of local infection or bacteremia. Patients with symptomatic B-cell abnormalities are usually given monthly therapy with concentrated human gamma globulin that has been screened for hepatitis B and HIV.[29] Prior to instituting dental treatment, the gamma globulin level should be checked to ensure that it is at least 200 mg/dL. When oral surgery is necessary, an extra dose of gamma globulin should be administered the day before surgery, in a dose usually between 100 and 200 mg/kg of body weight.[30,31]

Unusual transfusion reactions occur in patients with primary immunodeficiency and must be taken into account when using blood replacement therapy. Patients with B-cell defi-

ciency resulting in the absence of particular immunoglobulins may experience severe transfusion reactions when receiving blood from a patient who has normal immunoglobulin levels. The immunoglobulin acts as a foreign protein and causes an allergic response. For this reason, the patient with selective IgA deficiency must be given IgA-depleted blood.[32]

Another problem in administering a transfusion to a patient with primary immunodeficiency is the development of GVHD. The immunocompetent cells in the transfused blood will react against the tissues of the immunodeficient recipient. Only fresh blood in which the immunocompetent lymphocytes have been destroyed can be used.

Dental infections in patients with primary immunodeficiencies must be treated vigorously. A culture and sensitivity for bacteria and fungi should be taken prior to instituting antibiotic therapy. Few dentists do this routinely for normal patients with abscesses, but it is particularly important for immunodeficient patients because these patients get unusual infections with fungi and gram-negative bacteria.[33]

▼ SECONDARY IMMUNODEFICIENCIES

Secondary immunodeficiencies can be caused by immunosuppressive drug therapy, HIV infection, malignancy or granulomatous disease of the lymphoid system, or protein-depleting disorders. Specific diseases that result in secondary immunodeficiency include leukemia, Hodgkin's disease, non-Hodgkin's lymphoma, acquired immunodeficiency syndrome (AIDS), nephrotic syndrome, multiple myeloma, and sarcoidosis. (These disorders are discussed in detail in other chapters of this text. This section confines itself to a discussion of the immunologic aspects of these diseases. HIV infection and AIDS are discussed in Chapter 20, "Infectious Diseases.")

Leukemia

Infection is the major cause of death in patients with leukemia; thus, it poses a major clinical management problem. The majority of these infections are caused by microorganisms that rarely cause fatal illness in normal individuals (eg, gram-negative bacilli, fungi, and herpesviruses)[34] (Figure 18-2).

Infections in patients with acute leukemia are caused by a severe decrease in mature functioning granulocytes. Signs of an infection may be present although typical findings of a purulent infection or inflammatory response is muted in patients with severe granulocytopenia. The function of the B lymphocytes and T lymphocytes appears to be intact until cytotoxic chemotherapy is initiated. Studies of neutrophils from patients with acute leukemia show both an impaired ability to migrate and diminished bactericidal and chemotactic functions.

Chronic lymphocytic leukemia involves B lymphocytes in most cases, affecting the humoral antibody response and resulting in hypogammaglobulinemia with secondary bacterial infection, particularly respiratory infection. Infections with encapsulated bacteria (pneumococci, *Haemophilus influenzae*, and group A streptococci) are common, presumably because

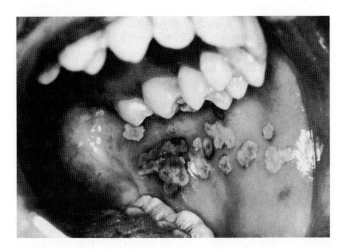

FIGURE 18-2 Extensive recurrent herpes simplex lesions of the buccal mucosa and palate of a patient receiving chemotherapy for leukemia.

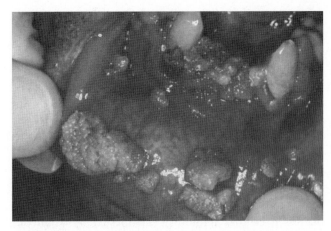

FIGURE 18-3 Extensive condyloma acuminatum from human papillomavirus infection in a patient receiving chemotherapy for non-Hodgkin's lymphoma.

of the patient's inability to produce antibodies. Serum immunoglobulin levels are frequently low, and the circulating antibody response to vaccines is impaired, but delayed hypersensitivity reactions to recall antigens are usually intact.

Patients with chronic myelogenous leukemia have a lower incidence of infection, consistent with laboratory studies that show a good antibody response in these patients (see Chapter 16, "Hematologic Diseases").

Hodgkin's Disease

Patients with Hodgkin's disease have a loss of T-lymphocyte function that worsens as the disease progresses. The radiotherapy and chemotherapy used to treat the disease further suppress normal immune function.

Studies of patients with advanced Hodgkin's disease reveal changes consistent with the deficient T-cell response, including unresponsiveness to skin tests with previously encountered antigens and prolonged skin graft survival time. In vitro studies of lymphocytes from patients with Hodgkin's disease show an abnormal response to antigens. The major clinical infections seen in patients with Hodgkin's disease are fungal, viral, and protozoal. The most common fungal infections are histoplasmosis and infections with *Cryptococcus neoformans*, *Candida albicans*, and actinomycetes. The viral infections are with herpes simplex virus, varicella-zoster virus, and *Cytomegalovirus*. The protozoal infections include toxoplasmosis and infections with *Pneumocystis carinii*. Chemotherapy and radiotherapy may suppress neutrophil and antibody function for years, increasing the patient's susceptibility to bacterial infection (see Chapter 16, "Hematologic Diseases").

Non-Hodgkin's Lymphoma

Some patients with non-Hodgkin's lymphoma have a deficiency of the B-cell or T-cell system, caused by the disease itself or by chemotherapy. This deficiency becomes more severe late in the course of the disease. Lymphoma patients

have an increased rate of infections with bacteria, viruses, and fungi (Figure 18-3) (see Chapter 16, "Hematologic Diseases").

Nephrotic Syndrome

Patients with nephrotic syndrome lose large amounts of serum protein through the destroyed or damaged glomeruli, which causes secondary hypogammaglobulinemia. Bacterial infections secondary to hypogammaglobulinemia have been described as a cause of death in children with nephrotic syndrome. The common sites of infection in these patients are the oropharynx, the skin, and the lungs. The prophylactic use of gamma globulin and antibiotics has decreased the incidence of infection dramatically (see Chapter 15, "Renal Disease").

Multiple Myeloma

Multiple myeloma is a malignancy of plasma cells, the cells primarily responsible for the humoral antibody response. These defective plasma cells produce large quantities of myeloma proteins instead of the normal immunoglobulins. The myeloma proteins offer no protection against infection, and repeated bouts of bacterial infection, particularly pneumococcal pneumonia, are common. Bone marrow suppression by malignant plasma cells and chemotherapy further increases the patient's susceptibility to infection. A viral infection that occurs with increased frequency in multiple myeloma patients is varicella-zoster virus infection, which may occur as localized herpes zoster or as generalized varicella (see Chapter 16, "Hematologic Diseases").

Sarcoidosis

Sarcoidosis is a systemic granulomatous disease that primarily affects the lungs and the lymphatic system but can also affect mucocutaneous surfaces, the eyes, and the salivary glands. The diagnosis is established when clinical and radiographic lesions are supported by histologic evidence of noncaseating epithelioid granulomas in more than one organ system and when other disorders that are known to cause granulomatous disease are excluded. Sarcoidosis commonly affects young and middle-aged adults (between 20 and 40 years of age) and frequently presents with bilateral hilar lymphadenopathy, pulmonary infiltration, and ocular and skin lesions.

Although the cause of sarcoidosis remains unknown, there is evidence that it results from the exposure of genetically susceptible hosts to specific environmental agents.[35] Frequently observed immunologic features are depression of cutaneous delayed-type hypersensitivity and a heightened helper T cell type 1 (Th1) immune response at sites of disease. Circulating immunocomplexes, along with signs of B-cell hyperactivity, may also be found.[36]

Sarcoidosis is characterized by distinctive laboratory abnormalities, including hyperglobulinemia, an elevated level of serum angiotensin-converting enzyme, evidence of depressed cellular immunity (manifested by cutaneous anergy), and occasionally, hypercalcemia and hypercalciuria. Systemic steroids remain the mainstay of therapy when treatment is required although other anti-inflammatory agents are being used increasingly often. (See Chapter 12, "Diseases of the Respiratory System.")

▼ CONNECTIVE-TISSUE DISEASES

Connective-tissue diseases are customarily grouped together under names such as collagen disease, collagen vascular disease, hyperimmune disease, or autoimmune disease. They include systemic lupus erythematosus, rheumatoid arthritis, scleroderma (progressive systemic sclerosis), dermatomyositis, and polyarteritis nodosa. Rheumatic fever is also sometimes classified with these disorders.

The term "autoimmune" has been used to describe this group of diseases because autoantibodies that react with normal tissue in vitro have been detected in significant quantities in patients with these diseases. This term appears to be justified when it is used to describe pemphigus or Hashimoto's thyroiditis, diseases in which autoantibodies appear to cause direct and specific damage to tissues.

In connective-tissue diseases, the term "immunocomplex" more accurately describes the source of most of the tissue damage although autoantibodies appear to cause some hematologic changes. In immunocomplex disease, a non-specific inflammatory response results from the accumulation of antigen-antibody complexes rather than from specific destruction by antibodies. When immunocomplexes form, they activate the complement system, which attracts neutrophils and macrophages. Vasculitis and tissue damage result when immunocomplexes are present in sufficient quantity. Serum sickness, a generalized allergic reaction, is a classic example of a self-limiting disease caused by circulating immunocomplexes.

The stimulus that causes the formation of the abnormal antibodies that trigger the immunocomplexes is unknown, but some investigators believe that viruses or other microorganisms are responsible.

Systemic Lupus Erythematosus

Systemic lupus erythematosus (SLE) is the prototypical autoimmune disease characterized by the production of numerous autoantibodies. Organ injury is secondary to either the direct binding of autoantibodies to self-antigens or the deposition of immunocomplexes in vessels or tissues. It is estimated that 15 to 17% of lupus cases occur prior to the age of 16 years,[37] with the peak incidence being in the age range of 20 to 40 years. SLE occurs ten times more frequently in females and has a higher incidence among black people. The autoantibodies of SLE may be directed against nucleoproteins, erythrocytes, leukocytes, platelets, coagulation factors, and organs such as the liver, the kidneys, or the heart. SLE therefore has a variety of clinical manifestations.

NOMENCLATURE (SUBTYPES)

Over the years, the classification of lupus has been modified to include additional forms. Discoid lupus erythematosus (DLE) is confined to the skin and mucosa; only approximately 10 to 20% of patients with DLE develop systemic manifestations later in the course of the disease. The skin lesions of DLE begin as erythematous scaling lesions with sharp borders that slowly expand forming telangiectasias and (eventually) depigmented scars. Follicular plugging that extends down into the skin follicles can be observed when the scale is removed. The malar or so-called butterfly rash is common, but does not always occur and is not pathognomonic for DLE as it is also seen in other dermatologic diseases such as seborrheic dermatitis.

Chronic cutaneous lupus erythematosus and subacute cutaneous lupus erythematosus are mainly dermatologic diseases that are almost always restricted to the skin (most often the face and scalp) and to the oral mucosa.

Neonatal lupus erythematosus is most often a transient self-limited disease. Dermatologic, hepatic, and hematologic involvement usually disappears at the age of about 6 months, in parallel with the decline in maternal antibodies in the neonatal circulation.

Drug-induced lupus erythematosus has many features in common with SLE and characteristically develops in people who have no history of systemic rheumatic disease. By far, the drugs with the highest risk are procainamide and hydralazine, with incidences of approximately 20% for procainamide and 5 to 8% for hydralazine. The risk for developing lupuslike disease with other drugs is much lower: quinidine can be considered a moderate-risk drug, whereas sulfasalazine, chlorpromazine, penicillamine, methyldopa, carbamazepine, acebutalol, isoniazid, captopril, propylthiuracil, and mincycline are relatively low-risk drugs.[38]

ETIOLOGY AND PATHOGENESIS

The specific etiology of SLE is not known with certainty, but immunocomplexes, autoantibodies, and genetic, infectious, environmental, and endocrine factors play significant roles.

Genetic Factors.   Familial clustering and an increased rate among identical twins (24 to 57%) demonstrate the important role of genetic susceptibility. Relatives of SLE patients have higher incidences of autoantibodies, immunodeficiency, and connective-tissue disease. Genes that increase the risk of SLE have been identified (specifically, *HLA-DR2* and *HLA-DR3*). Genetic linkage analyses yield consistent findings for linkage of SLE on chromosome 1.[39]

Infectious and Environmental Factors. Viruslike particles of ribonucleic acid (RNA) viruses have been detected in tissues of SLE patients and are thought by some to initiate the abnormal immune response. Epstein-Barr virus, *Cytomegalovirus*, varicella-zoster virus, and other endogenous/exogenous retroviruses have been reported to occur with increased frequency in patients with SLE. This association could result from the intrinsic susceptibility of lupus patients to these infections, or virus-infected individuals may simply be prone to developing lupus.

Endocrine Factors. A hormonal component to SLE is suggested by its high incidence in women in their childbearing years, the many reports of remission during pregnancy, and the finding of increased estrogen levels in SLE patients.

Immunocomplexes and Autoantibodies. Immunocomplexes consisting chiefly of nucleic acid and antibody account for the majority of the tissue damage seen in SLE. These complexes set off immunologic reactions that activate complement and attract neutrophils and macrophages. The result is vasculitis, fibrosis, and tissue necrosis. Patients with increased circulating immunocomplexes have more severe disease, particularly of the kidney. Immunocomplexes also account for tissue damage in the central nervous system, skin, and lungs.

The autoantibodies in SLE patients could be the actual pathogenic agents of tissue destruction, or they could be the consequence of tissue damage.[40,41] Autoantibodies are a cause of the hemolytic anemia, thrombocytopenia, and lymphopenia seen in SLE patients. The formation of autoantibodies is thought to be related to the decreased functioning of suppressor T lymphocytes and hyperreactive B lymphocytes.

A unified theory that accounts for many of the findings described above has been developed. In this theory, many factors acting together result in SLE. An individual with a genetic predisposition develops a chronic viral infection that releases nucleic acid antigens. Sunburn or damage from chemicals may also contribute to antigen release. A lack of normal suppressor T-lymphocyte function and B-lymphocyte hyperactivity leads to the formation of autoantibodies and immunocomplexes; widespread tissue damage results.

CLINICAL MANIFESTATIONS

SLE is a disease with multiorgan involvement. Immunocomplex deposition causes small-vessel vasculitis, which then leads to renal, cardiac, hematologic, mucocutaneous, and central nervous system destruction. In addition, inflammation of the serous membranes results in joint, peritoneal, and pleuropericardial symptoms. As there is no typical pattern of presentation, one patient may present with dermatitis and kidney disease whereas another may present with arthritis, anemia, and pleurisy. Thus, whenever a patient demonstrates signs and symptoms of mul-

tiorgan involvement, SLE should be considered in the differential diagnosis, especially for a female who is 20 to 40 years of age. The following is a brief overview of the most frequently encountered clinical manifestations.

Renal Manifestations. Kidney involvement in the form of glomerular destruction is seen in approximately 50% of patients. The glomerulonephritis results from the deposition of complement and immunocomplexes in the basement membrane of the glomerulus. Five to twenty-two percent of SLE patients progress to end-stage renal disease and require hemodialysis or transplantation.[42] Nephrotic syndrome results from massive destruction and is a common cause of death in SLE patients. The severity of kidney disease is often a good indication of the overall prognosis of the patient.

Cardiac Manifestations. Accelerated atherosclerosis and valvular heart disease constitute the primary cardiac manifestations of SLE. The most common of all cardiac lesions in SLE patients involves the endocardium and was originally described (by Libman and Sacks) as verrucous valvular lesions. Lupus-related valvular pathoses can include valve leaflet thickening, with or without regurgitation.

Hematologic Manifestations. The primary hematologic diseases among SLE patients are leukopenia, anemia, and thrombocytopenia. Leukopenia ($< 4{,}000/mm^3$) is common and usually reflects lymphopenia but can also be due to immunosuppressive therapies. Anemia of chronic disease occurs in most patients during periods of disease activity but is also often due to hemodialysis. Hemolytic anemia occurs in a small proportion of patients with positive Coombs' test results. Thrombocytopenia ($< 100{,}000/mm^3$) results from increased phagocytosis of autoantibody-coated platelets by spleen, liver, bone marrow and lymph node macrophages and can occur in up to 25% of patients. When antiphospholipid antibodies or the lupus anticoagulant and anticardiolipin antibodies are present, patients are prone to episodic thrombosis, thrombocytopenia, and spontaneous abortion.

Mucocutaneous Manifestations. The cutaneous manifestations of SLE include photosensitive rashes, alopecia, periungual telangiectasias, Raynaud's phenomenon, and skin ulceration secondary to vasculitis (Figure 18-4). Cutaneous involvement does not necessarily correlate with increased systemic disease. The malar or "butterfly" rash (which affects fewer than half of SLE patients) and the discoid rash are the two most characteristic rashes of SLE. The malar rash is a fixed flat or raised erythematous rash over the cheeks and bridge of the nose, often involving the chin and ears (Figure 18-5). It is usually exacerbated by ultraviolet light. A more diffuse maculopapular rash, mainly in sun-exposed areas, is also common. Vasculitic skin lesions include subcutaneous nodules, ulcers, and infarcts of skin or digits. Oral mucosal lesions can be found as annular leukoplakic areas and/or erythematous erosions or chronic ulcerations, often resembling lichen planus.

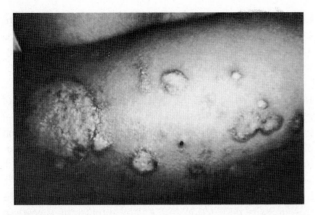

FIGURE 18-4 Skin lesions in a patient with systemic lupus erythematosus. (Courtesy of Dr. George Ehrlich)

Musculoskeletal Manifestations.   Arthritis and arthropathies are the primary musculoskeletal disorders associated with SLE. Arthralgia with morning stiffness is the most common initial manifestation of SLE. More than 75 % of SLE patients develop a true arthritis, which is symmetrical and non-erosive and which usually involves the hands, wrists, and knees. Deforming arthritis is uncommon in SLE patients.

Central Nervous System Manifestations.   Significant neuropsychiatric signs and symptoms are found in 10 to 20% of patients who have SLE.[43] Diffuse and focal cerebral dysfunctions (including psychoses, seizures, and cerebrovascular accidents) in addition to peripheral sensorimotor neu-

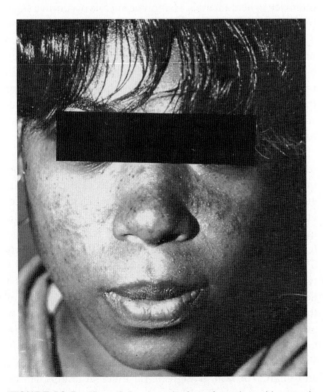

FIGURE 18-5 "Butterfly" rash on the face of a patient with systemic lupus erythematosus. (Courtesy of Dr. Robert Arm)

ropathies, account for more than 60% of neuropsychiatric manifestations.[44] Central nervous system involvement is a poor prognostic sign.

DIAGNOSIS AND LABORATORY EVALUATION

The most important diagnostic laboratory test for SLE is the test for antinuclear antibody (ANA) in the serum, which is positive for 96 to 100% of patients with SLE. The clinician should remember that the ANA test is also positive in a minority of patients with scleroderma or rheumatoid arthritis; therefore, the diagnosis must be made on the total clinical picture, not on a single laboratory test. In addition, SLE is characterized by the production of numerous autoantibodies, including ANAs, anti–native DNA, rheumatoid factor, antibody to Smith (Sm) antigen, antibody to Ro (SS-A) antigen, and antibody to La (SS-B) antigen. Many of these autoantibodies produce specific laboratory and clinical abnormalities and can also be seen in a variety of other rheumatologic diseases. An individual with elevated ANA and anti–native DNA most likely has lupus (Table 18-1).

Important findings on routine laboratory tests include anemia, thrombocytopenia, (which may occasionally be severe enough to cause purpura), increased levels of globulins, and a biologic false-positive result on the serologic test for syphilis (STS). Depressed complement levels (particularly C3 and C4), are also common.

ORAL MANIFESTATIONS

Patients with SLE are affected by a variety of orofacial disorders, including characteristic oral lesions, nonspecific ulcerations, salivary gland disease, and temporomandibular disorders. The reported incidence of these manifestations varies considerably, depending on the criteria of the investigators. The first report of oral manifestations of SLE in the American dental literature was in 1931, by the dermatologist Monash, who reported a 50% incidence of oral lesions.[45] More recently, Rhodus and Johnson reported a higher incidence (81.3 to 87.5%) of various oral lesions, including ulceration, angular cheilosis, mucositis,

TABLE 18-1 Proportion of Autoantibodies Associated with Lupus Erythematosus and Other Rheumatic Diseases

Autoantibody Type	Presence in Autoimmune Disease (% of Cases)			
	SLE	RA	SS	Diffuse Scleroderma
Antinuclear antibodies	96–100	30–60	95	80–95
Anti–native DNA	60	0–5	0	0
Rheumatoid factor	20	72–85	75	25–33
Anti-Sm	10–25	0	0	0
Anti-Ro	15–20	0–5	60–70	0
Anti-La	5–20	0–2	60–70	0

Adapted from De Rossi SS, Glick M.[43]

Anti-Sm = antibody to Smith antigen; Anti-Ro = antibody to Ro (SS-A) antigen; Anti-La = antibody to La (SS-B) antigen; DNA = deoxyribonucleic acid; RA = rheumatoid arthritis; SLE = systemic lupus erythematosus; SS = Sjögren's syndrome.

and glossitis. They also reported a high incidence (75.0 to 87.5%) of signs and symptoms of oral conditions, including glossodynia, dysgeusia, dysphagia, and dry mouth.[46]

The oral lesions of SLE are caused by vasculitis and appear as frank ulceration or mucosal inflammation. Some individuals with SLE or discoid lupus have discoid-appearing oral lesions.[47] The lip lesions often have a central atrophic and occasionally ulcerated area with small white dots, surrounded by a keratinized border composed of small radiating white striae (Figure 18-6). The intraoral lesions are somewhat different because of the thinner epithelium; they are composed of a central depressed red atrophic area surrounded by a 2 to 4 mm elevated keratotic zone that dissolves into small white lines (Figures 18-7 and 18-8).

The oral lesions of SLE are easily confused with the lesions of lichen planus, both clinically and histologically. The World Health Organization established criteria for the histologic diagnosis of oral SLE, but these criteria often do not adequately distinguish lupus from lichen planus. Karjalainen and Tomich[48] compared 17 cases of SLE with 17 cases of lichen planus and described five histologic criteria to distinguish these two disorders by light microscopy: (1) vascularization of keratinocytes, (2) subepithelial presence of patchy periodic acid–Schiff (PAS)-positive deposits, (3) edema in the upper lamina propria, (4) PAS-positive thickening of blood vessel walls, and (5) severe deep or perivascular inflammatory infiltration. Sanchez and colleagues demonstrated that the inflammatory infiltrate in the oral lesions of SLE consists primarily of helper or inducer T lymphocytes.[47]

Direct fluorescent antibody staining of biopsy specimens has become an important aid in the diagnosis of the mucosal or skin lesions of SLE. More than 90% of patients with either DLE or SLE have deposits of immunoglobulin and C3 in the basement membrane zone. This lupus band test is an excellent means of differentiating lupus lesions from lichen planus, which is often clinically and histologically indistinguishable from other forms of leukoplakia. Immunoglobulin deposits are detected in oral lesions of SLE and of DLE

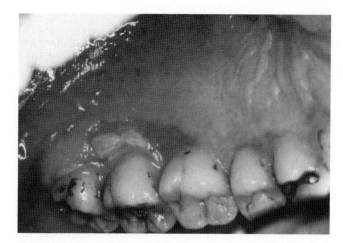

FIGURE 18-7 A chronic palatal lesion (the initial sign of systemic lupus erythematosus in this patient).

whereas those deposits are rare in lichen planus or leukoplakia. There are a small number of cases, however, in which DLE and lichen planus overlap.

Another oral sign of SLE is xerostomia secondary to Sjögren's syndrome.[49] Xerostomia can significantly increase the occurrence of dental caries and candidiasis, especially when patients are being treated with steroids or immunosuppressive agents.

Temporomandibular-joint involvement commonly occurs in SLE patients sometime during the course of their disease and may cause pain and mechanical dysfunction.

TREATMENT

With regard to the management of the oral lesions of SLE, there have been no reports involving the treatment of a large series of patients. In general, the oral ulcerations of SLE are transient, occurring with acute lupus flares. Symptomatic lesions can be treated with high-potency topical corticosteroids or intralesional steroid injections.

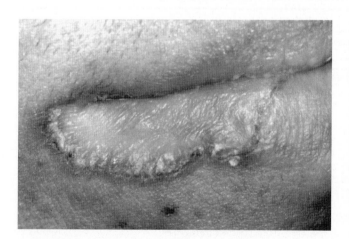

FIGURE 18-6 Discoid lupus lesions on the lower lip.

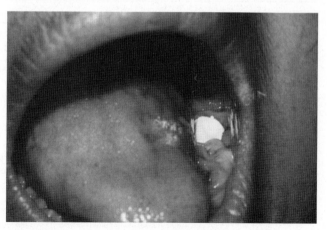

FIGURE 18-8 Chronic lesion of the dorsal tongue in a patient with systemic lupus.

DENTAL CONSIDERATIONS

Because SLE can be a widespread disease affecting many organ systems, the dental management of an SLE patient requires a good understanding of general medicine. The more common problems seen in SLE patients are discussed below.

Adrenal Suppression. Patients with SLE may be taking adrenal-suppressive doses of corticosteroids, which makes these patients susceptible to shock. Glucocorticosteroid therapy will cause adrenal suppression that affects adrenal function for up to 12 months, but the patient's stress response will return within 14 to 30 days. There is no need for replacement therapy for dental treatment in patients who have not taken glucocorticosteroids during the preceding 30 days. Patients who are receiving alternate-day therapy can be treated on an "off" day without supplementation if they have been on the alternate-day regimen for at least 2 weeks. Patients who are receiving daily low-dose corticosteroid therapy (< 30 mg hydrocortisone equivalent) will not need replacement therapy. Patients who are receiving daily high-dose corticosteroid therapy (> 30 mg hydrocortisone equivalent) should be treated as if they were completely adrenally suppressed and were without a normal stress response. The dose will need to be doubled on the day of treatment. The patient's primary care physician should be consulted if the replacement dosage is uncertain or when highly stressful procedures are to be done (eg, general anesthesia)[50] (Table 18-2).

Infection. Patients who are taking cytotoxic or immunosuppressive agents are at an increased risk of infection. Patients with an absolute neutrophil count of between 500 and 1,000 cells/mm^3 will need perioperative prophylactic antibiotics. Although infection due to opportunistic pathogens should be considered in patients who are on high steroid dosages (especially patients who are on adjuvant immunosuppressive therapy), no protocol has been established for the prophylactic use of antibiotics.

Hematologic Abnormalities. Patients with SLE can frequently develop normochromic normocytic anemia, hemolytic anemia, leukopenia, and thrombocytopenia. The presence of an elevated partial thromboplastin time can result from circulating anticoagulant. Prior to any extensive dental procedures, a preoperative complete blood count can screen for thrombocytopenia, anemia, and leukopenia, and a prothrombin time/partial thromboplastin time measurement can screen for a coagulopathy.

Cardiac Disease. Libman-Sacks vegetations under the mitral-valve leaflets may occur in patients with SLE. These vegetations rarely affect function but can lead to bacterial endocarditis. Patients with SLE and heart murmurs should have antibiotic prophylaxis prior to dental treatment that is likely to cause bacteremia.

Renal Disease. Renal disease is common in SLE patients and ranges from an asymptomatic state to frank renal failure; therefore, the dentist should be aware of the patient's renal function (ie, creatinine clearance, serum creatinine, and blood urea nitrogen). Patients who are undergoing hemodialysis should receive dental treatment on nondialysis days.[51]

Exacerbation by Surgery. The dentist should proceed with caution in performing elective surgery or dental procedures, especially in patients who have a history of postsurgery lupus flares.

Exacerbation by Drug Therapy. Drugs that have been related to acute lupus flares include penicillin, sulfonamides, and nonsteroidal anti-inflammatory drugs (NSAIDs) with photosensitizing potential. All of these should be used judiciously.

TABLE 18-2   Protocol for Supplementation of Patients on Glucocorticoid Therapy Who Are Undergoing Dental Care

Dental Procedure	Previous Systemic Steroid Use	Current Systemic Steroid Use	Daily Alternating Systemic Steroid Use	Current Topical Steroid Use
Routine procedures	If prior usage lasted for > 2 weeks and ceased < 14–30 days ago, give previous maintenance dose	No supplementation needed	Treat on steroid dosage day; no further supplementation needed	No supplementation needed
	If prior usage ceased > 14–30 days ago, no supplementation needed			
Extractions, surgery, or extensive procedures	If prior usage lasted > 2 weeks and ceased < 14–30 days ago, give previous maintenance dose	Double daily dose on day of procedure	Treat on steroid dosage day, and give double daily dose on day of procedure	No supplementation needed
	If prior usage ceased > 14–30 days ago, no supplementation needed	Double daily dose on first postoperative day when pain is anticipated	Give normal daily dose on first postoperative day when pain is anticipated	

Adapted from De Rossi SS, Glick M.[51]

Scleroderma

Scleroderma is a multisystem connective-tissue disease that involves hardening of the skin and mucosa, smooth-muscle atrophy, and fibrosis of internal organs. The prevalence of scleroderma is estimated to be about 250 per million, with women being affected significantly more frequently than men.[52] Several US studies have suggested that black patients have a higher age-specific incidence rate and more severe disease than have white patients.[53]

NOMENCLATURE (SUBTYPES)

Localized scleroderma refers to scleroderma primarily involving the skin, with minimal (if any) systemic features. Only rarely have patients with localized scleroderma developed systemic sclerosis. Three major types of localized scleroderma exist: morphea, generalized morphea, and linear scleroderma. Morphea begins with violaceous skin patches that enlarge, become indurated, and eventually lose hair and the ability to sweat. Later in the course of the disease, the lesion "burns out" and appears as a hypo- or hyperpigmented area depressed below the level of the skin.[54] A small number of patients develop numerous larger lesions that coalesce, and these patients are said to have generalized morphea (Figure 18-9). Patients with either type of morphea usually have a benign course characterized by the softening of the lesions over time. Linear scleroderma is a form of the localized disease that may develop during childhood and that usually involves the arms, legs, or head. This form of the disease develops as a thin band of sclerosis that may run the entire length of an extremity,

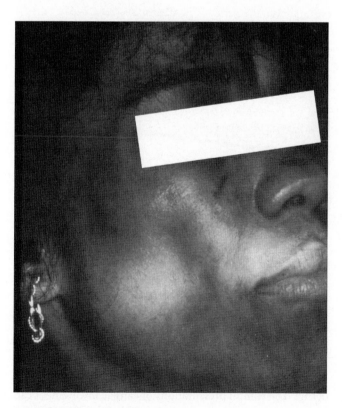

FIGURE 18-9 Morphea of the face.

involving underlying muscle, bones, and joints. When the disease crosses a joint, limitation of motion is possible, along with growth abnormalities. The lesion of linear localized scleroderma of the head and face is called en coup de sabre, and these lesions may result in hemiatrophy of the face. Scleroderma localized to the hands is called acrosclerosis.

Progressive systemic sclerosis (PSS) is a multisystem disease characterized by the inflammation and fibrosis of many organs. PSS occurs three to four times more frequently in females, with its highest incidence occurring between the ages of 25 and 50 years. There are two major subsets: limited cutaneous scleroderma (previously called calcinosis cutis, Raynaud's phenomenon, esophageal dysmotility, sclerodactyly, and telangiectasia [CREST syndrome]) and diffuse cutaneous scleroderma. The major difference between limited and diffuse scleroderma is the pace of the disease. Patients with limited scleroderma often have a long history of Raynaud's phenomenon before the appearance of other symptoms. They have skin thickening limited to hands and frequently have problems with digital ulcers and esophageal dysmotility. Although generally a milder form of disease than diffuse scleroderma, limited scleroderma can have life-threatening complications. Diffuse scleroderma patients have a more acute onset, with constitutional symptoms, arthritis, carpal tunnel syndrome, and marked swelling of the hands and legs. They also characteristically develop widespread skin thickening (progressing from the fingers to the trunk) as well as internal organ involvement (including gastrointestinal and pulmonary fibrosis) and potentially life-threatening cardiac and renal failure. Other possible variants are an overlapping syndrome with SLE, Sjögren's syndrome, rheumatoid arthritis, and dermatomyositis.

ETIOLOGY AND PATHOGENESIS

The etiology of PSS is unclear, but the pathogenesis is characterized by vascular injury as well as the overproduction of normal collagen. Vascular wall fibrosis of small and medium-size arterioles is a prominent alteration in PSS and likely plays a crucial role in the pathogenesis of pulmonary hypertension, renal crisis, myocardial dysfunction, and digital gangrene in this disease.[55] Excessive collagen deposition in affected tissues is also a central event in the pathogenesis of PSS and is responsible for most of the clinical manifestations of this disease. The up-regulation of collagen gene expression in PSS fibroblasts and the aberrant expression of cytokines that positively or negatively influence fibroblast collagen synthesis appear to be critical events in the development of the pathologic tissue fibrosis that is characteristic of PSS.[55] A role for environmental factors in the pathogenesis of PSS is suggested by an increased rate of PSS and PSS-like disease detected in individuals who are exposed to silica dust, vinyl chloride, benzene, and tryptophan.[56]

CLINICAL MANIFESTATIONS

PSS sclerosis is a chronic multisystem disorder characterized by intense fibrosis involving the skin, vasculature, synovium, skeletal muscles, and internal organs. The following is an overview of frequently encountered clinical manifestations.

Raynaud's Phenomenon.   Raynaud's phenomenon, a paroxysmal vasospasm of the fingers that results in a change in the color of the fingertips as a response to cold or emotion, is the most common finding of PSS. More than 95% of scleroderma patients eventually experience the characteristic digital cyanosis and blanching that results from intimal hyperplasia.[57] Raynaud's phenomenon may be nothing more than a nuisance, but some patients have recurrent episodes that are associated with digital pitting scars, nail fold infarcts, or digital ulcers.

Cutaneous Manifestations.   The thickening of the skin of PSS patients always begins in the fingers. Early skin changes, starting with pitting edema, often involve the whole hand and the extremities. In several months, the edema is replaced by a tightening and hardening of the skin, which results in difficulty in moving the affected parts. Hyperpigmentation, telangiectases (Figure 18-10), and subcutaneous calcifications may also occur, leading to deformity and severe cosmetic problems (Figure 18-11).

Musculoskeletal Manifestations.   Polyarthralgias and morning stiffness affecting both small and large joints are frequent in patients with scleroderma. Inflammatory joint pain with markedly swollen fingers often appears to be true synovitis and can lead to the premature diagnosis of rheumatoid arthritis.

Gastrointestinal Manifestations.   Distal esophageal motor dysfunction is the most frequent gastrointestinal finding; it results from weakness and incoordination of esophageal

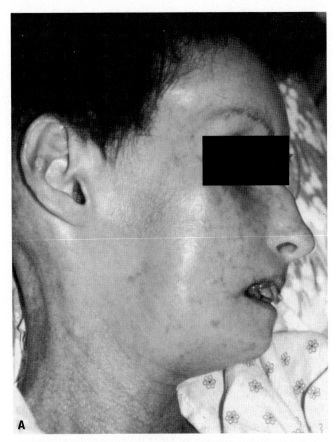

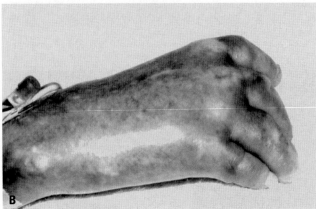

FIGURE 18-11   Manifestations of scleroderma. **A,** Severe tightening of the skin and narrowing of the oral aperture of a patient with scleroderma. **B,** Extensive involvement of the fingers and hand of the same patient causes a lack of mobility and the resorption of phalanges.

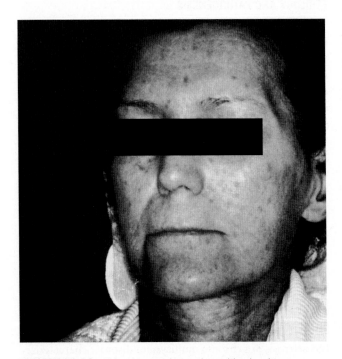

FIGURE 18-10   Telangiectases in a patient with scleroderma.

smooth muscle and leads to distal dysphagia. Intestinal fibrosis leading to severe intestinal malabsorption can also occur.

Cardiac Manifestations.   Clinical evidence of myocardial involvement in scleroderma cases is uncommon, but such involvement is more frequent in patients with diffuse scleroderma. The clinical presentations of cardiac involvement can include pericarditis, conduction problems, and congestive heart failure. Patchy replacement of the myocardium and the conduction system by fibrous tissue occurs in most patients.

Pulmonary Manifestations.   Pulmonary interstitial fibrosis is now the most frequent cause of death in patients with scleroderma since renal disease has become a treatable complication. Patients with either limited or diffuse scleroderma can develop interstitial disease although it tends to be more severe in patients with diffuse scleroderma. In patients with severe fibrosis, the greatest damage occurs during the first 5 years of illness, often when there are no pulmonary symptoms. Pleural thickening, pleural effusions, and pneumothorax are less frequent manifestations of lung disease in patients with scleroderma.[58]

Renal Manifestations.   Until recently, renal involvement was the most dreaded and deadly complication of scleroderma. The use of high-dose corticosteroids for the treatment of scleroderma has been implicated in precipitating renal crisis in some patients. In addition, pathologic changes due to the disease itself typically show alterations resembling hypertensive nephrosclerosis as well as mucinoid hyperplasia and vascular fibrinoid necrosis in the interlobar arteries. Renal crisis is characterized by malignant hypertension, which can rapidly progress to renal failure. The use of angiotensin-converting enzyme inhibitors has helped to make renal disease due to scleroderma a very treatable condition.

LABORATORY EVALUATION

ANAs are present in approximately 90% of scleroderma patients and are characteristically antinucleolar or anticentromere antibodies. There are a few other important ANAs that are specific for scleroderma but are not yet commercially available. Anti-ribonucleic acid (RNA) polymerase III may be the most common antibody found in patients with scleroderma. Other laboratory findings include anemia, an elevated erythrocyte sedimentation rate, and hypergammaglobulinemia.

TREATMENT

The treatment of PSS depends on the extent and severity of skin and organ involvement. D-penicillamine, a drug effective for both rheumatoid arthritis and Wilson's disease, has shown promise in the management of PSS by decreasing both skin thickening and organ involvement. This drug has two mechanisms of action: interference with cross-linking of collagen and immunosuppression. Nifedipine is a calcium channel blocker that has been shown to be effective in managing Raynaud's phenomenon and myocardial perfusion.[59] Extracorporeal photochemotherapy has also shown promise in reversing cutaneous sclerosis in patients in the early stages of PSS.[60]

ORAL FINDINGS

The clinical signs of scleroderma of the mouth and jaws are consistent with findings elsewhere in the body. The lips become rigid, and the oral aperture narrows considerably.[61] Skin folds are lost around the mouth, giving a masklike appearance to the face. The tongue can also become hard and rigid, making speaking and swallowing difficult. Involvement of the esophagus causes dysphagia.[62] Oral telangiectasia is equally prevalent in both limited and diffuse forms of PSS and is most commonly observed on the hard palate and the lips.[63] When the soft tissues around the temporomandibular joint are affected, they restrict movement of the mandible, causing pseudoankylosis.[64]

The linear form of localized scleroderma may involve the face as well as underlying bone and teeth. Dental radiographic findings have been reported and widely described; these classic findings (which include uniform thickening of the periodontal membrane, especially around the posterior teeth) are found in less than 10% of patients (Figure 18-12). Other characteristic radiographic findings include calcinosis of the soft tissues around the jaws. The areas of calcinosis will be detected by dental radiography and may be misinterpreted as radiographic intrabony lesions. A thorough clinical examination will demonstrate that the calcifications are present in the soft tissue.

When the facial tissues and muscles of mastication are extensively involved, the pressure exerted will cause resorption of the mandible. This resorption is particularly apparent at the angle of the mandible at the attachment of the masseter muscle. The coronoid process, condyle, or area of attachment of the digastric muscles may also be damaged by the continual pressure.[65]

Patients may also have oral disease secondary to drug therapy or xerostomia. Gingival hyperplasia can result from the use of calcium channel blockers; pemphigus, blood dyscrasias, or lichenoid reactions may result from penicillamine use. Salivary

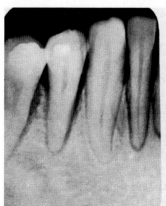
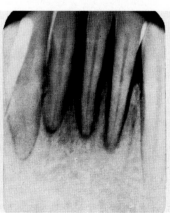
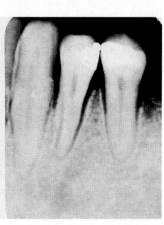

FIGURE 18-12 Radiographs showing thickening of the periodontal membrane in a patient with scleroderma.

gland hypofunction that frequently correlated with kerato-conjunctivitis sicca occurred in 14 of 32 patients studied by Nagy and colleagues.[61] Although some such patients have overlapping Sjögren's syndrome and have anti–SS-A antibody and a lip biopsy which shows inflammation, most simply have fibrotic glands that cause the lack of saliva or tears. Xerostomia results in an increased susceptibility to dental caries, *Candida* infections, and periodontal disease.

DENTAL MANAGEMENT

The most common problem in the dental treatment of scleroderma patients is the physical limitation caused by the narrowing of the oral aperture and rigidity of the tongue. Procedures such as molar endodontics, prosthetics, and restorative procedures in the posterior portions of the mouth become difficult, and the dental treatment plan may sometimes need to be altered because of the physical problem of access. The oral opening may be increased an average of 5 mm by stretching exercises. One particularly effective technique is the use of an increasing number of tongue blades between the posterior teeth to stretch the facial tissues. In addition, mechanical devices that assist the patient in performing the stretching exercises are available. If these approaches are insufficient, a bilateral commissurotomy may be necessary.

When treating a patient with diffuse scleroderma, the extent of the heart, lung, or kidney involvement should be considered, and appropriate alterations should be made before, during, and after treatment.

Patients with extensive resorption of the angle of the mandible are at risk for developing pathologic fractures from minor trauma, including dental extractions. Patients with Sjögren's syndrome should have daily fluoride treatments and make frequent visits to the oral hygienist.

Dermatomyositis

Dermatomyositis (DM) is a rare inflammatory degenerative disease characterized by skin lesions and progressive muscle atrophy. The disease occurs most frequently during childhood and between the fourth and sixth decades of life. The true incidence and prevalence are difficult to ascertain because of the rarity of the disease and the lack of consistent diagnostic criteria. Most studies have found a preponderance of female patients over male patients. Skin manifestations have been identified in 30 to 40% of adult patients and in 95% of affected children.[66] DM is classified with the connective-tissue diseases because of many overlapping clinical features and the fact that it is frequently seen together with scleroderma, SLE, rheumatoid arthritis, or Sjögren's syndrome.

NOMENCLATURE (SUBTYPES)

The three types of idiopathic inflammatory myopathies are DM, polymyositis (PM), and inclusion body myositis. Specific subtypes of DM or PM can be categorized as adult idiopathic, juvenile, or amyopathic DM. There is also a form of DM that is associated with connective-tissue disease or malignancy.

ETIOLOGY AND PATHOGENESIS

The etiology of DM is unknown, but genetic, immunologic, and environmental factors are likely to play an important role. Studies of histocompatibility antigen prevalence have demonstrated that human leukocyte antigens HLA-B8, HLA-B14, and HLA-DR3 are associated with dermatomyositis, but these studies have failed to link HLA haplotype with disease.[67] Immune mechanisms play a significant role in the onset of the disease, particularly circulating immunocomplexes, cellular immunity, and autoantibodies to skeletal-muscle myoglobin or myosin. The onset of the disease has been associated with infections such as influenza, hepatitis, coxsackie virus infection, and infection with the protozoan *Toxoplasma gondii*. DM has also been linked to drug therapy and cancer.

CLINICAL MANIFESTATIONS

DM usually begins with a symmetric and painless weakness of the proximal muscles of the arms, legs, and trunk. The weakness is progressive and characteristically spreads to the face, neck, larynx, pharynx, and heart. Muscle involvement may become severe enough to confine the patient to bed or to cause death due to failure of the respiratory muscles.

The primary classic skin lesion is a violaceous macular erythema distributed symmetrically. As the disease progresses, the erythema may become progressively indurated due to mucin deposition. The pathognomonic skin manifestations, occurring in approximately 70% of patients, are Gottron's papules, which are violaceous papules overlying the dorsal elbow, knee, or interphalangeal or metacarpophalangeal joints. Facial changes may take on the "butterfly" distribution associated with SLE or may primarily involve the eyelids and the forehead. Other skin changes are nonspecific diffuse erythema, erythematous plaques, macules, papules, telangiectases, and Raynaud's phenomenon. Diagnosis from skin lesions alone is rarely possible.

Noncutaneous manifestations of DM include interstitial lung disease, cardiac conduction abnormalities, conjunctival edema, and renal damage.

DIAGNOSIS AND LABORATORY EVALUATION

A diagnosis of definite PM or DM is given if any four of the following criteria are met:

1. Proximal symmetric muscle weakness, progressing from weeks to months
2. Evidence of an inflammatory myopathy on muscle biopsy
3. Elevation of serum muscle enzymes
4. Electromyographic features of myopathy
5. Cutaneous eruption that is typical of DM

A diagnosis of probable PM or DM is given if three criteria are met, and a diagnosis of possible PM or DM is given if two criteria are fulfilled.

Laboratory reports show evidence of muscle destruction by elevated levels of aspartate aminotransferase (formerly called serum glutamic-oxaloacetic transaminase), lactate dehydrogenase, alanine aminotransferase (formerly called serum glutamic-pyruvic transaminase), and creatine phosphokinase.

TREATMENT

An underlying carcinoma should be ruled out in all cases of DM since it is present in 10 to 25% of patients. Initial therapy consists of bed rest combined with high doses of systemic corticosteroids. In resistant cases, plasmapheresis or immunosuppressive drugs such as methotrexate or azathioprine have been helpful.[68]

ORAL FEATURES

Oral involvement is rarely a part of the disease process of DM. The most common clinical manifestations in the head and neck include weakness of the pharyngeal and palatal muscles, which causes difficulty in swallowing (dysphagia) and nasal speech (dystonia). The muscles of mastication and the facial muscles may also be involved, causing difficulty in chewing. Involvement of the oral mucosa has been described, but the lesions are not diagnostic. These lesions include shallow ulcers, erythematous patches, and telangiectasis. More characteristic are the facial skin lesions, which may present as a "butterfly" rash (similar to the lesions of SLE) or as a swelling of the eyelids, face, or lips. Lilac-colored eyelids secondary to stasis of blood in multiple telangiectasias is also a common finding. Calcinosis of the soft tissues is seen, especially in children. These calcified nodules may appear in the face and may show up on dental radiographs, leading to misinterpretation. The tongue may also become rigid due to severe calcinosis.

DENTAL MANAGEMENT

The disease process of DM poses no significant challenge to the dentist. The same precautions as are necessary for all patients who are taking high-dose long-term steroids and antimetabolites should be taken.

Rheumatoid Arthritis

Rheumatoid arthritis (RA) is a disease characterized by inflammation of the synovial membrane. Women are approximately three times more likely to be affected than men, and 80% of people with RA develop signs and symptoms of the disease at between 35 and 50 years of age. Epidemiologic studies suggest that the incidence of the disease is declining in younger age groups because of unknown environmental factors.[69]

Unlike degenerative joint disease (osteoarthritis), which is localized to the joints in middle-aged and elderly individuals, rheumatoid arthritis affects people of all age groups and affects other organs, including muscles and the hematopoietic system. Although this disease is called arthritis, there are frequent extra-articular manifestations.

NOMENCLATURE (SUBTYPES)

Several variations of RA exist. Felty's syndrome accounts for less than 5% of the total cases. In addition to having the usual

manifestations of RA, patients with Felty's syndrome also have splenomegaly and leukopenia, with neutrophils showing the greatest decrease. In severe cases, recurrent bacterial infection is a common cause of death.

Another variant is juvenile RA (Still's disease), which is thought by some rheumatologists to be a separate disease and not just a simple variation of adult RA.[70] Systemic extra-articular symptoms are prominent, including fever, lymphadenopathy, hepatosplenomegaly, carditis, and rash. Visual impairment secondary to iridocyclitis (inflammation of the iris and ciliary body) may also occur. In 50% of patients, growth and sexual maturation are delayed during active stages of the disease.

ETIOLOGY AND PATHOGENESIS

The pathogenesis of RA is unknown, but it appears to be multifactorial, involving genetic, immune, and infectious etiologies.

Genetic Factors. Studies of identical twins demonstrate that genetic factors play an important role in the pathogenesis of RA. This is confirmed by the findings of the HLA-DR4 major histocompatibility complex in up to 70% of RA patients.

Immune Factors. Most of research into the cause of RA involves studies of the immune system. The inflammatory response that causes joint and other injury is immune in nature. RA is believed to be a T-lymphocyte-driven disease in which a sudden influx of T cells into the affected joint(s) is followed by an increased number of macrophages and fibroblasts. The initiating factor of this immune response is unknown. The evidence of immune features in this disease includes the following:

1. The presence of rheumatoid factors (antigammaglobulin antibodies that form soluble complexes, measured in the serum by coating latex particles with IgG and testing the agglutinating properties of the patient's serum) in the serum and synovial fluid of affected patients
2. Extensive collections of plasma cells and lymphocytes found on histologic examination of affected tissues
3. Decreased complement levels in the synovial fluid of affected patients (suggests complement use during hypersensitivity reactions)
4. The overlap of RA with SLE and other diseases suspected of an immune pathogenesis.

Infectious Factors. Several infectious agents (including both bacteria such as streptococci and *Mycoplasma*, as well as viruses such as Epstein-Barr virus) have been suggested to cause the initial T-cell influx.

CLINICAL MANIFESTATIONS

The initial symptom in a majority of patients with RA is nonspecific weakness and fatigue, which may precede joint symptoms by several months. This is followed by symmetric polyarthritis characterized by a complaint of stiffness and a finding of a spindle-shaped swelling of the involved joints.

The proximal interphalangeal joints of the fingers and metacarpophalangeal joints of the hands are most commonly involved (Figure 18-13); the wrists, elbows, knees, and ankles also are frequently affected (Figure 18-14). In some patients, all joints may be involved, including the temporomandibular joint and the cricoarytenoid joint of the larynx. The joints that are affected with RA become red, swollen, and warm to the touch. Muscle atrophy around the affected joint is common.

Extracapsular manifestations include subcutaneous nodules (Figure 18-15) (especially over pressure points), which occur in 20 to 25% of patients; enlargement of the lymph nodes and spleen; chronic skin ulcers from a diffuse arteritis; pleural effusion; and pulmonary fibrosis. Rheumatoid granulomas may affect the heart, the eyes, or the brain.

Some patients may have a short course of nondisabling disease whereas others have an unrelenting downhill course of crippling and severe disability. A fluctuating course of remissions and exacerbations is seen in many patients, and this unpredictable course makes the choice of therapeutic regimens difficult.

DIAGNOSIS AND LABORATORY EVALUATION

In 1987, The American College of Rheumatology revised the criteria for the diagnosis of RA. The diagnosis is based on satisfying at least four of the following seven criteria: (1) morn-

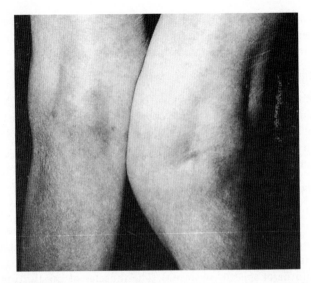

FIGURE 18-14   Rheumatoid arthritis in the knees. (Courtesy of Dr. George Ehrlich)

ing stiffness, (2) arthritis of three or more joint areas, (3) arthritis of the joints of the hand, (4) symmetric arthritis, (5) rheumatoid nodules, (6) serum rheumatoid factor, and (7) radiographic changes. The first four criteria must be present for at least 6 weeks, and the second through fifth must be observed by a physician.[71]

Autoantibodies (such as ANA and rheumatoid factor) are respectively found in 30 to 60% and 72 to 85% of adult patients. However, these autoantibodies are not specific to RA and are found in patients who have a number of other conditions, such as SLE and scleroderma. Rheumatoid factor, particularly in high titers, adds weight to the diagnosis of RA and is associated with more destructive disease and a worse prognosis (see Table 18-1).

Other associated laboratory findings include an elevated erythrocyte sedimentation rate and normochromic normocytic anemia. Some tests may be helpful in excluding RA by indicating an alternative diagnosis. For example, antibodies to DNA would indicate SLE whereas anti-Ro (SS-A) or anti-La

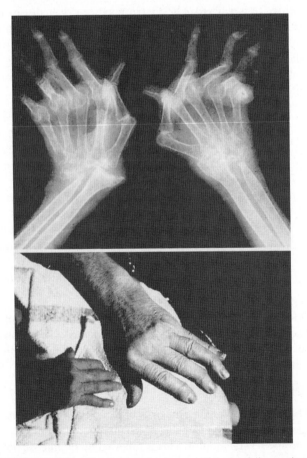

FIGURE 18-13   Characteristic involvement of the hands in a patient with rheumatoid arthritis. (Courtesy of Dr. George Ehrlich)

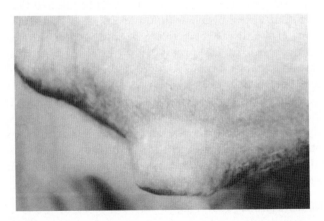

FIGURE 18-15   Subcutaneous nodules of the arm in a patient with rheumatoid arthritis. (Courtesy of Dr. George Ehrlich)

(SS-B) antibodies suggest Sjögren's syndrome. Conversely, the absence of such antibodies favors a diagnosis of RA.

ORAL SIGNS

The treatment of RA can cause oral manifestations. The long-term use of methotrexate and other antirheumatic agents such as D-penicillamine and NSAIDs can cause stomatitis. Cyclosporine may cause gingival overgrowth.

Direct effects of the disease are also seen. Patients with long-standing active RA have an increased incidence of periodontal disease, including loss of alveolar bone and teeth. Similarities in the host immune responses of RA and periodontal disease, involving reduced cellular and enhanced humoral activity, have been reported[72] although the increased dental and periodontal disease may be chiefly related to a decreased ability to maintain proper oral hygiene. Sjögren's syndrome is a common complication of RA (see Chapter 9, "Salivary Gland Disease"). RA of the temporomandibular joint (Figure 18-16) was discussed earlier (see Chapter 10).

DENTAL MANAGEMENT

The most common complication that affects dental treatment relates to the toxicity of the drugs used to treat RA. It is imperative that the dentist knows the drugs the patient is currently taking and their possible side effects and interactions with other drugs. The most common adverse effects of NSAIDs involve the gastrointestinal (GI) tract and the kidneys. In addition, many patients take aspirin at dosages approaching 5 g per day or take an equivalent dosage of NSAIDs. These drugs affect platelet function, causing a prolongation of the bleeding time and possible hemorrhage after surgery.

Intramuscular doses of gold salts are used for some patients who are refractory to other forms of treatment. The side effects of this therapy include stomatitis, blood dyscrasias, and nephrotic syndrome. Other refractory patients respond to D-penicillamine, a drug that may cause bone marrow depression as well as renal toxicity, heptotoxicity, or drug-induced pemphigus. Therefore, any patient who is taking either of these drugs should have a complete blood count and chemistry prior to dental treatment. Corticosteroids and immunosuppressive drugs are still used for some refractory patients; therefore, appropriate measures should be taken with these patients prior to dental care (see "Dental Considerations" under "Systemic Lupus Erythematosus," above).

Patients with severe RA who have had joints surgically replaced with prosthetic joints may require prophylactic antibiotic therapy before invasive dental procedures. No prophylaxis is indicated for otherwise healthy patients 2 years after placement of a prosthesis. However, patients should receive prophylactic antibiotics after the 2 years if they are on immunosuppressive agents or have had postoperative joint infections. Antibiotic prophylaxis should be considered for patients who will be undergoing dental procedures that are associated with a higher incidence of bacteremia. Such procedures include dental extractions, periodontal surgery, implant placement, replacement of avulsed teeth, endodontic therapy beyond the apex, intraligamentary local anesthetic injections, placement of orthodontic bands, and any procedure in which bleeding is anticipated[73] (Table 18-3).

Patients with Sjögren's syndrome may require additional instruction in personal oral care, instruction on diet and dietary modifications, home clinical fluoride therapy treatment for xerostomia, more frequent recall visits and radiography, and more conservative treatment plans.[74]

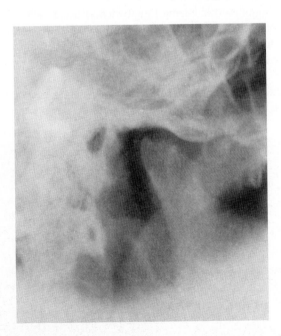

FIGURE 18-16 Evidence of flattening of the condylar articular surface with deepening radiolucency in a patient with rheumatoid arthritis. Note the lack of depth of temporal bone fossa.

TABLE 18-3 Indications for Antibiotic Prophylaxis for Dental Patients with Total Joint Replacements and Suggested Antibiotic Regimens

Dental procedures for which antibiotic prophylaxis is indicated
    Dental extractions
    Periodontal procedures
    Dental implant placement
    Reimplantation of avulsed teeth
    Endodontic instrumentation beyond apex, or endodontic surgery
    Initial placement of orthodontic bands (not brackets)
    Intraligamentary injections of local anesthetic
    Prophylactic cleaning of teeth or implants when bleeding is anticipated

Suggested antibiotic prophylaxis regimens
    Patient not allergic to penicillin: cephalexin, cephradine, or amoxicillin, 2 g PO 1 hour before dental procedure
    Patient not allergic to penicillin and unable to take oral medications: cefazolin (1 g) or ampicillin (2 g) IM or IV 1 hour before dental procedure
    Patient allergic to penicillin: clindamycin, 600 mg PO 1 hour before dental procedure
    Patient allergic to penicillin and unable to take oral medications: clindamycin, 600 mg IV 1 hour before dental procedure

Adapted from Treister N, Glick M.[74]

IM = intramuscularly; IV = intravenously; PO = orally.

The dentist should determine if the RA patient has a form of the disease that affects the bone marrow (such as Felty's syndrome) since such patients have an increased risk of developing infection due to neutropenia and hemorrhage secondary to thrombocytopenia.[75]

Mixed Connective-Tissue Disease

The term "mixed connective-tissue disease" (MCTD) was coined in 1972 to denote a condition that has the combined clinical features of SLE, PSS, and DM. Clinicians have suggested a variety of terms to describe the clinical disease in patients who exhibit the clinical features of multiple rheumatologic diseases. Such descriptive phrases include overlap syndrome, sclerodermatomyositis, rheumatoid arthritis and systemic lupus erythematosus (RUPUS), mixed collagenosis, and systemic lupus erythematosus and scleroderma (lupoderma).

The cause of MCTD, as with other rheumatologic diseases, is unknown. The prevalence of MCTD is also unknown, but MCTD is believed to occur more commonly than DM, less often than SLE, and as frequently as PSS. Most MCTD patients are women, and the average age at the time of diagnosis is 37 years.[76]

Common clinical features of MCTD include Raynaud's phenomenon, polyarthritis, sclerodactyly, and inflammatory myositis. Generalized lymphadenopathy has been observed in 50% of patients with MCTD. Pericarditis, renal disease, and pulmonary disease are also common.[77]

Using HLA type to predict the differentiation of MCTD, some investigators have suggested that MCTD is an intermediate stage in a genetically determined progression to a recognized connective-tissue disease and that those whose disease remains undifferentiated might be considered a distinct subset.[78] Black suggested in 1992 that the concept of MCTD as a distinct disease entity is better replaced by the term "undifferentiated autoimmune rheumatic/connective-tissue disorder" because the condition of many of these patients later converts to PSS or SLE.[79]

A prerequisite for the diagnosis of MCTD is the presence of high titers of autoantibodies against small nuclear ribonucleoprotein (SnRNP) antigen. The characteristic laboratory abnormalities in MCTD cases include high titers (> 1:1,000) of speckled ANAs, high levels of antibody to ribonuclease (RNase)-sensitive extractable nuclear antigen, and the presence of snRNP antigen antibody.[80]

Little has been reported concerning the oral manifestations of MCTD. The oral manifestations of conditions such as xerostomia and a decreased mandibular range of movement are possible features although few reports are available.

▼ ALLERGY

The modern dentist uses a wide variety of drugs to treat patients, including antibiotics, hypnotics, and anesthetics. All practitioners who use these medications must know how to manage reactions to them. In this section, acute allergic reac-

tions and their management is discussed. Stomatitis associated with allergy is discussed in Chapter 4.

Acute allergic reactions are caused by an immediate-type hypersensitivity reaction. A good model for understanding this mechanism is anaphylaxis. A patient previously exposed to a drug or other antigen has antibody (primarily IgE) fixed to basophils and mast cells. When the antigen (in the form of a drug, food, or an airborne substance) is re-introduced into the body, it will react with the fixed antibody, bind complement, and open mast cells, releasing active mediators such as histamine and slow-reacting substance of anaphylaxis (SRS-A). These substances cause vasodilation and increased capillary permeability, which result in fluid and leukocytes leaving the blood vessels and accumulating in the tissues and forming areas of edema. Constriction of bronchial smooth muscle results when IgE is bound in the pulmonary region. The anaphylactic reaction may be localized and lead to urticaria and angioneurotic edema, or a generalized reaction may result, causing anaphylactic shock (Figure 18-17).

Localized Anaphylaxis

A localized anaphylactic reaction involving superficial blood vessels results in urticaria (hives). Urticaria begins with pruritus in the area of the release of histamine and other active substances. Wheals (welts) then appear on the skin as an area of localized edema on an erythematous base. These lesions can occur anywhere on the skin or mucous membranes. Urticaria of the lips and the oral mucosa occurs most frequently after food ingestion by an allergic individual. Common food allergens include chocolate, nuts, shellfish, and tomatoes. Drugs such as penicillin and aspirin may cause urticaria, and cold, heat, or pressure may cause the reaction in susceptible individuals.

Angioneurotic edema (angioedema) occurs when blood vessels that are deeper in the subcutaneous tissues are affected, producing a large diffuse area of subcutaneous swelling under normal overlying skin. This reaction may be caused by contact with an allergen, but a significant number of cases are idiopathic. A recurrent form is inherited as an autosomal dominant trait. Hereditary angioneurotic edema is fatal in approximately

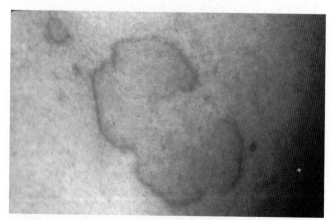

FIGURE 18-17 Urticaria resulting from use of a nonsteroidal anti-inflammatory drug.

one-quarter of cases because of severe laryngeal edema. The mechanism of the hereditary form of the disease is a deficiency of a C1 esterase inhibitor, which normally acts as an inhibitor of the first component of complement and kallikrein.

Angioedema commonly occurs on the lips and tongue and around the eyes (Figure 18-18). It is temporarily disfiguring but is not serious unless the posterior portion of the tongue or larynx compromises respiration. The patient who is in respiratory distress should be treated immediately with 0.5 mL of epinephrine (1:1,000) subcutaneously or 0.2 mL of intravenous epinephrine, injected slowly. When the immediate danger has passed, 50 mg of diphenhydramine hydrochloride (Benadryl [Pfizer, Parsippany, N.J.]) should be given four times a day until the swelling diminishes.

Serum Sickness

Serum sickness is named for its frequent occurrence after the administration of foreign serum, which was given for the treatment of infectious diseases before the advent of antibiotics. The reaction is presently less common but still occurs as a result of the susceptible patient's being given tetanus antitoxin, rabies antiserum, or drugs that combine with body proteins to form allergens. Penicillin, a drug commonly prescribed by dentists, occasionally causes serum sickness.

The pathogenesis of serum sickness differs from that of anaphylaxis. Antibodies form immunocomplexes in blood vessels with administered antigens. The complexes fix complement, which attracts leukocytes to the area, causing direct tissue injury.

Serum sickness and vasculitis usually begin 7 to 10 days after the administration of the allergen, but this period can vary from 3 days to as long as 1 month. Unlike other allergic diseases, serum sickness may occur during the initial administration of the drug.

Major symptoms consist of fever, swelling, lymphadenopathy, joint and muscle pains, and rash. Less common manifestations include peripheral neuritis, kidney disease, and myocardial ischemia. Serum sickness is usually self-limiting, with spontaneous recovery in 1 to 3 weeks. Treatment is symptomatic; aspirin is given for arthralgia, and antihistamines are given for the skin rash. Severe cases should be treated with a short course of systemic corticosteroids, which significantly shortens the course of the disease. Although this reaction is rare, the dentist who is prescribing penicillin should be aware of the possibility of serum sickness occurring weeks after use of the drug.

Generalized Anaphylaxis

Generalized anaphylaxis is an allergic emergency. The mechanism of generalized anaphylaxis is the reaction of IgE antibodies to an allergen that causes the release of histamine, bradykinin, and SRS-A. These chemical mediators cause the contraction of smooth muscles of the respiratory and intestinal tracts, as well as increased vascular permeability.

The following factors increase the patient's risk for anaphylaxis:

1. History of allergy to other drugs or food
2. History of asthma
3. Family history of allergy
4. Parenteral administration of the drug
5. Administration of high-risk allergens such as penicillin

Anaphylactic reactions may occur within seconds of drug administration or may occur 30 to 40 minutes later, complicating the diagnosis. The symptoms of generalized anaphylaxis should be known so that prompt treatment may be initiated. For example, patients have been diagnosed as allergic to local anesthetics when a psychic reaction to an injection or a reac-

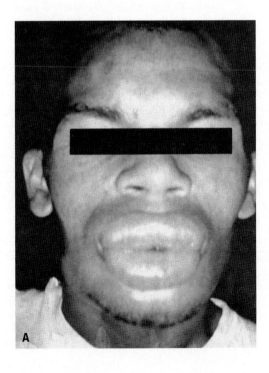

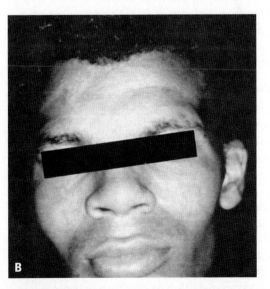

FIGURE 18-18 **A,** Angioneurotic edema of an allergic reaction to intramuscularly administered penicillin. **B,** Same patient 48 hours later, after therapy with epinephrine and antihistamine agents.

tion to epinephrine have occurred. Such an erroneous diagnosis will make future dental management difficult.

The generalized anaphylactic reaction may involve the skin, the cardiovascular system, the intestines, and the respiratory system. The first signs often occur on the skin and are similar to those seen in localized anaphylaxis (eg, urticaria, angioedema, erythema, and pruritus). Pulmonary symptoms include dyspnea, wheezing, and asthma. GI tract disease (eg, vomiting, cramps, and diarrhea) often follows skin symptoms. If these are untreated, symptoms of hypotension appear as the result of the loss of intravascular fluid; if untreated, this leads to shock. Patients with generalized anaphylactic reactions may die from respiratory failure, hypotensive shock, or laryngeal edema.

The most important therapy for generalized anaphylaxis is the administration of epinephrine. All clinicians who administer drugs should have a vial of aqueous epinephrine (at a 1:1,000 dilution) and a sterile syringe easily accessible. For adults, 0.5 mL of epinephrine should be administered intramuscularly or subcutaneously; smaller doses of from 0.1 to 0.3 mL should be used for children, depending on their size. If the allergen was administered in an extremity, a tourniquet should be placed above the injection site to minimize further absorption into the blood. The absorption can be further reduced by injecting 0.3 mL of epinephrine (1:1,000) directly into the injection site. The tourniquet should be removed every 10 minutes.

Epinephrine will usually reverse all severe signs of generalized anaphylaxis. If improvement is not observed in 10 minutes, re-administer epinephrine. If the patient continues to deteriorate, several steps can be taken, depending on whether the patient is experiencing bronchospasm or edema. For bronchospasm, slowly inject 250 mg of aminophylline intravenously, over a period of 10 minutes. Too rapid an administration can lead to fatal cardiac arrhythmias. Do not give aminophylline if hypotensive shock is a part of the clinical picture. Inhalation sympathomimetics may also be used to treat bronchospasm, and oxygen should be given to prevent or manage hypoxia. For the patient with laryngeal edema, establish an airway. This may necessitate endotracheal intubation; in some cases, a cricothyroidotomy may be necessary.

Latex Allergy

The increased use of protective gloves has led to numerous undesirable cutaneous and mucosal reactions. Unfortunately, the number of objective methods for verifying immediate dermal and mucosal irritation is rather small. While studies repeatedly uncover high prevalence rates, the nonspecific nature of the symptoms and the lack of knowledge about latex allergy result in missed diagnoses in many sensitized persons who are at risk for the progression of serious allergic reactions.[81] Originally, urticaria, rhinitis, and eyelid edema were identified as immediate manifestations of latex allergy. Severe systemic reactions (such as asthma and anaphylaxis), which may result in permanent disability or even death, have now been recognized.[81]

In the health care setting, the two major strategies for management are (1) the safe care of the latex allergic patient and (2) the prevention and treatment of occupational latex allergy in employees. In managing a patient with latex sensitivity, the distinction between an immediate hypersensitivity reaction to latex and an allergic contact dermatitis due to other irritants must be established. At initial evaluation, latex allergy status should be established by the history and documented clearly on the chart. Any history of an immediate hypersensitivity reaction to latex necessitates a latex-free environment for that person. The operatory should include nonlatex products; "hypoallergenic" latex gloves or latex-containing products (such as blood pressure cuffs and disposable tourniquets) should not be worn or used in the vicinity of persons who are allergic to latex. Premedication with antihistamines, steroids, and histamine H_2 blocking agents is sometimes carried out in operating rooms, but anaphylactic reactions have occurred despite such pretreatment.

Workers who are irritated by gloves should change the type of gloves worn or change the type of soap used for scrubbing. In addition, the use of cotton liners and emollients may effectively prevent sensitivity reactions. In cases of true latex allergy, the avoidance of all latex products is the only measure that can avert a serious allergic reaction.

All persons with latex hypersensitivity should carry an epinephrine autoinjection kit and wear MedicAlert identification. Acute systemic reactions to latex should be treated in the same manner as other anaphylactic reactions are treated (ie, airway and circulation assessment, administration of oxygen, and administration of epinephrine and steroids as needed). In the course of resuscitation, all latex contact must be avoided.[82]

▼ REFERENCES

1. Fearon DT, Locksley RM. The instructive role of innate immunity in the acquired immune response. Science 1996;272:50–3.
2. Alam R. A brief review of the immune system. Primary Care 1998;25:727–38.
3. Haynes BF, Fauci AS. Introduction to the immune system. In: Wilson JD, Braunwald E, Isselbacker KJ, editors. Harrison's principles of internal medicine. 14th ed. New York: McGraw-Hill; p. 1753–76.
4. Roitt IM. Primary immunodeficiency. In: Roitt IM, Brostoff J, Male D, editors. Clinical immunology. 5th ed. London: Mosby, 1998. p. 285–92.
5. Heraszewsli RA, Webster ADB. Primary hypogammaglobulinemia: a survey of clinical manifestations and complications. QJM 1993;86:31.
6. Harrison LF, Shearer WT. Evaluation and management of B and T cell abnormalities. Allergy Proc 1991;12:25-30.
7. Tsukada S, Saffran DC, Rawlings DJ, et al. Deficient expression of a B-cell cytoplasmic tyrosine kinase in human X-linked agammaglobulinemia. Cell 1993;72:279–90.
8. Mohamed AJ, Nore BF, Christensson B, Smith CI. Signalling of Bruton's tyrosine kinase Btk. Scand J Immunol 1999;49:113-8.
9. Mamlock RJ. Primary immunodeficiency disorders. Primary Care 1998;25:739–58.
10. Nononyama S. Recent advances in the diagnosis of X-linked agammaglobulinemia. Intern Med 1999;38:687.
11. Liese JG, Wintergerst U, Tympner KD, Belohradsky BH. High-vs low-dose immunoglobulin therapy in the treatment of X-linked agammaglobulinemia. Am J Dis Child 1992;146:335-9.

12. Secondary immunodeficiency. In: Roitt IM, Brostoff J, Male D, editors. Clinical immunology. 5th ed. London: Mosby, 1998. p. 293.

13. Cunningham-Rundles C. Disorders of the IgA system. In: Stiehm ER, editor. Immunologic disorders in infants and children. 4th ed. Philadelphia: W.B. Saunders; 1996.

14. Burrows PD, Cooper MD. IgA deficiency. Adv Immunol 1997;65:245-76.

15. Hong R. The DiGeorge anomaly. Clin Rev Allergy Immunol 2001;20:43-60.

16. Hillebrand G, Siebert R, Simeoni E, Santer R. DiGeorge syndrome with discordant phenotype in monozygotic twins. J Med Genet 2000;37:E23.

17. Weissman IL, Shizuru J. Immune reconstitution. N Engl J Med 1999;341:1227-9.

18. Rogers MH, Lwin R, Fairbanks L, et al. Cognitive and behavioral abnormalities in adenosine deaminase deficient severe combined immunodeficiency. J Pediatr 2001;139:44-50.

19. Siegfried EC, Prose NS, Friedman NJ, Paller AS. Cutaneous granulomas in children with combined immunodeficiency. J Am Acad Dermatol 1991;25:761-6.

20. Savitsky K, Bar-Shira A, Gilad S, et al. A single ataxia telangiectasia gene with a product similar to PI-3 kinase. Science 1995;268:1749-53.

21. Lavin MF. Radiosensitivity and oxidative signalling in ataxia telangiectasia: an update. Radiother Oncol 1998;47:113–23.

22. Norhagen GE, Engstrom PE, Hammarstrom L, et al. Oral and intestinal microflora in individuals with different immunoglobulin deficiencies. Eur J Clin Microbiol Infect Dis 1990;9:631-3.

23. Greenberg MS. Oral herpes simplex infections in immunosuppressed patients. Compend Suppl 1988;9:S289–91.

24. Porter AR, Scully C. Orofacial manifestations in the primary immunodeficiency disorders. Oral Surg Oral Med Oral Pathol 1994;78:4–13.

25. Spickett GP, Misbah SA, Chapel HM. Primary antibody deficiency in adults. Lancet 1991;337:281-4.

26. Tolo K. Periodontal disease mechanisms in immunocompromised patients. J Clin Periodontol 1991;18:431-5.

27. Porter AR, Scully C. Orofacial manifestations in primary immunodeficiencies: IgA. J Oral Pathol Med 1993;22:117–9.

28. Porter AR, Scully C. Orofacial manifestations in primary immunodeficiencies: common variable immunodeficiencies. J Oral Pathol Med 1993; 22:157–8.

29. Buckley RH. Advances in the diagnosis and treatment of primary immunodeficiency diseases. Arch Intern Med 1986;146:377-84.

30. Huston DP, Kavanaugh AF, Rohane PW, Huston MM. Immunoglobulin deficiency syndromes and therapy. J Allergy Clin Immunol 1991;87:1-17.

31. Steihm ER. Appropriate therapeutic use of immunoglobulin. Transfus Med Revi 1996;10:203.

32. Yu Z, Lennon VA. Mechanism of intravenous immune globulin therapy in antibody mediated autoimmune diseases. N Engl J Med 1999;340:227-8.

33. Heimdahl A, Nord CE. Oral infections in immunocompromised patients. J Clin Periodontol 1990;17:501-3.

34. Greenberg MS, Cohen SG, McKitrick J, Cassileth P. The oral flora as a source of septicemia in patients with leukemia. Oral Surg Oral Med Oral Pathol 1982;53:32-4.

35. Joint Statement of the American Thoracic Society, the European Respiratory Society, and the World Association of Sarcoidosis and Other Granulomatous Disorders. Statement on sarcoidosis. Am J Respir Crit Care Med. 1999;160:736–55.

36. Jones RE, Chatham WW. Update on sarcoidosis. Curr Opin Rheumatol 1999;11:83-7.

37. Arkachaisri T, Lehman TJ. Systemic lupus erythematosus and related disorders of childhood. Curr Opin Rheumatol 1999;11:384-92.

38. Rubin RL. Etiology and mechanisms of drug-induced lupus. Curr Opin Rheumatol 1999;11:357–63.

39. McCurdy D. Genetic susceptibility to the connective tissue diseases. Curr Opin in Rheumatol 1999;11:399-407.

40. Naparstek Y, Plotz PH. The role of autoantibodies in autoimmune disease. Ann Rev Immunol 1993;11:79–104.

41. Evans J. Antinuclear antibody testing in systemic autoimmune disease. Clin Chest Med 1998;19:613–25.

42. Mojcik CF, Klippel JH. End stage renal disease and systemic lupus erythematosus. Am J Med 1996;101:100–7.

43. De Rossi SS, Glick M. Lupus erythematosus: considerations for dentistry. J Am Dent Assoc 1998;129:330-9.

44. Bluestein HG. The central nervous system in systemic lupus erythematosus. In: Lahita RD, editor. Systemic lupus erythematosus. New York: Churchill Livingstone; 1992. p. 639.

45. Monash S. Oral lesions of lupus erythematosus. Dent Cosmos 1931;73:511.

46. Rhodus NL, Johnson DK. The prevalence of oral manifestations of systemic lupus erythematosus. Quintessence Int 1990;21:461-5.

47. Sanchez R, Jonsson R, Ahlfors E, et al. Oral lesions of lupus erythematosus patients in relation to other chronic inflammatory oral diseases: an immunologic study. Scand Dent Res 1988;96:569-78.

48. Karjalainen TK, Tomich CE. A histopathologic study of oral mucosal lupus erythematosus. Oral Surg Oral Med Oral Pathol 1989;67:547-54.

49. Andonopoulos AP, Skopouli FN, Dimou GS, Drosos AA. Sjögren's syndrome in systemic lupus erythematosus. J Rheumatol 1990;17:201-4.

50. Glick M. Glucocorticosteroid replacement therapy: a literature review and suggested replacement therapy. Oral Surg Oral Med Oral Pathol 1989;67:614–20.

51. De Rossi SS, Glick M. Dental considerations for the patient with renal disease receiving hemodialysis. J Am Dent Assoc 1996;127:211–9.

52. Mayes MD. Scleroderma epidemiology. Rheum Dis Clin North Am 1996; 22:751–64.

53. Laing TJ, Gillespie BW, Toth MB, et al. Racial differences in scleroderma among Michigan women. Arthritis Rheum 1997;40(4):734-42.

54. Callen JP. Collagen vascular diseases. Med Clin North Am 1998;82:1217–37.

55. Jimenez SA, Hitraya E, Varga J. Pathogenesis of scleroderma: collagen. Rheum Dis Clin North Am 1996;22:647–74.

56. Silver RM, Heyes MP, Maize JC, et al. Scleroderma, fasciitis and eosinophilia associated with the ingestion of tryptophan. N Engl J Med 1990;322:874-81.

57. Steen VD. Clinical manifestations of systemic sclerosis. Semin Cutan Med Surg 1998;17:48–54.

58. Steen VD, Conte C, Owens GR, et al. Severe restrictive lung disease in systemic sclerosis. Arthritis Rheum 1994;37:1283–9.

59. Rademaker M, Meyric K, Thomas RH, et al. The anti-platelet effect of nifedipine in patients with systemic sclerosis. Clin Exp Rheumatol 1992;10:57.

60. Rook AH, Freundlich B, Jegasothy BV, et al. Treatment of systemic sclerosis with extracorporeal photochemotherapy: results of a multicenter trial. Arch Dermatol 1992;128:337-46.

61. Nagy G, Kovacs J, Zeher M, et al. Analysis of the oral manifestations of systemic sclerosis. Oral Surg Oral Med Oral Pathol 1994;77:141–6.

62. Montesi A, Pesaresi A, Cavalli ML, et al. Oropharyngeal and esophageal function in scleroderma.Dysphagia 1991;6:219-23.

63. Callen JP. Oral manifestations of collagen vascular disease. Semin Cutan Med Surg 1997;16:323–7.

64. Rubin MM, San Filippo RJ. Resorption of the mandibular angle in progressive systemic sclerosis: case report. J Oral Maxillofac Surg 1992;50:75-7.

65. Wood KE, Lee P. Analysis of the oral manifestations of systemic sclerosis. Oral Surg Oral Med Oral Pathol 1988;65:172.

66. Dalakas MC. Polymyositis, dermatomyositis, and inclusion body myositis. N Engl J Med 1999;325:1487–98.

67. Kovacs SO, Kovacs SC. Dermatomyositis. J Am Acad Dermatol 1998;39:899–920.

68. Villalba L, Adams EM. Update on therapy for refractory dermatomyositis and polymyositis. Curr Opin Rheumatol 1996;8:544–51.

69. Michet C. Update in the epidemiology of the rheumatic diseases. Curr Opin Rheumatol 1998; 10:129–35.

70. Gallagher KT, Bernstein B. Juvenile rheumatoid arthritis. Curr Opin Rheumatol 1999;11:372–6.

71. Arnett FC, Edworthy SM, Bloch DA, et al. The American Rheumatism Association 1987 revised criteria for the classification of rheumatoid arthritis. Arthritis Rheum 1988;31:315-24.

72. Kaber UR, Gleissner C, Dehne F, et al. Risk for periodontal disease in patient with longstanding rheumatoid arthritis. Arthritis Rheum 1997;40:2248–51.

73. American Dental Association and American Academy of Orthopedic Surgeons. Antibiotic prophylaxis for dental patients with total joint replacements. J Am Dent Assoc 1997;128:1004–8.

74. Treister N, Glick M. Rheumatoid arthritis: a review and suggested dental care considerations. J Am Dent Assoc 1999; 130:689–98.

75. Rosenstein ED, Kramer N. Felty's and pseudo-Felty's syndromes. Semin Arthritis Rheum 1991;21:129–42.

76. Sharp GC, Singsen BH. Mixed connective tissue disease. In: McCarty DJ, editor. Arthritis and allied conditions: a textbook of rheumatology. 11th ed. Philadelphia: Lea and Febiger, 1989. p. 1080–91.

77. Prakash UBS. Respiratory complications in mixed connective tissue disease. Clin Chest Med 1998;19:733–46.

78. Gendi NS, Welsh KI, Van Venrooij WJ, et al. HLA type as a predictor of mixed connective tissue disease differentiation. Ten year clinical and immunogenetic follow up of 46 patients. Arthritis Rheum 1995;38:259–66.

79. Black C, Isenberg DA. Mixed connective tissue disease: goodbye to all that. Br J Rheumatol 1992;31:695–700.

80. Burdt MA, Hoffman RW, Deutscher SL, et al. Long-term outcome in mixed connective tissue disease: longitudinal clinical and serologic findings. Arthritis Rheum 1999;42:899–909.

81. Kujala V. A review of current literature on epidemiology of immediate glove irritation and latex allergy. Occup Med 1999;49:3–9.

82. Reddy S. Latex allergy. Am Fam Physician 1998;71:93–100.

19

TRANSPLANTATION MEDICINE

THOMAS P. SOLLECITO, DMD

Organ transplants are mainly used to treat various life-threatening end-stage diseases. As an increasing number of surgeons have mastered the surgical procedures involved in organ transplantation, it is becoming a norm rather than an exception in many medical institutions. Technologies such as cold ischemia and preservation solutions allow for approximately 6 hours of "nonfunctioning" time for hearts and other organs, and 24 hours (or longer) for kidneys.[1] Medical management of patients receiving a transplant is also continuously improving, which also allows for longer-term successful outcomes. The main limitation to even greater usage of transplantation as a treatment modality for end-stage organ damage is the relative paucity of available organs.

Attempts at organ and bone marrow transplantation date back to the 1800s. In more recent history, Dr. Joseph Murray performed the first human renal transplantation in 1954. He successfully transplanted a kidney from an identical twin to his brother. This procedure was well tolerated, as there was no rejection by the genetically identical recipient. The first successful allogeneic (not genetically identical) transplantation was a kidney transplantation performed in 1959 in which the recipient was "conditioned" (immunosuppressed to prevent rejection) by total body irradiation. In 1962, a successful cadaveric donor renal transplant was achieved; and, in 1966, a pancreas transplantation was successfully performed. In the following year, the first human liver transplantation was performed, resulting in a 13-month survival. In the same year, a heart was transplanted. In 1968, a genetically related bone marrow transplantation (BMT, today referred to as a hematopoietic cell transplantation [HCT]) was performed; in 1973 a genetically unrelated HCT was performed. Lung transplantation has also been performed both as a single procedure and in combination with a heart transplantation. The first heart-lung transplantation in the United States was done in 1981, and the first single lung transplantation in Canada was performed in 1983. Other organs that have been successfully transplanted include the small bowel, the skin, various limbs, and components of the human eye.

In the past 20 years, significant advances including tissue typing and the development of immunosuppressive medications have increased the success of transplantation. Overall, long-term patient survival has also significantly increased over the past 30 years, both in solid organ and HCT recipients. Most transplant clinicians consider the discovery of the immunosuppressive agent cyclosporine to be the most significant advance in transplantation medicine. This medication was approved for use in 1983.[2]

Both solid organ and nonsolid organ transplants are becoming more routine throughout the world. In the beginning of the twenty-first century, over 71, 000 patients in the United States alone were waiting for a solid organ transplant. In 1999, just over 21,000 solid organs were transplanted (Table 19-1). Presently, in the United States, there are over 800 transplantation programs performing various types of solid organ transplants.[2]

As the process of solid organ transplantation becomes more routine, the need for solid organ donation continues to increase. The limitation of available donor organs will hopefully become less of an issue with increased awareness of organ donation and perhaps with alternative organ procurement methods including xenografts or stem cell–derived tissue.

The likelihood of a dentist having the opportunity to treat a transplanted patient is increasing, as many of these transplant recipients resume normal ways of life after the transplantation. This chapter reviews different aspects of transplantation medicine pertinent for the dentist.

▼ CLASSIFICATION

When describing a transplantation, most clinical classification systems employ both the type of tissue transplanted and the genetic relationship of the donor tissue to the recipient. It is extremely important for the clinician to know exactly what type of transplant was performed, as both the management and the prognosis are intimately related. This will become evident as it is discussed later in this chapter.

Some authorities broadly divide clinical transplants as being either a solid organ/tissue or an HCT. Virtually all types of solid organs/tissues have been attempted to be transplanted, including hearts, lungs, kidneys, livers, intestines, pancreas, skin, eye components, and limbs. Another type of transplant frequently used to treat various hematologic and nonhematologic malignancies/disorders is known as HCT. HCT poses special management concerns to the clinician, which are detailed later in this chapter.

Classification of transplants can also be based broadly on the genetic relationship of the recipient to the donor. For the purpose of this chapter, the transplanted cell, tissue, or organ is referred to as the "graft." A transplant to and from one's self (autograft) is known as an "autologous transplant." A transplantation from an identical twin (identical genetic make-up) is known as an "isograft," with the process of this type of transplantation known as "isogeneic or syngeneic transplantation." Most transplants are from donors that are not genetically identical to the recipient (allografts). These types of transplants are known as "allogeneic transplants." Finally, transplants from donors of one species to recipients of another species (xenografts) are known as "xenogeneic transplants"[3] (Table 19-2).

Due to the scarcity of isografts and the obvious limitations to autografts, allogeneic transplants are most commonly used today. The success of allogeneic transplantation relies on sophisticated mechanisms for identifying and matching specific genetic markers between the donor and the recipient, as well as suppressing the recipient's immune system to prevent transplant rejection. These are the concepts that serve as the basic foundation in transplantation medicine. In the future, these concepts may be extended and improved to allow transplantation across species. Tissue xenografts, which have been treated to reduce their immunogenicity, have been a successfully used treatment modality in some applications (ie, porcine heart valves), but whole organ xenografts have been unsuccessful. Research regarding genetically altered xenografts is ongoing. When the important immunologic barriers to xenogeneic transplantation are eliminated, the use of animal donors may possibly alleviate the relative paucity of available organs. Of course, significant ethical questions, as well as transplant longevity and transmissible infectious diseases from animals, are questions that must be entertained before these types of transplants become commonplace.[4–6] Perhaps genetically derived tissues/organs may someday be fabricated in vitro and transplanted back into the patient.

TABLE 19-1 Waiting Lists and Transplanted Solid Organs in the United States, 1999*

Organ	Transplants Awaited	Transplants Performed
Liver	> 15,000	< 4,600
Kidney	> 46,000	< 12,400
Lung	> 3,500	< 800
Heart	> 4,100	< 2,100

Adapted from the 1999 annual report of the USSRTROPTN.[2]

*Note these numbers do not equal those cited in the text since other organs, including small intestine and pancreas, are not included in this table.

TABLE 19-2 Types of Transplants

Type of Graft	Type of Transplantation Procedure	Description
Autograft	Autologous	Transplant from self
Isograft	Syngeneic	Transplant between genetically identical individuals (monozygotic twin)
Allograft	Allogeneic	Transplant from a genetically different individual of the same species
Xenograft	Xenogeneic	Transplants between different species

▼ TRANSPLANTATION IMMUNOLOGY

Transplantation immunology encompasses most aspects of the human immune response. When a donor's and a recipient's genetic compositions are not identical, a grafted organ stimulates an immune response. Transplantation medicine would be grossly unsuccessful if this concept were not appropriately appreciated and manipulated. To appreciate the intricacies of organ transplantation, a basic understanding of immunologic concepts is helpful.

Lymphocytes, particularly T lymphocytes (T cells), are instrumental in transplantation failure and are stimulated during rejection. A donor's major histocompatibility complex (MHC), a genetic region found on the short arm of chromosome number 6 of all mammalian cells, codes for products (antigens) that allow immune cells to identify "self" from "non-self." In humans, the "self-antigens" encoded by the MHC include the human leukocyte antigen (HLA) system. Although there are many other gene products, from more than 30 histocompatibility gene loci, that can stimulate graft rejection, it is the HLA system that produces the strongest immunologic response.[3]

MHC genes are inherited from each parent; every child has components of both mother's and father's HLAs on their cell surfaces. The MHC/HLA system is broadly divided into regions. MHC class I and class II regions are those significantly involved in rejection. MHC class I regions include HLA-A, -B, -C, -E, -F, and -G. (The present role of the E, F, and G regions in transplantation is not well understood.) MHC class II regions include HLA-DR, -DQ, -DP, -DO, and -DN. MHC class II genes have two chains, allowing for four different gene products for each locus.

The MHC has extensive polymorphism, allowing remarkable diversity among genes of the HLA system.[7] There are over 180 different class I alleles in the HLA-B region alone and over 220 class II alleles in just one loci of the HLA-DR region that have been recognized in humans. Today, deoxyribonucleic acid (DNA)–based typing (see below) has led to a more specific and detailed classification of the transplantation genes, such that the HLA alleles are related to their DNA sequences.[7]

HLA class I antigens are expressed on most nucleated cells and on red blood cells, whereas class II antigens are expressed only on certain cells known as antigen-presenting cells (APCs). APCs include macrophages, B cells, dendritic cells, and some endothelial cells. The expression of these MHC gene products (antigens) on a cell's surface is regulated by various cytokines such as interferon-γ (IFN-γ) and tumor necrosis factor (TNF).

Transplanted foreign MHC molecules activate the immune response by stimulating the recipient's T cells to respond to foreign antigens. The interaction of the MHC of the donor cells with the recipient's T-cell receptor initiates the immune reaction. T cells can be activated either by the donor's or the recipient's APCs, resulting in expression and production of lymphokines and cytokines that promote activation of cytotoxic T cells, activation of B cells, and activation of natural killer cell activity as well as promote enhanced expression of MHC and increased macrophage activity. This, in turn, causes further immune reactions that result in direct tissue damage and damage to the vascular endothelium of the graft, which may ultimately result in graft rejection.

Transplantation is unsuccessful if rejection is the overwhelming outcome. Rejection, even with the most sophisticated management of the recipient's immune system (see below), does occur. It may be an acute process occurring within days to weeks of the transplantation surgery. This acute process is related to the primary activation of T cells and usually can be reversed by changing the immunosuppressive medication or the medication regimen.

Chronic rejection of the transplanted organ is also a significant problem leading to organ failure. This type of rejection is slow and insidious and cannot be reversed. It probably occurs by continued, albeit muted, cell-mediated toxicity that results in vascular changes to the transplanted organ (as well as other actions, which have not been fully elucidated), leading ultimately to graft rejection.[8]

Another type of rejection is known as "hyperacute rejection"; this occurs within minutes to hours after a transplant procedure. This pattern of rejection occurs in patients who have undergone previous transplantations, patients who have had multiple pregnancies, and patients who have had multiple blood transfusions. It is caused by "preformed" antidonor antibodies that activate complement, resulting in a severe attack of the graft, which often cannot be reversed[9,10] (Table 19-3).

▼ CLINICAL INDICATIONS

The clinical indications for transplantation vary, but the disease outcome is usually fatal without the transplant (except perhaps for renal, pancreatic, eye, skin, or limb), regardless of the transplant indication. The more common indications for transplant are listed in Table 19-4.

Other indications can also be added to this list when quality of life can be improved by transplantation. For example, HCT may ameliorate the affects of systemic lupus erythematosus or other autoimmune disorders.[11] More recently, HCT has been cited as a possible treatment for the management of various solid tumors, including metastatic breast cancer.[12] Other potential uses for hematopoietic stem cell therapy in various other disorders, such as diabetes and amyloidosis, are also being considered.[13–16]

TABLE 19-3 Rejection

Type of Rejection	Description
Acute	Usually occurs within days to weeks due to primary activation of the T-cell response
Chronic	Usually occurs months to years after transplantation; probably occurs by continued, albeit muted, cell-mediated toxicity and other unclear causes
Hyperacute	Usually occurs minutes to hours after transplantation and is caused by preformed antidonor antibodies activating complement

TABLE 19-4 Major Indications for Transplantation*

Type of Transplant	Indications
Kidney	End-stage renal disease Glomerulonephritis Pyelonephritis Congenital abnormalities Nephrotic syndrome
Liver	End-stage liver disease Primary biliary cirrhosis Biliary atresia (children) Chronic hepatitis Sclerosing cholangitis
Pancreas	Severe diabetes leading to renal disease
Intestinal	Massive short-bowel syndrome
Heart	Cardiomyopathy Severe coronary artery disease Congestive heart failure
Heart and lung	Multiorgan end-stage disease Congenital abnormalities Amyloidosis
Lung	Primary pulmonary hypertension COPD/emphysema Pulmonary fibrosis Cystic fibrosis
Hematopoietic cell	Acute myelogenous leukemia Acute lymphoblastic leukemia Chronic myelogenous leukemia Aplastic anemia Multiple myeloma Lymphoma (Hodgkin's and non-Hodgkin's) Various solid tumors Primary immunodeficiencies ? SLE/autoimmune disorders

COPD = chronic obstructive pulmonary disorder; SLE = systemic lupus erythematosus.
* Partial listing only.

▼ MEDICAL MANAGEMENT

Medical management of the transplant candidate focuses on successfully preventing rejection. When the donor and recipient tissue are genetically identical (autologous), the outcome of the transplantation is dependent solely upon the surgical success of the procedure. When tissue from genetically different sources is transplanted, a sophisticated means of preventing rejection must be instituted to ensure graft survival. Transplantation surgeons and oncologists have mastered the surgical procedures for various transplants; medical management to achieve longer-term successful grafts and longer-term overall patient survival has been quite successful, yet it still is fraught with complications. The success of an allogeneic transplantation relies on the ability to identify and match certain genetic markers between the donor and the recipient, while suppressing the recipient's immune system in order to prevent rejection.

Blood and Tissue Typing

Blood and tissue matching are used today for all allogeneic transplants. Standard ABO and Rh ± blood typing are performed to prevent red blood cell agglutination. In addition to blood typing, some method of tissue typing is usually performed (as timing allows) before solid allogeneic transplantations take place and always before allogeneic HCT. Tissue typing allows for matching of the HLA system of antigens found on donor and recipient cells. There is significant variation in HLA testing, depending on the methods employed. Furthermore, based on the type of organ to be transplanted, there is variation in the extent of testing needed to safely transplant the organ. For example, typing is mandatory in allogeneic HCT, but it may be less important in first renal transplantations and for graft survival in liver or heart transplantations.[17] Tissue typing generally can be performed by serologic or DNA-based testing methods. Serologic testing methods for HLA class I antigen identification can be performed by adding antisera of known HLA specificity with complement to a donor sample. Death of the donor cells confirms that they carried the specific HLA antigen. This test usually can be conducted in a couple of hours.[3]

Another test used to specifically determine HLA class II antigens is the mixed lymphocyte culture (MLC) reaction, in which test lymphocytes are incubated with cells expressing known HLA. This results in either proliferation of the stimulated cell or no reaction if the HLA region is the same. This test is time consuming, and because of the short viability of the donor organ/tissue, it is not practical to confirm HLA compatibility in some solid organ transplant.[7]

DNA-based testing for tissue typing is being used more commonly today. Polymerase chain reaction (PCR) is used to identify the DNA in the HLA genes of both the donor and recipient cells. As DNA-based techniques become a more common method for tissue typing, HLA nomenclature will probably change to reflect DNA sequences rather than names that have been serologically defined previously.

Matching for all known HLA alleles is not practical. However, matching for specific MHC class I and class II antigens, especially HLA-A, -B, and -DR (and perhaps -DQ), is important for transplant success in HCT and renal transplantation.

Cross-matching (crossing recipient serum with donor lymphocytes) is usually done to prevent hyperacute rejection in allogeneic solid organ transplants. This is a basic serologic test that is regarded as necessary in those allogeneic transplant recipients who have previously experienced massive immune challenges such as a prior transplantation, multiple pregnancies, or multiple blood transfusions. Since transplantation of solid organs (heart, lung, liver) often requires some expediency, time-consuming complex cross-matching or tissue typing cannot be performed. Instead, absence of antibodies to a panel of cells (defined in advance and known as "panel-reactive antibodies" [PRAs]) is usually adequate for heart and lung transplantation.[18] Interestingly, MHC compatibility in liver transplantation seems negligible in achieving better outcomes.[17] This is fortunate because the timing of liver transplantation often precludes HLA typing.[19]

Immunosuppression

Immunosuppressive regimens vary among transplant centers and among transplantation (organ-specific) programs. Since tissues in allogeneic transplants are not genetically identical, medications used to mute the immune response are essential for graft survival.[20,21] All allogeneic transplantations initially require immunosuppression if the transplanted organs are not to be acutely rejected. Furthermore, most allogeneic solid organ transplant recipients require lifelong maintenance immunosuppression. This may not always be the case with HCT. Additionally, more intensive immunosuppressive regimens are employed later in the post-transplantation period in cases of acute rejection episodes.

Most immunosuppressive medications are nonspecific and cannot prevent a specific component of the immune response. More sophisticated and directed medications are being developed currently; these will allow for graft tolerance while allowing the body to still react to infectious and other detrimental antigens.

Arguably, the most significant advances in transplantation have been made in pharmacotherapeutic immunosuppression. As there is improved understanding of how graft rejection transpires, there is improvement in the specificity of the immunomodulator. The most frequently used contemporary medication classes are discussed in this chapter, with a brief review of some promising formulations (Table 19-5).

CYCLOSPORINE ANALOGUES

Cyclosporine (CSA) is a cyclic polypeptide macrolide medication derived from a metabolite of the fungus *Beauveria nivea*. It is indicated for the prevention of graft rejection because of its immunosuppressive effects. It specifically and reversibly inhibits immunocompetent lymphocytes in the G_0 and G_1 phase of the cell cycle. CSA binds with an intracellular protein, cyclophilin, and inhibits calcineurin. Calcineurin activates a nuclear component of T cells that is thought to initiate gene transcription for the formation of interleukin (IL)-2. Presumably, CSA inhibits IL-2 by preventing the expression of its gene. CSA also reduces the expression of IL-2 receptors. T- helper and, to some extent, T-suppressor cells are preferentially suppressed.[22,23] This medication has some effect on humoral immunity but not on phagocytic function, neutrophil migration, macrophage migration, or direct bone marrow suppression. Absorption of this drug is variable, and frequent blood levels must be drawn to ensure that the drug is in the therapeutic range. A microemulsion formulation is used to enhance the drug's bioavailability.[24]

TACROLIMUS

Tacrolimus (FK-506) (Prograf, Fujisawa Healthcare Inc, Deerfield, IL) is a macrolide immunosuppressant produced by *Streptomyces tsukubaensis* that is used to prevent organ rejection. This medication is similar to CSA in that it suppresses cell-mediated reactions by suppressing T-cell activation. Tacrolimus inhibits calcineurin by interacting with an intracellular protein known as the FK-binding protein. Consequently, T cells are not activated, and cell-mediated cytotoxicity is impeded.[23] There may be a lower incidence of rejection with the use of tacrolimus as compared with the use of CSA in liver, kidney, and lung transplantations. Overall graft and patient survival rates in kidney transplantations do not seem to differ significantly with the use of this medication.

SIROLIMUS

Sirolimus (Rapamycin) (Rapamune, Wyeth-Ayerst Pharmaceuticals, Philadelphia, PA) is another macrolide immunosuppressive agent; it was discovered more than 25 years ago in the soil of Easter Island and is produced by *Streptomyces hygroscopicus*. It is used for prophylaxis against acute rejection of various organs[25–28] and may be appropriate for use in chronic rejection.[29] Sirolimus's mechanism of action is somewhat unique. Sirolimus inhibits the activation of a particular cellular kinase (target of rapamycin), which then interferes with intracellular signaling pathways of the IL-2 receptor, thereby preventing lymphocyte activation. The response of T cells to IL-2 and other cytokines is inhibited. Specifically, the overall effect is interference of T-cell activation during the cells' G_1 to the S phase. Sirolimus is recommended to be used in conjunction with CSA and corticosteroids. This medication has been shown to reduce acute rejection in the first 6 months following renal transplantation, compared with rejection rates when azathioprine is used.[30, 31]

AZATHIOPRINE

Azathioprine (AZA) is an antimetabolite that inhibits ribonucleic acid (RNA) and DNA synthesis by interfering with the purine synthesis that results in decreased T- and B-cell proliferation. It does not interfere with lymphokine production but has significant anti-inflammatory properties. AZA can be bone marrow suppressive, leading to pancytopenia, and it can also cause significant liver dysfunction. Significant drug interactions with allopurinol[32] and ACE inhibitors have been reported. AZA has been used for many years in conjunction with CSA and corticosteroids as triple immunosuppressive therapy. Today, mycophenolate mofetil (MMF), a newer purine analogue, is being tested as an alternative to AZA, as it may have a more specific action against T cells.

MYCOPHENOLATE MOFETIL

MMF, an ester of mycophenolic acid, is an antimetabolite that is used for prophylaxis against graft rejection, and that may have some action in reversing ongoing acute rejection. It inhibits inflammation by interfering with purine synthesis. Both T cells and B cells, which are dependent on this synthesis for their proliferation, are prevented from reproducing. Additionally, MMF interferes with intercellular adhesion of lymphocytes to endothelial cells. It does not inhibit IL-1 or IL-2 but may inhibit medial smooth-muscle proliferation. Based on a multicenter trial, it is thought that this medication can replace AZA in a triple-drug regimen in kidney and heart transplantation.[33] Although the incidence of graft rejection episodes is less with MMF, 1-year renal transplant-graft and patient survival have not been significantly improved by the use of MMF.[34]

TABLE 19-5 Major Immunosuppressive Agents*

Drug	Type	Indications	Major Side Effects†	Dental Implications†
Cyclosporine	Macrolide immunosuppressant Calcineurin inhibitor	Prophylaxis against organ rejection	Hepatotoxicity Nephrotoxicity Elevation of blood pressure	Immunosuppressant‡ P-450 metabolized§ Gingival hyperplasia Monitor CV system May effect renal elimination of some drugs Risk of neoplasm
Tacrolimus	Macrolide immunosuppressant Calcineurin inhibitor	Prophylaxis against organ rejection	Hepatotoxicity Neurotoxicity Nephrotoxicity Post-transplant diabetes mellitus Elevation of blood pressure	Immunosuppressant‡ P-450 metabolized§ Monitor CV system May effect renal elimination of some drugs Risk of neoplasm
Sirolimus	Macrolide immunosuppressant	Prophylaxis against acute and perhaps chronic organ rejection	Hyperlipidemia Hypertriglyceremia	Immunosuppressant‡ P-450 metabolized§ Monitor CV system May effect renal elimination of some drugs Risk of neoplasm
Azathioprine	Antimetabolite	Prophylaxis against organ rejection	Bone marrow suppression Hepatotoxicity	Immunosuppressant‡ Risk of neoplasm
Mycophenolate mofetil	Antimetabolite	Prophylaxis against organ rejection and possible agent to reverse ongoing acute rejection	Leukopenia	Immunosuppressant‡ Absorption is altered by antibiotics, antacids, and bile acid binders Risk of neoplasm
ATG/ALG	Polyclonal antibody	Conditioning agents used prior to transplant	Leukopenia Pulmonary edema Renal dysfunction	Immunosuppressant‡
Muromonab-CD3	Monoclonal antibody	Reversal of acute organ rejection, including steroid-resistant acute rejection	Cytokine release syndrome	Immunosuppressant‡ Interacts with indomethacin
Daclizumab and basiliximab	Monoclonal antibodies	Reversal of acute organ rejection	Pulmonary edema Renal dysfunction	Immunosuppressant‡ Risk of neoplasm
Corticosteroids	Nonspecific immunosuppressant	Reversal of acute organ rejection	Multiple#	Broad nonspecific immunosuppressant‡ Avoid NSAIDs and ASA Monitor CV system Poor wound healing Risk of neoplasm Steroid supplement may be needed with stressful procedures

ASA = acetylsalicylic acid; ATG/ALG = antithymocyte globulin/antilymphocyte globulin; CV = cardiovascular; NSAIDs = nonsteroidal anti-inflammatory drugs.

*Major mechanisms of action are outlined in the text.

†Partial listing only.

‡Use of an immunosuppressant results in an increased risk of infection.

§Dental/oral pharmacotherapeutics that are metabolized by the liver's cytochrome P450 3A system alter this drug's serum levels. This group of medications includes, but is not limited to, erythromycin, clarithromycin, "azole" antifungals, benzodiazepines, carbamazepine, colchicines,, prednisolone, and metronidazole.

#See Table 19-6.

MUROMONAB-CD3

Muromonab-CD3 (Orthoclone OKT-3, Ortho Biotech Products, L.P., Raritan, NJ) is a murine monoclonal antibody (IgG2A) to the CD3 receptor on mature human T cells. It is indicated for reversal of acute allograft rejection and cases of corticosteroid-resistant acute rejection. Monoclonal antibodies in general are effective immunosuppressants. They act by various mechanisms including cell depletion (via opsonization or complement fixation) and antigenic modulation. Cell depletion occurs by phagocytosis or cell lysis. Cell surface coating acts to interfere with cell-to-cell interaction. Antigenic modulation works via redistributing antigen/antibody complexes on the cell surface by internalizing certain receptors or shedding them. OKT3 blocks the generation and function of cytotoxic/mature T cells. This drug is effective for approximately 1 week; approximately 3 days after administration, the patient has no detectable circulating mature T cells. There may be some neutralizing antibodies to OKT3.

ANTITHYMOCYTE AND ANTILYMPHOCYTE GLOBULIN

Polyclonal antilymphocyte sera, antilymphocyte globulin (ALG), and antithymocyte globulin (ATG) are part of the same medication class. These agents are produced by immunizing animals with human lymphoid cells; the animals then produce antibodies to reduce the number of circulating T cells. Individually, these agents affect lymphocyte immunosuppression by reacting with common T-cell surface markers, then coating (opsonizing) the lymphocyte—marking it as foreign for phagocytosis. Polyclonal antibodies are used as conditioning agents prior to transplant.

DACLIZUMAB AND BASILIXIMAB

Daclizumab and Basiliximab are newer agents (synthetic monoclonal antibodies) used for reversal of acute organ rejection. They may also have a significant role during induction immunosuppression.[35] These monoclonal antibodies bind the CD25 receptor (IL-2 receptor) on the surface of activated T cells (IL-2 receptor antagonists), preventing the expansion of CD4 and CD8 lymphocytes. They may be effective in conjunction with MMF and corticosteroids to eliminate the need for CSA use in the early post-transplant period.[35] Anti-CD25 agents have also been reported to be efficacious in treatment of corticosteroid-resistant graft-versus-host disease (GVHD).[36] Other promising targets for monoclonal antibody immunomodulation are being studied currently. The target receptors vary in their function, but development of target-specific medications will probably aid in selected immunosuppression.

CORTICOSTEROIDS

Corticosteroids are consistently used in all allogeneic transplantations for prophylaxis against graft rejection and for reversal of acute rejection. The mechanism of action of this medication is extremely nonspecific as it affects the immune system in many complex ways. Steroids have anti-inflammatory effects and are able to suppress activated macrophages. They also interfere with antigen presentation and reduce the expression of MHC antigens on cells. Steroids reverse the effect of INF-γ and alter the expression of adhesion molecules on vascular endothelium. These medications also have significant effects on IL-1 activity and block the IL-2 gene and its production.[37]

OTHER CYTOTOXIC AGENTS

Cytotoxic agents that are used in conditioning bone marrow prior to HCT include medications, specifically busulfan and/or cyclophosphamide, and also total body irradiation. They cause bone marrow suppression, resulting in pancytopenia (loss of cellular blood elements such as leukocytes and thrombocytes). Cytotoxic therapies are designed to destroy malignant cells, totally immunosuppress the recipient, and make room in the recipient's bone marrow for the HCT. As a result of these agents, the patient is not only highly susceptible to infection but is at a significantly high risk for bleeding.

NEWER IMMUNOSUPPRESSIVE STRATEGIES

Novel approaches to immunosuppression are currently being developed. The definitive immunosuppressive agent would be an agent that is able to destroy only the T cells that are involved with graft rejection, while leaving the remainder of the T cells and the immune system intact. Other monoclonal antibodies are currently under development, with promising immune modulation targets including more specific T cells and natural killer cells as well as endothelium-activated cells.[36]

FTY720 is a new immunosuppressive compound that may cause antigen-induced apoptosis (programmed cell death)[38] of cytotoxic T cells; it is presently being studied in clinical trials.[39] This agent exhibits no inhibition on the production of IL-2 or IL-3 but seems to act synergistically with CSA. Further study of this agent's mechanism of action is warranted.[40,41]

Another promising approach to chemically induced immunosuppression is via a class of agents called the "T-cell co-stimulatory pathway modifiers."[42] Studies have suggested that immune system function has significant self-regulatory capabilities. It is now well recognized that T-cell receptors (TCRs) must recognize MHC-presented antigens to activate a T-cell response. However, it is also thought that TCR recognition requires *two* specific signals to stimulate T-cell activation—that is, recognition of both the TCR signal and a co-stimulatory receptor(s) such as CD28 and/or CD40 ligand, both mandatory for T-cell activation. Blocking of the co-stimulatory signal is the basis of this novel approach to preventing rejection of an allogeneic transplant.

Another interesting finding that has been reported is that use of pravastatin during the early transplantation period may have some effect as an adjunct in immunosuppressive therapy via reduction in natural killer cell cytotoxicity.[43,44]

Although newer immunosuppressive agents have been developed and are being used, they have not shown any clear benefit in patient or organ survival over CSA or tacrolimus. The newer agents, however, have shown some promise in reducing the incidence and severity of rejection. These newer agents probably have a role in reducing the need for cortico-steroids as well as reducing the toxic profiles of CSA or tacrolimus.[45]

Clinical studies to prove a possible synergistic interaction between sirolimus and CSA in reducing renal graft rejection may, in the future, reduce the need for steroids and CSA.[30] Thus far, sirolimus has been approved as an adjuvant to CSA.[46] Ultimately, graft and patient survival profiles coupled with side effects will determine the best antirejection "cocktail" to be used in various transplantations.

A different strategy, aimed at reducing the need for profound immunosuppression, is pretreatment of the recipient with donor blood. This procedure may extend graft survival, as evidenced in some animal models,[47] by enhancing chimerism (ability of both donor and recipient immunocompetent cells to coexist). This concept of transplantation tolerance, whereby the recipient's immune system is first significantly stimulated and then muted, was initially described by Starzl in 1963.[48] The exact mechanism is speculative, but it has been verified in experiments. Starzl described low-level leukocyte chimerism in patients that received allografts and postulated that coexisting donor and recipient leukocyte populations lead to a down-regulated immune response to donor antigens. This is not to suggest that immunosuppression is not needed during the transplantation process but, rather, that if donor immunocompetent cells are transferred with the organ, they can take residence in the recipient's bone marrow and perhaps allow for coexistence and tolerance. Protocols have been developed to infuse donor bone marrow at the time of transplantation, and they are presently being explored.[48]

Antimicrobial Medication

In addition to immunosuppressive medication regimens, antimicrobial medication regimens are important in preventing infection in the transplant recipient. These regimens vary from center to center and from program to program. Patients with a transplant usually need prophylactic antibiotic, antifungal, and, in some cases, antiviral preparations. These medications may include sulfamethoxazole/trimethoprim, nystatin, fluconazole, acyclovir, ganciclovir, and others.

Recently, the Centers for Disease Control and Prevention (CDC) has published guidelines for preventing opportunistic infections among HCT recipients.[49] During the HCT process, all patients take multiple broad-spectrum antibiotics until their donated hematopoietic cells produce functional blood count levels. Additionally, most patients, especially those with a history of herpes simplex virus (HSV), take acyclovir.

Various protocols have been proposed based on the type of transplant, the time frame after transplant, and the signs and symptoms that a transplant patient may experience.[50] Antimicrobial medication coverage has proven to be effective in prevention of some of the transplant-associated infections,[51] especially in HCT, but it still requires further study.[52,53] Some have questioned whether antimicrobial agents are overused during the perioperative period in renal transplants.[54] The CDC offers guidelines for HCT patients based on the quality of the evidence supporting the recommendation.

The CDC also proposes guidelines for vaccination for HCT patients and for their family members/close contacts.[49] Vaccination against hepatitis B and varicella-zoster viruses is usually considered if the transplant recipient does not have antibodies to these diseases. Special consideration for vaccination must be taken into account in the pediatric population. It is of utmost importance for children to receive appropriate vaccination.[55]

▼ COMPLICATIONS

Complications with transplantation are still frequent and require close medical management. General complications can be broadly characterized into those caused by rejection, side effects from medication, and those induced by immunosuppression. Additionally, there are some organ-specific complications observed in certain types of transplantations.

Rejection

As previously mentioned, rejection of the transplanted organ remains a significant obstacle to long-term transplant graft and patient survival. The temporal relationship between the transplant and rejection episodes allows categorization of the particular rejection process (see Table 19-3). Rejection leads to end-organ damage and remanifestation of the various complications of a nonfunctioning organ. Clinically, rejection may be indicated in many ways, including an increased bleeding tendency (rejection of liver), a decreased metabolism or elimination of medications (rejection of liver/kidney), or even complete organ failure and death (rejection of lung/heart). In cases of end-organ disease (except those of kidney failure), retransplantation may be the only way to prevent death.

Rejection is continually monitored throughout the posttransplant period. Most chronic rejection is insidious and is monitored by frequent laboratory analysis and by organ biopsy. Biopsy of tissue from the transplanted organ provides a reliable means to assess rejection. An alternative approach to monitoring rejection in a transplanted heart is the use of pacemakers to record changes in ventricular evoked response amplitude (VERA). Subtle changes in VERA have been correlated with acute rejection of heart transplants.[56]

Medication-Induced Complications

The medications used to produce immunosuppression and prevent graft rejection have significant systemic side effects, which pose serious complications to the transplant recipient. Some of the major side effects are listed here; however, complete drug information can be obtained through an appropriate medication reference source.

CSA, a mainstay in immunosuppression, is nephrotoxic and may alter renal function. It is associated with hypertension and is hepatotoxic. CSA is metabolized via the P450 CYP

3A system of the liver; therefore, it has many drug interactions, including interactions with drugs frequently used in dentistry (see below).

Tacrolimus has also been associated with hypertension and hepatotoxicity. Also, it is nephrotoxic and neurotoxic. There are many other side effects associated with the use of this medication, one of which is the development of insulin-dependent post-transplant diabetes mellitus (PTDM). Its incidence appears to be higher with tacrolimus use than with CSA use in liver transplantations.[57] Tacrolimus is metabolized by the P450 CYP 3A system in the liver. It is 99% protein bound and requires titration. Tacrolimus also has significant interactions with medications used in dentistry (see below).

Sirolimus is hepatotoxic and may cause liver dysfunction. Sirolimus is also associated with a high incidence of hyperlipidemia owing to elevated triglyceride and cholesterol levels.[25–27] Being a substrate for P450 CYP 3A, sirolimus also interferes with the metabolism of other medications.

Azathioprine may cause bone marrow suppression resulting in pancytopenia, which leaves the patient not only susceptible to opportunistic infections but also at significant risk for bleeding.

MMF has significant drug interactions that are particularly important to the dentist. One interaction that is commonly cited occurs as a result of antibiotic regimens that can alter gastrointestinal flora, leading to dramatic changes in MMF drug levels. For example, if a patient is taking a broad-spectrum antibiotic for a dentoalveolar infection, the possibility and probability of an abnormal MMF level does exist. Other medications, such as antacids (containing magnesium or aluminum) and bile acid binders, may also interfere with absorption of MMF. MMF is usually well tolerated, without significant hepatotoxicity or nephrotoxicity, but hematologic alterations (mostly leukopenia) can be a side effect.

OKT3 can be associated with a severe reaction known as "cytokine release syndrome." Cytokines (including TNF) are rapidly released, resulting in significant medical issues including fever, chills, nephrotoxicity, vomiting, pulmonary edema, and, in a few instances, arterial thrombosis.[58] OKT3 has been reported to have interactions with indomethacin, including the potential development of encephalopathy.[59,60]

Both monoclonal and polyclonal antibodies have been associated with significant side effects (in addition to significant cytokine release), including a high risk of viral/fungal infection and an increased incidence of post-transplant lymphoproliferative disorders.[36]

Corticosteroids, another mainstay used in transplantation immunosuppression, can have multiple detrimental side effects, causing various disorders (Table 19-6).

Cytotoxic agents such as cyclophosphamide, busulfan, and total body irradiation cause bone marrow suppression resulting in pancytopenia.

Immunosuppression-Induced Complications

Immunosuppression used to prevent rejection of a transplanted organ also can pose serious complications to the recipient, including life-threatening infections and cancer.

Infections in this population are a significant problem.[61] The type of transplant and the time that transpires since the transplantation often predict the specific infection. For example, patients who have had an HCT usually have broad immunologic defects, either due to their underlying disease or to the induction chemotherapeutic regimen, resulting in profound immunosuppression of all "branches" of the immune system. These patients are at a significantly higher risk of infection than are those patients transplanted with solid organs. Additionally, transplants of certain organs are associated with a greater likelihood of a particular infection.

Timing following the transplantation may correspond with a specific infective process.[50] Bacterial infections are usually seen in the early postoperative period (immediately after transplantation) in solid organ transplantations. The type of bacteria varies with each specific organ. Infections may include both gram-positive and gram-negative bacterial species. Drug-resistant bacterial infections have been documented, such as staphylococcal infections associated with skin wounds, upper and lower respiratory infections (pneumonia), and tuberculosis. Infective endocarditis has also been seen in transplant recipients. In this population, endocarditis is often related to *Staphylococcus* or aspergillosis.[62]

Systemic viral infections are also a common problem in immunosuppressed patients. *Cytomegalovirus* (CMV) and herpes simplex viruses are often the etiologic viral agents involved. CMV infection is more commonly associated with solid organ transplants. Other viral agents, including adenovirus, hepatitis B and C viruses, varicella-zoster virus, Epstein-Barr virus, and human parvovirus B19, have also been implicated in causing disease in a transplant population.[63] Viral infections are also related to time following transplantation. Herpes simplex virus (HSV) infections usually occur at 2 to 6 weeks after organ transplantation, whereas CMV infections usually occur at 1 to 6 months after transplantation, and varicella-zoster virus infections usually occur between 2 and 10 months post transplantation.[64]

TABLE 19-6 Corticosteroid Side Effect Profile

Induces diabetes

Induces muscle weakness

Induces osteoporosis

Alters fat metabolism and distribution

Induces hyperlipidemia

Induces electrolyte imbalances

Induces central nervous system effects including psychological changes

Induces ocular changes—cataracts, glaucoma

Aggravates high blood pressure

Aggravates congestive heart failure

Aggravates peptic ulcer disease

Aggravates underlying infectious processes (eg, tuberculosis)

Suppresses the pituitary-adrenal axis, resulting in adrenal atrophy

Suppresses the stress response

Patients that are immunosuppressed are susceptible to local and systemic fungal infections. These infections vary from those of *Candida* species to deep fungal infections caused by *Aspergillus, Cryptococcus neoformans* phaeohyphomycosis, *Fusarium,* and *Trichosporon.* Deep fungal infections are usually seen later in the transplantation process. Systemic fungal infections are often difficult to treat in the immunosuppressed patient and require systemic antifungal agents.[50] Some have considered the role of macrophage colony-stimulating factor, a cytokine used to stimulate macrophages and monocytes, in the treatment of patients with fungal infections.[65–67]

Parasitic infections caused by *Toxoplasma gondii, Pneumocystis carinii* (now classified as a fungus species),[68] *Strongyloides stercoralis,* and others can be seen in immunosuppressed transplant recipients.

In addition to, and perhaps directly related to, infectious complications, immunosuppression renders the patient at a higher risk for the development of cancer. The immune system provides surveillance against antigens that may act as initiators or promoters of cancer. When the immune response is muted, so too is the surveillance system. Cancers most commonly associated with immunosuppression are squamous cell carcinomas of the skin,[69,70] lymphomas[71] (collectively referred to as post-transplant lymphoproliferative diseases [PTLDs]), and Kaposi's sarcoma. Squamous cell carcinoma of the skin may be related to the human papillomaviruses,[72] whereas human herpesvirus 8 has been implicated in Kaposi's sarcoma,[73] and Epstein-Barr virus in PTLDs.[71] PTLDs have been treated with decreased immunosuppression, antilymphocyte agents, conventional chemotherapy, radiotherapy, and IFN-α therapy.[74,75]

Specific Organ/Hematopoietic Cell Transplantation Complications

A significant medical complication seen in patients receiving solid organ transplants is accelerated advanced cardiovascular disease including coronary artery disease (CAD). The cause of this rapid CAD is thought to be either infectious (CMV), medication induced, or, more likely, both. Many investigators have explored the etiologic role of hypertension in CAD.[76] Probably in this population CAD is multifactorial. For instance, steroids, CSA, and sirolimus have been associated with hyperlipidemia, a condition associated with CAD.

Hypertension is also a common post-transplantation problem, often related to the immunosuppressive medication regimen.[77] In many transplantation facilities, hypertension is being treated by calcium channel antagonists. Some clinicians note that this group of medications may raise serum levels of CSA, thus decreasing the cost of immunosuppression.[78] Caution must be exercised with any drug affecting CSA metabolism; for this reason, most clinicians prefer to prescribe medications that do not alter CSA levels. Nifedipine is one such calcium channel antagonist, but it has adverse oral effects such as gingival overgrowth (see below).

Another significant condition associated with transplantation is post-transplant diabetes mellitus. This disorder is a frequent consequence of allogeneic organ transplantation. Experimental

and clinical observations both suggest this phenomenon is related to the immunosuppressive agents.[79] Post-transplant diabetes mellitus may cause both macro- and microvascular changes, which affect both graft and patient survival.[79]

Neurologic complications, such as neuropathies, can also be noted in transplant recipients.[80]

Re-infection with hepatitis C virus after transplant is high in recipients of liver transplants. This re-infection is associated with a high rate of mortality.[81]

The second most common long-term cause of morbidity and mortality (infection being the first) after lung transplantation is bronchiolitis obliterans. This disorder is an inflammation and constriction in bronchioles. It probably is related to chronic rejection and infection and perhaps altered microvasculature.[82]

Heart transplantation is also fraught with complications. As previously mentioned, post-transplant CAD is common in all transplantations, including heart transplants. Additionally, early after transplantation, the heart is denervated such that symptoms of angina may be absent and the heart may have diminished vagal response.[83,84] There is, however, evidence of sympathetic and possibly parasympathetic re-innervation later in the post-transplant period, suggesting that angina and heart rate changes to stress are regained.[83,85,86] Care of patients with cardiac transplants must recognize these cardiac abnormalities.[87] Mitral and tricuspid regurgitation has also been observed after heart transplantation.[88,89]

Perhaps the largest numbers of complications are those observed after an allogeneic HCT. Allogeneic transplantation often involves both administration of very high doses of myeloablative chemotherapy and total body irradiation. The major complications of allogeneic HCT include the following:

1. End-organ damage from the pretransplant therapy
2. Graft-versus-host disease (GVHD)
3. Infections

A significant complication seen in these patients prior to HCT occurs during the conditioning regimen. One such complication is known as veno-occlusive disease of the liver. This is caused by nonthrombotic occlusion of the central veins of the hepatic lobules. It is characterized by jaundice, hepatomegaly, and fluid retention. Treatment for this process is supportive.[90]

Perhaps the most frequently cited complication associated with HCT is GVHD, which is a complex immunologic phenomenon that occurs when immunocompetent cells from the donor are given to an immunodeficient host. The host, who possesses transplantation antigens foreign to the graft, stimulates an immune response by the newly engrafted immune cells. GVHD affects the entire gastrointestinal system, including the mouth, as well as the skin and the liver. This reaction can be lethal, and, in acute disease, needs to be reversed with increased immunosuppression. Chronic mucosal ulceration seen in GVHD may serve as an entry port for other infectious pathogens.[91] Chronic low-grade GVHD may be beneficial insofar as it could be considered as a graft-versus-leukemia reaction to kill persistent leukemic cells.[92]

▼ PROGNOSIS

Transplantation outcomes have improved over the past decade. In this chapter, the outcomes of patients who have received HCT are separated from outcomes of those receiving solid organ transplants. Furthermore, solid organ transplants are summarized and categorized by each specific organ. Data regarding clinical outcomes of solid organ transplantation must also be separated into *graft survival* as well as *patient survival* (Table 19-7). In the United States, total solid organ transplantation totaled just over 24,000 in 2001. The 1-year graft survival of renal transplantations performed was approximately 95% for a living donor transplant and 89% for a cadaveric kidney transplant. Liver transplant graft survival was 80%. Heart transplant graft survival was 84%, whereas lung and heart/lung graft survivals were 75% and 56%, respectively.[2]

One-year patient survival was 98% for those receiving a living donor renal transplant, 87% for a liver transplant, 85% for a heart transplant, and 76% for a lung transplant. Five-year graft and patient survival rates for solid organ transplants are lower. The 5-year graft survival rate for cadaveric donor kidney transplants was 61%, whereas the rate for living donor kidney transplants was 76%. Five-year liver graft survival was 64%, whereas heart and lung graft survivals were 68% and 40%, respectively. Patient survival rate at 5 years was 81% for cadaveric donor kidney transplant recipients and 91% for living transplant recipients. Five-year patient survival rates for liver, heart, and lung transplantations were 75%, 70%, and 43%, respectively.[2]

The number of patients on waiting lists for solid organ transplants significantly increased from 1989 to 1998. The deaths of patients awaiting kidney transplants increased slightly over the same period of time, whereas the death rates for patients awaiting for heart and liver transplants decreased.

The longest living adult recipient is solid organ transplants (patient survival) in the United States is approximately 37 years for a kidney transplant, 22 years for a liver transplant, 22 years for a heart transplant, and 11 years for a lung transplant.[2]

Current estimates of HCTs performed annually are 30,000 to 40,000 worldwide. The annual rate of growth of this procedure has been estimated to be 10 to 20%.[93] Improved HCT-related health care has resulted in less morbidity and lower mortality rates. Traditionally, HCTs for hematologic malig-

nancies were undertaken as salvage therapy for refractory cancers. Today, outcomes are actually better for patients who are treated with HCT soon after diagnosis rather than after multiple relapses of hematologic disease. Outcomes have improved in both autologous and allogeneic HCTs. There are various reasons that the success of HCT has improved. In the 1980s, CSA was introduced as an immunosuppressive agent. Currently, CSA is often used with other medications, including methotrexate and corticosteroids, in prevention of GVHD. The incidence of both acute and chronic GVHD after HLA-matched sibling allogeneic transplantations has decreased to approximately 30%. Additionally, CMV status prior to and after the transplant is more closely monitored. Screened "CMV-free" blood products are used for CMV-negative patients. CMV-positive patients are treated with a prophylactic or pre-emptive strategy and are given CMV prophylaxis. These procedures have decreased the mortality associated with CMV interstitial pneumonitis.[49] Post-transplant cell growth factors have also been cited as improving outcomes in HCT patients.[66] These growth factors allow for a speedier recovery after myeloablative chemotherapy. In allogeneic HCT, these advances have led to a decrease in overall mortality from 50% in 1974 to approximately 30% in 1994.[93–95] Transplant-related mortality following autologous transplantation is even lower—approximately 5%.[93] There are over 20,000 patients that have survived HCT for 5 years or greater, and the future holds even greater promise as the various transplant techniques become further refined.

Outcomes of recipients who have received *both* bone marrow and solid organ transplantation have also been reviewed.[94] Some of the patients in this review by Dey and colleagues had an HCT and subsequently developed end-organ damage as a complication of some aspect of the transplantation procedure. They were later treated with a solid organ transplant. Similarly, there were patients that received a solid organ transplant only to be subsequently diagnosed with a hematologic disorder, which was treated by an HCT. A total of 28 patients were studied: 21 had an HCT followed by a solid organ transplant whereas the other 7 received the solid organ transplant first. Eight patients died before they could be included in this review. None of those reported deaths were due to graft failure or rejection. Of the patients reviewed, 2 were cardiac transplant recipients. At the time of this review, 1 patient was noted to be leukemia free and free of congestive heart failure at 1 year, and

TABLE 19-7 Outcomes of Solid Organ Transplantations

Type of Survival	Type of Transplantation				
	Renal (Living Donor)	Renal (Cadaveric Donor)	Heart	Liver (Cadaveric)	Lung
1-year graft survival (%)	95	89	84	80	75
5-year graft survival (%)	76	61	68	64	40
1-year patient survival (%)	98	95	85	87	76
5-year patient survival (%)	91	81	70	75	43

Data from the 2001 annual report of the USSRTROPTN.[2] Accessed June 2002.

the other patient was disease free at 6 months. Three lung transplant survivors after HCT were noted at 9, 14, and 15 months. Five of 10 recipients of liver transplants after HCT died. One partial liver transplant recipient was reported as "doing well." Four kidney transplant recipients were noted to be "doing well"; they each had received a transplant of a kidney from the same person who had donated bone marrow to them.

Allogeneic HCTs were performed on 7 patients who had been treated with a renal or a liver transplantation. Four liver transplant recipients were noted to be doing well 2 years after their HCTs. One of 3 who underwent renal transplantation followed by HCT was "doing well" at 22 months post HCT.

There are many clinical and immunologic considerations that are highlighted by reviewing this unique patient population. Further study regarding the concept of immunologic tolerance/chimerism in these patients may provide clues for future studies or for consideration of routine treatment regimens including HCT with the transplanted solid organ. Close monitoring of these patients will allow a better understanding of the concept of chimerism.[94]

▼ ORAL HEALTH CONSIDERATIONS

Oral Lesions

Patients who have had an organ transplantation may present to their health care practitioner with oral complaints. Often these complaints are related to oral mucosal lesions or masses. These lesions can be broadly related to an infectious process or a noninfectious process. Oral mucosal lesions and masses need to be identified, diagnosed, and treated.

Comprehensive oral examination is paramount in the transplant recipient, given the fact that the patient is more susceptible to oral infections of bacterial, viral, and fungal origins. Signs of oral infection may be *muted* due to a decreased inflammatory response, or occasionally, the signs of infection may be *exaggerated*. The presentation of an oral infection is dependent upon the patient's level of immunosuppression and the patient's ability to mount an immune response. Oral infections must be diagnosed and treated, as local infections may spread quickly. Systemic infections may also manifest orally. It is also important to remember that in severely immunocompromised hospitalized patients, the infectious agent associated with oral ulceration may be one that is normally not associated with oral infections.[96,97] Culture and sensitivity testing of all types of infections is prudent.

Bacterial infections, including dentoalveolar abscesses, may not manifest in traditional patterns. Therefore, treatment of bacterial infections requires prompt antibiotic therapy. Culture and sensitivity should be considered in severe infections or in those not responding quickly to empiric antibiotic therapy.

Dental caries, a bacterial infection, has been associated with many end-stage diseases and is presumably related to the various therapies/medications required to treat those diseases. However, the precise cause of the increased rate of caries remains somewhat questionable. Children who have had an HCT for acute lymphoblastic leukemia have had a higher number of restored teeth.[98] Caries in limited numbers of kidney transplant recipients were studied in relation to salivary IgA. Low salivary IgA level (presumably related to immunosuppressive medications) was not associated with increased incidence of caries within 12 months post transplant. It should be noted that the relationship might differ in transplant recipients after the initial 12-month period.[99]

Periodontal health in this patient population is often compromised. Medications and their side effects have been related to periodontal disorders, particularly gingival overgrowth. The medication-induced gingival overgrowth seen in the transplant recipient seems to be related to the immunosuppressive agent CSA (Figure 19-1). Furthermore, CSA-associated gingival overgrowth may be exaggerated by the coadministration of nifedipine, a calcium channel blocker often used to treat hypertension in this patient population. Nifedipine is so often the drug of choice because it will not alter plasma levels of CSA, as do some other antihypertensive medications.

Biopsy should be performed on gingival overgrowth as case reports of malignant tumors have been associated with some of these growths.[100,101] Impeccable oral hygiene has been noted to be helpful in preventing gingival overgrowth.[102] Partial reversal of CSA-induced overgrowth has been reported upon discontinuation of the medication.[103] However, treatment of severe gingival overgrowth usually requires gingivectomy.

Viral infections are a common problem in immunosuppressed patients. HSV is the most common viral pathogen cultured from oral infections. Recurrent herpes simplex infections can be both of the labial and intraoral varieties. (Figures 19-2 to 19-4). Recurrent intraoral herpes may be chronic and difficult to diagnose based solely on clinical appearance (Figure 19-5). Varicella-zoster and Epstein-Barr viruses, as well as other viruses, have also been implicated in oral disease. Oral hairy leukoplakia has been seen in transplant recipients not infected with human immunodeficiency viruses.[104–106] Treatment of viral infections involves the appropriate antiviral agent. Occasionally, HSV mutants not responsive to acyclovir require treatment with foscarnet (an antiviral medica-

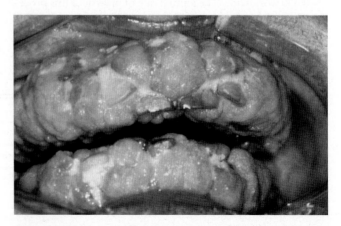

FIGURE 19-1 Gingival overgrowth in a kidney transplant recipient taking cyclosporine and nifedipine who also had poor oral hygiene.

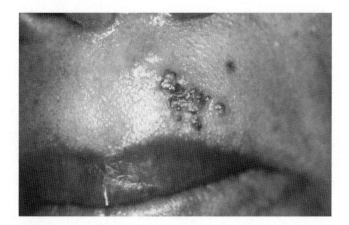

FIGURE 19-2 Recurrent herpes labialis.

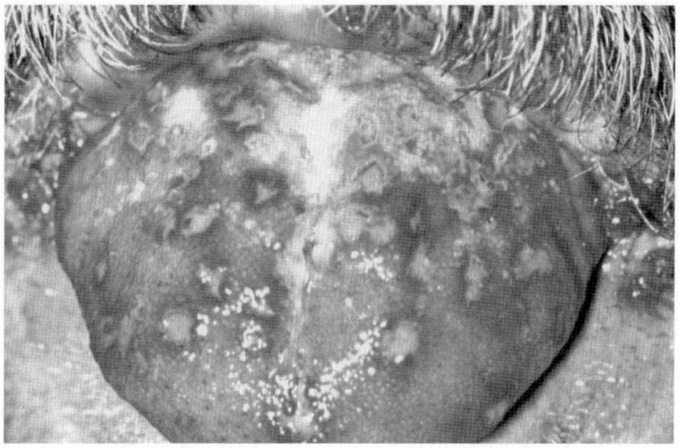

FIGURE 19-4 Recurrent intraoral herpes in a cardiac transplant recipient.

tion with a mechanism of action different than that of acyclovir).[107] Cases are now emerging of both acyclovir- and foscarnet-resistant oral HSV. Successful treatment of multiresistant HSV infection with cidofovir has been reported.[108]

Patients who are immunosuppressed are more susceptible to fungal infections. These infections vary from those of candidal species, including pseudomembranous candidiasis, to deep fungal infections including aspergillosis, cryptococcosis, mucormycosis, and blastomycosis (Figures 19-6 and 19-7). These infections may manifest in various presentations in the oral cavity. Candidiasis can present as the classic pseudomembranous form, or it can be atrophic or even hyperplastic (see Figures 19-6 to 19-9). Hyperplastic candidiasis is not removed by scraping the lesion and often requires biopsy for definitive diagnosis. Occasionally candidiasis is not responsive to the typical "azole-type" antifungal agents[109,110] and may require treatment with amphotericin B. It is important to note that candidal hyphae have been reported in CSA-induced gingival overgrowth.[111]

Deep fungal infections involving the upper respiratory tract/sinuses may manifest as necrotic plaques in the palatal areas of recipients of HCT (see Figure 19-7). These fungal infections are very difficult to treat and often require intravenous antifungal agents such as amphotericin B. In patients who are severely neutropenic, these infections may prove fatal, with the patient ultimately succumbing to a systemic deep fungal infection.

Noninfectious oral lesions are also common in the transplant recipients. Some of these lesions may represent neoplasms. The transplant recipient is at a higher risk of developing lymphoma and other cancers, such as Kaposi's sarcoma and squamous cell carcinoma of the skin (see above).[112] Lymphoma and Kaposi's sarcoma can be present in the mouth,[100,113,114] whereas epithelial malignancy often involves the lips.[115,116] One reported case describes a cutaneous squamous cell carcinoma metastasizing to the parotid gland.

Treatment of opportunistic post-transplant lymphoproliferative disorders may include decreased immunosuppression, antilymphocyte agents, conventional chemotherapy, radiotherapy, and IFN-α therapy.[74,75]

GVHD is a unique complication of HCT. In the oral cavity, this process clinically resembles lichenoid inflammation/lichen planus. Oral GVHD appears as an area of wispy hyperkeratosis on an erythematous base in various areas of the oral mucosa. In

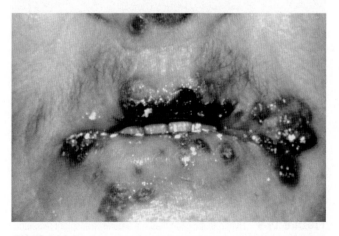

FIGURE 19-3 Recurrent herpes labialis in an immunocompromised patient.

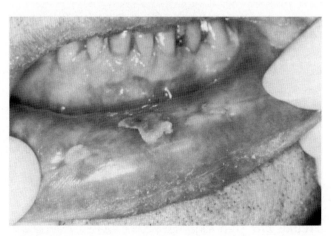

FIGURE 19-5 Chronic herpes simplex in a chronically immunosuppressed transplant recipient.

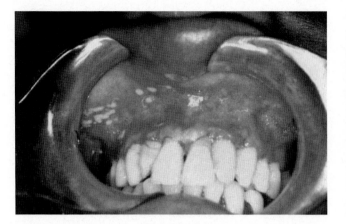

FIGURE 19-6 Pseudomembranous candidiasis.

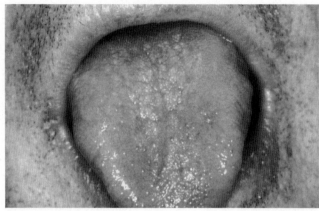

FIGURE 19-8 Atrophic candidiasis.

more severe GVHD, the lesions can appear significantly eroded and may be associated with chronic mucosal ulceration[117] (Figure 19-10). These ulcerations may serve as a systemic port of entry for oral pathogens. GVHD not only affects the mouth but the entire gastrointestinal system, as well as the skin and the liver. This reaction can be lethal, and, in acute disease, it needs to be reversed. However, chronic GVHD may be considered somewhat beneficial if it functions as a graft-versus-leukemia reaction, an immunologic process to kill persistent leukemic cells. GVHD in the oral mucous membrane is often difficult to treat locally and often requires a change in the immunosuppressive regimen.[117] Some have used topical CSA in a bioadhesive base with good results.[118] Ultraviolet B irradiation as well as ultraviolet A irradiation with oral psoralen (PUVA) has been reported to be effective.[119,120] A novel approach for treating oral GVHD involves the use of topical azathioprine.[121]

In addition to GVHD, a patient who has had an allogeneic HCT may also experience a nongingival soft-tissue growth, presumably related to the use of CSA. These lesions can be seen in the buccal mucosa, alveolar mucosa, and elsewhere[122] (Figure 19-11).

Oral mucositis is a common complaint of patients who have had chemotherapy.[123] Mucositis after HCT is usually related to the preconditioning regimen, and it is difficult to distinguish from an oral infection (Figure 19-12). Often mucositis is treated with palliative agents; a mixture of an anesthetic, an antihistamine, and a coating agent is commonly used. These agents tend to provide transient relief with no significant improvement in the mucositis. Palliative treatment with lidocaine has been associated with only minor systemic absorption.[124] Some have suggested the use of topical tretinoin prophylaxis to prevent HCT mucositis.[125] Newer agents with specific antimucositis indications are presently being explored.

Salivary gland dysfunction is also quite common in patients after HCT. This may be acutely related to the chemotherapeutic regimens used to rid the bone marrow of leukemic cells. Patients who have chronic GVHD also have diminution of salivary flow, presumably from a lymphocytic infiltrate of salivary tissue[126] (Figure 19-13).

Developmental tooth defects such as altered root formation and dentofacial alterations must also be considered, as

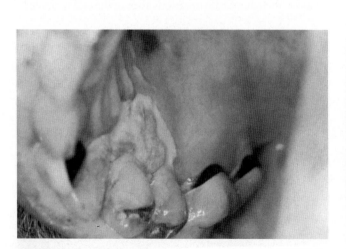

FIGURE 19-7 Deep fungal aspergillosis in a patient who underwent HCT. The patient succumbed to disseminated aspergillosis shortly after this photograph was taken.

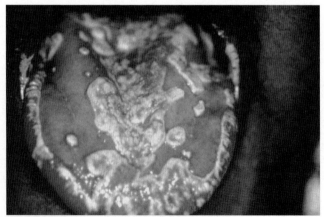

FIGURE 19-9 Hyperplastic candidiasis in a kidney transplant recipient. This infection did not respond to fluconazole.

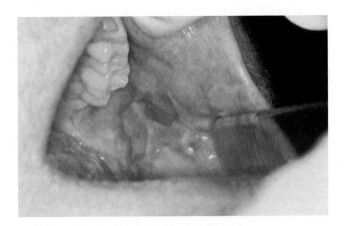
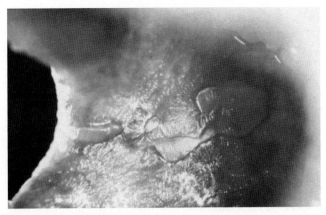

FIGURE 19-10 Graft-versus-host disease in a patient who had undergone HCT. Note the clinical resemblance to erosive lichen planus.

they have been reported in children who have undergone HCT[127] (Figure 19-14).

Dental Management

Dental treatment for patients who are preparing for transplantation or for those who have had a transplant should be coordinated with the performing physician. The patient may be a better candidate for elective dental treatment after the transplanted organ is stable. Often, however, the physician may consult the patient's general dentist before "listing" the patient for the transplantation. The nature of this consult is to assure that the patient does not have any acute (or potentially acute) dental/oral infection that could complicate the transplantation process. It is prudent for a transplant candidate to be examined by the dentist in the pretransplantation period.

A dentist treating members of this unique population must be aware of certain considerations regarding the medical health of the individuals; providing dental care is often challenging. Close and detailed communication between the health care workers is essential. Dental management for this patient population can be divided into as pretransplantation and posttransplantation issues (Table 19-8).

PRETRANSPLANTATION CONSIDERATIONS

Pretransplantation concerns include the fact that these patients are critically ill and have significant end-organ damage. Specific organ damage poses unique challenges. Patients with end-stage liver disease may have difficulties with excessive bleeding due to coagulopathy. These patients may have difficulty metabolizing medications (Table 19-9).

Patients awaiting a kidney transplant have end-stage renal disease and are usually receiving hemodialysis. These patients require antibiotic prophylaxis prior to dental treatment to prevent bacterial endocarditis. They also may be fluid overloaded and have hypertension; therefore, monitoring of the patient's blood pressure is usually prudent. When determining the blood pressure, the cuff must *not* be placed on the arm used for dialysis access. Occasionally, electrolyte balance may be altered. Variation of drug metabolism and excretion must also be considered in this population, as changing of the dose of various medications, including those used in dentistry, may be required[128] (see Table 19-9).

Patients awaiting a heart transplant are usually poor candidates for outpatient dental treatment. The majority of these

FIGURE 19-11 Nongingival soft-tissue growth.

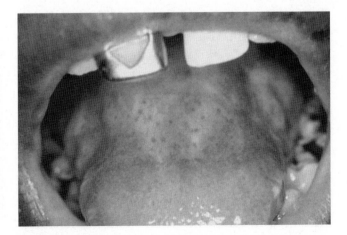

FIGURE 19-12 Mucositis shortly after induction chemotherapy for acute myelogenous leukemia.

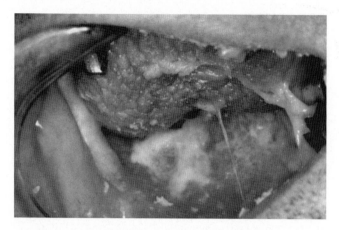

FIGURE 19-13   Salivary hypofunction.

patients have severe CAD or congestive heart failure. The cardiovascular reserve of these patients is small, rendering them much better candidates for elective dental treatment after they have undergone transplantation. Some patients awaiting heart transplants may not be discharged from the hospital until they receive their new heart.

Patients awaiting lung transplants are also critically ill. Most are on oxygen therapy and have difficulty breathing. Dental treatment should preclude the use of combustible sources near the patient if he or she is using oxygen therapy. Inhaled anesthetics are contraindicated in these patients. Narcotic medications that cause respiratory depression are also contraindicated.

Patients awaiting pancreatic transplants have significant problems in glucose management; therefore, considerations of serum glucose levels prior to initiating treatment must be made. These patients may be poor wound healers and may have "brittle insulin-dependent diabetes"; that is, these patients may experience sharp alterations in blood glucose levels and be prone to both ketoacidosis and insulin shock (see Chapter 21 on diabetes).

HCT candidates are frequently also significantly ill. Most have been through induction and have endured consolidation chemotherapy to treat a hematologic malignancy. Many of these patients are pancytopenic and are prone to infections and bleeding. They are therefore considered poor candidates for routine outpatient dental treatment. Other patients may have had a significant remission of their disease with normalizing blood counts, allowing emergency dental treatment prior to the HCT.

When treating patients who are transplantation candidates, the dentist must be familiar with the underlying disorder as well as laboratory evaluations pertinent to the particular disorder. Consultation with the patient's physician is mandatory.

A dentist caring for members of the pretransplantation population must not only consider providing/withholding care after considering the underlying disorders, he or she must consider the potential dental complications that can significantly impact the transplantation process. A detailed clinical examination of the dentition, periodontium, and oral mucosa as well as the head and neck areas, including the lymph nodes and salivary glands, is prudent. There has been some controversy as to the optimal radiographic examination regimen required to evaluate patients who will undergo HCT;[129] however, recent dental radiographs must be part of the evaluation.

Once the evaluation has been performed, a medical/dental risk assessment should be formulated. Generally speaking, elec-

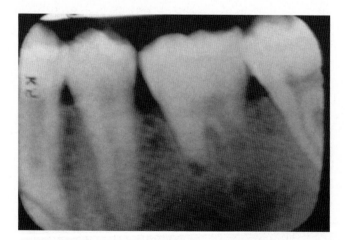

FIGURE 19-14   Dental root alteration as a result of childhood treatment for lymphoma.

TABLE 19-8   Dental Management Considerations

Pretransplantation considerations

   Significantly ill patient with end-organ damage

   Medical consultation required

   Consider postponing elective treatment

   Dental consultation prior to anticipated transplant:
      Rule out dental infectious sources, definitively
      Perform necessary treatment; this will require consultation with transplantation physician to determine medical risk-to-benefit ratio
      Obtain laboratory information/supplemental information as needed
      Become acquainted with specific management issues (eg, blood products, prophylactic antibiotics) that may need to be employed if treatment is rendered

Post-transplantation considerations

   Immediate post-transplantation period
      No elective dental treatment performed
      Emergency treatment only with medical consultation and consideration of specific management needs

   Stable post-transplantation period
      Elective treatment may be performed after medical consultation with the transplantation physician
      Issues of immunosuppression must be recognized
      Oral mucosal disease must be diagnosed and treated
      Supplemental corticosteroids (steroid boost) may be necessary
      Consideration of antibiotic prophylaxis needed
      Consideration of specific management needs

   Post-transplantation chronic rejection period
      Only emergency treatment
      Patients are very ill as they are immunosuppressed and have organ failure

TABLE 19-9   Medication Considerations in Patients with Liver or Kidney Failure*

Drug	Dose Change Required?	
	Kidney Failure[†]	Liver Failure
Acetaminophen	–	Avoid use
Acyclovir	+	–
Amoxicillin	+	–
Cephalexin	+	–
Clavulanic acid with amoxicillin	+	–
Clindamycin	–	+
Codeine	+	+
Diazepam	+	+
Erythromycin	–	+
Ibuprofen	–	Unknown
Ketoconazole	–	+
Lidocaine	–	–
Metronidazole	+	+
Minocycline	–	+
Naproxen	+	+
Penicillin	+	–
Salicylates	+/Avoid use	Avoid use
Tetracycline	+/Avoid use	Avoid use

Adapted from Byrne, BE. Therapeutics in renal hepatic disease. In: Ciancio S, editor. ADA guide to dental therapeutics. Chicago (IL): ADA publishing Co.; 1998. p. 432–40.

+ = May require a dose change and/or avoidance of use, depending on severity of renal or hepatic disease.

– = No dose change required.

*Includes only drugs commonly used in dentistry.

[†]Degree of function of renal system must be considered before dose change is determined.

tive dental treatment in patients with end-stage disease should be postponed as the patient will be more "medically stable" after the transplantation. However, whenever possible, it is important for the dentist to eliminate dental infections prior to the transplantation as the patient will be significantly immunosuppressed immediately and for some time after the transplantation. Dental treatment planning must therefore take into account the patient's laboratory evaluation, including such parameters as blood cell and platelet counts, serum chemistry to determine degree of organ dysfunction, and coagulation studies. In addition, other tests that are more specific for each particular organ function must be obtained and reviewed. A medical risk assessment is necessary to determine if a patient can systemically tolerate an extraction or other dental procedure. Some HCT and heart transplant candidates cannot withstand even emergency treatment. When risk assessment favors treatment, the most *definitive* treatment option should be considered (often extraction). Antibiotic prophylaxis prior to the dental treatment is often warranted in patients awaiting HCT or heart or kidney transplants. Patients awaiting HCT or liver transplants may need platelets, coagulation factors, or other supportive products prior to dental treatment.

POST-TRANSPLANTATION CONSIDERATIONS

Patients who have undergone transplantation also pose concerns to the treating dentist. The post transplantation period can be divided into the immediate post-transplantation period, the stable period, and the chronic rejection period. The immediate post-transplantation period is the time when the patient is most susceptible to both rejection and severe infection. This period of time begins immediately post transplantation and extends to when the grafted organ is functioning appropriately. Due to increased levels of immunosuppression used to foil rejection during this period, the dentist should *not* perform elective dental treatment, and emergency treatment should be provided only after consultation with the transplantation physician. Patients have shown benefit from chlorhexidine mouth rinses during this period of time.[130]

The stable post-transplantation period occurs when the grafted organ is stable. It is during this time that the problems of chronic rejection, immunosuppression, and side effects of immunosuppressive medications may become apparent. Dental treatment planning must consider these important factors. The length of time that a patient remains in this stage is variable. Generally, this period is the best time to perform elective dental treatment since the organ is functioning appropriately. In general, there are no absolute contraindications to any type of dental procedure in patients after a successful HCT.[131] Consultation with the transplantation physician is essential due to the delicate balance of rejection/immunosuppression and their implications in medical/dental risk assessment.

Antibiotic prophylaxis prior to dental treatment is often requested by the transplantation physician, although whether this is necessary requires further evidence-based research. Corticosteroid supplementation *may* also be required due to adrenal suppression associated with higher-dose chronic corticosteroid use. This supplementation may help to avoid cardiovascular collapse during stressful procedures, and it is recommended when the stress of the procedure or the patient's perception of the stress (pain) of the procedure is increased.[132] Some have questioned the need for supplementation when treating gingival overgrowth via gingivectomy under local anesthetic.[133]

Other considerations for the dental provider during the stable post transplant period involve medication interactions as several antirejection immunosuppressive medications have interactions with medications that a dentist may prescribe. For example, patients who are taking CSA as one of their antirejection medications may require the use of clindamycin instead of erythromycin. CSA levels are affected by anti-inflammatory drugs such as diclofenac, sulindac, and naproxen; antifungal medications such as itraconazole, fluconazole, and ketoconazole; and antibiotics such as clarithromycin and erythromycin. Reviewing potential interactions between the medications that the transplant patient is taking and those the dentist intends to prescribe is prudent. As the trends in immunosuppression change, the dentist will need to be familiar with the newer medications and the potential risk of interactions with the various medications used in dentistry.

The stable post-transplantation period ends and the chronic rejection period starts when a grafted organ begins to fail. Laboratory parameters indicate organ function failure, and biopsies are used to confirm this process. For dentists, these patients are often the most complicated to manage since the organ is failing and the patient is immunosuppressed. Only emergency dental treatment is indicated, and the transplantation physician's input is essential. The treating dentist must consider the ramifications of organ failure and make appropriate provisions.

▼ CONCLUSION

Oral considerations in the transplantation population are vast. The dentist needs an exceptionally strong knowledge base in medicine to minimize adverse outcomes secondary to provision of oral health care. As this unique population grows, so does the need for qualified dental practitioners. It is essential that the dentist familiarize himself or herself with the special needs of these patients. Their dental health is imperative; therefore, patients who have had an organ transplantation need to have routine dental examinations. It is incumbent on the dental practitioner to expediently diagnose and treat any oral infection. Gingival health in this population is extremely important and must be monitored regularly, particularly because CSA may induce gingival overgrowth, which precludes adequate home care and encourages further periodontal breakdown.

Arguably, patients undergoing allogeneic HCT should be evaluated more frequently than the general population owing to the decreased salivary flow, which may be associated with an increased caries rate.[134] Consideration should be given to providing patients with supplemental topical fluoride applications. These patients may also have oral ulceration from GVHD. These ulcers can serve as a portal of entry for any oral pathogen to infect the immunocompromised host.

The patient's medical history should be updated with each dental appointment. Close coordination with the transplantation physician is necessary as the patient's medical condition can change quickly.

As with all dental patients, excellent oral hygiene is difficult to achieve solely by the clinician's professional service. It is extremely important to provide oral hygiene instruction and to discuss with the patient the need for appropriate hygiene to prevent oral infection. These patients can be at high risk of serious complications, even from initially minimal dental infections. The patient should also be taught to perform an oral examination and encouraged to perform it frequently at home. This procedure enables the patient to constantly monitor his or her own oral condition and to aid the health care professional in early diagnosis of pathology.

▼ REFERENCES

1. Muhlbacher F, Langer F, Mittermayer C. Preservation solutions for transplantation. Transplant Proc 1999;31:2069–70.

2. 1999 annual report of the U.S. Scientific Registry of Transplant Recipients and the Organ Procurement and Transplantation Network: transplant data 1989–1998. Rockville (MD) and Richmond (VA): HHS/HRSA/OSP/DOT and UNOS; 2000 (accessed Feb 21, 2000).

3. Hutchinson I. Transplantation and rejection. In: Roitt I, Brostoff J, Male D, editors. Immunology. 5th ed. London: Mosby; 1998. p. 26.1–26.13.

4. McKenzie I, Loveland B, Fishman JA, et al. Xenotransplantation. In: Ginns LC, Cosimi AB, Morris PJ, editors. Transplantation. Malden (MA): Blackwell Science; 1999. p. 827–66.

5. Hammer C, Linke R, Wagner F, Diefenbeck M. Organs from animals for man. Int Arch Allergy Immunol 1998;116:5–21.

6. Allan JS. The risk of using baboons as transplant donors. Exogenous and endogenous viruses. Ann N Y Acad Sci 1998; 862:87–9.

7. Mickelson E, Petersdorf EW. Histocompatibility. In: Thomas ED, Blume KG, Forman SJ, editors. Hematopoietic cell transplantation. 2nd ed. Oxford, Malden (MA): Blackwell Science; 1999.

8. Wilhelm MJ, Kusaka M, Pratschke J, Tilney NL. Chronic rejection: increasing evidence for the importance of allogen-independent factors. Transplant Proc 1998;30:2402–6.

9. Crespo M, Delmonic F, Saidman S, et al. Acute humoral rejection in kidney transplantation. Graft 2000;3:12–7.

10. Kupiec-Weglinski JW. Graft rejection in sensitized recipients. Ann Transplant 1996;1:34–40.

11. Marmont AM. Stem cell transplantation for severe autoimmune disorders, with special reference to rheumatic diseases. Rheumatology 1997;48:13–8.

12. Peters WP, Baynes RD. Autologous hematopoietic cell transplantation in breast cancer. In: Thomas ED, Blume KG, Forman SJ, editors. Hematopoietic cell transplantation. 2nd ed. Oxford: Malden (MA): Blackwell Science; 1999. p. 1029–42.

13. Section VII. In: Thomas ED, Blume KG, Forman SJ, editors. Hematopoietic cell transplantation. 2nd ed. Oxford, Malden (MA): Blackwell Science; 1999. p. 1137–1204.

14. Ramiya VK, Maraist M, Arfors KE, et al. Reversal of insulin-dependent diabetes using islets generated in vitro from pancreatic stem cells. Nat Med 2000;6:278–82.

15. White SA, James RF, Swift SM, et al. Human islet cell transplantation—future prospects. Diabet Med 2001;18:78–103.

16. Comenzo RL. Hematopoietic cell transplantation for primary systemic amyloidosis: what have we learned. Leuk Lymphoma 2000;37:245–58.

17. Welsh K. Commentary of histocompatibility systems. In: Ginns LC, Cosimi AB, Morris PJ, editors. Transplantation. Malden (MA): Blackwell Science; 1999. p. 74–7.

18. Carpenter C. Histocompatibility systems. In: Ginns LC, Cosimi AB, Morris PJ, editors. Transplantation. Malden (MA): Blackwell Science; 1999. p. 60–74.

19. Powelson JA, Cosimi AB. Liver transplantation. In: Ginns LC,

Cosimi AB, Morris PJ, editors. Transplantation. Malden (MA): Blackwell Science; 1999. p.324–73.

20. O'Donnell M, Parmenter KL. Transplant medications. Crit Care Nurs Clin North Am 1996;8:253–71.

21. Braun F, Lorf T, Ringe B. Update of current immunosuppressive drugs used in clinical organ transplantation. Transpl Int 1998;11:77–81.

22. Physicians' Desk Reference 1997. 51st ed. Montvale (NJ): Medical Economics Data Production Company; 1997.

23. Chao N. Pharmacology and use of immunosuppressive agents after hematopoietic cell transplantation. In: Thomas ED, Blume KG, Forman SJ, editors. Hematopoietic cell transplantation. 2nd ed. Oxford: Malden (MA): Blackwell Science; 1999. p. 176–85.

24. Levy GA. Neoral/cyclosporine-based immunosuppression. Liver Transpl Surg 1999;5:537–47.

25. Kahan BD, Podbielski J, Napoli KL, et al. Immunosuppressive effects and safety of a sirolimus/cyclosporine combination regimen for renal transplantation. Transplantation 1998; 66:1040–6.

26. Groth CG, Backman L, Morales JM, et al. Sirolimus (rapamycin)-based therapy in human renal transplantation: similar efficacy and different toxicity compared with cyclosporine. Sirolimus European Renal Transplant Study Group. Transplantation 1997;67:1036–42.

27. Watson CJ, Friend PJ, Jamieson NV, et al. Sirolimus: a potent new immunosuppressant for liver transplantation. Transplantation 1999;67:505–9.

28. Longoria J, Roberts RF, Marboe CC, et al. Sirolimus (rapamycin) potentiates cyclosporine in prevention of acute lung rejection. Thorac Cardiovasc Surg 1999;117:714–8.

29. Kahan BD. Rapamycin: personal algorithms for use based on 250 treated renal allograft recipients. Transplant Proc 1998;30:2185–8.

30. Vasquez EM. Sirolimus: a new agent for prevention of renal allograft rejection. Am J Health Syst Pharm 2000;57:437–48.

31. Miller JL. Sirolimus approved with renal transplant indication. Am J Health Syst Pharm 1999;56:2177–8.

32. Kennedy DT, Hayney MS, Lake KD. Azathioprine and allopurinol: the price of an avoidable drug interaction. Ann Pharmacother 1996;30:951–4.

33. Rayhill SC, Sollinger HW. Mycophenolate mofetil: experimental and clinical experience. In: Ginns LC, Cosimi AB, Morris PJ, editors. Transplantation. Malden (MA): Blackwell Science; 1999. p. 147–66.

34. Halloran P, Mathew T, Tomlanovich S, et al. Mycophenolate mofetil in renal allograft recipients: a pooled efficacy analysis of three randomized, double-blind, clinical studies in prevention of rejection. The International Mycophenolate Mofetil Renal Transplant Study Groups [published erratum appears in Transplantation 1997;63:618]. Transplantation 1997;63:39–47.

35. Hong JC, Kahan BD. Use of anti-CD25 monoclonal antibody in combination with rapamycin to eliminate cyclosporine treatment during the induction phase of immunosuppression. Transplantation 1999;68:701–4.

36. Eason JD, Cosimi AB. Biologic immunosuppressive agents. In: Ginns LC, Cosimi AB, Morris PJ editors. Transplantation. Malden (MA): Blackwell Science; 1999. p. 196–224.

37. Walker RG. Steroids and transplantation. In: Ginns LC, Cosimi AB, Morris PJ, editors. Transplantation. Malden (MA): Blackwell Science; 1999. p. 115–26.

38. Suzuki S, Enosawa S, Kakefuda T, et al. A novel immunosuppressant, FTY720, with a unique mechanism of action, induces long-term graft acceptance in rat and dog allotransplantation. Transplantation 1996;61:200–5.

39. Senel F, Kahan BD. New small molecule immunosuppressive agents. In: Ginns LC, Cosimi AB, Morris PJ, editors. Transplantation. Malden (MA): Blackwell Science; 1999. p. 167–84.

40. Troncoso P, Kahan BD. Preclinical evaluation of a new immunosuppressive agent, FTY720. Clin Biochem 1998; 31:369–73.

41. Wang ME, Tejpal N, Qu X, et al. Immunosuppressive effects of FTY720 alone or in combination with cyclosporine and/or sirolimus. Transplantation 1998;65:899–905.

42. Harlan DM, Kirk AD. The future of organ and tissue transplantation: can T-cell costimulatory pathway modifiers revolutionize the prevention of graft rejection? JAMA 1999; 282:1076–82.

43. Kobashigawa JA, Katznelson S, Laks H, et al. Effect of pravastatin on outcomes after cardiac transplantation. N Engl J Med 1995;333:621–7.

44. Kobashigawa JA. Postoperative management following heart transplantation. Transplant Proc 1999;31:2038–46.

45. Jain A, Khanna A, Molmenti EP, et al. Immunosuppressive therapy. Surg Clin North Am 1999;79:59–76.

46. Hussar DA. New drugs of 1999. J Am Pharm Assoc (Wash) 2000;40:181–221.

47. Gammie JS, Pham SM. Simultaneous donor bone marrow and cardiac transplantation: can tolerance be induced with the development of chimerism? Curr Opin Cardiol 1999; 14:126–32.

48. Fung JJ. Toward tolerance: lessons learned from liver transplantation. Liver Transpl Surg 1999;5:S90–7.

49. Dykewicz CA, Jaffe HW, Kaplan JE, et al. Guidelines for preventing opportunistic infections among hematopoietic stem cell transplant recipients: recommendations of CDC, the Infectious Disease Society of America, and the American Society of Blood and Marrow Transplantation. MMWR Morb Mortal Wkly Rep 2000;49:1–128.

50. Pizzo PA. Fever in immunocompromised patients. N Engl J Med 1999;341:893–900.

51. Froland SS. Antimicrobial chemoprophylaxis in immunocompromised patients. Scand J Infect Dis 1990;70:130–40.

52. Momin F, Chandrasekar PH. Antimicrobial prophylaxis in bone marrow transplantation. Ann Intern Med 1995; 123:205–15.

53. Engels EA, Ellis CA, Supran SE, et al. Early infection in bone marrow transplantation: quantitative study of clinical factors that affect risk. Clin Infect Dis 1999; 28:256–66.

54. Midtvedt K, Hartmann A, Midtvedt T, Brekke IB. Routine perioperative antibiotic prophylaxis in renal transplantation. Nephrol Dial Transplant 1998;13:1637–41.

55. Neu AM, Fivush BA. Recommended immunization practices for pediatric renal transplant recipients. Pediatr Transplant 1998;2:263–9.

56. Eisen HJ. Noninvasive detection of cardiac transplant rejection using electronic monitoring. Curr Opin Cardiol 1999;14:151–4.

57. Klintmalm G. Tacrolimus. In: Ginns LC, Cosimi AB, Morris PJ, editors. Transplantation. Malden (MA): Blackwell Science; 1999. p. 127–46.

58. Jeyarajah DR, Thistlethwaite JR Jr. General aspects of cytokine-release syndrome: timing and incidence of symptoms. Transplant Proc 1993;25:16–20.

59. Chan GL, Weinstein SS, Wright CE, et al. Encephalopathy associated with OKT3 administration: possible interaction with indomethacin. Transplantation 1991;52:148–50.

60. Mignat C. Clinically significant drug interactions with new immunosuppressive agents. Drug Saf 1997;16:267–78.

61. Murphy OM, Gould FK. Prevention of nosocomial infection in solid organ transplantation. J Hosp Infect 1999;42:177–83.

62. Paterson DL, Dominguez EA, Chang FY, et al. Infective endocarditis in solid organ transplant recipients. Clin Infect Dis 1998;26:689–94.

63. Marchand S, Tchernia G, Hiesse C, et al. Human parvovirus B19 infection in organ transplant recipients. Clin Transplant 1999;13:17–24.

64. Rubin RH, Fishman JA. Infection in the organ transplant recipient. In: Ginns C, Cosimi AB, Morris PJ, editors. Transplantation. Malden (MA): Blackwell Science; 1999. p. 747–69.

65. Rodriguez-Adrian LJ, Grazziutti ML, Rex JH, Anaissie EJ. The potential role of cytokine therapy for fungal infections in patients with cancer: is recovery from neutropenia all that is needed? Clin Infect Dis 1998;26:1270–8.

66. Giles FJ. Monocyte-macrophages, granulocyte-macrophage colony-stimulating factor, and prolonged survival among patients with acute myeloid leukemia and stem cell transplants. Clin Infect Dis 1998;26:1282–9.

67. Nemunaitis J. Use of macrophage colony-stimulating factor in the treatment of fungal infections. Clin Infect Dis 1998; 26:1279–81.

68. Dei-Cas E, Cailliez JC, Palluault F, et al. Is *Pneumocystis carinii* a deep mycosis-like agent? Eur J Epidemiol 1992;8:460–70.

69. Dreno B, Mansat E, Legoux B, Litoux P. Skin cancers in transplant patients. Adv Nephrol Necker Hosp 1997;27:377–89.

70. Euvrard S, Kanitakis J, Pouteil-Noble C, et al. Skin cancers in organ transplant recipients. Ann Transplant 1997;2:28–32.

71. Haque T, Crawford DH. The role of adoptive immunotherapy in the prevention and treatment of lymphoproliferative disease following transplantation. Br J Haematol 1999;106:309–16.

72. Mueller N. Overview of the epidemiology of malignancy in immune deficiency. J Acquir Immune Defic Syndr Hum Retroviral 1999;21 Suppl 1:S5–10.

73. Iscovich J, Boffetta P, Franceschi S, et al. Classic Kaposi sarcoma: epidemiology and risk factors. Cancer 2000;88:500–17.

74. Davis CL, Wood BL, Sabath DE, et al. Interferon-alpha treatment of posttransplant lymphoproliferative disorder in recipients of solid organ transplants. Transplantation 1998; 66:1770–9.

75. Mamzer-Bruneel MF, Bourquelot P, Hermine O, et al. Treatment and prognosis of post-transplant lymphoproliferative disease. Ann Transplant 1997;2:42–8.

76. Fellstrom B, Backman U, Larsson E, Wahlberg J. Accelerated atherosclerosis in the transplant recipient: role of hypertension. J Hum Hypertens 1998;12:851–4.

77. Zeier M, Mandelbaum A, Ritz E. Hypertension in the transplanted patient. Nephron 1998;80:257–68.

78. Elliott WJ. Traditional drug therapy of hypertension in transplant recipients. J Hum Hypertens 1998;12:845–9.

79. Weir MR, Fink JC. Risk for posttransplant diabetes mellitus with current immunosuppressive medications. Am J Kidney Dis 1999;34:1–13.

80. Lee JM, Raps EC. Neurologic complications of transplantation. Neurol Clin 1998;16:21–33.

81. Vierling JM, Villamil FG, Rojter SE, et al. Morbidity and mortality of recurrent hepatitis C infection after orthotopic liver transplantation. J Viral Hepat 1997;4 Suppl 1:117–24.

82. McFadden PM, Emory WB. Lung transplantation. Surg Clin North Am 1998;78:749–62.

83. Akosah K, Olsovsky M, Mohanty PK. Dobutamine stress-induced angina in patients with denervated cardiac transplants: clinical and angiographic correlates. Chest 1995;108:695–700.

84. Shapiro PA, Sloan RP, Bigger JT Jr, et al. Cardiac denervation and cardiovascular reactivity to psychological stress. Am J Psychiatry 1994;151:1140–7.

85. Uberfuhr P, Frey AW, Reichart B. Vagal reinnervation in the long term after orthotopic heart transplantation. J Heart Lung Transplant 2000;19:946–50.

86. Doering LV, Dracup K, Moser DK, et al. Evidence of time-dependent autonomic reinnervation after heart transplantation. Nurs Res 1999;48:308–16.

87. Cotts WG, Oren RM. Function of the transplanted heart: unique physiology and therapeutic implications. Am J Med Sci 1997;314:164–72.

88. Stevenson LW, Dadourian BJ, Kobashigawa J, et al. Mitral regurgitation after cardiac transplantation. Am J Cardiol 1987;60:119–22.

89. Yankah AC, Musci M, Weng Y, et al. Tricuspid valve dysfunction and surgery after orthotopic cardiac transplantation. Eur J Cardiothorac Surg 2000;17:343–8.

90. Baron F, Deprez M, Beguin Y. The veno-occlusive disease of the liver. Haematologica 1997;82:718–25.

91. Lazarchik DA, Filler SJ, Winkler MP. Dental evaluation in bone marrow transplantation. Gen Dent 1995;43:369–71.

92. Horowitz MM, Gale RP, Sondel PM, et al. Graft-versus-leukemia reactions after bone marrow transplantation. Blood 1990;75:555–62.

93. Horowitz MM. Uses and growth of hematopoietic cell transplantation. In: Thomas ED, Blume KG, Forman SJ, editors. Hematopoietic cell transplantation. 2nd ed. Oxford Malden (MA): Blackwell Science; 1999. p. 12–8.

94. Dey B, Sykes M, Spitzer TR. Outcomes of recipients of both bone marrow and solid organ transplants: a review. Medicine 1998;77:355–69.

95. Faderl S, Talpaz M, Estrov Z, Kantarjian HM. Chronic myelogenous leukemia: biology and therapy. Ann Intern Med 1999;131:207–19.

96. Greenberg MS, Cohen SG, McKitrick JC, Cassileth PA. The oral flora as a source of septicemia in patients with acute leukemia. Oral Surg Oral Med Oral Pathol 1982;53:32–6.

97. Galili D, Donitza A, Garfunkel A, Sela MN. Gram-negative enteric bacteria in the oral cavity of leukemia patients. Oral Surg Oral Med Oral Pathol 1992;74:459–62.

98. Pajari U, Ollila P, Lanning M. Incidence of dental caries in children with acute lymphoblastic leukemia is related to the therapy used. J Dent Child 1995;62:349–52.

99. Benderli Y, Erdilek D, Koray F, et al. The relation between salivary IgA and caries in renal transplant patients. Oral Surg Oral Med Oral Pathol Oral Radiol Endod 2000;89:588–93.

100. Bowie SA Jr, Bach D. Oral Kaposi's sarcoma in a non-AIDS patient. Gen Dent 1999;47:413–5.

101. Saito K, Mori S, Tanda N, Sakamoto S. Expression of p53 protein and Ki-67 antigen in gingival hyperplasia induced by nifedipine and phenytoin. J Periodontol 1999;70:581–6.

102. Kantarci A, Cebeci I, Tuncer O, et al. Clinical effects of periodontal therapy on the severity of cyclosporin A–induced gingival hyperplasia. J Periodontol 1999;70:587–93.

103. Somacarrera ML, Lucas M, Acero J. Reversion of gingival hyperplasia in a heart transplant patient upon interruption of cyclosporine therapy. Spec Care Dentist 1996;16:18–21.

104. Triantos D, Porter SR, Scully C, Teo CG. Oral hairy leukoplakia: clinicopathologic features, pathogenesis, diagnosis, and clinical significance. Clin Infect Dis 1997;25:1392–6.

105. King GN, Healy CM, Glover MT, et al. Prevalence and risk factors associated with leukoplakia, hairy leukoplakia, erythematous candidiasis, and gingival hyperplasia in renal transplant recipients. Oral Surg Oral Med Oral Pathol 1994;78:718–26.

106. Wurapa AK, Luque AE, Menegus MA. Oral hairy leukoplakia: a manifestation of primary infection with Epstein-Barr virus? Scand J Infect Dis 1999;31:505–6.

107. Darville JM, Ley BE, Roome AP, Foot AB. Acyclovir-resistant herpes simplex virus infections in a bone marrow transplant population. Bone Marrow Transplant 1998;22:587–9.

108. LoPresti AE, Levine JF, Munk GB, et al. Successful treatment of an acyclovir- and foscarnet-resistant herpes simplex virus type 1 lesion with intravenous cidofovir. Clin Infect Dis 1998; 26:512–3.

109. Marr KA, White TC, van Burik JA, Bowden RA. Development of fluconazole resistance in Candida albicans causing disseminated infection in a patient undergoing marrow transplantation. Clin Infect Dis 1997;25:908–10.

110. Marr KA, Lyons CN, Rustad TR, et al. Rapid, transient fluconazole resistance in Candida albicans is associated with increased mRNA levels of CDR [published erratum appears in Antimicrob Agents Chemother 1999;43:438]. Antimicrob Agents Chemother 1998;42:2584–9.

111. Khocht A, Schneider LC. Periodontal management of gingival overgrowth in the heart transplant patient: a case report. J Periodontol 1997;68:1140–6.

112. Christiansen TN, Freije JE, Neuburg M, Roza A. Cutaneous squamous cell carcinoma metastatic to the parotid gland in a transplant patient. Clin Transplant 1996;10:561–3.

113. Bencini PL, Marchesi L, Cainelli T, Crosti C. Kaposi's sarcoma in kidney transplant recipients treated with cyclosporin. Br J Dermatol 1988;118:709–14.

114. Maxymiw WG, Wood RE, Lee L. Primary, multi-focal, non-Hodgkin's lymphoma of the jaws presenting as periodontal disease in a renal transplant patient. Int J Oral Maxillofac Surg 1991;20:69–70.

115. Seymour RA, Thomason JM, Nolan A. Oral lesions in organ transplant patients. J Oral Pathol Med 1997;26:297–304.

116. Harris JP, Penn I. Immunosuppression and the development of malignancies of the upper airway and related structures. Laryngoscope 1981;91:520–8.

117. Schubert MM, Sullivan KM. Recognition, incidence, and management of oral graft-versus-host disease. NCI Monogr 1990; 9:135–43.

118. Epstein JB, Truelove EL. Topical cyclosporine in a bioadhesive for treatment of oral lichenoid mucosal reactions: an open label clinical trial. Oral Surg Oral Med Oral Pathol Oral Radiol Endod 1996;82:532–6.

119. Elad S, Garfunkel AA, Enk CD, et al. Ultraviolet B irradiation: a new therapeutic concept for the management of oral manifestations of graft-versus-host disease. Oral Surg Oral Med Oral Pathol Oral Radiol Endod 1999;88:444–50.

120. Epstein JB, Nantel S, Sheoltch SM. Topical azathioprine in the combined treatment of chronic oral graft-versus-host disease. Bone Marrow Transplant 2000;25:683–7.

121. Redding SW, Callander NS, Haveman CW, Leonard DL. Treatment of oral chronic graft-versus-host disease with PUVA therapy: case report and literature review. Oral Surg Oral Med Oral Pathol Oral Radiol Endod 1998;86:183–7.

122. Woo SB, Allen CM, Orden A, et al. Non-gingival soft tissue growths after allogeneic marrow transplantation. Bone Marrow Transplant 1996;17:1127–32.

123. Sonis ST. Mucositis as a biological process: a new hypothesis for the development of chemotherapy-induced stomatotoxicity. Oral Oncol 1998;34:39–43.

124. Elad S, Cohen G, Zylber-Katz E, et al. Systemic absorption of lidocaine after topical application for the treatment of oral mucositis in bone marrow transplantation patients. J Oral Pathol Med 1999;28:170–2.

125. Cohen G, Elad S, Or R, et al. The use of tretinoin as oral mucositis prophylaxis in bone marrow transplantation patients: a preliminary study. Oral Dis 1997;3:243–6.

126. Nagler RM, Sherman Y, Nagler A. Histopathological study of the human submandibular gland in graft versus host disease. J Clin Pathol 1999;52:395–7.

127. Uderzo C, Fraschini D, Balduzzi A, et al. Long-term effects of bone marrow transplantation on dental status in children with leukaemia. Bone Marrow Transplant 1997;20:865–9.

128. De Rossi SS, Glick M. Dental considerations for the patient with renal disease receiving hemodialysis. J Am Dent Assoc 1996;127:211–9.

129. Bishay N, Petrikowski CG, Maxymiw WG, et al. Optimum dental radiography in bone marrow transplant patients. Oral Surg Oral Med Oral Pathol Oral Radiol Endod 1999;87:375–9.

130. Rutkauskas JS, Davis JW. Effects of chlorhexidine during immunosuppressive chemotherapy. A preliminary report. Oral Surg Oral Med Oral Pathol 1993;76:441–8.

131. Curtis JW Jr. Implant placement and restoration following bone marrow transplantation for chronic leukemia: a case report. Int J Oral Maxillofac Implants 1996;11:81–6.

132. Glick M. Glucocorticosteroid replacement therapy: a literature review and suggested replacement therapy. Oral Surg Oral Med Oral Pathol 1989;67:614–20.

133. Thomason JM, Girdler NM, Kendall-Taylor P, et al. An investigation into the need for supplementary steroids in organ transplant patients undergoing gingival surgery. A double-blind, split-mouth, cross-over study. J Clin Periodontol 1999;26:577–82.

134. Dens F, Boogaerts M, Boute P, et al. Caries-related salivary microorganisms and salivary flow rate in bone marrow recipients. Oral Surg Oral Med Oral Pathol Oral Radiol Endod 1996;81:38–43.

135. Johnson KJ, Chensue SW, Ward PA. Immunopathology. In: Rubin E, Farber JR, editors. Pathology. 3rd ed. Philadelphia: Lippincott-Raven Publishers; 1999.

20

INFECTIOUS DISEASES

JOHN A. MOLINARI, PHD
MICHAEL GLICK, DMD

▼ BACTERIAL INFECTIONS
  Tuberculosis
  Legionella
▼ PROTOZOAL INFECTION:
  CRYPTOSPORIDIUM
  Microbial Characteristics
  Epidemiology and Transmission
  Clinical Syndrome
  Treatment and Control
▼ VIRAL INFECTIONS
  Hepatitis C Virus
  HIV Infection

In the early 1960s, Sir MacFarlane Burnet proclaimed, "One can think of the middle of the twentieth century as the end of one of the most important social revolutions in history, the virtual elimination of the infectious disease as a significant factor in social life."[1] This was not an uncommon sentiment among the medical community and resulted in a decrease in awareness, research, and funding to combat emerging, re-emerging, and drug-resistant infections. Consequently, the medical community was ill prepared when diseases thought to be conquered, and new diseases, started to emerge in the 1980s and 1990s. In a recent report from the Institute of Medicine, six major factors were identified as contributors to the emergence and re-emergence of infectious disease, as follows:[2]

1. Changes in human demographics and behavior
2. Advances in technology and changes in industry practices
3. Economic development and changes in land use patterns
4. Dramatic increases in volume and speed of international travel and commerce
5. Microbial adaptation and change
6. Breakdown of public health capacity required to handle infectious diseases

Although the number of deaths from infectious diseases has decreased dramatically in the United States during the twentieth century, there was a temporary increase between 1980 and 1995, mainly due to human immunodeficiency virus (HIV) disease.[3] HIV and other emerging and re-emerging infectious diseases are recognized as significant health hazards and have become the focus of many federal and academic health initiatives. Efforts in controling infectious diseases have addressed sanitation and hygiene, vaccination, the use of antibiotics and other antimicrobial medications, and improved technology in detection and monitoring. Oral health care providers are not excluded from these efforts, as many of these endeavors impact directly on dental care.

This chapter highlights a few infectious diseases that are of importance to dentistry. Some of these diseases are well established, whereas others are emerging and may become important sources of both contamination and transmission in dental settings. Oral health care providers need to be able to assess and evaluate patients who are carriers of infectious diseases with the purpose of providing appropriate and safe dental care.

▼ BACTERIAL INFECTIONS

Tuberculosis

There is a well-known phrase that states, "The more things change, the more they stay the same." This expression continues to apply to tuberculosis (TB), a widespread infectious disease scourge traced back to the earliest of centuries. As a result of a resurgence of TB cases in the United States during the 1980s, attention refocused on the factors associated with the observed reversal of a previous declining disease trend; transmission modes of *Mycobacterium tuberculosis*, occupational infection risks associated with health care, and airborne-hazard infection control precautions.[4–8] Despite dramatic improvements in public health measures associated with *M. tuberculosis* infection and disease, such as living conditions, nutrition, and antimicrobial chemotherapy, that resulted in an observed dramatic decline in the incidence of TB in the United States and certain other countries during the past century, TB remains a major public health concern for much of the world's population.[9,10] Evidence supporting this statement includes the following:

1. TB is the most common cause of death from a single microbial agent.
2. TB is responsible for almost 1 in 4 preventable deaths in the world.
3. The World Health Organization estimates that worldwide there are approximately 20 million active TB cases.
4. Approximately 3 million people die each year from TB, with 80% of this total occurring in developing countries.

In short, many problems associated with tuberculosis as a significant world health problem 100 years ago remain as this debilitating illness continues to be an even greater infectious disease concern at the end of the twentieth century.

The United States witnessed a dramatically different pattern of TB incidence from much of the rest of the world, documenting a three-decade decline through to 1984 (Table 20-1). Based on that rate of decline, the Centers for Disease Control and Prevention (CDC) projected that TB would be eliminated within the United States by the year 2010. These optimistic predictions were quietened in 1985, when the number of reported cases showed a smaller decrease compared to the previous 2 years. In 1986, the number of reported cases actually exceeded

TABLE 20-1 Summary of Reported Cases of Tuberculosis in the United States by Year

Year	Total Number of Cases
1954	79,775
1967	45,647
1970	37,137
1975	33,989
1980	27,749
1985	22,201
1986	22,768
1990	25,701
1992	26,673
1993	25,313
1994	24,361
1995	22,860
1996	21,337
1997	19,851
1998	18,361
1999	16,607
2000	12,942

CDC. Reported tuberculosis in the United States, 2000. Surveillance Reports; 2001.

the 1985 figure. This trend continued until the peak year of 1992 (26,673 cases). With the development and institution of appropriate infection control policies and procedures aimed at minimizing airborne spread of *M. tuberculosis*, continued decrease in new TB cases has been noted in each subsequent year.[11,12]

ETIOLOGY AND PATHOGENESIS

The genus *Mycobacterium* contains a variety of species, ranging from human pathogens to relatively harmless organisms. As the major cause of TB, a chronic communicable disease, *M. tuberculosis* is by far the most historically prominent member of this group of bacteria. In addition to their very slow growth on special enriched media, these aerobic slender rods are characterized by their acid-fast staining feature. The unusually high lipid content of the cell wall confers the organisms with an ability to strongly retain a red dye (carbolfuchsin) after treatment with an acid-alcohol solution. This unique structure also allows the bacteria to survive outside a host's body, suspended in airborne microdroplet nuclei for extended periods of time.

Contrary to a perception believed through the ages, *M. tuberculosis* is not a highly contagious bacterium. It does not synthesize potent exotoxins or extracellular enzymes, and it is not surrounded by an antiphagocytic capsule. Onset of infection appears to be related to the ability of tubercle bacilli to multiply within host cells and tissues while at the same time resisting host defenses. Infection with *M. tuberculosis* typically requires prolonged close contact of a susceptible host with an infectious source. The closeness of the contact with aerosolized bacilli and the degree of infectivity of the mycobacterial source are the most important considerations for infection. The overwhelming majority of primary human infections involve inhalation of mycobacteria-laden respiratory microdroplets.[13,14] The diameter of these aerosolized droplets ranges from 1 to 5 microns. Dispersal of *M. tuberculosis* occurs via these droplets as a result of coughing, sneezing, or even speaking. Microdroplet nuclei are small enough to bypass protective host bronchial mucocilliary defenses, leading to mycobacteria subsequently replicating in both free alveolar spaces and within phagocytic cells (Figure 20-1). Repeated prolonged exposure to air that has been contaminated by droplets from a person with TB predisposes others to infection. This rationale is illustrated by the fact that people who live in the same home with an infected individual, or close friends or co-workers who routinely breathe the same mycobacteria-contaminated air from an undiagnosed or untreated person with pulmonary TB, have a high risk of acquiring infection. The organisms' oxygen requirement predisposes the lungs as primary infection sites, with the potential for subsequent dissemination to other tissues. Cross-infection or spread of tubercle bacilli does not result from casual or sporadic exposure.

Onset of clinical disease is characterized by gradual infiltration of neutrophils, macrophages, and T lymphocytes. Distinctive granulomatous TB lesions called tubercles may appear anywhere in the lung parenchyma; however, they are most evident in the periphery (Figure 20-2). Because TB is the prototype microbial infection for inducing protective cellular immunity, the immunocompetence of the affected host plays a significant role in controlling the extent and severity of resultant disease.[15,16] It is important to remember that most people infected with *M. tuberculosis* develop a positive type IV hypersensitive skin test reaction when challenged (Figure 20-3) but do not progress to clinical disease. For those infected individuals who develop clinical symptoms, fatigue, malaise, weight loss, night sweats, and fever are most commonly noted

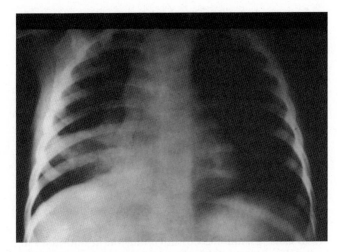

FIGURE 20-2 Chest radiograph of lungs in a patient with primary symptomatic tuberculosis. Multiple areas of disease are visible, with radiographic evidence of chronic granulomatous tubercles.

in addition to positive chest radiograph manifestations. Pulmonary manifestations most frequently are chest pain, bloody sputum, and the presence of a prolonged productive cough of greater than 3 weeks' duration.

Initial mycobacterial infection may progress to several different states depending on the extent of *M. tuberculosis* exposure and resistance of the patient. These include (1) asymptomatic primary tuberculosis, (2) symptomatic primary tuberculosis, (3) progressive primary tuberculosis, and (4) reactivation tuberculosis. A major risk factor for progression of initial infection with tubercle bacilli to more severe disease stages is the absence of an adequate host acquired cellular immune response to mycobacterial antigens. The ability of an infected individual to develop dual cellular and humoral immune responses against *M. tuberculosis* antigens thus greatly influences disease onset and progression.

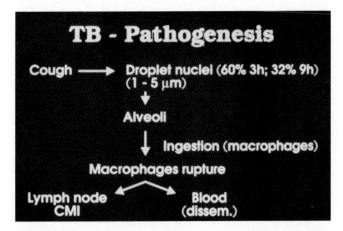

FIGURE 20-1 Sequence of infection from a *Mycobaterium tuberculosis*–laden microdroplet in a susceptible person.

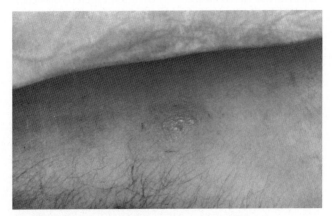

FIGURE 20-3 Positive 48-hour skin test following purified protein derivative intradermal challenge of a person with primary asymptomatic tuberculosis. No evidence of clinical disease was present, and the patient remained asymptomatic following a prolonged course of isoniazid chemotherapy.

Asymptomatic Primary Tuberculosis. Individuals may be infected with *M. tuberculosis* without apparent clinical manifestations. When skin tested, individuals with asymptomatic primary tuberculosis display a positive tuberculin reaction indicating that they have been infected and have developed cell-mediated immunity against the bacteria. This protective immune response prevents the continued multiplication and dissemination of the bacteria, but it does not destroy all of the bacteria present. The remaining bacteria are sequestered within tubercles in the affected tissues and may be the source of bacteria that initiate reactivation tuberculosis.

Symptomatic Primary Tuberculosis. In symptomatic primary tuberculosis, *M. tuberculosis* is spread via the lymphatics to cause granulomatous inflammation in both the lung periphery and hilar nodes, and it is accompanied by respiratory symptoms. The usual result is one of healing and development of cell-mediated immunity. The Ghon complex, a remnant of this infection, most often occurs in infants and children and is comprised of small calcified lung nodules and lymphadenopathy of the hilar lymph nodes.

Progressive Primary Tuberculosis. A much more serious disease may develop in those individuals who are less resistant to tubercle bacilli. In these patients, microorganisms may spread throughout the body either (1) by means of the blood, resulting in miliary tuberculosis; (2) via the respiratory tissues, inducing a bronchopneumonia; or (3) through the gastrointestinal tract as a result of the organisms being coughed up. In miliary tuberculosis, foci of infection occur in distant organs and tissues but most frequently develop in the meninges, lungs, liver, and renal cortex. Although cell-mediated immunity may develop in some patients, others may not react (anergy) when skin tested with tuberculin protein preparations. Anergic patients have a poor prognosis for recovery and often die without rapid treatment.

Reactivation Tuberculosis. Reactivation tuberculosis occurs in individuals who have developed primary tuberculosis and who are asymptomatic, but who still carry the bacteria within tubercles. These patients exhibit positive tuberculin skin tests and thus demonstrate cellular immunity. Reactivation of disease is thought to be due to the activation of persistent bacteria in the tubercles of a previous infection, which become activated by some alteration in host resistance. Infection is characterized by tubercle formation, caseation, fibrosis, and further extension of the lesion. Progression may advance into a bronchus, leading to cavitation of the lung and secretion of an infectious sputum.

ORAL MANIFESTATIONS

Oral manifestations of tuberculosis occur in approximately 3% of cases involving long-standing pulmonary and/or systemic infection.[17,18] The bacteria can infect oral tissues and lymph nodes (scrofula) (Figure 20-4). Within the oral cavity, lesions can occur in the soft tissues and supporting bone

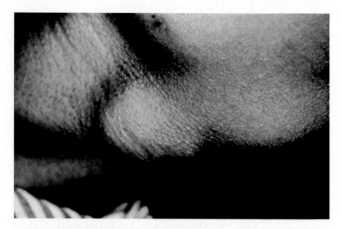

FIGURE 20-4 Cervical tuberculosis lymphadenitis (scrofula) secondary to pulmonary tuberculosis in a 16-year-old male.

(Figure 20-5) and in tooth extraction sites, and may even affect the tongue and floor of the mouth (Figure 20-6).

When reviewing this information, it becomes apparent that progression of infection with tubercle bacilli to more severe disseminated stages occurs in the absence of adequate cellular immunity to infection. Thus, the ability of an infected individual to develop a dual immune response against *M. tuberculosis* antigens greatly influences disease onset and progression. These crucial protective responses are (1) acquired immunity to infection and (2) development of tuberculin hypersensitivity.

DIAGNOSIS

A diagnosis of infection with *M. tuberculosis* relies on (1) development of a positive delayed hypersensitivity (tuberculin) skin reaction to purified protein derivative (PPD), a mycobacterial antigen isolated from bacterial cultures, and (2) demonstration of acid-fast mycobacteria in clinical specimens. Information obtained while collecting a patient's medical history can provide evidence for suspicion of TB (Table 20-2).

RISK FACTORS

The re-emergence of *M. tuberculosis* infection as a significant US public health problem appears to be the result of a combination of changing host susceptibility factors and declining societal conditions for particular population groups. Among

TABLE 20-2 Patient History Prompting Suspicion of Active Tuberculosis

1. Productive cough (> 3 wk)— pulmonary tuberculosis
2. Other symptoms (eg, fever, chills, night sweats, fatigue)
3. Extrapulmonary tuberculosis (occurs in 15% of cases)
4. Patients with tuberculosis and HIV infection—40–75% have extrapulmonary tuberculosis and pulmonary tuberculosis
5. History of tuberculosis exposure and/or previous tuberculosis infection (active disease)

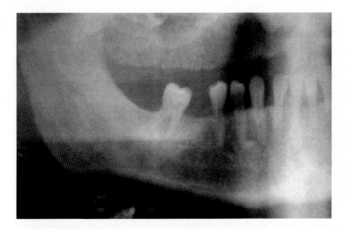

FIGURE 20-5 Partially calcified oral tuberculosis localized in the soft tissue at the angle of the mandible.

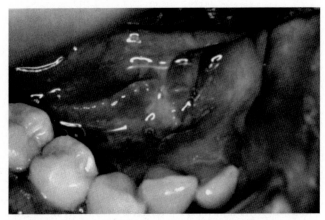

FIGURE 20-6 Oral tuberculosis in the soft tissue of mandible.

the most frequently noted risk factors is infection with HIV.[19–23] The suppressive effect of HIV infection on cell-mediated immunity increases host susceptibility to a variety of microbial pathogens that are normally controlled by these defense mechanisms. It should be noted, however, that current information does not suggest HIV-infected persons are more susceptible to *M. tuberculosis* infection, but they can present with earlier clinical manifestations of the disease. Increased immigration of people to the United States from countries with high TB prevalence rates adds to the reservoir for mycobacterial transmission.[24] Unfortunately, funding for TB research, screening programs, and epidemiologic tracking lagged in the 1980s as attention focused on other infectious diseases, such as those caused by herpesviruses, hepatitis B, and HIV/acquired immunodeficiency syndrome (AIDS). These factors, together with documented societal tragedies such as increased parenteral drug abuse, homelessness, malnutrition, and crowding, especially in larger US cities, have exacerbated the potential for the spread of TB (Table 20-3).[13]

TREATMENT

Prior to the advent of antimicrobial chemotherapy, approximately 50% of persons with active TB died within 2 years after

onset of symptoms.[24] Regimens of multiple antibiotics are currently used to treat patients with active TB to ensure tissue penetration and minimize emergence of resistant organisms. General guidelines for appropriate TB chemotherapy include necessity for long-term treatment interval (up to 2 years), initiation of treatment if sputum smear is positive for acid-fast bacilli, and patient compliance (a major factor in determining chemotherapy success).

Isoniazid (INH) is the antimycobacterial therapy cornerstone and is included in all routine drug regimens. People who develop a positive tuberculin skin reaction but do not have active disease, as well as close contacts of patients who develop TB, are placed on INH for 6 months to 1 year.

For treatment of patients with active TB, combinations of three or more drugs are chosen based on the nature and site of disease (Table 20-4). In addition to INH, rifampin, pyrazinamide, and ethambutol are the most frequently applied drug combinations unless a specific instance of mycobacterial resistance is noted.[25,26] Hepatotoxicity is a frequent adverse effect noted with prolonged administration of antimycobacterial chemotherapy.

Unfortunately, a major complication preventing successful elimination of acid-fast organisms in TB patients is noncompliance to the prolonged drug regimens. Patients often notice a substantial decline in symptoms within a few weeks of therapy and prematurely discontinue their medications. Consequently, bacterial strains causing multidrug-resistant tuberculosis (MDR-TB) have emerged and spread throughout the world.[27–30]

TABLE 20-3 Persons at High Risk for Contracting Tuberculosis

1. Persons with HIV infection
2. Persons with close contacts with infectious patients
3. Persons with medical conditions that increase risk of contracting TB
4. Persons from countries with high rates of TB
5. Persons in low-income populations
6. Alcoholics
7. Intravenous drug abusers
8. Prisoners
9. Nursing home residents
10. Health care workers in certain work settings (local risk)

TB = tuberculosis

TABLE 20-4 Chemotherapy for Tuberculosis

Combination therapy: usually 3–4 drugs to prevent resistance, chosen from the following: isoniazid, rifampin, ethambutol, rifabutin, streptomycin, pyrazinamide

Prolonged therapy—6 mo minimum— indicated for slow growth rate of bacteria, increasing incidence of *Mycobacterium tuberculosis* drug resistance

TUBERCULOSIS VACCINES

Bacille Calmette-Guérin (BCG), an attenuated strain of *Mycobacterium bovis*, has been used for more than 80 years to protect humans against TB. The original mycobacterial isolates were responsible for causing TB in cattle. Calmette and Guerin attenuated these bacteria by culturing, passaging, and maintaining them in specialized growth media for more than 10 years. Humans began receiving the BCG preparations in 1921, with resultant protection observed in vaccinated children. Most countries currently vaccinate children against TB, and this preventive approach has been shown to result in a 60 to 80% reduction in disease in treated individuals.[31] Unfortunately, the vaccine is much less effective in adults, for reasons that are still unexplained. With adults comprising the major sources of infection, the expected worldwide success of the BCG vaccine has not been accomplished. The successful sequencing of the complete *M. tuberculosis* genome has provided new opportunities for vaccine development. Ongoing efforts are being directed at using combinations of established approaches to vaccine composition, with newer deoxyribonucleic acid (DNA) technologies that look at the roles of host and mycobacterial genetic factors, to better ascertain the development of protective immune responses.[32]

ORAL HEALTH CONSIDERATIONS

The risk of TB transmission from patients to dental care providers is considered to be minimal.[33] Responding to reports and confirmation of *M. tuberculosis* transmission in institutional settings occurring the 1980s, the CDC developed a series of guidelines for prevention of the spread of TB in health care environments. Special emphasis within the document was directed at the heightened TB risks for those persons living with HIV infection or AIDS as a result of virus-induced suppression of cellular immune defenses. As more clinical data and scientific input were obtained from health care and public sources, the CDC incorporated that information in updated draft recommendations. The finalized document released in 1994 provided the following:

1. Guidance for assessing potential TB risks in a variety of health care facilities
2. Detailed description of administrative procedures, infection control practices, engineering controls, and respiratory personal equipment appropriate for minimizing airborne microbial transmission
3. Suggestions for ongoing health care worker (HCW) training and education.[34]

Specific considerations for dentistry were delineated within this document and provided well-thought out administrative and infection control practice for the range of possible dental exposure categories.

The efforts of the CDC have been very effective, yet they represent only one component of the governmental response to the public health threat posed by mycobacterial infection and TB. The Labor Coalition to fight TB in the Workplace submitted a request to Occupational Safety and Health Administration (OSHA) in December 1992 to issue national enforcement guidelines to protect workers against *M. tuberculosis* exposure. This was followed by the coalition of labor unions petitioning OSHA in 1993 to develop a permanent set of rules to protect workers (mostly in patient care facilities) from occupational TB transmission. Serious concern was expressed by these groups about the emergence of cases of MDR-TB, along with the contention that nonmandatory recommendations and guidelines would not be fully implemented or enforced appropriately in many workplaces. The final OSHA-proposed rule incorporated many of the components of the 1994 CDC guidelines but also added a number of mandatory regulations that have stirred considerable controversy within the CDC, among numerous hospital-based infection-control professionals, and infection-control groups. A few of the areas of contention include (1) overstatement of the current TB risk to HCWs in lieu of the effectiveness of the 1994 CDC TB control guidelines; (2) elimination of the CDC-recommended facility TB risk assessment protocol; (3) additional respirator fit-testing requirements; (4) more frequent skin-testing requirements for employees, including TB skin testing within 30 days of job termination; and (5) increased facility costs to implement new regulations.

OSHA's rationale for mandatory TB controls stemmed from the assessment that TB is still endemic in certain population groups, and HCWs and other employees who come into contact with persons manifesting active TB may have significantly increased infection risks above that of the general population. The agency also made a preliminary determination that the portions of the standard directing engineering, work practice, and administrative controls, respiratory protection, training, and medical surveillance are technologically and economically feasible for affected workplaces. Few OSHA proposals for worker protection in any American workplace have sparked as much debate and resistance as the proposed rules regarding tuberculosis. The issue may have been resolved in favor of continuing the successful adherence to the 1994 CDC guidelines in early 2001, but the Institute of Medicine then published a report that critically reviewed the proposed standard and found numerous problems with some of mandatory aspects of the legislation.[35]

Legionella

Scientists, clinicians, and the public officially became acquainted with *Legionella pneumophila* as a result of the outbreak of "legionnaires' disease" in a Philadelphia hotel housing the 1976 American Legion convention. As a result of the first reports of sudden severe pneumonia among conventioneers, multiple epidemiologic groups were rapidly mobilized in an effort to determine both the cause(s) and contributory factors responsible for the 221 total cases and 34 illness-associated deaths.[36]

MICROBIAL CHARACTERISTICS

When the elusive etiologic bacterium was eventually isolated in 1977, using lung tissue from patients in the

TABLE 20-5 Bacteriologic Characteristics of *Legionella pneumophila*

Family: Legionellaceae

Morphology: gram-negative non-spore-forming motile unencapsulated bacilli

Physiology: aerobic and nutritionally fastidious; does not grow on standard bacteriologic media; requires charcoal yeast extract at pH 6.9; L-cysteine is essential nutrient

Ecology: natural habitat: rivers, lakes, streams, thermally polluted waters; can survive water treatment processes; chlorine tolerant; proliferates in man-made water habitats (cooling towers, water distribution systems)

Philadelphia epidemic, it became apparent that the aerobic gram-negative bacillus represented a previously unrecognized species. Table 20-5 summarizes representative bacteriologic features of this organism.[37–39]

One of the early surprises stemming from these studies was that *L. pneumophila* had actually first been isolated from the blood of a patient with respiratory illness in 1947.[40] Improved more-sensitive research technologies provided better cultural and serologic methodologies for isolation and characterization. As a result, scientists began to appreciate (1) the ubiquity of *L. pneumophila* and related species in man-made waterborne environments, (2) the role of this bacterial species as one of the three most common microbial etiologies of community-acquired pneumonia, and (3) the multiple forms of disease that can develop in immunocompetent and immunocompromised individuals. *L. pneumophila* serogroup 1 is still the most clinically important pathogenic species, causing the overwhelming majority of illnesses after exposure to contaminated water.

MAJOR HABITATS

Legionella species are found extensively in natural bodies of water. Most samples from colonized rivers, lakes, and other sources typically contain only low concentrations of *L. pneumophila*. However, the species is remarkably chlorine tolerant. This feature appears to allow for microbial survival during treatment procedures, leading to subsequent entrance and proliferation in water distribution systems.

Multiple studies have shown that the presence of amebae and other waterborne microbes offers *L. pneumophila* a unique opportunity for initial parasitism, leading to ultimate survival and proliferation. Amebae appear to serve as primary natural hosts for the bacteria in man-made water environments such as water distribution systems.[41–43] This intracellular parasitic characteristic allows the legionellae to thrive and replicate, protected from adverse external surroundings. When the infected amebae die and lyse, both the water source and other susceptible single-cell organisms are then exposed to a much higher concentration of *Legionella*.

CLINICAL SYNDROME

Clinical conditions caused by *L. pneumophila* and other *Legionella* species are grouped under the term "legionellosis."

With regard to virulence factors, neither exotoxins nor destructive enzymes have been associated with the pneumonia caused by *L. pneumophila*. The acute inflammatory infiltration and febrile nature of clinical illness appear to be consistent with the biologic manifestations of released endotoxin in tissues.

MODES OF TRANSMISSION

Legionella infections differ from other kinds of pneumonia-inducing conditions in that the bacteria are not transmitted from person to person but from contaminated environmental reservoirs. Evidence accumulated from outbreaks of the disease and experimental investigations suggests that *Legionella* species may be passed to susceptible hosts via multiple routes: aspiration, aerosolization, and instillation into the lungs. Aspiration of contaminated water appears to be the major means of human infection.[44] In one study, passage of microorganisms via this mechanism appeared to be exceptionally serious in patients after surgery for head and neck cancer because of the patients' frequency of aspiration of fluids.[45] Aerosolization of contaminated water occurs from such sources as humidifiers, nebulizers, and cooling tower air conditioners. Because the organisms are resistant to destruction in moist environments, it is believed that exposure to legionellae is common. Reports in the literature in recent years have implicated potable water harboring *L. pneumophila* as an important source of community-acquired pneumonia. As a result, investigation of legionellosis cases now includes examination of water supplies in patients' rooms, homes, and workplaces.[46–48]

CLINICAL FEATURES

Two disparate forms of clinical disease can develop after *Legionella* infection. The most common manifestation, known as Pontiac fever, presents as an acute influenza-like illness without any evidence of pneumonia. There is a 24- to 48-hour incubation period, and many patients experience fever, chills, malaise, and headaches. Patients typically recover from this self-limiting illness within 7 to 10 days.[49] Although the attack rate for Pontiac fever among exposed persons is high (Tables 20-6 and 20-7), many cases of legionellosis are never diagnosed because symptoms are either absent or mild.

Published reports suggest that dental professionals may have a significant occupational exposure to *Legionella* from aerosolization of contaminated dental-unit water, resulting in the formation of anti-*Legionella* antibodies.[50,51] Individuals similarly exposed in a variety of environments may have subsequently developed Pontiac fever and not been aware of it.

The second, more publicized, type of legionellosis is a potentially life-threatening illness termed "legionnaires' disease." The incubation period (2 to 10 days) is longer than that for Pontiac fever. An individual may abruptly exhibit fever, chills, headache, and other nonspecific signs of acute infection. Subsequently, multisystem involvement becomes evident with pneumonia as the pathognomonic feature.[52] If untreated, this form of severe pneumonia can result in a 15%

TABLE 20-6   Clinical Conditions Caused by _Legionella_

Characteristic	Conditions	
	Legionnaires' Disease	Pontiac Fever
Epidemiology		
Attack rate	< 5%	> 90%
Person-to-person spread	No	No
Clinical manifestations		
Incubation period	2–10 d	1–2 d
Clinical features	Pneumonia is dominant feature; spectrum from mild cough to stupor with multisystem failure; cough initially mild; only slightly productive	Acute self-limiting influenza-like illness; no pneumonia; fever, malaise, myalgia, chills, and headache are predominant symptoms
Course	Requires antibiotic therapy (eg, erythromycin)	Self-limiting
Mortality	15–20%; higher if diagnosis is delayed	< 1%

or higher patient mortality rate (see Tables 20-6 and 20-8). Legionnaires' disease in healthy immunocompetent persons appears infrequently because of efficient innate and specific host defenses. Most patients diagnosed with legionnaires' disease present with previous immunosuppressive disorders. Investigation of nosocomially acquired legionnaires' disease suggests that patients recovering from surgery may be at greatest risk of contraction.[53–55] Other conditions identified as legionellosis risk factors include advanced age, cigarette smoking, chronic obstructive pulmonary disease, neoplasia, and immunosuppressive therapy.

TREATMENT

Erythromycin was the historic antibiotic of choice for treatment of legionnaires' disease. Timely appropriate chemotherapy can dramatically reduce the mortality rate of legionnaires' disease, with many patients showing signs of recovery within 3 to 5 days. With the advent of later-generation macrolides, azithromycin has replaced erythromycin because of azithromycin's lower toxicity potential in a range of infected patients.[52] Quinolones also have been shown to be effective antimicrobial agents in studies of patients with community-acquired pneumonia who are suspected of having _L. pneumophila_ legionnaires' disease.[56,57] Antibiotic therapy is not indicated for patients diagnosed with Pontiac fever because of the self-limiting nature of the infection.

▼ PROTOZOAL INFECTION: _CRYPTOSPORIDIUM_

Although first isolated and identified in 1907,[58] the protozoan genus _Cryptosporidium_ was not associated with human disease until 1976.[59] Only a few cases of cryptosporidiosis were reported over the next few years, with those occurring in persons having severely compromised immune defenses. Since the early 1980s, however, _Cryptosporidium parvum_ has emerged as a major etiology of persistent diarrhea in people of developing countries, of severe life-threatening diarrhea in persons with AIDS and other immunosuppressive conditions, and in previously healthy individuals, as well as an increasingly serious threat to the safety of the US water supply.

Microbial Characteristics

Among the most common of human pathogens, the diversity of members within the protozoa has required their classification to be accomplished via disparate criteria, including phylogeny, epidemiology, and clinical manifestations. Protozoa such as _Plasmodium_, _Entamoeba_, and _Trypanosoma_ have long been recognized as leading causes of human disease and mortality in many parts of the world. The dramatic increase in numbers of individuals with less-than-adequate immune defenses throughout the world, in part related to HIV infection with subsequent progression to AIDS, has also been related to significant increases in other protozoan infections, such as those caused by _Cryptosporidium_ species.[60–65]

TABLE 20-7   Characteristics of Pontiac Fever

Acute self-limiting influenza-like illness

24- to 48-hour incubation period

Malaise, myalgia, fever, chills, headache

> 90% of those exposed develop symptoms

Only symptomatic treatment necessary

Complete recovery within 1 wk

Most cases undiagnosed

TABLE 20-8   Characteristics of Legionnaires' Disease

Early influenza-like symptoms—initial cough

2- to 10-day incubation period

Chest pain may be prominent

Pneumonia is dominant finding

Spectrum from mild cough to stupor with multisystem failure

Treatment: erythromycin and other macrolides

The type-species of this genus is *C. parvum*, which measures approximately 2.5 μm in diameter, about the same size and shape as yeast cells. It is capable of infecting and causing disease in both humans and mammals. The infectious form of *C. parvum* is a thick-walled oocyst that is excreted in feces from infected hosts. Oocysts are resistant to standard municipal chlorination procedures, and this feature is important in distinguishing cryptosporidia from many other unicellular waterborne organisms. Because the oocysts can be found in numerous natural water sources, they can readily cause large cryptosporidiosis outbreaks when water treatment is less than optimal and community supplies become contaminated. Cryptosporidia are also unlike many other single-celled waterborne organisms in that they are highly resistant to the chlorine treatments used in municipal water facilities. In addition, they are difficult to filter out because of their small size, and thus they can escape the standard water treatment processes.

Epidemiology and Transmission

As awareness of the potential threat of cryptosporidiosis has increased, so have efforts to investigate water sources for evidence of contamination. Unfortunately, accumulated data suggest that *Cryptosporidium* is found in numerous municipal water supplies, public pools, nursing homes, and hospitals. It is also highly infectious, with an inoculum of 30 to 100 oocysts capable of initiating infection.[66,67] Numerous outbreaks have been demonstrated over the past 20 years. With the development of better detection techniques, some important epidemiologic features have become apparent (Table 20-9). Most cases in the United States have occurred as a result of environmental water contamination related to treatment facility failures.[68–71]

As reports of the wide distribution of this pathogen accumulate, so have the number of cryptosporidiosis cases with life-threatening acute diarrhea, mostly seen in immunocompromised persons but also in previously healthy individuals. A dramatic rise in the number of large outbreaks and individual cases has been noted since 1982, corresponding to the early days of the AIDS epidemic. Multiple reports have shown persons with AIDS to be among the most susceptible immunocompromised groups.[63–65]

The largest documented outbreak occurred in 1993, involving the entire city of Milwaukee, in which over 400,000 people became ill after drinking parasite-contaminated water. Defective filtration of the city's water supply was determined to be the prime factor responsible for the epidemic, which resulted in the death of a number of severely immunocompromised patients.[68] Other instances of waterborne

TABLE 20-9 Epidemiology of *Cryptosporidium* Infection

C. parvum is a highly infectious enteric pathogen.

The protozoa are ubiquitous in many mammals.

Infections can occur worldwide.

It is the leading cause of persistent diarrhea in developing countries.

C. parvum infection have been traced back to ingestion of water from oocyst-contaminated swimming pools and amusement park wave pools.[70]

A second mode of parasite infection is person-to-person spread. Fecal-oral transmission of oocysts within day care centers, hospitals, and households is probably much more common than accumulated statistics suggest.[72–74] The route of microbial passage can place child care workers, children in day care facilities, and other health care providers, who come into direct contact with feces while attending to cryptosporidiosis patients, at increased risk for acquiring the infection.

The ability of *C. parvum* to infect and colonize a variety of mammals has also led to investigation of suggested animal-to-person cryptosporidiosis. Multiple investigations have shown protozoal transmission from calves to humans, and these have triggered intense study of potential risks for those persons who have constant close contact on dairy farms.[75]

The least proven risk factor for cryptosporidiosis involves food. Although the CDC confirmed an outbreak in children in 1994 traced to fresh-pressed apple cider unknowingly contaminated with animal feces, contaminated hands were also thought to have substantially contributed to oocyst cross-infection.[76]

Clinical Syndrome

The complex *C. parvum* life cycle occurs within a single host.[77] Symptoms of cryptosporidiosis may develop within 2 to 10 days after a person has swallowed environmentally contaminated water. The most common manifestations of *C. parvum* infection are a profuse watery diarrhea, accompanied by fever, severe abdominal cramping, and pain. Rapid dehydration of patients is a major concern for physicians, as onset of diarrhea can be quite sudden and can last for over 2 weeks. Gastrointestinal symptoms abate in many patients with healthy immune systems in about 2 weeks, although some may suffer a relapse of the syndrome.[78] The infection is typically more protracted and severe in immunocompromised hosts, however, as extensive dehydration and weight loss may occur over a prolonged period of longer than 2 weeks. In some cases, multiple intravenous infusions of fluids are required to replace body fluids lost owing to diarrhea. Even after symptoms of cryptosporidiosis diminish or disappear, the patient can still transmit infectious parasites to others for months via contaminated stools (fecal-oral transmission). Infected individuals with debilitated immune systems can remain infectious much longer.

Treatment and Control

Currently, there is no generally accepted antimicrobial agent available to treat cryptosporidiosis, and thus, supportive care of patients remains the treatment of choice.[77] As expected, this problem is a major area of research, with certain experimental antibiotic regimens showing some promise. Because the thick-walled oocyst portion of the *C. parvum* life cycle is so resistant to chlorine, new approaches to control the spread of these infectious particles are also being pursued. Reverse osmosis, better filtration techniques, and other efficient procedures are under investigation.

▼ VIRAL INFECTIONS

Hepatitis C Virus

Traditional health care concerns about viral hepatitis focused primarily on hepatitis B virus (HBV) from the late 1940s to the early 1980s. Yet, despite accumulated evidence for the documented occupational risks for HBV over a three-decade period, significant voids from other potentially serious hepatitis challenges continue to require definition. Although the routine application of specific serologic tests was valuable in screening and diagnosing infections caused by hepatitis A virus (HAV) and HBV, a number of reports, written beginning in 1975, described a form of bloodborne post-transfusion hepatitis that could not be attributed to any known microorganism.[79,80] Since diagnosis of this type of hepatitis was based on abnormal liver function in the absence of positive blood markers for HAV, HBV, and other viruses known to cause hepatitis, the term "non-A, non-B hepatitis" (NANBH) was introduced. Most of the risk factors associated with NANBH transmission were identified prior to recognition and characterization of its viral etiology. These included blood transfusion, parenteral drug use, health care worker exposure in clinical settings, sexual transmission from a person with a history of hepatitis, and low socioeconomic status. Significant advances in recombinant DNA technology were instrumental in the later isolation and cloning of the responsible microorganism in 1989—the hepatitis C virus (HCV).[81] A initial diagnostic serologic assay was also developed for detection of antibodies to HCV (anti-HCV) produced by infected persons against a recombinant viral antigen c100-3.[82] Later generations of more sensitive immunoassays have been implemented since 1990. Currently, at least six viral agents appear to account for the majority of viral hepatitis cases (Table 20-10), with new information emerging to expand this list.

VIROLOGY

HCV is a single-stranded positive-sense ribonucleic acid (RNA) virus whose structure appears closely related to the genera *Flavivirus* and *Pestivirus*. Because of the similarities to these viral types, HCV is currently classified as a separate genus in the family Flaviviridae. Detailed molecular biologic studies have shown that different HCV strains can have substantial differences in genome sequencing. These are due to the ability of the virus to mutate and modify surface components during replication within an infected host. As a result, several genotypes, or quasi-species, have been described that can exhibit significant differences throughout the RNA genome[83–85] and contribute to the observed alarming high rate of chronic infection.

EPIDEMIOLOGY AND TRANSMISSION

HCV has a primary bloodborne mode of transmission and is a dominant cause of chronic liver disease throughout the world. Data using anti-HCV as a marker have been used to approximate both worldwide infection prevalence and HCV incidence in various geographic areas, in an attempt to better define infection and disease patterns.[86] Infection with HCV is also the most common chronic bloodborne infection in the United States. Current estimates range from 2.7 (1.3%) to 3.9 (1.8%) million HCV-infected persons in the United States (Table 20-11).[87,88]

Approximately 2.7 million people are thought to have persistent chronic hepatitis C infection, and thus are classified as potentially infectious viral carriers. Mortality in the United States from all forms of hepatitis C infection is believed to occur in 8,000 to 10,000 people each year. With the advent of widespread use of anti-HCV assays and increased awareness of documented risks and changing viral transmission patterns, the incidence of new cases of acute hepatitis C has declined by greater than 80% since 1989.

Statistics acquired during the 1970s and 1980s indicated that parenteral NANBH was responsible for nearly 90% of the reported US transfusion-associated hepatitis cases. Accumulated data suggested that approximately 150,000 persons (5 to 10%) of 3,000,000 who received transfusions developed acute NANBH.[89,90] With the advent of routine testing using sensitive anti-HCV tests, however, the current risk for acquiring transfusion-associated hepatitis C is 1/100,000 per unit transfused.[91] According to CDC national surveillance data, parenteral drug use was the most common risk factor reported by patients with NANBH between 1990 and 1992. Injection-drug use remains the primary risk factor for new cases of HCV infection. In addition, persons with hemophilia who routinely received factor VIII or IX before 1987 and chronic hemodialysis patients have also been considered at risk. Occasionally, health care workers who have frequent contact with blood and personal contact with others who may be infected have been documented to have an increased incidence for hepatitis C compared with that of the general population.[91,92] A summary of these and other epidemiologic estimates is presented in Table 20-12. In recent years, other serologic surveys have revealed a large previously undetected group of persons at risk for HCV: military veterans, especially Vietnam-era veterans. Testing at multiple Veterans Administration (VA) hospitals found an 8 to 10% HCV prevalence rate, which is over four times that of the general population. Other reports indicate that more than half of the patients receiving liver transplants in VA medical centers were diagnosed with HCV infections.[93–95] Unfortunately, even with improved epidemiologic tracking, published studies continue to report that greater than 40% of the hepatitis C patients do not have any identifiable risk factors.[91] Evidence of sexual transmission and of perinatal passage from HCV-infected mothers to their offspring suggest possible, but not efficient, modes of viral exposure. In summary, transmission data still strongly implicate parenteral exposure as the primary mechanism for HCV transmission.

SEROLOGY

In May 1990, the US Food and Drug Administration (FDA) licensed two anti-HCV screening tests.[96] Almost immediately, blood donation centers began testing for HCV infection

TABLE 20-10 Comparison of Major Microbiologic and Clinical Features of Hepatitis Viruses

Feature	Hepatitis A Virus (HAV)	Hepatitis B Virus (HBV)	Hepatitis C Virus (HCV)	Hepatitis D Virus (HDV)	Hepatitis E Virus (HEV)	Hepatitis G Virus (HGV)
Family characteristics	Picornaviridae; non-enveloped single-stranded RNA	Hepadnaviridae; double-stranded DNA	Flaviviridae; enveloped single-stranded RNA	Satellite; non-enveloped single-stranded RNA	Caliciviridae; RNA	Flaviviridae; RNA
Incubation period	15–40 d	50–180 d	1–5 mo	21–90 d	2–9 wk	NA
Onset	Usually acute	Usually insidious	Usually insidious	Usually acute	Usually acute	Acute disease spectrum unknown
Prodrome: arthritis/rash	Not present	Sometimes	Sometimes	Unknown	Not present	NA
Transmission	Fecal-oral; poor sanitation	Parenteral; sexual contact; perinatal; other secretions (eg, saliva)	Usually parenteral; sexual contact less common; perinatal	Usually parenteral; sexual contact less common	Fecal-oral; waterborne (common in developing countries)	Parenteral; perinatal frequent co-infection with HCV
Carrier state	No	Yes (5–10%)	Yes (> 85%)	Yes	No	Yes
Possible manifestations	None reported	Hepatocellular carcinoma; cirrhosis	Hepatocellulair carcinoma; cirrhosis	Hepatocellular carcinoma; cirrhosis	None reported	None reported
Mortality rate (%)	0.1–0.2	1–2; higher in adults > 40 yr	1–2	2–20	1–2 in gen population; 20 in pregnant women	NA
Homologous immunity	Anti-HAV	Anti-HBsAg	Not defined	Anti-HBsAg	Anti-HEV	Anti-HGV

Adapted from Krugman S. Viral hepatitis: A, B, C, D, and E—infection. Pediatr Rev 1992;13:203; Molinari JA. Hepatitis C virus infection. Hepatitis C virus infection. Dent Clin North Am 1996;40:309–25.
DNA = deoxyribonucleic acid; HBsAg = hepatitis B surface antigen; NA = not applicable; RNA = ribonucleic acid.

TABLE 20-11 Hepatitis C Incidence in the United States

Approximately 3.9 million HCV-infected persons (1.8% of population)

4 times HIV infection incidence

2.7 million chronic potentially infectious carriers

10,000 HCV-related deaths/yr

80% decline in new cases since 1989

> 50% new cases related to IV-drug users

Incidence of transfusion cases is declining rapidly.

Most cases are mild to asymptomatic.

Many cases still have no risk factors.

HCV = hepatitis C virus; HIV = human immunodeficiency virus; IV = intravenous.

as a component of their routine donor screening. In a noteworthy positive outcome, the use of this radioimmunoassay was found to yield positive anti-HCV results in 80 to 90% of specimens from potential donors thought to be infectious for HCV.[97] Unfortunately, false-negative results are possible at early stages of HCV infection since development of detectable antibody could be delayed for months post viral infection. This prolonged delay in seroconversion suggests that some potentially infectious donors could pass undetected through screening, and their blood subsequently administered to patients. In addition, false-positive test results are possible for those donors with certain immunopathologic conditions, such as hypergammaglobulinemia, liver disease, or autoimmune connective-tissue disorders.[98] More recently, blood tests have used other recombinant HCV synthetic peptide antigens, and these assays have increased sensitivity and specificity (Table 20-13).[91] As a result, the incidence of transfusion-associated hepatitis C has become increasingly uncommon.

PATHOGENESIS

Presentation of viral hepatitis in patients ranges from asymptomatic illness to a fulminant chronic form in which severe sequelae and high mortality rates are seen. Many chronic hepatitis carriers are also at increased risk for hepatocellular carcinoma. For those individuals who develop icteric manifestations of acute viral hepatitis, symptomatologies may vary in intensity; yet they can be strikingly similar in their spectrum, regardless of the etiology. Disease presentations may include jaundice, malaise, fever, anorexia, nausea, abdominal pain, dark ("stormy," "foamy") urine, chalky gray stools, rash, and arthritis.

The clinical features of HCV infection can be variable, in patterns reminiscent of those observed for other hepatitis viruses. Less than one-third of HCV-infected individuals

TABLE 20-12 Estimated Average Prevalence of Hepatitis C Virus Infection in the United States*

Characteristic	Infection Prevalence		Prevalence of Persons with Characteristic (%)
	%	Range %	
Persons with hemophilia treated with products made before 1987	87	74–90	< 0.01
Injection-drug users			
Current	79	72–86	0.5
History of prior use	No data	—	5
Persons with abnormal alanine aminotransferase levels	15	10–18	5
Chronic hemodialysis patients	10	0–64	0.1
Persons with multiple sex partners (lifetime)			
≥ 50	9	6–16	4
10–49	3	3–4	22
2–9	2	1–2	52
Persons reporting a history of sexually transmitted diseases	6	1–10	17
Persons receiving blood transfusions before 1990	6	5–9	6
Infants born to infected mothers	5	0–25	0.1
Men who have sex with men	4	2–18	5
General population	1.8	1.5–2.3	NA
Health care workers	1	1–2	9
Pregnant women	1	—	1.5
Military personnel	0.3	0.2–0.4	0.5
Volunteer blood donors	0.16	—	5

NA = not applicable.

*By various characteristics and estimated prevalence of persons with these characteristics in the population.

TABLE 20-13   Tests for Hepatitis C Virus Infection

Test/Type	Applications	Comments
Hepatitis C virus antibody (anti-HCV) EIA (enzyme immunoassay); supplemental assay (ie, recombinant immunoblot assay [RIBA])	Indicates past or present infection but does not differentiate between acute, chronic, or resolved infection All positive EIA results should be verified with supplemental assay	Sensitivity ≥ 97% EIA alone has low positive-predictive value in low-prevalence populations
HCV RNA (hepatitis C virus ribonucleic acid) Qualitative tests *†: reverse transcriptase polymerase chain reaction (RT-PCR) amplification of HCV RNA by in-house or commercial assays (eg, Amplicor HCV)	Detect presence of circulating HCV RNA Monitor patients on antiviral therapy	Detect virus as early as 1–2 wk after exposure Detection of HCV RNA during course of infection might be intermittent; single negative RT-PCR is not conclusive False-positive and false-negative results might occur
Quantitative tests *†: RT-PCR amplification of HCV RNA by in-house or commercial assays (eg, Amplicor HCV Monitor) Branched-chain DNA (bDNA) assays (eg, Quantiplex HCV RNA Assay)	Determine concentration of HCV RNA Might be useful for assessing the likelihood of response to antiviral therapy	Less sensitive than qualitative RT-PCR Should not be used to exclude the diagnosis of HCV infection or to determine treatment end point
Genotype *†: several methodologies available (eg, hybridization, sequencing)	Group isolates of HCV on the basis of genetic differences into 6 genotypes and > 90 subtypes With new therapies, length of treatment might vary based on genotype	Genotype 1 (subtypes 1a and 1b) most common in United States and associated with lower response to antiviral therapy
Serotype*: EIA based on immunoreactivity to synthetic peptides (eg, Murex HCV Serotyping 1–6 Assay)	No clinical utility	Cannot distinguish between subtypes Dual infections often observed

DNA = deoxyribonucleic acid; HCV = hepatitis C virus.

*Currently not approved by US Food and Drug Administration; lack standardization.

†Samples require special handling (eg, serum must be separated within 2–4 h of collection and stored frozen [-20˚C or -70˚C]; frozen samples should be shipped on dry ice).

manifest jaundice after receiving contaminated units of blood.[99,100] They may appear healthy with normal liver function and no pathologic sequelae, or develop acute and/or chronic disease manifestations. Although acute hepatitis C can resemble hepatitis A and hepatitis B clinically, HCV infection often induces less hepatic inflammatory reactions and thus usually manifests milder symptoms. Serologic demonstration of anti-HCV often does not occur for weeks to months after viral infection, thereby providing a prolonged undetected period during which the patient continues to be infectious. As occurs with HBV infection, pathologic sequelae can occur in persons who have chronic HCV infection, often with life-threatening ramifications. Unfortunately, as many as 50% of long-term chronic hepatitis C cases may progress to chronic hepatitis C liver disease. This develops far more often than the 5 to 10% carrier rate observed with HBV infection. Persons with chronic hepatitis C can present with few initial clinical manifestations of liver disease and remain so as inactive viral carriers, or persistent viral infection can predispose a person later to increased risk for hepatic failure and hepatocellular carcinoma.[101] Patients with pre-existent immunosuppressive conditions, such as those with HIV infection and others undergoing kidney or liver transplantation, also have been found to have higher hepatitis C morbidity. Transmission here is most probably due to the patients' potential to experience frequent parenteral exposure to HCV via blood transfusion or intravenous drug use. High-risk sexual activity may also be a factor.

At the present time, the demonstration and characterization of a protective host immune response against HCV have not been accomplished. Presence of anti-HCV in a person's blood does not distinguish between cases of acute or chronic hepatitis C, nor can a positive test for this immunoglobulin discriminate between a person who has recovered from infection with natural active immunity from one who has developed chronic hepatitis C.

OCCUPATIONAL RISKS TO HEALTH CARE PROFESSIONALS

Health care workers are at risk for exposure to patient blood and possible subsequent infection from bloodborne diseases, such as those caused by members of the hepatitis virus group. Early observation that a form of NANBH has a bloodborne etiology spurred intense occupational-risk investigations by clinical scientists. Accidental injuries from contaminated sharps have been associated with resulting onset of both hepatitis B and hepatitis C. Information describing occupational HCV transmission in hospital settings was investigated and published even before cloning of the virus was accomplished. Multiple investigations documented HCV transmission to health care workers and to other patients following percutaneous accidents involving blood (Table 20-14).[102–106]

TABLE 20-14 Modes of Transmission of Hepatitis C Virus in Health Care Settings

Accidental needlesticks

Blood splashes into eyes

Blood transfusion (incidence declining rapidly)

Association with contaminated immune globin

Organ/tissue transplantation

Infected cardiac surgeon to patients

Infected patient to anesthesia assistant to other patients

Patient to patient via colonoscope

Relatively few studies have looked at HCV transmission in dental treatment facilities. Initial reports showed oral surgeons had a significantly higher incidence of positive anti-HCV results than did general dentists and the general population, owing to greater potential exposures to blood.[107] These and other data have been summarized by Cleveland and colleagues.[108] When taken together, accumulated findings suggest that although hepatitis C remains a bloodborne infection of occupational concern, the long-term application of universal infection-control precautions targeting HBV as the most infectious bloodborne pathogen has significantly lowered the dental provider's risks for contracting HCV infection.

The most hazardous type of exposure that can increase the possibility of HCV acquisition is an on-the-job needlestick injury. A second primary characteristic of HCV risks to health care workers is related to the virus life cycle and the titers of infectious particles in blood. HCV is present in concentrations ranging from only a few virions to 100,000 or more particles per milliliter of a patient's blood. Although this reinforces HCV's position as being a greater occupational infectious risk than HIV, the concentrations fall far below those routinely seen in HBV-infected persons. Thus, the substantially lower HCV titer in blood offers less opportunity for occupational transmission per exposure incident. Table 20-15 puts this into perspective by summarizing potential transmission risks to health care workers for HBV, HIV, and HCV, by comparing viral concentrations found in blood and calculated infection rates following needlestick accidents.[109]

TABLE 20-15 Risks of Transmission to Health Care Workers

Pathogen	Concentration/mL of Serum/Plasma	Transmission Rate (%)*
HBV	1,000,000–100,000,000	6.0–30.0
HCV	10–1,000,000	2.7–6.0
HIV	10–1,000	0.30

Adapted from Lanphear BP.[109]

HBV = hepatitis B virus; HCV=hepatitis C virus; HIV = human immunodeficiency virus.

*As a result of a needlestick accident.

Infection control precautions against bloodborne disease have correctly focused on prevention of hepatitis B transmission in health care facilities, in large part because of the high HBV concentrations that can be reached in the blood of infected patients and the high potential of infection after exposure to certain contaminated body fluids. With regard to hepatitis C, sizable volumes of HCV-contaminated blood, such as those used for blood transfusion, can readily cause infection. Despite apparent lower risks from sharps, however, HCV infection carries with it the increased possibility of chronic liver disease. The progression from persistent viral infection to either hepatic cirrhosis in about one-quarter of infected persons or to hepatocellular carcinoma in others presents real challenges to infection control for care providers.

HCV THERAPY AND PREVENTIVE APPROACHES

Preliminary studies began appearing in the literature in the mid-1980s that suggested that a prolonged course of therapy with interferon-α could have beneficial effects for persons with chronic hepatitis C.[110,111] These beneficial effects occurred rapidly during therapy, with alanine aminotransferase (ALT) levels eventually falling to within the normal range. Follow-up testing after completion of the regimen unfortunately found the ALT decline to be transient in most of the patients. Later investigations involving larger numbers of HCV-infected persons led to FDA approval of a recombinant form of this antiviral agent for treatment of chronic hepatitis C in 1991.[112] Additional studies have attempted to further refine therapeutic dosages and drug regimen intervals.[113]

Combination of chemotherapeutic agents has shown promising results in recent years. Currently, a daily regimen of interferon α-2b plus ribavirin for 6 to 12 months has demonstrated a significant improvement in patient biochemical and virologic responses when compared with interferon monotherapy. Approximately 50% of treated patients have a sustained beneficial response, compared with response rates of 15 to 25% using interferon alone.[114] Future therapies will probably include additional multidrug approaches, such as other forms of interferon and specific HCV enzyme inhibitors.[115]

An effective vaccine for hepatitis C is not yet commercially available. Multiple factors have hindered research efforts directed at prophylactic strategies. Two principal factors are the failure to define a protective host immune response against HCV infection, and the antigenic heterogeneity described for different viral strains. Until scientists ascertain how host resistance develops during recovery from hepatitis C, and against what antigen(s) the immunity is directed, vaccine studies will continue to be limited. At present, routine use of universal precautions during patient care and anti-HCV screening of potential blood donors appears to be successful in reducing health care provider, patient, and public exposures.

HIV Infection

Since the early 1980s, HIV has been recognized as one of the most devastating infectious diseases of the twentieth century. By the end of the century, almost 60 million people worldwide had been infected with the virus, and the rate of infection continued unabated.[116] The vast majority of exposed and at-risk individuals had no access to effective medications to combat the virus or its associated opportunistic infections. Even in the early stage of the twenty-first century, there are few indications that there soon will be any effective and affordable vaccines or anti-HIV medications available for most people afflicted by this disease. This chapter explores many different aspects of HIV disease and emphasizes oral health considerations, which impact on the overall health of HIV-infected individuals.

EPIDEMIOLOGY

In June and July of 1981, the Centers for Disease Control published two reports on several clusters of young homosexual men who developed opportunistic infections that were chiefly detected in severely immunodeficient individuals.[117,118] It was not clear what caused this apparent immunodeficiency, and the disease was initially referred to as "gay-related immune deficiency," or "GRID." Several theories focusing on the lifestyle of homosexual and bisexual men were put forth to explain the cause of this illness. However, soon after, it became clear that there were other groups in society who also developed this rapidly evolving disease and that the cause was most probably an infectious pathogen and not sexual preference.[119–125]

It became evident that finding a causative agent, developing an accurate test to detect this pathogen, and elucidating the modes of transmission were imperative to slow down the quickly expanding epidemic. The etiologic agent of this disease, now termed "human immunodeficiency virus," was recognized within 2 years of the first reported cases.[126,127] Due to the severe immunosuppression observed in affected individuals, this disease was eventually given the name "acquired immunodeficiency syndrome." The CDC quickly put a surveillance system in place. This surveillance system was based on standard case definitions. Due to the changing nature of this disease, the original case definition from 1985 was expanded in 1987 and again in 1993 to better incorporate specific illnesses in different populations as well as reflect changes in infected individuals' immune status[128] (Table 20-16). AIDS, the stage of HIV disease when individuals start to develop opportunistic infections or have severe immunosuppression, is a reportable condition in all 50 states, the District of Columbia, and the US territories. At the time of this writing, HIV infection is not a reportable condition in all states. The number of total accumulated cases of AIDS and the rate of AIDS in the United States are reported by the CDC on a biannual basis[129] (Table 20-17). Although the number of total accumulated cases of AIDS changes over time, the ranking of states and metropolitan areas remains fairly stable. More important than the actual number of cases and rates is the trend of change. The directions of these trends reflect the course of the HIV epidemic. Between June 1999 and June 2000, there were an additional 42,563 persons who developed AIDS in the United States. However, this represented a decrease of 7.6% of new cases from 1998 to 1999. Also, the rate of AIDS per 100,000 population decreased by 8.2%. A decrease of 8.6% in new cases

among males and a decrease of 3.4% in new cases among females were noted for the same period. Thus, even though new cases were reported, there was a marked decrease in the rate of new AIDS cases. Taking into consideration that there are between 40,000 to 50,000 new HIV infections annually in the United States, the decreasing number of AIDS cases suggests that infected individuals are remaining healthier and that the disease is progressing more slowly over time. Since the introduction of more potent anti-HIV medications in the middle 1990s, an initial dramatic decrease in the rate of death of persons with AIDS has been observed (Table 20-18).[129] However, this trend has tapered off due to factors such as increased resistance to medications and patients reaching the limits of extending survival with these medications. By the end of the 1990s, it was estimated that there were 650,000 to 900,000 HIV-infected persons in the United States; approximately 500,000 of these persons were aware of their HIV infection, and an estimated 335,000 of these received medical care.[130]

There are two different types of HIV: HIV-1 and HIV-2. Both viruses cause immune deterioration and AIDS, but HIV-2 has been associated with a more indolent course and a less efficient transmission. The median time from infection to AIDS has been reported to be approximately 10 years for those infected with HIV-1 but almost 20 years for those with HIV-2. The vast majority of HIV infections are caused by HIV-1, except in particular geographic areas, such as the western parts of Africa. Unless specified, "HIV" in this chapter refers to HIV-1.

Mainly through phylogenic analyses, it has been possible to extrapolate that HIV-1, HIV-2, and the simian immunodeficiency virus (SIV) may have originated from the same source in Africa and started to separate into different viruses in the beginning of 1900s. It is not clear when HIV was introduced into the human host, but it likely happened in the 1920s or 1930s, with a more rapid sustained spread around the mid-1940s. The prevailing theory suggests that the human variant of this immunodeficiency virus originated from different types of primates. It is assumed that SIV from chimpanzees (SIV_{CPZ}) is the source of HIV-1, whereas HIV-2 originated from monkeys, predominantly sooty mangabeys (SIV_{SM}).[131,132] The earliest reported cases of AIDS in Europe were observed in the 1950s; approximately 10 years later, AIDS was reported in the United States. HIV is transmitted sexually through contaminated blood and products, and vertically from mother to child. It is important to realize that since the recognition of HIV disease, the modes of transmission have not changed and are not likely to change in the future. Although extraordinary cases of HIV transmission by other means have been reported, they are extremely rare or are based on faulty documentation. There has never been any documented case of occupational transmission of HIV from patients to dental health care workers. In one celebrated case from 1990, an HIV-infected dentist was implicated in transmitting the virus to several of his patients. Although this case was thoroughly investigated by CDC and other agencies, how the transmission occurred was never fully elucidated.[133]

TABLE 20-16   1993 Revised Classification System for HIV Infection and Expanded Surveillance Case Definition for AIDS among Adolescents and Adults

CD4+ T-Lymphocyte Categories

The lowest accurate CD4+ T-lymphocyte count should be used for classification purposes, even though more recent and possibly different counts may be available.

Clinical Categories

Clinical category A
  Conditions:
      Asymptomatic human immunodeficiency virus (HIV) infection
      Persistent generalized lymphadenopathy (PGL)
      Acute HIV infection with accompanying illness or history of acute HIV infection
  Conditions listed in category B and category C must not have occurred.

Clinical category B
  Symptomatic conditions in HIV-infected adolescents or adults that are not included in clinical category C and meet at least one of the following criteria: (a) the conditions are attributed to HIV infection or are indicative of a defect in cell-mediated immunity; (b) the conditions are considered by physicians to have a clinical course or to require management that is complicated by HIV infection.

  Examples of, but not limited to, the following conditions:
      Bacillary angiomatosis
      Candidiasis, oropharyngeal (thrush)
      Candidiasis, vulvovaginal; persistent, frequent, or poorly responsive to therapy
      Cervical dysplasia (moderate or severe)/cervical carcinoma in situ
      Constitutional symptoms, such as fever (38.5°C) or diarrhea lasting > 1 mo
      Herpes zoster (shingles) involving at least two distinct episodes or more than one dermatome
      Idiopathic thrombocytopenia purpura
      Listeriosis
      Oral hairy leukoplakia
      Pelvic inflammatory disease, particular if complicated by tubo-ovarian abscess
      Peripheral neuropathy

Clinical category C
  Conditions:
      Candidiasis of bronchi, trachea, or lung
      Candidiasis, esophageal
      Cervical cancer, invasive
      Coccidioidomycosis, disseminated or extrapulmonary
      Cryptococcosis, extrapulmonary
      Cryptosporidiosis, chronic intestinal (> 1 mo duration)
      Cytomegalovirus disease (other than liver, spleen, or nodes)
      Cytomegalovirus retinitis (with loss of vision)
      Encephalopathy, HIV related
      Herpes simplex: chronic ulcer(s) (> 1 mo duration); or bronchitis, pneumonitis, or esophagitis
      Histoplasmosis, disseminated or extrapulmonary
      Isosporiasis, chronic intestinal (> 1 mo duration)
      Kaposi's sarcoma
      Lymphoma, Burkitt's (or equivalent term)
      Lymphoma, immunoblastic (or equivalent term)
      Lymphoma, primary, of brain
      Mycobacterium avium-intracellulare complex or *Mycobacterium kansasii,* disseminated or extrapulmonary
      Mycobacterium tuberculosis, any site (pulmonary or extrapulmonary)
      Mycobacterium, other species or unidentified species, disseminated or extrapulmonary
      Pneumocystis carinii pneumonia
      Pneumonia, recurrent
      Progressive multifocal leukoencephalopathy
      Salmonella septicemia, recurrent
      Toxoplasmosis
      Wasting syndrome due to HIV infection

CD4+ T Cells/mm³ or CD4+ Percentage	Clinical Categories		
	A: Asymptomatic Acute HIV or PGL	B: Symptomatic, no A or C Conditions	C: AIDS-Indicator Conditions
≥ 500 or ≥ 29%	A1	B1	C1*
200–499 or 14–28%	A2	B2	C2*
< 200 or < 14%	A3*	B3*	C3*

Adapted from Centers for Disease Control and Prevention.[128]

* Expanded acquired immunodeficiency syndrome (AIDS) surveillance case definition.

TABLE 20-17 Ranking of AIDS Cases and Rates per 100,000 Population*

Area of Residence	Total Cases
New York	139,248
California	117,521
Florida	78,043
Texas	52,667
New Jersey	41,245
Illinois	24,425
Puerto Rico	24,061
Pennsylvania	23,678
Georgia	22,197
Maryland	20,833

Area of Residence	Rates
District of Columbia	189.4
New York	39.4
Virgin Islands, US	37.6
Florida	33.4
Maryland	27.2
Puerto Rico	26.4
Delaware	26.3
Massachusetts	24.4
New Jersey	23.6
South Carolina	20.9

Metropolitan Area of Residence	Total Cases
New York, NY	117,792
Los Angeles, CA	42,394
San Francisco, CA	27,567
Miami, FL	23,521
Washington, DC	22,321
Chicago, IL	21,173
Houston, TX	18,735
Philadelphia, PA	18,348
Newark, NJ	16,739
Atlanta, GA	15,524

Metropolitan Area of Residence	Rates
New York, NY	68.1
Miami, FL	58.3
Fort Lauderdale, FL	56.9
San Francisco, CA	52.6
West Palm Beach, FL	50.5
Jersey City, NJ	43.2
Newark, NJ	40.3
Columbia, SC	39.7
Baltimore, MD	35.9
Washington, DC	35.8

Adapted from Centers for Disease Control and Prevention.[129]

*In the United States reported through June 2000.

PATHOGENESIS

Early in the HIV epidemic, it was recognized that this disease was caused by a virus that gradually destroyed a host's immune defenses, making virtually all infected individuals susceptible to opportunistic infections. The particular immunodeficiency in HIV disease was attributed to CD4+ lymphocyte depletion, enabling the development of specific opportunistic infections that were associated with a high degree of morbidity and mor-

tality. More than 20 years after the recognition of this disease and its causative agents, it has been possible, with the help of improved and new molecular biologic tools and methods, to explain in more detail the pathogenesis of HIV disease.

HIV is a retrovirus harboring its genetic information in two copies of a single-stranded RNA. The viral genome is contained within a protein core, which also contains the enzyme reverse transcriptase. Surrounding the core particle is a lipid membrane. Embedded within this membrane are two envelope glycoproteins, gp 41 and gp 120, both essential for the recognition and binding of target cells. These two glycoproteins are subunits generated by the cleavage of the gp 160 precursor. HIV targets cells expressing CD4 molecules, particularly CD4+ T lymphocytes, monocytes, and macrophages, taking advantage of the affinity between the viral gp 120 and the cellular CD4 receptor. The binding of gp 120 to CD4 receptors causes a conformational change in gp 120, which exposes and stabilizes a cellular chemokine receptor called CCR5. These interactions activate gp 41, resulting in fusion of the viral membrane with the cellular membrane, which allows the viral RNA and reverse transcriptase to enter into the target cell. The reverse transcriptase transcribes the viral RNA into DNA, which integrates into the target cell's genome. With the successful integration of viral DNA into the cellular genetic material, an infection has occurred.

HIV gains entry into the body directly through the blood or at mucosal surfaces. The virus establishes itself within lymphoid tissues, where it replicates, makes itself available to the cells of the immune system (such as T lymphocytes, monocytes, and macrophages), and slowly brings about destruction of the lymphoid tissue. Mucosal surfaces have an abundance of dendritic cells, such as Langerhans' cells, that trap the virus and enable the uptake of the virus into lymphoid aggregates below the surface. Contact between mucosal surfaces and HIV can result in infection of Langerhans' cells after only a couple of hours. Within a few days, the virus can be detected in regional lymph nodes.

The rapid replication of HIV results in an initial viremia causing seeding of the virus to lymphoid tissue throughout the body. It is estimated that more than 10 billion virions, with a half-life of approximately 1.6 days, are produced daily in infected individuals.[134,135] This continuous turnover of viruses results in one-half of the circulating viruses being replaced with newly formed virions every day. Furthermore, almost 2 billion CD4+ lymphocytes are destroyed and replaced every day.

Activated CD4+ lymphocytes express high levels of chemokine receptors and are primary targets of HIV. However, although these activated cells usually die within a few days, a latent reservoir of HIV is established among CD4+ cells. An extremely high viral titer can be detected in the blood during the primary stage of HIV infection, but, over time, infectious virions became undetectable in the plasma. The initial control of viral replication is associated with antibody-dependent cellular cytotoxicity activity and HIV-specific cytotoxic T lymphocytes. However, neutralizing antibodies also develop.

TABLE 20-18   Estimated Deaths and Rate of Change of Death of Persons with AIDS, in the United States

Measure	1993	1994	1995	1996	1997	1998	1999
Estimated number of deaths	45,381	49,869	50,610	37,787	21,923	17,930	16,273
Change (%)	—	+9.9	+1.5	−25.3	−42.0	−18.2	−9.2

Unfortunately, HIV replication is associated with a very high mutation rate, resulting in a great genetic diversity of HIV quasi-species in individual patients.[136] This heterogeneity increases over time. Consequently, it is important to initiate viral suppression as early as possible after infection. This will accomplish a decrease in viral diversity, resulting in more effective immune control and less drug resistance. Even a single nucleotide change in the HIV-1 transcriptase gene is enough to confer high levels of drug resistance to particular anti-HIV medications.[137]

The hallmark of HIV disease is the progressive loss of CD4+ lymphocytes. Without intervention, an average of 60 to 80 cells/mm^3 are lost every year; this loss is highly variable and occurs in periods of more stability and rapid decline.[138] An estimation of the plasma level of these cells (a CD4 cell count) indicates an individual's immune status. Normal CD4 cell counts are usually above 500 to 600 cells/mm^3, whereas levels below 200 cells/mm^3 are considered to indicate severe immune suppression. The lower the CD4 cell count, the more susceptible is a patient to develop opportunistic infections. As part of the latest AIDS definition, a patient has an AIDS diagnosis when the CD4 cell count drops below 200 cells/mm^3 (see Table 20-16). At this level the patient is at very high risk of developing specific major opportunistic infections, such as *Pneumocystis carinii* pneumonia (PCP), and prophylactic medications are administered to ward off these infections. Although the CD4 cell count was used for many years as a marker for HIV disease progression, other biologic indicators, such as the level of plasma viral RNA, or viral load, have since proven to be more reliable and accurate.[139] Today, CD4 cell counts are mainly used to assess a patient's immune status, to determine when to institute antiretroviral medications, to determine when to institute prophylaxis against opportunistic infections, and as an indicator for AIDS. Recent advances in molecular biology have enabled detection of HIV RNA in plasma and within different tissues.[140] The most common method used for clinical HIV care is reverse transcription coupled to the polymerase chain reaction (RT-PCR). This method uses a PCR-based assay to assess the presence, as well as measure the quantity, of HIV RNA. Numerous retrospective studies have determined the progression of HIV disease, as well as the prognosis, based on the quantity of plasma HIV-1 RNA[139] (Table 20-19). Many of these studies show surprising consistency.[141–144] According to these studies, the risk for disease progression and death is reduced by 30% when the viral load is halved, by 55% with a four-fold reduction in viral load, and by 65% with a 10-fold reduction in viral load.

As viral load significantly corresponds with changes in disease progression, this measure has also been used to assess the efficacy of antiretroviral medications.[145] Effective drug therapy is reflected in reduced viral loads; no or little viral load change suggests less effective therapy. This association has created new standards of care for patients with HIV. Acute HIV infection occurs 2 to 6 weeks after exposure. During the acute stage of the disease, affected individuals develop high plasma levels of the virus. An antibody response can only be detected approximately 2 to 3 months after exposure. Twenty to 90% of exposed individuals develop a self-limited nonspecific illness characterized by fever, lymphadenopathy, myalgia, arthralgia, sore throat, and occasional rashes and oral ulcerations. This illness has sometimes been described as a "mononucleosis-like" syndrome and is referred to as the acute seroconversion syndrome or acute retroviral syndrome. Identification of individuals at this stage of the disease is important for several reasons. Of primary importance is the potential for further transmission. As affected individuals have very high viral loads, they are highly infectious and can unwittingly transmit the virus to unsuspected partners.[146] There is epidemiologic evidence that suggests that recently infected individuals are responsible for a high percentage of transmissions.[147] Evaluation of individuals during the acute retroviral syndrome needs to include both a virologic test and an antibody test. A positive HIV RNA test, together with a negative HIV-antibody test, is diagnostic for primary HIV infection. Due to the possible false-positive result from an HIV RNA PCR-based assay, a true positive result is considered when the viral load is above 100,000 copies/mL. Results below 5,000 copies/mL are more likely to be false-positive than true positive.[148]

Another benefit of early recognition of HIV infection is the potential to achieve viral suppression during this stage of the disease. This may facilitate a more effective immune response and diminish viral diversity. Institution of antiretroviral therapy during this stage of the disease has been shown to enhance the immune system's ability to destroy infected cells and to diminish CD4 cell depletion.[149–151]

After the acute retroviral syndrome, most individuals remain asymptomatic for many years. However, the deteriorating immune system eventually gives way, and opportunistic infections develop. Without treatment, the median time from primary infection to AIDS is approximately 10 years.[152]

In most industrialized countries, individuals with HIV have access to antiretroviral therapy. Consequently, the epidemiology of HIV disease has changed dramatically since the mid-1990s. At that point, new and more potent antiretroviral medications were introduced that decreased the incidence of opportunistic infections and death rate[153] (see Tables 20-18 and 20-20). Unfortunately, the rate of decline in the inci-

TABLE 20-19   Prediction of Immune Deterioration, HIV Disease Progression, and AIDS by HIV-1 RNA

HIV-1 RNA Copies/mL	Decrease in Yearly CD4+ Cell Count/mm^3	Individuals Developing AIDS Within 6 Years (%)	Individuals Dying Within 6 Years (%)
< 500	36.3	5.4	0.9
501–3,000	44.8	16.6	6.3
3,001–10,000	55.2	31.7	18.1
10,001–30,000	64.8	55.2	34.9
> 30,000	76.5	80.0	69.5

Adapted from Coffin JM.[136]

AIDS = acquired immunodeficiency syndrome; HIV-1 = human immunodeficiency virus type 1; RNA = ribonucleic acid.

dence of opportunistic infections, AIDS incidence, and AIDS-related deaths has slowed down. These latest trends are most probably related to the development of resistance to antiretroviral drugs, transmission of HIV-resistant strains, and the inability to maintain complete viral suppression for extended periods of time in all individuals. Furthermore, several new opportunistic syndromes have been described in patients given antiretroviral medications.[154] It is possible that this phenomenon, termed "reversal syndromes," is due to a rebounding immune system that initially does not have the same antigenic divergence as developing naïve CD4+ lymphocytes. This immune dysfunction may facilitate the development of latent opportunistic infections or unmask an undiagnosed opportunistic infection.

Apparently, not all individuals exposed to HIV become infected. Furthermore, the rate of HIV disease progression in individuals is highly variable. Some infected persons may progress from infection to AIDS within months, whereas others have no signs of opportunistic infections or immune suppression even after 15 to 20 years. Approximately 10% of HIV-infected persons progress to AIDS within the 2 to 3 years after infection, whereas 10 to 17% of infected individuals may not develop AIDS even 20 years after infection.[155] Obviously, these subgroups of infected persons are of great interest, as they may provide invaluable information regarding the variables associated with infection, progression, and even immunity to HIV, and subsequent treatment.

Numerous studies have focused on the ability and inability of HIV to enter into target cells, and the capability of the immune system to rid the body of the virus. During the earliest stages of HIV infection, the virus particularly seeks out and infects macrophages and memory T lymphocytes, using, in addition to these cells' CD4 receptors, the cells' chemokine receptors. The chemokine receptor used in these cells as a co-receptor for HIV is CCR5. At this stage of the disease it is common that the virus is referred to as "macrophage-tropic," or "M-tropic." M-tropic viruses do not have the ability to form syncytia in vitro; they are therefore also referred to as "non–syncytia-inducing isolates." In addition, due to the virus's predilection for cells expressing CCR5, the virus is referred to as an "R5 isolate." Investigations of chemokine receptors have indicated that individuals with a homozygous mutation of CCR5 may be almost completely resistant to HIV. This specific mutation has been referred to as "CCR5 δ 32," indicating a characteristic 32 base-pair deletion in the gene encoding CCR5. Individuals with a heterozygous mutation of CCR5 δ 32, one normal and one altered allele, tend to progress more slowly to AIDS and live longer than individuals without this mutation.[156,157] Furthermore, a promoter mutation in CCR5 has also been associated with a slower progression to AIDS.[158] Interestingly, persons harboring these chemokine receptor changes do not exhibit any pathologic effects due to these polymorphisms. Unfortunately, very few individuals, approximately 1% of Caucasians, exhibit homozygous deletion of the 32 base pair; 10% are heterozygotes. CCR5 δ 32 is rare among Africans, Native Americans, and East Asians.

All chemokine receptors have natural ligands, cytokines that bind to the receptor. Three main cytokines have been identified that bind to and block the CCR5 receptor: MIP-1-α, MIP-1-β and RANTES. Interestingly, these cytokines are generated by CD8+ T lymphocytes, which are cells that have been implicated in releasing factors suppressing HIV infection.[159] Selective blockage of CCR5 with these cytokines has been shown to occur.

During the later stages of HIV disease, the virus predominantly infects T lymphocytes expressing CD4 receptors and a chemokine co-receptor designated CXCR4. These T-tropic viruses can cause multinucleated syncytia formation in vitro and are therefore referred to as "syncytia-inducing isolates" and "X4 isolates." The use of the CXCR4 receptor by HIV is associated with a more rapid depletion of CD4+ T lymphocytes and disease progression.[160] Chemokines SDF-1-α and SDF-1-β have been identified as ligands to CXCR4 and can selectively inhibit T-tropic HIV-1 strains.

TABLE 20-20   Decrease in Rate of Opportunistic Infections in HIV-Positive Individuals

Disease	Rate of Decrease	
	1992–1995	1996–1998
Pneumocystis carinii pneumonia	–3.4	–21.5
Mycobacterium avium-intracellulare complex	–4.7	–39.9
Esophageal candidiasis	–0.2	–16.7

Adapted from Kaplan JE et al.[153]

Use of these chemokine receptors is not exclusive, and about 40% of HIV-positive individuals use CXCR4 instead of, and sometimes in addition to, CCR5.[161] These viral isolates are referred to as "R5X4." Unfortunately, several other chemokine receptors are involved in HIV's selection of target cells, increasing the complexity of all HIV–target cell interactions (Table 20-21).[161–163]

MEDICAL TREATMENT

A better understanding of the pathogenesis of HIV disease has, in recent years, changed many of the treatment paradigms for infected individuals during the course of their illness. The recognition that there exist different individual responses to HIV infection, and even resistance, has provided clues to intervention strategies based on more accurate predictions of disease progression. Furthermore, better knowledge of the mechanisms for viral entry into target cells, integration, transcription, and subsequent viral replication has enabled a more varied and focused treatment strategy. Although the mainstay of HIV therapy is based on trying to slow down viral replication with antiretroviral medications, an important part of treatment for patients with HIV disease is also the prevention and treatment of opportunistic infections. HIV-infected individuals therefore take many different medications, some which impact on oral health and provision of dental care (Table 20-22).

The first antiretroviral drug was introduced in 1997. This medication, AZT or zidovudine (ZDV), belongs to a group of medications called nucleoside reverse transcriptase inhibitors (NRTIs). These medications competitively inhibit the reverse transcriptase from converting the viral RNA into viral DNA. Other nucleoside analogues are abacavir (ABC), didanosine (ddI), lamivudine (3TC), stavudine (d4T), and zalcitabine (ddC). A similar group of medications that also inhibits reverse transcriptase is the non-nucleoside reverse transcriptase inhibitors (NNRTIs). NNRTIs include efavirenz (EFV), delaviridine (DLV), and nevirapine (NVP). In the mid-1990s, a new class of antiretroviral medications was introduced—protease inhibitors. These powerful medications prevent the breakdown of viral proteins into appropriate building blocks for viral replication. Included in these medications are amprenavir (APV), indinavir (IDV), nelfinavir (NFV), ritonavir (RTV), and saquinavir (SQV). Due to the high level of toxicity and the rapid development of drug resistance, antiretroviral medications are given as double or triple therapy. This combination therapy is referred to as highly active antiretroviral therapy, or HAART. Antiretroviral therapy is usually instituted when a patient's CD4 cell count drops below a critical value and/or when a patient's viral load exceeds a critical level. These predetermined values vary as better scientific information regarding the pathogenesis of HIV disease is elucidated and depending on how patients react and respond to new and better combinations of medications.

Prophylaxis against opportunistic infections is instituted according to a patient's immune status. Usually patients with CD4 cell counts below 200 cells/mm^3 are considered for prophylaxis to prevent *Pneumocystis carinii* pneumonia, and, at even lower levels, prophylaxis is instituted against various fungal and mycobacterial infections. Knowledge about the type of medications used to treat and prevent opportunistic infections helps the dental provider to attain additional insight into a patient's health status.

ORAL HEALTH CONSIDERATIONS

Oral health considerations for persons infected with HIV focus on provision of dental care and oral conditions associated with their underlying disease.[164–166] An appropriate work-up for an HIV-infected patient needs to ascertain a patient's overall health, immune status, prognosis, presence and history of opportunistic infections, risk for developing more severe opportunistic infections and oral lesions, current medications, and chance for long-term survival (Figure 20-7). The patient may be able to provide all necessary information, but it is appropriate to have the patient sign a consent form that enables the provider to obtain more medical information from the patient's primary care physician (Figure 20-8).

As a general rule, no dental modifications are required for patients based on their HIV status. Most individuals presenting for outpatient dental care are sufficiently healthy to tolerate all types of dental procedures, ranging from scaling to implants.[167] Also, numerous studies have indicated that patients with HIV disease are not more susceptible to complications after dental care, regardless of CD4 cell count.[168,169]

As with other medically complex patients, the major concerns are impaired hemostasis, susceptibility to dentally induced infections, drug actions and interactions, and the patient's ability to withstand the stress and trauma of dental procedures. Few patients present with increased bleeding tendencies, unless they have concomitant liver disease or idiopathic thrombocytopenic purpura.[170] Even when patients' CD4 cell counts are very low, they are not more susceptible to dentally induced bacteremia. Thus, there are no indications for routine use of antibiotic prophylaxis based on patients' HIV status. However, patients with neutrophil counts below 500 to 750 cells/mm^3 require antibiotic prophylaxis. Furthermore, some patients may be at an increased risk for developing sub-

---

TABLE 20-21 Characteristics of Individuals with Slow Disease Progression

Attenuated virus
   Reduced replication kinetics
   Low viral load

Effective cellular immune response
   Strong HIV-1–specific cytotoxic T lymphocytes
   Effective antibody-dependent cellular cytotoxicity
   Increased levels of CD8+ T lymphocytes
   Increased divergence of the CD4+ T-lymphocyte repertoire, possibly due to exposure to greater viral diversity

Polymorphisms and inhibition/blockage of chemokine receptors
   Homozygote CCR5-δ 32 genotype
   Heterozygote CCR5-δ 32 genotype
   Inhibition/blockage by MIP-1-α, MIP-1-β, RANTES generated by CD8+ T cells

Data from Berger EA et al;[161] Learmont J et al;[162] Klein MR et al.[163]

TABLE 20-22 Impact of Treatments for HIV Infection

Drug Name*	Type of Drug	Adverse Effects of Significance for Dentists	Co.†
(+)-calanolide A*	NNRTI	Dysgeusia	12
3TC or lamivudine, Epivir; also in Combivir and Trizivir	NRTI	Peripheral neuropathy	9
Abacavir (ABC), Ziagen; also in Trizivir	NRTI	Associated with liver damage	9
ABC, see abacavir			
AG1661* or HIV-1 Immunogen* or Salk vaccine*, Remune*	IBT	Not known	2
Agenerase, see amprenavir			
Aldesleukin or interleukin-2 (IL-2), Proleukin	IBT	Not known	6
Amprenavir (APV), Agenerase	PI	Associated with hyperglycemia, dygeusia, and paraoral tingling sensations Do not use with the following medications: midazolam, triazolam, ergotamine, tricyclic antidepressants, vitamin E Avoid use with the following medications: erythromycin, benzodiazepine, or itraconazole	9
APV, see amprenavir			
AZT or zidovudine, Retrovir; also in Combivir and Trizivir	NRTI	Associated with seizures, rapid, uncontrollable eye movements, decreased coordination, liver damage, and peripheral neuropathy	9
BCH-10652* or dOTC*	NRTI	None	3
Bis(POC) PMPA*, see tenofovir disoproxil fumarate*			
BMS-232632*	PI	Not known	5
Capravirine* (CPV) Coactinon*, see emivirine*	NNRTI	Dysgeusia	2
Combivir combination of zidovudine + lamivudine	NRTI	Associated with liver damage and peripheral neuropathy	9
Coviracil*, see emtricitabine* and FTC*			
CPV*, see capravirine*			
Crixivan, see indinavir			
d4T or stavudine, Zerit	NRTI	Peripheral neuropathy	5
DAPD*	NRTI	Not known	13
ddC or zalcitabine, Hivid	NRTI	Associated with oral ulcerations, liver damage, and peripheral neuropathy	11
ddl or didanosine, Videx or Videx EC (delayed-release capsules)	NRTI	Associated with xerostomia, liver damage, and peripheral neuropathy Do not take the following medications within 2 hours of ddl: tetracycline, doxycycline, minocycline, and ciprofloxacin Take the following medications at least 2 hours before ddl: ketoconazole and itraconazole	5
Delaviridine (DLV), Drescriptor	NNRTI	Do not use with orange and cranberry juice Do not use with the following medications: clarithromycin, dapsone, ergotamine, alprazolam, midazolam, triazolam, carbamazepine, phenobarbital, and cimetidine	2
Didanosine, see ddl			
DLV, see delaviridine			
DMP-450*	PI	Not known	13
DOTC* or BCH-10652*	NRTI	Not known	3
Drescriptor, see delavirdine			
Droxia, see hydroxyurea			
Efavirenz (EFV), Sustiva	NNRTI	Associated with confusion, abnormal behavior, or hallucinations Do not use together with the following medications: midazolam and triazolam	7

Continued

TABLE 20-22 Impact of Treatments for HIV Infection (Continued)

Drug Name*	Type of Drug	Adverse Effects of Significance for Dentists	Co.†
EFV, see efavirenz			
Emivirine* (EMV), Coactinon*	NNRTI	Not known	13
Emtricitabine* or FTC*, Coviracil*	NNRTI	Not known	13
EMV*, see emivirine*			
Epivir, see lamivudine or 3TC			
Fortovase, see saquinavir (soft gel cap)	PI		11
FTC*, see emtricitabine*			
GW-420867X*	NNRTI	Not known	9
GW-433908* or VX-175*	PI	Associated with hyperglycemia, dysgeusia, and paraoral tingling sensations Do not use with the following medications: midazolam, triazolam, ergotamine, tricyclic antidepressants, or vitamin E Avoid use together with the following medications: erythromycin, benzodiazepine, or itraconazole	9
HIV-1 Immunogen* or Salk vaccine* or AG1661*Remune*	IBT	Not known	2
Hivid, see zalcitabine or ddC			
HU, see hydroxyurea			
Hydroxyurea (HU), Droxia	CI	Oral ulcerations; associated with bleeding and bruising	5
IDV, see indinavir			
Indinavir (IDV), Crixivan	PI	Do not use with the following medications: midazolam, triazolam, or ergotamine Avoid use with the following medications: ketoconazole and dexamethasone	10
Interleukin-2 (IL-2), or aldesleukin, Proleukin	IBT	Not known	6
Invirase, see saquinavir (hard gel cap)			
Kaletra, see lopinavir + ritonavir			
Lamivudine or 3TC, Epivir; also in Combivir and Trizivir	NRTI	Peripheral neuropathy	9
Lopinavir + ritonavir, Kaletra	PI	Associated with hyperglycemia Do not use with the following medications: midazolam or triazolam Avoid use with metronidazole	1
Nelfinavir (NFV), Viracept	PI	Do not use with the following medications: midazolam, triazolam, or ergotamine	2
Nevirapine (NVP), Viramune	NNRTI	Associated with liver damage	4
NFV, see nelfinavir			
Norvir, see ritonavir			
NVP, see nevirapine			
PNU-140690* or tipranavir*	PI	Not known	4
Proleukin, see aldesleukin or interleukin-2			
Remune,* see HIV-1 Immunogen* or Salk vaccine* or AG1661*			
Retrovir, see zidovudine			
Ritonavir (RTV), Norvir; also in Kaletra	PI	Do not use with the following medications: ergotamine, diazepam, midazolam, triazolam, meperidine, piroxicam, or propoxyphene Avoid use with the following medications: phenobarbital, dexamethasone, or metronidazole	1
RTV, see ritonavir			
Salk vaccine* or HIV-1 Immunogen* or AG1661*, Remune*	IBT	Not known	2
Saquinavir (SQV) (HGC) (hard gel cap), Invirase	PI	Associated with liver damage, peripheral neuropathy, and oral ulcerations Do not use with the following medications: midazolam, triazolam, or ergotamine Avoid use with the following medications: clarithromycin, phenobarbital, carbamazepine, dexamethasone, ketoconazole, itraconazole, or clindamycin	11

Continued

TABLE 20-22   Impact of Treatments for HIV Infection (Continued)

Drug Name*	Type of Drug	Adverse Effects of Significance for Dentists	Co.†
Saquinavir (SQV) (SGC) (soft gel cap), Fortovase	PI	Associated with liver damage, peripheral neuropathy, and oral ulcerations Do not use with the following medications: midazolam, triazolam, or ergotamine Avoid use with the following medications: clarithromycin, phenobarbital, carbamazepine dexamethasone, ketoconazole, itraconazole, or clindamycin	11
SQV, see saquinavir			
Stavudine or d4T, Zerit	NRTI	Peripheral neuropathy	5
Sustiva, see efavirenz			
T-20*	EI	Not known	14
TDF*, see tenofovir disoproxil fumarate*			
Tenofovir disoproxil fumarate* (TDF)	NtRTI	Not known	8
Tipranavir* or PNU-140690*	PI	Not known	4
Trizivir, see abacavir + zidovudine +lamivudine			
Videx, see didanosine or ddl			
Videx EC, see didanosine or ddl			
Viracept, see nelfinavir			
Viramune, see nevirapine			
SVX-175* or GW-433908*	PI	Associated with hyperglycemia, dygeusia, and paraoral tingling sensations Do not use with the following medications: midazolam, triazolam, ergotamine, tricyclic antidepressants, or vitamin E Avoid use with the following medications: erythromycin, benzodiazepine, or itraconazole	9
Zalcitabine or ddC, Hivid	NRTI	Associated with oral ulcerations, liver damage, and peripheral neuropathy	11
ZDV, see zidovudine			
Zerit, see stavudine or d4T			
Ziagen, see abacavir			
Zidovudine (ZDV) or AZT, Retrovir; also in Combivir and Trizivir	NRTI	Associated with seizures, rapid uncontrollable eye movements, decreased coordination, liver damage, and peripheral neuropathy	9

CI = cellular inhibitor; EI = entry inhibitor (also fusion inhibitor); IBT = immune-based therapy; NNRTI = non-nucleoside reverse transcriptase inhibitor; NRTI = nucleoside reverse transcriptase inhibitor; NtRTI = nucleotide reverse transcriptase inhibitor; PI = protease inhibitor.

*Drug not approved by US Food and Drug Administration.

†Pharmaceutical companies: 1-Abbott Laboratories; 2-Agouron Pharmaceuticals; 3-BioChem Pharma; 4-Boehringer Ingelheim ; 5-Bristol-Myers Squibb; 6-Chiron Corporation; 7-DuPont Pharmaceuticals; 8-Gilead Sciences; 9-Glaxo Wellcome; 10-Merck & Co.; 11-Roche Laboratories; 12-Sarawak Medichem; 13-Triangle Pharmaceuticals; 14- Trimeris.

acute bacterial endocarditis if they are former intravenous drug users.[171]

Most side effects from medications used to treat HIV disease are associated with xerostomia. Drug interactions with medications commonly used in a dental setting also exist (see Table 20-22). Patients with HIV disease have been shown to survive longer and are therefore more susceptible to develop complications, particularly from drug side effects. A trend suggesting increased frequency of cardiovascular disease has been noticed and should be considered in patients who have taken protease inhibitors for long periods of time.

Treatment planning for HIV-positive patients needs to address numerous considerations. The vast majority of patients have some degree of xerostomia, ranging from very mild to severe. Thus, when performing simple restorative pro-

cedures or fabricating fixed or removable prosthodontics, the type of restorative material, long-term use, and maintenance of a restoration need to be taken into consideration.

ORAL LESIONS

There are no oral lesions that are unique to HIV-infected individuals. All lesions found among HIV-positive patients also occur with other diseases associated with immune suppression. It is therefore not surprising to find a clear correlation between the appearance of oral lesions and a decreased immune system. Several lesions such as oral candidiasis, oral hairy leukoplakia, necrotizing ulcerative periodontal disease, and Kaposi's sarcoma are strongly suggestive of impaired immune response with CD4 cell counts below 200 cells/mm^3.[172–174] Using oral lesions for markers of immune

Date:

Personal and demographic data (including other care providers):

Chief complaint:

History of chief complaint:

Past medical history (including last visit to primary care provider):

HIV test with dates:

    First HIV test—

    Last negative HIV test—

    First positive HIV test—

Reason for HIV test:

Risk factor(s) for HIV:

History of HIV disease (illnesses, signs and symptoms):

CD4 cell count with dates:

    Initial count—

    Lowest count—

    Latest count—

Viral load and dates:

    Highest rate—

    Lowest rate—

    Latest rate—

Complete blood cell count with a differential:

Medications with dosage and schedules:

    Antiretrovirals—

    Anti-infectives—

    Other—

Allergies and drug sensitivity:

Hepatitis (type and status):

Sexually transmitted diseases (type and status):

Tuberculosis (date of test[s] and present status):

Tobacco use (history and present status):

Alcohol use (history and present status):

Recreational drug use (history and present status):

FIGURE 20-7   HIV-relevant history questionnaire.

Name and address of person permitted to disclose information:

....

....

Name and address of individual or organization to which the disclosure is to be made:

....

....

Name and address of patient:

....

....

Purpose of disclosure:

....

....

Information to be disclosed:

....

....

I, ..., hereby give my permission for the above mentioned individual and/or organization/hospital/clinic/laboratory to disclose pertinent medical records to the individual/organization listed above.

I further understand that I may revoke this consent at anytime. Unless revoked earlier by me, this consent expires ....

Patient signature: .... Date..........................

Witness signature: .... Date..........................

FIGURE 20-8   Consent for transmittal of HIV-related information.

suppression and HIV disease progression is important and can impact on medical intervention and treatment strategies.

T-lymphocyte depletion renders affected individuals more susceptible to fungal infections, viral infections, and neoplastic growth. Some immune surveillance is also diminished, enabling bacterial infections to flourish. Thus, it is not surprising to find oral infections of these types in patients with HIV disease.

Fungal Infections. Candidiasis. Intraoral candidiasis,[175,176] which is mainly caused by *Candida albicans*, is the most common oral manifestation in patients with HIV disease. Although it is not in itself pathognomonic for HIV disease, oral candidiasis may be an indication of immune deterioration.[177] A tentative diagnosis of oral candidiasis is usually based on clinical appearance but should be confirmed by laboratory tests. These tests include cytologic smears with potassium hydroxide, biopsy for periodic acid–Schiff and Gram staining for tissue infiltration by spores and hyphae, or culture.[178] In general, oral candidiasis has four different clinical presentations, as follows:

1. Pseudomembranous candidiasis, or thrush. This condition is a common type of oral candidiasis. It manifests as white or yellowish single or confluent plaques that can easily be rubbed off from the oral mucosa (Figure 20-9). It is found on all oral surfaces and may leave an erythematous or even bleeding underlying mucosa. Most patients are not aware of the presence of this form of candidiasis as pseudomembranous candidiasis is predominantly asymptomatic. The condition is noticed most commonly when CD4 cells counts drop below 400 cells/mm^3.

2. Erythematous or atrophic candidiasis. This condition appears on any mucosal surface as a reddish macular lesion, atrophic patches, or depapillation on the dorsum of tongue (Figure 20-10). Erythematous candidiasis may be present alone or in combination with the pseudomembranous type. Patients may complain of an occasional burning sensation in the mouth. Long-standing lesions may even present as mucosal ulcerations.

3. Hyperplastic or chronic candidiasis. This form of candidiasis is relatively uncommon and is found mainly in persons who are severely immunocompromised. Hyperplastic candidiasis, manifesting as white or discolored plaques that may be solitary or confluent and cannot be wiped off the mucosa, may be confused with oral hairy leukoplakia when located on the tongue only (Figure 20-11). Complaints of a burning sensation, dysphagia, and a feeling of having a large piece of cotton in the mouth are not unusual. This type of oral candidiasis is often present with esophageal candidiasis.

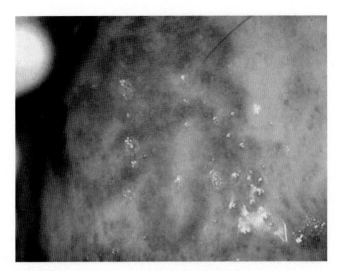

FIGURE 20-10 Erythematous or atrophic candidiasis on the hard palate. These erythematous lesions are usually asymptomatic.

4. Angular cheilitis. This condition, which is predominantly a mixed infection involving *C. albicans* and *Staphyloccocus aureus*, manifests itself as red fissures originating from the labial commissures of the mouth (Figure 20-12). Angular cheilitis may be present with intraoral candidiasis. Concurrent oral dryness also is not uncommon. Angular cheilitis has been associated with vitamin B deficiency and decreased vertical dimension of occlusion from either periodontal disease or ill-fitting dentures. Therefore, it is important to address concurrent conditions as antifungal treatment is instituted.

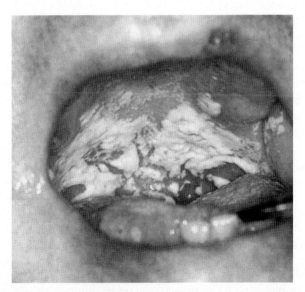

FIGURE 20-11 Hyperplastic or chronic candidiasis on the soft and hard palate of a severely debilitated HIV-infected patient. These lesions cannot be wiped off and do not respond well to topical antifungal medications. This type of candidiasis is almost exclusively seen in patients with extremely low CD4 cell counts and diminished salivary flow.

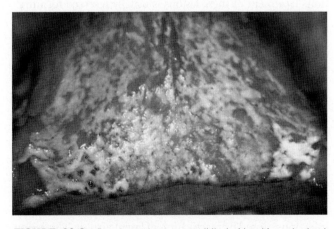

FIGURE 20-9 Pseudomembranous candidiasis (thrush) on the hard and soft palate in a patient with HIV disease. These white plaques can be wiped off, leaving an erythematous mucosa.

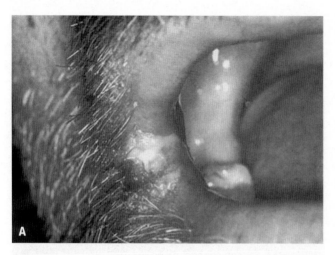
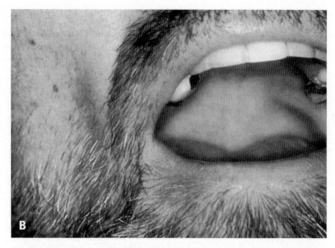

FIGURE 20-12   A, Angular cheilitis is commonly caused by *Candida albicans*. This lesion usually manifests with an ulcer at the corner of the mouth, with erythematous fissures radiating from the ulcer. A pseudomembrane sometimes covers the ulcers. **B,** Treatment with topical antifungal medications and antibiotics, for bacterial superinfections, is usually efficacious.

Treatment of oral candidiasis includes topical and systemic antifungal medications. Appropriate treatment should be instituted to reduce symptoms ranging from localized discomfort to significant dysphagia. Topical therapies include mouth rinses, troches, ointments, and creams. These formulations should be used concurrently with systemic agents to resolve the infection when there is a risk of esophageal candidiasis. Since there is a high sucrose content in these preparations, which predisposes patients to develop dental caries, a strict oral hygiene program and daily flouride treatment should be instituted while the patient is taking topical antifungal medications. Topical antifungal therapies are most efficacious in patients with CD4 counts above 150 to 200 cells/mm³. In patients with atrophic candidiasis, troches should be used with care since they may aggravate existing ulcerations through mechanical abrasion against the lesions.[179]

Common topical treatments include nystatin oral suspension (100,000 units/mL; 10 mL swished and swallowed four to five times per day) and nystatin troche (dissolved in the mouth four to five times per day). Ointments and creams such as 1% clotrimazole ointment, 2% ketoconazole cream, or nystatin cream are efficacious in treating angular cheilitis.

The efficacy of systemic antifungal medications may be significantly reduced by impaired gastric acid secretion and by drug interactions with medications such as rifampin. Furthermore, there exists a potential for liver toxicity that needs to be addressed. Common systemic antifungals include ketoconazole (200 mg tablets; one tablet twice a day with food), fluconazole (100 mg tablets; 200 mg on day 1, followed by 100 mg daily for 14 days),[4] and itraconazole (100 mg tablets; 200 mg daily with food). Resistance to fluconazole has been reported to occur in patients with severe immune deficiency. Treatment of patients who are resistant to fluconazole with a combination of fluconazole and terbinafine has been successful.[180] It is also possible to increase the fluconazole dosage to 600 to 700 mg/d in order to improve efficacy. Another approach to treat fluconazole-resistant fungal infections is to add a topical medication such as clotrimazole troches. This is successful if the resistance is owing to the emergence of *Candida krusei*, a species resistant to fluconazole but susceptible to clotrimazole. Protease inhibitor therapy has been associated with a decreased incidence of oral candidiasis.[177,181] This is owing mainly to improved immune status but may also be a direct result of the protease inhibitors.

Deep-Seated Infections.   Intraoral manifestations of deep-seated fungal infections, caused by *Cryptococcus neoformans*, *Histoplasma capsulatum*, *Geotrichum candidum*, and *Aspergillus* spp, are uncommon and are usually an indication of a disseminated disease.[182,183] Intraoral lesions associated with cryptococcosis, histoplasmosis, and aspergillosis have been reported as being ulcerative, nodular, or necrotic in nature, whereas geotrichosis lesions are described as being pseudomembranous. Since oral lesions of this category are nonspecific, definitive diagnosis requires histologic verification. Treatment of these lesions is usually reserved for intravenous amphotericin B.

Viral Infections.   Although there are no specific oral lesions caused by HIV infection, a patient can display oral manifestations as an early sign of HIV infection. Such oral symptoms may include nonspecific oral ulcerations, sore throat, exudative pharyngitis, and oral candidiasis during the initial acute infection state.[179] These nonspecific manifestations disappear after the acute phase.

Herpesvirus.   Oral herpes simplex virus (HSV) presents both as a local and a disseminated infection. The presence of intraoral HSV-associated lesions is usually the result of recurrent infections caused by reactivation of latent viruses. This lesion is not specifically related to HIV; it is also a fairly common occurrence among non-HIV infected individuals. However,

HSV infections among immunocompromised individuals may be more severe and manifest differently than what is noticed in immunocompetent patients. Although ulcerations caused by HSV-1 and HSV-2 are clinically indistinguishable, HSV-1 is more frequently associated with oral lesions. However, oral lesions caused by HSV-2 appear to have a higher recurrence rate and are associated with a higher incidence of resistance to acyclovir.[164]

HSV in the oral cavity manifests as single or coalescent crops of vesicles with subsequent ulceration and healing. The ulcers are small, shallow, and round to elliptical. In general, recurrent HSV infections occur primarily on more keratinized epithelium such as the gingiva. However, there are numerous reports of oral ulcerations caused by HSV infections on nonkeratinized epithelium in HIV-infected patients. HSV-associated ulcerations are usually accompanied by increased pain during the acute stage, which can affect an individual's nutritional intake. These ulcerations tend to heal in 7 to 10 days, although this may be extended in immunocompromised patients. In this particular patient population, lesions tend to be larger and occur with increased frequency. Furthermore, in these patients, recurrent HSV may exhibit clinical signs and symptoms that are similar to those of primary HSV infection, such as malaise, cervical lymphadenopathy, and intensely painful linear gingival erythema.[164]

Oral manifestations of HSV can be mistaken for other viral infections such as *Cytomegalovirus* and varicella-zoster virus, infection or for aphthous ulcers, and a definitive diagnosis should be made based on the clinical history and laboratory tests, such as cytologic staining for Tzanck cells, viral culture from the ulcer, biopsy, or HSV-1 detection via monoclonal-antibody testing. Treatment for HSV-1 infections usually consists of acyclovir (200 mg orally five times daily). Although famciclovir can also be used, valacyclovir is a poor alternative because it may cause severe side effects in immunocompromised patients. Foscarnet may be used for resistant infections.[184]

Cytomegalovirus. Oral manifestation of *Cytomegalovirus* (CMV) infection is only observed in patients with CD4 counts below 100 cells/mm^3. Lesions associated with CMV are non-specific ulcerations that usually appear as a single ulcer, without preceding vesicles, on any oral mucosal tissue. These ulcers are painful and tend to heal poorly. Differential diagnosis should include recurrent aphthous ulcers and HSV-associated lesions. A definitive diagnosis must include a biopsy specimen that shows basophilic intranuclear inclusions of CMV, or CMV identification via monoclonal-antibody assay or in situ hybridization.[185] A recommended regimen for intraoral lesions is high-dose acyclovir therapy (800 mg orally five times a day) for a minimum of 2 weeks. Oral manifestations of CMV may be associated with disseminated disease, and the patient needs to be evaluated for ophthamologic and other CMV-associated diseases once an oral diagnosis is confirmed.[186]

Epstein-Barr Virus. Epstein-Barr virus (EBV) infections have been associated with numerous manifestations, including infectious mononucleosis, Burkitt's lymphoma, nasopharyngeal carcinoma, and oral hairy leukoplakia. Oral hairy leukoplakia was initially described in individuals with HIV disease, but it has since been found in many other patient populations. This lesion may be present in all phases of HIV disease, but it is most commonly found in individuals with CD4 cell counts below 200 cells/mm^3. It manifests as an asymptomatic white lesion, most frequently with vertical hyperkeratotic striae that are usually seen on the lateral borders of the tongue[187] (Figure 20-13). The lesion may vary from linear striae to white patches that cannot be wiped off, and they often have white hyperkeratotic hairlike projections. Because of its clinical characteristics, differential diagnosis should include hyperplastic candidiasis. Although it is not thought that *Candida albicans* contributes to the clinical appearance of oral hairy leukoplakia, *C. albicans* may be present in more than 50% of oral hairy leukoplakia lesions. When definitive diagnosis of oral hairy leukoplakia needs to be established, it is necessary to verify the presence of EBV in the superficial layers of the involved epithelium. Owing to the significant association between this lesion and HIV, a biopsy is necessary to rule out oral hairy leukoplakia in patients yet to be tested for HIV. In HIV-positive individuals, an empiric diagnosis can be inferred when a clinical lesion resembling oral hairy leukoplakia does not respond to antifungal medications.

It is important to assure the patient that the presence of oral hairy leukoplakia has not been associated with person-to-person transmission of EBV.

Treatment of this lesion usually is not indicated unless the patient complains of esthetic disfiguration or masticatory functional impairment. Antiviral therapy (acyclovir 800 mg orally five times a day) is effective to achieve resolution of the

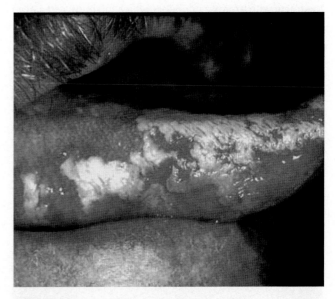

FIGURE 20-13 Oral hairy leukoplakia is an asymtomatic white lesion, caused by Epstein-Barr virus, that is usually found on the tongue. It is rare to find this lesion on other sites in the oral cavity. The lateral borders of the tongue are most commonly affected.

lesion within 2 weeks. Prophylactic therapy with 800 mg acyclovir per day may be necessary to prevent recurrence.

Varicella-Zoster Virus. There have been reports of increased incidence of human varicella-zoster virus (HZV) infections among HIV-infected persons, relative to increased age and degree of immunosuppression. Complications associated with HZV in immunocompromised patients are common and can be severe, especially for those individuals with CD4 counts fewer than 200 cells/mm³.[188] Clinically, oral HZV infection presents as vesicles that quickly rupture, resulting in ulcerations. The ulcers are multiple, shallow, and small, with an erythematous base, and are characteristically distributed unilaterally along a division of the fifth cranial nerve. Patients frequently complain of pain, neuropraxia, and tenderness. Although clinical presentation is distinct for HZV infection, a definitive diagnosis should be confirmed by laboratory tests such as histologic staining for multinucleated giant cells with intranuclear inclusions, direct immunofluorescence, and cytology smears taken from the lesion.

Treatment usually is focused on supportive care and is centered on the prevention of postherpetic neuralgia and dissemination. High doses of oral acyclovir (800 mg orally five times a day), famciclovir (500 mg orally three times a day), or valacyclovir (500 mg orally three times a day) have been efficacious in treating HZV infection. Caution is needed when using valacyclovir in severely immunosuppressed patients as this medication has been associated with hemolysis in this particular patient population. For greatly immunosuppressed patients, intravenous acyclovir therapy may be more appropriate. Foscarnet also may be useful for acyclovir-resistant herpes zoster.[189] It has been reported that there are high incidences of herpes zoster in patients shortly after they start treatment with protease inhibitors, which might suggest a need for prophylaxis for those at increased risk for developing herpes zoster infection.[190]

Human Herpesvirus 8. Recently, human herpesvirus 8 (HHV8) has been linked to the etiology of Kaposi's sarcoma (KS).[191] Most intraoral KS lesions are found on the hard and soft palates, manifesting as red-blue or purple-blue macules or nodules (Figure 20-14). The lesions are initially asymptomatic, but due to trauma and secondary ulcerations, they can become symptomatic as they get larger in size. Large lesions may interfere with the individual's ability to speak, swallow, and masticate. Lesions on the gingiva and tongue are also common; however, extrapalatal lesions are associated with a more rapid progression of KS, as well as HIV disease.

Oral KS is usually seen in patients with CD4 counts below 200 cells/mm³ but can be seen in all stages of HIV disease. The macular lesions can be confused with physiologic pigmentation; a differential diagnosis should also include bacillary (epithelioid) angiomatosis, lymphoma, and trauma.[192] As KS is an AIDS-defining lesion, a definitive diagnosis requires a biopsy.

Treatment for KS includes radiation (800 to 2,000 rad), surgical excision, and intralesional injections with chemotherapeutic agents such as vinblastine sulfate (0.1 mg/mm²) or sodium tetradecyl sulfate (0.1 mg/mm²). Intralesional injections are most effective for small nodular lesions and as an adjuvant to radiation. It is important to realize that most of these treatments do not result in a cure but are used to reduce the size and number of lesions.[193] Recent studies show some efficacy with antiangiogenesis agents, such as thalidomide, and oral 9-*cis* retinoic acid.[194] No antiherpetic medications have shown any benefit as prophylaxis or treatment for KS.

Human Papillomavirus. Oral manifestations with papillomaviruses are similar to human papillomavirus (HPV) infections at other sites. Infections with HPV may cause different distinct appearances, including oral squamous cell papilloma, verruca vulgaris, focal epithelial hyperplasia, and condyloma acuminatum (Figure 20-15). Each lesion has a specific expression of an identified HPV genotype. Oral

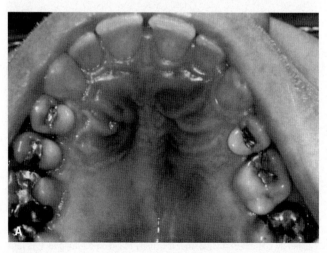
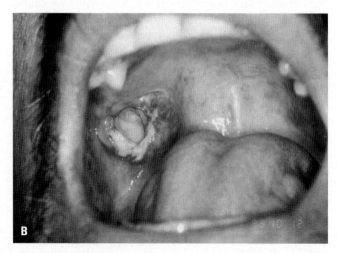

FIGURE 20-14 A, Initial lesions of Kaposi's sarcoma are usually found on the hard and soft palates. These lesions are commonly bluish-red macules. **B,** Long-standing palatal lesions may become nodular and even ulcerative.

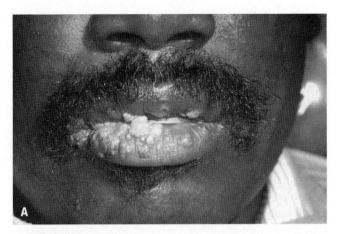
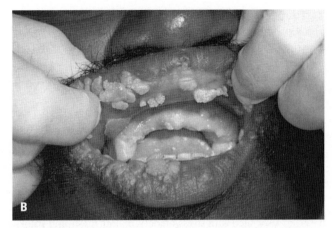

FIGURE 20-15 Human papillomavirus has become more common in individuals whose immune system is undergoing changes, such as reconstitution after severe CD4 cell depletion. Florid lesions may affect the lips **(A)** and intraoral mucosa **(B)**.

squamous cell papillomas may present as exophytic pedunculated papules with a cauliflower-like appearance. Verruca vulgaris (the common wart) is a firm, sessile, exophytic, and whitish lesion. This form of HPV presentation also has a hyperkeratinized superficial epithelium with a slight invagination of the center of the lesion. Focal epithelial hyperplasia (Heck's disease) may present as a single or multiple, smooth or pebble-like, hyperplastic leukoplakic lesion. Focal epithelial hyperplasia is commonly found on keratinized tissues such as the alveolar mucosa and the lips. Condyloma acuminatum presents as small white-to-pink nodules with a pebbled surface and is most commonly found on the soft and hard palates and the tongue.[195] The presence of HPV-associated lesions is not pathognomonic for HIV infection or progression. However, an increase in the prevalence of oral HPV infections among HIV-infected persons has been reported since the introduction of protease inhibitors.

Although most of oral HPV manifestations are asymptomatic, unless lesions are induced by trauma, they can interfere with mastication and may raise cosmetic concerns. Treatments for HPV include surgical removal, laser ablation, cryotherapy, and topical application of keratinolytic agents. For smaller lesions, topical application of 25% podophyllum resin may be used to reduce the size. A more novel approach has been the use of intralesional injection of antiviral agents. Interferon-α in intralesional injections (1,000,000 IU/cm² once weekly) and subcutaneous injections (3,000,000 IU/cm² twice weekly) have been shown to be effective in long-term resolution of lesions.[196]

Bacterial Infection. *Periodontal Disease.* The most common oral manifestations of bacterial origin are associated with periodontal conditions. These conditions are usually categorized by their clinical appearance and include linear gingival erythema (LGE), necrotizing ulcerative gingivitis (NUG), and necrotizing ulcerative periodontitis (NUP). It has also been noted that HIV-seropositive patients with previous periodontal disease may show faster rates of conventional periodontal deterioration as compared with those of HIV-seronegative persons. Lamster and colleagues have suggested that the progression of periodontal disease in HIV-infected persons is dependent on the immunologic competency of the host and local host response to typical and atypical microorganisms related to periodontal disease.[197] Thus, the level of immune suppression, as demonstrated by decreasing number of T-cell lymphocytes, in combination with the degree of plaque accumulation, may explain these conditions in HIV-infected patients.[173]

Linear gingival erythema is an atypical gingivitis that is depicted as a 2 to 3 mm distinct band of fiery redness at the marginal gingiva around the teeth (Figure 20-16). Such erythema is not proportional to the plaque accumulation and seems to only affect the soft tissue, without any ulcerations, increased pocket depths, or any attachment loss. Patients with this condition are usually asymptomatic. The true prevalence of LGE is difficult to determine due to variable diagnostic criteria that have been put forth.

Differential diagnosis should include a localized erythema due to dry mucosa associated with mouth breathing, lichen planus, mucous membrane pemphigoid, or an allergic reaction. The most recent theory regarding the pathogenesis of this lesion implicates subgingival candida infection as a possible cause.[197]

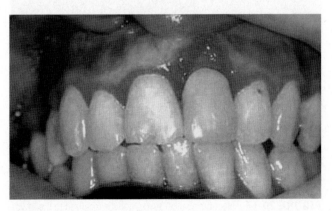

FIGURE 20-16 Linear gingival erythema of the gingival margin.

Treatments include improved oral home care and conventional dental scaling and root planing, along with the use of chlorhexidine gluconate (0.12%) mouth rinses (15 mL swished and expectorated twice a day) for up to 3 months. Additionally, concomitant use of topical antifungal medications may be beneficial.

Manifestations of *NUG* and *NUP* are triggered by changes in the immune status, most probably aggravated by intraoral bacteria. The two entities may present as a continuum of the same disease but also may appear as separate entities. NUG is limited to the gingiva (Figure 20-17), whereas NUP is characterized by localized to generalized aggressive alveolar bone and attachment destruction (Figure 20-18). Occurrence of NUG has been associated with stress, anxiety, malnutrition, and smoking. Patients with NUG complain of spontaneous gingival bleeding and mild to moderate gingival pain. NUP is associated with complaints of deep-seated bone pain, spontaneous gingival bleeding, halitosis, and tooth mobility. Clinically, these conditions are presented with initial lesions of limited craterlike necrosis of gingival papillae. When untreated, NUP may progress at a rate of 1 to 2 mm of soft- and hard-tissue destruction per week. NUP is mostly seen with severe immune suppression, with CD4 counts below 100 cells/mm³.[173]

A definitive diagnosis is based on clinical evaluation and radiologic evaluation with panoramic radiographs or specific periapical dental radiographs. Specific laboratory tests may be needed to rule out conditions and lesions such as bullous lesions of benign mucous membrane pemphigoid, erythema multiforme, acute forms of leukemia, and major aphthous ulceration.

Treatment for both NUG and NUP consists of débridement of necrotic soft and hard tissue, antibiotic therapy with metronidazole or tetracycline (500 mg four times a day) for a week, and a follow-up with scaling and débridement.[173] Due to the high risk for fungal infections in these patients, an antifungal regimen may be prescribed together with the antibiotics. Chlorohexidine gluconate (0.12%) mouth rinses are recommended as maintenance therapy. Metronidazole should be used with caution in patients who are taking lopinavir and retonavir.

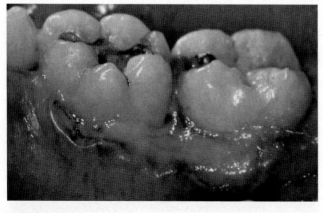

FIGURE 20-17 Necrotizing ulcerative gingivitis localized to the lower first and second molars.

Tuberculosis. Intraoral lesions associated with TB may present as single nonhealing caseating granulomatous ulcerations that are accompanied by deep-seated pain. The lesions have been noted on the tongue, the palate, the buccal mucosa, and the angles of the mouth.[198] Diagnosis by clinical presentation alone is difficult and needs to be complemented with demonstration of acid-fast TB bacilli within the lesion.[199] Treatment is locally palliative as an adjunct to systemic TB therapy.

Syphilis. Clinical presentation of syphilis includes chancres, snail-track ulcers, and gumma formation.[200] Chancres are mostly asymptomatic indurated ulcers with a brown crusted appearance that are usually seen on the lips, oral mucosa, tongue, palate, and posterior pharyngeal wall. Secondary syphilis is characterized by highly infectious mucosal ulcers with an appearance of white lesions surrounded by an erythematous base. Frank ulceration is most common in tertiary syphilis as a result of gummatous destruction. It is usually seen on the palate and tongue.

Differential diagnosis should include herpetic cold sores, deep-seated fungal infections, mycobacteria-associated ulcer, malignant ulcers, and trauma. A definitive diagnosis is made by dark-field microscopy that demonstrates the etiologic agent, *Treponema pallidum*. Treatment is based on appropriate systemic antibiotic therapy.

Nonspecific Ulcerations. *Necrotizing Stomatitis.* Necrotizing stomatitis is a localized acute painful ulcerative lesion on mucosal surfaces overlying bone (Figure 20-19). This condition eventually leads to necrosis of tissue and subsequent bone exposure. No specific microbial agent or mechanism has been linked to its etiology. This condition is seen in patients with CD4 cells fewer than 100 cells/mm³.[168] Differential diagnosis includes aphthous ulcer and NUP. Treatment consists of careful débridement, local or systemic steroid therapy, antibiotics, and institution of a soft-tissue stent to protect the affected area from further trauma and for delivery of topical medications.[201]

Aphthous Ulcers. Recurrent aphthous ulcerations (RAUs) are idiopathic oral ulcerations. There are three disease entities of RAUs: minor, major, and herpetiform. Diagnosis of RAUs is a diagnosis of exclusion; the clinical impression should be confirmed with histologic examination and by response to treatment.[179]

Minor (recurrent) aphthous ulcerations are smaller than 10 mm in diameter, well-circumscribed, round, sometimes covered by a yellow-gray pseudomembrane, and surrounded by an erythematous halo. The erythematous halo may be absent in severely immunocompromised patients due to their lack of an intact inflammatory response. Minor aphthous ulcerations are usually confined to the nonkeratinized oral mucosa and tend to recur, often at the same site. Their duration is about 1 to 2 weeks, and healing occurs without scarring. Minor aphthous ulcerations are prevalent in both non–HIV-infected populations and HIV-infected populations.

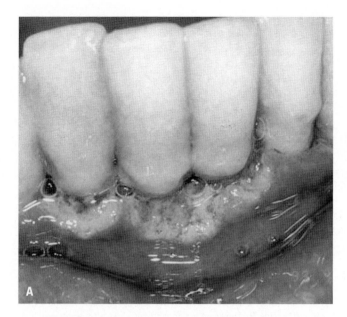

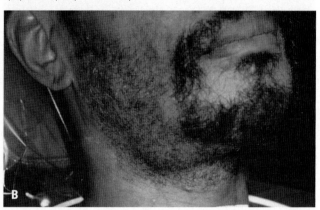

FIGURE 20-18 Necrotizing ulcerative periodontitis of the lower anterior region. **A,** Both gingival and alveolar bone are affected. **B,** Submandibular lymphadenopathy can also be present.

Differential diagnosis includes recurrent HSV infection. Treatment is focused to provide symptomatic relief. An analgesic mouth rinse, such as 2 to 4% viscous lidocaine solution (10 mL swished and expectorated), is most commonly instituted for relief.

Major (recurrent) aphthous ulcerations are larger than 10 mm in diameter, well-circumscribed, round, and shallow or deep with indurated margins (Figure 20-20). A gray pseudomembrane covering the lesion may sometimes be present. Major aphthous ulcerations can occur on any area of the oral mucosa. They are usually single ulcerations, but in immunosuppressed individuals, groups of up to 10 lesions have been observed. These ulcers tend to persist for more than 3 weeks and to heal with a scar formation. In patients with

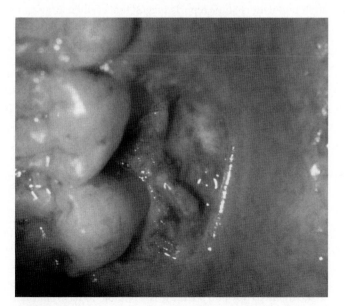

FIGURE 20-19 Necrotizing stomatitis on the palatal area of the upper first and second molars.

HIV, major aphthous ulcers have been associated with severe immune suppression, with CD4 counts below 100 cells/mm^3, and are markers for HIV disease progression.[202]

Treatment for major aphthous ulcerations includes administration of systemic corticosteroids. Topical formulations of clobetasol or fluocinonide gel applied directly to the lesion, dexamethasone elixir mouth rinses (0.5 mg/5 mL), and systemic administration of 60 to 80 mg of prednisone per day for 10 days have been used successfully. For steroid-resistant patients, alternative therapy of 100 to 200 mg thalidomide may be used. Thalidomide needs to be used with caution because of its severe adverse side effects. However, despite its severe side effects, thalidomide has been used with some success to treat both oral and esophageal ulcerations. Refractory cases may be treated with other agents including colchicine or levamisole.[203] Antibiotics and antifungal agents may be used concurrently when appropriate to prevent bacterial or fungal superinfections.

Herpetiform ulcers are the least common type of aphthous ulcers. These ulcers are pinpoint (smaller than 1 mm in diameter) and round, with perilesional erythema. They are usually found in batches of up to 100, appearing on nonkeratinized mucosa such as the ventral surface of the tongue and soft palate. Healing occurs without scarring. Treatments are similar to those for minor aphthous ulcers and include symptomatic relief, suppression of the local pathologic immune reaction, and treatment of any concomitant superinfection.

Drug-Induced Ulcerations. Several medications that are frequently used for HIV-infected patients have been associated with the development of oral ulcerations.[204–206] These medications include zidovudine, zalcitabine, foscarnet, interferon, and ganciclovir.[207] Drug-induced ulcerations are mainly seen on nonkeratinized mucosa, but they tend to affect keratinized mucosa in more severely immunocompromised patients.

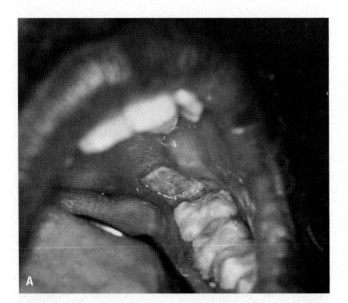 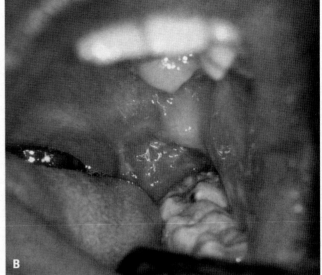

FIGURE 20-20   A, Major aphthous ulcer in the retromolar region in an HIV-infected patient. **B,** The same major aphthous ulcer, after treatment.

Certain antiretroviral therapies induce neutropenia and are thereby linked to the occurrence of oral ulcerations. Administration of a growth factor such as granulocyte-macrophage colony-stimulating factor has shown to be successful in resolving ulcerations associated with neutropenia.[208]

Xerostomia.   Xerostomia, or dry mouth, is a subjective symptomatic complaint that is frequently noted by HIV-infected patients. It has been reported that reduced salivary flow occurs in 2 to 10% of HIV-infected individuals.[207] However, the true prevalence is 80 to 90% of all patients taking HAART. The effect of oral dryness on quality of life is profound, and many patients with severe xerostomia sometimes opt to change or stop their antiretroviral medications in order to regain better salivary functions.

The most common cause of decreased salivary flow in HIV-infected patients is side effects of pharmocotherapeutic agents. Many medications, such as antiretroviral medications (including nucleoside transcriptase inhibitors, protease inhibitors) as well as antihistamines, anticholinergics, antihypertensives, decongestants, narcotic analgesics, and tricyclic antidepressants, have been associated with xerostomia. In addition, xerostomia may be a result of HIV-associated salivary gland disease in this population. The parotid glands are most frequently affected; however, minor salivary glands can also be affected by viral infection such as with CMV.[209] Another cause of reduced salivary flow is radiation therapy to the head and neck area, causing functional impairment of salivary glands in the radiated area.

Treatment for xerostomia focuses on symptomatic relief by encouraging patients to hydrate themselves frequently and to minimize the intake of caffeine and alcohol, which act as diuretics. Patients are also recommended to use commercially available artificial saliva substitutes (Xero-lube, Sali-synt, Moi-stir, Orex) to achieve relief. The use of pilocarpine and bethanechol to stimulate salivary flow can also be useful.

Ultimately, discontinuation or substitution of xerostomia-inducing drugs may be necessary.

Oral Lesions in the Pediatric Population.   HIV-infected children may also develop a spectrum of oral lesions. These lesions can affect children more severely than adults and can be a significant source of pain with subsequent limitation of oral intake of nutrition and medications.

The most common oral manifestation in immunocompromised children is candidiasis.[210] The presence of oral candidiasis in HIV-infected infants, as well as other clinical symptoms, is used as a clinical marker for disease progression in a prognosis-based clinical staging system. Clinical presentation of oral candidiasis in the pediatric population is similar to that of the adult population. Some reports suggest that erythematous candidiasis is more common than the pseudomembranous type in HIV-infected children.[211] A definitive diagnosis should be accompanied by laboratory tests, as described previously.

Both topical and systemic treatment with antifungal medications can be used to treat oral candidiasis. Several reports have shown that there are subtypes of *Candida* that are isolated in candidal lesions.[211,212] Therefore, it is not unreasonable to determine a specific subtype of *Candida* and to select a specific antifungal agent directed toward the subtype. A report has shown that fluconazole suspension (6 mg/kg loading dose followed by 3 mg/kg/d) has been highly effective and is superior to routine nystatin rinses.[213] In children who are fed by bottle, it is possible to place the antifungal medication inside the nipple, as well as to cover the nipple with a thin layer of topical medication.

Several of the medications used by children are made to taste better by the addition of sugar formulations, which also make them syrupy and sticky. It is advisable to have children rinse their mouths with water after administration of these medications in order to reduce the incidence of tooth decay.

▼ REFERENCES

1. Burnet M. Natural history of infectious disease. Cambridge: Cambridge University Press; 1962.

2. Institute of Medicine. Emerging infections: microbial threats to health in the United States. Washington: National Academy Press; 1992.

3. Centers for Disease Control and Prevention. Achievements in public health, 1990–1999: control of infectious diseases. MMWR Morb Mortal Wkly Rep 1999;48:621–9.

4. Centers for Disease Control and Prevention. Tuberculosis and acquired immunodeficiency syndrome—Florida. MMWR Morb Mortal Wkly Rep 1986; 35:587.

5. Centers for Disease Control and Prevention. Tuberculosis morbidity in the United States: final data, 1990. MMWR Morb Mortal Wkly Rep 1991;40(SS-3):23.

6. Bernardo J. Tuberculosis: a disease of the 1990's. Hosp Pract 1991;26:195.

7. Centers for Disease Control and Prevention. Tuberculosis morbidity—United States, 1997. MMWR Morb Mortal Wkly Rep 1998;47:253.

8. American Thoracic Society. Control of tuberculosis in the United States. Am Rev Respir Dis 1992;146:1623.

9. Dolin PJ, Raviglione MC, Kochi A. Global tuberculosis incidence and mortality during 1990–2000. Bull World Health Org 1994;72:213.

10. World Health Organization. Report on the tuberculosis epidemic. Geneva, Switzerland: WHO; 1997.

11. Centers for Disease Control and Prevention. Summary of notifiable diseases—1998. MMWR Morb Mortal Wkly Rep 1999;47:70.

12. Centers for Disease Control and Prevention. World TB day—March 24, 2001. MMWR Morb Mortal Wkly Rep 2001;50:201.

13. Centers for Disease Control and Prevention. Core curriculum on tuberculosis. 3rd ed. Atlanta: US Department of Health and Human Services; 1994.

14. Bates JH, Stead WW. The history of tuberculosis as a global epidemic. Med Clin North Am 1993;77:1205.

15. Orme IM, Anderson P, Boom WH. T cell response to *Mycobacterium tuberculosis*. J Infect Dis 1993;167:1481.

16. Ellner JJ. The immune response in human tuberculosis: implications for tuberculosis control. J Infect Dis 1997;176:1351.

17. Mani NJ. Tuberculosis initially diagnosed by asymptomatic oral lesions. J Oral Med 1985;40:39.

18. Molinari JA, Chandrasekar PH. Mycobacteria. In: Willett NP, White RR, Rosen S, editors. Essential dental microbiology. Norwalk: Appleton and Lange; 1991. p. 181.

19. Selwyn PA, Hartel D, Lewis VA, et al. A prospective study of the risk of tuberculosis among intravenous drug users with human immunodeficiency virus infection. N Engl J Med 1989;320:545.

20. Reider HL, Jereb JA, Frieden TR, et al. Epidemiology of tuberculosis in the United States. Epidemiol Rev 1989;11:79.

21. Theuer CP, Hopewell PC, Elias D, et al. Human immunodeficiency virus infection in tuberculosis patients. J Infect Dis 1990;162:8.

22. Small PM, Schecter GF, Goodman PC, et al. Treatment of tuberculosis in patients with advanced human immunodeficiency virus infection. N Engl J Med 1991;324:289.

23. Barnes PF, Bloch AB, Davidson PT, et al. Tuberculosis in patients with human immunodeficiency virus infection. N Engl J Med 1991;324:1644–50.

24. Styblo K. Recent advances in epidemiological research in tuberculosis. Adv Tuberc Res 1980;20:1.

25. Van Scoy RE, Wilkowske CJ. Antituberculous agents. Mayo Clin Proc 1992;67:179.

26. Centers for Disease Control and Prevention. Initial therapy for tuberculosis in the era of multidrug resistance: recommendations of the Advisory Council for the Elimination of Tuberculosis. J Am Med Assoc 1993;270:696.

27. Cohen ML. Epidemiology of drug resistance: implications for a post-antimicrobial era. Science 1992;257:1050.

28. Frieden TR, Sterling T, Pablos-Mendez A, et al. The emergence of drug-resistant tuberculosis in New York City. N Engl J Med 1993;328:521.

29. Shearer BG. MDR-TB: another challenge from the microbial world. J Am Dent Assoc 1994;125:43.

30. Raviglione MC, Dye C, Schmidt S, et al. Assessment of worldwide tuberculosis control. WHO global surveillance and monitoring project. Lancet 1997;350:624.

31. Luelmo F. BCG vaccination. Am Rev Respir Dis 1982;125:70.

32. Jacobs JR Jr. Advances in mycobacterial genetics: new promises for old diseases. Immunobiol 1992;184:147.

33. Cleveland JL, Gooch DF, Bolyard EA, et al. TB infection control recommendations from the CDC, 1994: considerations for dentistry. J Am Dent Assoc 1995;126:593.

34. US Department of Health and Human Services, Centers for Disease Control and Prevention. Guidelines for preventing the transmission of *Mycobacterium tuberculosis* in healthcare facilities. MMWR Morb Mortal Wkly Rep 1994;43(RR-13):1.

35. Field MJ, editor. Tuberculosis in the workplace. Washington (DC): National Academy Press; 2001.

36. Fraser DW, Tsai TR, Orenstein W, et al. Legionnaires' disease: description of an epidemic of pneumonia. N Engl J Med 1977;297:1189.

37. Centers for Disease Control and Prevention. Follow-up on respiratory illness—Philadelphia. MMWR Morb Mortal Wkly Rep 1977; 26:9.

38. McDade JE, Shepard CC, Fraser DW, et al. Legionnaires' disease: isolation of a bacterium and demonstration of its role in other respiratory disease. N Engl J Med 1977;297:1197.

39. Brenner DJ, Steigerwalt AG, McDade JE. Classification of the legionnaires' disease bacterium: *Legionella pneumophila*, genus *novum*, species *nova*, of the family *Legionellaceae*, family *nova*. Ann Intern Med 1978;90:656.

40. McDade JE, Brenner DJ, Bozeman FM. Legionnaires' disease bacterium isolated in 1947. Ann Intern Med 1979;90:659.

41. Rowbotham TJ. Current views on the relationship between amoebae, legionellae, and man. Isr J Med Sci 1986;22:1218.

42. Rowbotham TJ. Isolation of *Legionella pneumophila* from clinical specimens via amoebae, and the interaction of those and other isolates with amoebae. J Clin Pathol 1983;36:978.

43. Stout JE, Yu VL, Best M. Ecology of *Legionella pneumophila* within water distribution systems. Appl Environ Microbiol 1985;49:221.

44. Muder R, Yu VL, Woo A. Mode of transmission of *Legionella pneumophila*: a critical review. Arch Intern Med 1986;146:1607.

45. Johnson JT, Yu VL, Best M, et al. Nosocomial legionellosis uncovered in surgical patients with head and neck cancer: implications for epidemiologic reservoir and mode of transmission. Lancet 1985;2:298.

46. Stout JE, Yu VL, Muraca ME, et al. Potable water as a cause of sporadic cases of community-acquired pneumonia. N Engl J Med 1992;326:151.

47. Shands K, Ho J, Meyer R, et al. Potable water as a source of legionnaires' disease. J Am Med Assoc 1985;253:1412.

48. Stout JE, Yu VL, Muraca P. Legionnaires' disease acquired within the homes of two patients: link to the home water supply. J Am Med Assoc 1987;257:1215.

49. Kaufman AF, McDade J, Patton C, et al. Pontiac fever: isolation of the etiologic agent (*Legionella pneumophila*) and demonstration of its mode of transmission. Am J Epidemiol 1981;114:337.

50. Fotos PG, Westfall HN, Snyder IS, et al. Prevalence of *Legionella*–specific IgG and IgM antibody in a dental clinic population. J Dent Res 1985;64:1382.

51. Reinthaler FF, Mascher F, Stunzer D. Serological examinations for antibodies against *Legionella* species in dental personnel. J Dent Res 1988;67:942.

52. Yu VL. *Legionella pneumophila* (legionnaires' disease). In: Mandell GL, Bennett JE, Dolin R, editors. Principles and practice of infectious diseases. 5th ed. Churchill Livingstone; 2000. p. 2424.

53. Centers for Disease Control and Prevention. Sustained transmission of nosocomial legionnaires' disease—Arizona and Ohio. MMWR Morb Mortal Wkly Rep 1997;46:416.

54. Lowry PW, Tompkins LS. Nosocomial legionnellosis: a review of pulmonary and extrapulmonary syndromes. Am J Infect Control 1993;21:21.

55. Kirby BD, Snyder KM, Meyer RD, et al. Legionnaires' disease: report of sixty-five nosocomially-acquired cases and review of the literature. Medicine 1980;59:188.

56. Seu P, Winston DJ, Olthoft KM, et al. Legionnaires' disease in liver transplant recipients. Infect Dis Clin Pract 1993;2:109.

57. Singh N, Muder RR, Yu VL, et al. *Legionella* infection in liver transplant recipients: implications for management. Transplantation 1993;56:1549.

58. Tyzzer EE. A sporozoan found in the peptic glands of the common mouse. Proc Soc Exp Biol Med 1907;5:12.

59. Nime FA, Burek JD, Page DL, et al. Acute gastroenterocolitis in a human being infected with the protozoan *Cryptosporidium*. Gastroenterol 1976;70:592.

60. Current WL. Human cryptosporidiosis. N Engl J Med 1983;309:1325.

61. Peterson C. Cryptosporidiosis in patients infected with the human immunodeficiency virus. Clin Infect Dis 1992;15:903.

62. Laughon BE, Druckman DA, Vernon A, et al. Prevalence of enteric pathogens in homosexual men with and without acquired immunodeficiency syndrome. Gastroenterol 1988;94:984.

63. Smith PD, Lane HC, Gill VJ, et al. Intestinal infections in patients with the acquired immunodeficiency syndrome. Ann Intern Med 1988;108:328.

64. Pederson C, Danner S, Lazzarin A, et al. Epidemiology of cryptosporidiosis among European AIDS patients. Genitourin Med 1996;72:128.

65. Vakil NB, Schwartz SM, Buggy BP, et al. Biliary cryptosporidiosis in HIV-infected people after the waterborne outbreak of cryptosporidiosis in Milwaukee. N Engl J Med 1996;334:19.

66. Haas CN, Rose JB. Reconciliation of microbial risk models and outbreak epidemiology: the case of the Milwaukee outbreak. Proc Am Water Works Assoc 1994;517.

67. Fricker C, Crabb J. Waterborne cryptosporidiosis: detection methods and treatment options. Adv Parasitol 1998;40:242.

68. MacKenzie WR, Hoxie NJ, Proctor ME, et al. A massive outbreak in Milwaukee of *Cryptosporidium* infection transmitted through the public water supply. N Engl J Med 1994;331:161.

69. Hayes EB, Matte TD, O'Brien TR, et al. Large community outbreak of cryptosporidiosis due to contamination of a filter public water supply. N Engl J Med 1989;320:1372.

70. McAnulty JM, Fleming DW, Gonzalez AH. A community-wide outbreak of cryptosporidiosis associated with swimming at a wave pool. J Am Med Assoc 1994;272:1597.

71. Goldstein ST, Juranek DD, Ravenholt O, et al. Cryptosporidiosis: an outbreak associated with drinking water despite state-of-the-art water treatment. Ann Intern Med 1996;124:459.

72. Newman RD, Zu S-X, Wuhib T, et al. Household epidemiology of *Cryptosporidium parvum* infection. Ann Intern Med 1994;120:500.

73. Cordell RL, Addiss DG. Cryptosporidiosis in child care settings: a review of the literature and recommendations for prevention and control. Pediatr Infect Dis 1994;13:311.

74. Koch RL, Phillips DJ, Aber RC, et al. Cryptosporidiosis in hospital personnel. Ann Intern Med 1985;102:593.

75. Miron D, Kenes J, Dagan R. Calves as a source of an outbreak of cryptosporidiosis among young children in an agricultural closed community. Pediatr Infect Dis 1991;10:438.

76. Millard PS, Gensheimer KF, Addiss DG, et al. An outbreak of cryptosporidiosis from fresh-pressed apple cider. J Am Med Assoc 1994;272:1592.

77. Ungar BLP. *Cryptosporidium*. In: Mandell GL, Bennett JE, Dolan R, editors. Principles and practice of infectious diseases. 5th ed. New York: Churchill Livingstone; 2000. p. 2903.

78. Dupont H, Chappell C, Sterling C, et al. The infectivity of *Cryptosporidium parvum* in healthy volunteers. N Engl J Med 1995;332:885.

79. Alter HJ, Holland PV, Purcell RH. The emerging pattern of post-transfusion hepatitis. Am J Med Sci 1975;270:329.

80. Alter HJ, Purcell RH, Holland PV, et al. Clinical and serological analysis of transfusion-associated hepatitis. Lancet 1975;2:838.

81. Choo Q-L, Kuo G, Weiner, et al. Isolation of a cDNA clone derived from a blood-borne non-A, non-B viral hepatitis genome. Science 1989;244:359.

82. Kuo G, Choo Q-L, Alter HJ, et al. An assay for circulating antibodies to a major etiologic virus of human non-A, non-B hepatitis. Science 1989;244:362.

83. Bukh J, Miller RH, Purcell RH. Genetic heterogeneity of hepatitis C virus: quasispecies and genotypes. Semin Liver Dis 1995;15:41.

84. Cha T-A, Beall E, Irvine B, et al. At least five related, but distinct, hepatitis C viral genotypes exist. Proc Natl Acad Sci U S A 1992;89:7144.

85. Chan S-W, McOmish F, Holmes EC, et al. Analysis of a new hepatitis C virus type and its phylogenetic relationship to existing variants. J Gen Virol 1992;73:1131.

86. Rall CJN, Dienstag JL. Epidemiology of hepatitis C virus infection. Semin Gastrointest Dis 1995;6:3.

87. Alter MJ, Kruszon-Moran D, Nainan OV, et al. The prevalence of hepatitis C virus infection in the United States, 1988 through 1994. N Engl J Med 1999;341:556.

88. Seeff LB. Natural history of viral hepatitis, type C. Semin Gastrointest Dis 1995;6:20.

89. Dienstag JL. Non-A, non-B hepatitis. I. Recognition, epidemiology, and clinical features. Gastroenterology 1983;85:439.

90. Koretz RL, Abbey H, Coleman E, et al. Non-A, non-B post-transfusion hepatitis: looking back on the second decade. Ann Intern Med 1993;119:110.

91. Centers for Disease Control and Prevention. Recommendations for prevention and control of hepatitis C virus (HCV) infection and HCV-related chronic diseases. MMWR Morb Mortal Wkly Rep 1998;47(RR-19):1.

92. Ohto H, Terazawa S, Sasaki N, et al. Transmission of hepatitis C virus from mothers to infants. N Engl J Med 1994;330:744.

93. Liang JT, Rhermann J, Seeff LB, et al. NIH conference: pathogenesis, natural history, treatment, and prevention of hepatitis C. Ann Intern Med 2000;132:296.

94. Armstrong GL, Alter MJ, McQuillan GM, et al. The past incidence of hepatitis C virus infection: implications for the future burden of chronic liver disease in the United States. Hepatology 2000;31:777.

95. American Health Consultants. Fasten your seat belts: hospitals face a bumpy ride as hepatitis C cases peak. Hosp Infect Cont 2000;27:129.

96. Food and Drug Administration. New blood screening tests for hepatitis C. FDA Drug Bull 1990; October: 9.

97. Roth WK, Lee JH, Ruster B, et al. Comparison of two quantitative hepatitis C virus reverse transcriptase PCR assays. J Clin Microbiol 1996;34:261.

98. Alter MJ, Hadler SC, Judson FN, et al. The natural history of community-acquired hepatitis C in the United States. N Engl J Med 1992;327:1899.

99. Aach RD, Stevens CE, Hollinger FB, et al. Hepatitis C infection in post-transfusion hepatitis: an analysis with first- and second-generation assays. N Engl J Med 1991;325:1325.

100. Tremolada F, Casarin C, Alberti A, et al. Long-term follow-up of non-A, non-B (type C) post-transfusion hepatitis. J Hematol 1992;16:273.

101. Alter HJ, Seeff LB: Recovery, persistence and sequelae in hepatitis C infection: a perspective on long-term outcome. Semin Liver Dis 2000;20:17.

102. Kiyosawa K, Sodeyama T, Tanaka E, et al. Hepatitis C in hospital employees with needlestick injuries. Ann Intern Med 1991;115:367.

103. Lanphear BP, Linneman CC Jr, Cannon CG, et al. Hepatitis C virus infection in healthcare workers: risk of exposure and infection. Infect Control Hosp Epidemiol 1994;15:745.

104. Schlipkoter U, Roggendorf M, Cholmakow K, et al. Transmission of hepatitis C (HCV) from a hemodialysis patient to medical staff member. Scand J Infect Dis 1990;22:757.

105. Vaglia A, Nicolin R, Puro V, et al. Needlestick hepatitis C seroconversion in a surgeon. Lancet 1990;336:1315.

106. Ippolito G, Puro V, Petrosillo N, et al. Simultaneous infection with HIV and hepatitis C virus following occupational conjunctival blood exposure. J Am Med Assoc 1998;280:28.

107. Klein RS, Freeman K, Taylor PE, et al. Occupational risk for hepatitis C infection among New York City dentists. Lancet 1991;338:1539.

108. Cleveland JL, Gooch BF, Shearer BG, et al. Risk and prevention of hepatitis C infection: implications for dentistry. J Am Dent Assoc 1999;130:641.

109. Lanphear BP. Trends and patterns in the transmission of bloodborne pathogens to health care workers. Epidemiol Rev 1994;16:437.

110. Hoofnagle JH, Mullen KD, Jones DB, et al. Treatment of chronic non-A, non-B hepatitis with recombinant human alpha interferon: a preliminary report. N Engl J Med 1986;315:1575.

111. Thomson BJ, Doran M, Lever AML, et al. Alpha-interferon therapy for non-A, non-B hepatitis transmitted by gamma-globulin replacement therapy. Lancet 1987;1:539.

112. Food and Drug Administration. Interferon alfa-2b approved for hepatitis C. FDA Med Bull 1991;21(2):5.

113. National Institute of Health Consensus Development Conference Panel Statement. Management of hepatitis C. Hepatology 1997;26 Suppl 1:28.

114. Alter MJ, Mast EE, Moyer LA. Hepatitis C. Infect Dis Clin North Am 1998;12:13.

115. Keeffe E. Hepatitis C: current and future treatment. Infect Med 2000;17:603.

116. AIDS epidemic update: December 2000. UNAIDS/WHO; 2000.

117. Centers for Disease Control and Prevention. *Pneumocystis* pneumonia—Los Angeles. MMWR Morb Mortal Wkly Rep 1981;30:250.

118. Centers for Disease Control and Prevention. Kaposi's sarcoma and *Pneumocystis* pneumonia among homosexual men—New York City and California. MMWR Morb Mortal Wkly Rep 1981;30:305.

119. Centers for Disease Control and Prevention. A cluster of Kaposi's sarcoma and *Pneumocystis carinii* pneumonia among homosexual male residents of Los Angeles and Orange counties, California. MMWR Morb Mortal Wkly Rep 1982;31:305.

120. Jaffe HW, Choi K, Thomas PA, et al. National case-control study of Kaposi's sarcoma and *Pneumocystis carinii* pneumonia in homosexual men: part 1, epidemiologic results. Ann Intern Med 1983;99:145.

121. Centers for Disease Control and Prevention. Immunodeficiency among female sexual partners of males with acquired immune deficiency syndrome (AIDS)—New York. MMWR Morb Mortal Wkly Rep 1983;31:697.

122. Harris C, Small CB, Klein RS, et al. Immunodeficiency in female sexual partners of men with the acquired immunodeficiency syndrome. N Engl J Med 1983;308:1181.

123. Centers for Disease Control and Prevention. *Pneumocystis carinii* pneumonia among persons with hemophilia A. MMWR Morb Mortal Wkly Rep 1982;31:365.

124. Centers for Disease Control and Prevention. Possible transfusion-associated acquired immune deficiency syndrome (AIDS)— California. MMWR Morb Mortal Wkly Rep 1982;31:652.

125. Centers for Disease Control and Prevention. Unexplained immunodeficiency and opportunistic infections in infants—New York, New Jersey, and California. MMWR Morb Mortal Wkly Rep 1982;31:665.

126. Barre-Sinoussi F, Chermann JC, Rey F, et al. Isolation of a T-lymphotropic retrovirus from a patient at risk for acquired immune deficiency syndrome (AIDS). Science 1983;220:868.

127. Gallo RC, Salahuddin SZ, Popovic M, et al. Frequent detection and isolation of cytopathic retroviruses (HTLV-III) from patients with AIDS and at risk for AIDS. Science 1984;224:500.

128. Centers for Disease Control and Prevention. 1993 revised classification system for HIV infection and expanded surveillance case definition for AIDS among adolescents and adults. MMWR Morb Mortal Wkly Rep 1992;41:1.

129. Centers for Disease Control and Prevention. HIV/AIDS surveillance report. 2000;12:1.

130. Bozzette S, Berry SH, Duan N, et al. The care of HIV-infected adults in the United States. N Engl J Med 1998;339:1897.

131. Gao F, Bailes E, Robertson DL, et al. Origin of HIV-1 in the chimpanzee *Pan troglodytes*. Nature 1999;396:437.

132. Hahn BH, Shaw GM, De Cook KM, et al. AIDS as a zoonosis; scientific and public health implications. Science 2000;287:6076.

133. Ciesielski CA, Marianos DW, Schochetman G, et al. The 1990 Florida dental investigation. The press and the science. Ann Intern Med 1994;121:886.

134. Piatak M, Saag MS, Lang LC, et al. High levels of HIV-1 in plasma during all stages of infection determined by competitive PCR. Science 1993;259:1749.

135. Perelson AS, Neumann AU, Markowitz M, et al. HIV-1 dynamics in vivo: virion clearance rate, infected cell life-span, and viral generation time. Science 1996;271:1582.

136. Coffin JM. HIV population dynamics in vivo: implications for genetic variation, pathogenesis, and therapy. Science 1995;267:483.

137. Schuurman R, Nijhuis M, van Leeuwen R, et al. Rapid changes in human immunodeficiency virus type 1 RNA load and appearance of drug-resistant virus populations in persons treated with lamivudine (3TC). J Infect Dis 1995;171:1411.

138. Stein DS, Korvick JA, Vermund SH. CD4+ lymphocyte cell enumeration for prediction of clinical course of human immunodeficiency virus disease: a review. J Infect Dis 1992;165:352.

139. Mellors JW, Munoz A, Giorgi J, et al. Plasma load and CD4+ lymphocytes as prognostic markers of HIV-1 infection. Ann Intern Med 1997;126:946.

140. Mulder J, McKinney N, Christopherson C, et al. A rapid and simple PCR assay for quantification of HIV-1 RNA in plasma: application to acute retroviral infection. J Clin Microbiol 1994;32:292.

141. Welles SL, Jackson JB, Yen-Lieberman B, et al. Prognostic value of plasma human immunodeficiency virus type 1 (HIV-1) RNA levels in patients with advanced HIV-1 disease and with little or no prior zidovudine therapy. J Infect Dis 1996;174:696.

142. Coombs RW, Welles SL, Hooper C, et al. Association of plasma human immunodeficiency virus type 1 RNA level with risk of clinical progression in patients with advanced HIV infection. J Infect Dis 1996;174:704.

143. O'Brien WA, Hartigan PM, Martin D, et al. Changes in plasma HIV-1 RNA and CD4+ lymphocyte counts and the risk of progression to AIDS. N Engl J Med 1996;334:425.

144. Katzenstein DA, Hammer SM, Hughes MD, et al. The relation of virologic and immunologic markers to clinical outcomes after nucleoside therapy in HIV-infected adults with 200 to 500 CD4 cells per cubic millimeter. N Engl J Med 1996;335:1091.

145. Marschner IC, Collier AC, Coombs RW, et al. Use of changes in plasma levels of human immunodeficiency virus type-1 RNA to assess the clinical benefit of antiretroviral therapy. J Infect Dis 1998;177:40.

146. Quinn TC, Wawer MJ, Sewankambo N, et al. Viral load and heterosexual transmission of human immunodeficiency virus type 1. N Engl J Med 2000;342:921.

147. Jacquez J, Koopman J, Simon C, et al. Role of the primary infection in epidemics of HIV infection in gay cohorts. J Acquir Immune Defic Syndr 1994;7:1169.

148. Rich JD, Merriman NA, Mylonakis E, et al. Misdiagnosis of HIV infection by HIV-1 plasma viral load testing: a case series. Ann Intern Med 1999;130:37.

149. Musey L, Hughes J, Schacker T, et al. Cytotoxic-T-cell responses, viral load, and disease progression in early human immunodeficiency virus type 1 infection. N Engl J Med 1997;337:1267.

150. Rosenberg ES, Billingsley JM, Caliendo AM, et al. Vigorous HIV-1-specific CD4+ T-cell responses associated with control of viremia. Science 1997;278:1447.

151. Daar ES, Little SJ, Pitt JA, et al. Protease inhibitor (PI)- and non-PI-containing antiretroviral therapy (ART) compared to no treatment in primary HIV infection (PHI) [abstract402]. Program and abstracts of the 8th Conference on Retroviruses and Opportunistic Infections; 2001 Feb 4–8; Chicago, Illinois.

152. Lifson AR, Rutherford TW, Jaffe HW. The natural history of human immunodeficiency virus infection. J Infect Dis 1988;158:1360.

153. Kaplan JE, Hanson D, Dworkin MS, et al. Epidemiology of human immunodeficiency virus-associated opportunistic infections in the United States in the era of highly active antiretroviral therapy. Clin Infect Dis 2000;30:S5.

154. Michelet C, Arvieux C, François C, et al. Opportunistic infections occurring during highly active antiretroviral treatment. AIDS 1998;12:1815.

155. Haynes BF, Pantaleo G, Fauci AS. Toward an understanding of the correlates of protective immunity to HIV infection. Science 1996;271:324.

156. Dean M, Carrington M, Winkler C, et al. Genetic restriction of HIV-1 infection and progression to AIDS by a deletion allele of the CKR5 structural gene. Hemophilia Growth and Development Study, Multicenter AIDS Cohort Study, Multicenter Hemophilia Cohort Study, San Francisco City Cohort, ALIVE Study. Science 1996;273:1856.

157. Horuk R. Chemokine receptors and HIV-1: the fusion of two major research fields. Immunol Today 1999;20:89.

158. McDermott DH, Zimmerman PA, Guignard F, et al. CCR5 promoter polymorphism and HIV-1 disease progression. Lancet 1998;352:866.

159. Levy JA, Mackewicz CE, Barker E. Controlling HIV pathogenesis: the role of the noncytotoxic anti-HIV response of CD8(+) T cells. Immunol Today 1996;17:217.

160. Richman DD, Bozzette SA. The impact of the syncytium-inducing phenotype of human immunodeficiency virus on disease progression. J Infect Dis 1994;169:968.

161. Berger EA, Murphy PM, Farber JM. Chemokine receptors as HIV-1 coreceptors: roles in viral entry, tropism, and disease. Ann Rev Immunol 1999;17:657.

162. Learmont J, Geczy A, Raynes-Greenow C, et al. The Sydney Blood Bank Cohort infected with attenuated quasispecies of HIV-1: long-term nonprogression [abstract 13350]. XII World AIDS Conference; 1998 June 28–July 3; Geneva, Switzerland.

163. Klein MR, VanBaalen CA, Holwerden AM, et al. Kinetics of Gag-specific cytotoxic T lymphocyte responses during the clinical course of HIV-1 infection: a longitudinal analysis of rapid progressors and long-term asymptomatics. J Exp Med 1995;181:1365.

164. Glick M. Dental management of patients with HIV. Carol Stream (IL): Quintessence Publishing Co, Inc.; 1994.

165. Abel SN, Croser D, Fischman SL, et al. Dental Alliance for AIDS/HIV Care (DAAC): principles of dental management for the HIV-infected patient. Dental Alliance for AIDS/HIV Care; 1999.

166. Patton LL, Glick M. Clinician's guide to treatment of HIV-infected patients. 3rd ed. American Academy of Oral Medicine; 2001.

167. Glick M, Abel S. Dental implants and HIV disease. Implant Dent 1993;2:149.

168. Dodson TB, Perrott DH, Gongloff RK, et al. Human immunodeficiency virus serostatus and the risk of postextraction complications. Int J Maxillofac Surg 1994;2:100.

169. Glick M, Abel S, Muzyka B, et al. Dental complications after treating patients with AIDS. J Am Dent Assoc 1994;125:296.

170. Patton LL, Shugars DC. Immunologic and viral markers of HIV-1 disease progression: implications for dentistry. J Am Dent Assoc 1999;130:1313.

171. Glick M. Intravenous drug users: a consideration for infective endocarditis in dentistry? [editorial] Oral Surg Oral Med Oral Pathol Oral Radiol Endod 1995;80:125.

172. Glick M, Muzyka BC, Lurie D, et al. Oral manifestations associated with HIV disease as markers for immune suppression and AIDS. Oral Surg Oral Med Oral Pathol 1994;77:344.

173. Glick M, Muzyka BC, Salkin LM, et al. Necrotizing ulcerative periodontitis: a marker for immune deterioration and a predictor for the diagnosis of AIDS. J Periodontol 1994;65:393.

174. Patton LL. Sensitivity, specificity, and positive predictive value of oral opportunistic infections in adults with HIV/AIDS as markers of immune suppression and viral burden. Oral Surg Oral Med Oral Pathol Oral Radiol Endod 2000;90:182.

175. Glick M, Berthold P. Oral manifestations and conditions found in individuals with HIV infection. In: Buckley RM, editor. HIV infection in primary care. Philadelphia (PA): W. B. Saunders; [In press]

176. Muzyka BC, Glick M. A review of oral fungal infections and appropriate therapy. J Am Dent Assoc 1995;126:63.

177. Patton LL, McKaig R, Strauss R, et al. Changing prevalence of oral manifestations of human immunodeficiency virus in the era of protease inhibitor therapy. Oral Surg Oral Med Oral Pathol Oral Radiol Endod 2000;89:299.

178. Barr CE, Glick M. Diagnosis and management of oral and cutaneous lesions in HIV-1 disease. Oral Maxillofac Surg Clin North Am 1998;1:25.

179. Kademani D, Glick M. Oral ulcerations in individuals infected with human immunodeficiency virus: clinical presentations, diagnosis, management, and relevance to disease progression. Quintessence Int 1998;29:523.

180. Ghannoum MA, Elewski B. Successful treatment of fluconazole resistant oropharyngeal candidiasis by a combination of fluconazole and terbinafine. Clin Diagn Lab Immunol 1999;6:921.

181. Diz Dios P, Ocampo A, Miralles C, et al. Frequency of oropharyngeal candidiasis in HIV-infected patients on protease inhibitor therapy. Oral Surg Oral Med Oral Pathol Oral Radiol Endod 1999;87;437.

182. Glick M, Cohen SG, Cheney RT, et al. Oral manifestations of disseminated Cryptococcus in a patient with acquired immunodeficiency syndrome. Oral Surg Oral Med Oral Pathol 1987;64:454.

183. Heinic GS, Greenspan D, MacPhail LA, et al. Oral Geotrichum candidum infection associated with HIV infection. A case report. Oral Surg Oral Med Oral Pathol 1992;73:726–8.

184. MacPhail LA, Greenspan D, Shiodt M, et al. Acyclovir-resistant, foscarnet-sensitive oral herpes simplex type 2 lesion in a patient with AIDS. Oral Surg Oral Med Oral Pathol 1989;67:427.

185. Heinic GS, Northfelt DW, Greenspan JS, et al. Concurrent oral CMV and HSV infection in association with HIV infection: a case report. Oral Surg Oral Med Oral Pathol 1993;75:488.

186. Glick M, Cleveland DB, Salkin LM, et al. Intraoral Cytomegalovirus lesion and HIV-associated periodontitis in a patient with acquired immunodeficiency syndrome. Oral Surg Oral Med Oral Pathol 1991;72:716.

187. Kabani S, Greenspan D, deSouze Y, et al. Oral hairy leukoplakia with extensive oral mucosal involvement. Oral Surg Oral Med Oral Pathol 1989;67:411.

188. Glesby MJ, Moore RD, Chaisson RE. Clinical spectrum of herpes zoster in adults infected with human immunodeficiency virus. Clin Infect Dis 1995;21:370.

189. Breton G, Fillet AM, Katlama C, et al. Acyclovir-resistant herpes zoster in human immunodeficiency virus–infected patients: results of foscarnet study. Clin Infect Dis 1998;27:1525.

190. Martinez E, Gatell J, Moran Y, et al. High incidence of herpes zoster in patients with AIDS soon after protease inhibitor therapy. Clin Infect Dis 1998;27:1510.

191. Ensoli B, Sgadari C, Barillari G, et al. Biology of Kaposi's sarcoma. Eur J Cancer 2001;1251.

192. Glick M, Cleveland DB. Oral mucosal bacillary (epithelioid) angiomatosis in a patient with AIDS-associated with rapid alveolar bone loss: a case report. J Oral Pathol Med 1993;22:235.

193. Muzyka BC, Glick M. Sclerotherapy for the treatment of nodular intraoral Kaposi's sarcoma in patients with AIDS [correspondence]. N Engl J Med 1993;328:210.

194. Yarchoan R. Therapy for Kaposi's sarcoma: recent advances and experimental approaches. J AIDS 1999;21:S66.

195. Itin PH, Latenschlager S. Viral lesions of the mouth in HIV-infected patients. Dermotology 1997;194:1.

196. Lozada-Nur F, Glick M, Shubert M, et al. Use of intralesional interferon-alpha for the treatment of recalcitrant oral warts in patients with AIDS: report of 4 cases. Oral Surg Oral Med Oral Pathol Oral Radiol Endod. [In press]

197. Lamster IB, Grbic JT, Mitchell-Lewis D, et al. New concepts regarding the pathogenesis of periodontal disease in HIV infection. Ann Periodontol 1998;3:62.

198. Dimitrakopolous I, Zouloumis L, Lazaridis N, et al. Primary tuberculosis of the oral cavity. Oral Surg Oral Med Oral Pathol 1991;72:712.

199. Eng HL, Lu SY, Yang CH, et al. Oral tuberculosis. Oral Surg Oral Med Oral Pathol Oral Radiol Endod 1996;81:415.

200. Ficarra G, Zaragoza AM, Stendardi L, et al. Early oral presentation of lues maligna in a patient with HIV infection. Oral Surg Oral Med Oral Pathol 1993;75:728.

201. Muzyka BC, Glick M. Necrotizing stomatitis and AIDS. Gen Dent 1994;42:66.

202. Muzyka BC, Glick M. Major aphthous ulceration in patients with HIV disease. Oral Surg Oral Med Oral Pathol 1994;77:116.

203. Glick M, Muzyka BC. Alternative therapies for major aphthous ulcers in AIDS patients. J Am Dent Assoc 1992;123:61.

204. Gilquin J, Weiss L, Kazatchkine MD. Genital and oral erosions induced by foscarnet. Lancet 1990;335:287.

205. McLeod GX, Hammer SM. Zidovudine: five years later. Ann Intern Med 1992;117:487.

206. McNeely MC, Yarchoan R, Broder S, et al. Dermatologic complications associated with administration of 2'3'-dideoxycytidine in patients with human immunodeficiency virus. J Am Acad Dermatol 1989;21:1213.

207. Shiodt M. Less common oral lesions associated with HIV infection: prevalence and classification. Oral Dis 1997;3:S208.

208. Luzzi GA, Jones BJ. Treatment of neutropenic oral ulceration in human immunodeficiency virus infection with G-CSF. Oral Surg Oral Med Oral Pathol Oral Radiol Endod 1996;81:53.

209. Greenberg MS, Glick M, Nghiem L, et al. Relationship of *Cytomegalovirus* to salivary gland dysfunction in HIV-infected patients. Oral Surg Oral Med Oral Pathol Oral Radiol Endod 1997;83:334.

210. Flaitz CM, Hicks MJ. Oral candidiasis in children with immune suppression: clinical appearance and therapeutic considerations. ASDC J Dent Child 1999;66:161.

211. Nicolatou O, Theodoridou M, Mostrou G, et al. Oral lesions in children with perinatally acquired human immunodeficiency virus infection. J Oral Pathol Med 1999;28:49.

212. Velegraki A, Nicolatou O, Theodoridou M, et al. Paediatric AIDS-related linear gingival erythema: a form of erythematous candidiasis? J Oral Pathol Med 1999;28:178.

213. Flynn PM, Cunningham CK, Kerkering T, et al. Oropharyngeal candidiasis in immunocompromised children: a randomized, multicenter study of orally administered fluconazole suspension versus nystatin. J Pediatr 1995;127;322.

21

DIABETES MELLITUS

BRIAN MEALEY, DDS, MS

Diabetes mellitus is a metabolic disease characterized by dysregulation of carbohydrate, protein, and lipid metabolism. The primary feature of this disorder is elevation in blood glucose levels (hyperglycemia), resulting from either a defect in insulin secretion from the pancreas, a change in insulin action, or both. Sustained hyperglycemia has been shown to affect almost all tissues in the body and is associated with significant complications of multiple organ systems, including the eyes, nerves, kidneys, and blood vessels. These complications are responsible for the high degree of morbidity and mortality seen in the diabetic population.

▼ EPIDEMIOLOGY AND CLASSIFICATION

About 16 million Americans have diabetes (between 6 and 7% of the total US population).[1] Around the world, the prevalence of diabetes is expected to double between 1994 and 2010, at which time about 240 million people will have the disease.[2] In the United States, the incidence of diabetes rises as the population ages and as the prevalence of obesity increases. Unfortunately, about half of those Americans with diabetes are presently unaware that they have the disease. Most dental practices have a significant number of diabetic patients in their population. Based on US prevalence data, an "average" practice would have between 60 and 70 diabetic individuals for every 1,000 patients, and 30 to 35 of these patients would be undiagnosed.[3]

The American Diabetes Association provided the most recent classification of diabetes mellitus, in 1997[4] (Table 21-1). The most common forms of diabetes are termed type 1 and type 2. Type 1 diabetes was previously called insulin-dependent diabetes or juvenile diabetes while type 2 diabetes was formerly known as non-insulin-dependent diabetes or adult-onset diabetes. The older terminology was often confusing

TABLE 21-1   Classification of Diabetes Mellitus

Type 1 (insulin-dependent diabetes; juvenile diabetes)

Type 2 (non-insulin-dependent diabetes; adult-onset diabetes)

Gestational diabetes (pregnancy diabetes)

Other types of diabetes

   Genetic defects affecting beta-cell function or insulin action

   Pancreatic diseases or injuries (pancreatic cancer, pancreatitis, traumatic injury, cystic fibrosis, pancreatectomy)

   Infections (congenital rubella, *Cytomegalovirus* infection)

   Drug-induced diabetes (steroid hormones [glucocorticoids], thyroid hormone)

   Endocrine disorders (hyperthyroidism, Cushing's syndrome, glucagonoma, acromegaly, pheochromocytoma)

   Other genetic syndromes (with associated diabetes)

Reproduced with permission from American Diabetes Association.[4]

since both insulin-dependent and non-insulin-dependent diabetic individuals may take insulin as part of their management regimen. The difference is that type 1 patients are truly dependent on insulin therapy whereas type 2 patients may benefit from insulin therapy but are not dependent on it for survival. The new classification system minimizes this confusion because it is based on the pathophysiology of the different disease types, rather than on the treatment methodology used.

Gestational diabetes occurs during pregnancy and usually resolves after delivery. Other types of diabetes may occur in individuals with certain genetic disorders, pancreatic diseases, infections, injuries to the pancreas, and endocrine diseases. Drug therapy with certain agents may also induce a diabetic state.

▼ PATHOPHYSIOLOGY

An understanding of the pathophysiology of diabetes rests upon knowledge of the basics of carbohydrate metabolism and insulin action.[3] Following the consumption of food, carbohydrates are broken down into glucose molecules in the gut. Glucose is absorbed into the bloodstream elevating blood glucose levels. This rise in glycemia stimulates the secretion of insulin from the beta cells of the pancreas. Insulin is needed by most cells to allow glucose entry. Insulin binds to specific cellular receptors and facilitates entry of glucose into the cell, which uses the glucose for energy. The increased insulin secretion from the pancreas and the subsequent cellular utilization of glucose results in lowered of blood glucose levels. Lower glucose levels then result in decreased insulin secretion.

If insulin production and secretion are altered by disease, blood glucose dynamics will also change. If insulin production is decreased, glucose entry into cells will be inhibited, resulting in hyperglycemia. The same effect will be seen if insulin is secreted from the pancreas but is not used properly by target cells. If insulin secretion is increased, blood glucose levels may become very low (hypoglycemia) as large amounts of glucose enter tissue cells and little remains in the bloodstream.

Following meals, the amount of glucose available from carbohydrate breakdown often exceeds the cellular need for glucose. Excess glucose is stored in the liver in the form of glycogen, which serves as a ready reservoir for future use. When energy is required, glycogen stores in the liver are converted into glucose via glycogenolysis, elevating blood glucose levels and providing the needed cellular energy source. The liver also produces glucose from fat (fatty acids) and proteins (amino acids) through the process of gluconeogenesis. Glycogenolysis and gluconeogenesis both serve to increase blood glucose levels. Thus, glycemia is controlled by a complex interaction between the gastrointestinal tract, the pancreas, and the liver.

Multiple hormones may affect glycemia (Table 21-2). Insulin is the only hormone that lowers blood glucose levels. The counter-regulatory hormones such as glucagon, catecholamines, growth hormone, thyroid hormone, and glucocorticoids all act to increase blood glucose levels, in addition to their other effects.

Type 1 Diabetes

The underlying pathophysiologic defect in type 1 diabetes is an autoimmune destruction of pancreatic beta cells.[4] Following this destruction, the individual has an absolute insulin deficiency and no longer produces insulin. Autoimmune beta cell destruction is thought to be triggered by an environmental event, such as a viral infection.[2] Genetically determined susceptibility factors increase the risk of such autoimmune phenomena.

The onset of type 1 diabetes is usually abrupt. It generally occurs before the age of 30 years, but may be diagnosed at any age. Most type 1 diabetic individuals are of normal weight or are thin in stature. Since the pancreas no longer produces insulin, a type 1 diabetes patient is absolutely dependent on exogenously administered insulin for survival. People with type 1 diabetes are highly susceptible to diabetic ketoacidosis. Because the pancreas produces no insulin, glucose cannot enter cells and remains in the bloodstream. To meet cellular energy needs, fat is broken down through lipolysis, releasing glycerol and free fatty acids. Glycerol is converted to glucose for cellular use. Fatty acids are converted to ketones, resulting in increased ketone levels in body fluids and decreased hydrogen ion concentration (pH). Ketones are excreted in the urine, accompanied by large amounts of water. The accumulation of

TABLE 21-2   Hormonal Regulation of Blood Glucose

Hormone	Main Site of Hormone Production	Effect on Blood Glucose Levels
Insulin	Pancreas (beta cells)	Decrease
Glucagon	Pancreas (alpha cells)	Increase
Growth hormone	Pituitary gland	Increase
Thyroid hormone	Thyroid gland	Increase
Catecholamines (epinephrine)	Adrenal gland (medulla)	Increase
Glucocorticoids	Adrenal gland (cortex)	Increase

ketones in body fluids, decreased pH, electrolyte loss and dehydration from excessive urination, and alterations in the bicarbonate buffer system result in diabetic ketoacidosis (DKA). Untreated DKA can result in coma or death.

Many patients with type 1 diabetes are initially diagnosed with the disease following a hospital admission for DKA. In a known diabetic patient, periods of stress or infection may precipitate DKA. More often, however, DKA results from poor daily glycemic control. Patients who remain severely hyperglycemic for several days or longer due to inadequate insulin administration or excessive glucose intake are prone to developing DKA.

Type 2 Diabetes

About 90% of diabetic Americans have type 2 diabetes.[4] The prevalence of type 2 diabetes is higher in African Americans, Native Americans, Hispanics, and Pacific Islanders than it is in Caucasians. Most type 2 diabetes patients are overweight, and most are diagnosed as adults. The genetic influence in type 2 diabetes is greater than that seen with type 1.[5] While concordance rates between monozygous twins for type 1 diabetes are about 30 to 50%, the rate is approximately 90% for type 2 diabetes.[4,5] Although the genetic predisposition to type 2 diabetes is strong, no single genetic defect has been found.[6] In addition to genetic influences, acquired risk factors for type 2 diabetes include obesity, advancing age, and an inactive lifestyle.

The underlying pathophysiologic defect in type 2 diabetes does not involve autoimmune beta-cell destruction. Rather, type 2 diabetes is characterized by the following three disorders: (1) peripheral resistance to insulin, especially in muscle cells; (2) increased production of glucose by the liver; and, (3) altered pancreatic insulin secretion. Increased tissue resistance to insulin generally occurs first and is eventually followed by impaired insulin secretion. The pancreas produces insulin, yet insulin resistance prevents its proper use at the cellular level. Glucose cannot enter target cells and accumulates in the bloodstream, resulting in hyperglycemia. The high blood glucose levels often stimulate an increase in insulin production by the pancreas; thus, type 2 diabetic individuals often have excessive insulin production (hyperinsulinemia). Over the years, pancreatic insulin production usually decreases to below normal levels. In addition to hyperglycemia, type 2 diabetic patients often have a group of disorders that has been called "insulin resistance syndrome" or syndrome X[7,8] (Table 21-3).

TABLE 21-3 Disorders Associated with Type 2 Diabetes (Insulin Resistance Syndrome or Syndrome X)

Hyperglycemia

Hypertension

Dyslipidemia
  Elevated triglycerides
  Decreased high-density lipoprotein

Central (abdominal) obesity

Atherosclerosis

Obesity contributes greatly to insulin resistance, even in the absence of diabetes.[9] In fact, weight loss is a cornerstone of therapy for obese type 2 diabetic patients. Insulin resistance generally decreases with weight loss. Obesity also may explain the dramatic increase in the incidence of type 2 diabetes among young individuals in the United States in the past 10 to 20 years. Once considered a disease of adults, type 2 diabetes has increased among America's youth in direct correlation with the increase in the average weight of children and young adults during that time period.

Type 2 diabetes usually has a slow onset and may remain undiagnosed for years.[3,7] Approximately half of those who have type 2 diabetes are unaware of their disease. Unfortunately, the insidious nature of the disease allows prolonged periods of hyperglycemia to begin exerting negative effects on major organ systems. By the time many type 2 diabetic patients are diagnosed, diabetic complications have already begun. Type 2 diabetic patients do not require exogenous insulin for survival since they still produce insulin. However, insulin injection is often an integral part of medical management for type 2 diabetes. Unlike type 1 diabetic patients, individuals with type 2 diabetes are generally resistant to DKA because their pancreatic insulin production is often sufficient to prevent ketone formation. Severe physiologic stress may induce DKA in those with type 2 diabetes. Long periods of severe hyperglycemia may result in hyperosmolar nonketotic acidosis. Hyperglycemia results in the urinary excretion of large amounts of glucose, with attendant water loss. If fluids are not replaced, the dehydration can result in electrolyte imbalance and acidosis.

Gestational Diabetes

Gestational diabetes occurs in approximately 4% of pregnancies in the United States.[10] It usually develops during the third trimester and significantly increases perinatal morbidity and mortality.[11] The proper diagnosis and management of gestational diabetes improves pregnancy outcomes.[12] As with type 2 diabetes, the pathophysiology of gestational diabetes is associated with increased insulin resistance. Most patients with gestational diabetes return to a normoglycemic state after parturition; however, about 30 to 50% of women with a history of gestational diabetes will develop type 2 diabetes within 10 years.

Impaired Glucose Tolerance and Impaired Fasting Glucose

The conditions known as impaired glucose tolerance (IGT) and impaired fasting glucose (IFG) represent metabolic states lying between diabetes and normoglycemia.[7] People with IFG have increased fasting blood glucose levels but usually have normal levels following food consumption. Those with IGT are normoglycemic most of the time but can become hyperglycemic after large glucose loads. IGT and IFG are not considered to be clinical entities; rather, they are risk factors for future diabetes.[13] The pathophysiology of IFG and IGT is related primarily to increased insulin resistance whereas endogenous insulin secretion is normal in most patients.

Approximately 30 to 40% of individuals with IGT or IFG will develop type 2 diabetes within 10 years after onset.

▼ CLINICAL PRESENTATION, LABORATORY FINDINGS, AND DIAGNOSIS

The onset of type 1 diabetes is usually abrupt whereas type 2 diabetes is often present for years without overt signs or symptoms. Patients with undiagnosed diabetes may present with one or more signs and symptoms (Table 21-4). The diagnosis of diabetes is based on the presence of clinical signs and symptoms, along with specific laboratory findings. The most recent diagnostic guidelines were established by the American Diabetes Association in 1997 (Table 21-5).[14] These guidelines provide for the use of fasting glucose and casual (nonfasting) glucose levels for diagnosis and restrict routine use of the oral glucose tolerance test. The diagnosis of diabetes is not made until the patient has exceeded threshold glucose levels on two separate occasions. Urinary glucose analysis is no longer used in establishing the diagnosis of diabetes.

Both the fasting and casual plasma glucose tests provide a determination of glucose levels at a single moment in time, namely, at the time the blood sample is collected. It is often useful to assess the long-term control of glycemia, especially in known diabetic patients. The glycated (or glycosylated) hemoglobin assay (also called the glycohemoglobin test) allows the determination of blood glucose status over the 30 to 90 days prior to collection of the blood sample. As glucose circulates in the bloodstream, it becomes attached to a portion of the hemoglobin molecule on red blood cells. The higher the plasma glucose levels are over time, the greater is the percentage of hemoglobin that becomes glycated. There are two different glycated hemoglobin assays: the hemoglobin A_1 (HbA_1) test and the hemoglobin A_{1c} (HbA_{1c}) test. Because these tests measure two different portions of the hemoglobin molecule, the normal ranges for the test results differ.[15] The normal HbA_1 value is less than approximately 8% whereas the normal HbA_{1c} value is less than 6.0 to 6.5%. These tests are not cur-

rently standardized across all laboratories; therefore, glycated hemoglobin values must be interpreted in the context of normal ranges for the specific laboratory performing the test. The American Diabetes Association recommends that individuals with diabetes attempt to achieve a target HbA_{1c} value of less than 7% whereas an HbA_{1c} value of more than 8% suggests that a change in patient management may be needed to improve glycemic control.[16] The glycated hemoglobin assay is not currently recommended as a screening tool or as an initial test for the diagnosis of diabetes. It is used to monitor glycemic control in patients with previously diagnosed diabetes.

Another assay that can be used to determine long-term glucose control is the fructosamine test.[17] This test is not used as widely as the glycated hemoglobin assay but is often helpful in managing women with gestational diabetes. The fructosamine assay assesses glycemic control over the 2 to 4 weeks preceding the test. The normal range for fructosamine is 2.0 to 2.8 mmol/L. This test may become more widely used in the future, since at-home testing is now available.

Self–blood glucose monitoring (SBGM) has revolutionized patient management of diabetes.[18] The development of small handheld glucometers has allowed the diabetic individual to take much greater control of his or her disease. Glucometers use a small drop of capillary blood from a fingerstick sample to assess glucose levels within seconds. Almost all insulin-using diabetic patients (and many who are on oral agents) have glucometers. There are many different glucometers available, and the frequency with which the patient tests his or her blood glucose depends on that patient's individual treatment regimen. Some patients test once a day or even less often. Others, especially those taking insulin, test many times each day. As a general rule, more intensively managed diabetic patients use SBGM more frequently than less intensively managed individuals.

▼ COMPLICATIONS

The major cause of the high morbidity and mortality rate associated with diabetes is a group of microvascular and macrovascular complications affecting multiple organ systems (Table 21-6).[3] People with diabetes have a greatly increased risk for blindness, kidney failure, myocardial infarction, stroke, necessary limb amputation, and a host of other maladies. The onset and progression of these complications is strongly linked to the presence of sustained hyperglycemia. The complication rate and the severity of complications increase as the duration of diabetes increases. Other disorders (such as hypertension and dyslipidemia) commonly seen in people with diabetes increase the risk for microvascular and macrovascular complications. There may also be genetic determinants of risk for diabetic complications.

The vascular complications result from atherosclerosis and microangiopathy.[19–21] Increased lipid deposition and atheroma formation is seen in the larger blood vessels, along with increased thickness of arterial walls. Proliferation of endothelial cells, alterations in endothelial basement mem-

---

TABLE 21-4 Signs and Symptoms of Undiagnosed Diabetes

Polydipsia (excessive thirst)

Polyuria (excessive urination)

Polyphagia (excessive hunger)

Unexplained weight loss

Changes in vision

Weakness, malaise

Irritability

Nausea

Dry mouth

Ketoacidosis*

*Ketoacidosis is usually associated with severe hyperglycemia and occurs primarily in type 1 diabetes.

TABLE 21-5 Laboratory Diagnostic Criteria for Diabetes

Diagnosis is by any of the following three methods and *must be confirmed on a subsequent day* by any one of the same three methods.

1. Presence of diabetes symptoms plus casual (nonfasting) plasma glucose ≥ 200 mg/dL (casual glucose may be drawn at any time of day without regard to time since last meal)

2. Fasting plasma glucose* ≥ 126 mg/dL (fasting is defined as no caloric intake for at least 8 hours)

3. Two-hour postprandial glucose[†] ≥ 200 mg/dL during an oral glucose tolerance test using a glucose load containing the equivalent of 75 g of anhydrous glucose dissolved in water[‡]

Reproduced with permission from Lester E.[14]

*Categories of fasting plasma glucose are as follows: < 110 mg/dL = normal; ≥ 110 mg/dL and < 126 mg/dL = impaired; ≥ 126 mg/dL = provisional diagnosis of diabetes (must be confirmed on a subsequent day, as described above).

[†]Categories of 2-hour postprandial glucose are as follows: < 140 mg/dL = normal glucose tolerance; ≥ 140 mg/dL and < 200 mg/dL = impaired glucose tolerance; ≥ 200 mg/dL = provisional diagnosis of diabetes (must be confirmed on subsequent day, as described above).

[‡]This method is not recommended for routine use.

branes, and changes in the function of endothelial cells induce microvascular damage.

The pathophysiology of diabetic complications is complex. There is considerable heterogeneity within the diabetic population in regard to the development and progression of diabetic complications. While poor glycemic control is clearly a major risk factor for complications, not all poorly controlled diabetic patients develop complications. Conversely, some individuals develop complications despite relatively good glycemic control. Hyperglycemia plays a major role in both microvascular and macrovascular disease. Hyperglycemia dramatically alters the function of multiple cell types and their extracellular matrix. This results in structural and functional changes in the affected tissues. Research has recently focused on lipoprotein metabolism and on the glycation of proteins, lipids, and nucleic acids as possible common links between the different diabetic complications.

TABLE 21-6 Complications of Diabetes

Retinopathy
  Vision changes
  Blindness

Nephropathy (renal failure)

Neuropathy
  Sensory
    Loss of sensation in hands and feet (other areas may be affected as well)
    Impotence
    Other sensory dysfunction
  Autonomic
    Gastroparesis (affects stomach emptying and other gastrointestinal functions)
    Changes in cardiac rate, rhythm, conduction
    Other autonomic dysfunction

Macrovascular disease (accelerated atherosclerosis)
  Peripheral vascular disease
  Cardiovascular (coronary artery disease)
  Cerebrovascular (stroke)

Alterations in wound healing

The function of cell membranes is determined largely by their phospholipid bilayers; thus, changes in lipid metabolism can have major effects on cell function. The oxidation of circulating low-density lipoprotein (LDL) in hyperglycemic individuals increases oxidant stress within the vasculature.[22] This induces chemotaxis of monocytes and macrophages into the vessel walls, where oxidized LDL causes changes in cellular adhesion and increased production of cytokines and growth factors. Growth factor–induced stimulation of smooth-muscle cell proliferation increases vessel wall thickness. Other changes include increased atheroma formation and development of microthrombi in large blood vessels and alterations in vascular permeability and endothelial cell function in the microvasculature.

The glycation of proteins, lipids, and nucleic acids increases with sustained hyperglycemia. The microvasculature of the retina, renal glomerulus, and endoneurial areas, as well as the walls of the larger blood vessels, accumulate deposits of glycated proteins called advanced glycation end products (AGEs).[23,24] While all people form AGEs, the accumulation of AGEs is much greater in individuals with diabetes, especially when the diabetic state is poorly controlled. AGE formation alters the structural and functional properties of the affected tissues. For example, AGE formation on collagen macromolecules impairs their normal homeostatic turnover. In the walls of the large blood vessels, AGE-modified collagen accumulates, thickening the vessel wall and narrowing the lumen. AGE-modified arterial collagen immobilizes circulating LDL, contributing to atheroma formation. Accumulation of AGEs causes increased basement membrane thickness in the microvasculature of the retina and around the nerves and increased thickness of the mesangial matrix in the glomerulus. The cumulative effect of these changes is a progressive narrowing of the vessel lumen and decreased perfusion of affected tissues.

AGE formation also has major effects at the cellular level, causing modifications in extracellular matrix components and changes in cell-to-matrix and matrix-to-matrix interactions.[25,26] The binding of AGEs to specific cellular receptors that have been identified on the surface of smooth-muscle cells, endothelial cells, neurons, monocytes, and macrophages results in increased vascular permeability and thrombus formation, proliferation of smooth muscle in vessel walls, and phenotypic alteration in monocytes and macrophages. This last result causes hyper-responsiveness of monocytes and macrophages upon stimulation, with resultant increases in the production of proinflammatory cytokines and certain growth factors. These cytokines and growth factors contribute to the chronic inflammatory process in the formation of atherosclerotic lesions. They also significantly alter wound-healing events. Increased production of proinflammatory mediators results in increased tissue destruction in response to antigens such as the bacteria that cause periodontal disease.

These changes in protein and lipid metabolism, induced by the elevated plasma glucose levels characteristic of diabetes, may thus provide a common connection between the various diabetic complications. However, these metabolic changes vary among individuals.[23,24] For example, AGEs form in both diabetic and nondiabetic people, but their accumulation is greater in those with diabetes. There is significant heterogeneity in AGE formation even within the diabetic population, and it is thought that this heterogeneity may explain (at least, in part) the variation in the incidence and progression of diabetic complications.

▼ MANAGEMENT

Primary treatment goals for diabetes patients include the achieving of blood glucose levels that are as close to normal as possible and the prevention of diabetic complications.[17] Other goals are normal growth and development, normal body weight, the avoidance of sustained hyperglycemia or symptomatic hypoglycemia, the prevention of diabetic ketoacidosis and nonketotic acidosis, and the immediate detection and treatment of long-term diabetic complications.

Diet, exercise, weight control, and medications are the mainstays of diabetic care. Obesity is very common in type 2 diabetes and contributes greatly to insulin resistance. Weight reduction and exercise improve tissue sensitivity to insulin and allow its proper use by target tissues. The primary medication used in type 1 diabetes management is insulin, on which the type 1 diabetic patient is dependent for survival. Type 2 diabetic individuals frequently take oral medications although many also use insulin to improve glycemic control.

Medical management and the goals of therapy for diabetes have changed since the publication of the Diabetes Control and Complications Trial (DCCT) in 1993.[27–29] This prospective randomized controlled multicenter clinical trial compared the effects of intensive insulin therapy aimed at achieving the near normalization of glycemia with the effects of conventional insulin therapy on the initiation and progression of complications in patients with type 1 diabetes. The conventional control group took 1 or 2 insulin injections each day while the intensive control group took 3 or 4 injections daily or used a subcutaneous insulin infusion pump. The results showed that the intensive group had much better glycemic control during the 3- to 9-year follow-up period. The risk of developing retinopathy decreased by 76% in intensively managed patients when compared to conventional control group patients. Clinical and laboratory signs

and symptoms of nephropathy and neuropathy decreased by 54 to 60%. Macrovascular complications also decreased significantly. The dramatic benefits of intensive insulin therapy led the American Diabetes Association to issue a position statement declaring that the primary treatment goal in type 1 diabetes should be to attain blood glucose control "at least equal to that in the intensively treated cohort" of the DCCT.[30]

Several recent studies have also shown reductions in diabetic complications for intensively managed type 2 diabetic patients.[31–33] In one 6-year study, maintenance of near-normal glycemia resulted in a decrease of 54 to 70% in the risk of microvascular and macrovascular complications for these patients, compared to conventional controls.[31] Since type 2 diabetic patients make up about 90% of all diabetic Americans, these studies have the potential to affect millions of people. Diabetic patients are increasingly motivated to improve their glycemic control, and physicians have intensified diabetic management in response to recent research.

Oral Agents

A number of different oral agents are available for treating diabetes; most of these are taken by those with type 2 diabetes (Table 21-7).[34] The first-generation sulfonylureas, once the only drugs available for treating type 2 diabetes, are not used much today. They have been replaced with second-generation agents that are more potent, have fewer drug interactions, and produce less significant side effects. Sulfonylureas stimulate pancreatic insulin secretion. The increased quantity of secreted insulin helps counteract the qualitative decrease in tissue sensitivity to insulin, allowing greater glucose entry into target cells and thereby lowering blood glucose levels. Sulfonylureas generally have a relatively long duration of action of 12 to 24 hours, depending on the drug, and are taken once or twice per

---

TABLE 21-7   Oral Agents for Management of Diabetes

Sulfonylurea agents
  First generation
    Chlorpropamide
    Tolazamide
    Tolbutamide
  Second generation
    Glyburide
    Glipizide
    Glimepiride

Nonsulfonylurea insulin secretagogues
  Repaglinide

Biguanides
  Metformin

Thiazolidinediones
  Troglitazone
  Rosiglitazone
  Pioglitazone

α-Glucosidase inhibitors
  Acarbose

day. Hypoglycemia is a major side effect of sulfonylureas. In patients taking these agents, food intake must be adequate to prevent glucose levels from falling too low.

Like the sulfonylureas, repaglinide stimulates pancreatic insulin secretion. However, its pharmacodynamic properties and mechanism of action are different from those of the sulfonylureas. Repaglinide is rapidly absorbed, reaches peak plasma levels in 30 to 60 minutes, and is then rapidly metabolized. The drug is taken with meals and lowers the peaks of postprandial plasma glucose common with type 2 diabetes to a much greater degree than the sulfonylureas are able to do.

Metformin is a biguanide agent that lowers plasma glucose mainly by preventing glycogenolysis in the liver. Metformin also improves insulin use, counteracting the insulin resistance seen with type 2 diabetes. Because metformin does not stimulate increased insulin secretion, hypoglycemia is much less common with this drug.

The thiazolidinedione agents troglitazone, rosiglitazone, and pioglitazone act to increase tissue sensitivity to insulin, thus increasing glucose utilization and decreasing blood glucose levels. These drugs also decrease hepatic gluconeogenesis. Like metformin, the thiazolidinediones generally do not cause hypoglycemia.

Acarbose has a mechanism of action that is unlike that of the other agents used in diabetes management. Acarbose is taken with meals, and it slows the digestion and uptake of carbohydrates from the gut. This serves to lower postprandial plasma glucose peaks. Acarbose does not cause hypoglycemia, but if the delayed carbohydrate absorption occurs in a patient whose plasma insulin levels are increasing due to the injection of insulin or the use of a sulfonylurea, the level of glucose in the bloodstream will not be sufficient to prevent hypoglycemia.

Insulin

All type 1 diabetic patients use exogenous insulin, as do many with type 2 diabetes. Insulin is taken via subcutaneous injection, most often with a syringe.[3,18] Insulin infusion pumps deliver insulin through a subcutaneous catheter. There are a variety of insulin preparations available; they vary in their onset, peak, and duration of activity and are classified as long-, intermediate-, short-, or rapid-acting (Table 21-8). Although beef and pork insulin species are still available, most individuals use human insulin preparations today.

Ideally, the use of exogenous insulin provides an insulin profile similar to that seen in a nondiabetic individual, with a continuous basal level of insulin availability augmented by increased availability following each meal. There is no single insulin preparation that can achieve this goal with only one or two injections per day. Combinations of different insulin preparations taken three or more times daily or the use of a subcutaneous infusion pump more closely approximate the ideal profile, but even with such regimens, blood glucose levels are often unstable.[27]

Ultralente insulin is the longest-acting insulin. Commonly called "peakless" insulin, Ultralente has a very slow onset of action, minimal peak activity, and a long duration of action. It is usually taken to mimic the basal metabolic rate of insulin secreted from a normally functioning pancreas. The intermediate-acting insulins (lente and neutral protamine Hagedorn [NPH]) take several hours after injection to begin having an effect. Peak activity varies among individuals and sites of injection but generally occurs between 4 and 10 hours after injection. Thus, a patient who injects intermediate-acting insulin in the early morning will reach peak plasma insulin levels at about lunchtime. Regular insulin is short acting, with an onset of activity at about 30 minutes to 1 hour after injection and a peak activity at 2 to 3 hours. The rapid-acting insulin called lispro insulin is rapidly absorbed, becomes active about 15 minutes after injection, and is at peak activity at 30 to 90 minutes. Rapid- and short-acting insulins are usually taken just prior to or during meals. Thus, regular insulin taken prior to breakfast will peak at about midmorning; when taken prior to lunch, it will peak during the midafternoon. Some examples of common insulin regimens are given in Table 21-9.

The most common complication of insulin therapy is hypoglycemia, a potentially life-threatening emergency. While hypoglycemia may occur in patients who are taking oral agents such as sulfonylureas, it is much more common in those who are using insulin. Intensified treatment regimens for diabetes increase the risk of hypoglycemia. Thus, the long-term benefit of reduced diabetic complications seen with intensive treatment must be weighed against the increased risk of symptomatic low blood glucose. In the DCCT, the incidence of severe hypoglycemic events in which the patient became unconscious or required the assistance of another person was three times greater in the intensively

TABLE 21-8 Types of Insulin

Type	Classification	Onset of Activity (h)	Peak Activity (h)	Duration of Activity (h)
Ultralente	Long acting	6–10	12–16	20–30
Lente	Intermediate acting	3–4	4–12	16–20
NPH	Intermediate acting	2–4	4–10	14–18
Regular	Short acting	0.5–1.0	2–3	4–12
Lispro	Rapid acting	0.25	0.5–1.5	< 5

NPH = neutral protamine Hagedorn.

TABLE 21-9   Common Insulin Regimens

Description	Characteristics
Single injection of intermediate-acting insulin (early morning)	Peak insulin activity at midday Can provide enough insulin for midday meals only Hyperglycemia common upon rising and following breakfast and dinner
Single injection of mixture of intermediate-acting and regular or lispro insulin (early morning)	Peak insulin activity at both midmorning (from regular or lispro insulin) and midday (from intermediate-acting insulin) Can provide enough insulin for breakfast and midday meals Hyperglycemia common upon rising and from late afternoon until next morning
Twice-daily injection of intermediate-acting insulin (prior to breakfast and dinner)	Peak insulin activity at both midday (from morning injection) and late evening (from dinner injection) Can provide enough insulin for lunch and sometimes dinner; often prevents early-morning high blood glucose levels Hyperglycemia common after breakfast and shortly after dinner
Twice-daily injection of mixture of intermediate-acting insulin and regular or lispro insulin (prior to breakfast and dinner)	Peak insulin activity after breakfast (from morning regular or lispro insulin), after lunch (from morning intermediate-acting insulin), after dinner (from dinnertime regular or lispro insulin), and late evening or early morning (from dinnertime intermediate-acting insulin) Can provide enough insulin for all meals; often prevents early-morning high blood glucose levels
Three daily injections of regular or lispro insulin (prior to each main meal) and one injection of intermediate-acting insulin (bedtime)	Peak insulin activity after breakfast, lunch, and dinner (from regular or lispro insulin before each meal), and late evening or early morning (from dinnertime intermediate-acting insulin) Can provide enough insulin for all meals; often prevents early-morning high blood glucose levels Often provides better glycemic control than once- or twice-daily injection regimens
Three daily injections of regular or lispro insulin (prior to each main meal) and one injection of Ultralente insulin (morning)	Peak insulin activity after breakfast, lunch, and dinner (from regular or lispro insulin before each meal); insulin activity in late evening or early morning (from morning Ultralente insulin) Can provide enough insulin for all meals; often prevents early-morning high blood glucose levels Often provides better glycemic control than once- or twice-daily injection regimens
Use of insulin infusion pump with regular or lispro insulin; basal metabolic rate set to provide continuous delivery of small amounts of insulin (bolus of insulin programmed prior to each meal)	Provides on-demand insulin with meals Basal metabolic rate most closely mimics normal pancreatic function Often (but not always) provides better glycemic control than any injection regimen

managed cohort than in the conventional control group.[35,36] One-third of the severe hypoglycemic episodes resulted in seizure or loss of consciousness. In addition, 36% of the episodes occurred with no warning symptoms for the patient.

The phenomenon known as "hypoglycemia unawareness" is more common in diabetic patients with good glycemic control than in those with poor control.[35] Hypoglycemia unawareness is characterized by an inability to perceive the warning symptoms of hypoglycemia until the blood glucose drops to very low levels. Signs and symptoms of hypoglycemia are most common when blood glucose levels fall to < 60 mg/dL, but they may occur at higher levels in diabetic patients with chronic poor metabolic control.[18] In people with hypoglycemia unawareness, glucose levels can fall to 40 mg/dL or lower before an individual "feels" hypoglycemic.

▼ ORAL DISEASES AND DIABETES

Oral conditions that are seen in individuals with diabetes may include burning mouth, altered wound healing, and an increased incidence of infection. Enlargement of the parotid glands and xerostomia can occur; both are conditions that may be related to the metabolic control of the diabetic state.[37] Medications that diabetic patients often take for related or unrelated systemic conditions may have significant xerostomic effects. Thus, the xerostomia seen in individuals with diabetes may result more from medications than from the diabetic condition itself.

Neuropathy of the autonomic system can also cause changes in salivary secretion since salivary flow is controlled by the sympathetic and parasympathetic pathways.[38] Dry mucosal surfaces are easily irritated and are associated with "burning mouth" syndrome; they also provide a favorable environment for the growth of fungal organisms. Some studies have shown an increased incidence of oral candidiasis in patients with diabetes whereas other studies have not.[39,40]

The effect of diabetes on the dental caries rate is unclear. Some studies have demonstrated increased caries in people with diabetes, which has been associated with xerostomia or increased gingival crevicular fluid glucose levels.[41] Other studies have shown similar or decreased caries rates in people with diabetes.[42,43] Since most diabetic individuals limit their intake of fermentable carbohydrates, the less cariogenic diet may limit caries incidence. In recent studies of type 2 diabetic patients and nondiabetic control subjects, no differences were seen in salivary flow rates, organic constituents of saliva, salivary counts of acidogenic bacteria, salivary counts of fungal organisms, or coronal and root caries rates.[38,44] These findings suggest that diabetic individuals as a group are similar to nondiabetic people in regard to these oral conditions.

Periodontal Health and Diabetes

Strong evidence suggests that, unlike the conditions discussed above, diabetes is a risk factor for the prevalence and severity of gingivitis and periodontitis.[45,46] Diabetes is associated with increased gingival inflammation in response to bacterial plaque, but the degree of glycemic control is an important variable in this relationship. In general, well-controlled diabetic individuals and nondiabetic people have similar degrees of gingivitis, with the same level of plaque. Conversely, poorly controlled diabetic subjects have significantly increased gingivitis, compared to either well-controlled diabetic or nondiabetic individuals.[47–49]

In large epidemiologic studies, diabetes has been shown to significantly increase the risk of attachment loss and alveolar bone loss approximately threefold when compared to nondiabetic control subjects.[50,51] These findings have been confirmed in meta-analyses of multiple studies in various diabetic populations.[45] Diabetes increases not only the prevalence and severity of periodontitis but also the progression of bone loss and attachment loss over time.[52]

Periodontitis is similar to the classic complications of diabetes in its variation among individuals. Just as retinopathy, nephropathy, and neuropathy are more likely to be seen in diabetic patients with poor glycemic control, progressive destructive periodontitis is also more common in those with poor control.[53,54] However, some poorly controlled diabetic patients do not develop significant periodontal destruction, just as some do not develop the classic diabetic complications. Conversely, well-controlled diabetes places the person at a lower risk for periodontal disease, similar to the risk of nondiabetic individuals; yet, well-controlled diabetic patients may still develop periodontitis, just as nondiabetic individuals do. Other risk factors for periodontitis, such as poor oral hygiene and smoking, play a similar deleterious role in both diabetic and nondiabetic individuals.

The mechanisms by which diabetes influences the periodontium are similar in many respects to the pathophysiology of the classic diabetic complications. There are few differences between the subgingival microbiota of diabetic patients with periodontitis and nondiabetic patients with periodontitis.[55,56] This lack of significant differences in the primary bacteriologic agents of periodontal disease suggests that differences in host response may play a role in the increased prevalence and severity of periodontal destruction seen in patients with diabetes.

Hyperglycemia results in increased gingival crevicular fluid glucose levels, which may significantly alter periodontal wound-healing events by changing the interaction between cells and their extracellular matrix within the periodontium.[57,58] Vascular changes seen in the retina, glomerulus, and perineural areas also occur in the periodontium.[59,60] The formation of AGEs results in collagen accumulation in the periodontal capillary basement membranes, causing membrane thickening.[61] AGE-stimulated smooth-muscle proliferation increases the thickness of vessel walls. These changes decrease tissue perfusion and oxygenation. AGE-modified collagen in gingival blood vessel walls binds circulating LDL, which is frequently elevated in diabetes, resulting in atheroma formation and further narrowing of the vessel lumen.[62] These changes in the periodontium may dramatically alter the tissue response to periodontal pathogens, resulting in increased tissue destruction and diminished repair potential.

Diabetes results in changes in the function of host defense cells such as polymorphonuclear leukocytes (PMNs), monocytes, and macrophages. PMN adherence, chemotaxis, and phagocytosis are impaired.[63,64] Defects in this first line of defense against periodontopathic microorganisms may significantly increase periodontal destruction. Monocytes and macrophages in diabetic individuals are often hyper-responsive to bacterial antigens.[65] This up-regulation results in a significantly increased production of proinflammatory cytokines and mediators.[66,67] The net effect of these host defense alterations is an increase in periodontal inflammation, attachment loss, and bone loss.

Collagen is the primary structural protein in the periodontium. Changes in collagen metabolism in diabetic individuals contribute to wound-healing alterations and periodontal destruction.[68] The production of matrix metalloproteinases (MMPs) such as collagenase is increased in many diabetic patients. Increased collagenase production readily degrades newly formed collagen. Conversely, AGE modification of existing collagen decreases its solubility. The result of these changes in collagen metabolism is a rapid dissolution of recently synthesized collagen by host collagenase and a preponderance of older AGE-modified collagen. Thus, diabetes induces a shift in the normal homeostatic mechanism by which collagen is formed, stabilized, and eventually turned over; this shift alters healing responses to physical or microbial wounding of the periodontium. Tetracycline antibiotics and chemically modified tetracycline agents reduce host collagenase production and collagen degradation through mechanisms that are independent of their antimicrobial activity.[69] These drugs may have benefits in managing conditions such as periodontitis, arthritis, diabetes, osteoporosis, and others in which collagen metabolism is altered.

Effects of Periodontal Infection on Glycemic Control

Not only does diabetes affect the periodontium, but evidence also suggests that periodontal infection may adversely affect glycemic control of diabetes.[3,46] Diabetic subjects with severe periodontal disease often have a worsening of glycemic control over time, compared to diabetic subjects without periodontitis. Periodontal infection increased the risk of poor glycemic control by sixfold in one study.[70] Periodontitis is also associated with an increased risk for other diabetic complications, such as nephropathy and macrovascular disease. In one study, 82% of diabetic patients with severe periodontitis had at least one major cardiovascular, cerebrovascular, or peripheral vascular event during the 1- to 11-year study period, compared to only 21% of diabetic subjects with little or no periodontal disease.[71]

In diabetic patients with periodontitis, periodontal treatment may have beneficial effects on glycemic control. Several well-controlled studies of diabetic subjects with severe periodontal disease have shown improvements in glycemic control following a combination of mechanical débridement (scaling and root planing) and systemic doxycycline antibiotic therapy.[72–74] Other studies in which patients received only mechanical therapy or in which the subject population already had good glycemic control prior to periodontal treatment showed no significant effect on glycemic control.[75,76] The mechanisms by which adjunctive systemic antibiotics, when combined with subgingival mechanical débridement, may induce positive changes in glycemic control are presently unclear. Changes may result from more complete elimination of the subgingival pathogens in patients receiving antibiotics[73,74] or from the suppression of collagenase production and AGE formation.[69]

▼ DENTAL MANAGEMENT OF THE DIABETIC PATIENT

General Dental Treatment

Overall, diabetic patients respond to most dental treatments similarly to the way nondiabetic patients respond. Responses to therapy depend on many factors that are specific to each individual, including oral hygiene, diet, habits such as tobacco use, proper dental care and follow-up, overall oral health, and metabolic control of diabetes. For example, the diabetic patient with poor oral hygiene, a history of smoking, infrequent dental visits, and a high fermentable-carbohydrate intake is more likely to experience oral diseases such as caries and periodontitis and to respond poorly to dental treatment than a diabetic patient without these factors. Glycemic control appears to play an important role in the response to periodontal therapy. Well-controlled diabetic patients with periodontitis have positive responses to nonsurgical therapy, periodontal surgery, and maintenance that

are similar to those of people without diabetes.[74–77] However, poorly controlled diabetic patients respond much less favorably, and short-term improvements in periodontal health are frequently followed by regression and by recurrence of disease.[78] It is imperative that the dental practitioner have a clear understanding of each diabetic patient's level of glycemic control prior to initiating treatment.

Patients may present to the dental office with oral conditions that suggest an undiagnosed diabetic state. An example is severe rapidly progressing periodontitis that exceeds what would be expected given the patient's age, habit history, oral hygiene, and level of local factors (plaque, calculus) (Figures 21-1 and 21-2). Other findings seen in some undiagnosed diabetic patients include enlarged gingival tissues that bleed easily upon manipulation and the presence of multiple periodontal abscesses (Figures 21-3, 21-4, and 21-5).

If the clinician suspects an undiagnosed diabetic state, the patient should be questioned to elicit a history of polydipsia, polyuria, polyphagia, or unexplained weight loss (see Table 21-4). The patient should be questioned about a family history of diabetes. If diabetes is suspected, laboratory evaluation and physician referral are indicated (see Table 21-5). A patient with previously diagnosed but poorly controlled diabetes may present with oral findings similar to those of the undiagnosed diabetic individual. The dental practitioner must establish the level of glycemic control early in the treatment process; this can be done by physician referral or by a review of the patient's medical records. Patients who perform SBGM may be asked to bring their glucose log to the dental office for review by the dental team.

The clinician should determine the patient's recent glycated hemoglobin values since this test provides a measure of glycemic control over the preceding 2 to 3 months. HbA_{1c} values of less than 8% indicate relatively good glycemic control; values greater than 10% indicate poor control. Physician

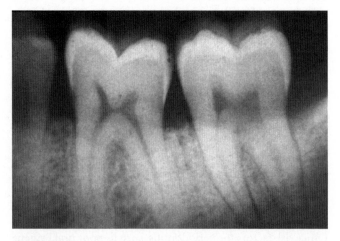

FIGURE 21-1 Radiograph of area 18-19 in a 35-year-old male with a 4-year history of type 1 diabetes. The patient had generalized moderate plaque levels but minimal alveolar bone loss. He rarely used dental floss. Widening of the periodontal ligament (space 18) was due to occlusal trauma, which was treated by occlusal adjustment.

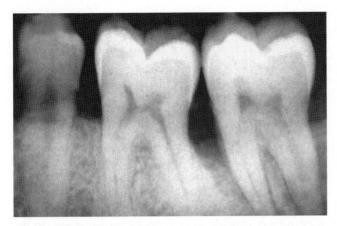

FIGURE 21-2 Radiograph of area 18-19 in the same patient shown in Figure 21-1 at 39 years of age and with an 8-year history of poorly controlled type 1 diabetes (HbA$_{1c}$ values were 10.2 to 11.3%). There is a rapid progression of bone loss, the severity of which exceeds that expected from plaque and calculus levels.

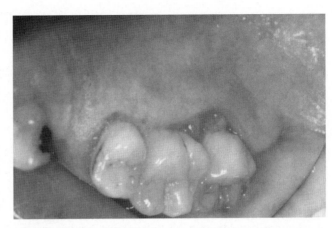

FIGURE 21-4 Palatal view of the maxillary right sextant in the same patient shown in Figure 21-3. An abscess can be noted on the palatal aspect of tooth 2.

referral is appropriate any time glycemic control is in question. The issue of glycemic control should be addressed often by the dental team since dental treatment outcomes may be dependent partly on good metabolic control of the underlying diabetic state. Other key dental treatment considerations for diabetic patients include stress reduction, treatment setting, the use of antibiotics, diet modification, appointment timing, changes in medication regimens, and the management of emergencies.

Endogenous production of epinephrine and cortisol increase during stressful situations. These hormones elevate blood glucose levels and interfere with glycemic control. Adequate pain control and stress reduction are therefore important in treating diabetic patients.[46,79] Profound anesthesia reduces pain and minimizes endogenous epinephrine release. The small amounts of epinephrine in dental local anesthetics at 1/100,000 concentration have no significant effect on blood glucose. Conscious sedation should be considered for extremely anxious patients. Most practitioners who use intravenous sedation elect to use fluids without dextrose, such as normal saline. However, fluids such as D5W (a 5% solution of dextrose in water) in small amounts should not produce wide fluctuations in glycemia in most patients.

Most diabetic patients can easily be managed on an outpatient basis in the dental office.[46] Patients with very poor glycemic control, severe head and neck infections, other systemic diseases or complications, and dental-treatment needs that will require long-term alteration of medication regimens or diet may be considered for treatment in a more controlled medical environment.

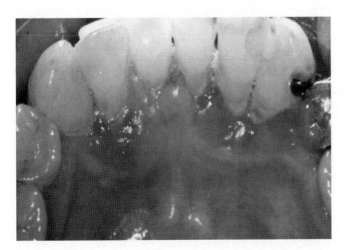

FIGURE 21-3 Lingual view of mandibular incisors of a 60-year-old female with poorly controlled type 2 diabetes. The HbA$_{1c}$ value at initial examination was 13.9%. Multiple periodontal abscesses (teeth 22, 23, 25, 26, and 27) with severe inflammation and bone loss can be seen.

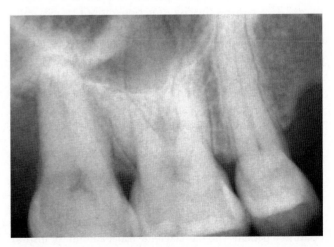

FIGURE 21-5 Radiograph of the same sextant shown in Figure 21-4. Severe bone loss can be noted on tooth 2.

The use of systemic antibiotics for routine dental treatment is not necessary for most diabetic patients. Antibiotics may be considered in the presence of acute infection. Some clinicians prefer to prescribe prophylactic antibiotic coverage prior to surgical therapy if the diabetic patient's glycemic control is poor. This usually applies to emergency situations since elective procedures are generally deferred until glycemic control improves. In patients with severe periodontitis, adjunctive use of tetracycline antibiotics in conjunction with mechanical periodontal therapy may have beneficial effects on glycemic control as well as on periodontal status.

Dental treatment can result in postoperative discomfort. This may necessitate changes in the diet, especially in cases of extensive dental therapy.[3,46] Because diet is a major component of diabetes management, diet alterations that are made because of dental treatment may have a major impact on the patient. Whereas some patients are very knowledgeable about their diabetic condition and can adjust for changes in diet, this may not be the case with others. The clinician may need to consult the patient's physician prior to therapy, to discuss diet modifications and required changes in medication regimens. Another diet change occurs when patients are placed on orders to take nothing by mouth (NPO) before dental treatment, a common recommendation before conscious sedation. Consultation with the patient's physician may be needed to adjust the dose of insulin or oral agents in this situation; however, some patients are able to make these adjustments themselves. Physicians often recommend reducing the insulin dose that immediately precedes lengthy or extensive dental procedures.

Appointment timing for the diabetic patient is often determined by the individual's medication regimen. Conventional wisdom holds that diabetic patients, like other medically compromised individuals, should receive dental treatment in the morning. While this may be true for some patients, it is not true for others. It is generally best to plan dental treatment to occur either before or after periods of peak insulin activity.[18,46] This reduces the risk of perioperative hypoglycemic reactions, which occur most often during peak insulin activity. For those who take insulin, the greatest risk of hypoglycemia will thus occur about 30 to 90 minutes after injecting lispro insulin, 2 to 3 hours after regular insulin, and 4 to 10 hours after NPH or Lente insulin (see Table 21-8). For those who are taking oral sulfonylureas, peak insulin activity depends on the individual drug taken. Metformin and the thiazolidinediones rarely cause hypoglycemia.

The main factor to consider in determining appointment times is the peak action of insulin and the amount of glucose being absorbed from the gut following the last food intake. Questions such as those listed in Table 21-10 allow the clinician to assess the risk of hypoglycemia. The greatest risk would occur in a patient who has taken the usual amount of insulin or oral agent but has reduced or eliminated a meal prior to dental treatment. For example, if the patient takes the usual dose of regular insulin before breakfast but then fails to eat or eats less than the usual amount, the patient will be at increased risk for hypoglycemia during a morning dental appointment. Patients with good long-term glycemic control and patients with a previous history of severe hypoglycemic episodes are at greater risk for future hypoglycemia.

Often, it is not possible to plan dental treatment so as to avoid peak insulin activity. This is particularly true for patients who take frequent insulin injections (see Table 21-9). In these instances, the clinician must be aware that the patient is at risk for perioperative hypoglycemia. It is helpful to check the pretreatment blood glucose level (using the patient's glucometer) and to have a source of carbohydrates readily available. When treating patients with a history of asthma or angina, dentists usually have the patients bring their inhaler or nitroglycerine with them to dental appointments. In the same way, diabetic patients should be encouraged to bring their glucometer with them to the dental office. Before dental treatment begins, the patient may check his or her blood glucose. If the level is near the lower end of the normal range, a small amount of pretreatment carbohydrate may prevent hypoglycemia during the appointment. Having the glucometer available also allows rapid determination of blood glucose levels should the patient experience signs and symptoms of hypoglycemia.

Diabetic Emergencies in the Dental Office

The most common diabetic emergency in the dental office is hypoglycemia (Table 21-11), a potentially life-threatening complication that must be managed accordingly.[80] Signs and symptoms include confusion, sweating, tremors, agitation, anxiety, dizziness, tingling or numbness, and tachycardia.[3,18] Severe hypoglycemia may result in seizures or loss of consciousness.

As soon as a patient experiences signs or symptoms of possible hypoglycemia, he or she should check the blood glucose with a glucometer. If a glucometer is unavailable, the condition should be treated presumptively as a hypoglycemic episode. The dental practitioner should give the patient approximately 15 g of oral carbohydrate in a form that will be absorbed rapidly (Table 21-12). If the patient is unable to

---

TABLE 21-10   Determining Risk of Hypoglycemia: Questions to Patient

1. Have you ever had a severe hypoglycemic reaction before?

2. How often do you have hypoglycemic reactions?

3. How well controlled is your diabetes? What was your last glycated hemoglobin* level?

4. What diabetic medication(s) do you take?
    —Did you take them today?
    —When did you take them? Is that the same time as usual?
    —How much of each medication did you take?
    —Is this the same amount you normally take?

5. What did you eat today before you came to the dental office?
    —What time did you eat? Is that when you normally eat?
    —Did you eat the same amount you normally eat for that meal?
    —Did you skip a meal?

*Hemoglobin A_1 or A_{1c}.

TABLE 21-11 Factors That Increase Risk of Hypoglycemia

Skipping or delaying food intake

Injection of too much insulin

Injection of insulin into tissue with high blood flow (eg, injection into thigh after exercise such as running)

Increasing exercise level without adjusting insulin or sulfonylurea dose

Alcohol consumption

Inability to recognize symptoms of hypoglycemia

Anxiety, stress

Denial of warning signs or symptoms

Past history of hypoglycemia

Hypoglycemia unawareness

Good long-term glycemic control

take food by mouth and an intravenous line is in place, 25 to 50 mL of a 50% dextrose solution (D50) or 1 mg of glucagon can be given intravenously. If an intravenous line is not in place, 1 mg of glucagon can be injected subcutaneously or intramuscularly at almost any body site. Glucagon injection causes rapid glycogenolysis in the liver, releasing stored glycogen and rapidly elevating blood glucose. Following treatment, the signs and symptoms of hypoglycemia should resolve in 10 to 15 minutes. The patient should be observed for 30 to 60 minutes after recovery. Evaluation by glucometer can ensure that normal blood glucose levels have been achieved before the patient is released.

In some instances, marked hyperglycemia may present with symptoms mimicking hypoglycemia.[18,79] If a glucometer is not available, these symptoms must be treated as hypoglycemia (see Table 21-12). If the event was actually hyperglycemia, the small amount of extra glucose derived from treatment will generally not have a significant effect. On the other hand, if glucose-elevating emergency treatment was withheld from a patient in a mistaken belief that the emergency was related to elevated glucose levels when hypoglycemia was in fact present, severe adverse outcomes are possible. The best means of determining the true nature of a glucose-related emergency is to check the blood glucose level with a glucometer.

TABLE 21-12 Treatment of Hypoglycemia

1. If patient is awake and able to take food by mouth, give 15 g oral carbohydrate in one of the following forms:
   —4–6 oz fruit juice or soda
   —3–4 tsp table sugar
   —hard candy
   —cake frosting

2. If patient is unable to take food by mouth and IV line is in place, give 25–30 mL D50 or 1 mg glucagon.

3. If patient is unable to take food by mouth and IV line is not in place, give 1 mg glucagon subcutaneously or intramuscularly.

D50 = 50% dextrose solution; IV = intravenous; oz = ounce; tsp = teaspoon.

Because hyperglycemic emergencies develop more slowly than does hypoglycemia, they are less likely to be encountered in the dental office. Diabetic ketoacidosis and hyperosmolar nonketotic acidosis require immediate medical evaluation and treatment. In the dental office, care is limited to activating the emergency medical system, opening the airway and administering oxygen, evaluating and supporting circulation, and monitoring vital signs. The patient should be transported to a hospital as soon as possible.

▼ CONCLUSION

Diabetes mellitus is a metabolic condition affecting multiple organ systems. The oral cavity frequently undergoes changes that are related to the diabetic condition, and oral infections may adversely affect metabolic control of the diabetic state. The mechanisms underlie the oral effects of diabetes share many similarities with the mechanisms that are responsible for the classic diabetic complications. The intimate relationship between oral health and systemic health in individuals with diabetes suggests a need for increased interaction between the dental and medical professionals who are charged with the management of these patients. Oral health assessment and treatment should become as common as the eye, foot, and kidney evaluations that are routinely performed as part of preventive medical therapies. Dental professionals with a thorough understanding of current medical treatment regimens and the implications of diabetes on dental care are able to help their diabetic patients achieve and maintain the best possible oral health.

▼ REFERENCES

1. National Diabetes Data Group. Diabetes in America. 2nd ed. Bethesda (MD): National Institutes of Health; 1995. NIH Publication No 95-1468.
2. Mandrup-Poulsen T. Recent advances — diabetes. BMJ 1998;316:1221–5.
3. Mealey BL. Diabetes mellitus. In: Rose LF, Genco RJ, Mealey BL, Cohen DW, editors. Periodontal medicine. Toronto, Canada: BC Decker Inc.; 2000.
4. American Diabetes Association. Report of the Expert Committee on the Diagnosis and Classification of Diabetes Mellitus. Diabetes Care 1997;20:1183–97.
5. Newman B, Selby JV, Slemenda C, et al. Concordance for type 2 (non-insulin-dependent) diabetes mellitus in male twins. Diabetologia 1987;30:763–8.
6. Ghosh S, Schork NJ. Genetic analysis of NIDDM. Diabetes 1996;45:1–14.
7. Edelman SV. Type II diabetes mellitus. Adv Intern Med 1998;43:449–500.
8. Reaven GM. Role of insulin resistance in human disease. Diabetes 1988;37:1595–607.
9. Bogardus C, Lillioja S, Mott DM, et al. Relationship between degree of obesity and in vivo insulin action in man. Am J Physiol 1985;248:E286–E91.
10. Engelgau MM, Herman WH, Smith PJ, et al. The epidemiology of diabetes and pregnancy in the U.S., 1988. Diabetes Care 1995;18:1029–33.

11. Magee MS, Walden CE, Benedetti TJ. Influence of diagnostic criteria on the incidence of gestational diabetes and perinatal morbidity. JAMA 1993;269:609–15.

12. Langer O, Rodriguez DA, Xenakis EMJ, et al. Intensified versus conventional management of gestational diabetes. Am J Obstet Gynecol 1994;170:1036–47.

13. Charles MA, Fontboune A, Thibult N, et al. Risk factors for NIDDM in white populations: Paris Prospective Study. Diabetes 1991;40:796–9.

14. Lester E. The clinical value of glycated haemoglobin and glycated plasma proteins. Clin Biochem 1989;26:213–9.

15. Tsuji I, Nakamoto K, Hasegawa T, et al. Receiver operating characteristic analysis of fasting plasma glucose, HbA1c, and fructosamine on diabetes screening. Diabetes Care 1991;14:1075-7.

16. American Diabetes Association. Self-monitoring of blood glucose (consensus statement). Diabetes Care 1993;16:60-5.

17. American Diabetes Association. Standards of medical care for patients with diabetes mellitus. Diabetes Care 1998;21 Suppl 1:s23–31.

18. Mealey BL. Impact of advances in diabetes care on dental treatment of the diabetic patient. Compend Contin Educ Dent 1998;19:41–58.

19. Steinberg D. Diabetes and atherosclerosis. In: Porte D, Sherwin RS, editors. Diabetes mellitus. 5th ed. Stamford (CT): Appleton & Lange; 1997.

20. Steffes MW. Pathophysiology of renal complications. In: Porte D, Sherwin RS, editors. Diabetes mellitus. 5th ed. Stamford (CT): Appleton & Lange; 1997.

21. Klein R. Retinopathy and other ocular complications in diabetes. In: Porte D, Sherwin RS, editors. Diabetes mellitus. 5th ed. Stamford (CT): Appleton & Lange; 1997.

22. Brunzell JD, Chait A. Diabetic dyslipidemia: pathology and treatment. In: Porte D, Sherwin RS, editors. Diabetes mellitus. 5th ed. Stamford (CT): Appleton & Lange; 1997.

23. Brownlee M. Glycation and diabetic complications. Diabetes 1994;43:836–41.

24. Bierhaus A, Hofmann MA, Ziegler R, Nawroth PP. AGEs and their interaction with AGE-receptors in vascular disease and diabetes mellitus. I. The AGE concept. Cardiovasc Res 1998;37:586–600.

25. Vlassara H, Bucala R. Recent progress in advanced glycation and diabetic vascular disease: role of advanced glycation end product receptors. Diabetes 1996:45 Suppl 3:s65–6.

26. Schmidt AM, Yan SD, Wautier JL, Stern D. Activation of receptor for advanced glycation end products. A mechanism for chronic vascular dysfunction in diabetic vasculopathy and atherosclerosis. Circ Res 1999;84:489–97.

27. Diabetes Control and Complications Trial Research Group. The effect of intensive treatment of diabetes on the development and progression of long-term complications in insulin-dependent diabetes mellitus. N Engl J Med 1993;329:977–86.

28. Diabetes Control and Complications Trial Research Group. Progression of retinopathy with intensive versus conventional treatment in the Diabetes Control and Complications Trial. Ophthalmology 1995;102:647–61.

29. Diabetes Control and Complications Trial Research Group. Effect of intensive diabetes management on macrovascular and microvascular events and risk factors in the Diabetes Control and Complications Trial. Am J Cardiol 1995;75:894–903.

30. American Diabetes Association. Position statement. Implications of the Diabetes Control and Complications Trial. Diabetes Spectrum 1993;6:225–7.

31. Ohkubo Y, Kishikawa H, Araki E, et al. Intensive insulin therapy prevents the progression of diabetic microvascular complications in Japanese patients with non-insulin-dependent diabetes mellitus: a randomized prospective 6-year study. Diabetes Res Clin Pract 1995;28:103–17.

32. U.K. Prospective Diabetes Study (UKPDS) Group. Intensive blood-glucose control with sulphonylureas or insulin compared with conventional treatment and risk of complications in pateints with type 2 diabetes (UKPDS 33). Lancet 1998;352:837–53.

33. U.K. Prospective Diabetes Study (UKPDS) Group. Effect of intensive blood-glucose control with metformin on complications in overweight patients with type 2 diabetes (UKPDS 34). Lancet 1998;352:854–65.

34. Scheen AJ, Lefebvre PJ. Oral antidiabetic agents. A guide to selection. Drugs 1998;55:225–36.

35. Diabetes Control and Complications Trial Research Group. Epidemiology of severe hypoglycemia in the Diabetes Control and Complications Trial. Am J Med 1991;90:450–9.

36. Diabetes Control and Complications Trial Research Group. Hypoglycemia in the Diabetes Control and Complications Trial. Diabetes 1997;46:271–86.

37. Sreebny LM, Yu A, Green A, Valdini A. Xerostomia in diabetes mellitus. Diabetes Care 1992;15:900–4.

38. Meurman JH, Collin HL, Niskanen L, et al. Saliva in non-insulin-dependent diabetic patients and control subjects. The role of the autonomic nervous system. Oral Surg Oral Med Oral Pathol Oral Radiol Endod 1998;86:69–76.

39. Fisher BM, Lamey PJ, Samaranayake LP, et al. Carriage of *Candida* species in the oral cavity in diabetic patients: relationship to glycaemic control. J Oral Pathol 1987;16:282–4.

40. Phelan JA, Levin SM. A prevalence study of denture stomatitis in subjects with diabetes mellitus or elevated plasma glucose levels. Oral Surg Oral Med Oral Pathol 1986;62:303–5.

41. Jones RB, McCallum RM, Kay EJ, et al. Oral health and oral health behavior in a population of diabetic clinic attenders. Community Dent Oral Epidemiol 1992;20:204–7.

42. Tenovuo J, Alanen P, Larjava H, et al. Oral health of patients with insulin dependent diabetes mellitus. Scand J Dent Res 1986;94:338–46.

43. Tavares M, DePaola P, Soparkar P, Joshipura K. Prevalence of root caries in a diabetic population. J Dent Res 1991; 70:979–83.

44. Collin HL, Uusitupa M, Niskanen L, et al. Caries in patients with non-insulin-dependent diabetes mellitus. Oral Surg Oral Med Oral Pathol Oral Radiol Endod 1998;85:680–5.

45. Papapanou PN. 1996 World Workshop in Clinical Periodontics. Periodontal diseases: epidemiology. Ann Periodontol 1996;1:1–36.

46. Mealey BL. 1996 World Workshop in Clinical Periodontics. Periodontal implications: medically compromised patients. Ann Periodontol 1996;1:256–321.

47. Gusberti FA, Syed SA, Bacon G, et al. Puberty gingivitis in insulin-dependent diabetic children. J Periodontol 1983; 54:714–20.

48. Ervasti T, Knuuttila M, Pohjamo L, Haukipuro K. Relation between control of diabetes and gingival bleeding. J Periodontol 1985;56:154–7.

49. Karjalainen KM, Knuuttila MLE. The onset of diabetes and poor metabolic control increases gingival bleeding in children and adolescents with insulin-dependent diabetes mellitus. J Clin Periodontol 1996;23:1060–7.

50. Emrich LJ, Shlossman M, Genco RJ. Periodontal disease in non-insulin-dependent diabetes mellitus. J Periodontol 1991;62:123–30.

51. Shlossman M, Knowler WC, Pettitt DJ, Genco RJ. Type 2 diabetes mellitus and periodontal disease. J Am Dent Assoc 1990;121:532–6.

52. Taylor GW, Burt BA, Becker MP, et al. Non-insulin dependent diabetes mellitus and alveolar bone loss progression over 2 years. J Periodontol 1998;69:76–83.

53. Seppala B, Seppala M, Ainamo J. A longitudinal study on insulin-dependent diabetes mellitus and periodontal disease. J Clin Periodontol 1993;20:161–5.

54. Tervonen T, Oliver RC. Long-term control of diabetes mellitus and periodontitis. J Clin Periodontol 1993;20:431–5.

55. Zambon JJ, Reynolds H, Fisher JG, et al. Microbiological and immunological studies of adult periodontitis in patients with non-insulin dependent diabetes mellitus. J Periodontol 1988;59:23–31.

56. Sastrowijoto SH, Hillemans P, van Steenbergen TJ, et al. Periodontal condition and microbiology of healthy and diseased periodontal pockets in type 1 diabetes mellitus patients. J Clin Periodontol 1989;16:316–22.

57. Ficara AJ, Levin MP, Grower MF, Kramer GD. A comparison of the glucose and protein content of gingival crevicular fluid from diabetics and nondiabetics. J Periodontal Res 1975;10:171–5.

58. Nishimura F, Takahashi K, Kurihara M, et al. Periodontal disease as a complication of diabetes mellitus. Ann Periodontol 1998;3:20–9.

59. Frantzis TG, Reeve CM, Brown AL. The ultrastructure of capillary basement membranes in the attached gingiva of diabetic and non-diabetic patients with periodontal disease. J Periodontol 1971;42:406–11.

60. Seppala B, Sorsa T, Ainamo J. Morphometric analysis of cellular and vascular changes in gingival connective tissue in long-term insulin-dependent diabetes. J Periodontol 1997;68:1237–45.

61. Schmidt AM, Weidman E, Lalla E, et al. Advanced glycation endproducts (AGEs) induce oxidant stress in the gingiva: a potential mechanism underlying accelerated periodontal disease associated with diabetes. J Periodontal Res 1996;31:508–15.

62. Iacopino AM. Diabetic periodontitis: possible lipid-induced defect in tissue repair through alteration of macrophage phenotype and function. Oral Dis 1995;1:214–29.

63. Manoucher-Pour M, Spagnuolo PJ, Rodman HM, Bissada NF. Comparison of neutrophil chemotactic response in diabetic patients with mild and severe periodontal disease. J Periodontol 1981;52:410–5.

64. McMullen JA, Van Dyke TE, Horoszewicz HU, Genco RJ. Neutrophil chemotaxis in individuals with advanced periodontal disease and a genetic predisposition to diabetes mellitus. J Periodontol 1981;52:167–73.

65. Offenbacher S. Periodontal diseases: pathogenesis. Ann Periodontol 1996;1:821–78.

66. Salvi GE, Collins JG, Yalda B, et al. Monocytic TNF-α secretion patterns in IDDM patients with periodontal diseases. J Clin Periodontol 1997;24:8–16.

67. Salvi GE, Yalda B, Collins JG, et al. Inflammatory mediator response as a potential risk marker for periodontal diseases in insulin-dependent diabetes mellitus patients. J Periodontol 1997;68:127–35.

68. Birkedal-Hansen H. Role of matrix metalloproteinases in human periodontal disease. J Periodontol 1993;64:474–84.

69. Golub LM, Lee H-M, Ryan ME. Tetracyclines inhibit connective tissue breakdown by multiple non-antimicrobial mechanisms. Adv Dent Res 1998;12:12–26.

70. Taylor GW, Burt BA, Becker MP, et al. Severe periodontitis and risk for poor glycemic control in patients with non-insulin-dependent diabetes mellitus. J Periodontol 1996;67:1085–93.

71. Thorstensson H, Kuylensteirna J, Hugoson A. Medical status and complications in relation to periodontal disease experience in insulin-dependent diabetics. J Clin Periodontol 1996;23:194–202.

72. Miller LS, Manwell MA, Newbold D, et al. The relationship between reduction in periodontal inflammation and diabetes control: a report of 9 cases. J Periodontol 1992;63:843–8.

73. Grossi SG, Skrepcinski FB, DeCaro T, et al. Response to periodontal therapy in diabetics and smokers. J Periodontol 1996;67:1094–12.

74. Grossi SG, Skrepcinski FB, DeCaro T, et al. Treatment of periodontal disease in diabetics reduces glycated hemoglobin. J Periodontol 1997;68:713–9.

75. Aldridge JP, Lester V, Watts TLP, et al. Single-blind studies of the effects of improved periodontal health on metabolic control in type 1 diabetes mellitus. J Clin Periodontol 1995; 22:271–5.

76. Christgau M, Palitzsch KD, Schmalz G, et al. Healing response to non-surgical periodontal therapy in patients with diabetes mellitus: clinical, microbiological, and immunological results. J Clin Periodontol 1998;25:112–24.

77. Westfelt E, Rylander H, Blohme G, et al. The effect of periodontal therapy in diabetics. Results after 5 years. J Clin Periodontol 1996;23:92–100.

78. Tervonen T, Karjalainen K. Periodontal disease related to diabetic status. A pilot study of the response to periodontal therapy in type 1 diabetes. J Clin Periodontol 1997;24:505–10.

79. Rees TD. The diabetic dental patient. Dent Clin North Am 1994;38:447–63.

80. American Academy of Periodontology. Diabetes and periodontal diseases. Position paper. J Periodontol 1999;70:935–49.

22

ENDOCRINE DISEASE

Susan F. Silverton, MD, PhD

▼ HYPOTHALAMUS AND ANTERIOR PITUITARY

Pituitary disease can present with either overt disease or subtle findings to the oral health clinician. Patients with hormonal dysfunctions caused by pituitary disease may be found to have significant abnormalities on head and neck examination. Large pituitary adenomas frequently present with changes in vision and loss of visual-field integrity, and the oral health clinician may be the first medical professional to note these diseases. For example, in active Graves' disease (one of the conditions causing excessive function of the thyroid), defects in the motor function of cranial nerves III, IV, and VI may be observed. In acromegaly and in Cushing's disease, pituitary adenomas secrete active hormones, causing gradual changes in facial features and orofacial structures. In addition to the changes an oral health clinician can observe and document on physical examination, patients with disease caused by pituitary adenomas often have alterations in the blood levels of several circulating hormones.[1] Notably, abnormal hormone levels may also be the result of previous medical or surgical therapy for underlying pituitary disease. Normally, blood levels of hormones secreted by the pituitary are exquisitely regulated.[2] Disruption of pituitary function can produce life-threatening conditions, adversely affecting the safety of patients during all but the most minor clinical interventions. Prompt recognition of pituitary dysfunction can prevent complications of dental treatment and can provide a safe setting for clinical and therapeutic interventions in these patients. Even after definitive medical or surgical treatment of pituitary disease, patients may require lifelong replacement of several hormones. Replacement therapy may be indicated after partial resection or partial destruction of pituitary tissue.[1] As a result of the destruction of specialized cells, the pituitary may no longer capable of secreting selected hormones. Replacement hormone therapy may interfere with standard preoperative instructions before dental surgery or treatment and may require the oral health care clinician, in consultation with the patient's physician, to alter the medical regimen or the preoperative instructions in order to insure a safe outcome. A general understanding of the pathophysiology of pituitary function and of the relationship of pituitary function to the regulation of endocrine function will help the clinician recognize new presentations of endocrine disease. Understanding endocrine function and the regulatory role of the pituitary will allow the clinician to avoid complications during the treatment of these patients with complex disease.

Pathophysiology

Current understanding of hypothalamic peptide release and of the role of the anterior pituitary hormones in the regulation of endocrine function is a work in progress. Four characteristic elements in the regulation of pituitary hormone levels have been identified. Specific hypothalamic neurons release small peptides into the anterior pituitary.[3] Secretory cells in the pituitary coordinate the release of larger peptides into the systemic circulation.[4] Resultant changes in specific endocrine organs, which act as a target tissue for the pituitary hormones, have been linked to specific pituitary hormones. A well-documented negative feedback by the hormone product of the target organ has been demonstrated upon the secretory pituitary cell and upon hypothalamic neuronal secretions.[3–7] In the central nervous system, peptidergic neurons in the hypothalamus release small peptides (3–8 amino acids) that specifically signal secretory cells in the pituitary to produce and release larger peptides (20 to > 1,000 amino acids) into the systemic circulation (Figure 22-1).

Within the pituitary, the specific transcription factors PROP1 and PIT1 have been described and studied.[8,9] PROP1 is required for anterior pituitary organogenesis, and PIT1 is essential for the synthesis and release of several pituitary hormones.[8] PIT1 is required for the production of three pituitary hormones—growth hormone (GH), thyroid stimulating hormone (TSH), and prolactin (PRL)—and is normally produced by the specific pituitary cell types secreting these three peptides.[9] Historically, the small peptides from the hypothalamus and larger peptides from the pituitary were linked to the endocrine functions of separate glands; thus, the nomenclature identifies the endocrine gland to which the releasing factor was originally thought to be targeted. In the case of the thyroid and the adrenal glands, the specific pituitary hormones released, TSH and adrenocorticotrophic hormone (ACTH), are taken up by specialized endocrine glands in the body (thyroid and adrenal glands, respectively) (Figure 22-2).

The thyroid and the adrenal glands release specific hormones; these are thyroxine (or thyroid hormone) from the thyroid and cortisol (along with several other related steroids) from the adrenal cortices. The adrenal medulla also releases other hormones, including angiotensin and aldosterone, but these adrenal products are regulated more

effectively by direct neural pathways than by circulating anterior pituitary hormones.[6,7,10–13] The hormones released from the thyroid and adrenal glands are circulated to many of the tissues of the body, causing changes in cell metabolism and function. Thyroid hormone (called T4 because of the presence of four iodine molecules in the mature hormone) and cortisol also provide negative feedback to the pituitary and to the hypothalamus. In early research on the hypothalamic-pituitary-thyroid axis, a small hypothalamic peptide most specific to thyroid function was characterized and named thyrotropin-releasing hormone (TRH). TSH, a larger peptide from the pituitary, is predominantly associated with thyroid function. Together, these peptides control three major functions of the thyroid: the production of thyroid hormone (T4), the growth and proliferation of thyroid cells, and the production of thyroglobulin (a large protein that acts as a binding, storage, and maturation protein for T4). As a consequence of driving thyroid hormone production with TSH, circulating systemic blood levels of T4 are elevated. The increased blood levels of T4 result in decreased pituitary secretion of TSH, forming a negative feedback loop. The negative feedback mechanism causes decreases in the specific releasing and stimulating hormones of the hypo-

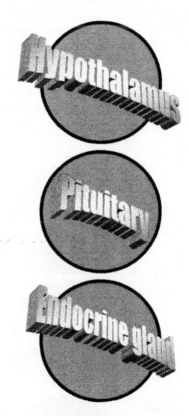

FIGURE 22-1 The hypothalamic-pituitary-endocrine axes control the major endocrine glands in the human. Peptidergic neurons in the hypothalamus release small peptides near the pituitary secretory cells. Specialized pituitary cells respond to the small peptides and release larger peptides into the systemic circulation. The endocrine gland is the target of specialized pituitary peptides.

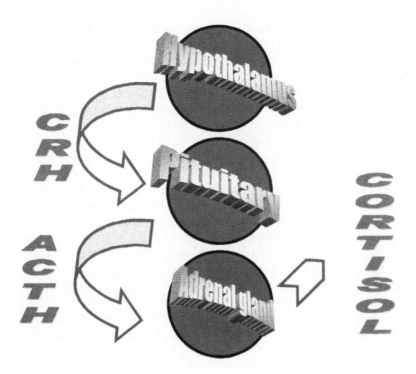

FIGURE 22-2 Corticotropin-releasing hormone (CRH) is released near the pituitary by peptidergic neurons in the hypothalamus. CRH stimulates secretory cells of the pituitary to release adrenocorticotrophic hormone (ACTH) into the systemic circulation. ACTH stimulates the adrenal glands, located above each kidney, to release cortisol into the blood.

thalamus and pituitary.[1,3,5,14,15] In a similar manner, rising concentrations of cortisol results in decreases in corticotropin-releasing hormone (CRH). Decreases in the pituitary production of the corresponding stimulating hormones, TSH and ACTH, result in the down-regulation of the hormone produced by the specific endocrine gland, T4 and cortisol (Figure 22-3). For TRH, the physical mechanism proposed as the hypothalamic signaling system is a mesh of small blood vessels with fenestrated capillaries located in the floor of the hypothalamus and resting in intimate con-

tact with the anterior part of the pituitary, where the cells producing TSH are found.[3]

TRH secretion from the hypothalamus is decreased by increasing T4 levels in the blood, but research on the hypothalamic levels of releasing hormones in cerebrospinal fluid surrounding the brain and spinal cord has made confirmation of the negative feedback at the hypothalamic level more difficult to investigate. A recent set of experiments showed that transgenic mice with no TRH expression exhibit only mild hypothyroidism whereas a human case described with a dys-

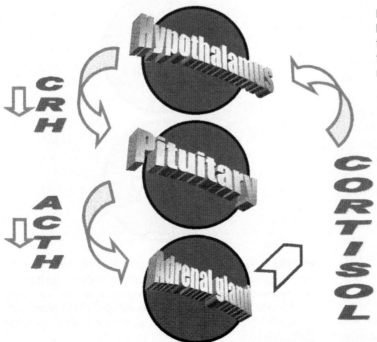

FIGURE 22-3 Cortisol, released by the adrenal glands into the blood, circulates throughout the body. Cortisol provides a negative feedback on the hypothalamus, decreasing the release of CRH from hypothalamic peptidergic neurons. The decrease in CRH release results in a decrease in ACTH secreted from the pituitary.

functional pituitary cell TRH receptor had mainly symptoms of short stature and delayed bone maturation.[3] These two observations suggest that while TRH secretion may up-regulate TSH and thyroid gland function, there is probably a basal secretion of TSH capable of maintaining basal thyroid function in the absence of TRH functionality.

Molecular Pathophysiology of the Hypothalamic-Pituitary-Thyroid Axis

The pituitary TRH receptor protein has been identified as a member of the family of G proteins; it has a molecular weight of 44.5 kDa and contains seven transmembrane segments.[3] G proteins are a common type of transmembrane receptor and include adrenergic and cyclic nucleotide receptors as well. Functional TRH receptors in the pituitary bind to TRH and are rapidly and extensively internalized by clathrin-coated vesicles. Some recent research has focused on the properties of the TRH and T4 signaling system within the hypothalamus and on the TSH receptor on the thyroid.[3,14] Specific TRH-degrading enzymes have been shown to provide significant control over TRH action on the pituitary. The conclusions of this research fit in with the partial dependence of TSH secretion on T4 and the partial independence from TRH secretion found in the previously described transgenic mouse with an absent TRH phenotype.

In most clinical cases in dentistry, practitioner knowledge of thyroid diseases can be based on an understanding of the classic hypothalamic-pituitary-thyroid axis as shown in Figure 22-4. With this knowledge and laboratory data, the practitioner can use the data in Table 22-1 to understand the current thyroid status of the patient. The interpretation of thyroid laboratory values is discussed further in the section on thyroid disease, below.

Pathophysiology of the Hypothalamic-Pituitary-Adrenal Axis

In the case of the hypothalamic-pituitary-adrenal axis, the small hypothalamic peptide thought to be specific to adrenal function was CRH. A larger peptide from the pituitary, associated specifically with adrenal function, is ACTH. ACTH is part of a much larger peptide, pro-opiomelanocortin (POMC), which also includes melanocyte-stimulating hormone and β-endorphins. Together, CRH and ACTH control the major functions of the adrenal cortex: the production of the stress hormone, cortisol, and several other related steroid hormones.[5,16] ACTH is also permissive for medullary adrenal function and for the production of renin and aldosterone, mineralocorticoids that are active in controlling blood volume and blood pressure.[12] The consequence of driving cortisol production with ACTH is an elevation of circulating levels of cortisol in the systemic blood. The increased levels of cortisol result in decreased pituitary secretion of ACTH, forming a negative feedback loop (see Figure 22-3). CRH levels are also decreased, but confirmation of the negative feedback at the hypothalamic level, as with the thyroid axis, has been more difficult to investigate.

For clinical dentistry, cortisol deficiency or excess is overwhelmingly an iatrogenic disease, caused either by treatment of the patient with glucocorticoids or by patient withdrawal from previous glucocorticoid treatment.[17] These circumstances and the clinical consequences of glucocorticoid therapy are discussed below in the section on adrenal disease.

PATHOPHYSIOLOGY OF GH-RH–GH–IGF-I

The hormonal axis associated with growth hormone (GH) differs from the previous two hormonal axes (the hypothalamic-pituitary-thyroid axis and the hypothalamic-pituitary-

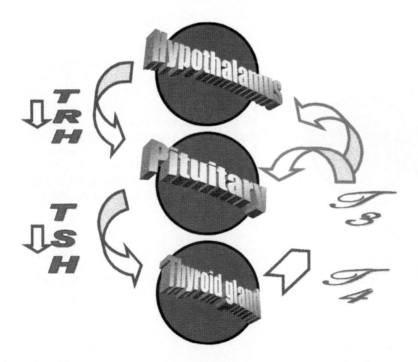

FIGURE 22-4 Thyrotropin-releasing hormone (TRH) is released near the pituitary by peptidergic neurons in the hypothalamus. TRH stimulates secretory cells of the pituitary to release thyroid-stimulating hormone (TSH) into the systemic circulation. TSH stimulates the thyroid gland, located in the neck, to synthesize and release thyroid hormone (T4) into the blood. The intracellular form of thyroid hormone (T3) provides negative feedback to both the hypothalamus and the pituitary. T3 decreases the release of TRH from hypothalamic peptidergic neurons. The decrease in the release of TRH, combined with the direct effect of T3 on the pituitary, results in a decrease in the secretion of TSH.

TABLE 22-1   Thyroid Status as Determined by Laboratory Testing for Hypothyroidism and Hyperthyroidism

Thyroid Status	Laboratory Tests	T4	TSH	Goiter*	Eye Signs/Orbitopathy
Hyperthyroid	Free T4; TSH	Above normal	Below normal	May be present	May be present and may progress
Normal, or subclinical thyroid disease	—	1. Normal[†] 2. High;[†] TSH normal 3. Low;[†] TSH normal	1. Normal 2. Low; free T4 normal 3. High; free T4 normal	—	May be only presenting signs of subclinical thyroid disease
Hypothyroid	Free T4; TSH	Below normal	Above normal	May be present	May be present
Other thyroid disease	—	Normal	Normal	Goiter nodules or asymmetric enlargement may be present	May be present from previous hyperthyroid disease

T4 = thyroid hormone; TSH = thyroid-stimulating hormone.

*Thyroid two times larger than normal size.

[†]Free T4.

adrenal axis). There is a similar release of a growth hormone–releasing hormone (GH-RH) from the hypothalamus. However, an additional peptide produced by the hypothalamus, somatostatin, inhibits the secretory cells in the pituitary from releasing GH. The pituitary releases GH in pulsatile bursts, with the maximal secretion occurring at night.[18] GH is active in many cells, leading to specific receptor binding on cell surfaces and to the production of insulin-like growth factor I (IGF-I). Along with increased cellular proliferation, cell growth and increased deposition of extracellular matrix proteins and mucopolysaccharides are the results of IGF-I action. Several binding proteins have been identified as IGF-I carriers. IGF-I is secreted from the liver, along with a liver specific binding protein, and circulates to other cells in the body, including those of the pituitary, where a negative feedback on GH is postulated to occur (Figure 22-5). Recent studies indicate that growth factor–binding protein 3 can be used to diagnose GH deficiencies and GH replacement therapy, usually in combination with circulating IGF-I levels.[18]

Generally, patients presenting to the dental practitioner with GH-related disease or therapy will be either children of short stature who are being treated with recombinant growth hormone or patients with acromegaly, a disease in which excess GH is secreted by the pituitary.

Acromegaly is a life-threatening disease because of GH effects on the cardiovascular system.[1] These pathologic changes include heart muscle hypertrophy and an excessive deposition of mucopolysaccharides around heart muscle fibers. Excess GH also decreases glucose tolerance in acromegalic patients, leading to mild to moderate diabetes mellitus and to the attendant accelerated atherosclerosis.[19] The accelerated aging of the arterial vessels is associated with increased blood levels of glucose. Elevation of glucose levels in the blood leads to increases in the non-enzymatic chemical combination of glucose with blood proteins, leading to increases in abnormal glycoproteins such as hemoglobin A_{1c}. Levels of this blood glycoprotein are used to assess the efficacy of intervention therapies for diabetes mellitus.

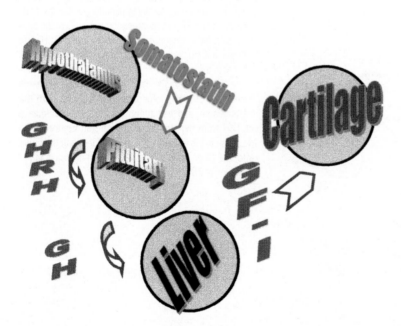

FIGURE 22-5   Growth hormone–releasing hormone (GH-RH) is released near the pituitary by peptidergic neurons in the hypothalamus. GH-RH stimulates the secretory cells of the pituitary to release growth hormone (GH) into the systemic circulation. GH stimulates the production of insulin-dependent growth factor I (IGF-I) by the liver. The liver releases IGF-I, bound to IGF-I–binding proteins, into the blood. IGF-I is responsible for growth in many cell types, including cartilage cells. Somatostatin, an antagonist of GH-RH, is also released from the hypothalamus.

One of the target tissues for GH and for IGF-I is growth cartilage.[20] In children, growth cartilage is found at the epiphyseal plate (an anatomic location in long bones, where new cartilage cells proliferate and form the long cartilage cell columns that will lead to long-bone lengthening and longitudinal growth).[18] One of the signs of excess GH before puberty is gigantism. In adults, there are fewer sites where growth cartilage is present; one notable site is the mandible. Patients with acromegaly show a gradual change in facial structure, with increasing length and breadth of the mandible, nose, and ears being the most prominent change. Patients with diagnosed acromegaly and patients with undiscovered acromegaly may present to the dental practitioner for orthodontic treatment as a result of these changes in facial structures.

Excess GH results in increased stature in prepubertal patients, by the action of GH and IGF-I on the growth cartilage of long bones. Even prompt treatment of this disorder cannot reverse the effects on bone lengthening or cartilage growth, but another sign of the disease, increased subcutaneous tissue (including mucopolysaccharides), regresses after definitive treatment, leaving the longer jaw, nose, and ears in place but partially diminishing the typical broadening of these features seen in active disease. Modern treatment of pituitary tumors secreting GH is to (1) surgically debulk large tumors, (2) remove small pituitary adenomas through trans-sphenoidal surgery, or (3) medically control small tumors either with dopamine agonists such as bromocryptine or with somatostatin analogues such as octreotide.[1] Older patients or patients who were treated previously may have had radiation therapy to the tumor in the past and may have multiple recurrences of their disease. Recently, a new agent, pegvisomant, a GH receptor antagonist, has shown to produce a reduction of IGF-I. Concentrations of IGF-I were significantly reduced after 2 weeks of treatment on as little as 10 mg/d of pegvisomant per day.[21] In this study, significant clinical improvement in four out of five clinical parameters was shown after 12 weeks on 20 mg/d of pegvisomant per day.[21] Frequently, patients with diagnosed acromegaly are on continuing medication for their disease.[1] However, some patients with evident facial signs of acromegaly have had curative resection or medication or have had a spontaneous resolution of the excessive GH secretion. In adults, bilateral growth of the mandible and new onset of diabetes mellitus should suggest acromegaly to the oral health practitioner.

▼ ADRENAL DISEASES AND CONDITIONS

Patients with ACTH-secreting pituitary tumors have Cushing's disease whereas those with similar symptoms (central obesity, cutaneous atrophy, easy bruising, muscle wasting, osteoporosis, hypertension, diabetes mellitus, immunosuppression, and psychiatric symptoms) from iatrogenic glucocorticoids, from adrenal tumors, or from ectopic secretion of ACTH have Cushing's syndrome. Cushing's disease is rare and occurs five times more often in women than in men, with a peak incidence

between 20 to 50 years of age.[1] Rarely, ectopic production of ACTH occurs, usually in a malignant tumor of pulmonary origin, leading to the classic symptoms of Cushing's syndrome. The usual cause of Cushing's syndrome is overwhelmingly the result of glucocorticoid therapy for another underlying disease. For the oral health care practitioner, the clinical complications of glucocorticoid therapy are manifest both during therapy with the glucocorticoid and after the glucocorticoid therapy is withdrawn.[17] In essence, the patient on corticosteroid therapy is at risk for the complications associated with Cushing's syndrome whereas the patient who has been withdrawn from corticosteroid therapy is at risk for complications associated with adrenal insufficiency. The dual risk for the patient is the result of the negative feedback of glucocorticoids on the pituitary secretion of ACTH and associated POMC peptides and on the hypothalamic secretion of CRH (see Figure 22-3). Chronic suppression of ACTH and CRH results in decreased adrenal production of glucocorticoids (Figure 22-6) and decreases the ability of the adrenal cortex to respond appropriately to ACTH and to produce endogenous glucocorticoids in adequate amounts.[15,22,23] The inadequate response of the suppressed adrenal glands to ACTH compromises the patient's ability to mount a stress response and impairs the normal stress response to systemic infections.[22,24–27] The suppressive effects of glucocoticoids on the stress response to endogenous ACTH are usually associated with high dose and chronic glucocorticoid therapy. But dose-related suppressive effects of exogenous glucocorticoids have also been detected (by sensitive measures of basal adrenal activity) with the recommended doses of inhaled glucocorticoids in children with asthma.[15]

Pathophysiology

The release of CRH and ACTH is governed by multiple stimuli other than cortisol (see "Hypothalamus and Anterior Pituitary," above). For example, leptin, a peptide hormone secreted by adipocytes, contributes to the regulation of CRH expression in the hypothalamus. Physiologically, leptin mediates the complex response of the body to starvation.[28] Leptin levels in blood reflect the proportion of body fat mass, rising in obese subjects and decreasing during weight loss, starvation, and malnutrition. But the levels of leptin are also related to meals and to ACTH diurnal rhythms. An inverse relationship has been demonstated between continuous 24-hour plasma levels of ACTH and leptin in normal subjects. Furthermore, exogenous glucocorticoids in pharmacologic doses produce a sustained rise in circulating leptin in both normal and obese subjects. This observation suggests a continuing inverse relationship between ACTH and leptin, extending into the pharmacologic range.[28] In addition to leptin, thymic peptides have been shown to stimulate the production of ACTH.[29] These peptides are produced by the thymus, which is the site of maturation of T lymphocytes. Thymulins have been postulated to act as thymic hormones, circulating to the pituitary and acting on secretory cells to increase ACTH release. The net effect of thymulins on the pituitary-adrenal axis is to augment the adrenal production of glucocorticoids. An additional finding

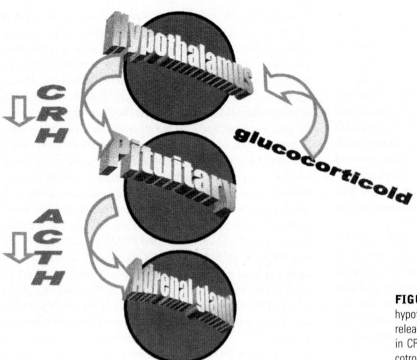

FIGURE 22-6 Exogenous glucocorticoids act on the hypothalamus, inhibiting the production of corticotropin-releasing hormone (CRH) by peptidergic neurons. Decreases in CRH cause a concomitant decrease in the adrenocorticotropic hormone (ACTH) secreted by the pituitary.

is that ACTH has been shown to produce reciprocal up-regulation of thymic peptides.[29] This intriguing observation suggests a positive feedback mechanism in which thymulins and ACTH reinforce each other after being activated during stress. Indeed, in the case of chronic adrenal insufficiency, in which ACTH is very high (Figure 22-7), the pronounced hypersecretion of thymulin is reversed by the administration of glucocorticoid replacement therapy.[29]

As part of the systemic response to stress, the activation of the immune system is accompanied by tightly regulated increases in glucocorticoid production by the adrenal glands. The effectors of stress-related glucocorticoid increases are cytokines acting on the pituitary and the hypothalamus.[27] Specifically, interleukin-1 (IL-1), interleukin-6 (IL-6), and tumor necrosis factor-α (TNF-α) have all been implicated as cytokines that participate in this process. In recent experiments,

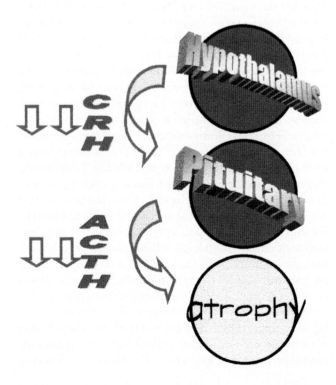

FIGURE 22-7 Withdrawal of glucocorticoids after therapy for inflammatory disease increases the release of corticotropin-releasing hormone (CRH) from hypothalamic peptidergic neurons. The pituitary is stimulated to increased adrenocorticotropic hormone (ACTH) secretion into the blood. After glucocorticoid therapy, however, the adrenal glands may be atrophied and incapable of responding appropriately to increased ACTH. The inappropriate response of the adrenals is called adrenal insufficiency. Clinical manifestations of adrenal insufficiency are hypotension, tachycardia, sweating, nausea, symptoms of cardiovascular collapse, shock, and death.

anti-CRH antibodies were able to block the cytokine effects on ACTH and glucocorticoids.[27] In contrast, glucocorticoids have been identified with severe immunosuppression. Even relatively modest doses of glucocorticoids (eg, 100 mg of hydrocortisone) have been shown to suppress neutrophil function.[22] Correspondingly, the beneficial effect of glucocorticoid therapy on chronic inflammatory diseases such as pulmonary fibrosis, rheumatoid arthritis, and pemphigoid is related to the ability of these agents to decrease the production of T lymphocytes, which contribute to the progress of autoimmune disease. Glucocorticoids have also been shown to decrease the production of cytokines, including IL-1, interleukin-2 (IL-2), IL-6, and TNF-α.[27] Furthermore, experiments have shown that timely glucocorticoid administration is important for avoiding the development of autoimmune disease in the Lewis rat (an animal model of chronic arthritis).[27] Gender differences in concentrations of ACTH and glucocorticoids have been documented in rodents, with females demonstrating higher levels and stronger glucocorticoid responses to IL-1.[27] The sex differences have been linked to the effects of estrogen and testosterone on the adrenal secretion of cortisol and have been demonstrated in humans as well as in experimental animals.

Glucocorticoid levels in the blood of normal subjects have been shown to increase with age in both men and women.[11] Some authors have suggested that the deleterious effects of glucocorticoids on the central nervous system, and specifically on memory and learning, are most evident at very low and very high levels of glucocorticoids.[16] There are other well-recognized effects of glucocorticoids on central nervous system function. Clinically evident to the practitioner who sees patients on moderate or high-dose glucocorticoid therapy is the euphoria associated with elevated glucocorticoid levels. Unfortunately, subsequent withdrawal of these psychoactive medications can produce dysphoria and depression. The mental disturbances associated with glucocorticoid withrawal are difficult for the patient and for the practitioner to manage in cases of chronic disease requiring intermittent glucocorticoid therapy. These symptoms occur in addition to the memory and learning deficits that have been suggested more recently. Some studies now suggest possible neurotoxic effects of glucocorticoids in primates, but the significance of these findings for humans is unknown.[13]

Clinical and Laboratory Findings and Diagnosis

The clinical findings of Cushing's syndrome are identical to the typical manifestations of moderate to high-dose glucocorticoid therapy. These signs and symptoms include central obesity, cutaneous atrophy, easy bruising, muscle wasting, osteoporosis, hypertension, diabetes mellitus, immunosuppression, and psychiatric symptoms (Table 22-2). Laboratory findings are usually unhelpful in diagnosing exacerbations of iatrogenic disease, except in the case of elevated glucose associated with diabetes mellitus. Cortisol levels may be high, normal, or low, depending on the interference with the cortisol assay produced by the therapeutic glucocorticoid employed. The underlying state of adrenal insufficiency secondary to the exoge-

neous administration of glucocorticoids is equally difficult to assess. In the normal subject, plasma cortisol levels during the daytime range from 100 to 300 nmol/L, but morning (8:00 am) peaks of > 400 nmol/L are expected because of the pulsatile secretion of ACTH at night.[15] This normal diurnal variation of cortisol may mask the diagnosis of adrenal insufficiency. Urinary free cortisol levels are often used to diagnose Cushing's disease, in which the elevation of urinary cortisol is due to a pituitary adenoma secreting ACTH. But urinary free cortisol levels may not be suppressed by inhaled glucocorticoids, even though plasma cortisol may not rise appropriately in response to a pharmacologic dose of ACTH, suggesting that adrenal insufficiency may coexist with apparently normal levels of urinary free cortisol. As rule of thumb, an 8:00 am plasma cortisol level of > 200 nmol/L would be unlikely to be found if adrenal insufficiency was present.[15]

Management

The clinical manifestation of adrenal insufficiency usually occurs when a patient on glucocorticoids is being withdrawn from glucocorticoid therapy or when a patient with a previous history of glucocorticoid therapy is challenged by a stressful event. Stress may occur in the form of an invasive surgical procedure, the onset of infection, an exacerbation of an underlying disease, or a serious life event such as the death of a family member. During stress in normal individuals, plasma cortisol levels may double, suggesting an inherent ability of the adrenal glands to increase cortisol production by 100%. In the patient with adrenal insufficiency, adrenal function is inadequate to produce adequate cortisol in the face of stress, and the patient may experience severe hypotension, nausea, cardiovascular events, stroke, coma, and death (see Table 22-2). Known severe adrenal insufficiency usually requires the premedication of the patient with 100 mg of hydrocortisone acetate intramuscularly 30 minutes before an invasive procedure.[30] Patients with a history of adrenal insufficiency are

TABLE 22-2 Signs and Symptoms of Glucocorticoid Excess and Adrenal Insufficiency

Glucocorticoid Excess	Adrenal Insufficiency
Decreased levels of cortisol	Decreased levels of 8:00 am cortisol
Decreased levels of ACTH	Increased levels of ACTH
Moon facies, central obesity	Anorexia, wasting
Muscle wasting, loss of subcutaneous tissue	Nausea
Poor wound healing, fungal infections	Stress-induced hypotension
Euphoria	Dysphoria
Increase in blood glucose, increase in insulin requirements	Stress-induced shock and cardiovascular collapse
Immunocompromised patient	—

ACTH = adrenocorticotropic hormone

often aware of the risk of stress and may self-medicate and increase or double their usual chronic dose of oral glucocorticoids before a procedure. Subclinical adrenal insufficiency may be suspected after as little as 5 days of high-dose glucocorticoid therapy (> 60 mg of prednisone). Dose equivalents for currently prescribed glucocorticoids are stated in the *Physicians' Desk Reference*.[31] Four of the most common equivalents are shown in Table 22-3. Many patients with chronic inflammatory diseases such as pulmonary fibrosis, rheumatoid arthritis, and severe asthma are on an alternate-day dosage regimen for glucocorticoids. The alternate-day regimen is usually reserved for stable chronic disease and permits the reactivation of adrenal and pituitary function on the days during which no oral glucocorticoid is given. For patients on long-acting glucocorticoids, especially the most potent agents, no stimulation of adrenal and pituitary function may occur on the off-therapy day because of a long drug half-life. Pituitary ACTH production takes place mainly at night. If circulating glucocorticoid levels are still elevated in the evening hours, the ACTH produced will be insufficient to stimulate the adrenal glands, even during "off" days. This is a particular problem with multiple daily dosing with glucocorticoids such as dexamethasone, which are most potent and which have long half-lives. Alternate-day therapy, as a strategy for limiting adrenal insufficiency, is best managed by using a high morning dose of prednisone or another short-acting glucocorticoid. Initially, the total dose for the 2 days should be additive; if 20 mg is given every day, then 40 mg will be required on the "on" day. Physicians usually initiate alternate-day therapy by gradually increasing the "on" day dosage while tapering the "off" day dosage, thus maintaining the total dose as a constant. In patients with recognized adrenal insufficiency, alternate-day dosage can be life threatening if significant stress occurs on the "off" day. If the patient cannot respond to stress and does not increase the oral glucocorticoid dosage, then severe hypotension, nausea, and shock may result. The problem of an adequate response to stress is even more significant in children with severe asthma, in whom inhaled glucocorticoid therapy has been shown to cause acute adrenal insufficiency.[23]

Prognosis

The course of iatrogenic Cushing's syndrome follows the course of glucocorticoid therapy for the underlying disease.

TABLE 22–3   Prednisone Dose Equivalents for Several Common Glucocorticoids

Medication	Equivalent Dose (mg)
Prednisone	5
Dexamethasone	0.75
Triamcinolone	4
Prednisolone	5
Hydrocortisone	20
Cortisone	25

During remissions of the underlying disease, as glucocorticoid doses are lowered, patients will have decreased symptoms associated with the glucocorticoid use; instead, the symptoms of glucocorticoid withdrawal will be evident. Additionally, symptoms of adrenal insufficiency may be unmasked as glucocorticoid therapy is withdrawn. Long-standing chronic disease with long-standing glucocorticoid therapy leads to adrenal insufficiency and a patient who requires exogenous glucocorticoids.

Patients with Cushing's syndrome are considered to be immunocompromised and may have unusual infections. Patients on increasing doses of glucocorticoids will also present with oral candidiasis and the reactivation of latent herpes zoster and herpes simplex virus infection.

Treatment

Treatment of patients with iatrogenic Cushing's syndrome must take into account the underlying chronic disease for which the patient is receiving glucocorticoids. Treatment of these patients should also follow the guidelines for the treatment of other immunocompromised patients, including appropriate antibiotic prophylaxis, careful attention to wound healing, and prompt intervention if infection occurs. For those patients with known or suspected adrenal insufficiency, consultation with the patient and the physician can decrease the risk of complications associated with inadequate adrenal function during invasive procedures associated with dental care.

Oral Health Considerations

HEMOSTASIS

Patients who are on chronic glucocorticoid therapy have decreases in subcutaneous collagen and the production of other extracellular proteins by fibroblasts. This lack of collagen fibrils and other proteins has been postulated to explain the tendency of patients with Cushing's syndrome to bleed and to bruise easily. There may also be related defects in the walls of small blood vessels, resulting in defective constriction of these vessels during bleeding. Wound healing is also impaired, and scar formation is less timely and less vigorous than in a normal subject.

SUSCEPTIBILITY TO INFECTION

Patients who are on chronic glucocorticoid therapy are considered to be immunocompromised and more than normally susceptible to infection.[32] Antibiotic prophylaxis is decided on the basis of the underlying disease, however, and not on the basis of glucocorticoid therapy. Patients with Cushing's syndrome are also more likely to have *Candida* and fungal infections, possibly due to abnormal flora on the skin and mucosa.

DRUG ACTIONS AND INTERACTIONS

Drug actions and interactions have been described in the above section that deals with the iatrogenic origin of most cases of Cushing's syndrome seen by the oral health care practitioner. The severe effects of adrenal insufficiency, which can be caused by previous or coexistent glucocorticoid therapy in the presence of stress, infection, or an invasive surgical procedure, are the likely consequence of not recognizing this syndrome.

ABILITY TO WITHSTAND DENTAL CARE

The stable patient with chronic inflammatory disease who is receiving low-dose glucocorticoid therapy will withstand dental care well as long as the potential consequences of adrenal insufficiency are avoided. Those patients on higher doses of glucocorticoids often exhibit the signs and symptoms of Cushing's syndrome and are thus subject to difficulties with wound healing and to minor difficulties with hemostasis and immunosuppression that may complicate oral health care delivery.

▼ THYROID DISEASE

General Description, Incidence, and Etiology

After diabetes mellitus, thyroid disease is the most common endocrine problem in the general population.[33] Many signs and symptoms of thyroid disease are observable during examination of the orofacial complex. Furthermore, under- or overactivity of the thyroid gland can cause life-threatening cardiac events. Consequently, the dental practitioner must be knowledgeable about thyroid pathophysiology and the treatment of thyroid conditions. Thyroid diseases often require long-term treatment, are frequently intermittent diseases, and worsen during life stresses such as childbirth or depression.[34–36] Thyroid diseases occur more often in women and most often in women older than 50 years of age. It has been estimated that the lifetime risk of thyrotoxicosis (eg, clinically significant hyperfunction of the thyroid gland) is 5% for women and 1% for men.[37,38] Routine screening for thyroid disease in an older (> 50 years of age) population of women will detect an unsuspected symptomatic thyroid dysfunction in 1 in 71 women.[35]

The second most common thyroid disease is found in the neonatal population.[39,40] Congenital hypothyroidism is caused by a clinically significant defect in thyroid hormone production at birth. Congenital hypothyroidism occurs in 1 in 3,500 newborns, affects females twice as often as males, and is one of the common preventable causes of mental retardation.[37] In the newborn with hypothyroidism, no clinical features are specific, but there is an inverse relationship between the age at which treatment is started and the degree of mental retardation. State-funded newborn screening programs for congenital hypothyroidism have had a significant effect on this common cause of mental retardation.

For adults, the most common signs and symptoms of hyperthyroidism and hypothyroidism are shown in Table 22-4. The signs and symptoms of hyperthyroidism are the result of increased secretion of T4 by the thyroid gland, but many are identical to the signs and symptoms of anxiety. In the dental patient in pain, signs of hyperthyroidism may coexist with and exacerbate the patient's normal response to pain and anxiety. In addition, routine examination of the head and neck may disclose signs of thyroid disease, including changes in oculomotor function, protrusion of the eyes, excess sweating,

TABLE 22-4 Signs and Symptoms of Hyperthyroidism and Hypothyroidism

Hyperthyroidism	Hypothyroidism
Anxious appearance	Lethargic appearance
Tachycardia	Low hoarse voice
Excess sweating	Slow pulse rate
Warm moist skin	Dry skin
Heat intolerance	Cold intolerance
Atrial fibrillation	Elevated blood cholesterol levels
Muscle wasting	Increase of subcutaneous tissue
Goiter	Goiter
Fine tremor of outstretched hands	Decreased hearing
Some weight loss	Some weight gain

enlargement of the thyroid or the tongue, lingual thyroid tissue, and difficulty in swallowing. Treatment of thyroid disease can accelerate the protrusion of the eyes and can cause agranulocytosis.[33] Atrial fibrillation, increasing thyroid size, and swings in thyroid hormone levels to symptomatic hypothyroid or hyperthyroid status are also possible during medical therapy for underlying thyroid disease.

Pathophysiology

The thyroid is a unique endocrine gland that depends on dietary iodine intake to produce the hormone thyroxine. Thyroxine regulates the pace of metabolism in all cells through interactions with mitochondrial, nuclear and extramitochondrial processes.[41] Dietary iodine intake modulates the functional activity of the thyroid gland, directly altering thyroid sensitivity to TSH as well as producing an inhibitory effect on thyroid function independent of TSH.[42] In the United States, bread and salt contain supplemental iodine, and the thyroid diseases that are most commonly seen have autoimmune etiologies. In many other countries, iodine deficiency results in increases in thyroid gland size (goiter) and hypothyroidism.

The major circulating form of thyroid hormone is T4, but T3, the tri-iodinated variation of thyroxine, is the active intracellular form of the hormone.[41] The location of the thyroid gland (at the base of the neck, just superior to the sternal notch) permits easy observation and examination by the oral healthcare practitioner. Autoimmune disease and the excess production of TSH by a pituitary adenoma also causes goiter. The two most common autoimmune diseases of the thyroid are Graves' disease and Hashimoto's thyroiditis.[43,44] Graves' disease presents most often with hyperthyroidism, goiter, and eye symptoms, which are linked to the etiology of the disease, namely, the production of autoantibodies that mimic the action of TSH at the TSH receptor on the cellular membrane of the thyroid cell.[45] An antigenically related site that interacts with anti-TSH receptor antibodies is also present in orbital muscle tissue.[43,46–48] Hashimoto's thyroiditis, which may present clinically with either hypothyroid or hyperthyroid symptoms and laboratory results, is an intermittent disease that is often exacerbated by intercurrent viral infection.[49] Sjögren's syndrome has been suggested to have the same immunologic etiology and to coexist with autoimmune thyroid disease.[50] In animal models, the NOD mouse and the BB rat spontaneously develop autoimmune thyroid disease along with diabetes mellitus. The co-incident diseases suggest that related immune defects may contribute to a common etiology.[43] In addition, environmental factors have been linked to autoimmune thyroid diseases.[49,51]

Thyroglobulin, a protein synthesized in the thyroid, not only binds T4 but also acts as a storage and maturation protein.[52] Thyroglobulin is recycled through the follicular lumen of the thyroid gland until the poorly iodinated prohormone bound to the protein is further matured; T4, containing four iodine molecules, is the major product.[52] This macromanagement of hormone production by protein transportation within the gland is unique to the thyroid and represents an additional layer of control of prohormone trafficking. Animal models of autoimmune thyroid disease have been useful for studying the onset of thyroid dysfunction, and researchers have used circulating thyroglobulin levels as an indicator of disease progression.[43] The control of thyroid hormone maturation by thyroglobulin is disrupted in thyroid cancer cells. Patients with thyroid cancer have abnormalities of prohormone maturation and a defective iodine interaction with thyroglobulin, which can be demonstrated in the thyroid cancer cells.[42]

Clinical and Laboratory Findings

Screening for thyroid disease can be divided into two categories: (1) screening of newborns for congenital hypothyroidism and (2) screening of adult patients seen for non-thyroid-related reasons, using the 1998 primary care guidelines formulated by the American College of Physicians.[37] Screening for neonatal hypothyroidism relies on TSH testing; an abnormally high TSH result requires follow-up by a T4 determination to confirm the hypothyroid condition (see Table 22-1). Screening for thyroid dysfunction in adults can identify four disease conditions: overt hypothyroidism and hyperthyroidism and subclinical hypothyroidism and hyperthyroidism. For adults, the primary screen is the TSH level, which, if abnormal, is followed by a determination of free T4 (ie, circulating T4 that is not bound to serum proteins).[35] If the TSH level is abnormally low, clinically significant hyperthyroid disease would be confirmed by an elevated level of free T4. If the TSH level is abnormally high, a subnormal level of free T4 would indicate clinically significant hypothyroidism. Subclinical disease for hypothyroidism is diagnosed by the combination of a high TSH level and a normal T4 level whereas a low TSH level and a normal T4 level represents subclinical hyperthyroidism. Screening is indicated for women over 50 years of age and for all patients presenting with any of the following signs or symptoms: thyroid enlargement, eye signs compatible with thyroid disease, new onset of atrial fibrillation, and a history of previous thyroid disease and new symptoms of either hypo- or hyperthyroidism (see Table 22-4 for a list of symptoms of hypo- and hyperthyroidism).[35] A new finding of asymmetry of the thyroid gland on routine examination of the head and neck requires referral and follow-up by an internist or endocrinologist. Whether the cause of the abnormality is multinodular goiter, nonfunctioning thyroid nodules or cysts, or thyroid cancer, the prognosis is good for early intervention and treatment in all cases except those of anaplastic thyroid carcinomas, which have a 10-year survival rate of 2%.[53] Diagnosis of a pathologic lesion in an abnormal gland is often a noninvasive procedure using fine-needle biopsy with aspiration cytology of the affected region.[54] Other diagnostic methods include ultrasonography, computed tomography, magetic resonance imaging, and nuclear scintigraphy with radioactive iodine.[55] Classification of thyroid cytology from fine-needle aspiration biopsy specimens is well developed and is often diagnostic. Papillary thyroid cancer is the most common epithelial tumor and accounts for 80% of all thyroid cancers.[53] Thyroid cancers are treated by excision and by radiation. Recurrence of the cancer after excision or radiation therapy may be followed with serum or tissue thyroglobulin determinations.[56] Rarely, thyroid cancers are metastatic. Metastases are seen especially with medullary thyroid cancer, a cancer linked to a rare autosomally dominant inherited defect of the *RET* proto-oncogene, which causes the familial syndromes that are called multiple endocrine neoplasia.[53] More common than thyroid cancer, solitary benign nodules of the thyroid are a frequent final diagnosis after the clinical finding of thyroid gland asymmetry. The treatment of these lesions is controversial and may include long-term T4 therapy.[57] Patients on T4 therapy for suppression of a thyroid nodule may never have had a history of either hypothyroidism or hyperthyroidism.

Differential Diagnosis

Knowledge of the differential diagnosis of thyroid disease insures the practitioner that planned oral health care does not pose a risk to the affected patient. For example, it is not uncommon for patients with an intermittent hyperthyroid condition such as Hashimoto's thyroiditis or for patients on medical therapy for Graves' disease to have an elevated blood pressure and heart rate, atrial fibrillation or severe symptoms of anxiety. Consultation with the treating internist or endocrinologist may allow additional therapy, such as β-blockers, to be added to the patient's regimen to decrease the symptoms of thyroid disease. This intervention will allow the oral health treatment plan to be carried out while the patient is still in treatment for the thyroid disorder. Patients with thyroid cancer may have surgery or radiation therapy to the neck, affecting the tissues of the head and neck area. As with the complications of other head and neck cancer therapies, postsurgical or postradiation complications may require special oral health care measures, depending on the patient's presentation. Tooth loss, diminished mandibular bone density, decreased salivary flow, difficulty in swallowing, and breakdown of skin and mucosa are the effects of previous radiation therapy.

The detection of hypothyroidism in the neonate is critical, but patients of all ages may present with hypothyroidism as a consequence of hypothalamic or pituitary disease (which interferes with TRH or TSH production) or as a consequence of previous hyperthyroid disorders.[35,39,40] Thyroid hormone replacement in the form of T4 is the recommended therapy for clinical hypothyroidism although some practitioners have used a combination of T4 and T3.[35] Hypothyroid patients require thyroid hormone supplements continuously and will often have follow-up laboratory studies of TSH levels while they are on T4 replacement therapy. Discontinuation of replacement thyroid hormone in a hypothyroid patient leads to an elevation of TSH level and to symptoms of hypothyroidism after 4 to 6 weeks. The elderly patient who is on inadequate thyroid replacement therapy is particularly at risk. Progression of the hypothyroidism can lead to impaired cardiac function, depression, increased deafness, fatigue, and skin changes. Blood levels of serum cholesterol increase as the hypothyroidism progresses, and renal function may also decrease.

Management

In addition to the management issues discussed above, thyroid-associated orbitopathy and thyroid-dependent bone loss may also be a result of thyroid disease in the patient presenting to the oral health care practitioner. Also, patients on lithium therapy for psychiatric disorders or on amiodarone for cardiovascular disease may have thyroid disorders associated with either medical therapy. In addition, the treatment of hyperthyroidism with methimazole or propylthiouracil may result in agranulocytosis.[33] Finally, in the Framingham study, a well-known longitudinal study of cardiovascular disease in a normal population, the incidence of atrial fibrillation was found to be inversely related to the level of TSH. The inverse relationship suggests a linkage (in a general population) between atrial fibrillation and the first subclinical manifestation of hyperthyroidism, decreasing TSH.[33]

Thyroid-associated orbitopathy is the most frequent extrathyroidal manifestation of Graves' disease. Two characteristic abnormalities are present microscopically: (1) excess glycosaminoglycans and (2) a marked chronic inflammatory infiltration of orbital connective tissue, fatty tissue, and extraocular muscles, with macrophages and T lymphocytes (usually cluster designation 3 [CD3] negative, CD8 positive [+], and CD4+) predominating.[48] TSH receptor protein has been detected in messenger ribonucleic acid and in protein from orbital fibroblasts in patients with Graves' disease.[58] Consistent with the etiology of Graves' disease, in which antibodies that mimic TSH action are postulated to interact with TSH receptors on the thyroid gland, it is presumed that the TSH receptor proteins in the orbital fibroblasts are stimulated by the same TSH mimics.[46,47,58] In 20% of patients who experience eye disease associated with Graves' disease, the orbitopathy appears before the symptoms of hyperthyroidism, and in 40% of patients, eye signs occur along with the diagnosis of hyperthyroidism. In the remaining 40% of patients with Graves' ophthalmopathy, signs of the disease may occur with radioiodine therapy or later in the disease process.[33] Less progression of eye disease is seen in Graves' disease patients who are treated with methimazole, and less progression is seen when radioiodine therapy is accompanied by a 3-month course of prednisone.[35] Smoking is known to exacerbate thyroid-associated orbitopathy. A combined analysis of studies of the effects of smoking on the progression of thyroid-associated orbitopathy showed an odds ratio of 7.7 (range, 4.3 to 13.7) for smokers compared to nonsmokers.[59] Most patients with thyroid-associated orbitopathy do not require surgery. Only in extreme cases with exposure keratopathy, globe subluxation, or compressive optic neuropathy is surgical decompression of the orbit required.[60] For many years, the most popular surgical approach was the removal of the medial orbital wall and orbital floor. More recent decompression methods are the removal of orbital fat, an endoscopic approach with total ethmoidectomy, and lateral wall decompression with lag screw fixation and reduction of the greater wing of the sphenoid.[60] The repertoire of surgical techniques may be individualized for the needs of the patient.

Bone mineral density and both exogenous and endogenous thyroxine excess have been extensively investigated.[33] With either replacement doses or doses used to suppress thyroid function (usually in the case of thyroid nodules), significant bone mineral density losses were reported in postmenopausal women but not in premenopausal women.[33] In a meta-analysis of all studies of thyroid replacement and suppression, premenopausal women showed bone loss from suppressive therapy whereas postmenopausal women showed bone loss from replacement therapy.[33] This result is consistent with the usual age of the women treated with these two thyroid conditions. Postmenopausal women are more likely to be hypothyroid and thus to require thyroid hormone replacement. Younger (premenopausal) women are more likely to be on thyroid medication for the suppression of nodule growth. Another analysis of the studies in the literature recommended that the bone density of both premenopausal and postmenopausal women on thyroid replacement or suppression be followed.[61] The influence of thyroid hormone on bone loss may be less significant in men than in women; however, there are fewer studies in the literature on the treatment of thyroid disease in men, and there is a lower incidence of thyroid disease in men.[61]

Lithium, used for the treatment of manic-depressive disorders, can interfere with thyroid hormone secretion. At high doses, lithium therapy can cause clinical hypothyroidism and result in increases in TSH and decreases in T4.[62] Amiodarone, an antiarrhythmic agent used in therapy for cardiovascular disease, is almost 40% iodide. This large dose of iodine transiently decreases T4 production. In most patients, normal thyroid function is restored within 3 months of amiodarone therapy.[33] Finally, for the oral health care practitioner who treats patients undergoing medical therapy for hyperthyroidism, the medications used to treat Graves' disease may cause low leukocyte counts. If their leukocyte counts decrease, patients on these medications should be referred immediately to an internist or endocrinologist, who will confirm or rule out agranulocytosis.

Prognosis

The prognosis is good for the benign thyroid diseases, including hyperthyroidism and hypothyroidism. Hyperthyroidism may follow an intermittent course, with exacerbations causing increasing serum levels of thyroid hormone. In addition, patients who have been treated for hyperthyroidism with radioiodine have an increased risk of hypothyroidism in the 10 to 20 years after therapy. Notably, changes in the dose of thyroid hormone may affect the metabolism of other medications. An internist or endocrinologist should monitor hypothyroid patients upon the initiation of thyroid hormone replacement and should be consulted in regard to interactions with other medications. For example, serum concentrations of warfarin sodium (Coumadin) or digoxin can be altered by changes in metabolism during the adjustment of thyroid hormone replacement therapy.

Oral Health Considerations

In hyperthyroidism, exophthalmoses, goiter, lid lag, and oculomotor defects are seen. Facial myxedema, an enlarged tongue, and a hoarse voice are observed in the hypothyroid state.

HEMOSTASIS

Patients with hyperthyroidism may have elevated blood pressure and heart rates on the basis of the effects of thyroid hormone on sympathetic nervous system activity. Patients with high arteriolar pressures may require increased attention and a longer duration of local pressure to stop bleeding. Hyperthyroidism patients who are on warfarin (Coumadin) may have an increased metabolism of this drug, leading to decreases in previously therapeutic coagulation indices.

Patients with long-standing hypothyroidism may have increased subcutaneous mucopolysaccharides due to decreases in the degradation of these substances. The presence of excess subcutaneous mucopolysaccharides may decrease the ability of small vessels to constrict when cut and may result in increased bleeding from the infiltrated tissues, including mucosa and skin. Local pressure for an extended time will probably adequately control the small-vessel bleeding.

SUSCEPTIBILITY TO INFECTIONS

Patients with hypothyroidism may have delayed wound healing due to decreased metabolic activity in fibroblasts. Delayed wound healing may be associated with an increased risk for infection because of the longer exposure of the unhealed tissue to pathogenic organisms. Hypothyroid patients are not considered to be immunocompromised.

DRUG ACTIONS AND INTERACTIONS

Drug interactions may result from the increased metabolic rate associated with hyperthyroidism or the decreased metabolic rate associated with hypothyroidism (see "Management" and "Prognosis," above, for more details). Well-controlled hyperthyroidism and hypothyroidism should not present an excess risk to the patient undergoing dental care. A complete history and physical examination of the patient with thyroid disease is necessary to define the particular thyroid disease and determine the stability of the individual patient. Consultation with the physician of the patient at risk is advised when history and physical examination indicate undiagnosed, untreated, or unstable disease.

▼ REFERENCES

1. Freda PU, Wardlaw SL. Clinical review 110: diagnosis and treatment of pituitary tumors. J Clin Endocrinol Metab 1999;84:3859–66.
2. MacArthur L, Eiden L. Neuropeptide genes: targets of activity-dependent signal transduction. Peptides 1999;17:721–8.
3. Bauer K, Schomberg L, Heuer H, Schafer MK. Thyrotropin releasing hormone (TRH), the TRH receptor and the TRH-degrading ectoenzyme; three elements of a peptidergic signaling system. Results Probl Cell Differ 1999;26:13–42.
4. Maurer RA, Kim KE, Schoderbek, WE, et al. Regulation of glycoprotein hormone alpha-subunit gene expression. Recent Prog Horm Res 1999;54:455–84.
5. Bugajski J. Social stress adapts signaling pathways involved in stimulation of the hypothalamic-pituitary-adrenal axis. J Physiol Pharmacol 1999;50:367–79.
6. Figlewicz DP. Endocrine regulation of neurotransmitter transporters. Epilepsy Research 1999;37:203–10.
7. Koob GF. Corticotropin-releasing factor, norepinephrine, and stress. Biol Psychiatry 1999;46:1167–80.
8. Pfaffle RW, Blankenstein O, Wuller S, Kentrup H. Combined pituitary hormone deficiency: role of Pit-1 and Prop-1. Acta Paediatr Suppl 1999;88:33–41.
9. Tatsumi K, Amino N. PIT1 abnormality. Growth Horm IGF Res 1999;9:18–23.
10. Mortensen LH. Endothelin and the central and peripheral nervous systems: a decade of endothelin research. Clin Exp Pharmacol Physiol 1999;26:980–4.
11. Perry HM III. The endocrinology of aging. Clin Chem 1999;45:1369–76.
12. Reichardt HM, Tronche F, Berger S, et al. New insights into glucocorticoid and mineralocorticoid signaling: lessons from gene targeting. In: Hormones and signaling. Boston: Academic Press; 2000. p. 1–21.
13. Sapolsky R. Stress, glucocorticoids, and damage to the nervous system. The current state of confusion. Stress 1996;1:1–16.
14. Russo D, Arturi F, Chiefari E, Filetti S. Thyrotropin receptor: a role for thyroid tumorigenesis? Forum (Genova) 1999; 9:166–75.
15. Wolthers OD, Honour JW. Measures of hypothalamic-pituitary-adrenal function in patients with asthma treated with inhaled glucocorticoids: clinical and research implications. J Asthma 1999;36:477–86.
16. Sapolsky RM. Glucocoticoids, stress and their adverse neurological effects: relevance to aging. Exp Gerontol 1999;34:721–32.
17. DeRossi SS, Glick M. Lupus erythematosus: considerations for dentistry. J Am Dent Assoc 1998;129:330–9.
18. Wood AJJ. Growth hormone therapy in adults and children. N Engl J Med 1999;341:1206–16.
19. Johannsson G, Bengtsson BA. Growth hormone and the metabolic syndrome. J Endocrinol Invest 1999;22(5 Suppl):41–6.
20. Pirinen S. Endocrine regulation of craniofacial growth. Acta Odontol Scand 1995;53:179–85.
21. Trainer PJ, Drake WM, Katznelson L, et al. Treatment of acromegaly with the growth hormone-receptor antagonist pegvisomant. N Engl J Med 2000;342:1171–7.

22. Abraham E. Corticosteroids and the neutrophil: cutting both ways. Crit Care Med 1999;27:2583–4.

23. Gordon AC, McDonald CF, Thomson SA, et al. Dose of inhaled budesonide required to produce clinical suppression of plasma cortisol. Eur J Respir Dis 1987;71(1):10–4.

24. Hunter JA, Blyth TH. A risk-benefit assessment of intra-articular corticosteroids in rheumatic disorders. Drug Saf 1999;21:353–65.

25. Jeffcoate W. Assessment of corticosteroid replacement therapy in adults with adrenal insufficiency. Ann Clin Biochem 1999;36:151–7.

26. Kapur S, Kupfer Y, Tessler S. Glucocorticoids for chronic obstructive pulmonary disease [letter]. N Engl J Med 1999; 34:1772–3.

27. Da Silva JA. Sex hormones and glucocorticoids: interactions with the immune system. Ann N Y Acad Sci 1999;876:102–17.

28. Casanueva FF, Dieguez C. Neuroendocrine regulation and actions of leptin. Front Neuroendocrinol 1999;20:317–63.

29. Dardenne M. Role of thymic peptides as transmitters between the neuroendocrine and immune systems. Ann Med 1999;31 Suppl 2:34–9.

30. Ferri F. The care of the medical patient. 4th ed. St. Louis: Mosby; 1998. p. 377.

31. Physicians' Desk Reference. 2000 Montvale (NJ): Medical Economics Company; 2000. Prednisone equivalents. http://www.pdr.net.

32. McEvoy CE, Niewoehner DE. Adverse effects of corticosteroid therapy for COPD: a critical review. Chest 1997;111:732–43.

33. Hanna FWF Lazarus JH, Scanlon MF. Fortnightly review: controversial aspects of thyroid disease. BMJ 1999;319:894–9.

34. Harris B. Postpartum depression and thyroid antibody status. Thyroid 1999;9:699–703.

35. Woeber KA. The year in review; the thyroid. Ann Intern Med 1999;131:959–62.

36. Nobuyuki A, Tada H, Hidaka Y. Postpartum autoimmune thyroid syndrome: a model of aggravation of autoimmune disease. Thyroid 1999;9:705–13.

37. Anonymous. Clinical guideline part 1. Screening for thyroid disease. American College of Physicians. Ann Intern Med 1998;129:141–3.

38. Maussier M, D'Errico G, Putignano P, et al. Thyrotoxicosis: clinical and laboratory assessment. Rays 1999;24:263–72.

39. LaFranchi S. Congenital hypothyroidism: etiologies, diagnosis and management.Thyroid 1999;9:735–40.

40. Weetman AP. Hypothyroidism: screening and subclinical disease. BMJ 1997;314:1175–8.

41. Oppenheimer JH. Evolving concepts of thyroid hormone action. Biochimie 1999;81:539–43.

42. Filetti S, Bidart J-M, Arturi F, et al. Sodium/iodide symporter: a key transport system in thyroid cancer cell metabolism. Eur J Endocrinol 1999;141:443–57.

43. Krogh Rasmussen A, Hartoft-Nielsen ML, Feldt-Rasmussen U. Models to study the pathogenesis of thyroid autoimmunity. Biochimie 1999;81:511–5.

44. Segni M, Leonardi E, Mazzoncini B, et al. Special features of Graves' disease in early childhood. Thyroid 1999;9:871–7.

45. Di Cerbo A, Corda D. Signaling pathways involved in thyroid hyperfunction and growth in Graves' disease. Biochimie 1999;81:415–24.

46. Heufelder AE, Bahn RS. Evidence for the presence of a functional TSH receptor in retroocular fibroblasts. Exp Clin Endocrinol 1992;100:62–7.

47. Heufelder A, Wenzel B, Bahn R. Cell surface localization of a 72 kilodalton heat shock protein in retroocular fibroblasts from patients with Graves' ophthalmopathy. J Clin Endocrinol Metab 1992;74:732–6.

48. Heufelder AE, Kahaly GJ. Thyroid-associated orbitopathy. Exp Clin Endocrinol & Diabetes 1999;107 Suppl:S152–57.

49. Wiersinga WM. Environmental factors in autoimmune thyroid disease. Exp Clin Endocrinol Diabetes 1999;107:S67–70.

50. Kohriyama K, Katayama Y, Tsurusako Y. Relationship between primary Sjogren's syndrome and autoimmune thyroiditis. Nippon Rinsho 1999;57:1878–81.

51. Baccarelli A. [Occupational agents and endocrine function: updating of experimental and human data.] Med Lav 1999;90:650–70.

52. Dunn JT, Dunn AD. The importance of thyroglobulin structure for thyroid hormone biosynthesis. Biochimie 1999; 81:505–9.

53. Udelsman R, Chen H. The current management of thyroid cancer. Adv Surgery 1999;33:1–27.

54. Fadda G, LiVolsi VA. Histology and aspiration cytology of benign thyroid diseases. Rays 1999;24:182–96.

55. Meller J, Becker W. Scintigraphy with 99mTc-pertechnetate in the evaluation of functional thyroidal autonomy. Q J Nucl Med 1999;43:179–87.

56. Pacini F, Pinchera A. Serum and tissue thyroglobulin measurement: clinical applications in thyroid disease. Biochimie 1999;81:463–7.

57. Walsh RM, Watkinson JC, Franklyn J. The management of the solitary thyroid nodule: a review. Clin Otolaryngol 1999; 24:388–97.

58. Warwar RE. New insights into pathogenesis and potential therapeutic options for Graves orbitopathy. Curr Opin Opthalmol 1999;10:358–61.

59. Mann K. Risk of smoking in thyroid-associated orbitopathy. Exp Clin Endocrinol Diabetes 1999;107 Suppl 5:164–7.

60. Graham SM, Chee L, Alford MA, Carter KD. New techniques for surgical decompression of thyroid-related orbitopathy. Ann Acad Med Singapore 1999;28:494–7.

61. Greenspan SL, Greenspan FS. The effect of thyroid hormone on skeletal integrity. Ann Intern Med 1999;130:750–8.

62. Johnston AM, Eagles JM. Lithium-associated clinical hypothyroidism. Prevalence and risk factors. Br. J Psychiatry 1999; 175:336–9.

63. Meier CA. [Hyperthyroidism — advantages and disadvantages of medical, surgical therapy and treatment with radioactive iodine.] Ther Umsch 1999;56:364–8.

23

NEUROMUSCULAR DISEASES

KATHARINE N. CIARROCCA, DMD, MSEd
MARTIN S. GREENBERG, DDS
ADI GARFUNKEL, DDS

Diseases that affect both nerve and muscle tissue encompass a broad range of symptoms that often have profound implications for the successful management of the dental patient. The diseases discussed in this chapter include only those that affect the orofacial region or that have a significant effect on dental practice.

▼ CEREBROVASCULAR DISEASE

Cerebrovascular disease includes all disorders that cause damage to the blood vessels supplying the brain, thereby producing neurologic damage. "Stroke" and "cerebrovascular accident" (CVA) are terms used to describe an acute neurologic injury resulting from a severe interruption in the flow of blood to the brain. Complete cessation of the flow may render an irreversible cerebral infarct within a period of 3 or 4 minutes. General symptoms following stroke include variable motor paralysis, sensory loss, visual difficulties, and speech impairment.

Epidemiologic studies have shown that cerebrovascular disease is the third leading cause of death in developed countries, with a prevalence of 0.8% of the total population affected. It is estimated that more than 400,000 individuals are affected by stroke annually in the United States. The majority of patients are over 60 years of age. The overall mortality rate following stroke is 25% in the first month and 50% within 5 years.

Cerebrovascular Accident or Stroke

Approximately 80% of strokes are associated with the development of atherosclerosis leading to cerebral ischemia and infarction. The remaining 20% of cases are caused by cerebral hemorrhage.[1] Deposition of atheromas in artery walls predisposes a patient to the development of thrombosis and embolus formation, which results in infarction of the area of the brain supplied by the occluded vessel. A thrombus is a clot in the vasculature that forms from the constituents of blood and may be occlusive or attached to a vessel without obstructing the lumen. An embolus is a clot, composed of a detached thrombus, mass of bacteria, or other foreign body, that originates from a distant site in the body and occludes a vessel. Atheromas commonly develop in the branching portions of the arterial system, particularly at the origin of the internal carotid artery. Additional sites of thrombus formation associated with stroke include the vertebral, basilar, and middle cerebral arteries.

LACUNAR INFARCTION

Lacunar infarcts are small lesions (usually < 5 mm in diameter) that occur in the distribution of the short penetrating arterioles in the basal ganglia, circle of Willis, pons, cerebellum, anterior limb of the internal capsule, and (less commonly) deep cerebral white matter. Lacunar infarcts are associated with poorly controlled hypertension or diabetes. Symptoms usually include unilateral motor or sensory deficit without visual field deficit or disturbance of consciousness or language. The neurologic deficit produced by the lacunar infarct may progress over 24 to 36 hours before stabilizing; however, the prognosis for recovery from the deficit produced by a lacunar infarct is usually good, with partial or complete resolution occurring over the following 4 to 6 weeks in many instances.

CEREBRAL INFARCTION

A cerebral infarction occurs when there is ischemia and necrosis of an area of the brain after a reduction of blood supply to a level below the level necessary for cell survival. The two major causes of cerebral infarction are thrombosis and embolism, often the result of atherosclerosis. Emboli frequently originate in atherosclerotic plaques in any vessel of the neck, such as the carotid artery. The emboli break off, pass through the vasculature, and ultimately occlude an intracranial vessel, thus causing a stroke. Thrombosis of an intracranial vessel may also lead to stroke.

The resulting deficit depends on the particular vessel involved and the extent of any collateral circulation. Carotid artery atherosclerosis, for example, will most frequently cause infarction in the region of the brain supplied by the middle cerebral artery. Occlusion of this artery results in contralateral signs such as facial weakness, head and eye deviation, flaccid hemiparesis or hemiplegia, and hemisensory loss.

Thromboembolic cerebral infarction also occurs as a complication of other diseases. Many of the emboli that occlude intracranial vessels arise from thrombi that have formed in the left side of the heart. Emboli originating from the heart are often the result of thrombus formation after acute myocardial infarction, chronic atrial fibrillation, or rheumatic heart disease. Hypertension is an important risk factor in the development of thrombosis, particularly at the carotid bifurcation. Treatment of severe hypertension is essential for the prevention of stroke since it is estimated that the risk of stroke increases sevenfold in individuals with uncontrolled hypertension. Septic emboli may result from bacterial endocarditis, particularly when the mitral valve is involved.

Other causes of ischemia and infarction of the brain include decreased blood flow secondary to sudden severe hypotension, acute hypertension causing spasm of the cerebral vessels, and hematologic abnormalities such as thrombocytosis, anemia, and cavernous sinus thrombosis.

CEREBRAL HEMORRHAGE

Hemorrhage of intracranial vessels may also cause stroke. The two most common reasons for hemorrhage are (1) rupture of an aneurysm and (2) an arteriovenous malformation (AVM) that hemorrhages spontaneously, often secondary to hypertension or following the administration of anticoagulant medication.

The majority of cases are aneurysmal. Aneurysms are localized dilations of arteries, caused by structural weakness of vessel walls. True aneurysms are found in arteries with normal wall structures that have been damaged by conditions such as atherosclerosis, mycotic infections, and syphilis. False aneurysms occur after the traumatic rupture of arteries and their subsequent repair by fibrous tissue. The size of the aneurysm is important in determining its tendency to rupture, a tendency that is aggravated by smoking, alcohol consumption, or strenuous exercise. The sequelae of hemorrhage from ruptured aneurysms are usually sudden and severe, ranging from seizures and coma to death. In the acute situation, it is vital to distinguish ischemic stroke from hemorrhagic stroke by the use of computed tomography (CT) without contrast.

CLINICAL MANIFESTATIONS AND TREATMENT OF STROKE

Strokes due to ischemia may be classified clinically either as a stroke in evolution or as a completed stroke. "Stroke in evolution" is a descriptive term used to indicate a condition in which symptoms associated with cerebral ischemia become progressively worse while the patient is under observation. The etiology is often related to the propagation of a thrombus in the carotid artery. Treatment should be immediate and consists of controlling severe hypertension (> 185/110). However, decreasing milder hypertension may actually increase infarction in a patient with acute thrombosis. The use of thrombolytic agents such as recombinant tissue plasminogen activator may decrease the severity of a stroke in carefully selected patients, but intracranial hemorrhage complicates this therapy. This regimen attempts to minimize the extent of permanent neurologic damage due to ischemia. Anticoagulants (such as heparin) or antiplatelet therapy with aspirin may also be used. Daily low doses of aspirin are recommended to decrease the incidence of thromboembolic strokes.[2]

A completed stroke caused by a thrombus often evolves slowly, and the full neurologic picture may take hours or even days to emerge. This clinical picture commonly includes hemiplegia, aphasia, and cranial nerve defects involving nerves V, VII, IX, and X. Symptoms of stroke caused by an embolus develop suddenly. It is not preceded by transient ischemic attacks (see below); rather, the stroke itself evolves rapidly because the clot originates elsewhere and suddenly blocks a cerebral vessel. Whatever the cause of the neurologic damage, the resultant infarct may enlarge for a period of 4 to 5 days because of cerebral edema. Repair is dependent on good collateral circulation and is accomplished by the formation of fibrogliotic scar tissue. Significant clinical improvement may occur after 3 weeks, when the cerebral edema has subsided.[3]

After a completed stroke, treatment focuses on the prevention of further neurologic damage, through the reduction of underlying risk factors and by rehabilitation procedures, including speech and physical therapy.

An intracranial hemorrhage should also be treated as a medical emergency of airway maintenance and requires the transfer of the patient to an intensive care unit with close monitoring. Blood pressure should be maintained in the 140/90 range. Fluid intake should be limited. Treatment with fibrinolytic drugs such as tranexamic acid might reduce new episodes of bleeding. Cerebral edema may be treated with dexamethasone and diuretics. The surgical treatment of a hemorrhaging aneurysm or an AVM consists of closing off the blood vessels that supply the area and removing the abnormality. This procedure has generally yielded high success rates.

Transient Ischemic Attack

A transient ischemic attack (TIA) is a sudden but reversible neurologic deficit that lasts from a few minutes to 24 hours. Approximately 30% of individuals with a history of TIA experience a completed stroke within a 5-year period.[4] The frequency of TIAs varies considerably, ranging from multiple daily attacks over an extended period to only a few attacks before a true stroke occurs.

ETIOLOGY

An important cause of transient cerebral ischemia is embolization. In many patients who experience these attacks, a source is readily apparent in the heart or a major extracranial artery to the head, and emboli sometimes are visible in the retinal arteries. Cardiac causes of embolic ischemic attacks include rheumatic heart disease, mitral valve disease, cardiac arrhythmia, infective endocarditis, and mural thrombi complicating myocardial infarction. An ulcerated plaque on a major artery to the brain may also serve as a source of emboli. Hematologic causes of ischemic attacks include polycythemia, sickle cell disease, and hyperviscosity syndromes.

CLINICAL MANIFESTATIONS

The symptoms of TIAs vary markedly among patients; however, the symptoms in a given individual tend to be constant in type. Onset is abrupt and without warning, and recovery usually occurs rapidly, often within a few minutes. During the attack, a wide variety of neurologic signs and symptoms can develop, depending on which site of the brain is affected by ischemia. Repeated short periods of arm and hand weakness are associated with focal ischemia in the contralateral frontal lobe. If the vertebrobasilar arterial system is involved, short episodes of dizziness, diplopia, dysarthria, facial paresthesia, and headache are common symptoms.

TREATMENT

Treatment of TIAs should be initiated as soon as the diagnosis is established and should be directed toward the correction of the immediate pathologic problem (eg, embolism). In addition, measures to control the primary underlying problem (eg, hypertension or coagulopathy) should be undertaken. Anticoagulant therapy with either heparin or coumadin is often used, but there is little convincing evidence that anticoagulant drugs are of value. Treatment with aspirin, however, significantly reduces the frequency of TIAs and the incidence of stroke in high-risk patients. Dipyridamole is also used but is not as effective; when added to aspirin, it offers no advantage over the use of aspirin alone for stroke prevention.[5]

Vascular surgical endarterectomy is now often used as an alternative treatment of TIAs caused by carotid stenosis. After surgery, a reduction in the frequency of TIAs and their progression to stroke has been observed.[4]

Oral Health Considerations

As the first line of medical management of stroke patients is often anticoagulant therapy, the patient may have a predisposition to excessive bleeding. A thorough medical history with an accurate medication list that includes dosages is essential. In addition, it may be necessary to confer with the patient's physician to obtain current coagulation values (ie, PT, INR) so as to ensure that the patient is stable for more invasive dental treatment.

Xerostomia is a common side effect of the medications used in the management of cerebrovascular disease and related disease processes. Patients who are thus affected can then be susceptible to a higher caries rate. Meticulous oral hygiene, more frequent recalls, saliva substitutes, and fluoride application can aid in the maintenance of the dentition.[6]

Stroke patients can also have physical disabilities, which can affect the orofacial area and can alter the provision of dental care. Patients with hemiplegia or hemiparesis may need additional help in home care. Patients with weakness in the muscles of the orofacial area may have poor control of oral secretions, a reduced gag reflex, and changes in their ability to masticate, leading to poor nutrition. Patients with apraxia affecting the orofacial region may have impaired voluntary movements, such as protruding the tongue, expectorating, and lip puckering.

In general, dental treatment should not present major problems for most poststroke patients. Careful history taking, checking of blood pressure prior to treatment, avoidance of lengthy appointments, and general reassurance are all important factors in the provision of dental treatment for patients with a history of stroke.

▼ CAVERNOUS SINUS THROMBOSIS

Cavernous sinus thrombosis, usually secondary to dental, nasal, or ocular infections, is a rare but severe complication because of its possible fatal outcome. Infections of the maxillary dentition may spread to the cavernous sinus through openings in the cranial bones or through emissary veins connecting the extra- and intracranial systems. Venous propagation begins with the facial vein and proceeds through the ophthalmic vein, which is an affluent of the cavernous sinus. In most cases, patients experience rapid swelling of the face and eyelids. The classic neurologic signs of acute cavernous sinus thrombosis are exophthalmos, periorbital edema, retinal vein thrombosis, and involvement of the ophthalmic division of the trigeminal nerve and trochlear and abducent nerves, leading to ptosis, dilated pupils, and lack of corneal reflexes. Treatment consists of immediate antibiotic therapy and the removal of the source of infection whenever possible.

▼ MULTIPLE SCLEROSIS

Multiple sclerosis (MS) is a chronic neurologic disease associated with the demyelination of axons within the central nervous system. The disease occurs more frequently among women. The average age of onset is during the fourth decade of life, but MS may occur at any age. The disease presents in the form of recurrent attacks; in some cases, the attacks are

years apart. The most common symptoms following an acute exacerbation include impairment of vision, muscular incoordination, and bladder dysfunction. The general histologic features are multiple disseminated plaques or areas of demyelination within the central nervous system.

Etiology and Epidemiology

The specific etiology of MS has not been clearly determined. An immunologic basis is strongly suggested by the presence of activated T lymphocytes and autoantibodies to glycoproteins detected in MS lesions. In addition, it is considered probable that both genetic and environmental factors are involved, with infection as the major environmental agent. Both viral and bacterial infections can initiate or precipitate attacks of MS. Evidence that implicates certain viruses in the initiation of the disease has been documented; increased antibody titers against measles virus, rubella virus, mumps virus, Epstein-Barr virus, herpes simplex viruses 1 and 2, and human herpesvirus 6 (HHV-6) have been found in the cerebrospinal fluid and serum. To date, none of these viruses has been isolated from the lesions of MS, and no specific relationship between MS and a specific microorganism has been proven. Further data supportive of an infectious etiology for MS include the observation that MS has occurred in clusters in specific populations, the prime example being the increased incidence of MS in the population of the Faroe Islands following foreign troop occupation during World War II.[7]

Genetic influences also appear to play a significant role in the development of MS. Studies of identical twins have shown that if one twin suffers from MS, there is a 26% chance that the other twin will also be affected by the disease. A preponderance of specific human leukocyte antigen (HLA) types has also been noted in MS patients.[8,9]

The most accepted general finding related to the etiology of MS is the fact that disease prevalence increases with distance from the equator; for example, MS is most common in northern Europe, Canada, and New Zealand. There are no obvious reasons for this geographic difference in disease prevalence.

Clinical Manifestations

The clinical signs and symptoms of MS depend on the site of the demyelinating lesion. The lesions may occur almost anywhere in the central nervous system, but they have a predilection for certain areas. More than 60% of individuals with MS have visual disturbances caused by demyelinating lesions of the second cranial nerve. The loss of vision usually occurs over a period of several days, with partial recovery within 1 month. Other ophthalmic symptoms include "color blindness" and diplopia caused by involvement of the third, fourth, and sixth cranial nerves. Uhthoff's sign, found in MS, is characterized by rapid vision loss following a body temperature increase that is associated with strenuous exercise. Another important sign of ocular disturbance associated with MS is Marcus Gunn's pupillary sign, which can be elicited in patients with unilateral optic neuritis in the following manner: a bright light is shone into each eye separately; when this light is moved from the normal to the affected eye, the pupil of the latter dilates rather than constricts.

Weakness or paresthesia of the extremities, with an increase in the deep tendon reflexes, is another common early finding in cases of MS. An important feature of motor nerve function in MS patients is the relative fluctuation of symptoms on a daily basis. These symptoms may remit for long periods and then suddenly reverse, leading to paraplegia. Other common signs of the disease include bladder dysfunction, euphoria, ataxia, vertigo, and generalized incoordination.

The majority of cases of MS are chronic and are characterized by exacerbations and remissions over a period of many years. During acute episodes, severe neurologic involvement is evident. This slowly resolves, but some permanent neurologic involvement remains after each episode. The extent and severity of the permanent involvement varies considerably from patient to patient. In mild cases, little permanent effect is noted, and patients may have a normal life span. In severe acute cases, total paralysis may occur within months. Overall, it has been found that approximately 70% of patients with MS live for more than 25 years after the onset of the disease.

Diagnosis

The diagnosis of MS is clinical and is based on the age of the patient, the presence of neurologic signs that cannot be explained by a single lesion, the progressive nature of the disease, and a history of exacerbations and remissions. There are no definitive laboratory tests for MS, but demyelinating changes can be seen on magnetic resonance imaging (MRI) in more than 90% of cases.[4] The presence of increased immunoglobulins (specifically immunoglobulin G [IgG]) in the cerebrospinal fluid without infection is another diagnostic indicator of the disease.

Treatment

Evidence suggests that high doses of intravenous corticosteroids may arrest the progress of MS; about 85% of patients with relapsing-remitting MS show objective signs of neurologic improvement during treatment with intravenous corticosteroids. Long-term treatment with immunosuppressants may reduce the frequency of relapse in patients with MS. Azathioprine is probably the safest drug in this category and has reduced relapse to 70% of study patients in 3 years, compared to 80% of patients in the placebo group. Administration of methotrexate appears to be the best therapy for slowing deterioration in patients with chronic progressive MS. The use of interferon-γ-1b and -1a has shown promise; both have been shown to reduce clinical attacks and lesions detectable by contrast-enhanced MRI by approximately 30% when compared to placebo. Other nonpharmacologic measures, such as total lymphoid irradiation, plasmapheresis, and immunoglobulin therapy, have had marginal benefit.[10]

Oral Health Considerations

Certain clinical manifestations of MS affect the orofacial region; three are of particular interest to the dentist: trigem-

inal neuralgia, sensory neuropathy of the trigeminal nerve, and facial palsy.[11]

Trigeminal neuralgia (TGN) is present in about 2% of cases of MS and is an initial manifestation in 0.3% of cases.[12] In those cases in which MS is associated with TGN, there appears to be an earlier age of onset, and symptoms are commonly bilateral. Pain is normally severe and lancinating, but trigger zones may be absent. In time, the pain often becomes less severe but more continuous. Effective drug therapy includes the use of carbamazepine, baclofen, gabapentin, or phenytoin. When medication proves inadequate, thermocoagulation, surgical sectioning of the nerve, or alcohol injection may be considered.

Sensory neuropathy secondary to MS can be progressive and difficult to diagnosis. It most often affects the second and third divisions of the trigeminal nerve, has a sudden onset, and is painful. Neuropathy to the mental nerve can cause numbness of the lower lip and chin.

Facial paralysis appears later in the course of the disease. It may be difficult to distinguish between the paralysis caused by MS and that due to Bell's palsy, but up to 24% of MS sufferers may experience facial paralysis.[11]

▼ AMYOTROPHIC LATERAL SCLEROSIS

Amyotrophic lateral sclerosis (ALS), also known as Lou Gehrig disease and motor neuron disease, belongs to a group of degenerative diseases affecting both the upper and the lower motor neurons of the central nervous system. The principal symptoms are weakness and wasting, which normally begin in the upper extremities and are invariably unilateral at onset. The estimated prevalence of ALS in the United States is reported as 2 to 7 per 100,000 persons, with slightly more males than females affected. The average age of onset is between the fourth and sixth decades of life. The etiology is unknown, although the disease is familial in 10% of cases when it is inherited as an autosomal dominant or autosomal recessive trait.[1] The degenerative changes of ALS can be seen in the corticospinal tracts (upper motor neurons), the motor cells of the brainstem, and the anterior horn cells of the spinal cord (lower motor neurons).

Clinical Manifestations

In the most typical form of ALS, stiffness of the fingers, awkwardness in tasks requiring fine finger movements, and slight weakness or wasting of the hand muscles are the first indications of the disease. Cramping and fasciculation of the muscles of the forearm, upper arm, and shoulder girdle also appear. Before long, the triad of atrophic weakness of the hands and forearms, light spasticity of the arms and legs, and generalized hyperreflexia (in the absence of sensory changes) leaves little doubt as to the diagnosis. After some time, the disease affects all regions, including the muscles of mastication, facial expression, and tongue, leading to difficulties in mastication and speech. Dysfunction of the temporomandibular joint and the development of malocclusion may also occur as the disease progresses. Aspiration pneumonia is the cause of death in most patients with ALS.

Treatment

There is no effective treatment for this disease, and the course is one of progressive deterioration, with a mean survival of 3 years. Ceftriaxone, gabapentin, guanidine hydrochloride, gangliosides, interferons, and cyclophosphamide are a few of the long list of agents that have all proven to be ineffective. Only supportive measures can be used.[13]

Oral Health Considerations

Muscles of the orofacial area can be affected by the disease process of ALS. The most striking physical effect of ALS relates to the declining function of the muscles used for breathing. As the patient may not be able to cough or clear the throat, a reclining position for dental treatment is contraindicated due to the increased risk of aspiration.[14]

In addition, a hyperactive gag reflex can pose a problem. Although it provides assurance that no dental debris will be aspirated, every effort must be made not to induce gagging or vomiting. Topical anesthetics should be avoided, patients should be nil per os (NPO) for 12 hours prior to treatment, and the dentist should avoid contact with soft-tissue areas that may induce gagging. Topical fluoride may also induce nausea.

Finally, patients with ALS may have difficulty with oral hygiene. Not only will these patients be challenged with physical disabilities that limit their effectiveness in maintaining oral hygiene, they are also faced with a loss of the natural clearing ability of the oral cavity because of decreased muscular activity of the tongue and the perioral musculature.[14] Mechanical toothbrushes, fluoride rinses, and more frequent periodontal recall may benefit these patients greatly.

▼ PARKINSONISM: PARKINSON'S DISEASE (PARALYSIS AGITANS)

Parkinsonism is a neurodegenerative disorder characterized by rigidity, tremors, bradykinesis, and impaired postural reflexes. The most common form of parkinsonism is Parkinson's disease (paralysis agitans), but parkinsonism is seen in a variety of disorders such as postencephalitic parkinsonism, arteriosclerotic parkinsonism, and post-traumatic parkinsonism following closed head injury. Parkinson's disease was first described by James Parkinson in 1817. It is an idiopathic disease that mainly affects adults in middle or late life. The reported prevalence rate in the general population is 130 in 100,000 persons; however, among those who are older than 60 years of age, the rate is considerably higher.[15,16]

Etiology and Pathogenesis

In idiopathic parkinsonism, dopamine depletion due to degeneration of the dopaminergic nigrostriatal system in the brainstem leads to an imbalance of dopamine and acetylcholine, neurotransmitters that are normally present in the corpus striatum. Experiments to reduce dopamine levels in animals have clearly shown that the classic symptoms of Parkinson's disease can be observed following this procedure. Thus, a low dopamine level will result in hypokinesia whereas a high level will lead to hyperkinesia. Symptoms similar to parkinsonism may also be induced by drugs that cause a reduction of dopamine in the brain, the most common of the drugs being phenothiazine derivatives. When drugs such as these are terminated, symptoms also quickly subside. Although a definite etiology has not been established, the most likely explanation is that the disease results from a combination of accelerated aging, genetic predisposition, exposure to toxins, and an abnormality in oxidative mechanisms.[15,16]

Clinical Manifestations

Tremor, rigidity, bradykinesia, and postural instability are the cardinal features of parkinsonism and may be present in any combination. The tremor is most conspicuous at rest, is enhanced by emotional stress, and tends to be less severe during voluntary activity. Rigidity (an increase in resistance to passive movement) is responsible for the characteristically flexed posture seen in many patients. The most disabling symptoms are due to bradykinesia, manifested as a slowness of voluntary movement and a reduction in automatic movements such as the swinging of the arms while walking.

The onset of the disease is generally insidious. Mild stiffness of the muscles of the extremities and tremor of the hands are frequently early signs. The typical hand tremor is often called a "pill-rolling" movement, characterized by the rubbing of the thumb against the fingers, and is particularly pronounced when the patient is otherwise at rest. The general stiffness progresses slowly until significant disability is noted by the patient. Walking becomes more difficult, and the patient develops a slow shuffling gait with a stooped position. As the ability to perform voluntary movements decreases, patients usually experience an inability to coordinate separate or independent movements.

Many of the signs of Parkinson's disease are found in the head and neck. The typical "masklike" facial appearance with infrequent blinking and lack of expression is caused by bradykinesia. The muscle rigidity also causes difficulty in swallowing, resulting in drooling. Speech becomes labored because of the lack of muscle control, and mandibular tremor results in masticatory difficulties, especially in those with removable dental appliances. Abnormalities in oral behavior, such as purposeless chewing, grinding, and sucking movements, are also well recognized in patients with Parkinson's disease and make dental treatment especially difficult.

Treatment

MEDICAL MEASURES

Drug treatment is often not required early in the course of parkinsonism. Patients with mild symptoms but no disability may be helped by amantadine. This drug improves all of the clinical features of parkinsonism, but its mode of action is unclear. Anticholinergics are more helpful in alleviating tremor and rigidity than in alleviating bradykinesia, but these drugs have many side effects. Levodopa, a dopamine precursor that can cross the blood-brain barrier, improves all the major features of parkinsonism. This drug is used solely as replacement therapy for the underlying dopamine deficiency; it will neither halt nor reverse the degenerative process affecting brainstem neurons. Side effects associated with this drug therapy may be minimized by using a combination of levodopa and carbidopa. Carbidopa prevents the destruction of levodopa in the bloodstream, enabling lower (and therefore less toxic) dosages to be prescribed.

Dopamine agonists act directly on dopamine receptors, and their use in the treatment of parkinsonism is associated with a lower incidence of the response fluctuations and dyskinesias that occur with long-term levodopa therapy. The two most widely used agonists are bromocriptine and pergolide, which are equally effective ergot derivatives. Pramipexole and ropinirol are two newer dopamine agonists that are not ergot derivatives; they are more selective, have fewer side effects, and may produce a longer-lasting response than the older ergot derivatives.[17]

GENERAL MEASURES, SURGICAL MEASURES, AND BRAIN STIMULATION

Physical therapy or speech therapy can help many patients. Surgical procedures, such as thalamotomy or pallidotomy, may be helpful for patients who become unresponsive to medical treatment or who experience intolerable side effects from medications. Finally, high-frequency thalamic stimulation is effective in suppressing the rest tremor of Parkinson's disease. Because electrical stimulation of the brain has the advantages of being reversible and of causing minimal or no damage to the brain, its use is being explored.[17]

Oral Health Considerations

Patients with Parkinson's disease can pose a multitude of challenges to the dental practitioner. Patients must often be treated in the upright position, making access to certain areas of the oral cavity difficult for the dentist. In addition, anxiety in a Parkinson's disease patient can increase both the tremor and the degree of muscle rigidity. Due to dysphagia and an altered gag reflex, special precautions must be taken to avoid the aspiration of water or materials used during dental procedures. In patients who suffer with hypersialorrhea, maintaining a dry field in procedures that require such can be especially difficult.[18] Xerostomia, on the other hand, is a common side effect of antiparkinsonism medications; the consequent root caries and recurrent decay must be diligently treated. Patients also often have difficulty maintaining their dentition because of their physical disability. For all of these reasons, more frequent recall may be necessary. When dental treatment is finished, the patient should be warned to take care when moving from a supine position to a standing position since levodopa has a significant orthostatic hypotensive effect.

▼ HUNTINGTON'S DISEASE (HUNTINGTON'S CHOREA)

Huntington's disease is a hereditary degenerative disease of the central nervous system, characterized by chorea (involuntary movements) and dementia. It is inherited in an autosomal dominant manner and occurs throughout the world and in all ethnic groups, with a prevalence rate of about 5 per 100,000. Clinical onset is usually between 30 and 50 years of age. The disease is progressive and usually leads to a fatal outcome within 15 to 20 years The gene responsible for the disease has been located on the short arm of chromosome 4.[19]

Clinical Manifestations

The earliest manifestation of the disease consists of depression or irritability, coupled with a slowing of cognition. There are subtle changes in coordination and minor choreiform movements appear. The main clinical manifestation is progressively worsening choreic movements that can be observed in the face, tongue, and head. With time, the hyperkinesia becomes aggravated, and movements can become violent, with difficulty in speech and in swallowing.

Treatment

There is no cure for Huntington's disease; progression cannot be halted, and treatment is purely symptomatic. Treatment is usually dependent on dopamine receptor blocking agents such as haloperidol and phenothiazines, which temporarily reduce the hyperkinesis and the behavior disturbances.[19]

Oral Health Considerations

Dysphagia and choreic movement of the face and tongue will make dental treatment especially challenging. Sedation with diazepam may be considered. Whenever possible, dentures should be avoided because of the danger of fracture or the accidental swallowing of the dentures.[18]

▼ CEREBRAL PALSY

The term "cerebral palsy" refers to a group of disorders with motor manifestations due to nonprogressive brain damage occurring before or after birth. The incidence of cerebral palsy (CP) is 2 to 6 in every 1,000 live births. There are a multiplicity of causes of CP. Anoxia and ischemia during labor have been implicated, but congenital infections such as toxoplasmosis, rubella, *Cytomegalovirus* disease, herpes simplex, syphilis, and influenza have also been associated with CP or mental retardation.[1,20]

Clinical Manifestations

The clinical manifestations of CP can be spastic, dyskinetic, ataxic, or a combination affecting one or all four limbs. The spastic forms of CP are the most common, and the legs are most commonly affected. Speaking problems are prevalent, with dysarthria, chewing, and swallowing difficulties. Drooling is both a functional and esthetic inconvenience. In hemiplegic cases of CP, the right side is more often involved. Sometimes, there are seizures associated with mental retardation. The dyskinetic type is characterized by athetotic purposeless movement, involving both agonist and antagonist muscles, that is increased by voluntary activity. During either natural or induced sleep, the movements cease. Head movements and facial grimacing are characteristic. One should not be misled by the appearance of the patient since most CP patients are intellectually normal.

Treatment

With improved perinatal care, both anoxia and perinatal infections have been markedly reduced, thus leading to a reduction in the incidence of CP. The key to success in the management of CP is teamwork and a planned approach to the individual child's problem. Many children with CP have normal intelligence and should not be penalized because of dysarthria or involuntary movements. Physiotherapy should be instituted as early as possible in order to prevent contractures, and orthopedic surgery has been used occasionally with some degree of success.[21] If the patient suffers from seizures, appropriate drug therapy is instituted (see "Epilepsy," later in this chapter).

Oral Health Considerations

Children with CP show an increased incidence of enamel defects, the cause of which is not clear. A much more bothersome finding is the sialorrhea and drooling experienced by CP patients. This develops in the absence of orofacial and neck muscle coordination. One treatment, sialodocholoplasty (the relocation of salivary gland ducts into the tonsillar fossa and the removal of the sublingual salivary glands), has been shown to be effective.[22] Less invasive management of sialorrhea includes a systemic medication such as glycopyrolate and anticholinergic agents.[23]

▼ BELL'S PALSY

Bell's palsy is recognized as a unilateral paresis of the facial nerve. The dysfunction has been attributed to an inflammatory reaction involving the facial nerve. A relationship has been demonstrated between Bell's palsy and the isolation of herpes simplex virus 1 from nerve tissues.[24–26] Bell's palsy must be differentiated from other causes of facial nerve palsy, including Lyme disease, herpes zoster of the geniculate ganglion (Ramsay Hunt syndrome), and tumors such as acoustic neuromas.[27]

Clinical Manifestations

Bell's palsy begins with slight pain around one ear, followed by an abrupt paralysis of the muscles on that side of the face. The eye on the affected side stays open, the corner of the mouth drops, and there is drooling. As a result of masseter weakness, food is retained in both the upper and lower buccal and labial folds. The facial expression changes remarkably, and the creases of the forehead are flattened. Due to impaired blinking, corneal ulcerations from foreign bodies can occur. Involvement of the chorda tympani nerve leads to loss of taste

perception on the anterior two-thirds of the tongue and reduced salivary secretion.

Treatment

The only medical treatment that may influence the outcome is the administration of systemic corticosteroids within the first few days after the onset of paralysis, but this therapy should be avoided if Lyme disease is suspected. Combining steroids with antiherpetic drugs such as acyclovir may decrease the severity and length of paralysis.[28]

It is also helpful to protect the eye with lubricating drops or ointment and a patch if eye closure is not possible. When paralysis-induced eye opening is permanent, intrapalpebral gold weights are inserted, thus closing the upper eyelid. Facial plastic surgery and the creation of an anastomosis between the facial and hypoglossal nerves can occasionally restore partial function and improve appearance for patients with permanent damage.

▼ GUILLAIN-BARRÉ SYNDROME

Guillain-Barré syndrome (acute idiopathic polyneuropathy)is an acute symmetrical ascending polyneuropathy, often occurring 1 to 3 weeks (and occasionally up to 8 weeks) after an acute infection. The Guillain-Barré syndrome often follows a nonspecific respiratory or gastrointestinal illness but has also been described after a few specific infections (such as with *Cytomegalovirus*, Epstein-Barr virus, *Enterovirus*, *Campylobacter jejuni*, or *Mycoplasma*) and after immunization. There is a worldwide incidence of 1.6 to 1.9 cases per 100,000 population per year.[29] The disorder probably has an immunologic basis, but the precise mechanism is unclear.

Clinical Manifestations

The syndrome often begins with myalgia or paresthesias of the lower limbs, followed by weakness, which often ascends to involve abdominal, thoracic, and upper-limb muscles. In severe cases, respiration is compromised. Involvement of the autonomic nervous system by the disease process may induce changes in blood pressure and pulse rate. From an oral medicine perspective, the interesting feature of this disease is the fact that impaired swallowing or paresthesias of the mouth and face may be early signs of the disease. The seventh cranial nerve is frequently involved, and bilateral facial weakness is common. Involvement of other cranial nerves may result in ptosis or facial myokymia. Dysarthria, dysphagia and diplopia may develop in severe cases.

Treatment and Prognosis

The paralysis in Guillain-Barré syndrome may progress for about 10 days and may then remain relatively unchanged for about 2 weeks. The recovery phase is much slower and may take from 6 months to 2 years for completion. Permanent signs of neurologic damage can persist in some patients.

Treatment with prednisone is ineffective and may actually affect the outcome adversely by prolonging recovery time.

Plasmapheresis is of value; however it is best performed within the first few days of illness and is best reserved for clinically severe or rapidly progressive cases.[1]

▼ MYASTHENIA GRAVIS

Myasthenia gravis (MG) is a disease characterized by progressive muscular weakness on exertion, secondary to a disorder at the neuromuscular junction. Acetylcholine normally transmits the impulse from nerve to muscle at the neuromuscular junction, and cholinesterase hydrolyzes acetylcholine. In patients with MG, autoantibodies that combine with and may destroy the acetylcholine receptor sites at the neuromuscular junction are present, preventing the transmission of nerve impulses to the muscle. The origin of the autoantibodies is unknown, but other findings linking MG to autoimmunity include the incidence of thymoma in MG patients, the improvement of symptoms after thymectomy, and the association of MG with other diseases involving abnormal immune phenomena, such as pemphigus, pemphigoid, systemic lupus erythematosus, and rheumatoid arthritis. The disease occurs more frequently in women than in men, particularly during the third and fourth decades of life.[30]

Clinical Manifestations

The initial signs of this disease commonly occur in areas innervated by the cranial nerves (frequently, the eye muscles). Patients present with ptosis, diplopia, difficulty in chewing or swallowing, respiratory difficulties, limb weakness, or some combination of these problems. In some patients, the disease remains confined to the eye muscles, but in most cases, it progresses to other cranial nerves as well as to the shoulders and limbs. MG follows an unpredictable course, and exacerbations and remissions occur frequently. In severe advanced cases, respiratory difficulty arises.

Diagnosis is made initially on the basis of clinical presentation. The inability of a patient to continually blink the eyes voluntarily is highly suggestive of MG. The clinical diagnosis can be confirmed by the dramatic improvement of symptoms with the administration of a short-acting anticholinesterase; it will antagonize the effect of cholinesterase on acetylcholine, allowing increased levels of this chemical at the neuromuscular junction. Specific tests for detecting the antiacetylcholine receptor antibody are now available for confirmation of diagnosis.

Treatment

Anticholinesterase drugs such as neostigmine and pyridostigmine bromide provide symptomatic benefit without influencing the course of the disease.[30] In patients with more severe disease, remission may be achieved by thymectomy. In other cases, long-term cortico-steroids and immunosuppressive drugs are necessary. Plasmapheresis has been of temporary value in patients with severe exacerbations of MG.

Oral Health Considerations

Oral and facial signs are an important component of the clinical picture of MG. The facial muscles are commonly involved, giving the patient an immobile and expressionless appearance. This has led to the incorrect diagnosis of psychiatric disease in MG patients. Tongue edema may also be present in MG, making eating difficult for patients.[31] Patients whose muscles of mastication are weakened can also experience consequent difficulty in chewing; these patients will be unable to finish chewing a bolus of food because of the easy fatigability of the muscles. It is essential to be aware that this may be an early sign of disease. The patient's masticatory muscles may become so tired that the mouth remains open after eating. An important indication of MG is a patient who must hold his jaws closed with his hand.

When treating known MG patients, the dentist must be aware that a respiratory crisis may develop from the disease itself or from overmedication. If a patient is at risk for developing a respiratory crisis, dental treatment should be performed in a hospital where endotracheal intubation can be performed. The airway must be kept clear because aspiration may occur in patients whose swallowing muscles are involved. Adequate suction and the use of a rubber dam are aids in these cases.

The dentist should avoid prescribing drugs that may affect the neuromuscular junction, such as narcotics, tranquilizers, and barbiturates. Certain antibiotics, including tetracycline, streptomycin, sulfonamides, and clindamycin, may reduce neuromuscular activity and should be avoided.

▼ MUSCULAR DYSTROPHY

Muscular dystrophy (MD) is a genetic disease characterized by muscle atrophy that causes severe progressive weakness. The primary biochemical defect has not been identified, but evidence is accumulating to implicate an enzymatic dysfunction at the muscle surface membrane.

Clinical Manifestations

The various forms of MD are genetically determined myopathies characterized by progressive muscular weakness and the degeneration of muscle fibers. The muscular dystrophies are classified according to mode of inheritance, age at onset, and clinical features.

DUCHENNE'S MUSCULAR DYSTROPHY

Duchenne's muscular dystrophy is the most common form of MD and is seen almost exclusively in young males. This type of MD is a result of a mutation of the dystrophin gene located on the short arm of the X chromosome.[32] Clinical manifestations begin during the first 3 years of life. Affected children appear normal at birth and may be extremely placid. Early signs are difficulty in walking, frequent falling, and the inability to run. Symptoms progress as muscles continue to atrophy. Initially, the atrophy is marked although muscles may appear even larger than normal, primarily because of the fat deposition in the muscles. Pseudohypertrophy of muscles frequently occurs at some stage. Intellectual retardation is common, and there may be skeletal deformities, muscle contractures, and cardiac involvement. Serum levels of the enzyme creatine phosphokinase are elevated in affected males as well as in female carriers.

At the end of the first decade of life, the child will be unable to walk and will be bedridden. Respiratory muscles will begin to be affected, and most patients die in the late teenage years or early twenties. A better understanding of pulmonary problems and improved treatment of respiratory infections have increased the life span of these patients. The muscles of the pelvis and femoral region are most severely affected by the Duchenne form of MD, but the muscles of the face, head, and neck are not involved.

BECKER'S MUSCULAR DYSTROPHY

Becker's MD is a milder expression of the disease, caused by mutation of the *dystrophin* gene. There is a wide range of presenting symptoms that vary in severity from a slightly milder form of the disease resembling Duchenne's MD to an asymptomatic elevation of creatine kinase. The age of onset is between 5 and 25 years, with a mean age of 11 years.[32] The progression of Becker's MD is slow, and patients may have a normal life span.

FACIOSCAPULOHUMERAL DYSTROPHY

Facioscapulohumeral dystrophy is inherited as an autosomal dominant trait and affects both males and females. Symptoms do not usually begin until the second decade of life. It is not as universally devastating as the Duchenne form of MD, and some patients may live a normal life span with minimal physical disability. The muscles of the face and pectoral girdle are most severely involved, and these patients characteristically exhibit weakness of the arms, winging of the scapulae, and weakness of the muscles of the eyes and mouth.

LIMB-GIRDLE DYSTROPHY

Limb-girdle MD is inherited, usually as an autosomal recessive trait; however, it may also be sporadically or dominantly inherited. It affects both sexes and has its onset in the second and third decades of life. The weakness starts in either the shoulders or the pelvis but will eventually spread to both. This is characteristically a slowly progressing form of MD. Facial muscles are not involved.

OCULOPHARYNGEAL MUSCULAR DYSTROPHY

A rare form of MD, oculopharyngeal MD is inherited as an autosomal dominant trait and is characterized by the late onset of chronically progressive ptosis and dysphagia. Symptoms may begin at any age and consist of progressive weakness of levator palpebrae and chronic contraction of the frontalis muscle. The patient will maintain a chin-up head position and will have difficulty in swallowing solid food initially and liquids later. A late weakness of limb-girdle muscles may occur.

MYOTONIC DYSTROPHY

Myotonic dystrophy is a multisystem disorder inherited as an autosomal dominant trait through a locus on chromosome 19.[1] The signs and symptoms may appear at any time from birth to the age of 40 years, and the disease is characterized by progressive muscular weakness, myotonia, cataracts, cardiac abnormalities, hypogonadism, and frontal balding. The most severe involvement occurs in the muscles of the head and neck and in the distal extremities. Myotonia is the persistence of the contraction of muscles; in this form of MD, the patient is unable to relax the muscles after contraction. This symptom can be best observed in the forearm, thumb, and tongue. Wasting of muscles and subsequent weakness are as prominent as in other forms of MD. Involvement of the facial muscles and hands is especially striking. Cardiac abnormalities may include a prolapsed mitral valve and atrial flutter; patients with more advanced cases have severe cardiac fibrosis.[33]

Treatment

All forms of MD are incurable, and no satisfactory method of retarding the muscle atrophy exists. Corticosteroids have been shown to decrease the rate of muscle loss, but only in the short term. A physical therapy program will help to delay the development of joint contractures, and orthopedic procedures may help to counteract deformities. The ultimate outcome in severe forms of the disease is grave.[34]

Oral Health Considerations

Oral and facial signs are prominent in the facioscapulohumeral and myotonic forms of MD. Patients with the myotonic-type disease develop severe atrophy of the sternomastoid muscles, with a resultant difficulty in the ability to turn the head. The muscles of facial expression and mastication are also commonly affected, such that the patient has difficulty in chewing or in pursing the lips. Weakness of the facial muscles and enlargement of the tongue due to fatty deposits has been occasionally observed. Patients with the oculopharyngeal form of the disease have significant difficulty in swallowing.

Occlusal abnormalities have also been reported in patients with MD. This is thought to result from the lack of the proper muscle tension necessary to keep the teeth properly aligned in the dental arch. If the tongue is enlarged and the facial muscles are weak, the teeth will be pushed out. Other abnormalities include macroglossia, anterior open bite, and (occasionally) temporomandibular joint dysfunction.

▼ EPILEPSY

Epilepsy is a condition characterized by abnormal, recurrent, and excessive neuronal discharges precipitated by many different disturbances within the central nervous system. These aberrant discharges may cause episodes of sensory and motor abnormalities as well as loss of consciousness. Each episode of aberrant neurologic activity is referred to as a seizure. Epilepsy is common, affecting approximately 0.5% of the population in the United States.[35] Although the disease may occur at any stage of life, the age of the patient at the onset of seizures is closely associated with the various causes of epilepsy. Infants are much more likely to suffer from epilepsy after complications at birth, such as anoxia, intracranial injury, metabolic disorders, and congenital malformations. Predominant causes in children and adolescents include trauma and acute or febrile infections whereas young adults who have engaged in alcohol or drug abuse commonly suffer from generalized seizures after periods of severe abuse. Epilepsy in older adults may occur as a complication of any of the previously mentioned causes but is more often associated with cerebrovascular diseases such as stroke and tumor.

Classification of Seizures

Seizures can be categorized in various ways, but the descriptive classification proposed by the International League Against Epilepsy is clinically the most useful. Seizures are divided into those that are generalized and those that affect only part of the brain (partial seizures)[36] (Table 23-1). Simple partial seizures originate from one localized area of the brain and do not feature loss of consciousness. In contrast, complex partial seizures, often referred to as temporal lobe or psychomotor seizures, are associated with an impairment of consciousness. The majority of generalized seizures are called either absence (petit mal) seizures or tonic-clonic seizures (grand mal). The remaining generalized seizure types described in the classification (ie, myoclonic or infantile seizures and clonic, tonic, and atonic seizures) are usually found in childhood and carry a poorer prognosis for normal childhood development. "Status epilepticus" refers to a period of recurrent seizure attacks without recovery between each attack. All forms of seizure may progress to a period of status epilepticus.

Clinical Manifestations

Nonspecific changes such as headache, mood alterations, lethargy, and myoclonic jerking alert some patients to an impending seizure hours before it occurs. These prodromal symptoms are distinct from the aura that may precede a generalized seizure by a few seconds or minutes and that is itself a part of the attack, arising locally from a restricted region of the brain.

The most common type of seizure is the tonic-clonic or grand mal seizure; 90% of epileptics experience it alone or in combination with another type of seizure. A grand mal seizure characteristically begins with an aura. The aura may be experienced as epigastric discomfort, as an emotion, or as an hallucination of hearing, vision, or smell. The aura is followed seconds to minutes later by unconsciousness, a cry, and tonic muscle spasms; this rigid phase lasts about 30 seconds. Because of the spasm of the respiratory muscles, the patient does not breathe and becomes cyanotic during this period. The tonic phase is followed by a clonic phase composed of convulsive jerky movements, incontinence, and tongue biting (Figure 23-1). The patient may injure him- or herself seriously if he or she is near hard or sharp objects. A postictal state characterized by headache, confusion, lethargy, occasional temporary neurologic deficit, and deep sleep usually follows a grand mal seizure.

The number, severity, and duration of grand mal seizures vary considerably from one patient to another. Status epilepticus, a severe form of the disorder, occurs when a series of seizures follow each other before the patient is able to regain consciousness.

Absence or petit mal seizure is the second most common type of seizure, and it occurs without an aura and with few or no clonic or tonic movements. Absence seizures present almost exclusively in children and frequently disappear during the second decade of life. A single seizure lasts just seconds. The patient loses consciousness and appears to stare into space. He or she continues normal activity immediately after the seizure is over. Petit mal seizures may occur several times each day, and severe cases may interfere with school and social activities. Around puberty, approximately 50% of persons who experience petit mal seizures will develop tonic-clonic seizures.

Treatment of Seizures

For patients with recurring seizures, drug treatment is prescribed with the goal of preventing further attacks and is usually continued until there have been no seizures for at least 3 years.[35]

The drug with which treatment is best initiated depends on the type of seizures to be treated. The dose of the selected drug is gradually increased until seizures are controlled or until side effects prevent further increase. If seizures continue despite treatment at the maximal tolerated dose, a second drug is added. The second drug's dose is increased, depending on the patient's tolerance, and the first drug is then gradually withdrawn. In the treatment of partial and secondarily generalized tonic-clonic seizures, the success rate is higher with carbamazepine, phenytoin, or valproic acid than with phenobarbital or primidone. Gabapentin, topiramate, and lamotrigine are newer antiepileptic drugs that are effective adjunctive therapy for partial or secondarily generalized seizures. In most patients with seizures of a single type, satisfactory control can be achieved with a single anticonvulsant drug.[37,38]

The choice of medication is usually related to individual tolerance and efficacy, but it should be remembered that all of

---

TABLE 23-1   International Classification of Epileptic Seizures

Partial (focal) seizures
    Simple partial seizures
    Complex partial seizures
    Partial seizures leading to secondarily generalized seizures

Generalized Seizures
    Absence seizures
        Typical
        Atypical
    Myoclonic seizures
    Clonic seizures
    Tonic seizures
    Tonic-clonic seizures
    Atonic seizures (astatic seizures)

Adapted from Kelley WN, DeVita VT Jr, Dupont HL, Harris Ed Jr. Internal medicine for dentistry. 2nd ed. Philadelphia: J.B. Lippincott; 1992.

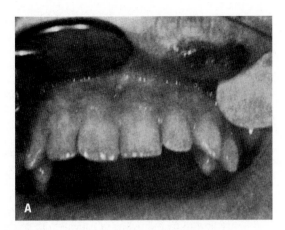
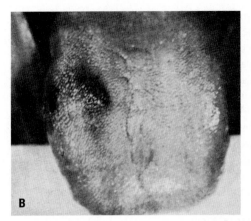

FIGURE 23-1 **A,** Bilateral human bites of the upper lip, received during an epileptic seizure. **B,** Traumatic injury (bite) to tongue occurred during an epileptic seizure.

these drugs produce significant but different side effects, including blood dyscrasias, anemia, and alteration of hepatic function.

Oral Health Considerations

Patients with epilepsy may be treated in the private dental setting. A thorough medical history should indicate what type of seizures the patient has, how well the seizures are controlled, the frequency and duration of seizures, the potential triggers for seizures, and what to expect if the patient has a seizure. Treatment planning may be altered, however, depending on the status of the seizure disorder. As a general rule, it is better to place a fixed prosthesis rather than a removable appliance because of the potential for removable appliances to become dislodged during a seizure.[39]

Patients who are taking anticonvulsant drugs are subject to gingival overgrowth. This overgrowth is most often associated with patients who are taking phenytoin (Figure 23-2). About half of the patients placed on phenytoin will show evidence of gingival enlargement, usually within 2 to 18 months after starting the medication. The etiology is still unknown, but there appears to be an increase in the number of fibroblasts in the connective tissues.[40] Gingival overgrowth may occur at any age but seems to affect younger patients to a greater degree than adults. Men and women are equally affected. There does not appear to be a correlation between dosage and the incidence of gingival overgrowth. There is strong clinical evidence of a correlation between poor oral hygiene and the amount of tissue enlargement.

Clinically, phenytoin gingival overgrowth starts in the interdental papillae and occurs only where teeth are present. The papillae enlarge buccally and lingually. The enlarged areas are firm, pink, and covered with normal mucosa. The severity of the hyperplasia varies. In some patients, the enlarged gingivae may involve just one or two papillae; in other cases, the crowns of the teeth are completely covered with gingival tissue. The best treatment of phenytoin gingival overgrowth begins with prevention. Little doubt remains that careful oral hygiene can prevent or at least minimize the gingival enlargement. Soon after being placed on anticonvulsant therapy, each patient should be referred to a dentist for oral hygiene instruction and gingival curettage. Patients who have not been properly managed and who develop gross gingival enlargement will require gingivectomy. Curettage

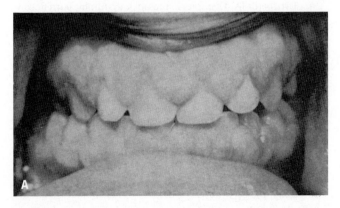
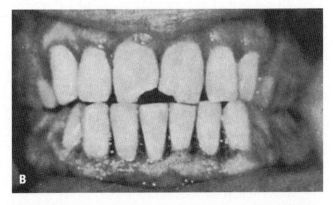

FIGURE 23-2 **A,** Phenytoin gingival overgrowth in a 17-year-old girl. The enlarged tissues are light pink and fibrous, and they show no evidence of edema, inflammation, or ulceration. **B,** Patient with phenytoin gingival overgrowth following electrocautery of enlarged gingival tissues. The excess maxillary gingival tissue had been removed 10 days previously. The excess mandibular gingival tissue had just been removed. Fractures of the mesioincisal angles of the maxillary first incisors occurred during a seizure.

and careful attention to oral hygiene must follow the surgery, or the hyperplastic tissue will return.

It is known that side effects other than gingival overgrowth also occur in patients taking phenytoin. This includes megaloblastic anemia, hirsutism, and lymphadenopathy. Changes in connective tissue and bone (including osteomalacia, thickening of the heel pad and of the calvarium, and coarse facies) have also been reported.[40] Routine dental treatment for patients with well-controlled epilepsy may be performed with no change from normal treatment. There is no reason to increase the dose of anticonvulsant therapy prior to dental treatment, and routine use of sedation is not indicated.

▼ REFERENCES

1. Gilroy J. Basic neurology. 3rd ed. New York: McGraw-Hill; 2000.
2. Adams HP Jr, Brott TG, Furlan AJ, et al. Guidelines for thrombolytic therapy for acute stroke: a supplement to the guidelines for the management of patients with acute ischemic stroke. Stroke 1996; 27:1711–8.
3. Wolf PA, Clagett GP, Easton JD, et al. Preventing ischemic stroke in patients with prior stroke and TIA: a statement for healthcare professionals from the stroke council of the American Heart Association. Stroke 1999;30:1991–4.
4. Victor M, Ropper AH. Adams and Victor's principles of neurology. 7th ed. New York: McGraw-Hill; 2001.
5. Feinberg WM, Albers GW, Barnett HJ, et al. Guidelines for the management of TIAs. From the Ad Hoc Committee on Guidelines for the Management of Transient Ischemic Attacks of the Stroke Council of the American Heart Association. Circulation 1994;89:2950–65.
6. Ostuni E. Stroke and the dental patient. J Am Dent Assoc 1994;125:721–7.
7. Kurtzke JF, Hellested K. Multiple sclerosis in the Faroe Islands: clinical and epidemiological features. Ann Neurol 1979;5:6.
8. Sadovnick AD, Ebers GC. Genetics in multiple sclerosis. Neurol Clin 1995;13:99–118.
9. Mumford CJ, Wood NW, Kellar-Wood H, et al. The British Isles survey of multiple sclerosis in twins. Neurology 1994;44:11–5.
10. Rudick RA, Cohen JA, Weinstock-Gutman B, et al. Management of multiple sclerosis. N Engl J Med 1997; 337:1604–11.
11. Chemaly D, Lefrancois A, Perusse R. Oral and maxillofacial manifestations of multiple sclerosis. J Can Dent Assoc 2000; 66:600–5.
12. Gale D, Prime S, Campbell MJ. Trigeminal neuralgia and multiple sclerosis, a complex diagnosis. Oral Surg Oral Med Oral Pathol Oral Radiol Endod 1995;79:398–401.
13. Houde SC, Mangolds V. Amyotrophic lateral sclerosis: a team approach to primary care. Clin Excell Nurse Prac 1999; 3(6):337–45.
14. Asher RS, Alfred T. Dental management of long-term amyotrophic lateral sclerosis: case report. Spec Care Dentist 1993;13(6):241–4.
15. Lang AE, Lozano AM. Parkinson's disease. Part 1. N Engl J Med 1998;339:1044–53.
16. Lang AE, Lozano AM. Parkinson's disease Part 2. N Engl J Med 1998;339:1130–43.
17. Olanow CW, Koller WC. An algorithm for the management of Parkinson's disease: treatment guidelines. Neurology 1998;50(3 Suppl 3):S1–57.
18. Kieser J, Jones G, Borlase G. Dental treatment of patients with neurodegenerative disease. N Z Dent J 1999;95(422):130-4.
19. Quinn N, Schrag A. Huntington's disease and other choreas. J Neurol 1998;245(11):709-16.
20. Bass N. Cerebral palsy and neurodegenerative disease. Curr Opin Pediatr 1999;11(6):504–7.
21. Dabney KW, Lipton GE, Miller F. Cerebral palsy. Curr Opin Pediatr 1997;9(1):81–8.
22. Becmeur F, Horta-Geraud P, Brunot B, et al. Diversion of salivary flow to treat drooling in patients with cerebral palsy. J Pediatr Surg 1996;31(12):1629–33.
23. Bachrach SJ, Walter RS, Trzcinski K. Use of glycopyrrolate and other anticholinergic medications for sialorrhea in children with cerebral palsy. Clin Pediatr 1998;37(8):485–90.
24. Murakami S, Mizobuchi M, Nakashiro Y, et al. Bell's palsy and herpes virus: identification of viral DNA in endoneurial fluid and muscle. Ann Intern Med 1996;124:27–30.
25. Sanchez Rodriguez A. Bell's palsy in association with herpes simplex virus infection. Arch Intern Med 1998;158(14):1577–8.
26. Nasatzky E, Katz J. Bell's palsy associated with herpes simplex gingivostomatitis: a case report. Oral Surg Oral Med Oral Pathol 1998;86(3):292–6.
27. Billue JS. Bell's palsy: an update on idiopathic facial paralysis. Nurse Pract 1997;22(8):88,97–100,102–5.
28. Adour KK. Bell's palsy treatment with acyclovir and prednisone compared with prednisone alone: a double-blind, randomized, controlled trial. Ann Otol Rhinol Laryngol 1996; 105:371–8.
29. Van der Meche FG, Aan Doorn PA, Meulstee J, et al. Diagnostic and classification criteria for the Guillain-Barre syndrome. Eur Neurol 2001;45(3):133–9.
30. Keesey J. Myasthenia gravis. Arch Neurol 1998;55(5):745–6.
31. Davison SP. Swollen tongue: a presentation of myasthenia gravis. Otolaryngol Head Neck Surg 1997;116(2):244–6.
32. Ptacek L. The familial periodic paralyses and nondystrophic myotonias. Am J Med 1998;104:58–70.
33. Arahata K. Muscular dystrophy. Neuropathology 2000 Sep; 20 Suppl:S34-41.
34. Urtizberea JA. Therapies in muscular dystrophy: current concepts and future prospects. Eur Neurol 2000;43(3):127–32.
35. Browne TR, Holmes GL. Epilepsy. N Engl J Med 2001; 344(15):1145–51.
36. Proposal for revised clinical classification of epileptic seizures. From the Commission on Class and Terminology of the International League Against Epilepsy. Epilepsia 1981;22:489–501.
37. Bradie MJ, Dichter MA. Antiepileptic drugs. N Engl J Med 1996;334:168–75.
38. Mattson RH. Medical management of epilepsy in adults. Neurology 1998;51 Suppl 4:515–20.
39. Sanders BJ, Weddell JA, Dodge NN. Managing patients who have seizure disorders: dental and medical issues. J Am Dent Assoc 1995;126:1641–7.
40. Perlik F, Kolinova M, Zvarova J, et al. Phenytoin as a risk factor in gingival hyperplasia. Ther Drug Monit 1995;17(5):445–8.

24

GERIATRICS

JONATHAN A. SHIP, DMD

The geriatric population is the most rapidly growing segment of the general population, a fact that will have dramatic implications for systemic and oral health in the future. In 1950, only approximately 10% of the US population was aged 65 years or older. This number increased to 13% in 1997 and is expected to reach 20% by the year 2030.[1] The number of adults aged 85 years or older in the United States will rise from 3.3 million in 1994 to 8.6 million in 2030 and will further increase to 19 million by 2050. In 1997, life expectancy was 76.5 years (79.4 years for females, 73.6 years for males), and over one-third of the population survived beyond the age of 85 years.[2] On the basis of mortality experienced in 1997, a person aged 65 years could expect to live an average of 17.7 more years, and a person aged 100 years could expect to live an additional 2.5 years on average. In comparison to statistics from 1900, the population has changed dramatically.[2] The median age of death has reached 80 years (in 1900, it was 58 years), and 1.5% of the population survives to age 100 years (in 1900, the proportion was 0.03%).

As more people live longer and become elderly, there will be an increase in chronic conditions and illnesses that will influence both oral and systemic health.[3,4] The most common causes of death in adults aged > 65 years in the United States are diseases of the heart, cancers, and cerebrovascular and pulmonary diseases (Table 24-1). The most common chronic diseases in elderly people are arthritis, hypertension, heart disease, sinus diseases, and diabetes mellitus (Table 24-2). All of these acute and chronic conditions have potential oral sequelae, particularly in an older and more medically compromised adult. Furthermore, the treatment of these diseases with medications, chemotherapy, and radiotherapy has implications for the maintenance of oral health (Table 24-3). Chronic impairments are also prevalent among elderly persons; hearing, visual, and orthopedic impairments and speech disorders are the most common of these (Table 24-4). Older adults experience other sensory impairments

TABLE 24-1 Leading Causes of Death in Adults Aged 65 Years and Older in the United States, 1996

Rank	Cause of Death	Rate/100,000 Persons
1	Diseases of the heart	1,808
2	Malignant neoplasms	1,131
3	Cerebrovascular diseases	415
4	COPD	270
5	Pneumonia and influenza	221
6	Diabetes mellitus	137
7	Accidents and adverse effects	91
8	Alzheimer's disease	62
9	Renal diseases	62
10	Septicemia	51

Adapted from National Center for Health Statistics. National vital statistics report. Vital Health Statistics; 1998.

COPD = chronic obstructive pulmonary disease.

such as olfactory and gustatory dysfunction, as well as oral motor problems including difficulty with mastication, speech, and swallowing.[5–7] These chronic impairments can directly affect oral health and impair dental treatment, and simple steps taken by dental professionals will help improve communication with these patients (Table 24-5).

Many of the systemic conditions that are common among elderly people (see Tables 24-1, 24-2, and 24-4) and that directly or indirectly affect oral health are discussed elsewhere in this book, with the exception of dementias. Dementias are a considerable problem among the elderly population. There are some estimates that the prevalence is ~1% at the age of 60 years and doubles every 5 years to reach more than 50% by the age of 85 years.[8–10] Dementia is characterized by both mental and physical decline. With increased severity of dementia, there is progressive cognitive and memory loss, development of social and behavioral problems, and inability to perform daily activities.[8,11] Dementias comprise more than 55 ill-

TABLE 24-2 Leading Chronic Conditions in Adults Aged 65 Years and Older in the Untied States, 1994

Rank	Chronic Conditions	Rate/1,000 Persons
1	Arthritis	502
2	Hypertension	364
3	Heart disease	324
4	Chronic sinusitis	151
5	Diabetes mellitus	101
6	Allergic rhinitis	80
7	Varicosities	75
8	Hernia	64
9	Hemorrhoids	62
10	Chronic bronchitis	61

Adapted from National Center for Health Statistics. National health interview survey, 1994. Vital Health Statistics; 1995.

nesses, with the most common being Alzheimer's disease and Parkinson's disease.[8] Estimates for the prevalence of Alzheimer's disease approach 50% in adults aged > 85 years in the community population.[9] Furthermore, US Census Bureau projections estimate 10.3 million persons with the disease by the year 2050.[12] The incidence of Parkinson's disease also increases steeply with advancing age,[13] reaching a prevalence of 5% in community-dwelling adults aged 85 to 89 years,[14] with a similar prevalence in nursing homes.[15] More than two-thirds of these patients have moderate to severe functional disability,[15] which will dramatically affect their oral health and the ability of dental professionals to deliver dental services to these patients. With the rapid growth of the elderly population and the retention of the natural dentition, there will be an increased need for dental care services for older adults with dementia.[16]

The progression of dementia is accompanied by a gradual inability to perform self-care, including adequate oral hygiene, due to self-neglect and loss of cognitive and motor skills.[17] Persons with dementia, even those living in the community and experiencing few medical problems, have impaired oral health as a result of poor oral hygiene.[18] For example, patients with Alzheimer's disease have more gingival plaque, bleeding, and calculus compared to age- and gender-matched adults,[19] and submandibular saliva output is impaired in nonmedicated persons with Alzheimer's disease.[20] Poor gingival health and oral hygiene have been found to increase with the severity of dementia.[21] The neuronal degeneration that accompanies Parkinson's disease also impacts negatively on oral health.[22] Insufficient and inadequate oral hygiene, impaired access to professional oral examination and treatment, and frequent medical management with psychotropic medications that cause salivary dysfunction all combine to negatively affect oral health and function.

Oral care, treatment planning, and behavioral management for persons with dementia must be designed with consideration of the severity of disease and must involve family members or caregivers.[17,23] Early in the disease process, aggressive preventive and interceptive steps need to be formulated to preserve existing stomatologic health. As dementia progresses, treatment becomes problem based, and short-acting benzodiazepines may be helpful for managing patients' behavior.[16] Frequent recall and preventive measures must be continued. The role of the caregiver becomes more critical in providing symptomatic and objective information as well as in performing daily oral hygiene. Complex and time-consuming dental treatment should be avoided in persons with severe dementia. The emphasis should be on keeping the patient free of pain and able to maintain adequate nutritional intake, particularly if the patient is no longer able or willing to wear removable prostheses. Intravenous sedation or general anesthesia can be considered for necessary dental care.[24] In summary, oral health care providers will be increasingly challenged with preserving the oral and nutritional health of these patients, to diminish pain and pathology, and to maintain their dignity and quality of life.

TABLE 24-3 Systemic Conditions in Elderly Patients: Oral Treatment Considerations

Systemic Condition	Causes	Oral Considerations	Treatment Considerations
Coagulation disorders	Anticoagulation therapy Chemotherapy Liver cirrhosis Renal disease	Increased bleeding risk	Alter anticoagulation therapy Limit dentoalveolar surgery Use topical anticoagulation methods
Immunosuppression	Alcoholic cirrhosis Chemotherapy Diabetes Medications Organ transplant therapy Renal disease	Microbial infections	Appropriate antimicrobial medications
Joint replacement	Accidents Osteoarthritis Rheumatoid arthritis	Increased risk for late prosthetic joint infections	Antibiotic prophylaxis
Radiation sequelae	Head and neck radiation	Salivary hypofunction Mucositis Osteoradionecrosis Increased caries risk Dysphagia Dysgeusia Difficulty with mastication Microbial infections Impaired denture retention	Regular fluoride use Salivary substitutes and stimulants Aggressive oral hygiene and recall Pain management
Steroid therapy	Autoimmune diseases Organ transplant therapy	Microbial infections Increased risk for adrenal insufficiency	Appropriate antimicrobial medications Steroid supplementation for dental procedures
Valvular damage, heart murmur	Acquired heart defects Congenital heart defects Valvular transplants	Increased risk for developing subacute bacterial endocarditis	Antibiotic prophylaxis

Another concern in the elderly population is access to medical and oral health care services. Overall, 4% of the older population lives in nursing homes; however, the prevalence increases dramatically with age. Approximately 1% of adults aged 65 to 74 years reside in nursing homes, compared with almost 20% of persons aged ≥ 85 years.[25] Furthermore, the percentage of community-dwelling individuals needing personal assistance with activities of daily living, including oral hygiene, increases with age. The estimated number of persons served by home health care agencies rose from 1.2 million in 1992 to 2.4 million in 1996, doubling in less than 5 years.[26] One-half of the population aged 65 years and receiving home health care requires help with personal hygiene, one-quarter requires assistance preparing meals, and nearly 10% needs assistance with eating. Therefore, the growing number of older adults with chronic medical problems and requiring assistance with activities of daily living will have a dramatic impact on geriatric dental health.

Oral health and function is commonly altered in older adults.[5] However, age alone does not seem to play a strong role in the impairments. Dental, periodontal, oral mucosal, and salivary diseases have a detrimental and compounding affect on oral health in elderly persons, yet oral disease is not necessarily a concomitant of growing older. Importantly, numerous medical problems, medications, and other medical treatments can adversely affect oral function in an older adult.[3,4,27] These disorders must be recognized and managed appropriately by health care practitioners to eradicate disease, restore function, and improve the quality of a person's life. Stomatologic diseases in medically, physically, behaviorally,

TABLE 24-4 Most Common Chronic Impairments in US Adults Aged 65 Years and Older

		Age Group (Yr)		
Rank	Chronic Impairments	65+	65–74	75+
1	Hearing*	376.5	324.7	450.4
2	Vision†	318.8	229.2	447.0
3	Orthopedic‡	198.4	182.7	221.0
4	Speech	90.1	90.1	90.0

Adapted from National Center for Health Statistics. National vital statistics report. Vital Health Statistics; 1995.

*Hearing impairment, tinnitus.

†Visual impairment, color blindness, cataracts, glaucoma.

‡Absence and paralysis of extremities; deformities of back and upper and lower extremities.

TABLE 24-5   Suggestions for Improving Communication with Patients Who Have Hearing, Vision, and Speech Impairments

Suggestion for Improving Communication	H	V	S
Make certain hearing aids are in place and working properly.	✔		
Know how to assist the patient with the hearing aid if necessary.	✔		
Avoid long sentences.	✔		
Avoid sudden topic changes.	✔		
For severely hearing-impaired patients, use special devices that fit into the ear and block out all extraneous sounds.	✔		
Speak in low tones when possible.	✔		
Do not distort your voice with hands, chewing gum, etc.	✔		
Speak clearly and loudly, but do not shout or overexaggerate the words.	✔		
Reduce glare.		✔	
Make certain the patient wears glasses when necessary.		✔	
Do not finish sentences or add words for patients.			✔
Ask questions slowly, with adequate response time.	✔		✔
Do not speak fast.	✔	✔	
Minimize outside noise.	✔	✔	
Get the person's attention before speaking (eg, tap on the shoulder).	✔	✔	
Use gestures when appropriate.	✔	✔	
Face the patient, and make eye contact.	✔	✔	
Write in bold letters, contrasting letters and paper when possible.	✔	✔	
Touch may be useful, unless disturbing to patient or practitioner.	✔	✔	
Avoid asking more than one question at a time.	✔	✔	✔
If explanations or instructions must be lengthy, review, point by point.	✔	✔	✔
Decrease speaking space if not disturbing to patient or practitioner.	✔	✔	✔
Discuss treatment needs in areas with decreased distractions and increased privacy.	✔	✔	✔
Avoid physical barriers (eg, desk) that can impose a psychological barrier.	✔	✔	✔
Do not speak to the patient as if speaking to a child.	✔	✔	✔
Provide complete explanations prior to making decisions or doing procedures.	✔	✔	✔
Keep the number of people in the clinical area to a minimum.	✔	✔	✔

Adapted from Scully C, Cawson RA. Medical problems in dentistry. 2nd ed. Bristol: Wright; 1987. Kiyak H. Psychological aspects of aging: implications for dental care of the older patient. In: Papas A, Niessen L, Chauncey H, editors. Geriatric dentistry—aging and oral health. St. Louis: Mosby-Year Book; 1991. p. 14–43.

H = hearing impairment; V = vision impairment; S = speech impairment.

and mentally compromised older adults can now be treated in a variety of patient care settings, including long-term care institutions,[28] which will have a positive impact on the quality of life of these patients.

Importantly, the effects of stomatologic diseases are not necessarily limited to the oral cavity. Oral diseases give rise to pathogens that can be bloodborne or aspirated into the lungs. These pathogens can cause immediate systemic complications (eg, aspiration pneumonia, bacteremia) or (by complex immunologic pathways) may be associated with long-term problems (eg, coronary heart disease and cerebrovascular disorders).[29–40]

This chapter is dedicated to geriatric oral medicine and attempts to summarize the effects of aging and the influence of systemic diseases and their treatment on a variety of vital oral health topics. Age-related changes in oral tissues (Table 24-6) and common oral conditions in the geriatric population are described (Table 24-7). Finally, an overview of the pre-vention and management of oral diseases in the geriatric population is provided.

TABLE 24-6   Summary of Oropharyngeal Processes in the Elderly Population

Process	Healthy Older People	Medically Compromised Older People
Taste	Unaffected	Diminished
Smell	Diminished	Diminished
Food enjoyment	Unaffected	Diminished
Salivary output	Unaffected	Diminished
Chewing efficiency	Slightly diminished	Diminished
Swallowing	Slightly diminished	Diminished

Adapted from Ship JA et al;[7] Ship JA. The oral cavity. In: Hazzard WR, Blass JP, Ettinger WH, et al, editors. Principles of geriatric medicine and gerontology. 4th ed. New York: McGraw-Hill; 1999. p. 591–602.

TABLE 24-7   Summary of Oral Disorders in Elderly Persons

Oral Tissue or Function	Disorders
Oral mucosa	Cancers Vesiculobullous diseases Ulcerative diseases
Oral and pharyngeal mucosa; dentition	Viral diseases Fungal diseases Bacterial diseases
Dentition	Root surface caries Coronal caries Attrition
Periodontium	Gingivitis Periodontitis Abscesses
Salivary glands	Obstructions Bacterial infections Hypofunction Cancers
Chemosensory function	Taste dysfunction Smell dysfunction
Swallowing	Delayed swallowing Aspiration
Edentulousness	Osteoporosis Atrophic mandible Denture difficulties Pain over the mental foramen
Pain sensation	Atypical facial pain "Burning mouth" syndrome Postherpetic neuralgia Trigeminal neuralgia

▼ AGE-RELATED CHANGES IN ORAL HEALTH

Oral Mucosa

The clinical appearance of the oral mucosa in many healthy older persons is indistinguishable from that of younger people. However, a lifelong history of oral mucosal trauma (eg, cheek biting), mucosal diseases (eg, lichen planus), oral habits (eg, smoking), and salivary disorders (eg, salivary hypofunction) can alter the clinical appearance and histologic character of the oral mucosa in an older adult. Histologically, there is evidence of epithelial thinning, less-prominent rete pegs, decreased cellular proliferation, loss of submucosal elastin and fat, and increased fibrotic connective tissues with degenerative alteration in collagen.[41] Clinically, these structural changes may be accompanied by dry thin smooth mucosal surfaces, with loss of elasticity and stippling. These changes may predispose the oral mucosa to trauma and infection, particularly when they are associated with denture use and salivary hypofunction.

Oral mucosal immunity is believed to undergo some age-related changes.[42] Wound healing and regeneration of tissue may be delayed in elderly individuals, yet older age plays only a minor role in the response of oral mucosa to injury.[43] It is not known if advanced age *per se* has a clinically significant adverse effect on the appearance and function of the oral mucosa. However, the concomitant effects of oral mucosal diseases with age-related structural and immunologic changes, local trauma, systemic diseases, medications, and poor nutritional status can cause significant oral mucosal changes in an older adult.

Dentition

Major epidemiologic changes have occurred over the past several decades in regard to retention of the dentition. Only about 30% of adults aged ≥ 65 years are completely edentulous, and between 1983 and 1993, the prevalence decreased by 10% in all older age groups.[44] These trends are expected to continue with improved oral health care, greater tooth preservation, and enhanced restorative techniques and materials.

Changes in the dentition due to aging can be attributed to normal physiologic processes and to pathologic changes in response to functional and environmental stresses. External tooth changes include discoloration (to a yellowish brown color) and loss of enamel due to attrition (Figure 24-1), abrasion, and erosion. Severe enamel wear will ultimately expose underlying dentin, which produces sclerotic and secondary dentin[45] in response to trauma, caries, and masticatory forces. Over time, dentin undergoes a reduction in thermal, osmotic, and electrical sensitivity and pain perception, and its susceptibility to caries decreases.[46] Cementum thickness[46] and pulp dimensions[47,48] are reduced with age. Secondary dentin deposition, pulpal calcifications, external root resorption, increased density and volume of pulpal collagen fibers, and diminished nerve supply all contribute to a progressive decrease in the size of the pulp. These age-related pulpal changes diminish tooth sensitivity and pain perception, reduce responsiveness to pulp testing, and usually decrease the need for local anesthesia for dental procedures.[49]

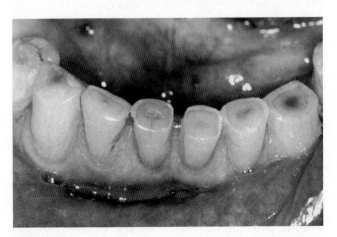

FIGURE 24-1   Exposed dentin and sclerosed pulpal chambers due to dental attrition.

The prevalence of coronal and root surface caries increases with age,[50] and greater than 30% of the population aged ≥ 65 years has untreated coronal and root caries.[44] Increases in caries are influenced by two trends: a greater retention of teeth among elderly persons, and a decline in caries among younger people.[51] Teeth are susceptible to new decay as well as recurrent caries around existing restorations. Due to gingival recession, these teeth are at risk for developing cervical or root surface caries. With extended retention of the natural dentition into older age, previously restored teeth are more prone to recurrent decay, due to defective restorations, fractured fillings, poor oral hygiene, and inaccessible restoration margins.

Dental plaque is the primary source of microorganisms (eg, *Streptococcus mutans* and lactobacilli) causing coronal and root surface caries in elderly people. Individuals of all ages are susceptible to the development of dental plaque. However, following abstention from daily oral care, older individuals form plaque more rapidly than do younger people.[52,53] This occurs as a result gingival recession, diminished salivary gland function, disturbances in oral motor function, and difficulty in performing oral hygiene. Since these factors are directly associated with dental caries, older patients are more susceptible to new and recurrent tooth decay. When detected early, caries can be restored with a variety of dental materials.[54] In most circumstances, untreated caries will progress to severe or even total loss of tooth structure and possibly to pain, abscess formation, cellulitis, and bacteremia.

Periodontium

The clinical appearance of periodontal tissues in an elderly individual reflects age-related changes and an accumulation of previous disease experiences and trauma over time. With increased age, gingival recession (Figure 24-2) and loss of periodontal attachment and alveolar bone are essentially universal; nearly 95% of dentate Americans over the age of 65 years have measurable attachment loss.[50] However, changes in the periodontium that are attribuable solely to age are not sufficient to lead to tooth loss, especially in a healthy adult.[55] Most frequently, periodontal changes over time lead to greater recession without significant increased periodontal pocket depth.[56]

Age-related immunologic changes[42] and histologic alterations in periodontal tissues[57,58] could alter the host response to dental plaque microorganisms,[52,53,58,59] affecting the patient's ability to respond to periodontal treatment. It has been reported that following periodontal therapy, younger patients in studies healed with a higher frequency of shallow pockets and a greater gain of probing attachment, compared to older patients.[60]

Several systemic conditions and medications that are more prevalent among older adults have been linked with periodontal disorders. Osteoporosis adversely affects collagen metabolism and bone mineralization, with a concomitant decrease in bone mass. There is some evidence that severe osteoporosis significantly reduces the bone mineral content of the jaws and that it may be associated with greater periodontal attachment loss and tooth loss.[61–63] Interestingly, estrogen replacement for the treatment for osteoporosis in older women has been associated with less gingival bleeding and may be beneficial in preventing tooth loss in postmenopausal women.[64] In older adults, diabetes is the sixth most common cause of death (see Table 24-1), the fifth most common chronic medical condition (see Table 24-2), and a risk factor for the development of periodontal diseases.[65,66] Several classes of medications that are frequently prescribed for older persons have been associated with gingival overgrowth or hyperplasia. These include calcium channel blockers, the antiseizure drug phenytoin, and the immunosuppressant cyclosporine.[67]

Finally, there are oral and sociobehavioral factors that influence the progression of periodontal disease in elderly people. Deep periodontal pocketing, irregular dental visits, smoking, psychosocial stress, and poor socioeconomic status all are predictors of periodontal attachment loss in older patients.[68–72]

Salivary Glands

Saliva plays a critical role in the maintenance of oral health, and diminished output can cause dental caries, oral mucosal infections, sensory disturbances, speech dysfunction, decreased nutritional intake, and difficulty in chewing, swallowing, and denture retention.[73] It was previously thought that changes in qualitative and quantitative salivary production were associated with normal aging. This may have been partly due to the common complaint of xerostomia (mouth dryness) in older people.[74,75] However, it is now accepted that significant changes in salivary flow are not observed in healthy elderly persons.[76,77] In addition, no age-related decreases in the secretion of certain salivary constituents (eg, total proteins, proline-rich proteins, lactoferrin, sodium, and potassium) are seen in a healthy population.[78]

Histologically, there are age-related alterations in the cellular makeup of salivary glands, with an increase in connective tissue and adipose deposition and a decrease in acinar cells.[79] This

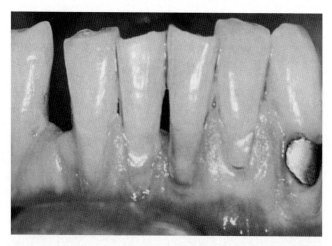

FIGURE 24-2 Gingival recession, exposing root surface cementum. Previous root surface caries have been restored with amalgam and composite materials.

loss of fluid-producing acinar cells increases the susceptibility of an older individual to salivary perturbations such as those caused by medications with anticholinergic side effects. However, in the absence of medical problems and their treatment in an older adult, it does not appear that these morphologic findings have a considerable impact on salivary secretions.

Taste and Smell

The chemosensory functions of smell and taste play a vital role in human physiology and in a patient's quality of life. Many older adults complain of diminished food recognition and enjoyment, as well as altered smell and taste function.[80] While gustatory function in healthy older adults remains remarkably intact,[81] olfaction undergoes dramatic age-related changes, even in healthy older adults.[82] The olfactory bulb and peripheral receptors are sensitive to a variety of environmental toxins, trauma, medications, and respiratory infections. Over the course of a lifetime, these common conditions cause a diminished sensitivity to olfactory cues and impair smell identification. Conversely, multiple taste buds that are located on the tongue, palate, and oropharynx, and innervation by three bilateral cranial nerves (VII, IX, and X) help produce a strong resistance to taste changes. Nevertheless, medications, chemo- and radiotherapy, trauma, surgery, and neurologic events can cause temporary or permanent taste changes in an older adult.

Other investigations have evaluated the more complicated problems of flavor perception, food recognition, and food preference. Although results are not uniform, older individuals do less well when performance is assessed in these tasks.[7] While older age *per se* has been associated with certain chemosensory alterations, many oral and systemic conditions have been linked more strongly to smell and taste dysfunction.[83] Therefore, age and oral and systemic disorders and their treatments can adversely affect smell and taste function, which could place an older adult at risk for developing nutritional deficits[84] and could adversely affect his or her quality of life.

Mastication and Swallowing

The oral motor functions of mastication and swallowing require the coordination of intricate neuromuscular activities that are necessary for the translocation of foods and fluids into the gastrointestinal tract. The most frequently reported oral motor disturbance in older people is related to altered mastication, and even fully dentate older persons are less able to prepare food for swallowing as efficiently as are younger individuals.[85] However, research data support the view that dentition, not age *per se*, has a direct influence on mastication.[7] Altered masticatory ability in older age can be exacerbated further in individuals who are partially or fully edentulous, have painful or mobile teeth due to caries or periodontal diseases, or have a decreased salivary output.

Following mastication, the food bolus is translocated to the pharynx. The oral phase of swallowing requires well-coordinated neuromuscular processing, an intact mucosal barrier, and adequate salivary production.[5] Alterations in any of these components can disturb deglutition and reduce nutri-

tional intake. Normal aging has been reported to have minor adverse effects on swallowing[86] although in the healthy older person, advanced age alone does not appear to cause any clinical dysfunction.[87,88] Conversely, systemic and oral disorders have an adverse effect on swallowing, which could place an older person at risk of choking or aspiration.[7,89,90] Cerebrovascular and neurologic diseases (eg, Parkinson's disease, Alzheimer's disease, and multiple sclerosis), head and neck cancer and its treatment (surgery and/or radiation), other systemic disorders (eg, arthritis and diabetes), and diseases and medications that decrease salivary output will adversely affect swallowing in older people.

Oral-Facial Pain

The presence of oral-facial pain in an older adult should not be attributed solely to the aging process. There is also no convincing evidence that age *per se* is a factor in treatment outcome for an older patient with pain.[91] However, oral, systemic, psychological, and behavioral problems are more likely to be major contributors to oral-facial pain. Epidemiologic surveys suggest that both acute pain and chronic oral-facial pain are significant problems among elderly people[92,93] and that they require a thorough multidisciplinary approach to diagnosis and management. Traditionally, it was accepted that there is a decrease in sensitivity to painful stimulation as persons get older. More recently, however, it has been shown that pain perception does not undergo dramatic changes with age[94] but that differences in the clinical presentation of disease may account for altered pain association.[95]

Some oral findings in older persons include a lower incidence of dentinal sensitivity and a diminished use of analgesics and local anesthesia. Altered pain sensation in elderly persons may be related to the diminished functional capability of neurophysiologic components associated with pain or to the alterations in neural pathways that are involved in nociception.[95] Aging and the incremental effects of dental wear, caries experience, trauma, previous restorative treatments, oral diseases, and oral hygiene practices can induce structural changes in teeth and periodontal tissues that can alter the perception of pain in elderly individuals.

Diagnosing pain in older adults may be challenging, especially for those patients who cannot respond to questions and who have difficulty communicating the nature of their problem.[96] The most prevalent pain in the oral-facial complex involves the teeth and periodontium. However, neuropathic pain, which can be a sequela of nerve injury, also affects elderly persons. Intraoral pain disorders affect teeth (eg, caries, root sensitivity), periodontium (eg, periodontal abscess), oral mucosa (eg, neoplasia, mucosal infection), and bone (eg, trauma, infection) and can also be idiopathic (eg, "burning mouth" syndrome). Extraoral pain disorders (exclusive of headaches) include disorders of the temporomandibular joint and of the muscles of mastication (eg, masticatory myalgia, internal joint disorder), neuralgias (eg, trigeminal or glossopharyngeal neuralgia), and atypical facial pain.[95] Regardless of the etiology, oral and craniofacial pain in an older person requires thorough examination and management, and may frequently involve multiple health care providers.

▼ COMMON ORAL CONDITIONS IN OLDER ADULTS

Oral Mucosal Diseases

Oral mucosal diseases and lesions are common in elderly people.[97] Many older adults have pigmented (varices, lingual varicosities, melanotic macules) and benign soft-tissue (fibromas, Fordyce granules) and hard-tissue conditions (exostoses, tori). Tongue conditions include geographic tongue, black hairy tongue, lingual varicosities (Figure 24-3), and atrophy of filiform and fungiform papillae.[27] The tongue may be fissured, coated, or enlarged (especially in edentulous individuals). A smooth, bald, or shiny tongue can indicate a nutritional or hematologic disorder (eg, iron or folate deficiency).

A variety of vesiculobullous and ulcerative mucosal conditions affect the elderly population. Many lesions are attributed to local trauma, such as denture-related irritation, accidental biting, and sharp dental and restorative surfaces. An ill-fitting denture can also cause inflammation (denture-induced stomatitis or papillary hyperplasia) and atrophy (resorption of residual alveolar ridges). Persistent low-grade irritation by an ill-fitting denture can induce a hyperplastic reaction, leading to the formation of an epulis fissuratum or traumatic hyperkeratosis.

Oral vesiculobullous diseases in older adults include lichen planus, pemphigus vulgaris, and cicatricial pemphigoid.[27] The most common condition is lichen planus (Figure 24-4), a recurrent, chronic, inflammatory, and autoimmune mucocutaneous disorder that affects approximately 1% of the population, of which about 35% are aged ≥ 50 years[98] (see also Chapter 4). Lichenoid mucosal lesions can also be caused by a variety of medications commonly prescribed in older patients (eg, acyclovir, gold salts, methyldopa, and thiazide diuretics). Pemphigus vulgaris is a potentially serious autoimmune vesiculobullous disorder that usually affects individuals in their fifth and sixth decades of life

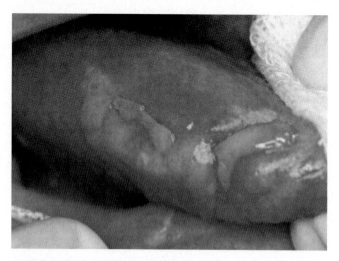

FIGURE 24-4 Lingual erosive lichen planus.

(see Chapter 4). Cicatricial pemphigoid is another immunologically mediated disorder; it affects primarily older women (see Chapter 4). The prolonged use of dentures in any of these conditions can cause exacerbation of oral mucosal lesions. Recurrent aphthous stomatitis is less common among elderly people; however, nutritional and hematologic deficiencies that are common in older adults can predispose to recurrent ulcers[99] (see Chapter 4). Although erythema multiforme is also an unusual occurrence among the elderly population, it can develop and can persist, especially in immunocompromised persons (see Chapter 4).

Oral cancer is the most significant oral mucosal disease in older adults (see Chapter 8). Incidence rates increase with age; over 95% of all oral cancers occur in individuals aged 45 years and older.[100] In the Untied States, 30,000 cases were diagnosed in 2000, with approximately 8,000 deaths.[101] The most common premalignant oral lesion is leukoplakia, and the incidence of leukoplakic lesions undergoing malignant transformation rises sharply with age. Mortality rates for oral cancer also increase with age and are high compared with those of other cancers, with overall 5-year survival rates of only 50%.[100] Typical sites of oral malignancy in elderly individuals include the tongue, lips, buccal mucosa, floor of mouth, and posterior oropharynx. The most common risk factors are increased age and the use of tobacco and alcohol. Approximately 90% of all oral cancers are squamous cell carcinomas, with the remaining 10% being salivary, bone, or lymphoid cancers.[102] These lesions can appear as exophytic, poorly demarcated, and ulcerated, erythroplakic and/or leukoplakic masses that metastasize to regional lymph nodes before involving distant organs. Excellent information is provided in numerous texts[102,103] and in Chapter 8.

Infectious Diseases

Due to numerous age- and disease-related changes in the oral and systemic immune systems, older adults are more susceptible to developing opportunistic oral infections. Viral, fungal, and bacterial organisms invade, infect, and become latent in

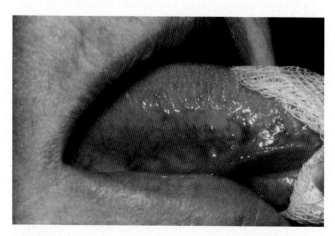

FIGURE 24-3 Lingual varicosities.

the hard and soft tissues of the oropharyngeal region, predisposing the person to disseminated systemic infections.[5]

The most common viral infections come from the herpes family (ie, herpes simplex virus [HSV] and varicella-zoster virus [VZV]). Initial infections typically occur in childhood; the viruses then remain dormant in sensory ganglia until reactivation occurs secondary to immunosuppression, trauma, stress, sunlight, gastrointestinal disturbances, or concurrent infections (see Chapter 4). The clinical presentation in an older adult will be similar to that in a younger person, but lesions may persist longer because of concomitant immunocompromising conditions. Shingles, a VZV infection, is an acute condition with very painful and frequently incapacitating oral-facial lesions (see Chapter 4). Its incidence exceeds 10 cases per 1,000 persons annually among adults aged 80 years and older, and it is most common in immunocompromised patients.[104] The VZV infection is acquired from exposure to chickenpox during childhood. It is then reactivated, causing vesicular eruptions on the skin and mucous membranes in the areas that follow the unilateral distribution of ophthalmic, maxillary, or mandibular divisions of trigeminal sensory nerves. Postherpetic neuralgia has dangerous sequelae, including blindness, facial paralysis, auditory deficits, and vertigo.[96] Postherpetic neuralgia occurs more frequently in older patients; more than 50% of zoster patients over 60 years of age will develop postherpetic neuralgia that may persist for months or even years.[104]

The most frequent oral fungal infection in older adults is caused by *Candida albicans*.[105] Several oral and systemic conditions in older adults lead to fungal proliferation and the subsequent development of infectious diseases. Removable dental prostheses (Figure 24-5), poor oral or denture hygiene, endocrine disorders (eg, diabetes), underlying immunosuppression, nutritional deficiencies, salivary gland hypofunction, and medications (eg, antibiotics, corticosteroids, immunosuppressants, and cytotoxic agents) have all been associated with oral fungal infections (see Chapter 5). The loss of vertical dimension, as well as drooling problems secondary to cerebrovascular accidents, creates a moist environment in the labial commissures that also favors yeast infection.

The bacteria that cause the most common infections are those associated with new and recurrent dental caries (*Streptococcus mutans*, *Lactobacillus*), periodontal diseases (*Porphyromonas gingivalis*, *Treponema denticola*), and acute and chronic salivary infections (*Staphylococcus aureus*, *Streptococcus viridans*).

Dental Disorders

Root surface caries result from an age-related condition[50] that develops on cementum following gingival recession (see Figure 24-2) or as an extension of existing coronal caries onto the root surface. Both new and recurrent root surface caries develop at the same rate.[106] Since cementum is less mineralized than enamel, it is more susceptible to decay. These lesions appear as well-defined and discolored defects on cementum or at the cementum-enamel junction (Figure 24-6). The prevalence of untreated root surface caries has been reported as 22% in an older population,[107] with an increased incidence in residents of facilities for long-term care.[108] Individuals who have multiple medical conditions, who are taking numerous medications, and who are undergoing medical procedures are at risk.[109] Other factors that predispose elderly individuals to root surface caries are a poor diet (with frequent sugar consumption), salivary gland hypofunction, insufficient fluoride exposure, gingival recession, oral-facial motor deficits, poor oral hygiene, and decreased access to regular dental treatment. A recent study also demonstrated that the presence of removable partial dentures are an independent risk factor for developing root surface caries in older adults.[110] Root surface caries are a diagnostic and restorative challenge since they are frequently located on interproximal surfaces, may not be visible by intraoral radiography, and can extend into subgingival regions.

Coronal caries are also quite prevalent among older persons,[50] and the risk factors are similar to those for root surface caries (with the exception of gingival recession). These enamel lesions present clinically as discolored defects on occlusal

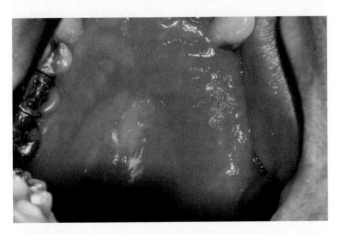

FIGURE 24-5 Denture stomatitis or erythemic candidiasis on the hard palate, beneath a partial removable prosthesis.

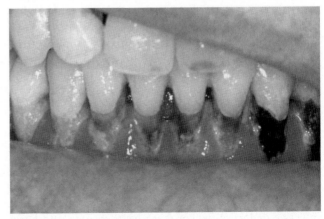

FIGURE 24-6 Unrestored root surface caries.

and/or proximal tooth surfaces and range from soft to rubbery in texture. Although rapidly progressing decay is soft and can be painful, slowly developing long-standing lesions are typically harder (from remineralization) and are asymptomatic. As a tooth ages, deposition of secondary and reparative dentin occurs, which can aid in increasing caries resistance and in decreasing dental sensitivity.

A lifelong history of dental restorations places the older person at risk for developing recurrent coronal decay. Of the reported cases of coronal caries in one study of geriatric patients, 86% were recurrent lesions.[106] Another study found that 31% of dentate individuals over the age of 70 years had clinically untreated coronal caries.[107] Decay developing around existing restorations is difficult to detect and more challenging to restore.

Periodontal Diseases

With the increasing retention of the natural dentition, the number of teeth in older adults at risk of developing periodontal disease is growing.[55] It is currently believed that only a small proportion of dentate older adults suffer from active advanced periodontal destruction. Conversely, gingivitis is much more likely to develop in older patients because of oral and systemic factors. Dental plaque, gingival bleeding, and calculus accumulations develop as a result of softer diets, reduced oral motor activity, and salivary gland hypofunction. Gingival recession, root caries, tooth furcation involvement, and tooth drifting and mobility increase the likelihood of developing gingivitis. Detriments in manual dexterity, vision, neuromuscular coordination, and physical, cognitive, and memory abilities (eg, as caused by arthritis, Parkinson's disease, cerebrovascular accidents, and Alzheimer's disease) can impair the daily performance of oral hygiene. Finally, older people (especially those living in extended-care institutions) are less likely to see dental professionals[5] and therefore have a greater risk of developing gingivitis and periodontitis.

Medications and medical problems that are common among older adults have an adverse effect on periodontal health.[111] For example, gingival hyperplasia has been associated with the use of phenytoin, cyclosporine, and calcium channel blockers.[67] Diabetes, even when well controlled, is associated with rapid periodontal breakdown due to impaired leukocyte function, altered collagen metabolism, and microvascular changes.[65,66,111] Oral mucocutaneous diseases such as erosive lichen planus and cicatricial pemphigoid will produce desquamative gingivitis.

The implications of age-related attachment loss and recession extend beyond periodontal concerns. Exposed cemental surfaces are more susceptible to root surface caries that can lead to tooth loss if untreated. Significant attachment loss and tooth mobility can cause tooth drifting and occlusal interferences. Finally, advanced periodontal diseases have been associated with non-oral diseases such as pneumonia, bacteremia, infective endocarditis, coronary heart disease, and brain abscesses, and they may interfere with the treatment of systemic diseases (eg, diabetes).[29–36]

Salivary Gland Dysfunction

Salivary gland dysfunction in older persons can be a result of local and systemic disease, head and neck radiation treatment, chemotherapy, immunologic disorders, and prescription and nonprescription medications.[112–114] Obstructions (due to mucous plugs or calcifications) and acute or chronic bacterial infections cause salivary dysfunction. Sjögren's syndrome is an autoimmune disease that affects exocrine glands (salivary and lacrimal), predominantly in older females, and salivary dysfunction is a common sequela along with associated dry eyes and dry mouth.[115] Other systemic conditions common in elderly people, such as Alzheimer's disease, diabetes, and dehydration, have been implicated in salivary gland hypofunction. Finally, numerous prescription and nonprescription medications frequently taken by older persons cause salivary hypofunction.[114] Many common drugs are antidepressants, antihypertensives, antiparkinsonian drugs, antipsychotics, and antihistamines, which have been reported to cause xerostomia and salivary dysfunction.

Extraoral manifestations of salivary gland dysfunction include candidiasis in the labial commissures and dry cracked lips (Figure 24-7). Parotid or submandibular gland enlargement with associated pain and suppuration may indicate infections or ductal obstructions. The intraoral sequelae of insufficient salivary production are dental caries, gingivitis, materia alba, candidiasis, poorly fitting dentures, dysphagia, dysgeusia, and altered mastication and deglutition.[112] These oral and pharyngeal problems can have serious consequences to an older adult. Impaired food and beverage intake can result in malnutrition and dehydration. Recurrent oral infections and impaired oral immunity can lead to aspiration pneumonia and systemic opportunistic infections.

Smell and Taste Dysfunction

The complaint of a smell or taste problem may be indicative of a chemosensory disorder, or it could be the manifestation

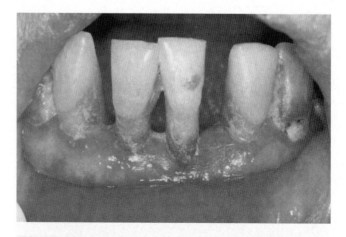

FIGURE 24-7 Results of salivary dysfunction secondary to multiple medications with anticholinergic sequelae. Dry lips and mucosal surfaces, xerostomia, calculus, dental plaque, and root surface caries have resulted from insufficient salivary output.

of an oral and/or systemic medical problem.[80] For example, the sudden loss of either smell or taste may be a sign of a brain tumor. However, older subjects are more likely to have chemosensory complaints due to chronic and long-term problems. These patients may require a multidisciplinary approach to the diagnosis and treatment of the disorder.[116,117] Since olfaction is more likely to undergo age-related decrements, compared to gustation, disorders that affect the sense of smell (such as sinus and respiratory diseases, head trauma, multiple systemic diseases, and disorders caused by medications) are more likely to adversely affect the sensation of flavor in an elderly person. Taste changes may be due to oral conditions (fungal infection, salivary hypofunction, gingivitis, halitosis, galvanism, poorly fitting prostheses, dentoalveolar abscess) and to systemic conditions (medications, medical problems, chemotherapy, radiotherapy) as well.

The most common medical conditions affecting smell and taste are neurologic (Alzheimer's disease, Parkinson's disease, multiple sclerosis), endocrine (diabetes), infectious (upper respiratory infection), and gastrointestinal (reflux, ulcers). These conditions and their treatment with multiple medications can impair the sensation of tastants and odorants. However, it is important to know that age-related losses in smell are gradual and are frequently undetected by the affected individual. Subjective changes in smell and/or taste may represent more than a "normal" aging phenomenon and require appropriate stomatologic and medical evaluation.

Swallowing Disorders

More than one-third of older adults in the general population complain of swallowing and esophageal problems,[118] and the prevalence of such disorders is probably even greater among institutionalized adults and those receiving parenteral and enteral nutrition.[119] Dysphagia in elderly persons can be caused by a variety of medical conditions; these include immunologic disorders (eg, arthritis, diabetes), neurologic or neuromuscular disorders (eg, Parkinson's disease, stroke), and psychological disorders, (eg, depression, dementia). Dysphagia in this population can also be caused by the environmental effects of certain conditions (eg, smoking, toxins) and by surgery (eg, for head and neck cancer).[87–90,120,121] A common oral condition that is associated with dysphagia in elderly people is salivary gland dysfunction, which can decrease the transit time of the food bolus from the mouth into the esophagus.[122] One study examined the influence of age and denture use on functional eating and swallowing and reported that denture use, not age, played the stronger role in impaired functional eating.[123] Therefore, good oral and systemic health (as well as an intact dentition) probably play a strong role in preventing swallowing problems.

The most serious sequela of dysphagia is aspiration, particularly in a neurologically impaired person.[120] An impaired or absent cough reflex is a strong indication that the airway cannot be protected even from oral and nasopharyngeal secretions. Oral motor weakness in the lips, tongue, and buccal mucosa are additional predictors of a poor swallow reflex. Lip weakness causes drooling from the lips, delaying the initiation of the oral phase of the swallow. Tongue weakness impairs the formation of a food bolus, and the food bolus then begins to drip down over the base of the tongue into the pharynx, pooling in the pharyngeal recesses. This is a frequent cause of aspiration after the swallow and can lead to pneumonia.

Edentulousness

A functional dentition plays an essential role in mastication, deglutition, phonation, facial aesthetics and expression, dietary selection, and the hedonic aspect of eating. Until recently, the loss of all teeth was considered a normal part of aging. With the increased retention of natural dentition by older adults,[51] the traditional perception of an edentulous older person (with or without dentures) is now changing. Tooth loss is directly linked to dental caries and periodontal disease but may also be related to systemic conditions such as osteoporosis and diabetes mellitus. However, despite the decline in tooth loss over the last 30 years, the prevalence of edentulism among the elderly population is still quite high; about 30% of adults aged 65 years or more are completely edentulous.[44]

Edentulous adults, even those with removable prostheses, have decreased masticatory forces and impaired chewing efficiency. Diminished oral motor function can induce masticatory muscle atrophy and deterioration of muscle contractile properties, further inhibiting chewing capability. Rapid alveolar bone resorption follows tooth loss and continues throughout life. In severe cases, alveolar ridge atrophy, especially in the mandible, can lead to significant problems in denture fabrication and retention and possibly to mandibular fracture. Furthermore, poorly fitting prostheses can accelerate the loss of alveolar bone.

▼ PREVENTION AND TREATMENT OF ORAL CONDITIONS IN THE OLDER POPULATION

Oral Mucosal Diseases

Prevention of oral cancer begins with the elimination of established risk factors (eg, the use of tobacco and alcohol). Early detection and recognition through regular comprehensive extra- and intraoral examinations in dentate and edentulous persons will enhance the prognosis and reduce the morbidity and mortality associated with cancer and its treatments.[102] Oral cancer is treated by surgery, chemotherapy, and radiotherapy, which also have significant oral sequelae including stomatitis, dysphagia, dysgeusia, pain, paresthesias, facial disfigurement, oral motor dysfunction, salivary hypofunction, and an increased risk of developing osteoradionecrosis. Comprehensive dental management before, during, and after treatment is essential to prevent complications. Importantly, older edentulous individuals are four times less likely to see a dentist than are dentate individuals,[124] and should therefore be targeted for regular annual examinations for head and neck cancer.[125,126]

Treatment of traumatic oral lesions begins with the elimination of underlying factors. To this end, the most common measure is the repair of an ill-fitting denture flange/base or the removal of an epulis fissuratum. Palliative topical medications (analgesics) are helpful, and antibiotic coverage to prevent secondary bacterial infection should be considered for the immunocompromised patient. For most oral vesiculobullous and erosive diseases, therapy depends on the severity of the condition and may range from mild topical steroids and oral rinses to strong topical steroids to systemic steroids, with or without immunosuppressant agents.[27] When high-dose steroids are considered, dentists should consult with the patient's physicians, especially if the older patient has concurrent medical problems such as diabetes, coronary heart disease, hypertension, osteoporosis, or depression. Procedures and medications for the prevention and management of oral mucosal diseases in elderly people are summarized in Table 24-8.

Infectious Diseases

Prevention of the spread of viral lesions in elderly patients can be accomplished by their avoiding individuals who have active infections. Herpes simplex and zoster lesions are usually self-limiting. Supportive measures are necessary to maintain adequate nutritional and fluid intake and to diminish pain. However, early diagnosis can diminish morbidity in older patients. In particular, immunocompromised adults are susceptible to recurrent herpes infections and require immediate and aggressive antiviral treatment in such cases. Patients with renal insufficiency should receive adjusted antiviral doses (acyclovir, valacyclovir, famciclovir). The treatment of older patients who have postherpetic neuralgia requires analgesics, tricyclic antidepressants, and (sometimes) steroids.[27]

Prevention of candidiasis involves meticulous oral and denture hygiene, the judicious use of antibiotics and immunosuppressants, and the elimination of underlying local and systemic etiologic factors (eg, salivary hypofunction, diabetes, or immunodeficiency). Comprehensive management of oral candidiasis with antifungal creams, rinses, and lozenges is usually successful, but persistent infections require systemic antifungal agents.[105,127] Dentures are frequent sources of fungal infections and require antifungal therapy with a 10- to 15-minute 1% sodium hypochlorite soak and antifungal creams during use. The prevention and treatment of common oral bacterial infections (eg, dental caries, periodontal diseases, and salivary gland infections) are discussed below.

Dental Disorders

Dental caries in elderly persons can be prevented by the rigorous maintenance of oral hygiene, including brushing and flossing after each meal. The use of fluoride-containing dentifrices and rinses can aid in the remineralization of existing decay and in the prevention of new carious lesions.[128,129] Lifelong exposure to fluoridated water has also been shown to diminish tooth loss and dental caries.[130] Traditionally, fluoride was recommended for the prevention of coronal caries, but there is considerable evidence that fluorides are also effective

TABLE 24-8 Prevention and Management of Oral Mucosal Diseases in Elderly Persons

Disease	Prevention	Treatment
Oral cancer	Eliminate established risk factors. Ensure early detection and recognition.	Surgery; chemotherapy; radiation therapy
Traumatic lesions	Eliminate underlying factors.	Oral rinses Viscous lidocaine HCL 2% Diphenhydramine elixir 12.5 mg/5 mL Dyclonine HCL 1% Sucralfate Systemic medications Penicillin VK tabs 500 mg qid Amoxicillin tabs 500 mg qid Erythromycin tabs 250 mg qid
Oral vesiculobullous and erosive diseases	Avoid drug hypersensitivity, trauma, and allergies.	Topical medications Fluocinonide gel 0.05% Triamcinolone acetonide gel 0.1% Clobetasol propionate gel 0.05% Oral rinses Dexamethasone elixir 0.5 mg/5 mL Diphenhydramine elixir 12.5 mg/5 mL Dyclonine HCL 1% Sucralfate Systemic medications Prednisone 5 mg dose pak or maintenance dose Azathioprine 50 mg 1–2 tabs qd Nutritional supplements; fluid intake

HCL = hydrochloride; qd = every day; qid = four times per day; tabs = tablets.

in remineralizing carious dentin.[131,132] The prevention and early treatment of dental caries requires regular dental visits for prophylaxis and examination. Since the bacterial acid production that causes tooth decay is precipitated by food intake, it is important to monitor the frequency of meals and snacking. Snacking on carbohydrate-rich foods and the consumption of sugar-containing beverages should be reduced.

The treatment of coronal and root surface dental caries has been facilitated by the development and perfection of numerous restorative materials. Enamel- and dentin-bonding techniques are helpful in restoring destroyed tooth morphology due to caries, abrasion, attrition, and erosion. Cosmetic dentistry has also made considerable advances that have implications for older adults. Conservative and esthetic restorative procedures have the potential to reverse the signs of dental aging, thereby making patients appear younger.[133] Traditionally reserved for younger patients, cosmetic enhancement of teeth and smiles can now be used in many older individuals.

Salivary gland dysfunction is a common predisposing factor to dental caries, and early recognition and management is thus vital to avoiding extensive restorative procedures, dentoalveolar abscesses, and tooth extraction. Patients affected with medical conditions that are known to cause salivary hypofunction (eg, Sjögren's syndrome, diabetes, head and neck irradiation, Alzheimer's disease) must be monitored more closely for new and recurrent dental caries. Similarly, patients who are taking medications associated with salivary hypofunction (eg, antidepressants, antihypertensives, anti-psychotics) should be on a more frequent recall to dental professionals. The older patient with salivary hypofunction requires rigorous oral hygiene practices with the addition of supplemental fluoride gels and rinses.

Caries prevention in elderly residents of facilities and institutions for long-term care requires daily assistance from caregivers, depending on the level of dependency of the individual.[134] An electric toothbrush can help patients with impaired manual dexterity and other motor disabilities maintain oral hygiene. Prescription fluoride gels (1.0 or 1.1% sodium fluoride or 0.4% stannous fluoride) and rinses and 0.12% chlorhexidine rinses are recommended for these patients. A more frequent dental recall schedule is also indicated for prevention of dental decay.

Periodontal Diseases

Periodontal maintenance and prevention regimens are similar for all age groups but may require additional time, equipment, and recall visits, depending on the functional and mental capacity of the individual. Periodontal health can be maintained with toothbrushing and flossing after each meal and with regularly scheduled professional dental examinations and cleanings. In the case of older medically, physically, and behaviorally compromised patients, especially those who are homebound or institutionalized, caregivers should assist these patients with daily oral hygiene.[134] Dental professionals must instruct caregivers on the proper use of oral and denture hygiene techniques for their patients. Electric toothbrushes,

floss holders, pulsed-jet water irrigators, and 0.12% chlorhexidine antimicrobial rinses are also extremely useful. Patients with arthritic deformities or minimal or no manual dexterity will benefit from the modification of toothbrush handles for easier manipulation.

Treatment of periodontal diseases in the elderly patient requires an assessment of the patient's attitudes and expectations, previous dental and/or periodontal treatments, current oral health status, oral hygiene practices, medical conditions, medication use, physical and mental capacity, and level of caregiver support (if necessary). For most elderly patients, a nonsurgical approach with scaling and root planing and meticulous daily oral hygiene is indicated. Gingival recession, furcation involvement, and large embrasure spaces make periodontal treatment and maintenance more difficult in the older patient. Systemic antimicrobial therapy (eg, metronidazole, tetracycline, clindamycin)[135] may be helpful, but the practitioner must ensure that these medications are not contraindicated (eg, by renal, liver, or gastrointestinal disorders). Older persons with local periodontal defects are also good candidates for the implantation of antimicrobial fibers and chips (eg, tetracycline, chlorhexidine gluconate). Advanced age is not a contraindication for periodontal surgery although certain systemic conditions (eg, congestive heart disease, diabetes) and medications (eg, anticoagulants, corticosteroids) may complicate surgical procedures. Nevertheless, the long-term results of nonsurgical and surgical periodontal therapy are similar in young and older persons, with plaque control being the key to success.[111]

If the periodontal disease is believed to arise from the patient's medical conditions and their treatment, then a systemic approach to oral health management is required. For example, stabilization of blood glucose levels in a patient with diabetes mellitus should be established prior to the initiation of extensive periodontal treatment. Drug-induced gingival hyperplasia (eg, from use of calcium channel blockers, cyclosporine, dilantin)[67] frequently requires surgical reduction with concomitant plaque control and the consideration of substitute medication. Finally, periodontal therapy often requires concurrent dental treatment to eliminate comorbid factors (defective restorations, poorly fitting prostheses, caries) commonly found in older patients.

Salivary Gland Disorders

Disorders of the salivary glands require accurate diagnosis to initiate therapy and to avoid long-term oral and pharyngeal complications.[73] Salivary gland infections require diagnostic culture and sensitivity tests and appropriate antibiotic therapy. Amoxicillin and clavulanic acid (clindamycin if the patient is allergic to penicillin) should be immediately prescribed and monitored until the culture and sensitivity report is received. Diagnosis and treatment of salivary gland obstructions may require imaging tests (radiography, sialography, technetium-99m-pertechnetate scanning) and subsequent removal of the obstruction. Systemic diseases (eg, Sjögren's syndrome) should be identified, managed, and controlled. In medication-associated xerostomia, elimination or reduction of the causative drug, in collaboration with the patient's physician, is the ideal solution.[114] However, if this cannot be achieved, the substitution of one xerostomia-causing medication with a similar drug that has fewer undesirable side effects or the alteration of medication dosing schedules should be considered. For patients receiving head and neck radiation therapy for oropharyngeal cancers, contralateral parotid gland preservation techniques are effective and can help diminish postirradiation xerostomia.[136]

Patients with salivary hypofunction who have some remaining viable salivary parenchymal tissue will respond to salivary stimulants; these include sugarless candies, mints, and gums; nonsugared beverages, used frequently;[73] cevemeline HCI (30 mg tid) and pilocarpine (5 to 7.5 mg three times daily [tid] and every night at bedtime [qhs]).[137,138] Pilocarpine and cevimeline are contraindicated for patients with narrow-angle glaucoma, congestive heart disease, and pulmonary disease, and their major side effects are sweating and diarrhea. If there is little or no remaining viable salivary gland tissue, saliva substitutes[139] and the frequent intake of nonsugared beverages are necessary. In dry climates, a humidifier may also help relieve xerostomic complaints. Finally, it is vital that precautions be taken to prevent the deleterious sequelae of salivary gland dysfunction. These precautions include frequent dental recall, daily use of fluorides, brushing and flossing after each meal, and rigorous prosthesis hygiene.

Smell and Taste Dysfunction

The primary step in treating smell and taste disturbances is identification of the etiology.[117] A variety of oral problems can cause chemosensory alterations, including oral mucosal infections (eg, candidiasis), poorly fitting removable prostheses, periodontal and dental diseases, dentoalveolar infections, oral mucosal diseases (eg, pemphigus), and poor tongue hygiene. These underlying disorders should be managed, and their treatment may improve smell and/or taste function. Medications, chemotherapy, radiotherapy, and a myriad of systemic conditions can also cause chemosensory loss, and these should be monitored.[80,83,140]

Unfortunately, many older people continue to suffer from chemosensory disorders despite thorough oral and medical evaluations. There are several ways to improve the smell, taste, and other sensory qualities of foods and beverages to prevent the development of subsequent nutritional deficiencies in these individuals. Improving the visual display of certain foods may be helpful. Flavor enhancers can counteract taste and smell deficits that can help in the maintenance of nutritional health.[141] Foods and beverages that are salty or sweet or that stimulate the trigeminal nerve (eg, black or red pepper, carbonation) may add another dimension to the eating experience. However, the use of sweet and salty additives may be contraindicated for individuals with certain medical disorders such as diabetes and hypertension.

Older people may not recognize the olfactory decline that accompanies aging, yet they are capable of recognizing flavor improvements caused by odor fortification (eg, by the use of additional herbs and spices). Therefore, patients with chemosensory deficits should be encouraged to use herbs and spices that will augment flavor perception without adding unnecessary calories, fats, sugars, or salts. Finally, eating in a social atmosphere can draw a person's attention away from food flavor and can enhance the enjoyment of a meal.

Masticatory and Swallowing Disorders

Many older individuals experience eating and swallowing disorders that could cause nutritional impairments such as dehydration and malnutrition. Therefore, masticatory and swallowing problems must be diagnosed, treated by appropriate specialists, and followed to ensure adequate stabilization. As previously discussed, the status of the dentition may have a direct influence on mastication. Therefore, dental and periodontal problems should be eradicated, and functionally stable removable prostheses should be constructed. While adequate nutrition can be maintained in an edentate adult, most individuals benefit functionally, aesthetically, and socially from adequately fitting dentures. Salivary dysfunction can alter denture use; therefore, treatment of salivary hypofunction in the denture-wearing older adult will also help improve mastication.

Masticatory deficiencies are likely to be managed by dental professionals, but the management of dysphagia may require a combination of dental and medical health care providers.[142,143] If salivary hypofunction is suspected, diagnosis and treatment must be initiated. Increasing the patient's salivary function immediately before or during mealtime (eg, with additional fluids or with 5 mg of pilocarpine or 30 mg of cevimeline HCL given 30 minutes before mealtime) may be effective. Older adults should be reminded to eat and swallow carefully and to avoid large ingestions of foods and fluids. Additional time spent sipping fluids between bites of food will aid in swallowing, especially with dry foods. Intubation and artificial nutrition may be required in some institutionalized older adults due to the high risk of developing dysphagia and aspiration.

Edentulousness

Removable dental prostheses are a poor substitute for the natural dentition; therefore, prevention of total tooth loss is recommended for people of any age. The prevention and early treatment of dental caries and periodontal diseases and the maintenance of daily oral hygiene and regular professional care require lifelong effort.

There is some evidence to support a relationship between osteoporosis and osteopenia with alveolar bone resorption and tooth loss.[61–63] Furthermore, it has been suggested that the medical treatment of osteoporosis with estrogen supplements will help prevent tooth loss and will delay the atrophy of the mandibular and maxillary ridges.[64] One study demonstrated that postmenopausal women with periodontally healthy dentition had greater bone mineral density than edentulous women.[144] It was concluded that sufficient masticatory function in dentate older women could possibly inhibit or delay the progress of osteoporotic change in skeletal bone or that edentulous women might be more susceptible to osteoporosis.[144]

In summary, there may be significant relationships between the systemic and oral manifestations of bone loss, and strategies to maintain or increase skeletal bone may prove useful in the retention of natural dentition and alveolar bone.

The fabrication of removable prostheses (when retention of natural dentition is not possible) requires thorough attention to retention, occlusion, aesthetics, and the extension of peripheral margins.[145] Regular assessment of dentures, denture-bearing ridges, and all mucosal surfaces is required to reduce the risk of developing denture stomatitis, traumatic ulcerations, angular cheilitis, hyperplastic or granulomatous tissue reactions, and (ultimately) alveolar atrophy. Denture adjustments and/or relines are may be necessary at regular intervals for the lifetime of the patient.

Endosseous dentoalveolar implants for partially or completely edentulous adults have achieved remarkable success in the past several decades and can be included in the treatment plan of most older persons.[146–148] Patients who have undergone surgery and radiotherapy for oral cancers have been reported to have 5-year survival rates of 90% for oral implants.[149] Exceptions for implant use are (1) severely medically compromised and immunosuppressed patients and (2) individuals with severely atrophic edentulous ridges (although bony ridge augmentation can be considered).[150]

Finally, there are additional issues pertinent to the edentulous older adult that are frequently neglected. Annual examinations for head, neck, and oral cancer screenings are required for older adults and are currently recommended by the American Cancer Society.[126] As mentioned previously, many older adults have salivary hypofunction that can predispose to poorly fitting dentures and denture stomatitis. Efforts to increase salivary output may enhance denture retention. Lastly, in institutional settings, identification markings should be placed on each denture to avoid their misplacement.

▼ SUMMARY

Older adults are the most rapidly growing segment of the population. In the absence of major medical problems and interventions, aging is associated with few dramatic and deleterious consequences to the health and function of the oral cavity. However, oral and systemic diseases concurrently interact to produce a myriad of oropharyngeal disorders. Many older persons will thus experience oral mucosal, dental, periodontal, and alveolar diseases and chemosensory, masticatory, salivary, and swallowing disorders. Most of these problems can be treated to diminish morbidity and mortality in this population. Therefore, health care practitioners must be able to identify, manage, and prevent these problems in order to enhance the quality of life of older adults.

▼ REFERENCES

1. Day JC. Population projections of the United States by age, sex, race, and Hispanic origin: 1995 to 2050. Washington (DC): US Department of Commerce; 1996.
2. Anderson RN. United States life tables, 1997. Hyattsville (MD): National Center for Health Statistics; 1999.
3. Ghezzi EM, Ship JA. Systemic diseases and their treatments in the elderly: impact on oral health. J Public Health Dent 2000;60(4):289–96.
4. Chavez EM, Ship JA. Sensory and motor deficits in the elderly: impact on oral health. J Public Health Dent 2000;60(4):297–303.
5. Shay K, Ship JA. The importance of oral health in the older patient. J Am Geriatr Soc 1995;43(12):1414–22.
6. Ship JA. Oral sequelae of common geriatric diseases, disorders, impairments. Clin Geriatr Med 1992;8:483–97.
7. Ship JA, Duffy V, Jones JA, Langmore S. Geriatric oral health and its impact on eating. J Am Geriatr Soc 1996;44(4):456–64.
8. Geldmacher DS, Whitehouse PJ. Evaluation of dementia. N Engl J Med 1996;335(5):330–6.
9. Evans DA, Funkenstein HH, Albert MS, et al. Prevalence of Alzheimer's disease in a community population of older persons. Higher than previously reported. JAMA 1989;262(18):2551–6.
10. Hendrie HC. Epidemiology of dementia and Alzheimer's disease. Am J Geriatr Psychiatry 1998;6(2 Suppl 1):S3–18.
11. Kawas CH. Alzheimer's disease. In: Hazzard WR, Blass JP, Ettinger WH Jr, et al, editors. Principles of geriatric medicine and gerontology. 4th ed. New York: McGraw-Hill; 1999. p. 1257–69.
12. Evans DA. Estimated prevalence of Alzheimer's disease in the United States. Milbank Q 1990;68(2):267–89.
13. Bower JH, Maraganore DM, McDonnell SK, Rocca WA. Incidence and distribution of parkinsonism in Olmsted County, Minnesota, 1976-1990. Neurology 1999;52(6):1214–20.
14. de Rijk MC, Tzourio C, Breteler MM, et al. Prevalence of parkinsonism and Parkinson's disease in Europe: the EUROPARKINSON Collaborative Study. European Community Concerted Action on the Epidemiology of Parkinson's Disease. J Neurol Neurosurg Psychiatry 1997;62(1):10–5.
15. Lapane KL, Fernandez HH, Friedman JH. Prevalence, clinical characteristics, and pharmacologic treatment of Parkinson's disease in residents in long-term care facilities. SAGE Study Group. Pharmacotherapy 1999;19(11):1321–7.
16. Ghezzi EM, Ship JA. Dementia and oral health. Oral Surg Oral Med Oral Path Oral Radiol Endod 2000;89(1):2–5.
17. Henry RG, Wekstein DR. Providing dental care for patients diagnosed with Alzheimer's disease. Dent Clin N Am 1997;41(4):915–44.
18. Ship JA, Puckett SA. Longitudinal study on oral health in subjects with Alzheimer's disease. J Am Geriatr Soc 1994;42:57–63.
19. Ship JA. Oral health in patients with Alzheimer's disease. J Am Dent Assoc 1992;123:53–8.
20. Ship JA, DeCarli C, Friedland RP, Baum BJ. Diminished submandibular salivary flow in dementia of the Alzheimer type. J Gerontol 1990;45(2):M61–6.
21. Warren JJ, Chalmers JM, Levy SM, et al. Oral health of persons with and without dementia attending a geriatric clinic. Spec Care Dentist 1997;17(2):47–53.
22. Persson M, Osterberg T, Granerus AK, Karlsson S. Influence of Parkinson's disease on oral health. Acta Odontol Scand 1992;50(1):37–42.
23. Niessen LC, Jones JA, Zocchi M, Gurian B. Dental care for the patient with Alzheimer's disease. J Am Dent Assoc 1985;110(2):207–9.

24. Ghezzi EM, Chavez EM, Ship JA. General anesthesia protocol for the dental patient: emphasis for older adults. Spec Care Dentist 2000;20(3):81–92.

25. Pamuk E, Makuc D, Heck K, et al. Health, United States, 1998 with socioeconomic status and health chartbook. Hyattsville (MD): National Center for Health Statistics; 1998.

26. Munson ML. Characteristics of elderly home health care users: data from the 1996 National Home and Hospice Care Survey. Hyattsville (MD): National Center for Health Statistics; 1999.

27. Ship JA, Mohammad AR. Clinician's guide to oral health in geriatric patients. 1st ed. Baltimore (MD): American Academy of Oral Medicine; 1999.

28. Berkey DB, Ela KM, Berg RG. Advances in portable and mobile equipment systems. Int Dent J 1993;43(5):455-65.

29. Loesche WJ, Schork A, Terpenning MS, et al. Assessing the relationship between dental disease and coronary heart disease in elderly U.S. veterans. J Am Dent Assoc 1998;129(3):301–11.

30. Loesche WJ, Schork A, Terpenning MS, et al. The relationship between dental disease and cerebral vascular accident in elderly United States veterans. Ann Periodontol 1998;3(1):161–74.

31. Loesche WJ. Association of the oral flora with important medical diseases. Curr Opin Periodontol 1997;4:21–8.

32. Beck JD, Offenbacher S. Oral health and systemic disease: periodontitis and cardiovascular disease. J Dent Educ 1998; 62(10):859–70.

33. Beck JD, Offenbacher S, Williams R, et al. Periodontitis: a risk factor for coronary heart disease? Ann Periodontol 1998;3(1):127–41.

34. Joshipura KJ, Rimm EB, Douglass CW, et al. Poor oral health and coronary heart disease. J Dent Res 1996;75(9):1631–6.

35. Garcia RI, Krall EA, Vokonas PS. Periodontal disease and mortality from all causes in the VA Dental Longitudinal Study. Ann Periodontol 1998;3(1):339–49.

36. Fourrier F, Duvivier B, Boutigny H, et al. Colonization of dental plaque: a source of nosocomial infections in intensive care unit patients. Crit Care Med 1998;26(2):301–8.

37. Arbes SJ Jr, Slade GD, Beck JD. Association between extent of periodontal attachment loss and self-reported history of heart attack: an analysis of NHANES III data. J Dent Res 1999;78(12):1777–82.

38. Beck JD, Pankow J, Tyroler HA, Offenbacher S. Dental infections and atherosclerosis. Am Heart J 1999;138(5 Pt 2):S528–33.

39. Slade GD, Offenbacher S, Beck JD, et al. Acute-phase inflammatory response to periodontal disease in the US population. J Dent Res 2000;79(1):49–57.

40. Wu T, Trevisan M, Genco RJ, et al. Examination of the relation between periodontal health status and cardiovascular risk factors: serum total and high density lipoprotein cholesterol, C-reactive protein, and plasma fibrinogen. Am J Epidemiol 2000;151(3):273–82.

41. Williams DM, Cruchley AT. Structural aspects of aging in the oral mucosa. In: Squier CA, Hill MW, editors. The effect of aging in oral mucosa and skin. Boca Raton (FL): CRC Press; 1994. p. 65–74.

42. Farthing PM, Walton LJ. Changes in immune function with age. In: Squier CA, Hill MW, editors. The effect of aging in oral mucosa and skin. Boca Raton (FL): CRC Press; 1994. p. 113–20.

43. Hill MW, Karthigasan J, Berg JH, Squier CA. Influence of age on the response of oral mucosa to injury. In: Squier CA, Hill MW, editors. The effect of aging in oral mucosa and skin. Boca Raton (FL): CRC Press; 1994. p. 129–42.

44. Kramarow E, Lentzner H, Rooks R, et al. Health and aging chartbook. Health, United States, 1999. Hyattsville (MD): National Center for Health Statistics; 1999.

45. Whittaker DK, Bakri MM. Racial variations in the extent of tooth root translucency in ageing individuals. Arch Oral Biol 1996;41(1):15–9.

46. Ketterl W. Age-induced changes in the teeth and their attachment apparatus. Int Dent J 1983;33(3):262–71.

47. Drusini AG, Toso O, Ranzato C. The coronal pulp cavity index: a biomarker for age determination in human adults. Am J Phys Anthropol 1997;103(3):353–63.

48. Morse DR, Esposito JV, Schoor RS. A radiographic study of aging changes of the dental pulp and dentin in normal teeth. Quintessence Int 1993;24(5):329–33.

49. Burke FM, Samarawickrama DY. Progressive changes in the pulpo-dentinal complex and their clinical consequences. Gerodontology 1995;12(12):57–66.

50. Miller AJ, Brunelle JA, Carlos JP, et al. Oral health of United States adults. Washington (DC): US Department of Health and Human Services, National Institutes of Health, Public Health Service; 1987.

51. Burt BA. Epidemiology of dental diseases in the elderly. Clin Geriatr Med 1992;8(3):447–59.

52. Holm-Pedersen P, Agerbaek N, Theilade E. Experimental gingivitis in young and elderly individuals. J Clin Periodontol 1975;2(1):14–24.

53. Holm-Pedersen P, Folke LE, Gawronski TH. Composition and metabolic activity of dental plaque from healthy young and elderly individuals. J Dent Res 1980;59(5):771–6.

54. Berkey DB, Shay K. General dental care for the elderly. Clin Geriatr Med 1992;8(3):579–97.

55. Burt BA. Periodontitis and aging: reviewing recent evidence. J Am Dent Assoc 1994;125(3):273–9.

56. Ship JA, Beck JD. A ten year longitudinal study of periodontal attachment loss in healthy adults. Oral Surg Oral Med Oral Pathol Oral Radiol Endod 1996;81:281–90.

57. Van der Velden U. Effect of age on the periodontium. J Clin Periodontol 1984;11(5):281–94.

58. Fransson C, Berglundh T, Lindhe J. The effect of age on the development of gingivitis. Clinical, microbiological and histological findings. J Clin Periodontol 1996;23(4):379–85.

59. Fransson C, Mooney J, Kinane DF, Berglundh T. Differences in the inflammatory response in young and old human subjects during the course of experimental gingivitis. J Clin Periodontol 1999;26(7):453–60.

60. Lindhe J, Socransky S, Nyman S, et al. Effect of age on healing following periodontal therapy. J Clin Periodontol 1985; 12(9):774–87.

61. Wactawski-Wende J, Grossi SG, Trevisan M, et al. The role of osteopenia in oral bone loss and periodontal disease. J Periodontol 1996;67(10 Suppl):1076–84.

62. Jeffcoat MK. Osteoporosis: a possible modifying factor in oral bone loss. Ann Periodontol 1998;3(1):312–21.

63. Kribbs PJ. Comparison of mandibular bone in normal and osteoporotic women. J Prosthet Dent 1990;63(2):218–22.

64. Paganini-Hill A. The benefits of estrogen replacement therapy on oral health. The Leisure World cohort. Arch Intern Med 1995;155(21):2325–9.

65. Taylor GW, Burt BA, Becker MP, et al. Glycemic control and alveolar bone loss progression in type 2 diabetes. Ann Periodontol 1998;3(1):30–9.

66. Taylor GW, Burt BA, Becker MP, et al. Severe periodontitis and risk for poor glycemic control in patients with non-insulin-dependent diabetes mellitus. J Periodontol 1996;67(10 Suppl):1085–93.

67. Meraw SJ, Sheridan PJ. Medically induced gingival hyperplasia. Mayo Clin Proc 1998;73(12):1196–9.

68. Genco RJ, Ho AW, Kopman J, et al. Models to evaluate the role of stress in periodontal disease. Ann Periodontol 1998;3(1):288–302.

69. Beck JD, Sharp T, Koch GG, Offenbacher S. A study of attachment loss patterns in survivor teeth at 18 months, 36 months and 5 years in community-dwelling older adults. J Periodontal Res 1997;32(6):497–505.

70. Beck JD, Slade GD. Epidemiology of periodontal diseases. Curr Opin Periodontol 1996;3:3–9.

71. Beck JD, Koch GG. Characteristics of older adults experiencing periodontal attachment loss as gingival recession or probing depth. J Periodontal Res 1994;29(4):290–8.

72. Axelsson P, Paulander J, Lindhe J. Relationship between smoking and dental status in 35-, 50-, 65-, and 75-year-old individuals. J Clin Periodontol 1998;25(4):297–305.

73. Atkinson JC, Wu A. Salivary gland dysfunction: causes, symptoms, treatment. J Am Dent Assoc 1994;125(4):409–16.

74. Baum BJ, Ship JA, Wu AJ. Salivary gland function and aging: a model for studying the interaction of aging and systemic disease. Crit Rev Oral Biol Med 1992;4:53–64.

75. Bergdahl M. Salivary flow and oral complaints in adult dental patients. Community Dent Oral Epidemiol 2000;28:59–66.

76. Ship JA, Nolan N, Puckett S. Longitudinal analysis of parotid and submandibular salivary flow rates in healthy, different aged adults. J Gerontol Med Sci 1995;50A:M285–9.

77. Ship JA, Baum BJ. Is reduced salivary flow normal in old people? Lancet 1990;336:1507.

78. Wu AJ, Atkinson JC, Fox PC, et al. Cross-sectional and longitudinal analyses of stimulated parotid salivary constituents in healthy different aged subjects. J Gerontol Med Sci 1993;48:M219–24.

79. Scott J, Flower EA, Burns J. A quantitative study of histological changes in the human parotid gland occurring with adult age. J Oral Pathol 1987;16(10):505–10.

80. Ship JA. The influence of aging on oral health and consequences for taste and smell. Physiol Behav 1999;66(2):209–15.

81. Weiffenbach JM, Bartoshuk LM. Taste and smell. Clin Geriatr Med 1992;8:543–55.

82. Ship JA, Pearson JD, Cruise LJ, et al. Longitudinal changes in smell identification. J Gerontol A Biol Sci Med Sci 1996;51A:M86–91.

83. Schiffman SS. Taste and smell losses in normal aging and disease. JAMA 1997;278(16):1357–62.

84. Murphy C. Nutrition and chemosensory perception in the elderly. Crit Rev Food Sci Nutr 1993;33:3–15.

85. Wayler AH, Muench ME, Kapur KK, Chauncey HH. Masticatory performance and food acceptability in persons with removable partial dentures, full dentures and intact natural dentition. J Gerontol 1984;39(3):284–9.

86. Kern M, Bardan E, Arndorfer R, et al. Comparison of upper esophageal sphincter opening in healthy asymptomatic young and elderly volunteers. Ann Otol Rhinol Laryngol 1999;108(10):982–9.

87. Robbins J. Normal swallowing and aging. Semin Neurol 1996;16(4):309–17.

88. Caruso AJ, Max L. Effects of aging on neuromotor processes of swallowing. Semin Speech Lang 1997;18(2):181–92.

89. Plant RL. Anatomy and physiology of swallowing in adults and geriatrics. Otolaryngol Clin North Am 1998;31(3):477–88.

90. Deron P. Dysphagia with systemic diseases. Acta Otorhinolaryngol Belg 1994;48(2):191–200.

91. Sorkin BA, Rudy TE, Hanlon RB, et al. Chronic pain in old and young patients: differences appear less important than similarities. J Gerontol 1990;45(2):64–8.

92. Riley JL 3rd, Gilbert GH, Heft MW. Health care utilization by older adults in response to painful orofacial symptoms. Pain 1999;81(1–2):67–75.

93. Lipton JA, Ship JA, Larach D. Prevalence of reported jaw joint, face, and burning mouth pain in the United States. J Am Dent Assoc 1993;124:115–21.

94. Heft MW, Cooper BY, O'Brien KK, et al. Aging effects on the perception of noxious and non-noxious thermal stimuli applied to the face. Aging (Milano) 1996;8(1):35–41.

95. Ship JA, Heft M, Harkins S. Oral facial pain in the elderly. In: Lomranz J, Mostofsky DI, editors. Handbook of pain and aging. 1st ed. New York: Plenum Publishing Co.; 1997. p. 321–46.

96. Heft MW. Orofacial pain. Clin Geriatr Med 1992;8(3):557–68.

97. Hand JS, Whitehill JM. The prevalence of oral mucosal lesions in an elderly population. J Am Dent Assoc 1986;112(1):73–6.

98. Scully C, Beyli M, Ferreiro MC, et al. Update on oral lichen planus: etiopathogenesis and management. Crit Rev Oral Biol Med 1998;9(1):86–122.

99. Ship JA, Chavez EM, Doerr PA, et al. Recurrent aphthous stomatitis. Quintessence Int 2000;31:95–112.

100. Natonal Cancer Institute. SEER Cancer Statistics Review, 1973–1996: Bethesda, MD: National Institutes of Health; 1996.

101. Greenlee RT, Murray T, Bolden S, Wingo PA. Cancer Statistics, 2000. CA Cancer J Clin 2000;50:7–33.

102. Silverman SJ. Oral cancer. 4th ed. Hamilton, Canada: The American Cancer Society, Inc.; 1998.

103. Million RR, Cassisi NJ. Management of head and neck cancer. 2nd ed. Philadelphia: J. B. Lippincott Co.; 1994.

104. Gershon AA. Epidemiology and management of postherpetic neuralgia. Semin Dermatol 1996;15(2 Suppl 1):8–13.

105. Peterson DE. Oral candidiasis. Clin Geriatr Med 1992;8(3):513–27.

106. Beck JD, Hunt RJ, Hand JS, Field HM. Prevalence of root and coronal caries in a noninstitutionalized older population. J Am Dent Assoc 1985;111(6):964–7.

107. Douglass CW, Jette AM, Fox CH, et al. Oral health status of the elderly in New England. J Gerontol 1993;48(2):M39–46.

108. Altieri JV, Vogler JC, Goldblatt R, Katz RV. The dental status of dentate institutionalized older adults: consideration of retained roots. Spec Care Dentist 1993;13(2):66–70.

109. Shay K. Root caries in the older patient: significance, prevention, and treatment. Dent Clin North Am 1997;41(4):763–94.

110. Steele JG, Walls AW, Murray JJ. Partial dentures as an independent indicator of root caries risk in a group of older adults. Gerodontology 1997;14(2):67–74.

111. Ship JA, Crow HC. Diseases of periodontal tissues in the elderly. Description, epidemiology, aetiology, and drug therapy. Drugs Aging 1994;5:346–57.

112. Fox PC. Management of dry mouth. Dent Clin North Am 1997;41(4):863–76.

113. Narhi TO, Meurman JH, Ainamo A. Xerostomia and hyposalivation: causes, consequences and treatment in the elderly. Drugs Aging 1999;15(2):103–16.

114. Sreebny LM, Schwartz SS. A reference guide to drugs and dry mouth—2nd edition. Gerodontology 1997;14(1):33–47.

115. Atkinson JC, Fox P. Sjogren's syndrome: oral and dental considerations. J Am Dent Assoc 1993;124(3):74–86.

116. Snow JBJ Jr, Doty RL, Bartoshuk LM. Clinical evaluation of olfactory and gustatory disorders. In: Getchell TC, Doty RL, Bartoshuk LM, Snow JB Jr, editors. Smell and taste in health and disease. 1st ed. New York: Raven Press; 1991. p. 463–70.

117. Ship JA. Gustatory and olfactory considerations in general dental practice. J Am Dent Assoc 1993;124:55–61.

118. Lindgren S, Janzon L. Prevalence of swallowing complaints and clinical findings among 50-79-year-old men and women in an urban population. Dysphagia 1991;6(4):187–92.

119. Howard L, Malone M. Clinical outcome of geriatric patients in the United States receiving home parenteral and enteral nutrition. Am J Clin Nutr 1997;66(6):1364–70.

120. Buchholz DW. Dysphagia associated with neurological disorders. Acta Otorhinolaryngol Belg 1994;48(2):143–55.

121. McConnel FM, O'Connor A. Dysphagia secondary to head and neck cancer surgery. Acta Otorhinolaryngol Belg 1994;48(2):165–70.

122. Caruso AJ, Sonies BC, Atkinson JC, Fox PC. Objective measures of swallowing in patients with primary Sjogren's syndrome. Dysphagia 1989;4(2):101–5.

123. Fucile S, Wright PM, Chan I, et al. Functional oral-motor skills: do they change with age? Dysphagia 1998;13(4):195–201.

124. Gift HC, Newman JF. How older adults use oral health care services: results of a National Health Interview Survey. J Am Dent Assoc 1993;124(1):89–93.

125. Guggenheimer J, Hoffman RD. The importance of screening edentulous patients for oral cancer. J Prosthet Dent 1994;72(2):141–3.

126. Smith RA, Mettlin CJ, Davis KJ, Eyre H. American Cancer Society guidelines for the early detection of cancer. CA Cancer J Clin 2000;50(1):34–49.

127. Shay K, Truhlar MR, Renner RP. Oropharyngeal candidosis in the older patient. J Am Geriatr Soc 1997;45(7):863–70.

128. Heifetz SB. Fluorides for the elderly. J Calif Dent Assoc 1994;22(3):49–54.

129. Winston AE, Bhaskar SN. Caries prevention in the 21st century. J Am Dent Assoc 1998;129(11):1579–87.

130. Stamm JW, Banting DW, Imrey PB. Adult root caries survey of two similar communities with contrasting natural water fluoride levels. J Am Dent Assoc 1990;120(2):143–9.

131. Hicks MJ, Flaitz CM, Garcia-Godoy F. Root-surface caries formation: effect of in vitro APF treatment. J Am Dent Assoc 1998;129(4):449–53.

132. ten Cate JM, Damen JJ, Buijs MJ. Inhibition of dentin demineralization by fluoride in vitro. Caries Res 1998;32(2):141–7.

133. Morley J. The role of cosmetic dentistry in restoring a youthful appearance. J Am Dent Assoc 1999;130(8):1166–72.

134. Ettinger RL. Oral care for the homebound and institutionalized. Clin Geriatr Med 1992;8(3):659–72.

135. van Winkelhoff AJ, Rams TE, Slots J. Systemic antibiotic therapy in periodontics. Periodontol 2000 1996;10:45–78.

136. Henson BS, Eisbruch A, D'Hondt E, Ship JA. Two-year longitudinal study of parotid salivary flow rates in head and neck cancer patients receiving unilateral neck parotid-sparing radiotherapy treatment. Oral Oncol 1999;35(3):234–41.

137. Johnson JT, Ferretti GA, Nethery WJ, et al. Oral pilocarpine for post-irradiation xerostomia in patients with head and neck cancer. N Engl J Med 1993;329(6):390–5.

138. Vivino FB, Al-Hashimi I, Khan Z, et al. Pilocarpine tablets for the treatment of dry mouth and dry eye symptoms in patients with Sjogren syndrome: a randomized, placebo-controlled, fixed-dose, multicenter trial. P92-01 Study Group. Arch Intern Med 1999;159(2):174–81.

139. Regelink G, Vissink A, Reintsema H, Nauta JM. Efficacy of a synthetic polymer saliva substitute in reducing oral complaints of patients suffering from irradiation-induced xerostomia. Quintessence Int 1998;29(6):383–8.

140. Schiffman SS. Drugs influencing taste and smell perception. In: Getchell TC, Doty RL, Bartoshuk LM, Snow JB, editors. Taste and smell in health and disease. New York: Raven Press; 1991. p. 845–8.

141. Schiffman SS, Warwick Z. Effect of flavor enhancement of foods for the elderly on nutritional status: food intake, biochemical indices, and anthropometric measures. Physiol Behav 1993;53(2):395–402.

142. Sonies BC. Swallowing disorders and rehabilitation techniques. J Pediatr Gastroenterol Nutr 1997;25 (Suppl 1):S32–3.

143. Broniatowski M, Sonies BC, Rubin JS, et al. Current evaluation and treatment of patients with swallowing disorders. Otolaryngol Head Neck Surg 1999;120(4):464–73.

144. Bando K, Nitta H, Matsubara M, Ishikawa I. Bone mineral density in periodontally healthy and edentulous postmenopausal women. Ann Periodontol 1998;3(1):322–6.

145. Ettinger RL. Managing and treating the atrophic mandible. J Am Dent Assoc 1993;124(7):234–41.

146. Roynesdal AK, Ambjornsen E, Stovne S, Haanaes HR. A comparative clinical study of three different endosseous implants in edentulous mandibles. Int J Oral Maxillofac Implants 1998;13(4):500–5.

147. Garg AK, Winkler S, Bakaeen LG, Mekayarajjananonth T. Dental implants and the geriatric patient. Implant Dent 1997;6(3):168–73.

148. Truhlar RS, Casino AJ, Cancro JJ. Treatment planning of the elderly implant patient. Dent Clin N Am 1997;41(4):847–61.

149. Mericske-Stern R, Perren R, Raveh J. Life table analysis and clinical evaluation of oral implants supporting prostheses after resection of malignant tumors. Int J Oral Maxillofac Implants 1999;14(5):673–80.

150. Chanavaz M. Patient screening and medical evaluation for implant and preprosthetic surgery. J Oral Implantol 1998;24(4):222–9.

INDEX